Brief Contents

Pediatric Nursing

A CASE-BASED APPROACH

Pediatric Nursing
A CASE-BASED APPROACH

Catherine Gannon Tagher, EdD, MSN, RN, APRN
Associate Dean and Associate Professor
College of Health and Human Services
Northern Kentucky University
Highland Heights, Kentucky

Lisa Marie Knapp, MEd, DNP, RN, CCRN
Registered Nurse III
Cincinnati Children's Hospital Medical Center
Cincinnati, Ohio

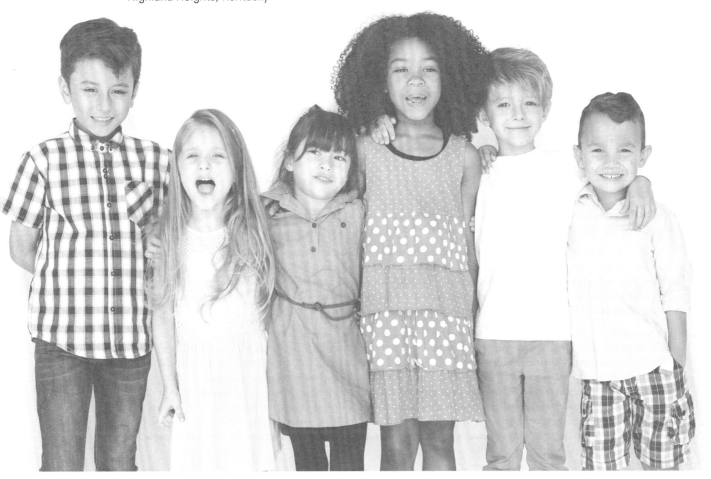

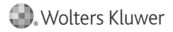. Wolters Kluwer

Philadelphia · Baltimore · New York · London
Buenos Aires · Hong Kong · Sydney · Tokyo

Vice President and Publisher: Julie K. Stegman
Director of Nursing Content Publishing: Renee Gagliardi
Acquisitions Editor: Michael Kerns
Director of Product Development: Jennifer K. Forestieri
Senior Development Editor: Meredith L. Brittain
Freelance Development Editor: David R. Payne
Editorial Coordinator: Tim Rinehart
Marketing Manager: Brittany Clements
Editorial Assistant: Molly Kennedy
Design Coordinator: Terry Mallon
Art Director, Illustration: Jennifer Clements
Production Project Manager: Barton Dudlick
Manufacturing Coordinator: Karin Duffield
Prepress Vendor: S4Carlisle Publishing Services

9 8 7 6 5 4 3 2 1

Printed in China (or the United States of America)

Library of Congress Cataloging-in-Publication Data

ISBN-13: 978-1-4963-9422-4

ISBN-10: 1-4963-9422-4

Library of Congress Control Number: 2019909542

---

shop.lww.com

CCS0819

Dedication

I would like to dedicate this book to my family and my parents. To my husband, in addition to being a loving husband and father, for supporting me through this journey while playing taxi driver, cook, and anything else that was needed. To my children, for putting up with their mom over the past few years. To my parents, for teaching me to have the courage to put myself out there and try something new. Finally, a special dedication to my dad, for always encouraging me to shoot for the moon. Thank you all for believing in me. I love you.

—Catherine Gannon Tagher

This book is dedicated to my family and friends. Without them in my life as I traveled this journey, I am sure I would not have been successful. To my husband, Nate, for not only taking over mom duties for our daughter when I was writing but also supporting me during late nights and long days sitting to accomplish this project. Being still is not easy for me, but your encouraging words and laughter made it bearable. To my daughter, Kasey Marie, for putting up with "just one more hour" of mommy writing the book. To my mom, for enduring my long phone calls about book-writing life. And finally, to my friends Lesha, Stephanie, and Jenni, for always answering with positive and encouraging words when I could not see the end in sight.

—Lisa Marie Knapp

About the Authors

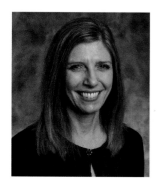

Catherine Gannon Tagher, EdD, MSN, RN, APRN

Catherine Gannon Tagher is the associate dean, associate professor, and chief nurse administrator for the College of Health and Human Services at Northern Kentucky University. She received her BSN from the University of Kentucky in 1997. As a registered nurse, she worked in pediatric oncology at Kentucky Children's Hospital and subsequently Cincinnati Children's Hospital. She earned her MSN from the University of Kentucky in 2001 and has been licensed as a pediatric nurse practitioner since. She has worked as a nurse practitioner in hematology/oncology and primary care. Her areas of expertise include pediatric growth and development and health promotion.

Dr. Tagher earned an EdD in educational leadership with a focus in nursing education from Northern Kentucky University in 2014. Her research focused on students' perceptions of stress in a high-stakes testing environment as well as helping students to view standardized testing as a challenge rather than a threat. She has published her research as well as presented at both national and international conferences. Additional research includes a longitudinal study, "Pathways to a Nursing Degree," which tracks students involved in early exposure to the nursing profession to determine whether they choose nursing for a major in college. Lastly, she is involved in a transdisciplinary research group at Northern Kentucky University, looking at innovative ways to approach the opioid crisis in Northern Kentucky through research and community partnerships.

Dr. Tagher has been a member of the faculty at Northern Kentucky University since 2005. She has taught pediatrics in the undergraduate BSN program as well as primary care of children with chronic illness and pediatric pharmacology in the MSN program. While teaching undergraduate nursing, she has used a flipped-classroom approach, teaching through cases and storytelling. She has served as the director of the BSN program and the chair of the Department of Nursing, overseeing the RN-BSN program, BSN program, MSN program, post-master's DNP program, and nurse anesthesia program.

Dr. Tagher is married to Dr. Robert Tagher, who is a primary care pediatrician in Northern Kentucky. Together they have three teenage children: Maggie, Mollie, and Andrew. They have two dogs and a cat. Dr. Tagher enjoys hiking, kayaking, paddleboarding, and anything to do with the ocean. She is learning to play the guitar in the hope that one day she will be able to entertain by the campfire.

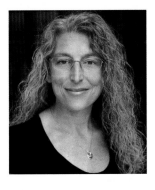

Lisa Marie Knapp, MEd, DNP, RN, CCRN

Lisa Marie Knapp is a registered nurse in the pediatric intensive care unit (PICU) at Cincinnati Children's Hospital Medical Center in Cincinnati, Ohio. She received her BSN from Hartwick College in 1997. As a registered nurse, she has worked her entire career at Cincinnati Children's Hospital Medical Center caring for critically ill pediatric patients in the intensive care unit. In 2002, she earned her MSN and MEd from Xavier University. Additionally, for many years, she worked part time as an RN in an adult intensive care unit and emergency room at Mercy Hospital, Cincinnati, Ohio. She was a member of the faculty at Northern Kentucky University from 2011 to 2016, teaching pediatric nursing, medical-surgical clinicals, advanced medical-surgical nursing, and several other undergraduate courses.

Dr. Knapp earned a DNP, with a focus on nurses' perceptions of parent participation in the pediatric hospital setting, from Northern Kentucky University in 2016. While completing her DNP, she spent a year as a trainee in the Leadership Education in Neurodevelopmental and Related Disabilities (LEND) program, immersed in learning about providing health and related services for children with neurodevelopmental disabilities and their families. During LEND, she collaborated with team members to continue a research project titled "Cincinnati Homelessness Study: The Family Point of View." Additionally, she completed an in-depth assessment of a community resource for those with developmental disabilities.

As an RN in the PICU, Dr. Knapp is responsible for direct patient care and management of the critically ill child and family including technical, psychosocial, educational, and emotional support using a variety of disciplines. As a PICU RN in a level I pediatric trauma center, she cares for critically ill patients with medical diagnoses including septic shock, respiratory failure, hematology/oncology disorders, congenital and chronic disease, and multiple system organ failure, as well as trauma patients and patients who are pre- and post-organ transplant, and post-surgery. She is a preceptor for new staff and an active member in house-wide shared governance. She also started a clinical coaching program in the PICU in which select, expert nurses work one-on-one with nurses who have been out of orientation for 6 months to 1 year and are ready to be challenged with more complex, critically ill patients and mentored in critical thinking, communication, and understanding the multiple complexities of severely ill children.

Dr. Knapp is married to Nathan Knapp. Together, they have a daughter, Kasey Marie. They live in the country, in a log cabin, and have a dog, two cats, and two gerbils. Dr. Knapp enjoys working out, running, backpacking in the wilderness, and being involved in Kasey's extracurricular activities including coaching soccer and being actively involved in Girl Scouts.

Contributors

Josie Bidwell, DNP, RN, FNP-C, DipACLM
Associate Professor
Department of Preventive Medicine
School of Medicine
University of Mississippi Medical Center
Jackson, Mississippi

Julie A. Hart, DNP, RN, CNE
Associate Professor
School of Nursing
College of Health and Human Services
Northern Kentucky University
Highland Heights, Kentucky

Lisa Marie Knapp, MEd, DNP, RN, CCRN
Registered Nurse III
Cincinnati Children's Hospital Medical Center
Cincinnati, Ohio

Laura Kubin, PhD, RN, CPN, CHES
Associate Professor
The Houston J. and Florence A. Doswell College of Nursing
T. Boone Pickens Institute of Health Sciences-Dallas Center
Texas Woman's University
Denton, Texas

Rebecca Logan, PhD, RN
Assistant Professor
Department of Nursing
Berry College
Mount Berry, Georgia

Jennifer L. Nahum, DNP, RN, PNP-BC, CPNP-AC
Clinical Assistant Professor
Rory Meyers College of Nursing
New York University
New York, New York

Anita Kay Williams-Prickett, PhD, RN
Retired Professor of Nursing
Jacksonville State University
Jacksonville, Alabama
Former Nurse
Children's Hospital of Alabama
Birmingham, Alabama

Karen A. Ripley, PhD, RN
Assistant Professor
School of Nursing
Loma Linda University
Loma Linda, California

Erin M. Robinson Ed.D, MSN, RN
Associate Director of Undergraduate Studies
School of Nursing
College of Health and Human Services
Northern Kentucky University
Highland Heights, Kentucky

Catherine Gannon Tagher, EdD, MSN, RN, APRN
Associate Dean and Associate Professor
College of Health and Human Services
Northern Kentucky University
Highland Heights, Kentucky

Trisha L. Wendling. DNP, APRN, CNP
Pediatric Nurse Practitioner
Education Consultant
Cincinnati Children's Hospital Medical Center
Cincinnati, Ohio

Cecilia Elaine Wilson, PhD, RN, CPN
Associate Clinical Professor
Texas Woman's University
Denton, Texas

For a list of the contributors for the ancillaries, please visit http://thepoint.lww.com/Tagher1e.

Reviewers

Daria Amato, RN, CNE, MSN
Associate Professor
Department of Nursing
Northern Virginia Community College
Annandale, Virginia

Josie H. Bidwell, DNP
University of Mississippi Medical Center
Jackson, Mississippi

Jutta Braun, RN, MS, CNE
Associate Professor
Department of Nursing
County College of Morris
Randolph, New Jersey

Susan J. Brillhart, PhD, RN, PNP-BC
Assistant Professor
Department of Nursing
Borough of Manhattan Community College
New York, New York

Kathleen Cahill, MS, RN, CNE
Instructor of Pediatrics
Department of Nursing
Saint Anselm College
Manchester, New Hampshire

Normajean Colby, PhD, RN, CNE, CPN
Associate Professor
School of Nursing
Widener University
Brookhaven, Pennsylvania

Hobie Etta Feagai, EdD, MSN, FNP-BC, APRN-Rx
Hawai'i Pacific University
Kaneohe, Hawaii

Niki Fogg, MS, RN, CPN
Associate Clinical Professor
College of Nursing
Texas Women's University
Allen, Texas

Jeffrey Fouche-Camargo, DNP, APRN, RNC-OB, WHNP-BC, C-EFM
Assistant Professor
Georgia Gwinnett College
Lawrenceville, Georgia

Ashley Gauthier, MSN, RN
Assistant Professor
Department of Nursing
AdventHealth University
Orlando, Florida

Belinda Gilbert, DNP, MSN-Ed, RNC-NIC
Instructor
Department of Nursing
Albany State University
Albany, New York

Tamara Hryshchuk, MS, RNC-NIC
Director of Nursing
School of Nursing and Health Professions
Langston University
Tulsa, Oklahoma

Lisa Jamerson, MSN, RN, NRP
Assistant Professor
Department of Nursing
Lynchburg College
Lynchburg, Virginia

Margaret Kennedy, MSN, RN, FNP-BC
Oakland University
Rochester, Michigan

Deborah Larson, RN, MSN, CPNP
Los Angeles Harbor College
Los Angeles, California

Francine Laterza, MSN, RN, PNP
Assistant Professor
Department of Nursing
Farmingdale State College
Bayside, New York

Preface

In today's world of healthcare, nurses care for complex pediatric patients in a myriad situations. Pediatric nurses are expected to provide care for children and families with multifaceted medical and social situations within inpatient, outpatient, and community settings. As a result of current drivers of curricular design, nursing faculty continue to devote less time to specialty nursing areas such as pediatrics in the nursing curriculum. However, the ability of students to apply pediatric concepts and analyze complex scenarios is a necessary skill to provide safe, quality care; to promote health; and to optimize growth and development for children of all ages and their families in a variety of healthcare settings.

Most students entering a pediatric nursing course have a base knowledge of medical-surgical principles. This textbook facilitates the application of these nursing concepts in the pediatric setting, allowing students to maximize learning within a limited amount of time. The book builds on students' prior knowledge to differentiate the care of children from that of adults. By using engaging, chapter-length case studies to highlight evidence-based practice, patient safety, prioritization of care, and interprofessional teamwork, the text helps students develop skills such as clinical judgment, patient advocacy, and patient education in any pediatric setting.

In addition to decreasing the amount of class time allotted to pediatric nursing, many programs are also reducing clinical time. Furthermore, many students start the pediatric clinical rotation before having any substantial didactic course time. As a way to help students prepare for clinical, the first unit of this book is made up entirely of fully developed case scenarios based on some of the most common types of problems seen in pediatric acute care or outpatient settings. These scenarios are start-to-finish case studies with concise explanations and rationales for interventions. The scenarios follow fictional pediatric patients from the home to the clinic to the emergency department and then through hospitalization, if needed, and discharge. Students learn health promotion, growth and development, and care of the pediatric patient. Nursing interventions, patient education, and safety are emphasized throughout each scenario, helping to promote clinical decision making. The information provided in these scenarios is expanded upon in later chapters of the textbook. In addition, characters introduced in these scenarios appear in later chapters to reinforce the principles of care for these children.

Organization

The book has a case-based theme. Patients are introduced in Unit 1, Scenarios for Clinical Preparation, and then threaded through the remainder of the book where appropriate to provide reinforcement and deeper learning of the material. Unit 2, Care of the Developing Child, provides an overview of growth and development. Unit 3, Care of the Hospitalized Child, is organized by body system.

Unit 1: Scenarios for Clinical Preparation

The first unit consists of the case-based scenarios. The purpose of this unit is to provide a clinical overview so that students are prepared to manage the pediatric patient in the concurrent clinical course. Common scenarios that are seen on general pediatric units or in outpatient settings, along with pertinent concepts of growth and development, are introduced here, early in the book. These cases enable students entering clinical to have a solid base for clinical practice. Every scenario is thorough enough to be used for clinical preparation. Clinical instructors can use the scenarios for discussion points in either the pre- or postconference setting. In addition, instructors can pull the end-of-chapter "Think Critically" questions from the scenario chapters to enhance the didactic portion of the course.

Each scenario introduces the story of a child at a certain age with a common medical diagnosis seen either on pediatric acute care units or in outpatient clinic settings. Relevant information regarding ethnicity, social background, growth and development, diagnosis, concepts of nursing care, and treatment is provided in a conversational tone that facilitates understanding the care of a pediatric patient within a contextual situation. When appropriate, cultural norms and preferences are discussed, enabling students to incorporate culturally sensitive, family-centered care into their nursing practice.

The scenarios begin outside of the hospital and continue through the clinic visit, the emergency department visit, and, if warranted, the hospitalization of the child, with discharge teaching and follow-up as indicated. Pertinent growth and development concepts are included based on the age of the child. The nursing care provided in the scenarios is based on current and accurate evidence. Only appropriate pharmacotherapy for the scenario is included, allowing students to focus only on the care of the child in the scenario.

The unique approach of Unit 1 allows problems to be discussed as a discrete entity. For example, programs implementing a concept-based curriculum could use the patient case on asthma in Chapter 2 as an exemplar in lieu of or in conjunction with covering the full chapter on alterations in respiratory function (Chapter 20).

Unit 2: Care of the Developing Child

The second unit discusses care of the developing child. This unit includes two major themes. The first theme is growth and development, which includes the concepts of growth, development, and health promotion. This information, although not exhaustive, incorporates normal growth and development and developmental concerns. This knowledge can be applied in any pediatric setting.

The second theme of this unit is common problems seen in an ambulatory setting. Chapters are organized by developmental stage: newborn and infant, toddler, preschooler, school-age child, and adolescent. The patients introduced in the first unit are referred to in chapters of this unit where appropriate when discussing the principles of growth and development, once again providing context and reinforcement of these principles to promote meaningful learning.

Unit 3: Care of the Hospitalized Child

The third unit is centered on the care of the hospitalized child. The chapters in this unit focus on body systems, including relevant problems in each. Each chapter begins by presenting body system–specific information related to pediatric assessment, variations in pediatric anatomy and physiology from those of an adult, and concept-based general nursing interventions for the conditions covered. This introductory content is followed in each chapter by sections covering conditions affecting the given body system that are commonly seen in children. Each condition section is further divided into the following standard subsections:

- Etiology and Pathophysiology
- Clinical Presentation
- Assessment and Diagnosis
- Therapeutic Interventions
- Evaluation
- Discharge Planning and Teaching

Pharmacological therapy (in addition to being presented in The Pharmacy feature, discussed in the User's Guide) is primarily covered in the Therapeutic Interventions subsection of the relevant condition rather than for the body system as a whole. Although this approach results in some repetition of pharmacology content, it also provides much-needed reinforcement of the drugs pertinent to the treatment of pediatric conditions and the nursing care involved in the administration of these drugs.

Once again, patients from the scenarios in the first unit are reintroduced in chapters of this unit on the basis of their diagnosis to reinforce priority nursing care, promote deeper learning, and enhance clinical judgment.

Features of This Book

Please refer to the User's Guide (which immediately follows this preface) for explanations of this book's features.

A Comprehensive Package for Teaching and Learning

To further facilitate teaching and learning, a carefully designed ancillary package has been developed to assist faculty and students.

Instructor Resources

Tools to assist you with teaching your course are available upon adoption of this book on thePoint® at http://thepoint.lww.com/Tagher1e.

- A **Test Generator** features National Council Licensure Exam (NCLEX)-style questions mapped to chapter learning objectives.
- An extensive collection of materials is provided for each book chapter:
  - **Pre-Lecture Quizzes** (and answers) allow you to check students' reading.
  - **PowerPoint Presentations** provide an easy way to integrate the textbook with your students' classroom experience; multiple-choice and true/false questions are included to promote class participation.
  - **Discussion Topics** (and suggested answers) can be used in the classroom or in online discussion boards to facilitate interaction with your students.
  - **Assignments** (and suggested answers) include group, written, clinical, and Web assignments to engage students in varied activities and assess their learning.
  - **Case Studies** with related questions (and suggested answers) give students an opportunity to apply their knowledge to a client case similar to one they might encounter in practice.
- **Answers to the Think Critically questions in the book** reinforce key concepts.
- Sample **Syllabi** are provided for 7-week and 15-week courses.
- **Maps Linking Cases with Chapters** provide a visual representation of the links between the content covered in Unit 1 with the content covered in Units 2 and 3.
- A **Quality and Safety Education for Nurses (QSEN) Competency Map** identifies content and special features in the book related to competencies identified by the QSEN Institute.
- A **Bachelor of Science in Nursing (BSN) Essentials Competency Map** identifies book content related to the BSN Essentials.
- An **Image Bank** lets you use the photographs and illustrations from this textbook in your course materials.
- An **ebook** serves as a handy resource.

- Access to all **Student Resources** is provided so that you can understand the student experience and use these resources in your course as well.

Student Resources

An exciting set of free learning resources is available on thePoint® to help students review and apply vital concepts in pediatric nursing. Multimedia engines have been optimized so that students can access many of these resources on mobile devices. Students can access all these resources at http://thepoint.lww.com/Tagher1e using the codes printed in the front of their textbooks.

- **NCLEX-Style Review Questions** for each chapter help students review important concepts and practice for NCLEX.
- **Journal Articles** offer access to current research relevant to each chapter and available in Wolters Kluwer journals to familiarize students with nursing literature.
- **Learning Objectives** from the book are provided for convenience.
- **Interactive Learning Resources** appeal to a variety of learning styles. Icons in the text direct readers to relevant resources:

  o **Practice & Learn Case Studies** present case scenarios and offer interactive exercises and questions to help students apply what they have learned.

  o **Watch & Learn Videos** reinforce skills from the textbook and appeal to visual and auditory learners.

Adaptive Learning Powered by PrepU

Lippincott's Adaptive Learning Powered by PrepU helps every student learn more while giving instructors the data they need to monitor each student's progress, strengths, and weaknesses. The adaptive learning system allows instructors to assign quizzes or students to take quizzes on their own that adapt to each student's individual mastery level. Visit http://thepoint.lww.com/prepU to learn more.

vSim for Nursing

vSim for Nursing, jointly developed by Laerdal Medical and Wolters Kluwer Health, offers innovative scenario-based learning modules consisting of Web-based virtual simulations, course learning materials, and curriculum tools designed to develop critical thinking skills and promote clinical confidence and competence. vSim for Nursing | Pediatric includes 10 of the 12 cases from the *Simulation in Nursing Education—Pediatric Scenarios*, authored by the National League for Nursing. Students can progress through suggested readings, pre- and postsimulation assessments, documentation assignments, and guided reflection questions and will receive an individualized feedback log immediately upon completion of the simulation. Throughout the student learning experience, the product offers remediation back to trusted Lippincott resources, including Lippincott Nursing Advisor and Lippincott Nursing Procedures—two online, evidence-based clinical information solutions used in healthcare facilities throughout the United States. This innovative product provides a comprehensive patient-focused solution for learning and integrating simulation into the classroom.

Contact your Wolters Kluwer sales representative or visit http://thepoint.lww.com/vsim for options to enhance your pediatric nursing course with vSim for Nursing.

Lippincott DocuCare

Lippincott DocuCare combines web-based academic electronic health record (EHR) simulation software with clinical case scenarios, allowing students to learn how to use an EHR in a safe, true-to-life setting while enabling instructors to measure their progress. Lippincott DocuCare's nonlinear solution works well in the classroom, simulation lab, and clinical practice.

Contact your Wolters Kluwer sales representative or visit http://thepoint.lww.com/DocuCare for options to enhance your pediatric nursing course with DocuCare.

A Comprehensive, Digital, Integrated Course Solution: Lippincott® CoursePoint+

The same trusted solution, innovation, and unmatched support that you have come to expect from *Lippincott CoursePoint+* is now enhanced with more engaging learning tools and deeper analytics to help prepare students for practice. This powerfully integrated digital learning solution combines learning tools, case studies, virtual simulation, real-time data, and the most trusted nursing education content on the market to make curriculum-wide learning more efficient and to meet students where they're at in their learning. And now, it's easier than ever for instructors and students to use, giving them everything they need for course and curriculum success!

Lippincott CoursePoint+ includes:

- Engaging course content provides a variety of learning tools to engage students of all learning styles.
- A more personalized learning approach, including adaptive learning powered by PrepU, gives students the content and tools they need at the moment they need it, giving them data for more focused remediation and helping to boost their confidence.
- Varying levels of case studies, virtual simulation, and access to Lippincott Advisor help students learn the critical thinking and clinical judgment skills to help them become practice-ready nurses.
- Unparalleled reporting provides in-depth dashboards with several data points to track student progress and help identify strengths and weaknesses.
- Unmatched support includes training coaches, product trainers, and nursing education consultants to help educators and students implement CoursePoint+ with ease.

User's Guide

Pediatric Nursing: A Case-Based Approach contains many accessible features to help students grasp the important content.

Case-Based Features

Chapter-length **Clinical Scenarios** make up Unit 1, as mentioned in the preface. Each of the 14 scenarios in Unit 1 presents the story of a different pediatric patient with one or several conditions related to a given body system, told from the point of view of the patient's parent (or, for a few of the older patients, from the patient's point of view). Together, the cases cover patients of a diverse range of ages, levels of growth and development, backgrounds, and conditions and body systems involved, as well as a variety of aspects of pediatric nursing assessment, diagnosis, and intervention.

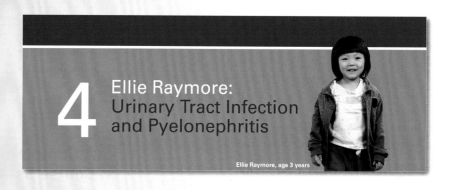

4 Ellie Raymore:
Urinary Tract Infection and Pyelonephritis

Ellie Raymore, age 3 years

In Chapter 4, Ellie Raymore presented with signs and symptoms of a urinary tract infection. What were these signs and symptoms? Was her assessment normal or abnormal? Why was further testing warranted in Ellie's case?

Greater breadth and depth of content emerge as the reader continues; Units 2 and 3, although still striving for compelling context, offer a more traditional textbook format, which provides a greater wealth of information. Through the case snippets in these units, which prompt students to recall patients from Unit 1, students can link these later units to those scenarios.

Unfolding Patient Stories, written by the National League for Nursing, are an engaging way to begin meaningful conversations in the classroom. These vignettes, which appear at the end of the first chapter in each unit, feature patients from Wolters Kluwer's *vSim for Nursing | Pediatric* (co-developed by Laerdal Medical) and DocuCare products; however, each Unfolding Patient Story in the book stands alone, not requiring purchase of these products.

Unfolding Patient Stories: Brittany Long • Part 1

Brittany Long is a 5-year-old diagnosed with sickle cell anemia who lives with her mother, 7-year-old sister, and grandmother. Her pain crises are mostly managed at home, and she has been hospitalized 3 times. How can the nurse help Brittany and her family cope with a long-term illness and the management of acute crises? How can the reactions of family members influence Brittany's adjustment to sickle cell disease? What effect can a long-term illness have on her sister, and what actions can support her sister's understanding and cooperation? (Brittany Long's story continues in Unit 3.)

Care for Brittany and other patients in a realistic virtual environment: *vSim for Nursing* (thepoint.lww.com/vSimPediatric). Practice documenting these patients' care in DocuCare (thepoint.lww.com /DocuCareEHR).

For your convenience, a list of all these case studies, along with their location in the book, appears in the "Case Studies in This Book" section later in this frontmatter.

The Nurse's Point of View feature in Unit 1 changes the narrator from the patient or the patient's parent to a knowledgeable nurse preceptor, who picks up the story from the nursing perspective, including information about how and why particular aspects of care are provided to a character.

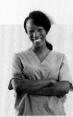

The Nurse's Point of View

Sarah: While I'm working triage, a man arrives carrying a young boy who appears to be nonresponsive. The man's name, I learn, is Kasim and the boy is Maalik. The boy's mother, Farrah, is also with them. I ask Kasim to lay Maalik on a bed so that I can assess him. Before he gets to the bed, however, Maalik vomits. The product of the emesis is mostly clear, with some mucus. I take a quick history on Maalik and realize that he is most likely very dehydrated.

Chapter-Beginning Features

Learning Objectives state clear and concise learning goals for each chapter.

Objectives

After completing this chapter, you will be able to:
1. Describe normal growth and development of the 7-year-old.
2. Discuss an appropriate teaching plan for a healthy 7-year-old.
3. Identify signs of diabetes type 1.
4. Explain the pathophysiology of diabetes type 1.
5. Identify signs and symptoms of diabetic ketoacidosis and hypoglycemia.
6. Relate insulin therapy to the treatment of diabetes type 1.
7. Discuss caloric needs of children diagnosed with diabetes type 1.
8. Create a nursing plan of care for a child newly diagnosed with diabetes type 1.

Key Terms are listed at the beginning of each chapter, boldfaced on first use in the chapter text, and included in a glossary at the back of the book.

Key Terms

Basal insulin
Bolus insulin
Diabetes type 1
Glucometer
Glycated hemoglobin A1c (HgbA1c)
Insulin pump

Diabetic ketoacidosis
Ketones
Polydipsia
Polyphagia
Polyuria

Features That Teach Skills and Concepts

For your convenience, a list of all the features that teach skills and concepts, along with their location in the book, appears in the "Special Features in This Book" section later in this frontmatter.

Growth and Development Check features throughout the book alert students to the importance of a child's age and developmental stage when using clinical judgment and implementing plans of care.

 Growth and Development Check 15.1

Delayed Verbal Skills

If an infant is not imitating sounds or babbling by 7 mo old, the infant has a delay in language development and further investigation is warranted. Problems with hearing are often the cause of speech delay. Infants who have had recurrent ear infections often have speech delay due to fluid in the middle ear (AAP, 2009b).

How Much Does It Hurt? 1.1

Chip's FLACC Score*

Chip's total FLACC (face, legs, activity, cry, and consolability) score is a 2, based on the following ratings:
- Face: 0
- Legs: 1
- Activity: 0
- Cry: 0
- Consolability: 1

*For a description of the FLACC scale, see Chapter 15.

How Much Does It Hurt? boxes incorporate principles of pediatric pain management.

Patient Safety 3.2

Monitoring for Signs of Complications

Complications of a fracture can include bleeding, impaired circulation, compartment syndrome, and neuropathy.

- **Bleeding:** assess heart rate, blood pressure, circulation, and bruising.
- **Impaired circulation:** assess capillary refill, skin temperature, and distal pulses.
- **Compartment syndrome:** monitor for the six Ps.
- **Neuropathy:** assess for tingling, numbness, and decreased or absent sensation distal to the injury.

Patient Safety reminders, as well as important signs and symptoms to which the nurse needs to pay attention, are highlighted as appropriate throughout the book.

Let's Compare boxes throughout the book differentiate between adult and pediatric anatomy, physiology, and assessment techniques.

Let's Compare 1.1   Airway Structures and Risk of Obstruction

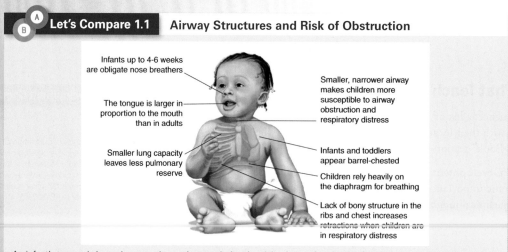

Infants up to 4-6 weeks are obligate nose breathers

The tongue is larger in proportion to the mouth than in adults

Smaller lung capacity leaves less pulmonary reserve

Smaller, narrower airway makes children more susceptible to airway obstruction and respiratory distress

Infants and toddlers appear barrel-chested

Children rely heavily on the diaphragm for breathing

Lack of bony structure in the ribs and chest increases retractions when children are in respiratory distress

An infant's tongue is larger in proportion to the mouth than in adults, increasing the risk for obstruction with narrowing of the airway. The trachea is cartilaginous and the neck is shorter in an infant, further increasing the risk for airway obstruction and collapse.

Because the bronchi and bronchioles are smaller in infants, they are more easily obstructed than those of adults. Infants also have fewer **alveoli** than adults, leaving even less room for air exchange when mucus is obstructing the bronchioles. Even slight obstruction can have a large impact on an infant's work of breathing.

Image adapted with permission from Ateah, C. A., Scott, S. D., & Kyle, T. (2012). *Canadian essentials of pediatric nursing* (1st ed., Fig. 19.1). Philadelphia, PA: Lippincott Williams & Wilkins.

Priority Care Concepts provide a quick overview of prioritization of care for pediatric patients.

Priority Care Concepts 8.1 — Monitoring Growth and Development

In the absence of underlying disease, the cause of failure to thrive is most likely decreased caloric intake (Romano et al., 2015; Vachani, 2018). Inadequate caloric intake affects not only an infant's weight but also his or her developmental milestones (Black et al., 2015). Therefore, it is essential that infants and children have adequate nutrition to meet developmental and cognitive milestones.

Goals
- Determine the infant's goal weight.
- Increase caloric intake on the basis of the goal weight.
- Reach developmental milestones appropriate for age.

Nursing Interventions
- Assess developmental milestones.
- Monitor growth and development.
- Monitor weight.
- Teach caregivers a way to help infants achieve developmental milestones.
- Teach caregivers methods for increasing caloric intake.
- Make referrals as appropriate:
  - The Special Supplemental Nutrition Program for women, infants, and children
  - Early intervention programs
  - Social work
  - Occupational therapy
  - Physical therapy

Whose Job Is It, Anyway? sections underscore roles of different members of the healthcare team.

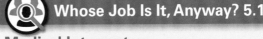

Whose Job Is It, Anyway? 5.1

Medical Interpreter

Most hospitals have access to interpreters for many different languages. These interpreters are trained in medical terminology and are often referred to as medical interpreters. Nurses are able to request an interpreter when families do not speak English or there is concern that a family may not understand instructions given to them. If there is any doubt whether a family fully understands their child's care and discharge instructions, enlist the help of an interpreter, if available, to prevent the child from harm.

Hospital Help boxes give tips for promoting the continued growth and development of children while they are in the hospital by addressing the unique needs and challenges of each stage.

Hospital Help 1.1

Building Infant Trust

Infants are in the Erickson stage of trust versus mistrust. When an infant is in the hospital, it is important to keep feeding routines the same as much as possible. Allowing parents and caregivers to hold an infant whenever they can helps the infant maintain a sense of trust. If parents or caregivers cannot stay at the hospital, they can leave a recording of themselves singing a song or talking to the infant. They can also leave an object, such as a blanket, that has their scent on it. If they cannot stay, it is important that the nurses make sure the infant's needs are met to continue to establish a sense of trust.

Analyze the Evidence 14.1

Influence of Peers on Diet and Exercise of Adolescents

A systematic review by Chung, Ersig, and McCarthy (2017) identified research studies that examined the influence of peers on diet and exercise. The review included 24 articles; 7 examined diet only, 14 examined exercise only, and 3 examined both. The results of the review indicated that the diet and exercise of adolescents were significantly associated with those of their peers. The association, however, depends on gender, type of exercise, and closeness of friends. The results of the review support the inclusion of peers in interventions that promote healthy diet and exercise.

Analyze the Evidence compares sometimes conflicting and contradictory research that supports or challenges current pediatric nursing practice.

Patient Teaching 15.1

Abnormal Stools

Teach the parent the differences between normal and abnormal stools. If the infant is having infrequent stools, such as every third day, yet the stools are soft and either pasty brown or seedy yellow, there is no cause for concern. Instruct the parent to call the healthcare provider if stools are hard, red, mucousy, frothy, or extremely foul smelling.

Patient Teaching includes important points nurses must cover with patients and their family to effectively educate them.

The Pharmacy provides must-know pharmaceutical information, including, where appropriate, drug classification, route of administration, action, and nursing considerations.

The Pharmacy 19.1 Fluoxetine

Classification	Route	Action	Nursing Considerations
Antidepressant	Oral	Inhibits serotonin reuptake in the central nervous system	• Assess for restlessness, hyperactivity, and agitation. • May cause nausea, vomiting, and diarrhea • Monitor for gastrointestinal bleeds. • Monitor for dizziness, headaches, and dry mouth. • Do not discontinue abruptly.

Adapted from Taketomo, C. R. (2015). *Pediatric & neonatal dosage handbook* (22nd ed.). Hudson, OH: Lexicomp.

In addition to the special boxes mentioned in this section, **Interactive Learning Tools** available online enrich learning and are identified with icons in the text:

Practice & Learn Case Studies present case scenarios and offer interactive exercises and questions to help students apply what they have learned.

Watch & Learn Video Clips reinforce skills from the textbook and appeal to visual and auditory learners.

Chapter-Ending Features

Think Critically offers short, often multipart questions requiring students to synthesize information found in the chapter. Suggested answers are available to instructors at http://thepoint.lww.com/Tagher1e.

Think Critically

1. Dezba piles her family into a pickup truck. What questions do you have surrounding this situation? What are the safety issues and how can nurses help with this?
2. What are other ways Mary could approach the subject of malnutrition with Dezba?
3. What are ways for caregivers to tell whether an infant is getting an adequate supply of breast milk?
4. Why might Dezba feel like a failure if she has to give Andrew formula? What can nurses do to alleviate this feeling?
5. Dezba relaxes when she senses the community health nurse is of American Indian Descent. Why is this?
6. How can nurses help ensure that Dezba and her family continue to have the resources they need to maintain health and wellness?

References cited are listed at the end of each chapter and include updated, current sources.

Suggested Readings include current evidence-based resources related to the key topics discussed in the chapter so that students can expand and deepen their understanding of the content.

References

American Academy of Pediatrics. (2018). *Starting solid foods.* Retrieved from https://www.healthychildren.org/English/ages-stages/baby/feeding-nutrition/Pages/Switching-To-Solid-Foods.aspx

Black, M. M., Pérez-Escamilla, R., & Rao, S. F. (2015). Integrating nutrition and child development interventions: Scientific basis, evidence of impact, and implementation considerations. *Advances in Nutrition, 6*, 852–859.

Eckhardt, C. L., Lutz, T., Karanja, N., Jobe, J. B., Maupome, G., & Rittenbaugh, C. (2014). Knowledge, attitudes, and beliefs that can influence infant feeding practices in American Indian mothers. *Journal of the Academy of Nutrition and Dietetics, 114*(10), 1587–1593.

Goss, C. W., Daily, N., Bair, B., Manson, S. M., Richardson, W. J., Nagamoto, H., & Shore, J. H. (2017). Rural American Indian and Alaska native veterans' telemental health: A model of culturally centered care. *Psychological Services, 14*(3), 270–278.

Homan, G. J. (2016). Failure to thrive: A practical guide. *American Family Physician, 94*(4), 295–299.

Kessler, D. O., Hopkins, O., Torres, E., & Prasad, A. (2015). Assimilating traditional healing into preventive medicine residency curriculum. *American Journal of Preventive Medicine, 49*(5S3), S263–S269.

Portman, T. A., & Garrett, M. T. (2006). Native American healing traditions. *International Journal of Disability, Development, and Education, 53*(4), 453–469.

Romano, C., Hartman, C., Privitera, C., Cardile, S., & Shamir, R. (2015). Current topics in the diagnosis and management of the pediatric non-organic feeding disorders (NOFEDs). *Clinical Nutrition, 34*, 195–200.

Sim, T. F., Hattingh, H. L., Sherriff, J., & Tee, L. B. (2014). Perspectives and attitudes of breastfeeding women using herbal galactogogues during breastfeeding: A qualitative study. *BMC Complementary and Alternative Medicine, 216*(14), 1–11.

Steyn, N., & Decloedt, E. H. (2017). Galactogues: Prescriber points for use in breastfeeding mothers. *Obstetrics and Gynaecology Forum, 27*(1), 16–18.

United States Department of Agriculture. (2015, February). *About WIC—WIC at a glance.* Retrieved from https://www.fns.usda.gov/wic/about-wic-wic-glance

Vachani, J. G. (2018). Failure to thrive: Early intervention mitigates long-term defects. *Contemporary Pediatrics, 35*(4), 13–120.

Suggested Readings

Centers for Disease Control and Prevention. (2017, August 21). *A look inside food deserts.* Retrieved from: https://www.cdc.gov/features/fooddeserts/index.html

Portman, T. A., & Garrett, M. T. (2006). Native American healing traditions. *International Journal of Disability, Development, and Education, 53*(4), 453–469.

United States Department of Health and Human Services, Indian Health Service. (2017, September 3). *Navajo Nation.* Retrieved from: https://www.ihs.gov/navajo/navajonation/

Contents

Unit 2
Care of the Developing Child   173

18 Care of the School-Age Child   244

19 Care of the Adolescent   267

Unit 3
Care of the Hospitalized Child   289

Case Studies in This Book

Cases in Unit 1 That Are Referred Back to in Later Units

Cases That Unfold Across Units

Special Features in This Book

Analyze the Evidence

Growth and Development Check

The Pharmacy

Priority Care Concepts

Whose Job Is It, Anyway?

Unit 1
Scenarios for Clinical Preparation

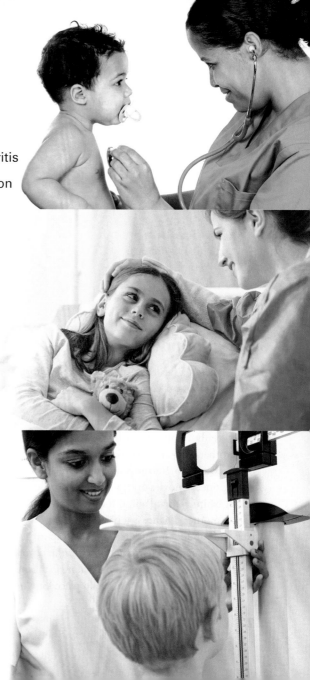

1

Chip Jones: Bronchiolitis

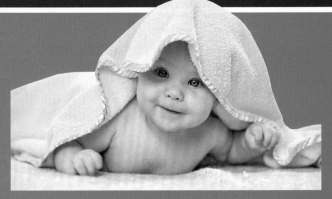

Objectives

After completing this chapter, you will be able to:
1. Describe normal growth and development of the 4-month-old.
2. Implement a teaching plan for a healthy 4-month-old.
3. Compare and contrast anatomic and physiologic characteristics of the respiratory systems of children and adults.
4. Relate pediatric assessment findings to the child's respiratory status.
5. Discuss the pathophysiology of bronchiolitis.
6. Identify various risk factors associated with bronchiolitis.
7. Outline the therapeutic regimen for bronchiolitis.
8. Create a nursing plan of care for an infant with bronchiolitis.

Key Terms

Alveoli
Anterior fontanelle
Anticipatory guidance
Antipyretic
Bronchioles

Grunting
Intercostal retractions
Nasal flaring
Posterior fontanelle
Temporal thermometer

Background

Chip Jones is a healthy 4-month-old male born at 38 weeks of gestation with no complications. He is the youngest of three siblings. He has a 3-year-old sister, Kate, who is in preschool and is not so thrilled to have another brother because she was really, really hoping for a little sister. Chip also has a 5-year-old brother, Tucker, who is in kindergarten. Tucker is excited to have another boy in the house so he doesn't have to watch any more princess movies or trip over any more high-heeled princess shoes. Chip's father, Paul, is the principal at a local high school. Chip's mother, Diane, is a paralegal. Diane went back to work part-time about a month ago, when Chip turned 12 weeks old.

Chip's parents were ready to put him in day care when Diane went back to work. There was an opening in the infant room where Kate is in preschool. Things were in place for Chip to start when

Paul's mother, who recently retired, offered to watch Chip at her house. This was a huge relief to Paul and Diane. Day cares do not usually take infants part-time, so Chip's parents would have had to pay the full-time rate, even though they would have only been using the day care 3 days a week. Money is scarce right now with them having three children and Diane only going back to work part-time, so Paul and Diane quickly accepted Grandma's offer.

The week before Diane started back to work, she began having doubts about Grandma watching Chip. Paul's mother smokes a pack of cigarettes per day. Diane knows that it is not healthy for babies to be around smokers, especially those who smoke inside the home (Patient Teaching 1.1). She decided to ask Grandma to only smoke on the deck and to wear a shirt or coat over her clothes while smoking that she can take off before she goes inside. Diane knows this is not ideal, but not having to pay for day care will help them save a lot of money.

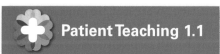

Patient Teaching 1.1 — The Effects of Exposure to Environmental Tobacco Smoke

It is important for parents and caregivers to understand the effects of exposure to environmental tobacco smoke (ETS) on infants and children, even if there are no smokers in their homes. ETS includes both secondhand smoke (SHS) and thirdhand smoke (THS). SHS is smoke that is inhaled directly from smokers. THS is exposure to nicotine-like contaminants that settle into furniture, carpets, rugs, food, and other household items. Infants and children with regular exposure to ETS are at increased risk for:

- Lower respiratory tract infections
- Otitis media (middle ear infection)
- Upper respiratory tract infections
- Overall decreased lung function
- Development of attention deficit hyperactivity disorder
- Decreased gross motor and fine motor function

Adapted from Evlampidou et al. (2015), Roberts et al. (2017), and Yeramaneni et al. (2015).

Inform parents and caregivers that the best way to decrease the risks to their children associated with exposure to ETS is for them to avoid any exposure to ETS at all. Just having someone smoke outside is not enough, as smoke particles can adhere to the smoker's clothing and be inhaled by the infant when he or she is held by the smoker. Similarly, when someone smokes inside the home, smoke particles can adhere to the carpet and furniture and later be inhaled by a child. If the parents of pediatric patients are smokers, tell them that the best way to keep their children healthy is to stop smoking. Even if you are not a smoker, family members and caregivers who smoke can still affect your baby. Tell them, too, to encourage family members, caregivers, and others who are around their children regularly to stop smoking. A list of resources to help with quitting smoking are available at the following website of the Centers for Disease Control and Prevention: http://www.cdc.gov/tobacco/quit_smoking/how_to_quit/resources/.

It has now been about a month since Diane went back to work. Things have been going well at Grandma's house. Diane was pleasantly surprised at how well Paul's mother accepted the request to smoke outside only. Diane is glad to have Chip with family rather than in a day care center, with all those germs.

Chip turns 4 months old this week. Diane remembers that she needs to make an appointment for his well-care visit. He had his 2-month-old immunizations on time, and she doesn't want him to fall behind on his 4-month-old immunizations. Also, Chip has only rolled over once from front to back, and she wants to make sure that he is on track developmentally (Growth and Development Check 1.1). She is concerned because her other two children seemed to roll over all the time once they figured out how.

Growth and Development Check 1.1 — Infant Milestones

Type of Development	Development Milestones at 2 mo	Development Milestones at 4 mo
• Social and emotional	• Has a purposeful and social smile • Focuses on the parent • Can calm self, briefly	• Smiles to get attention • Enjoys playing • Can calm self
• Speech	• Coos • Has different cries for different needs	• Babbles • May copy sounds
• Cognitive	• Follows objects with eyes • Can get bored	• Responds to affection • Indicates whether happy or upset • Recognizes people
• Gross and fine motor	• Can hold the head up when held • Begins to push up when on the stomach • Arm and leg movements are more coordinated	• May roll from front to back • Holds the head steady when sitting on a lap • Has the hand and eye coordination necessary to reach for objects • Pushes up on the elbows when lying on the stomach • Brings the hands to the mouth

Adapted from the Centers for Disease Control and Prevention. (2016, August 18). *Learn the signs. Act early. Developmental milestones.* Retrieved from https://www.cdc.gov/ncbddd/actearly/milestones/index.html

Growth and Development Check 1.2

Physical Growth

Age	Rate of Increase in Weight (oz/wk)	Rate of Increase in Length (in/mo)
Newborn to 6 mo	5–7	0.5–1
Six to 12 mo	3–5	0.5

Note: Infants typically double their birth weight by 6 mo and triple their birth weight by 1 y of age; they typically increase their birth length by 1½ times by 1 y of age.

Health Promotion

Diane is able to get Chip in quickly for his 4-month-old well-care visit. She is glad that the nurse practitioner, Laura, has an opening because Laura is gentle with babies. At birth, Chip weighed 7 lb 6 oz. Today, he weighs 13 lb 9 oz. His length at birth was 19.5 in. Today, his length is 23.5 in (Growth and Development Check 1.2).

Laura tells Diane, "Chip is right on track with his weight and length. Babies tend to double their birth weight at 5 to 6 months of age and triple their birth weight at 12 months. Are you still breastfeeding Chip since you've gone back to work?"

"I am," Diane says. "I pump while I'm at work and then take the bottles of breast milk to Grandma's house for Chip to have while he is there."

"So, tell me about Chip's gross motor development. How is he able to move his body now?"

"Well, he can hold his head steady, and he pushes up on his hands when he is on his belly. Also, he seems to want to stand up when you hold him upright on the floor."

"That's great," Laura says, typing some notes into Chip's electronic health record on her tablet. "Is there anything you're concerned about with his development?"

"Yes, actually," Diane says. "I'm a little worried because I've only seen him roll over once from lying on his front to lying on his back. My other kids were doing that all the time when they were his age."

"I don't think there's any cause for concern at this point. Babies tend to roll over between 4 and 5 months of age and should be able to roll both ways—from front to back and from back to front—by 6 months. If he's already rolled from front to back, then he's on track developmentally. And it's okay if he doesn't roll a lot; some babies just don't like to."

"How about smiling and talking?" Laura says. "Is he doing any of that?"

Diane laughs and says, "Are you kidding me? He can hardly stay quiet. He hears his brother and sister talking and tries to join in the conversation. He's so happy to see them when they get home in the afternoon—he has the biggest smile on his face."

"Wonderful," Laura says. "What about reaching out to grab things?"

"He does try to grab the toys that hang over his bouncy seat, but he can't quite reach them yet."

"Chip seems to be developing well. He's reaching milestones in all the domains we assess: gross motor, fine motor, speech/social, and cognitive/psychosocial."

Next, Laura completes Chip's physical exam. She listens to his chest with her stethoscope, and after a moment says, "His heart sounds are good, and his lungs sound nice and clear." She gently feels the top of his head and says, "The soft spot here, called the **anterior fontanelle**, is nice and soft and flat, which is perfectly normal. It typically closes between 12 and 18 months of age." She moves her hand to the back of his head and feels it. "Good—it feels like the soft spot in the back here, called the **posterior fontanelle**, is closed, as it should be. It usually closes between 2 and 3 months of age."

Laura finishes up the exam by assessing the ears, nose, and throat, which she says she saves for last because it irritates babies the most and she doesn't want to make Chip cry until she must.

When she's finished with the exam, Laura says, "Chip looks good. My only concern is that he does have some nasal congestion. Keep an eye on that, and if it gets worse or you're concerned, call the office and let us know."

"Oh—Okay," Diane says. How did she manage not to notice his congestion, she wonders. She worries about what could have caused it and feels a little guilty, although she's not sure why.

As usual, Laura completes the visit with some health promotion teaching and something she calls **anticipatory guidance**, which is explaining to Diane what to expect from Chip before their next well-care visit. If he stays healthy, Laura will not need to see Chip again until he is 6 months old. A big focus for Laura is safety.

"What kind of car seat are you using for Chip?" Laura asks (Box 1.1).

"I put him in a rear-facing car seat in the middle row of our van."

"Perfect. Another safety concern, now that Chip is rolling, is his home environment. There are many potential hazards in the home, especially with your older children around. Be careful not to set him down anyplace where he could injure himself by rolling over, such as on a bed or near open stairs. I recommend

Box 1.1 Child Car Seat Safety Recommendations and Laws

- The American Academy of Pediatrics recommends that infants stay in a rear-facing car seat with a five-point harness until 2 years of age (American Academy of Pediatric [AAP], 2014—Policy Statement).
- Car seat laws vary by state, but only four states (California, New Jersey, Pennsylvania, and Oklahoma) require children under the age of 2 to be in a rear-facing seat. You can find state car seat laws at http://www.ghsa.org/html/stateinfo/laws/childsafety_laws.html (Governor's Highway Safety Association, 2016).

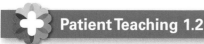

Patient Teaching 1.2

Protecting Infants Who Have Begun to Roll Over

Now that your baby can roll:
- Never leave your baby alone on a high surface, such as a bed, couch, or changing table
- Look for small objects on the floor that your baby could choke on
- Keep plastic bags away from your baby
- Keep hot liquids, such as a cup of coffee, out of your baby's reach

enlisting the help of Chip's siblings, Kate and Tucker, to help you make sure that the house is safe" (Patient Teaching 1.2).

"That's a great idea," Diane says. "They love helping me."

"Another danger to look out for is environmental tobacco smoke. I know you and Paul don't smoke, which is great, but you also need to avoid having Chip around smokers, because secondhand or thirdhand smoke can put him at risk for many things, including respiratory diseases and lower respiratory tract infections that could result in hospitalization" (Roberts, Wagler, & Carr, 2017).

"We're not around too many smokers," Diane says. "Except for Paul's mother. Grandma watches Chip 3 days a week while I'm at work." She sees a look of concern appear on Laura's face and quickly adds, "But we made her promise to not smoke in the house anymore, only outside."

Laura is quiet a moment and then says, "Smoking outside is definitely better than in the house, but it still poses a risk to the baby. Grandma is likely to still have smoke particles on her clothing and in her furniture, which still counts as exposure to environmental tobacco smoke. Is she your only option for child care?"

"Day care is so expensive," Diane says. She feels a vague sense of guilt coming over her and shudders. "Maybe I'll talk with Paul, to see what other options we might have."

"Great," Laura says. "Let's talk about feeding. I know you're an experienced mom. What is your game plan for starting Chip on solid food?"

"From what I recall, I should start him on baby food by the time he's 6 months old, right?"

"Exactly right. However, you shouldn't give him any honey or cow's milk until he is at least 1 year old."

"That's right," Diane says. "I remember that now. I've also heard recently that I shouldn't give him eggs or fish. Is that true?"

"Actually, no. There is no evidence to show that feeding your baby eggs or fish starting at 6 months of age will harm him, although I know that's a popular belief lately" (Analyze the Evidence 1.1).

After covering a few more points related to anticipatory guidance, Laura says, "Do you have any questions?"

Analyze the Evidence 1.1

Introduction of Solid Foods

The American Academy of Pediatrics recommends breastfeeding as the only source of nutrition until around 6 mo of age. However, many infants are ready to start solid foods between the ages of 4 and 6 mo. Although most healthcare providers recommend starting rice cereal first, followed by vegetables and then fruits, there is no medical evidence that the way in which solid foods are introduced matters. In fact, there is no evidence that introducing vegetables before fruits will ensure that children will like vegetables.

Healthcare providers also often recommend that infants should not have eggs or fish until 1 y of age due to the increased risk of allergies. However, there is no medical evidence that introducing these foods around 6 mo of age will increase a child's risk of allergies to them (AAP, 2017).

"No. Not right now."

"Okay. Well here's a sheet highlighting the important points about Chip's growth and development we've discussed, so that you'll have something to refer to at home" (Patient Teaching 1.3).

Patient Teaching 1.3

Anticipatory Guidance for 4-Month-Olds

Over the next 2 mo, you can expect your child to begin to:
- Recognize his or her name
- Enjoy playing, especially with parents
- String consonant sounds together while babbling
- Indicate joy and displeasure
- Eat pureed foods
- Reach for objects
- Roll both ways
- Sit in a tripod position without support
- Have teeth

As your child becomes more mobile, you will need to increase safety measures, such as the following:
- Either lock low cabinet doors or keep all breakable items and cleaning solutions in high cabinets
- Cover electrical outlets
- Make sure electrical cords are out of the way
- Never leave your child unattended on a high surface or on the floor
- Make sure all food is pureed, as your child will not be able to chew yet even if he or she has some teeth

"The last thing on the agenda for today's visit is immunizations," Laura says. "Chip will get the same immunizations today as he did at his 2-month-old visit." Laura explains that these include rotavirus; diphtheria, tetanus, acellular pertussis (DTaP); haemophilus influenzae type b (Hib); pneumococcal conjugate vaccine (PCV13); and inactivated polio vaccine (IPV; Patient Teaching 1.4). "How did Chip tolerate the 2-month-old immunizations?"

Patient Teaching 1.4

Immunizations for 4-Month-Olds

The immunizations that your baby will get at his or her 4-mo-old checkup are as follows:
- Diphtheria, tetanus, acellular pertussis (DTaP)
  - The DTaP vaccine protects against:
    - Diphtheria, a serious infection of the throat that can block the airway.
    - Tetanus, otherwise known as lockjaw, is a nerve disease.
    - Pertussis, otherwise known as whooping cough, is a respiratory infection that can have serious complications.
- *Haemophilus influenzae type b* (Hib)
  - The Hib vaccine protects against a type of bacteria that causes meningitis, mostly in children under the age of 5.
- Pneumococcal conjugate vaccine (PCV13)
  - The PCV13 vaccine protects against 13 types of pneumococcal bacteria, which can cause pneumonia, meningitis, and certain types of blood infections.
- Inactivated polio virus (IPV)
  - The IPV vaccine protects against polio, which can cause paralysis and death.
- Rotavirus (RV)
  - The RV vaccine protects against a virus that causes severe diarrhea in infants and that can lead to dehydration and even hospitalization.

Common Side Effects
After your baby gets immunizations, he or she may exhibit one or more of the following:
- Run a fever of up to around 102°F
- Have redness or a small amount of swelling at the injection site
- Be fussier in the 24 h after immunizations
- Sleep more in the 24 h after immunizations

When to Call the Healthcare Provider
- If your child has a fever of 105°F or higher
- If your child has a seizure
- If your child has uncontrollable crying for 3 h or longer

Adapted from the Centers for Disease Control and Prevention. (2017). *Provider resources for vaccine conversations with parents.* Retrieved from http://www.cdc.gov/vaccines/hcp/conversations/prevent-diseases/provider-resources-factsheets-infants.html

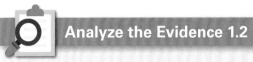

Analyze the Evidence 1.2

Antipyretics and Immunizations

It is common practice for healthcare providers to recommend that parents give an antipyretic either before or after the administration of immunizations to prevent fever. However, fever helps the body mount an antibody response against both viral and bacterial pathogens. The results from one study by Prymula et al. (2009) indicate that giving an antipyretic to infants receiving immunizations reduces the antigen response to the vaccine. Therefore, it might be best for the infant to only be given an antipyretic if necessary, such as in the case of a high fever or extreme fussiness.

In a more recent study, Saleh, Moody, and Walter (2016) further investigated the effects of antipyretics on immunization effectiveness. Saleh et al. (2016) found that the timing of the antipyretic played an important role in immunization effectiveness. Antipyretics given prophylactically reduced immunization effectiveness. Antipyretics given at least 4 h after the administration of an immunization had no effect on immunization effectiveness. Furthermore, antipyretics had no effect on immunization booster doses, no matter the timing of antipyretic administration.

"He slept more the day he got the immunizations and was a little fussier when he was awake, but otherwise he was fine," Diane says. "Oh—wait. He did have a temperature of 100.4°F that night. Could we give some acetaminophen before he gets the immunizations this time?"

"Actually, the fever helps his body create antibodies, which is a good thing, so unless Chip's temperature is high—say, above 103°F—or he is extremely uncomfortable, I'd prefer that we hold off on giving him the acetaminophen or any other **antipyretic**" (Analyze the Evidence 1.2; The Pharmacy 1.1).

Diane holds Chip while the nurse gives him the shots. Some of the immunizations are combined into one syringe, so he ends up only getting two shots, one in each thigh. Diane asks why Chip can't get the shots in his arm like her other children. The nurse tells her it is because infants do not have enough fat in their arms yet. Chip does well with his shots; he hardly cries. When Diane is on her way to the checkout window, Laura tells her that she will see her in 2 months for Chip's 6-month-old checkup.

At Home

Two days after his checkup, Chip wakes up with a stuffy nose. Diane checks his temperature with a **temporal thermometer**. It's 99.5°F, which is nothing really to worry about. Diane is supposed to go to work today, and she knows her husband, Paul, can't take the day off because it is midterm exam week at his school.

The Pharmacy 1.1 — Acetaminophen and Ibuprofen

Medication	Classification	Route	Action	Nursing Considerations

• Acetamin-ophen	• Analgesic
	• Antipyretic
		• PO
		• PR
		• IV
			• Analgesic: inhibits CNS prostaglandin synthesis and peripherally inhibits pain impulses
			• Antipyretic: inhibits the heat-regulating center of the hypothalamus
				• 10–15 mg/kg every 4–6 h
				• Do not exceed 4,000 mg/d
				• Metabolized by the liver
				• Can be hepatotoxic
				• Monitor with long-term use:
				  ○ Liver function
				  ○ Alanine aminotransferase
				• Aspartate aminotransferase
				• Monitor for s/s of liver toxicity

• Ibuprofen	• Analgesic
	• Antipyretic
	• Anti-inflammatory
		• PO
		• IV
			• Inhibits cyclooxygenase 1 and 2
			• Decreases prostaglandin precursors
				• 5–10 mg/kg every 6–8 h
				• Do not exceed 1,200 mg/d unless directed to by healthcare provider
				• Do not give to infants under 6 mo of age due to immature renal system
				• Excreted by the kidneys
				• Can be nephrotoxic
				• Monitor intake and output
				• Monitor with long-term use
				  ○ Blood urea nitrogen
				  ○ Creatinine
				• Monitor for s/s of:
				  ○ GI irritation
				  ○ GI bleeding
				• Increased bruising or bleeding due to decreased platelet adhesion

CNS, central nervous system; GI, gastrointestinal; IV, intravenous; PO, oral; PR, rectal; s/s, signs and symptoms.
Adapted from Taketomo, C. K., Hodding, J. H., & Kraus, D. M. (2018). *Pediatric & neonatal dosage handbook* (25th ed.). Hudson, OH: Lexicomp.

Although Diane knows that this temperature is not concerning, she can't remember whether it could be a side effect of the immunizations. Just to be sure, she calls the pediatrician's office.

After Diane tells the nurse who answers the phone her concerns, the nurse replies, "It's possible that his temperature is elevated from the immunizations, but if so, it should return to normal within the next 24 hours. However, his congestion is definitely not a side effect of the immunizations, and combined with the slight elevation in temperature, it could mean that he has an infection of some kind."

"I was afraid of that," Diane says. "What should I do?"

"Watch him closely for worsening symptoms, such as cough or difficulty breathing. He may also have more trouble nursing, because babies breathe through their noses until they are 4 months old, so when they're congested, they have trouble breathing and nursing or bottle-feeding at the same time" (Casey, 2015). "So, for the next few days, he may need to have more frequent feedings because he won't be able to take in as much at each feeding."

Diane is glad she called the pediatrician's office. She had forgotten about babies having trouble feeding while they are congested. She will need to remember to tell Grandma that Chip probably will not eat as much today because he is congested. She's also glad that Grandma is watching Chip. It is much more comforting knowing that he is being watched by a family member when he may be getting sick than having him at a day care. It really seems to be working out well. And Grandma has been keeping her word about not smoking in the house since Chip started coming there. At least it smells a lot less smoky lately than it used to. I'm just a little uptight, she thinks to herself. Chip will be fine.

That evening when Diane picks Chip up from Grandma's, Grandma tells her that Chip did eat less today. Normally, Grandma gives him three 5-oz bottles during the day. Today, he finished only 3 to 4 oz of each bottle. She also tells Diane that Chip was fussy most of the day and had trouble napping. She says it would have been nice to have a bulb syringe in the house so that she could have gotten some of the mucus out of Chip's nose before he ate (Fig. 1.1). Grandma asks Diane to bring one with her when she drops Chip off tomorrow.

Later that evening, Chip has trouble nursing. He keeps pulling off the breast because he is too congested. Diane tries to use the bulb syringe on his nose, and it really makes him mad. She gets some mucus out but not enough, and he continues to have trouble nursing. He is fussy all evening. When Diane puts him

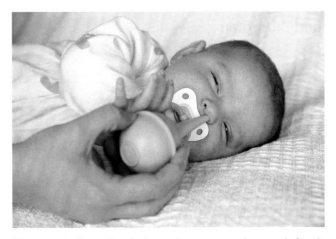

Figure 1.1. Use of a bulb syringe to suction an infant's nostrils. To use the bulb syringe, squeeze the bulb prior to inserting it in the nostril. Gently insert the tip of the syringe into the nostril and release the bulb. Empty the syringe into a tissue and wash the syringe after use.

to bed at 8:00, she takes his temperature. It is up to 100.8°F. She talks to Paul, and they decide to give Chip some Tylenol to help make him comfortable, so he can sleep. Tucker and Kate ask whether Chip is okay. Diane tells them that Chip seems to have a little cold but will be just fine.

Chip has a rough night and is up more than usual. The fussiness continues through the morning, but his temperature goes back down to 99.6°F. Diane considers calling in sick but Grandma convinces her to go to work. Once again, Diane drops Chip off at Grandma's. She gives her an extra bulb syringe but tells her it likely won't help very much.

When Diane returns to pick him up, Chip seems a little worse. Grandma says he ate less today than yesterday. Now he doesn't want to nurse at all. He is less fussy but more lethargic. His temperature at his 8:00 bedtime tonight is 101°F. Diane is not one to panic; after all, she has two older children and has been through illnesses like this before. She and Paul decide to see how Chip does through the night. If he is no better in the morning, Diane will make an appointment to see Laura. Diane is off tomorrow, so it works out well. She hopes that Chip is not getting an ear infection. Every time Tucker would get a cold, he would get an ear infection, although Tucker was in day care and around all those germs. Diane thinks that Chip is better off because Grandma is watching him, so there are fewer germs to contend with.

In the morning, Chip has a temperature of 101.5°F. He does not want to nurse at all, and Diane thinks that she hears some strange noises when he breathes. His nostrils also seem to be flaring out a lot when he takes a breath. She knows that this is definitely not normal and calls the pediatrician's office. The receptionist schedules a sick appointment with Laura for right before lunch.

At the Pediatrician's Office

By the time Diane gets to the appointment, she is starting to really worry about Chip. He still does not want to nurse, so she is pumping her breast milk. His temperature is still 101.5°F,

according to her temporal thermometer, but he just seems worse. His breathing is noisier and very fast.

The nurse calls Diane and Chip back to a room. Before they go into the room, they stop to get Chip's weight and vital signs. Chip weighs 13 lb 7 oz. That is odd, thinks Diane. Just 3 days ago at his checkup he weighed 13 lb 9 oz. He was naked both times, and he is on the same scale today as he was the other day. She will have to ask Laura about this. His temperature is 101.8°F, respiratory rate is 60 breaths/min, and apical heart rate is 150 beats/min (bpm). The nurse puts Diane and Chip in a room and says that Laura will be here in a minute.

Laura enters the room and says, "So what's been going with Chip?"

Diane recounts the story of how Chip has been since his visit 3 days ago. "I only gave him Tylenol once, the first night he was congested," she tells Laura. "He's barely eaten anything in the past 24 hours, and his weight is down 2 oz. I'm getting a little scared, to be honest."

Laura takes Chip from Diane, places him on the exam table, and examines him. "He's having trouble breathing," Laura says almost immediately. "See his **nasal flaring** and how the skin between his ribs pulls in when he breathes, which is called **intercostal retractions**? And do you hear those **grunting** sounds he makes with each breath?"

"What does that mean?" Diane says, feeling the anxiety rising up within her. "What do we do?"

"Let me check his oxygen saturation," Laura says. She sticks her head out the door and asks the nurse, "Pulse oximeter, please." Turning back to Diane, she says, "Chip's respiratory rate is high, and his nostril flaring, grunting, and intercostal retractions all indicate that he is in respiratory distress" (Box 1.2; Fig. 1.2).

Box 1.2 Signs of Respiratory Distress in Infants

Signs of mild respiratory distress include:
- Fussiness
- Congestion
- Decreased intake

Signs of moderate distress include:
- Nasal flaring
- Grunting
- Retractions
- Mild tachypnea
- Mild tachycardia

Signs of severe distress include:
- Cyanosis
- Diaphoresis
- Dehydration
- Severe tachypnea
- Severe tachycardia
- Exhaustion with respiratory effort

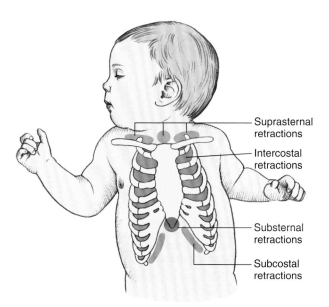

Figure 1.2. **Assessment of chest retractions.** Retractions can indicate respiratory distress in infants and children. During the focused respiratory assessment, note the location (subcostal, substernal, intercostal, or suprasternal) as well as the depth (mild or deep) of the retractions. Reprinted with permission from Gomella, L. G. (2007). *Nurse's 5-minute clinical consult: Signs & symptoms* (1st ed.). Philadelphia, PA: Lippincott Williams & Wilkins.

The nurse arrives with the pulse oximeter and attaches a sensor to his foot. She reports that Chip's O_2 saturation level is 89%.

"What does that mean?" Diane says. "Is that bad?"

"It means Chip does not have enough oxygen in his blood," Laura replies. "His body is trying to compensate for the low oxygen by breathing faster. The faster breathing causes Chip to lose more water. The increased respiratory rate, along with the decrease in breast milk intake, is why Chip has lost weight in the past few days."

"What causes the oxygen to be low, to begin with?" Diane asks.

"Most likely it's because he has mucus in his lungs that is clogging the **bronchioles** and preventing the lungs from properly oxygenating the blood. Babies' airways are much smaller and narrower than those in adults and can become obstructed more easily" (Let's Compare 1.1).

"I'm going to complete a focused respiratory assessment," Laura says. She examines the skin of his fingers and toes.

"His skin looks a little bluish," Diane says. "Is that because of the low oxygen?"

"Yes," Laura says. "It's not bad, though; he's not cyanotic." She pulls out her stethoscope and listens to his chest. "He has crackles in his lung bases bilaterally," she says, "And his peripheral pulses are two plus. He's lethargic but awake and responsive."

"What does all this mean?" Diane says, growing impatient.

Let's Compare 1.1 Airway Structures and Risk of Obstruction

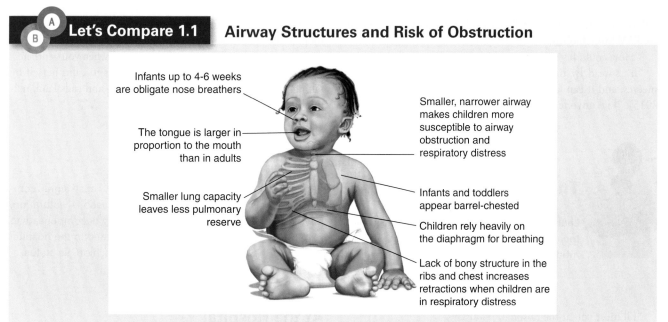

An infant's tongue is larger in proportion to the mouth than in adults, increasing the risk for obstruction with narrowing of the airway. The trachea is cartilaginous and the neck is shorter in an infant, further increasing the risk for airway obstruction and collapse.

Because the bronchi and bronchioles are smaller in infants, they are more easily obstructed than those of adults. Infants also have fewer **alveoli** than adults, leaving even less room for air exchange when mucus is obstructing the bronchioles. Even slight obstruction can have a large impact on an infant's work of breathing.

Image adapted with permission from Ateah, C. A., Scott, S. D., & Kyle, T. (2012). *Canadian essentials of pediatric nursing* (1st ed., Fig. 19.1). Philadelphia, PA: Lippincott Williams & Wilkins.

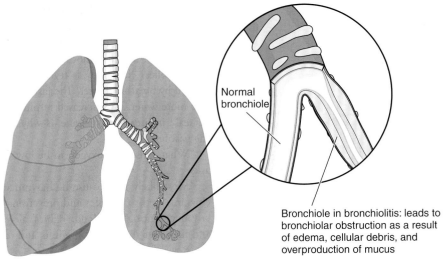

Normal bronchiole

Bronchiole in bronchiolitis: leads to bronchiolar obstruction as a result of edema, cellular debris, and overproduction of mucus

Figure 1.3. Bronchiolitis. Bronchiolitis is an infection that affects the small tubes that carry air in and out of the lungs. When infected, these tubes (called bronchioles) get swollen and inflamed, making it harder to breathe.

Laura hangs the stethoscope back around her neck and gently strokes Chip's cheek with the back of her hand. "I think he has bronchiolitis," she says after a moment. "It's a lower respiratory tract infection most commonly caused by RSV, which stands for respiratory syncytial virus. This virus causes the cells in the lining of the small airways, the bronchioles, to die and accumulate in the lower airway along with mucus, obstructing the smaller airways" (Fig. 1.3). "All of this is what is causing Chip to cough and have difficulty breathing" (Casey, 2015; Meissner, 2016). "This time of year, fall and winter, is the typical time to see RSV bronchiolitis."

"How could he have gotten this virus?" Diane asks.

"It's spread by tiny water droplets, such as when someone sneezes, and it can last up to 6 hours on hard surfaces" (Casey, 2015). "Has anyone else in your family been sick?"

"Kate came home from preschool with a runny nose a few days ago, but she's not *this* sick."

"Children over the age of two, like Kate, don't usually get as sick from bronchiolitis," Laura explains. "Chip's age, combined with the exposure to secondhand smoke, is the most likely reason he is having this much respiratory difficulty." Laura picks up Chip from the exam table and turns and hands him to Diane. Her expression is so serious that it gives Diane chills. "Chip needs to be admitted to the hospital," she says. "He is too sick to be observed at home. He needs oxygen, fluids, and observation. Take him to the emergency room at the children's hospital and tell them that he is a direct admit. The orders for admission will be waiting when you get there."

Clutching Chip in her arms, Diane tries to calm herself by taking some deep breaths. She begins to cry and calls Paul, telling him what is going on.

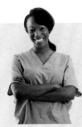

The Nurse's Point of View

Laura: I don't want to worry Diane and Paul too much, but Chip is showing signs of moderate respiratory distress such as nasal flaring, grunting, retractions, and lethargy. These signs, combined with his bilateral crackles and decreased O_2 saturation, have me concerned that Chip could quickly decompensate to respiratory failure. I want to get him admitted to the hospital quickly so the nurses can keep a close watch on his status.

"I'll meet you at the hospital," Paul says.

"No—wait," Diane says. "Someone needs to pick Kate and Tucker up from school."

"I'll ask my mom to get them and watch them. As soon as they're taken care of, I'll come to the hospital."

"Hurry, dear. I'm getting a little scared."

"Take a deep breath, Diane. It's going to be okay. Chip will be okay."

At the Hospital

Diane lugs Chip into the emergency room in his car seat carrier. She goes to the check-in desk and tells them Chip is a direct admit, just as Laura instructed her to do.

The clerk looks at her computer, finds Chip's name, and says, "Yes—we have his admission orders. An assistant will be down shortly to take you up to the pediatric unit."

"Could you please tell the assistant to hurry?" Diane says. "He's coughing more and more; I think he's getting worse."

Diane and Chip are quickly escorted to a private room on the pediatric inpatient unit, where Chip will be admitted. Diane takes him out of his carrier and sits and holds him while they wait. Chip is coughing a lot, and Diane tries to hold him upright and pats his back, hoping it will help. Really, though, she doesn't know what to do.

Soon a nurse comes in and says, "Hi. I'm Zac. I'll be admitting Chip and taking care of him until seven this evening. I have a student nurse with me; would it be okay with you if she helps me take care of Chip?"

"The more, the merrier," Diane says, trying to keep her spirits up.

Zac takes Chip from Diane, places him in the hospital crib, and puts an armband on him. He says, "Is this his correct name and birthdate?"

"Yes," Diane says.

Zac proceeds with Chip's admission orders.

"I'd like to begin with a quick assessment," Zac explains to his student. "Although we have a report from the patient's primary care provider, I want to make sure there have been no important changes in Chip's status since he left the pediatrician's office." Zac reports Chip's vital signs as follows:

- Temperature: 101.9°F (38.8°C)
- Apical pulse: 150 bpm
- Respiratory rate: 62 breaths/min
- Blood pressure: 80/40 mm Hg
- Blood O_2 saturation: 89% on room air

Chip continues to have grunting, nasal flaring, and intercostal retractions. Zac points out to his student that Chip is lethargic but fussy with the exam, has course crackles in the lung bases bilaterally, and is pale and mildly diaphoretic.

Zac asks Diane, "Would you take off Chip's clothes so that I can get an accurate weight?"

"But he was just weighed at the pediatrician's office," Diane says.

"Yes, but I need to get a baseline weight on the hospital scale because he will be measured on the same scale each day, for accuracy," Zac explains.

Zac weighs Chip and announces that his weight is 13 lb 7 oz on the hospital scale, or 6.1 kg, and then documents this in the chart.

"Why did you calculate the weight in kilograms?" the nursing student asks.

"All calculations for fluids and medication in children are weight-based, and kilograms are the standard unit of measure used to calculate correct doses," Zac replies.

"What's going to happen next?" Diane asks.

"Your nurse practitioner, Laura, sent orders that include starting intravenous, or IV, fluids, oxygen, and nasal suction, so I'll be getting all of that set up," Zac says (Box 1.3).

Zac and his student go through the orders together.

"Why is there no medication ordered?" The nursing student asks. "If bronchiolitis causes airway obstruction, shouldn't there

---

Box 1.3 Orders for Chip Jones

- Admit to A4 North with a diagnosis of bronchiolitis
- Implement respiratory (droplet) precautions
- Start a peripheral intravenous line
- Run normal saline at 25 mL/h
- Administer oxygen per nasal cannula and titrate to keep the O_2 saturation level at 92% or greater
- Check O_2 saturation every 2 h
- Perform nasotracheal suction prior to feeds
- Feed by mouth as tolerated
- Take daily weights

---

be a medication ordered to open the airway? I read that albuterol helps open the airway. Why wasn't it ordered for the patient?"

"The latest evidence indicates that medications do not decrease the length of stay in infants with bronchiolitis, nor do they improve the outcome," Zac says. "The mainstay of bronchiolitis treatment is supportive, hence the fluids and oxygen" (Analyze the Evidence 1.3).

Zac and his student set up the oxygen and nasal cannula. Zac explains that they are giving Chip oxygen at a rate of 3 L/min and that his blood O_2 saturation level currently is right at 92%, occasionally dropping to 91%.

"Do you know whether Chip's nose was suctioned at the pediatrician's office?" Zac asks Diane.

"No," she says. "Is that really necessary? Won't it make him mad?"

Analyze the Evidence 1.3

Bronchiolitis Guidelines

The latest guidelines from the American Academy of Pediatrics state that clinicians should not use albuterol, corticosteroids, or antibiotics in the treatment regimen of an infant with bronchiolitis. Furthermore, continuous O_2 saturation monitoring and chest physiotherapy have not been shown to be beneficial in the treatment of infants hospitalized with bronchiolitis. Numerous studies show hydration with isotonic intravenous fluids, feeding as tolerated with suction prior to feeds, and spot O_2 saturation checks to keep O_2 saturation above 90% to be adequate in the treatment of hospitalized infants with bronchiolitis.

Data from Makic, M. B. F., Rauen, C., Jones, K., & Fisk, A. C. (2015). Continuing to challenge practice to be evidence based. *Critical Care Nurse, 35*(2), 39-50; Moschino, L., Mario, F., Carraro, S., Visentin, F., Zanconato, S., & Baraldi, E. (2016). Is nasal suctioning warranted before measuring O2 saturation in infants with bronchiolitis? *Archives of Disease in Childhood, 101*(1), 114-115; Ralston, S. L., Lieberthal, A. S., Meissner, H. C., Alverson, B. K., Baley, J. E., Gadomski, A. M., . . . Hernandez-Cancio, S. (2014). Clinical practice guideline: The diagnosis, management and prevention of bronchiolitis. *Pediatrics, 134*(5), e1474 -e1502. doi:10.1542/peds.2014-2742.

"He probably won't be happy about it," Zac says. "But it can help clear his airway and improve his breathing, so that he'll require less supplemental oxygen and be able to nurse better."

"Why are we starting with the oxygen and suctioning instead of starting an IV line?" the nursing student asks.

"Infants develop respiratory distress very quickly, and Chip is already showing signs of moderate distress," Zac says. "To prevent him from decompensating, we need to attend to his respiratory status first" (Patient Safety 1.1).

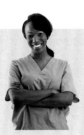

The Nurse's Point of View

Zac: I know that implementing interventions to improve Chip's respiratory status is my priority. I then need to continue monitoring his respiratory status throughout my shift. Chip's mother is scared, so I'll make sure to explain to her what I am doing and why. It's crucial that I'm aware of any slight changes indicating worsening respiratory status because he could decompensate to respiratory failure quickly. The concept of oxygenation is an important one for my student to learn. I think I'll quiz her at the end of the shift to make sure she understands oxygenation in infants and priority nursing interventions.

Zac explains to his student that they'll be using a size 6 French suction catheter and attaching it to the wall suction. Zac allows the student to carefully suction Chip's nostrils on both sides. Diane sees the student suction out a lot of thick, white mucus. Chip becomes extremely fussy.

"See—he doesn't like that," Diane says. "Poor kid is miserable enough, as it is."

"That's a normal reaction," Zac says. "It's actually a good thing, because it shows that he has enough energy and stamina to get mad." Zac reapplies the nasal cannula and reports that he is now able to get a steady blood O$_2$ saturation reading of 92% on 3 L of oxygen.

"Next, we're going to start the peripheral IV line," Zac tells his student. While they are placing the IV, Chip gets upset all

over again, but Zac again reassures Diane that the fussiness is a good sign. The IV goes in without incident and the normal saline line is primed and ready.

After Zac hooks the fluids up, he says to his student, "I'm setting the pump at 25 mL/h. Now, let's take a look at the IV site. What do you see?"

"It looks good," the student replies. "It's just a little pink with no evidence of infection or infiltration."

"Exactly," Zac says. "Now document that in the chart."

"Now that we've implemented the admission orders, we need to do a pain assessment," Zac tells the student, "Because the patient has not had surgery and is not on pain medication, we'll only need to conduct the pain assessment once per shift."

"How are we supposed to conduct a pain assessment on an infant?" the student asks. "It's not like he can tell us about his pain."

"Actually, there are a couple of ways to assess infant pain," Zac says. "The first is to ask the parents or caregivers. They are usually attuned to the different cries that babies have and know which one signals pain. The second is to use a pain scale. In this case, I'd like to use the FLACC infant pain scale, which assesses pain according to signs in five different areas: the face, legs, activity, cry, and consolability." Zac walks the student through assessing Chip's pain using this scale (How Much Does It Hurt? 1.1).

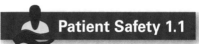

Monitoring Respiratory Status

Due to the narrow airways, cartilaginous trachea, short neck, and large tongue of infants, their respiratory status can decompensate very quickly. When an infant is admitted to the hospital with a respiratory illness, it is imperative that the respiratory status be monitored closely and any alterations in status, even the slightest change, be communicated to the healthcare provider in charge.

These changes include the following:
- Nasal flaring
- Grunting
- Retractions or change in location of retractions
- Increasing tachypnea
- Increasing tachycardia
- Decrease in O$_2$ saturation despite suction and oxygen administration
- Increased need for oxygen administration
- Increased irritability
- Decreased responsiveness
- Bradypnea
- Bradycardia

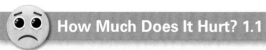

Chip's FLACC Score*

Chip's total FLACC (face, legs, activity, cry, and consolability) score is a 2, based on the following ratings:
- Face: 0
- Legs: 1
- Activity: 0
- Cry: 0
- Consolability: 1

*For a description of the FLACC scale, see Chapter 15.

"So, how's he doing?" Diane asks. "What's his pain level like?"

"Not bad," Zac says. "He seems to have settled down some. His score on the FLACC is a two, meaning he has mild discomfort, most likely from working so hard to breathe. His breathing is easier, though, after the suctioning and with the oxygen."

"So, what happens next?" Diane asks.

"The goal now is to let Chip rest," Zac says (Priority Care Concepts 1.1). "But you can hold him and nurse him as you would at home." He takes Chip and hands him to Diane. "We'll leave you alone for a bit, but we'll be checking in frequently. The call light is right here on the wall. Just push the button if you need anything."

The thought of being alone with Chip worries Diane, and she realizes only as he's about to leave how comforting it has been to have Zac there taking care of Chip. "Is there anything else I should be doing?" Diane asks.

"You're doing everything you can just by being here with Chip, holding him and feeding him," Zac says (Hospital Help 1.1).

Several hours later, after everything has calmed down, Paul finally makes it to the hospital.

"I'm so glad to see you!" Diane says, as Paul walks into the room and stoops next to her, where she is sitting and holding Chip. "I've been so stressed out, going through this alone."

Priority Care Concepts 1.1

Alteration in Respiratory Status

Goals

Prior to leaving the hospital, Chip will:
- Show no signs of respiratory distress, such as nasal flaring, grunting, or retractions
- Have decreased crackles bilaterally
- Have a respiratory rate and heart rate within normal limits
- Be able to nurse without difficulty
- Be back to his weight of 13 lb 9 oz, which he was at his 4-mo-old checkup

Nursing Interventions
- Place in a position of comfort to maximize respiratory effort
- Monitor vital signs to determine improvement in status or to detect early decompensation
- Assess lung sounds every 4 h to determine the presence of adventitious lung sounds
- Monitor O_2 saturation levels every 2 h and adjust the rate of oxygen administration as needed to keep the levels at 92% to ensure adequate oxygenation
- Monitor respiratory status for signs of decompensation to determine the need for further intervention
- Suction prior to feedings to increase oxygenation and provide easier feeding
- Record intake and output to determine hydration status
- Take daily weights as ordered to monitor nutritional and hydration status

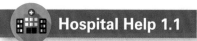

Hospital Help 1.1

Building Infant Trust

Infants are in the Erickson stage of trust versus mistrust. When an infant is in the hospital, it is important to keep feeding routines the same as much as possible. Allowing parents and caregivers to hold an infant whenever they can helps the infant maintain a sense of trust. If parents or caregivers cannot stay at the hospital, they can leave a recording of themselves singing a song or talking to the infant. They can also leave an object, such as a blanket, that has their scent on it. If they cannot stay, it is important that the nurses make sure the infant's needs are met to continue to establish a sense of trust.

Paul kisses her on the forehead and then gazes at Chip. "How you doing, there, little Chipper?" he says to his son. He asks his wife, "Okay if I hold him for a bit?"

"Sure," Diane says, holding Chip out to him. Paul takes him in his arms, stands, and rocks him from side to side. Paul seems so calm, so nonchalant. "What about Kate and Tucker?" Diane asks. "Who's watching them now?"

"They're at Grandma's," he says.

On hearing this, Diane feels overwhelmed and begins to cry.

"What's wrong, Di?" He says.

Diane is too distraught to talk and just cries harder.

Paul waits patiently as she cries it out, just like he always does. After a few moments, when she has calmed down, Paul ventures to say, "I know this has been stressful, and I'm sorry I couldn't get here sooner, but it seems like Chip is going to be just fine. They'll take good care of him here, I'm sure."

"It's all our fault that Chip is so sick," Diane says.

"What?" Paul says. "No. Why would you say a thing like that?"

"We shouldn't have let your mom keep him at her house. We should have just put him day care. Why were we so worried about saving the money? Why were we so stupid?"

"What are you talking about? What's wrong with him being at mom's? She takes good care of him."

"She smokes, Paul. It was the exposure to the smoke that made Chip sick, that made him prone to get this infection."

"I thought she had agreed to just smoke outside?"

Diane shook her head. "Doesn't matter. It's all in her clothes and her carpet and her furniture. It's everywhere."

Paul keeps rocking from side to side with Chip as he processes this.

"We can't let him go back there, Paul. Not unless she stops smoking altogether."

Paul is quiet. Out in the hall, a couple of nurses are discussing the shift schedule. Chip coughs a few times. "Okay, Di," Paul says at length. "I'll talk to mom about it."

Just then, Laura enters the room. "Hi, Diane," she says. "Hey, Paul. How are you all holding up?"

"Not great," Diane says.

"This has been a rough day for you all," Laura says. She walks over to Paul and smiles broadly at Chip. "Hey there, little guy." After a moment she turns back to Diane and Paul and says, "The good news is that Chip is already doing much better, according to the nurse's report here. Let me take a look at him myself."

Laura places Chip in the crib to examine him. "His grunting and nasal flaring have stopped, although he still has some intercostal retractions. He still has some crackles in his lungs, meaning there is still mucus and fluid. However, that may take a week or two to improve completely. I expect that tomorrow he will continue to improve and that he should be able to go home in about 48 hours, if all is well."

"What about nursing him?" Diane says. "He's had no interest today at all. What if I can't get him to nurse?"

"It's normal for infants in Chip's condition to refuse to feed," Laura says. "It should improve over the next couple of days. For now, I'd encourage you all to get some rest. There's a pull-out bed in the room, here, if one of you would like to stay in the room with him tonight. The night shift nurses here are just as great as the ones you met today, and they will keep a close eye on Chip overnight. I'll be back in the morning to see how he's doing."

Diane and Paul agree that she will stay with Chip overnight and that he'll pick up the other kids from Grandma's and take them home.

Zac and his nursing student come in later to check on Chip before the change of shift. "We're going to assess his oxygen saturation level and see whether we can start weaning him off the oxygen," Zac tells Diane. "To be discharged, Chip will need to be able to maintain his oxygen saturation at 92% or above on room air." Zac explains to his student that they are going to decrease Chip's oxygen rate from 3 to 2 L/min. They do so, and then monitor his O_2 saturation level for a time.

"It's going down," the nursing student says.

"That's not good, is it?" Diane says.

Zac shakes his head. "It's down to 90%. Looks like we'll need to keep him on 3 L/min through the night."

"Looks like we won't be headed home any time soon," Diane says. "How well does he have to be before he can be discharged?"

"Besides his oxygen saturation level being stable, he will also need to nurse without difficulty," Zac says. "I recommend that you call the night nurse to come and suction Chip when he is ready to nurse. That should make it easier for him. Beyond that, he'll need to demonstrate that he can breathe without difficulty, which means no nasal flaring or grunting and decreased retractions. However, he will most likely still be coughing, and his lung sounds probably will not be clear."

Zac and his student finish their assessments, and Zac says, "My shift ends now, but I'll be back in the morning. Do you need anything else before I leave?"

"No, I'm fine," she says. "Thanks for all you've done for Chip and me today. You've really helped calm some of my fears."

Before she goes to sleep, Diane calls home and tells Kate and Tucker goodnight and that she loves them very much.

The next morning, Zac enters the room and says good morning to Diane.

"Where's your student?" Diane asks.

"The students are only on the unit 1 day a week, so I'm flying solo today," Zac says. He looks over the report from the night nurse. "Looks like Chip had an uneventful night. He's still on 3 L of oxygen per minute via nasal cannula. He was suctioned twice, each time prior to nursing. Let's take a look at him."

Zac assesses Chip. After just a few minutes, Zac says, "I can already tell that Chip has improved."

"Really?" Diane says. She thinks Chip looks better, too, but she's been trying to not get her hopes up. "What makes you think so?"

"Well, he is no longer grunting, and his nasal flaring has decreased. His intercostal retractions are not as severe, and when I listened to his chest, I just heard fine crackles rather than course. His skin is pink and dry, and he is awake and alert."

"He's doing better with nursing, too," Diane says. "The first time Chip nursed during the night he was still having trouble latching well. However, the second time was much better; he nursed for 10 minutes on each side."

"That's wonderful to hear," Zac says. He goes on to report that Chip's vital signs this morning are as follows:

- Temperature: 100.2°F (37.9°C)
- Apical pulse: 140 bpm
- Respiratory rate: 50 breaths/min
- Blood pressure: 80/40 mm Hg
- Blood O_2 saturation: 94% on 3 L/min oxygen

"I'm really encouraged to see his oxygen saturation up to 94%," Zac says. "I'm going to try decreasing his oxygen to 2 L/min and will reassess his saturation level in 30 minutes or so to see if he is maintaining it at 92%. Do you need anything before I go?"

Chip is starting to get fussy, so Diane says, "Would you suction Chip so I can nurse him?"

"Sure." Zac suctions Chip's nares and then departs.

A few minutes later, Paul shows up with breakfast for Diane.

"Thanks for bringing breakfast," she says. "How are Kate and Tucker?"

"Doing fine. They understand that mommy needs to be with Chip. I dropped them off at school on the way over." Diane knows that later in their lives they won't really remember being away from their mother during this period, but it's still hard for her.

Chip nurses well this morning, 15 minutes on each side, and Diane is encouraged. As she is changing his diaper, Laura stops in.

"All the reports show that Chip is improving, as I hoped he would," Laura says with a smile. "If he keeps on this path, he will most likely be discharged tomorrow. The main hurdle now is to wean him off his oxygen."

Zac returns to reassess Chip's O_2 saturation level and reports that it is at 93% on 2 L/min of oxygen.

"Woo hoo!" Diane says.

Zac smiles and says, "Yes, this is a good sign." He weighs Chip and reports that he has gained an ounce. "It looks like

Chip is headed down the right path," Zac says. "I'll be back in 2 hours to recheck the saturation level."

The day continues in a positive direction. By the end of the day, Zac reports that he has weaned Chip down to 0.5 L/min of oxygen, with his O_2 saturation level holding steady at 92%. He also reports that Chip's breathing is easier and he no longer has any nasal flaring. His retractions continue to decrease in intensity and his lung sounds are improving with only occasional crackles bilaterally. He is nursing well and his FLACC score is 0. Chip appears content.

Once he completes his assessments, Zac tells Diane, "Well, I'm off tomorrow, and I most likely won't see you again, because I think Chip will probably go home before I'm back. Remember, though, that for Chip to be discharged, he still needs to be off his oxygen and to gain one more ounce, so that he is back to the weight he was at his 4-month-old checkup."

Overnight, the nurse weans Chip off of the remaining oxygen. She informs Diane that he is maintaining an O_2 saturation level of 93% on room air and that she is getting only a scant amount of mucus when she suctions.

In the morning, Laura writes orders to stop the IV fluids. She tells Diane that if Chip can maintain his O_2 saturation level at 92% or above on room air, he can be discharged after 3:00 p.m. with follow-up in the office in 48 hours. The nurse stops the IV fluids and weighs Chip. He is back to his weight of 13 lb 9 oz. He is awake, alert, and happy. He has no grunting or nasal flaring and only occasional intercostal retractions. The nurse reports that he continues to have an occasional wet cough with intermittent crackles bilaterally and that his vital signs this morning are as follows:

- Temperature: 99.6°F (37°F)
- Apical pulse: 120 bpm
- Respiratory rate: 38 breaths/min
- Blood pressure: 80/40 mm Hg
- Blood O_2 saturation: 94% on room air

Chip maintains his respiratory status throughout the day. Per Laura's orders, the nurse comes to the room at 3:15 p.m. to discharge Chip to home.

At Discharge

During the discharge instructions, the nurse reminds Diane that Chip will probably have a cough off and on for about 2 weeks. She may still see his muscles pulling in between his ribs, but this should decrease over the next few days. Further instructions include performing bulb suctioning before feedings, as needed, practicing good hand hygiene as a family, and avoiding secondhand smoke. The nurse tells Diane that she needs to call the pediatrician's office if Chip develops a fever of 100.5°F or greater, if he becomes lethargic, or if he exhibits any of the symptoms of respiratory distress that he had upon admission. Diane indicates that she understands the discharge instructions and signs the discharge paper. However, she wonders what they are going to do about child care because she knows that they can't send Chip back to Grandma's house.

Back at Home

Diane is happy to be home and very excited to see Kate and Tucker. They both have a lot of questions. She assures the children that Chip is okay but tells them they need to wash their hands well before they play with him.

Diane and Paul discuss what to do regarding day care. Paul tells Diane that they will be able to afford putting Chip in day care. He does not want to risk another illness like this one by exposing him to the environmental smoke at Grandma's house again. Diane is still not sure how she feels about day care. It seems that if Chip is exposed to all those germs that he will get sick again. Diane has to work, so she concludes that, compared with environmental smoke exposure, day care is the lesser of two evils.

That evening Grandma stops by for a visit. She apologizes to Diane and Paul, saying that she had no idea that she was putting Chip at risk of such a terrible illness. She wants to stop smoking and has considered smoking cessation programs. She knows it will be hard but is willing to try for the sake of her own health and that of her family.

Two days after they get home from the hospital, Diane takes Chip to the pediatrician's office for his follow-up appointment. Laura is happy to report that Chip continues to improve. Diane says that Chip still has a cough but that the nurse at the hospital said that is to be expected, and Laura agrees. She says Chip will most likely have a cough for about 2 weeks. Currently, his lungs are almost clear, so she does not feel the need to follow up again until his 6-month-old checkup unless other issues arise. Diane thanks Laura for all that she has done and says that she cannot wait until winter is over.

Think Critically

1. What is important anticipatory guidance for the parents of a 4-month-old?
2. How can breastfeeding play a role in the prevention of bronchiolitis?
3. What are the effects of environmental tobacco smoke exposure on an infant's respiratory system?
4. Why does respiratory syncytial virus affect infants differently than older children?
5. Why is there no medication ordered for bronchiolitis?
6. If Chip's O_2 saturation levels had continued to drop, what interventions would Zac have needed to implement?

Unfolding Patient Stories: Brittany Long • Part 1

Brittany Long is a 5-year-old diagnosed with sickle cell anemia who lives with her mother, 7-year-old sister, and grandmother. Her pain crises are mostly managed at home, and she has been hospitalized 3 times. How can the nurse help Brittany and her family cope with a long-term illness and the management of acute crises? How can the reactions of family members influence Brittany's adjustment to sickle cell disease? What effect can a long-term illness have on her sister, and what actions can support her sister's understanding and cooperation? (Brittany Long's story continues in Unit 3.)

Care for Brittany and other patients in a realistic virtual environment: **vSim** *for Nursing* (thepoint.lww.com/vSimPediatric). Practice documenting these patients' care in DocuCare (thepoint.lww.com /DocuCareEHR).

Unfolding Patient Stories: Eva Madison • Part 1

Eva Madison is a 5-year-old child who is diagnosed with bacterial gastroenteritis. How would the nurse prepare Eva and her parents for hospitalization? What nursing actions can promote a more favorable hospital experience in this age group? (Eva Madison's story continues in Unit 2.)

Care for Eva and other patients in a realistic virtual environment: **vSim** *for Nursing* (thepoint.lww.com/vSimPediatric). Practice documenting these patients' care in DocuCare (thepoint.lww.com /DocuCareEHR).

References

American Academy of Pediatrics. (2017). *Starting solid foods*. Retrieved from https://www.healthychildren.org/English/ages-stages/baby/feeding-nutrition/Pages/Switching-To-Solid-Foods.aspx

American Academy of Pediatrics, Committee on Injury, Violence, and Poison Prevention. (2014). Policy statement—child passenger safety. *Pediatrics, 127(4)*. Retrieved from www.pediatrics.org/cgi/doi/10.1542/peds.2011-0213

Centers for Disease Control and Prevention. (2016). *Smoking & tobacco use. Quit smoking resources*. Retrieved from http://www.cdc.gov/tobacco/quit_smoking/how_to_quit/resources/

Evlampidou, I., Bagkeris, M., Vardavas, C., Koutra, K., Patelarou, E., Koutis, A., . . . Kogevinas, M. (2015). Prenatal second-hand smoke exposure measured with urine cotinine may reduce gross motor development at 18 months of age. *The Journal of Pediatrics, 167*(2), 246–252. doi: 10.1016/j.jpeds.2015.03.006

Governor's Highway Safety Association. (2016). *Child passenger safety*. Retrieved from http://www.ghsa.org/html/stateinfo/laws/childsafety_laws.html

Meissner, H. C. (2016). Viral bronchiolitis in children. *The New England Journal of Medicine, 374*(1), 62–72.

Prymula, R., Siegrist, C. A., Chlibek, R., Zemlickova, H., M., Vackova, H., Smetana, J.,. . . . Schuerman, L. (2009). Effect of prophylactic paracetamol administration at time of vaccination on febrile reactions and antibody responses in children: Two open-label randomized controlled trials. *The Lancet, 374*, 1339–1350.

Saleh, E., Moody, A., & Walter, E. B. (2016). Effect of antipyretic analgesics on immune responses to vaccination. *Human Vaccines and Immunotherapeutics, 12*(9), 2391–2402.

Yeramaneni, S., Dietrich, K. N., Yolton, K., Parsons, P. J., Aldous, K. M., & Haynes, E. N. (2015). Secondhand tobacco smoke exposure and neuromotor function in rural children. *The Journal of Pediatrics, 167*(2), 253–259. doi: 10.1016/j.jpeds.2015.03.014

Suggested Readings

American Academy of Pediatrics. (2015). *Bronchiolitis*. Retrieved from https://www.healthychildren.org/English/health-issues/conditions/chest-lungs/Pages/Bronchiolitis.aspx

Casey, G. (2015). Bronchiolitis: A virus of infancy. *Kai Tiaki Nursing New Zealand, 21*(7), 20–24.

Roberts, C., Wagler, G., & Carr, M. M. (2017). Environmental tobacco smoke: Public perception of risks of exposing children to second-and third-hand tobacco smoke. *Journal of Pediatric Healthcare, 31*(1), e7–e13.

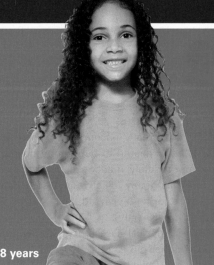

2 Mollie Sanders: Asthma

Mollie Sanders, age 8 years

Objectives

After completing this chapter, you will be able to:
1. Understand normal growth and development of the 8-year-old.
2. Implement a teaching plan for a healthy 8-year-old.
3. Compare and contrast anatomical and physiological characteristics of the respiratory systems of children and adults.
4. Relate pediatric assessment findings to the child's respiratory status.
5. Discuss the pathophysiology of asthma.
6. Identify various risk factors associated with asthma.
7. Outline the therapeutic regimen for asthma.
8. Identify priorities of nursing care for a child with asthma.

Key Terms

Airway resistance
Dyspneic
Intercostal retractions

Ventilation
Wheezing

Background

Mollie Sanders is an 8-year-old girl who was diagnosed with asthma at the age of 5 years after several episodes of **wheezing** and shortness of breath when playing soccer. Mollie is the middle child of five siblings. She has a 12-year-old sister, Annie, a 10-year-old brother, Adam, and twin younger brothers, Sam and Brian, who are 5 years old. Mollie lives with her mother, Susan, and father, Paul, in an older home, built in the 1930s, out in the country. Mollie and her family have a dog, which stays outside most of the time, and several fish. Mollie's older sister also has asthma. The other children in the home have no health issues or concerns.

Health Promotion

Several months ago, Susan took Mollie to her annual well-care visit with the nurse practitioner, Jessica. At that visit, Mollie began developing a rapport with Jessica, whom she also sees for

sick visits and visits related to asthma flare-ups. Mollie's last sick visit, which was over 9 months ago, was for increased work of breathing and increased use of her albuterol inhaler.

"So, Mollie," Jessica said as she was conducting her physical assessment, "Are you involved in any sports or fun activities this year?"

"Yes," Mollie replied. "I'm going to be on the soccer team, when it starts. And I love to jump rope with my friends."

"That sounds like fun," Jessica said.

"Yeah," Mollie said. "My best friend, Tara, and I play together with some other friends at recess. My favorite thing is to jump rope and sing jump rope songs. Tara likes reading chapter books in school. And she loves art class and music."

"Can you ride a bike?" Jessica asked.

"Yes!" Mollie said. "And I don't even need training wheels anymore!"

"Wow!" Jessica said. "That's wonderful." She glanced over at Susan as if for confirmation.

"That's right," Susan said. "She's growing up so fast."

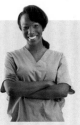

The Nurse's Point of View

Jessica: At Mollie's last well-care visit, I was really encouraged by my findings. She appeared to be in good health and was developing appropriately, meeting all milestones for an 8-year-old girl. She was highly talkative and demonstrated wonderful social skills for an 8-year-old. She is developing friendships and is physically active.

Mollie's physical assessment was within normal limits. Mollie weighed 58 lb (26.3 kg) and was 52 in (4.3 ft) tall (Growth and Development Check 2.1). She was still in the 50th percentile on the growth chart, which was great. Her vital signs, obtained by our medical assistant, were as follows: heart rate, 84 beats/min (bpm); respiratory rate, 20 breaths/min; temperature, 97.8°F (36.5°C); and blood pressure, 92/56 mm Hg. Her lungs were clear bilaterally with no signs of respiratory distress, her heart rate was regular and without murmurs, her abdomen was soft and flat with active bowel sounds, and her skin was warm and pink with brisk capillary refill.

All in all, she seems to be a healthy, happy girl.

Growth and Development Check 2.1

Physical Growth

The average weight for an 8-y-old girl is 57 lb (25.8 kg), and the average height is 50.5 in (4.2 ft). Given here are percentile values for weight and height for 8-y-old girls.

Weight

- 10th percentile: 44 lb (20 kg)
- 50th percentile: 56 lb (25.4 kg)
- 95th percentile: 78 lb (35.4 kg)

Height

- 10th percentile: 46 in (3.8 ft)
- 50th percentile: 50 in (4.2 ft)
- 95th percentile: 55 in (4.6 ft)

Adapted from the National Center for Health Statistics in collaboration with The National Center for Chronic Disease Prevention and Health Promotion. (2000). *2 to 20 years: Girls stature-for-age and weight-for-age percentiles.* Retrieved from https://www.cdc.gov/growthcharts/data/set1clinical/cj41l022.pdf

When she had completed her physical assessment of Mollie, Jessica said, "Everything looks fine. You're in good health, Mollie." Turning to Susan, she said, "Do you have any questions or concerns you'd like to talk over?"

"Actually," Susan said, "I have been a little concerned about Mollie's posture. As a teenager, I was treated for scoliosis, and I'd feel better if we checked her out."

"Absolutely," Jessica said. "Scoliosis is usually diagnosed in children between the ages of 10 and 12 years, but it can be seen in younger patients" (Horne, Flannery, & Usman, 2014). Jessica observed Mollie standing with her arms at her sides and bending forward with her arms hanging in front of her body (Fig. 2.1). She also watched Mollie walk heel to heel, walk heel to toe, walk on her toes, and hop.

"I don't find any signs of scoliosis at this time, but monitor her for uneven shoulders, altered gait, and back pain. As you probably already know, children of parents who had scoliosis are more likely to be diagnosed with the condition."

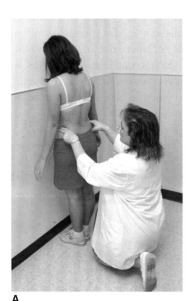

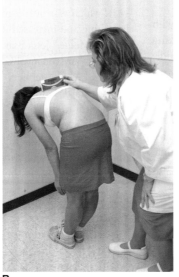

A **B**

Figure 2.1. Assessing for scoliosis. A. Assess for a lack of symmetry of the hips, scapula, or shoulders and for differences in skin creases and folds. **B.** Assess for curves or protrusions when the child is bending over. Reprinted with permission from Jensen, S. (2018). *Nursing health assessment: A best practice approach* (3rd ed., Fig. 21.10). Philadelphia, PA: Wolters Kluwer.

Yes, Susan thought. About 3 times more likely, actually (Horne et al., 2014).

Jessica discussed with Susan upcoming growth and development milestones for Mollie (Growth and Development Check 2.2), safety concerns, and tips on how to handle expected changes and issues that Mollie will face, something Jessica referred to as anticipatory guidance (Patient Teaching 2.1). She covered the appropriate use of car seats (Box 2.1), bicycle helmet use, firearm safety, and water safety. Regarding immunizations, Jessica informed Susan that Mollie was up to date according to the guidelines of the Centers for Disease Control and Prevention and therefore did not need to receive any immunizations at the well-care visit. Jessica also reminded Susan that

Growth and Development Check 2.2

School-Aged Milestones

School age is an important period for children who will need to acquire disease management skills such as caring for asthma. Children at this age can comprehend time and are developing logical thinking skills that will allow them to plan, problem-solve, and make decisions regarding their chronic diseases. School-aged children can also begin to understand the rationale, effects, and importance of consistent disease management. Given here are some other developmental milestones associated with this age.

Social/Emotional

- Develops hobbies, such as model building and working with crafts and yarn
- Thinks about the future
- Pays attention to friendships
- Wants to be liked and accepted by friends
- Focuses less on self and shows increased concern for others

Speech

- Talks through thoughts and feelings

Cognitive

- Reads
- Concentrates for increasingly longer periods of time
- Rapidly develops mental skills and use of judgment

Gross Motor/Fine Motor

- Learns to ride a bicycle
- Shows increased coordination
- Is skilled in running, jumping, skipping, hopping
- Throws objects with accurate aim and increased distance

Adapted from Centers for Disease Control and Prevention. (2017). *Middle childhood (6–8 years of age)*. Retrieved from https://www.cdc.gov/ncbddd/childdevelopment/positiveparenting/middle.html

Patient Teaching 2.1

Anticipatory Guidance for 8-Year-Olds

Safety

At this age, your child should do the following:

- Wear protective gear when playing sports.
- Wear a helmet at all times when biking and skating.
- Use a booster seat in the back seat of vehicles until he or she is 57 in tall or 8 y old.
- Know the family plan for exiting the home and meeting in the event of a fire.

To protect your child, you should do the following:

- Lock up guns and firearms.
- Supervise your child when near water, even if your child knows how to swim.
- Teach your child street safety: not to run after balls into the street, where it's safe to ride a bicycle, and how to cross the street.

Social

- To promote your child's social development, you should do the following:
- Meet and get to know your child's friends and their parents.
- Teach your child how to answer the phone and the door.
- Talk with your child about his or her friends and relationships with peers.
- Monitor for signs of bullying.

children around Mollie's age begin to develop a greater sense of independence and are more likely to give in to peer pressure, so Susan should regularly address safety issues at home.

Near the end of the well-care visit, Jessica reviewed the medications Mollie was currently taking, which included an albuterol inhaler, two puffs as needed for wheezing and difficulty breathing, and montelukast (Singulair) 5 mg each evening (The Pharmacy 2.1). Mollie knew the names of each

Box 2.1 Car Seat Safety

The American Academy of Pediatrics (AAP) recommends that children remain in an appropriate car seat or a booster seat until they are 8–12 y old. Specifically, the AAP promotes the use of belt-positioning booster seats until children reach 57 in (4.75 ft) and are 8–12 y old. Motor vehicle accidents are the most common cause of death from unintentional injury in the school-age population. Many of these deaths can be prevented when car seats and safety restraints are used appropriately.

You can find car seat laws at:

- http://www.ghsa.org/html/stateinfo/laws/childsafety_laws.html
- https://www.healthychildren.org/English/news/Pages/AAP-Updates-Recommendations-on-Car-Seats.aspx

The Pharmacy 2.1   Asthma Medications

Medication(s)	Classification	Route	Action	Nursing Considerations
Albuterol (Ventolin, ProAir, Proventil)	Beta$_2$-agonist short-acting bronchodilator	Metered-dose inhaler, nebulizer	• Decreases airway resistance • Dilates the lower airways • Increases expiratory flow in the smaller airways	• Monitor heart rate for tachycardia • May make the patient shaky after use • Monitor for signs of toxicity
Methylprednisolone, prednisone	Anti-inflammatory corticosteroid	IV, IM, PO	• Reduces inflammation in the airways • Decreases obstruction in the airways • Enhances bronchodilating effects of beta$_2$-agonists	Monitor: • Blood pressure for increases • Weight with long-term use • Electrolytes • Serum glucose • Growth with long-term use • Signs and symptoms of infection with long-term use
Montelukast (Singulair)	Leukotriene receptor antagonist	PO	• Reduces process that causes airway inflammation • Improves lung function • Decreases need for quick-relief medications, such as albuterol	
Salmeterol, formoterol	Beta$_2$-agonist long-acting bronchodilator	Inhalation, nebulizer	• Relaxes smooth muscle in the airways • Prevents exercise-induced bronchospasm	• May be used to reduce nocturnal symptoms • Clinical data are for children ≥12 y old • No studies in children <4 y old
Beclomethasone, budesonide, flunisolide, fluticasone, mometasone, triamcinolone	Anti-inflammatory	Metered-dose inhaler, nebulizer, dry powder inhaler	• Decreases airway inflammation by inhibiting inflammatory mediators such as histamine, leukotriene, and cytokines • Decreased inflammation reduces mucosal edema, secretions, and bronchoconstriction • Increases mucociliary action, promoting mobilization of mucous	• Do not abruptly stop taking • Ineffective in acute bronchospasm; not used as a rescue inhaler
Theophylline		PO, IV (in status asthmaticus)	• Relaxes muscles that constrict airways • Dilates airways • Sustained release for prevention of nocturnal symptoms	• Do not crush or chew tablets • Therapeutic level: 10–20 µg/L • Give at the same time each day • Avoid or limit caffeine intake • Monitor serum levels and adjust the dose for weight changes and therapeutic levels Monitor for side effects: • Tachycardia • Dysrhythmias • Hypotension • Tremors • Restlessness • Insomnia • Severe headaches • Vomiting • Diarrhea • Seizures

IM, intramuscular; IV, intravenous; PO, by mouth. Adapted from Taketomo, C. K. (2018). *Pediatric and neonatal dosage handbook* (25th ed). Hudson, OH: Lexicomp.

Asthma Action Plan

For: _____   Doctor: _____   Date: _____
Doctor's Phone Number _____   Hospital/Emergency Department Phone Number _____

GREEN ZONE

Doing Well
- No cough, wheeze, chest tightness, or shortness of breath during the day or night
- Can do usual activites

And, if a peak flow meter is used,
Peak flow: more than _____ (80% or more of my best peak flow)
My best peak flow is: _____

Take these long-term-control medicines each day (include an anti-inflammatory).

Medicine	How much to take	When to take it
_____	_____	_____
_____	_____	_____

Identify and avoid and control the things that make your asthma worse, like (list here):

_____   _____   _____
_____   _____   _____

Before exercise, if prescribed, take: □ 2 or □ 4 puffs _____   5 to 60 minutes before exercise

YELLOW ZONE

Asthma Is Getting Worse
- Cough, wheeze, chest tightness, or shortness of breath, or
- Waking at night due to asthma, or
- Can do some, but not all, usual activites

-Or-
Peak flow: _____ to _____
(50% to 79% of my best peak flow)

First Add: quick-relief medicine—and keep taking your GREEN ZONE medicine.

_____   □ 2 or □ 4 puffs, every 20 minutes for up to 1 hour
(short-acting beta₂-agonist)   □ Nebulizer, once

If applicable, remove yourself from the thing that made your asthma worse.

Second If your symptoms (and peak flow, if used) return to GREEN ZONE after 1 hour of above treatment:
Continue monitoring to be sure you stay in the green zone.
-Or-
If your symptoms (and peak flow, if used) do not return to GREEN ZONE after 1 hour of above treatment:
□ Take: _____   □ 2 or □ 4 puffs or □ Nebulizer
(short-acting beta₂-agonist)
□ Add: _____   mg per day For _____ (3-10) days
(oral corticosteroid)
□ Call the doctor: _____ , □ before/ □ within _____ hours after taking the oral corticosteroid.
(phone)

RED ZONE

Medical Alert!
- Very short of breath, or
- Quick-relief medicines have not helped, or
- Cannot do usual activites, or
- Symptoms are same or get worse after 24 hours in Yellow Zone

-Or-
Peak flow: less than _____
(50% of my best peak flow)

Take this medicine:

□ _____   □ 4 or □ 6 puffs or □ Nebulizer
(short-acting beta₂-agonist)
□ _____   mg
(oral corticosteroid)

Then call your doctor NOW. Go to the hospital or call an ambulance if:
- You are still in the red zone after 15 minutes AND
- You have not reached your doctor.

DANGER SIGNS
- Trouble walking and talking due to shortness of breath
- Lips or fingernails are blue

- Take □ 4 or □ 6 puffs of your quick-relief medicine AND
- Go to the hospital or call for an ambulance _____ NOW!
(phone)

Figure 2.2. **The stoplight asthma action plan.** Adapted from the National Heart, Lung, and Blood Institute. (2012). *Asthma care quick reference: Diagnosing and managing asthma* (NIH Publication No. 12-5075). Retrieved from https://www.nhlbi.nih .gov/files/docs/guidelines/asthma_qrg.pdf

of the medications and why she takes each one. Mollie was also able to tell Jessica when she should ask her mother or an adult to use her inhaler. Susan explained that they use the asthma stoplight plan at home and school for guidance in managing her asthma symptoms (Fig. 2.2; Analyze the Evidence 2.1). Jessica seemed impressed. Susan was proud of Mollie for remembering all she had been taught and for being so independent.

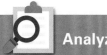

Analyze the Evidence 2.1

Use of Asthma Action Plans—Do They Improve Outcomes?

A key component in the self-management of asthma is education. The goal of an asthma action plan is to provide the patient, parent, and school personnel with a plan for decision making and immediate intervention when asthma symptoms deviate from the patient's baseline. National asthma treatment guidelines recommend the use of a written asthma action plan for anyone diagnosed with asthma. An example of a written asthma action plan is the Stoplight Tool (Fig. 2.2).

However, does the use of an asthma action plan improve outcomes? Do children who have an action plan achieve the goals of therapy, such as no activity limitations, normal lung function, and rare exacerbations requiring ER visits?

Kelso (2016) reports that healthcare providers should teach parents and children about symptoms, medications, proper use of an inhaler, and identifying and managing triggers rather than developing asthma action plans. According to a literature review by Kelso (2016), asthma action plans do not improve outcomes and may actually cause more harm. Unintended consequences of asthma action plans may include increased rates of hospitalization, higher costs, and greater medication usage. The conclusion of the literature review (Kelso, 2016) reiterates the need for verbal and written education at initial diagnosis and each time a child visits the healthcare provider, which takes minimal time but clearly makes a difference according to the articles reviewed.

Jessica ended the visit by encouraging Susan to monitor Mollie's use of the inhaler and provide guidance on appropriate technique. Jessica emphasized that for effective disease management in childhood, parents and children must share and balance the responsibility of the child's care (Martire & Helgeson, 2017).

At Home

April is now here, and the weather has been getting warmer. Mollie and her siblings have been spending more time outside after school playing on their swing set and riding bikes. Mollie also just started soccer in the spring league at her school. Susan has noticed Mollie sniffling more and rubbing her eyes when she comes in from being outside.

Tonight, Mollie has her second soccer practice of the season. It is 80°F (26.6°C) and muggy. After Susan reminds her, Mollie takes two puffs of her albuterol inhaler, using a spacer, 15 minutes before the start of practice (Fig. 2.3). During practice, Susan notices that Mollie is not keeping up with the others as they race down the field. About 30 minutes into practice, Mollie stops and talks to the coach. She looks short of breath. Sure enough, the coach sends her out to sit with her mother on the sidelines for several minutes until she "feels better." Mollie takes two more puffs of her albuterol inhaler. Later, Mollie is able to return to practice. She doesn't have any more trouble breathing during the remaining 45 minutes of practice.

Susan is surprised Mollie needed to use her inhaler because she has not used it in several months. However, as she thinks about Mollie's triggers (Patient Teaching 2.2), she realizes several of them are present at soccer practice. Later that evening, when playing outside with her siblings, Mollie again becomes short of breath and has to use her inhaler. The next morning, Susan calls the pediatrician and makes an appointment to check Mollie's breathing and discuss a plan for better managing her asthma.

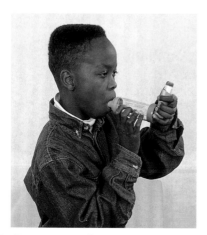

Figure 2.3. Proper use of a metered-dose inhaler with a spacer. Reprinted with permission from Hatfield, N. T., & Kincheloe, C. A. (2017). *Introductory maternity and pediatric nursing* (4th ed., Fig. 36-6B). Philadelphia, PA: Wolters Kluwer.

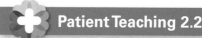

Patient Teaching 2.2

Triggers of Asthma

Knowing definitive and potential triggers of asthma is essential in preventing asthma flare-ups and successfully managing asthma. Triggers are often identified early by incidental exposure. For example, a child may go outside in the cold winter air and begin to wheeze and have difficulty breathing. The signs and symptoms of asthma may subside when the child leaves the cold air.

Common asthma triggers fall into several categories:

- Respiratory infections (including pneumonia, common cold, and bronchiolitis)
- Allergens (including dust, pollen, pet dander and furred animals, and weeds)
- Irritants (tobacco smoke, aerosol sprays, cleaning products, perfumes, and scented sprays)
- Exercise
- Cold air

Develop a plan with the parent and child to deal with asthma triggers. Optimally, they should avoid or extremely limit the child's exposure to triggers. For example, advise parents to quit smoking if tobacco smoke is a trigger. Even the parent smoking outside can trigger an asthma attack, because the smoke can be on the parent's clothes, hair, and skin. The only exception to trigger avoidance is exercise. Encourage exercise for all children. An asthma action plan is useful for children with exercise-induced asthma. Include in the plan the steps to prevent and treat exercise-related symptoms.

To help reduce triggers, tell parents and families to do the following:

- Remove carpets from bedrooms.
- Do not allow pets in the child's bedroom.
- Avoid smoking in, around, or near the child or his or her living quarters.
- Remove plants from the home.
- Cover the child's mattress and pillow in plastic covers to reduce accumulation of dust mites.
- Avoid toys that collect dust (stuffed animals, for example).
- Dehumidify moist climates, particularly in the child's bedroom.
- Keep homes in good repair to prevent entry of water and subsequent mold development.

Adapted from Miller, R. (2017). Patient education: Trigger avoidance in asthma (Beyond the basics). *UpToDate.* Retrieved from https://www.uptodate.com/contents/trigger-avoidance-in-asthma-beyond-the-basics

At the Pediatrician's Office

Later that morning, when she wakes up, Mollie has to use her albuterol inhaler again. She tells her mother on the way to the pediatrician's office that she feels like her chest is heavy sometimes. Susan is concerned because Mollie looks tired and pale and appears to be breathing a bit faster than she remembers.

At the pediatrician's office, the nurse obtains Mollie's heart rate and respiratory rate and does a spot check with the pulse oximeter. Susan asks the nurse how Mollie's doing. The nurse reports that Mollie's pulse is 84 bpm, her respiratory rate is 26 breaths/min, and her O_2 saturation is 93% on room air.

"I've had to use my inhaler a lot more than I usually do in the past couple of days," Mollie tells the nurse.

"I've heard Mollie wheezing a few times a day," Susan says, "but it stops when she takes a couple of puffs of her inhaler."

The nurse listens to Mollie's chest with a stethoscope. "Yes," the nurse says. "I'm hearing expiratory wheezing bilaterally. That means I hear a wheezing sound in both lungs when she breathes out. She has a slightly prolonged expiratory phase, or breathing-out time, and mild subcostal retractions and **intercostal retractions**, meaning her belly just below her ribs pulls in when she breathes."

Jessica, the nurse practitioner, walks into the exam room. "How are you feeling, Mollie?" she says.

"Okay," Mollie replies. "Yesterday I had a hard time breathing at soccer practice and when I was playing on my swing set at home. I used my inhaler a lot yesterday. And this morning, when I woke up, I felt like my chest was heavy, so mom made me use my inhaler again."

"Well, let's check you out," Jessica says.

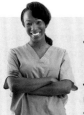

The Nurse's Point of View

Jessica: I begin the respiratory assessment by observing Mollie breathing while talking. I note Mollie has to take a few extra breaths when talking in sentences and appears **dyspneic**. Mollie's respiratory rate is increased, and I notice mild use of her subcostal muscles at times. I hear Mollie cough, and the cough sounds congested, but Mollie says that nothing comes up when she coughs. Upon auscultation, I hear bilateral expiratory wheezing in the right and left lower lobes of Mollie's lungs. I then ask the nurse to give Mollie an albuterol treatment using the nebulizer. Mollie has used the nebulizer mouthpiece in the past and remembers to place it in her mouth with her lips sealed around it and to breathe in through her mouth and out through her nose.

After the nebulizer treatment is complete, Jessica returns to check on Mollie. She reassesses her with the stethoscope. "Much better," Jessica says when she's done. I don't hear any more wheezing, and her respiratory rate has decreased to about 22 breaths/min, which is good. "How do you feel now, Mollie?" Jessica says.

"Way better," Mollie says. In fact, she's feeling so well that she proceeds to tell Jessica all about soccer and school and Tara and math class.

Jessica smiles at Susan and says, "Yep—she's definitely feeling better. Notice how she can say complete sentences now without taking a breath?"

"Yes," Susan says. "Back to normal." She laughs, but she's really relieved.

Jessica mentions that her pulse oximetry reading is up to 97% on room air. She discusses the triggers of this episode with Susan and Mollie, and they determine that the recent change in humidity, increase in pollen, and decrease in air quality, as well as starting soccer practice and increased activity, may have led to the asthma episode.

Jessica reviews with Susan and Mollie the signs of increased work of breathing and the need for using Mollie's albuterol inhaler (Patient Safety 2.1). Mollie even restates the symptoms she should

Patient Safety 2.1   Signs of Respiratory Distress in School-Aged Children

	Signs of Respiratory Distress		
Measure	**Mild**	**Moderate**	**Severe**
Behavior	Normal	Intermittent irritability	Increased irritability and/or lethargy
Respiratory rate	Normal or mildly increased	Increased	Increased or significantly decreased as the child tires
Retractions	None or minimal (subcostal, suprasternal)	Moderate (intercostal, supraclavicular)	Prominent chest retractions (intercostal, suprasternal, sternal, subcostal, supraclavicular)
Use of accessory muscles	None or minimal	Moderate (nasal flaring, forward posture)	Markedly increased
Color	Pink Appropriate for ethnicity	Pink or pale	Pale and/or cyanotic (O_2 saturation <85%)
Heart rate	Normal or slightly increased	Mildly increased	Significantly increased or bradycardia (late sign)
Blood pressure	Normal	Increased	Increased or decreased (late sign)

tell her mom about including a tight-feeling chest, pressure in her chest, feeling like she cannot catch her breath, noisy sounds when she breathes, feeling tired during the day, and coughing. Jessica also prescribes methylprednisolone 20 mg two times a day for 5 days.

Later in the evening, Susan becomes more worried about Mollie. Mollie has used her inhaler twice in the past hour.

At dinner, Mollie tells her mother, "I feel like I can't take a deep breath!" She has a look of panic on her face. Susan can

hear Mollie wheezing with each breath. Susan does as she was instructed by the nurse practitioner and takes Mollie to the emergency room (ER) at the nearby children's hospital.

At the Hospital

Mollie is quickly triaged and taken back to an exam room in the pediatric ER.

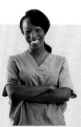

The Nurse's Point of View

Cecilia: In the ER, I observe Mollie for signs of respiratory distress as I obtain her vital signs, allergies, and a brief history. Mollie's vital signs are as follows:

- Heart rate: 110 bpm
- Respiratory rate: 32 breaths/min
- Temperature: 98°F (36.7°C)
- O_2 saturation: 89% on room air
- Blood pressure: 95/52 mm Hg

I can hear audible wheezing when Mollie exhales and inspiratory and expiratory wheezing on auscultation of her lungs (Let's Compare 2.1). Mollie has an occasional nonproductive cough. I ask Mollie to count to 10 without taking a breath. She can't do it. I note that Mollie is sitting forward with her shoulders hunched. I explain to Susan and Mollie that Mollie needs oxygen via a nasal cannula to help bring her O_2 saturation level up. I place Mollie on 2 L oxygen via nasal cannula. Her O_2 saturation level improves to 92%.

Let's Compare 2.1

Differences in Pediatric and Adult Respiratory Anatomy and Physiology

Variations in Anatomy and Physiology

A child's respiratory system constantly changes and continues to grow until about 12 y of age. Differences between the pediatric and adult airway can be summarized by comparing the upper airway differences and the lower airway differences (Fig. 2.4).

Comparing the Upper Airway

The upper airway comprises the nasopharynx and oropharynx and serves as the pathway for gas exchange during ventilation. **Ventilation** is the movement of oxygen into the lungs and of carbon dioxide out of the lungs. A child's airway is much shorter and narrower than an adult's airway. A smaller nasopharynx can lead to an easily occluded airway when secretions, edema, or foreign bodies enter the upper airway.

Children have small oral cavities and large tongues compared with that of adults. This can lead to an obstructed oropharynx when a child is lethargic, the throat is swollen, or there is a lack of head control. Children have long, floppy epiglottises, which can also lead to obstruction. A higher risk of aspiration is present in children as a result of a larynx and glottis that are higher in the neck in comparison to that of an adult. The cartilage supporting the neck and airways is much more flexible in children, and a child's head is larger in proportion to the body, which may lead to airway compression if the head and neck are

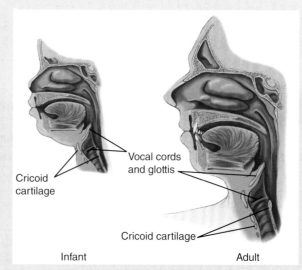

Figure 2.4. Comparison of the vocal cords and glottis of an infant with those of an adult. Reprinted with permission from Bowden, V., & Greenberg, C. S. (2013). *Children and their families* (3rd ed., Fig. 16-3). Philadelphia, PA: Wolters Kluwer Health/Lippincott Williams & Wilkins.

improperly supported. Narrower airways cause a greater increase in airway resistance. **Airway resistance** is the amount of force required to move air through the trachea

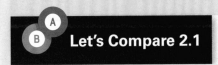

Let's Compare 2.1 | **Differences in Pediatric and Adult Respiratory Anatomy and Physiology (*continued*)**

into the lungs. Many conditions, such as croup, asthma, and epiglottitis, cause airway inflammation or edema, which can dramatically increase airway resistance (Fig. 2.5).

Comparing the Lower Airway

The larynx (voice box) divides the upper and lower airways. In a child, the right and left mainstem bronchi begin much higher and are at a steeper angle than in an adult airway. The trachea divides into the right and left mainstem bronchi at the level of the T3 vertebra, whereas in the adult, it divides at the level of the T6 vertebra (Fig. 2.6).

The number of alveoli in a full-term newborn is ~25 million, which may not be all fully developed. By ~32–36 weeks' gestation, a neonate has enough functioning alveoli to maintain gas exchange. Adults, in comparison, have about 300 million alveoli. Not until 8 y of age do the size and complexity of the alveoli begin to increase.

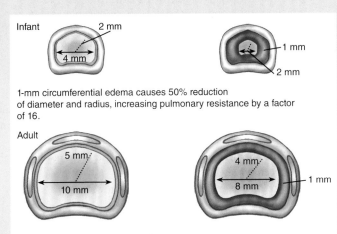

Infant

2 mm
4 mm
1 mm
2 mm

1-mm circumferential edema causes 50% reduction of diameter and radius, increasing pulmonary resistance by a factor of 16.

Adult

5 mm
10 mm
4 mm
8 mm
1 mm

1-mm circumferential edema causes 20% reduction of diameter and radius, increasing pulmonary resistance by a factor of 2.4.

Figure 2.5. Comparison of the effects of edema on airway diameter and resistance in an infant and an adult. Reprinted with permission from Kyle, T., & Carman, S. (2013). *Essentials of pediatric nursing* (2nd ed., Fig. 18.1). Philadelphia, PA: Wolters Kluwer Health/ Lippincott Williams & Wilkins.

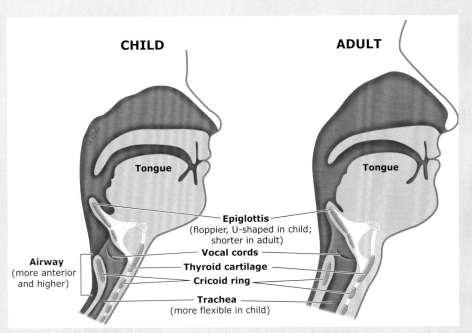

CHILD   ADULT

Tongue   Tongue

Epiglottis
(floppier, U-shaped in child;
shorter in adult)
Vocal cords
Airway
(more anterior
and higher)
Thyroid cartilage
Cricoid ring
Trachea
(more flexible in child)

Figure 2.6. Comparison of the trachea and other structures of the airway in a child and in an adult. Reproduced with permission from Nagler, J. (2019). Emergency airway management in children: Unique pediatric considerations. *UpToDate*. Retrieved from https://www.uptodate.com/contents/emergency-airway-management-in-children-unique-pediatric-considerations. Copyright © 2019 UpToDate, Inc. For more information visit www.uptodate.com

Box 2.2 Pathophysiology of Asthma

Asthma is the most common chronic disease in childhood. It affects about 7 million children in the United States and over 25 million Americans in total. There are three components to asthma: airway inflammation, airflow obstruction (bronchospasm), and airway hyperresponsiveness (National Asthma Education and Prevention Program [NAEPP], 2007). Airway inflammation can be acute or chronic and appear in varying degrees (Fig. 2.7). The principal cells identified in airway inflammation include mast cells, epithelial cells, macrophages, T lymphocytes, and eosinophils. Asthma results from many complex interactions among inflammatory cells, mediators, and airway cells and tissues (NAEPP, 2007). Multiple mechanisms and pathways contribute to airway inflammation.

Airflow obstruction can be caused by inflammation, bronchoconstriction related to spasms of the smooth muscles in the bronchi and bronchioles, airway edema, mucous plugging, and airway remodeling, which can result in permanent cellular changes (NAEPP, 2007). In a person without asthma, bronchial constriction is a normal reaction to foreign stimuli. However, in a person with asthma, bronchial constriction is severe and respiratory function becomes impaired.

Airway hyperresponsiveness is an exaggerated response to many exogenous and endogenous stimuli. However, inflammation appears to be a major factor in the degree of hyperresponsiveness. This exaggerated response results in varying degrees of bronchoconstriction. The degree of airway hyperresponsiveness correlates with the severity of clinical symptoms: the more severe the symptoms, the more severe the bronchoconstriction. Treating airway inflammation will reduce airway hyperresponsiveness and improve asthma symptoms as well as improve asthma control (NAAEP, 2007).

Soon after Cecilia assesses Mollie, the ER pediatrician, Dr. Matt, comes in to assess Mollie and introduces himself.

"So, what do you think brought on this event?" Dr. Matt asks Susan.

"We were just at the pediatrician's office yesterday for increased asthma symptoms, and the nurse practitioner thought the change in humidity, increased pollen level, and exercising outdoors triggered it," Susan explains (Box 2.2; Figs. 2.7 and 2.8).

"Has she been exposed to anyone who has a respiratory illness recently?" Dr. Matt asks.

"No," Susan answers. "Not that I know of."

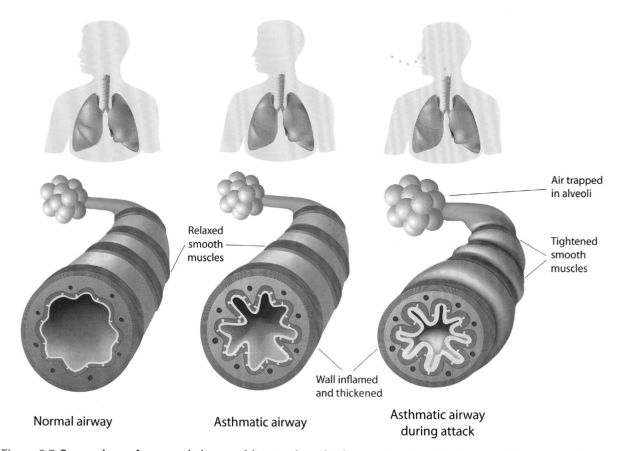

Figure 2.7. **Comparison of a normal airway with an asthmatic airway at rest and during an asthmatic attack.**

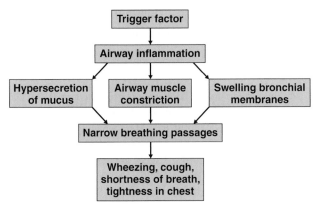

Figure 2.8. Steps in the asthmatic hypersensitivity response. Reprinted with permission from LaMorte, W. W., Boston University School of Public Health. (2017). *Respiratory health.* Available at http://sphweb.bumc.bu.edu/otlt/MPH-Modules/PH/RespiratoryHealth/

"Mollie needs back-to-back albuterol nebulizers," he says. "After that, I'll reassess her and see if she needs further treatment with continuous albuterol and other medications. The nebulizer treatments will help open the airways and reduce the bronchospasm associated with asthma."

The respiratory therapist, Ryan, comes in to set up and administer the albuterol nebulizer treatment. Ryan checks the physician's orders and verifies Mollie's first and last name as well as her birthdate. Mollie remains quiet while Ryan is in the room. She's never been to the ER before. Many people are coming in and out of her room.

"I'm scared!" Mollie tells her mom. She starts crying.

"It's okay, sweetie," Susan says, squeezing Mollie's hand. "All these people coming into your room are here to help you feel better. And I'm staying right here with you."

"Hey, there, Mollie," Ryan says. He's smiling at her and holding two colorful nebulizer masks. "Would you like the mask with the princess face on it or the one with the purple monster face?"

"Princess!" Mollie shouts.

After the back-to-back nebulizer treatments, Mollie's labored breathing has not improved. The nurse tells Susan that Mollie's O_2 saturation level is 89% on room air, and so she'll have to remain on the 2 L of oxygen via nasal cannula.

Dr. Matt comes in to reassess Mollie and tells the nurse that he is ordering continuous albuterol nebulization delivered via oxygen flow at 10 L/min, as well as methylprednisolone and a peripheral intravenous (IV) line to be started.

He turns to Susan, a serious look on his face. "We need to admit Mollie to the hospital."

Susan starts to cry. "Is there something I could have done to prevent this?"

"No, not all," Dr. Matt says. "You did all the right things. It's not your fault. Unless you have the ability to control the weather and pollen levels." He smiles, and Susan feels a little better.

The nurse returns to give Mollie methylprednisolone after verifying Mollie's name and birthdate. Before administration, the nurse explains that she has checked the ordered dose to ensure it is appropriate for Mollie's weight, because most pediatric medication dosing is based on weight. She also explains that the medication will help reduce the inflammation associated with asthma and will be administered every 12 hours while Mollie is in the hospital. Mollie just learned to swallow pills when her montelukast was changed from chewable tablets to the regular tablets after her recent well-care visit.

Cecilia sees that the admission orders for Mollie include the following:

- Admit to A6 North with diagnosis of asthma exacerbation
- Peripheral IV saline lock
- Flush peripheral IV with 3 mL of normal saline every 8 hours and prn
- Oxygen by facemask; titrate the oxygen to keep O_2 saturation levels greater than 92%
- Continuous pulse oximetry
- Diet: clear liquids as tolerated
- Medications:
  - Albuterol
  - Methylprednisolone
  - Singulair
- Begin asthma teaching protocol

Mollie is admitted to room A6N, room 26, which is near the nurses' station. The admitting nurse enters Mollie's room and says, "Hi, Mollie. I'm Brandy. Have you ever been in the hospital before?"

Mollie shakes her head no.

Brandy glances at Mollie's armband and asks Susan to state Mollie's full name and birthdate. "Great," Brandy says. "We have a match! I can take care of your admission orders now."

"This is the first admission for any of my children," Susan tells her. "Can I stay the night here with her?"

"Of course," Brandy says. "The sofa here has a pull-out bed. I can't vouch for how comfortable it is, though."

"I'm just going to do a quick head-to-toe assessment now to make sure nothing's changed since you were in the ER."

"She seems to be breathing fast," Susan remarks while Brandy assesses Mollie.

"Yes," Brandy replies. "Her respiratory rate is 32 breaths/min."

Mollie looks tired and has slight tremors in her hands. "Why are her hands shaking," Susan asks.

"It's a side effect of the continuous albuterol," Brandy says. "It can also cause increased heart rate, nausea, feeling jittery, and inability to sleep."

The nurse explains the plan of care and discharge criteria to Susan and Mollie. Mollie will remain on continuous albuterol until her asthma score is 3 or less using the Respiratory Clinical Score (Liu et al., 2004). The nurse briefly explains how the Respiratory Clinical Score helps clinicians assess how Mollie is progressing with treatment for this asthma episode.

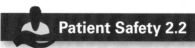

Patient Safety 2.2

Monitoring Respiratory Status

Owing to bronchospasm, inflammation, and increased mucus, a person with asthma can decompensate quickly. When a patient is admitted to the hospital with an asthma exacerbation, it is critical that the respiratory status be closely monitored and that any alterations in status, even slight changes, be reported to the healthcare provider in charge.

Changes in the respiratory status of a child with asthma may include the following:

- Feelings of "tightness" in the chest
- Feelings of being "unable to breathe"
- Decreased aeration to lung fields
- Increased wheezing (inspiratory, expiratory, or both)
- Increased coughing
- Increased need for oxygen
- Increased lethargy
- Increased tachypnea with short, shallow breaths

The nurse and respiratory therapist will assess Mollie's respiratory rate, work of breathing, and use of accessory muscles as well as auscultate her lungs to hear if and when she is wheezing (Patient Safety 2.2). The respiratory therapist will assess Mollie every hour or more frequently, if needed, until she is no longer on continuous albuterol nebulization. For now, Mollie can have clear liquids.

"But I'm hungry," Mollie says.

"Can't she have a little something to eat," Susan asks. It seems so unfair that with everything else she's going through she can't even eat, Susan thinks.

"I'm sorry," the nurse replies, "But until her breathing improves, she needs to just have clear liquids. Anything else might worsen her respiratory status or cause nausea and vomiting, which would put her at risk for aspiration."

Throughout the night, the nurse and respiratory therapist check on Mollie every hour. The hourly check includes listening to Mollie's lungs, watching her breath, and assessing for signs of distress. The nurse counts Mollie's respirations and watches for any signs of distress such as the position Mollie is sleeping in (knowing that an upright and leaning forward posture can indicate distress) and whether her expiratory phase is longer than her inspiratory phase. A prolonged expiratory phase indicates air trapping and difficulty exhaling, a nurse explains to her.

By 9:00 the next morning, Mollie is feeling better.

"I can breathe a lot better now," she tells her mom. "Can I go to school today?"

"No, I'm sorry, sweetie, but you'll miss school today," Susan says.

Mollie starts to cry. "A zookeeper is bringing animals to class today, and I won't get to see them." Susan consoles Mollie and sits next to her in bed. Mollie says, "I hate having asthma. I miss my friends at school."

The respiratory therapist, Caleb, arrives and assesses Mollie at 9:10 a.m. "Good news, Mollie," he says. "You don't have to wear the mask all the time anymore. What's wrong? You look sad."

Susan explains the conversation Mollie and she just had. Caleb sits down next to Mollie and says, "It's tough having asthma, isn't it?" Mollie nods vigorously. "Well, the good news is that most kids with asthma don't have to miss school very much, so you'll be back soon. And more good news is that we'll teach you and your mom how to manage your asthma so that it's not as bad. How does that sound?"

Mollie nods her head but says nothing. Susan catches a glimpse of smile, though, and is encouraged.

"Well, great then," Caleb says. Turning to Susan, he says, "She'll get another albuterol treatment in 1 hour. After that, the nurse, the doctor, and I will listen to her lungs and see how she's doing."

"When can I go home?" Mollie says.

"Not just yet," Caleb replies. "We'll know more after lunch time, when you've been off the continuous albuterol for several hours."

Throughout the day, Mollie's respiratory status improves. The child life intern visits Mollie and asks her what she would like to do while she is getting better in the hospital. Considering age-appropriate activities, the child life intern offers the following: color, paint, crafts, watch movies, work puzzles, read books, or draw. She explains to Mollie that she can bring things to her room for her to do. Mollie chooses crafts and movies. A short time later, the child life intern returns, as she told Mollie she would, with crafts and movies. Mollie smiles for the first time since admission.

At Discharge

The following morning, the nurse, Linda, tells Susan that Mollie has met all the discharge criteria and will be able to go home as soon as the care team rounds are over and discharge orders are written. Mollie squeals at the news, and Susan is relieved.

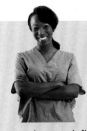

The Nurse's Point of View

Linda: Before discharge, I review several asthma education topics with Mollie and Susan. First, I ask Mollie to demonstrate how to use her peak flow meter. Mollie has used this tool before and accurately demonstrates how to perform a peak flow.

Next, I ask Mollie to demonstrate using her inhaler with a spacer. It is time for Mollie to have a dose of albuterol, so I allow Mollie to demonstrate while administering her own dose. Mollie demonstrates proper technique.

I then ask Mollie and Susan to list pertinent triggers that may lead to an asthma attack. Mollie tells me that running around outside during soccer when it is very hot or very cold often makes her feel as if she is having trouble breathing. I review the physician's orders, which include using two puffs of albuterol 15 to 30 minutes before soccer practice or engaging in physical activity. I ask Mollie and Susan to identify the signs and symptoms of worsening asthma. They name them all except for nighttime cough. I reiterate the importance of investigating a nighttime cough that is not associated with a cold or virus.

Given here is the discharge teaching checklist that I walk them through:

- Asthma triggers
- Asthma medications
- Use of inhaler and/or spacer
- Use of peak flow meter
- When to call the provider
- Returning to school

Mollie is discharged to home with her mother after completing the asthma discharge teaching.

Think Critically

1. Explain the three components of asthma and how these affect a child's ability to breathe.
2. You are teaching the parents of a child newly diagnosed with asthma ways to reduce triggers of asthma in the home. List five points of discussion for reducing triggers in the home.
3. Differentiate between the effects of albuterol and methylprednisolone on the pulmonary system. Why might a child with asthma need both medications during an acute flare-up?
4. You begin an assessment of a child who has been admitted with asthma. What signs and symptoms indicate that the child's condition is worsening?
5. During an education session with a 6-year-old newly diagnosed with asthma, the parents ask what the purpose of a peak flow meter is. Explain to the parent the rationale for a peak flow meter.

References

Horne, J. P., Flannery, R., & Usman, S. (2014). Adolescent idiopathic scoliosis: Diagnosis and management. *American Family Physician, 89*(3), 193–198.

Kelso, J. (2016). Do written asthma action plans improve outcomes? *Pediatric Allergy, Immunology, and Pulmonology, 29*(1), 2–5. doi:10.1089/ped.2016.0634

Liu, L., Gallaher, M., Davis, R., Rutter, C., Lewis, T., & Marcuse, E. (2004). Use of a respiratory clinical score among different providers. *Pediatric Pulmonology, 37*, 243–248.

Martire, L., & Helgeson, V. (2017). Close relationships and the management of chronic illness: Associations and interventions. *American Psychologist, 72*(6), 601.

National Asthma Education and Prevention Program (NAEPP). (2007). *Guidelines for the diagnosis and management of asthma*. Retrieved from https://www.nhlbi.nih.gov/health-pro/guidelines/current/asthma-guidelines/full-report

National Heart Lung and Blood Institute. (2007). *Asthma action plan*. Retrieved from https://www.nhlbi.nih.gov/files/docs/public/lung/asthma_actplan.pdf

Suggested Readings

American Academy of Allergy and Immunology. (n.d.). *Asthma*. Retrieved from http://www.aaaai.org/conditions-and-treatments/asthma

Centers for Disease Control and Prevention. (n.d.). *What is asthma?* Retrieved from https://www.cdc.gov/asthma/faqs.htm

National Heart, Lung and Blood Institute. (n.d.). *Asthma*. Retrieved from https://www.nhlbi.nih.gov/health/health-topics/topics/asthma

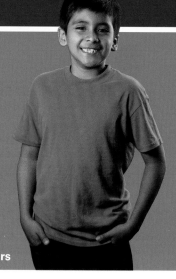

3 David Torres: Ulnar Fracture

David Torres, age 12 years

Objectives

After completing this chapter, you will be able to:

1. Understand normal growth and development of the 12-year-old.
2. Implement a teaching plan for a healthy 12-year-old.
3. Identify anatomical and physiological characteristics and concerns of the musculoskeletal system of preadolescent children.
4. Relate pediatric assessment findings to the child's musculoskeletal and circulatory status.
5. Discuss the pathophysiology of a fracture.
6. Identify various risk factors associated with pediatric fractures.
7. Outline the therapeutic regimen for a fracture.
8. Identify priorities of nursing care for a child with a fracture.

Key Terms

Buckle fracture
Compartment syndrome
Hemostasis

Physes
Poikilothermia

Background

David Torres is a healthy 12-year-old boy who is in the sixth grade and spends all his free time outside riding bikes and playing sports with his neighborhood friends. David lives with his mom, Alicia, stepdad, Santiago, and little sister, Elena, who is 2 years old. David's stepdad works the night shift in a factory, building car parts. David's mom stays at home and sells beauty products for additional income for the family. David's favorite sport is baseball. He recently made the travel baseball team after trials among many players. David recently started learning to do trick riding on his bike. One of his friends competes in bike trick-riding competitions.

Health Promotion

Two months ago, David had a well-care visit with his pediatrician, Dr. Juarez. At the visit, he and his mother learned that he weighed 92 lb (41.7 kg) and was 5 ft 1 in (61 in) tall, putting him in the 52nd percentile for weight and 75th percentile for height (Growth and Development Check 3.1). He received the flu vaccine, Tdap (tetanus, diphtheria, pertussis) vaccine, human papillomavirus (HPV) vaccine (the first of a two-shot series), and the meningococcal ACWY (MenACWY) vaccine. So, David is now up to date on his immunizations (Box 3.1).

The results of David's physical exam at his well-care visit were all within normal limits, according to the nurse. His vital signs

Box 3.1 Immunizations for 12-Year-Olds

The immunizations a child receives at his or her 12-y-old well-care visit include the following:

Tetanus, diphtheria, pertussis

The Tdap vaccine protects from tetanus, diphtheria, and pertussis. Tetanus is also known as lockjaw and leads to painful muscle tightening and stiffness. Diphtheria can lead to breathing problems, heart failure, paralysis, and death. Pertussis (known as whooping cough) causes severe coughing spells, difficulty breathing, and vomiting, as well as complications such as pneumonia. https://www.cdc.gov/vaccines/hcp/vis/vis-statements/tdap.html.

Human Papillomavirus

The human papillomavirus (HPV) vaccine prevents infection with HPV, which is associated with many cancers, such as cervical, vaginal, anal, throat, and penile cancers. It also prevents against genital warts. Most adolescents aged 9–14 y receive the HPV vaccine as a series of 2 doses separated by 6–12 mo. https://www.cdc.gov/vaccines/hcp/vis/vis-statements/hpv.html.

Meningococcal

Meningococcal (MenACWY) disease is a serious illness caused by *Neisseria meningitidis*, a type of bacteria. Meningococcal disease spreads quickly through close contact and can lead to meningitis and blood infections. Meningococcal disease kills 10–15 infected people out of 100. MenACWY can help prevent meningococcal disease caused by serogroups A, C, W, and Y. https://www.cdc.gov/vaccinesafety/vaccines/meningococcal-vaccine.html.

Adapted from Centers for Disease Control and Prevention. (2018). *Recommended immunization schedule for children and adolescents aged 18 years or younger.* Retrieved from https://www.cdc.gov/vaccines/schedules/hcp/imz/child-adolescent.html

 Growth and Development Check 3.1

Height and Weight Percentiles for a 12-Year-Old Boy

Percentile	Height, in (ft)	Weight, lb (kg)
10th	55 (4.6)	72 (32.7)
50th	59 (4.9)	90 (40.9)
90th	62 (5.2)	119 (54.09)

were age-appropriate. His heart rate was 72 beats/min (bpm), his blood pressure was 112/68 mm Hg, and his respiratory rate was 18 breaths/min.

Because of David's age, Dr. Juarez also took some time to discuss puberty. "David, I'd like to talk with you about puberty and some of the physical changes you may be experiencing. I know that can be a little embarrassing to talk about in front of your mother, so I'd like to give you the option of discussing it without her present. What do you think?"

Alicia suddenly felt incredibly awkward and even a little defensive sitting there. She'd always been present at her son's pediatrician visits, and the thought of being booted out upset and annoyed her. Still, she thought, David is growing up and changing, becoming a man. I need to respect his privacy.

"Actually, it's okay if she stays," David said. "Maybe she can help ask questions about some things I'm not sure about."

"Of course," said a relieved Alicia, grateful for her son's response. "I'd be happy to do that."

"Very well then," Dr. Juarez said. He went over some of the common changes in puberty and answered a few of Alicia's questions (Growth and Development Check 3.2). He also talked about David's friends and how he was getting along with kids at school and in extracurricular activities. David has always been an outgoing kid with many friends, so that was an easy conversation. Neither David nor his mother had concerns at that time about his social development.

At Home

One sunny Saturday evening, David returns from bike riding with his friends. His mother, Alicia, immediately notices that he is holding his right wrist in his left hand.

"What happened to your wrist?" she asks.

"Nothing," he says, letting go of his wrist and trying to act nonchalant. As soon as he lets go of it, though, he winces.

"What's wrong with your wrist?" she says. "Tell me the truth."

David sighs heavily and says, "Well, I was trying to do a trick off of this bike ramp we built and I guess I kind of crashed. I landed on my wrist when I tried to break my fall. I felt okay when I got up off the ground, but my wrist sort of hurt. I mean, it doesn't really hurt that bad; only when I move it."

Alicia puts some ice on his wrist and has him elevate it slightly above his heart while she finishes making dinner.

After dinner, Alicia takes another look at David's wrist and notices it is only slightly swollen and really is not even bruised. She wraps it in an elastic bandage and gives David some ibuprofen. David goes to bed.

In the morning, he tells his mother that his wrist still hurts and that the pain woke him twice during the night. His wrist does appear somewhat swollen, but there is no bruising that she can see. Alicia remembers her mother telling her that if a bone is broken, the area will be bruised. Still, she senses that something is just not right, so she calls David's pediatrician, Dr. Juarez, who encourages her to take David to the emergency room for an X-ray of his wrist.

Growth and Development Check 3.2

Male Adolescents (Young Teens, 12–14 Years Old)

Children grow taller, about 2.5 inches in a year, at a relatively consistent pace. Weight gain, typically 4 (1.8 kg) to 7 lb (3.2 kg) per year, occurs until puberty starts. Growth spurts occur at varying times throughout childhood and adolescence. It is possible for a child to rapidly lose and gain weight or suddenly add inches to height.

Physical

- Age-appropriate vital signs:
  - Heart rate: 60 to 110 bpm
  - Blood pressure: 100–135 (systolic)/65–85 (diastolic) mm Hg
  - Respiratory rate: 12–20 breaths/min
- Physical changes of puberty between ages 10 and 16 y
- Most rapid growth between ages 12 and 15 y
- Deepening of the voice
- Appearance of pubic hair, followed by underarm and facial hair
- Larynx cartilage (Adam's apple) gets bigger.
- Penis and testicles increase in size.
- Oily skin and/or acne

Social

- Focus on their own behavior and personal appearance (believe everyone is looking at them)
- Look more to peers than to parents
- Seek acceptance and trust
- Favor their own solutions and reject solutions from adults
- Question family values

Emotional

- Yearn for peer acceptance
- Want independence, yet want and need adult approval
- Compare self to others
- Seek privacy

Cognitive

- Think concretely; do not connect actions with future consequences
- Are developing skills in the use of logic
- Desire to explore the world outside of their own community

Safety

- Bicycle helmets
- Seatbelt use (especially when riding with teenaged drivers and friends)
- Guns and weapon safety

At the Hospital

Soon after they arrive at the local hospital emergency department, the triage nurse takes a brief history of David's health status and recent injury to his wrist. David rates his pain as a 6 on the numerical pain scale provided by the triage nurse (How Much Does It Hurt? 3.1). Alicia completes David's health history, indicating that he has no known allergies to medications, food, or dyes. The triage nurse performs what she calls a focused assessment on David's arm, explaining that it is to ensure that his circulation is not compromised and no bleeding is present (Let's Compare 3.1). The nurse then directs David and his mother to wait in the waiting room until they are called back to a room.

 ## How Much Does It Hurt? 3.1

Use of the Numerical Rating Scale for Pain Assessment

To adequately assess David's pain level, the nurse must use a pain scale that is appropriate for his age and stage of development. Because David is 12-y-old and of normal cognitive development, he should be able to describe, differentiate the characteristics of, and rate his pain. The nurse can use the mnemonic PQRST to determine the characteristics of the pain. The letters of this acronym stand for the following:

P = Provocation/palliation
Q = Quality/quantity
R = Region/radiation
S = Severity
T = Time

The Numerical Rating Scale is used to determine the severity of pain and is appropriate for use with David. The scale is from 0 to 10, with a score of 0 indicating no pain and a score of 10 indicating the worst pain possible.

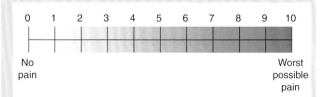

Image reprinted with permission from Morton, P. G., & Fontaine, D. K. (2017). *Critical care nursing* (11th ed., Fig. 5.1). Philadelphia, PA: Wolters Kluwer. Box adapted from *Validation of the numerical rating scale for pain intensity and unpleasantness in pediatric acute postoperative pain: Sensitivity to change over time.* Retrieved from https://doi.org/10.1016/j.jpain.2011.12.010

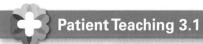

Let's Compare 3.1

The Musculoskeletal System

The musculoskeletal system of a child differs from that of an adult in several ways. First, children have a relatively greater amount of cartilage and collagen than do adults. This reduces the tensile strength of the bone, making propagation (growing of the crack or break) of fractures less likely in children. As a result of increased cartilage and collagen, fractures in children are often less identifiable on radiographs.

Second, children have **physes**, or growth plates. Growth plates are present at each end of a long bone and are where the bone grows. Growth plates are present until the child reaches skeletal maturity, which usually occurs between the ages of 13 and 15 y in girls and 15 and 17 y in boys. Once the child reaches skeletal maturity, the growth plates close and are replaced with solid bone.

Third, a child's bones are more elastic than an adult's bones, thus allowing for a greater degree of bend and deformation before a break actually occurs. In addition, a child's bones are much more porous than an adult's bones. Furthermore, the periosteal sleeve is much thicker in children than in adults. This characteristic acts as a restraint to the bone being displaced. Finally, the child's bones have an inherent potential to heal on their own as a result of the regeneration potential of the periosteum (Poduval, 2015).

Patient Teaching 3.1

Bicycle Helmet Safety

In the scenario, it is evident that David does not wear a helmet when he rides his bike. Bicycle helmet safety is a priority for this age. Adolescents are particularly resistant to consistently wearing a helmet. Bicycling is not only one of the most popular recreational sports among American children but it is also the leading cause of recreational sports injuries. Bicycle helmets are effective in preventing serious brain injuries. In fact, use of helmets can reduce serious brain injury by 88%.

Encourage parents and children to only buy helmets that meet the Consumer Product Safety Commission standards. Discuss with and present resources related to obtaining a properly fitting bicycle helmet to patients like David before discharge.

Useful information provided by the American Academy of Pediatrics can be found at:

https://www.healthychildren.org/English/safety-prevention/at-play/Pages/Bicycle-Helmets-What-Every-Parent-Should-Know.aspx

https://www.healthychildren.org/English/safety-prevention/at-play/Pages/Bicycle-Safety-Myths-And-Facts.aspx

http://pediatrics.aappublications.org/content/108/4/1030

After what seems like an eternity of waiting, David and Alicia are called back to an exam room in the emergency room. Soon, a woman who identifies herself as a patient care assistant (PCA) comes in and obtains David's vital signs. She has a gentle and patient manner, which Alicia appreciates. She explains that she is taking his blood pressure on his left arm to avoid any potential blood flow problems in the affected arm. As she completes each vital sign measurement, she reports them to David and Alicia. They are as follows:

- Heart rate: 92 bpm
- Respiratory rate: 22 breaths/min
- Temperature: 99.4°F (37.4°C)
- Blood pressure: 130/80 mm Hg
- Blood O_2 saturation (by pulse oximetry): 99% on room air

Just as she is finishing up, another woman enters the exam room.

"Hi," she says. "I'm Gabriella, your nurse. Can you tell me what happened with your arm, David?"

"Sure," he says. David tells her the entire story of the bike accident, leaving out the part about not wearing a helmet or any protective gear, Alicia notices (Patient Teaching 3.1).

Gabriella listens intently while David talks, occasionally typing in notes on her tablet. When he finishes, she pulls out a card with numbers and pictures on it representing different levels of pain and says, "On a scale from 0 to 10, with 0 being none and 10 being the worst pain you've ever felt, how would you rate the pain in your wrist, David?"

He looks at the card a moment and thinks. "Well, it doesn't hurt all the time."

"How about right now?" she says.

"It's about a 6, I guess," he says.

"I'll speak with the doctor to see if we can get an order for medication to treat the pain," Gabriella says. "Are you allergic to any medications?" She addresses this to David but glances over at Alicia.

David shrugs, and Alicia replies, "No. He's not allergic to anything that we know of."

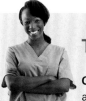

The Nurse's Point of View

Gabriella: David's injury is very typical for an active 12-year-old boy. On the basis of his report of the accident and the appearance of his arm, I'm guessing it's a fracture, but we'll have to wait for an X-ray and Dr. Singh's diagnosis to confirm that. In the meantime, I need to help alleviate David's pain and assess for any signs of possible complications related to a fracture. I ask the PCA to bring an ice pack for David and a pillow to elevate his arm with. Then I check the circulation in David's right arm and hand while comparing it with that of the left arm and

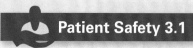

Patient Safety 3.1

Monitoring Circulation and Perfusion

Monitoring circulation and perfusion of the affected extremity is a priority for the nurse when caring for a patient with a fracture. If too much swelling occurs, compartment syndrome may develop. Compartment syndrome occurs when injured tissue swells within the fascia and pressure increases within the compartment, or area of injury and swelling. Decreased perfusion can lead to permanent damage related to ischemia of the affected tissues. One way to remember what to assess is to remember the "six Ps."

- **Pain:** increased intensity and unrelieved by elevation and pain medication
- **Pulse:** intensity (strong, diminished, or absent); delayed capillary refill, possibly an earlier sign of decreased circulation
- **Pallor:** pale and/or shiny skin distal to the injury
- **Paresthesia:** "pins and needles" sensation; numbness
- **Paralysis:** inability to move the limb distal to the injury
- **Poikilothermia:** difference in temperature between the injured limb and the uninjured limb; a cooler limb is a sign the injured limb is not able to thermoregulate (related to lack of perfusion).

hand (Patient Safety 3.1). I assess the pulse in each wrist and note they are equally strong and easy to palpate, which is reassuring. Next, I assess the color of each arm and note that the right wrist and hand seem slightly paler and have slight bruising on the lateral aspect compared with the left wrist and hand, which appear pink (Box 3.2). The reported pain level, swelling, and bruising all seem to point to a fracture; but, like I said, we'll have to wait for the X-ray to confirm.

Box 3.2   Pathophysiology of a Fracture

When a normally developed bone breaks, several anatomical and physiological responses occur. A fracture initiates an inflammatory response and **hemostasis**. A broken bone bleeds. Accumulating blood and edema cause pain in the affected area. Edema causes stretching of the periosteum of the bone and soft-tissue swelling. Spasms in the muscles surrounding the break can also occur, as the muscles attempt to hold the bone fragments together. Spasms can cause intense pain. Bradykinin and other chemical mediators are released and contribute to pain. Inflammation and swelling can also cause pain related to the pressure placed on the nerves near the affected area. Pain fibers in the nerve endings around the bone become irritated and can lead to increased pain.

"Do you have any unusual feelings in your right arm, wrist, or hand?" Gabriella asks.

"When I hold it down low," he says, moving his wrist down below the level of his heart, "it sometimes feels like I'm being poked with pins and needles."

"Can you wiggle all your fingers and your thumb for me?" David does so but winces.

"That hurts, doesn't it?" she asks. She also notes that David's right wrist and hand are slightly cooler than his uninjured left wrist and hand. She completes an SBAR report to give to Dr. Singh, the emergency room physician who will be seeing David (Box 3.3).

Later, after another long wait in the exam room, Gabriella returns. "Dr. Singh would like to order ibuprofen for your pain, but first we need to measure your current weight."

Box 3.3   Gabriella's SBAR Report to Dr. Singh

Situation

David, a 12-y-old boy, presents with pain to his right hand and wrist, which he rates a 6, on a scale of 0–10.

Background

David fell off his bicycle and landed on his wrist last night. Today, the pain was much worse and his mother called the pediatrician, who recommended he come to the emergency room for an X-ray and assessment for a possible fracture.

Assessment

The most recent assessment includes a circulation check, which reveals a slightly cool right wrist and hand with slight bruising on the lateral aspect, an easily palpable radial pulse, mild edema, and brisk capillary refill in the fingers of the right hand.

Recommendation

Treat the patient's pain with ice and pain medication. David has no known drug allergies, and his weight 2 mo ago at the pediatrician's office was 41.7 kg.

Analyze the Evidence 3.1 — Use of Codeine for Pain Control in Pediatrics

Recently, the American Academy of Pediatrics, the World Health Organization (WHO), and the U.S. Food and Drug Administration (FDA) strongly discouraged the use of codeine for pain control in the pediatric population. Historically, codeine was considered an optimal analgesic for treating acute pain in children because of the perception that it was a safe opioid analgesic and had limited risk of causing respiratory depression.

However, for codeine to work as an analgesic, it must be metabolized in the liver into morphine, which provides the analgesic effect. The problem is, ongoing investigations have shown a large variation in the conversion of codeine to morphine in the pediatric population. Hence, every child metabolizes the drug differently and therefore has varying levels of morphine in the body after conversion occurs. This is particularly important in the pediatric population because pediatric patients have greater susceptibility to the side effects of morphine (Benini & Barbi, 2014). There has been documented occurrence of unanticipated respiratory depression and death after children received codeine.

The FDA recently released a review of Adverse Event Reporting system data from 1965 to 2015 in children who used codeine or codeine-containing products. The review revealed a total of 64 cases of severe respiratory depression and 24 codeine-related deaths (Seymour, 2015). In light of this data, a study from 2011 reported that codeine was prescribed to >800,000 pediatric patients under the age of 11, more than any other opioid (Racoosin, 2011). Despite the evidence of potential harm with the use of codeine as an analgesic in the pediatric population, providers are still prescribing the medication. The FDA, WHO, Health Canada, and the European Medicines Agency have issued or are considering issuing a declaration of a contraindication for the use of codeine in the pediatric population for the treatment of pain and cough (used as an analgesic or antitussive).

"Why do you need to know my weight?" David says. "What does that have to do with anything?" He's cranky, Alicia thinks. The pain must really be getting to him.

"The dose of the medicine we'll be giving you depends on your weight," Gabriella explains. "The more you weigh, the bigger the dose needs to be for it to be effective."

The PCA leads David into the hall to weigh him, and they return a moment later. She reports his weight as 92.8 lb (42.1 kg). Gabriella tells them that she'll inform Dr. Singh of this so that he can write the order for the ibuprofen, which will be for 10 mg/kg oral for 1 dose (Analyze the Evidence 3.1; The Pharmacy 3.1).

The Pharmacy 3.1 — Analgesics

Medication	Classification	Route	Action	Nursing Considerations
Acetaminophen	• Analgesic • Antipyretic	• PO • PR • IV	• Analgesic: inhibits CNS prostaglandin synthesis and peripherally inhibits pain impulses • Antipyretic: inhibits the heat-regulating center of the hypothalamus	• Metabolized by the liver • Can be hepatotoxic • Monitor LFT, ALT, and AST with long-term use • Monitor for s/s of liver toxicity • PO dosing: 10–15 mg/kg every 4–6 h • Do not exceed 4,000 mg/d
Ibuprofen	• Analgesic • Antipyretic • Anti-inflammatory	• PO • IV	• Inhibits cyclooxygenase-1 and -2 • Decreases prostaglandin precursors	• Excreted by the kidneys • Can be nephrotoxic • Monitor intake and output • Monitor BUN and creatinine with long-term use • Do not give to infants younger than 6 mo due to immature renal system • Monitor for s/s of GI irritation • Monitor for s/s of increased bruising and bleeding due to decreased platelet adhesion

ALT, alanine transaminase; AST, aspartate transaminase; BUN, blood urea nitrogen; CNS, central nervous system; GI, gastrointestinal; IV, intravenous; LFT, liver function test; PO, oral; PR, rectal; s/s, signs and symptoms.
Adapted from Taketomo, C. K. (2018). *Pediatric & neonatal dosage handbook* (25th ed.). Hudson, OH: Lexicomp.

"I hope they can order that medicine soon," David tells Alicia after Gabriella has left the room. "My wrist is really hurting."

Fortunately, Gabriella is not gone long. When she returns, she says, "Okay. I have your medicine. I just need you to confirm your name and birthdate—it's just a precaution we take to make sure we are giving the right medication to the right person."

David answers her, and Gabriella goes on to explain to Alicia and David what the ibuprofen is for and how it should work to reduce inflammation, which will result in less pain.

Dr. Singh, the emergency room physician, arrives about 10 minutes after Gabriella gave David the ibuprofen. He asks David to explain what happened, and David relates again the story of his bike accident. Dr. Singh assesses David's pain level (which is still a 6), his ability to move his wrist and hand (David can move his fingers but has difficulty moving his wrist without feeling a lot of pain), and does a circulation check on his right arm and hand. Dr. Singh explains that David will need an X-ray of his wrist and writes an order for the X-ray.

The X-ray technologist arrives and introduces herself as Sarah. "I'm here to take you to have your X-ray done," she says. "Would you like your mom to come along?"

David is slow to respond but finally nods his head. Alicia can tell he's anxious about being in the emergency room. They go to radiography, and Sarah takes the X-rays. She then escorts them back to his room.

Gabriella returns and says, "How are you feeling now, David?"

"Better," he replies. "I think the ice is helping."

"How would you rate your pain now?" she asks.

"About a 3," he says.

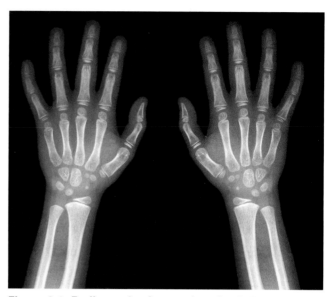

Figure 3.1. Radiograph of normal pediatric bones of the hand and forearm (ulna and radius).

Gabriella glances at her watch and says, "It's been about an hour since we gave you the ibuprofen, so the ibuprofen could be taking effect, too. It usually takes 30 to 45 minutes before it starts working to relieve pain. Keep your arm elevated near your heart with the pillow; that should help, too."

Dr. Singh comes in and says, "I have the results from your X-ray. You have a **buckle fracture** in your right ulna" (Figs. 3.1 and 3.2; Box 3.4). He flips a switch on the wall and shows

Box 3.4   Forearm Fractures in Childhood

Fractures of the lower forearm have been found to be the most common fractures in children, accounting for about 18% of childhood fractures (Naranje, Erali, Warner, Sawyer, & Kelly, 2016). Boys are more likely than girls to experience a fracture of the forearm. In a study to determine trends in pediatric wrist fractures, Shah, Buzas, and Zinberg (2015) found that bicycles accounted for 10% of pediatric wrist fractures.

A type of fracture that commonly occurs in the forearm (the type David, in the case scenario, has been diagnosed with) is the buckle fracture, or torus fracture. In a buckle fracture, one side of the bone buckles or bends inward in response to excessive pressure being applied to it. Buckle fractures are considered incomplete fractures of the shaft of the long bone and are characterized by bulging of the cortex of the bone. Buckle fractures (Fig. 3.2) occur when there is axial loading of the long bone and, in children, occur most commonly in the distal radius. Often, the fracture occurs as a result of an outstretched arm when a child tries to protect himself or herself during a fall.

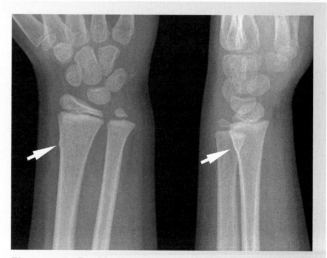

Figure 3.2. Buckle fracture. A radiograph of the wrist shows buckling of the cortex of the distal ulnar metaphysis *(arrows)*. Reprinted with permission from Siegel, M. J., & Coley, B. D. (2005). *The core curriculum: Pediatric imaging* (1st ed., Fig. 12.151). Philadelphia, PA: Lippincott Williams & Wilkins.

them a digital radiograph of David's right forearm. "See the little bulge in the bone there? That's it. You'll need to make an appointment with an orthopedic provider in the morning for further assessment and possible casting."

"A cast?" David says. "How long will I have the cast for?"

"I'm not sure," Dr. Singh replies. "The orthopedic provider will be able to give you details once he evaluates your X-rays and arm."

David looks worriedly at his mom and asks, "Does this mean I will miss baseball for the rest of the season?"

"I'm not sure, dear," she says. "But I'll make an appointment as soon as the orthopedic office opens in the morning."

Dr. Singh and Gabriella apply a splint and an elastic wrap to David's arm to keep it immobilized until he sees an orthopedic provider. Gabriella checks David's circulation after the application of the splint to ensure it is not too tight.

At Discharge

Before discharge, Gabriella gives David and his mother the following discharge instructions:

- Elevate the affected arm.
- Apply ice for 20 minutes 3 times a day.
- Wiggle the fingers every hour when awake.
- Notify the pediatrician or return to the emergency room if the hand becomes cold or dark in color; if pain is severe and unrelieved with rest, ice, elevation, and ibuprofen; and/or there is loss of sensation in the hand and fingers.
- Keep the splint clean and dry.
- Do not stick objects down the splint to scratch or rub the affected area.
- Make an appointment as soon as possible with an orthopedic provider.

Gabriella reviews the instructions with David and his mother and he is discharged from the emergency room.

At the Orthopedic Office

The next morning, Alicia makes an appointment to see a pediatric orthopedic specialist. David has been complaining of increased pain since he woke up.

"Would you like some ibuprofen?" she says.

"No, it's okay," he says. "I guess it's not really that bad."

"Just take the medicine, son," Alicia says. She's begun to lose patience with his complaining about his wrist. "The nurse said it would lessen the swelling, which will help reduce the pain." David reluctantly agrees.

Alicia and David arrive at the appointment as scheduled, at 10:00 a.m.

The medical assistant calls David and his mom back to the exam room. She asks David how he broke his arm, and he tells her his story.

"How's your pain level, on a scale of 0 to 10?" she asks.

"It's about a 7," he says, "especially when I hold my arm down by my waist."

Dr. Carter, the orthopedic physician, then comes in to assess David's hand and arm. He removes the splint that was placed in the emergency room the night before. After a thorough assessment of David's arm and looking at the X-rays obtained in the emergency room the night before, Dr. Carter says, "Yep, it's definitely a buckle fracture. You'll need a cast for 3 to 6 weeks. The good news is that this type of fracture does not require surgery and should heal with casting and rest." Alicia is relieved, but David does not look thrilled.

The casting nurse, Thomas, arrives and introduces himself. "I'll be setting up the room so Dr. Carter can cast your arm. You'll be getting a synthetic cast made of fiberglass."

"Fiberglass?" Alicia says. "When I broke my arm as a girl, I had a plaster cast."

"That's right," Thomas replies. "The fiberglass forms a hard, supportive layer. It's lighter weight and stronger than plaster, plus X-rays can penetrate it, so we can take X-rays with the cast in place."

Before applying the cast, Thomas applies a thin stocking or sock to David's arm and then a thick layer of cotton padding from his hand to just below his elbow. Finally, Dr. Carter applies the fiberglass casting material, which comes in a roll and must be dipped in water to soften it and make it pliable.

Following the application of the cast, Thomas returns to the exam room to give David and his mother follow-up instructions for cast care and safety, monitoring for complications and pain control, as well as the plan of care (Patient Teaching 3.2).

Patient Teaching 3.2

Cast Care and Safety

David and his parents will need to understand personal safety and how to care for the cast while the cast is in place. Teaching related to a cast should include the following:

1. *Keep the swelling down.*
2. *Recognize the warning signs of impaired circulation.*
3. *Safety: Do's and don'ts of caring for a cast*
   a. Never stick anything down the cast. This can lead to skin irritation, open areas of skin, and infection.
   b. Do not scratch or attempt to scratch itching skin under the cast. Avoid using powders or deodorants under the cast.
   c. Do not get the cast wet. Moisture can dampen the padding next to the skin and cause irritation.
   d. Avoid getting dirt, sand, or any powders in the cast. These can cause skin irritation.
   e. Never pull any of the padding out of the cast or splint. The cast or splint will not fit correctly if the padding is removed.

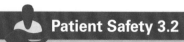

Patient Safety 3.2

Monitoring for Signs of Complications

Complications of a fracture can include bleeding, impaired circulation, compartment syndrome, and neuropathy.

- **Bleeding:** assess heart rate, blood pressure, circulation, and bruising.
- **Impaired circulation:** assess capillary refill, skin temperature, and distal pulses.
- **Compartment syndrome:** monitor for the six Ps.
- **Neuropathy:** assess for tingling, numbness, and decreased or absent sensation distal to the injury.

"With the cast on your arm," Thomas explains, "you are at risk for **compartment syndrome**, which occurs when severe swelling develops under the cast, which can lead to decreased blood flow and loss of oxygen to his wrist and fingers." Thomas reviews the signs and symptoms of compartment syndrome (Patient Safety 3.2).

"Elevate your arm to near or above heart level as often as you can," Thomas says. "And put an icepack on the cast over the wrist area for 10 to 20 minutes once each hour while awake for

the next 2 days. After that, apply ice at least 3 times a day for 10 to 20 minutes each time as long as there is swelling and pain is present. Finally, move your fingers on the injured hand often. This helps increase blood flow to the hand."

"Now that I've told you what to *do* with your cast, I'll tell you what *not to do*," Thomas says. "At some point, your arm will itch because the skin under a cast becomes moist, then dry, and eventually sloughs off. In fact, it will itch so bad that you'll be desperate to scratch it. Whatever you do, don't stick anything down in the cast to scratch your arm. The skin will be fragile and easy to injure, which can lead to an infection. And you don't want that, do you?"

David shook his head.

"You also need to avoid getting dirt or sand between the cast and your arm. This can also lead to infection. Again—bad. Finally, do not get the cast wet. Put a plastic bag over it or wrap your arm in several layers of plastic wrap when you shower. Understood?"

"Understood," David replies. Thomas has him repeat all the instructions a couple of times to make sure he understands. Smart man, Alicia thinks. He's dealt with 12-year-olds before.

David and his mom leave the orthopedic office with many instructions for taking care of the cast and helping his wrist to heal. David is excited that his friends will be able to sign his cast the next time he sees them.

Think Critically

1. What is important anticipatory guidance for the parents of a 12-year-old?
2. How did David's stage of growth and development affect the type of injury he sustained?
3. Why do members of David's healthcare team keep checking the circulation in his injured arm? What signs are they looking for? If these signs appeared, what would be the appropriate nursing action?
4. Why does wearing a cast put David at risk for developing compartment syndrome? What signs that would indicate this complication is occurring should he and his mom be looking for?
5. Why does David not receive a cast in the emergency room?
6. How effective is Thomas, the casting nurse, in communicating with David about his injury and recovery? Why?

References

Benini, F., & Barbi, E. (2014). Doing without codeine: Why and what are the alternatives? *Italian Journal of Pediatrics, 40*(1), 16. doi:10.1186/1824-7288-40-16

Naranje, S., Erali, R., Warner, W., Sawyer, J., & Kelly, D. (2016). Epidemiology of pediatric fractures presenting to emergency departments in the United States. *Journal of Pediatric Orthopedics, 36*(4), e45–e48.

Poduval, M. (2015). Skeletal system anatomy in children and toddlers. *Medscape*. Retrieved from http://emedicine.medscape.com/article/1899256-overview#showall

Racoosin, J., Roberson, D., Pacanowski, M., & Nielsen, D. (2013). New evidence about an old drug—Risk with codeine after adenotonsillectomy. *New England Journal of Medicine, 368*(23), 2155–2157.

Seymour, S. (2015, December 9). *Briefing document: Joint pulmonary-allergy drugs and drug safety and risk management advisory committee meeting.* Meeting of the Pulmonary-Allergy Drugs Advisory Committee, Silver Spring, MD. Retrieved from https://www.fda.gov/downloads/advisorycommittees/

committeesmeetingmaterials/drugs/pulmonary-allergydrugsadvisorycommittee/ucm482005.pdf

Shah, N., Buzas, D., & Zinberg, E. (2015). Epidemiologic dynamics contributing to pediatric wrist fractures in the United States. *Hand (N Y), 10*(2), 266–271.

Suggested Readings

American Academy of Orthopedic Surgeons. (2014). *Forearm fractures in children.* Retrieved from http://orthoinfo.aaos.org/topic.cfm?topic=a00039

American Society for Surgery of the Hand.

(2012). *Fractures in children.* Retrieved from http://www.assh.org/handcare/hand-arm-injuries/Fractures-in-Children

Hart, E., Albright, M., Rebello, G., & Grottkau, B. (2006). Broken bones: Common pediatric fractures—Part I. *Orthopedic Nursing, 25*(4), 251–256.

Hart, E., Grottkau, B., Rebello, G., & Albright, M. (2006). Broken bones: Common pediatric upper extremity fractures—Part II. *Orthopedic Nursing, 25*(5), 311–323; quiz 324–355.

4

Ellie Raymore: Urinary Tract Infection and Pyelonephritis

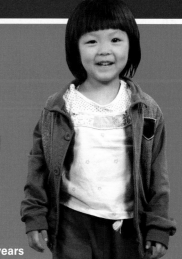

Ellie Raymore, age 3 years

Objectives

After completing this chapter, you will be able to:
1. Describe normal growth and development of the 3-year-old.
2. Discuss an appropriate teaching plan for a healthy 3-year-old.
3. Identify signs and symptoms of a urinary tract infection in infants and young children.
4. Explain the use of intravenous rehydration therapy in the treatment of dehydration.
5. Recognize the signs and symptoms of pyelonephritis.
6. Discuss special considerations when providing health care to a family with an adopted child.
7. Create a nursing plan of care for a toddler with pyelonephritis.

Key Terms

Pyelonephritis
Vesicoureteral reflux
Voiding cystourethrogram

Background

Ellie Raymore is a 3-year-old girl who loves playing with her dolls and sitting on her mother's lap while being read to. She lives with her adoptive parents, Sandy and Eric Raymore, and is their first and only child. They are in the process of adopting a child from Guatemala at the present time.

Sandy and Eric received little information regarding the prenatal care Ellie's biological mother received but were informed her mother was 17 years old when she delivered Ellie. The biological father's information is unknown. Ellie was in four different foster homes for the first 4 months of her life and was then placed in Sandy and Eric's home at about 5 months of age as a foster child. Her adoption was finalized when she was 16 months of age.

Ellie has adjusted well since she was placed in the Raymore's home. In the first few months, she did not gain weight as well as she should have, but by the age of about 11 to 12 months, she began to gain weight and grew in length. Ellie was not a good sleeper, only sleeping for 2 to 3 hours at a time when she first came to the Raymore's house. Again, however, by about the age of 12 months, she had developed a consistent sleeping pattern and was more consolable and playful during the day. Since coming to the Raymore's home, Ellie has been receiving regularly scheduled well-care visits at the pediatrician's office and is up to date on all her immunizations.

However, Ellie was diagnosed with grade 3 **vesicoureteral reflux** at the age of 11 months following a second urinary tract infection (UTI) within a 2-month period, which led her pediatrician to suspect vesicoureteral reflux (Fig. 4.1). To diagnose Ellie, the pediatrician ordered several tests and procedures, including a **voiding cystourethrogram**, a renal ultrasound, and laboratory tests such as blood urea nitrogen, creatinine, and renal function tests. Ellie takes a prophylactic antibiotic,

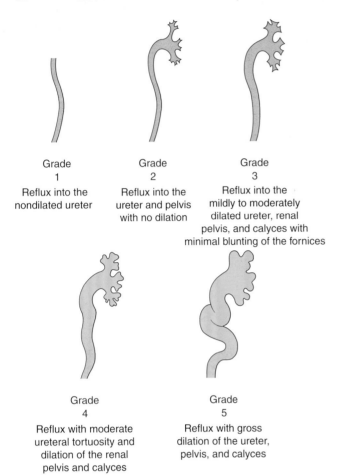

Grade
1

Reflux into the
nondilated ureter

Grade
2

Reflux into the
ureter and pelvis
with no dilation

Grade
3

Reflux into the
mildly to moderately
dilated ureter, renal
pelvis, and calyces with
minimal blunting of the fornices

Grade
4

Reflux with moderate
ureteral tortuosity and
dilation of the renal
pelvis and calyces

Grade
5

Reflux with gross
dilation of the ureter,
pelvis, and calyces

Figure 4.1. Vesicoureteral reflux, graded according to severity. In grade 1 vesicoureteral reflux, urine backs up into the ureter but does not dilate it. In grade 2, urine backs up into the ureter and renal pelvis but does not dilate them. In grades 3 to 5, urine backs up into the ureter, renal pelvis, and calyces and increasingly dilates them. Modified with permission from Marino, B. S., & Fine, K. S. (2013). *Blueprints pediatrics* (6th ed., Fig. 17.1). Philadelphia, PA: Wolters Kluwer Health/Lippincott Williams & Wilkins.

Box 4.1   Vesicoureteral Reflux

Vesicoureteral reflux occurs primarily in infants and young children but can be seen in adults. Vesicoureteral reflux can be primary or secondary. Primary vesicoureteral reflux is more common and is caused by a congenital defect in the functional valve between the bladder and the ureter that normally closes to prevent urine from flowing back into the ureter. The exact cause of vesicoureteral reflux is unknown, but it is thought to have a genetic component because the defect runs in families. Often, depending on the severity, as the child grows, the ureters grow longer and become straighter, which then improves valve function. Children diagnosed with grade 1 or 2 vesicoureteral reflux often outgrow it and have normal flow of urine. Children diagnosed with grade 3, 4, or 5 vesicoureteral reflux may have life-long reflux issues, requiring them to take prophylactic antibiotics, undergo annual testing for renal disease, and even have one or more surgeries to help reduce or correct the reflux severity. Secondary vesicoureteral reflux is caused by an obstruction or malfunction in the urinary tract, most commonly due to repeated infections that lead to scarring (National Institute of Diabetes and Digestive and Kidney Disorders, 2017).

sulfamethoxazole and trimethoprim (Bactrim), once a day to reduce the chances she will get a UTI.

Sandy and Eric have had a lot to learn about UTIs and vesicoureteral reflux (Box 4.1). When Sandy explains to family members what vesicoureteral reflux is, she tries to keep it simple. Essentially, she tells people, Ellie's urine flows backward instead of forward. Urine goes back into her ureters and possibly into her kidneys. This puts Ellie at high risk for UTIs, renal scarring, and **pyelonephritis**. If UTIs are not caught and treated quickly, Ellie could have permanently damaged kidneys because of repeated bouts of pyelonephritis.

Sandy and Eric enjoy watching Ellie grow and develop. Just recently, Ellie mastered a few puzzles and is so proud of herself she jumps up and down and claps her hands every time she tells someone about her puzzles. She recently started dressing herself in the mornings and changing into her pajamas without

help in the evening. She has also mastered riding her tricycle but takes her helmet off when Sandy and Eric are not looking. Despite her parents' many attempts at explaining why the helmet is important, Ellie still takes the helmet off. The rule at the Raymore house is that you have to wear a helmet when riding a bicycle or tricycle. Sandy and Eric model this behavior when they ride bicycles. Eric has begun taking the tricycle away from Ellie if she takes her helmet off. Ellie gets frustrated, cries, and throws a temper tantrum each time the tricycle is taken away. The "fit-throwing" (as Eric refers to the episodes) or temper tantrums are concerning to Sandy. She believes Ellie should be out of this phase.

Ellie has met several other milestones recently, as well (Growth and Development Check 4.1). She has been potty-trained since she was 28 months. She no longer has nighttime accidents now, either. Ellie likes to play in groups and seems to understand the meaning of "mine," "his," and "hers." She shares without prompting about 50% of the time she plays with children her age. Sandy is able to leave Ellie with family and familiar people as well as day care workers without signs of separation anxiety. Sandy has noticed that Ellie has begun running "like a normal kid" instead of being so wobbly like when she was a 2-year-old. Every day, it seems, a bit more of Ellie's personality appears and she discovers new words. She can carry on a conversation with others using one or two sentences and is very animated in her facial expressions when she talks.

Growth and Development Check 4.1

Three-Year-Old Milestones

Social/Emotional

- Copies adults and friends
- Takes turns when playing games
- Understands "mine," "his," and "hers"
- Separates easily from mom and dad

Speech

- Follows instructions with two or three steps
- Can name most familiar things
- Talks well enough to be understood by strangers most of the time
- Says first name, age, and sex
- Carries on a conversation using two or three sentences
- Can name a friend
- Uses "I," "me," "we," and some plural words correctly

Cognitive

- Does puzzles with three or four pieces
- Copies a circle with a pencil or crayon
- Turns pages in a book one at a time
- Can work toys with buttons, levers, and moving parts
- Turns door handles; screws and unscrews lids

Gross Motor/Fine Motor

- Dresses and undresses self
- Pedals a three-wheel bike (tricycle)
- Runs well
- Walks up and down stairs, one foot on each step
- Climbs with ease
- Uses scissors

Adapted from the Centers for Disease Control and Prevention. (2016). *Learn the signs. Act early.* Retrieved from https://www.cdc.gov/ncbddd/actearly/milestones/milestones-3yr.html

Health Promotion

Today, Sandy takes Ellie to the pediatrician, Dr. Engle, for her 3-year-old well-care visit. The nurse, Liz, helps Ellie step onto the scale to measure her weight and then measures her height. She then tells Sandy that Ellie weighs 32 lb (14.54 kg) and is 2.8 ft (37 in) tall. After tapping away on her tablet for a moment, Liz reports that, based on the growth chart and her body mass index (BMI), Ellie's weight is in the 63rd percentile and her height in the 37th percentile. She goes on to say that Ellie's BMI is 16.4, which is in the 70th percentile and normal, given that the healthy range for BMI is from the 5th percentile to the 85th percentile (Harriet Lane). Liz measures Ellie's head circumference with a tape measure and reports it to be 19 in (48.2 cm), which she says is within the normal range for a 3-year-old (18.25–20 in [46.3–50.8 cm] in is normal; Growth and

Growth and Development Check 4.2

Physical Growth

During the toddler years, physical growth is not as rapid as it was during infancy. Typically, the toddler gains 3–5 lb (1.36–2.27 kg) per year and grows about 3 in (7.62 cm) per year (AAP, 2017).

Development Check 4.2). Liz tells them that the doctor will be in to see them soon and then departs.

"Good morning, Ellie!" Dr. Engle says as he enters the exam room a few minutes later. "How are you doing today?"

"Okay," Ellie says, her eyes wide as she studies the pediatrician.

Dr. Engle greets Sandy, as well, and then looks over Ellie's health record on his tablet as he talks about the weather.

"Well, it looks like she's eating well and growing well," he says to Sandy. "Ellie won't receive any immunizations at this visit. She'll receive her next round when she turns 4." Dr. Engle sets his tablet down and says, "I'd like to talk with you about Ellie's development." He asks about her gross motor skills, cognitive skills, speech, and social skills.

"She's doing great," Sandy says. She proudly tells Dr. Engle that Ellie is potty-trained, is starting to share her toys, rides her tricycle, and runs without looking like she is going to fall anymore. Sandy also tells Dr. Engle that Ellie is working puzzles and proud of it, as well as dressing and undressing herself.

"Excellent!" Dr. Engle says. "Sounds like she's right on track socially and with her gross motor skills. How about her learning and speech?"

"I have some concerns, to be honest," Sandy says. She pauses a moment, reluctant to say her concerns out loud. Dr. Engle waits patiently. "Well, I read that Ellie should be copying circles and squares with a pencil or crayon by now and figuring out how to turn door handles and unscrew simple lids and containers."

"That's correct," Dr. Engle says.

"Well, she has no interest in using crayons and refuses to even hold one. If I hand her one, she just throws it. She also becomes frustrated and cries when she cannot get a lid open on one of her toys or open the door to go outside. And then there's her issue with speaking. I mean, Eric and I can always understand her, but other people often have trouble understanding her. She tends to only speak one or two sentences at a time, and only three or four words per sentence. At first, I wasn't overly concerned, but then I started noticing that several of my friends have 3-year-olds who talk much better and are easier to understand than Ellie. These things worry me, doctor."

"I understand your concern," Dr. Engle says. "But let me put your mind at ease a little. Ellie is meeting most of her other milestones. And children develop at different rates. Ellie may take a little longer in some of these areas, but that's okay. She'll still get there. I encourage you to keep offering her crayons, paper, and scissors and to demonstrate how to use them regularly. Is Ellie exposed to other children who may be performing these skills?"

"Not often," Sandy admits, feeling a twinge of guilt. "She's with Eric most of the time—he's a stay-at-home dad—so she doesn't go to day care. We don't have any family members in the area, and Ellie does not go to any play groups. About once or twice a month we take her to church functions where she gets to play with other kids her age."

"I recommend providing her with more exposure to other kids, because children this age tend to watch what their peers are doing and copy their behaviors, not just adults. As for her speech, I believe it will further develop in the next 6 months or so. If you don't notice a difference by then, bring Ellie back to the office and we'll discuss options for a speech evaluation."

Dr. Engle ends the visit by discussing safety concerns with 3-year-olds (Patient Teaching 4.1). He informs Sandy that the most common cause of death in children from 2 to 4 years of age is unintentional injury, such as burns, drowning, falls, poisoning, and traffic accidents (Centers for Disease Control and Prevention, 2017). He reinforces with Sandy the importance of Ellie wearing a helmet when riding the tricycle, of keeping Ellie away from the street and traffic, and of closely supervising her while she rides.

At Home

About a month after Ellie's well-care visit, Sandy notices that Ellie has been urinating every 1 to 2 hours when she is awake for the past 2 days. Today, she has been running to the potty yelling, "My pee hurts!" Sandy has also noticed that Ellie's panties are damp when she helps her wipe each time she goes to the potty. In addition, Sandy thought Ellie's urine smelled foul this morning. Sandy noticed that Ellie felt warm to the touch last night and was cranky and irritable. But the family had been out shopping and went to dinner, and Sandy just thought Ellie was tired and had had a long day. Thinking back, Sandy realizes that Ellie hasn't eaten very well in the past 2 days, either. Sandy calls the pediatrician's office, concerned that Ellie may have a UTI. It has been about 8 months since she last had a UTI. After Sandy explains her concerns to the office nurse, the nurse requests that Sandy make an appointment, considering that Ellie has the diagnosis of vesicoureteral reflux and is on prophylactic medications. Much to Sandy's relief, there is an appointment available at 3:00 this afternoon.

At the Pediatrician's Office

Sandy arrives at the pediatrician's office with Ellie at 3:00 p.m. Ellie fell asleep in the car. Luckily the office is not busy, and Sandy is able to take Ellie back to the exam room as soon as she has checked in.

Patient Teaching 4.1   Safety

Play
- Check outdoor playground equipment for loose screws and sharp edges.
- Water safety: teach children to swim, but always supervise children near water, including kiddie pools.
- Make sure children always wear a helmet when riding a tricycle.
- Supervise children when they are riding on a tricycle; keep them on the sidewalk and away from the street.

Preventing Falls
- Do not allow children to climb on furniture.
- Lock doors to dangerous areas.
- Supervise children on playground equipment.

Poisoning
- Keep all cleaning products out of reach, and use cabinet locks if kept in low cabinets.
- Keep all medications out of reach.
- Have the number for poison control easily accessible.

Preventing Choking
- Avoid giving children foods that can cause choking, such as the following:
  - Nuts
  - Hard candies
  - Hot dogs
  - Whole grapes
  - Marshmallows
- Supervise children while they are eating.
- Cut food into small bites.

Preventing Drowning
- Have a fence around backyard pools.
- Supervise children when they are around water.
- Do not leave buckets of water unattended.

Car Seats
- Children 2–4-y-old who have outgrown the height or weight limit of their rear-facing car seats may ride facing forward in a seat with a five-point harness.
- Children must remain in this type of seat until they are at least 4-y-old.

Adapted from Centers for Disease Control and Prevention. (2017). *Preschoolers (3-5 years of age)*. Retrieved from https://www.cdc.gov/ncbddd/childdevelopment/positiveparenting/preschoolers.html; Healthy Children.Org. *Safety for your child: 2 to 4 years*. Retrieved from https://www.healthychildren.org/English/ages-stages/toddler/Pages/Safety-for-Your-Child-2-to-4-Years.aspx

The nurse, Liz, greets them and says, "What brings you in today?"

"I think she has a UTI," Sandy explains. "She's been running to the potty every hour or two, was really cranky last night, and has damp panties in between using the potty."

Liz asks Ellie, who is now awake, "Does your tummy hurt?"

Ellie shakes her head no. She is being quite shy and just wants to sit on Sandy's lap and bury her head in Sandy's arms. Liz checks Ellie's temperature, listens to her heart with a stethoscope, checks the pulse at her wrist, and assesses her breathing. Liz reports her vital signs to Sandy: temperature, 101.8°F (38.7°C); heart rate, 128 beats/min (bpm); respiratory rate, 28 breaths/min.

"Has she had a fever or taken any medications for fever in the past 2 days?"

"I haven't taken her temperature," Sandy says, "But she did feel a bit warm last night when I put her to bed. I haven't given her any medications except for Bactrim, which I gave her yesterday evening before bed."

"Do you have any further concerns about Ellie's health at this time?"

Sandy shakes her head, and Liz leaves to get the doctor.

The pediatrician, Dr. Engle, comes in to see Ellie. "How is Ellie doing?" he asks Sandy.

"Not well," Sandy says. "I hope this is not another UTI. Ellie has been pretty sick in the past when she had a UTI."

Dr. Engle reviews the info the nurse obtained and begins to examine Ellie. She appears tired and closes her eyes when the doctor examines her. "Her lips and mucous membranes are moist," he reports to Liz, who enters the findings on her tablet. "Her nail beds are pink and her capillary refill is less than 2 seconds. Her apical pulse is strong, as are her radial and pedal pulses. Her lung sounds are clear bilaterally, and she does not appear to be in any respiratory distress. Her abdomen is soft." As he is pressing down on her lower abdomen, she starts to cry and says, "My pee hurts."

"I'd like to examine her genital area to check for redness and signs of drainage or infection," Dr. Engle says to Sandy. Sandy nods, and Dr. Engle, turning to Ellie, says, "No one except your mom or dad should ever touch you where your panties are. Doctors and nurses may sometimes need to look there, but your mom or dad should always be with you. Do you understand, Ellie?"

Ellie nods.

Dr. Engle examines Ellie while Sandy holds her hands, sings to her, and comforts her. "I see moderate redness at her urethral opening, but no rash or drainage. Her panties are just a bit damp, though."

"Yes," Sandy says. "I've noticed the same thing. I've been careful to wipe Ellie well each time she uses the potty, though."

"She may be having urgency and dribbling some urine," Dr. Engle says. "These are signs of a UTI" (Box 4.2).

Dr. Engle tells Liz, "I'd like a clean-catch urine specimen." Turning to Sandy, he says, "I'd like to check Ellie's urine for infection. I'm concerned she may have a UTI, despite the prophylactic antibiotic she has been taking for quite some time."

Box 4.2   Signs of Urinary Tract Infection in Young Girls

- Increased or frequent need to urinate even though only a small amount of urine may be passed
- Fever
- Abdominal pain in the area of the bladder
- Waking up at night to use the bathroom
- Stinging, burning, or pain when urinating
- Bed-wetting even when potty-trained
- Foul-smelling urine
- Cloudy and/or blood-tinged urine
- Poor appetite
- Irritability

Liz reviews with Sandy how to best collect the specimen and instructs Sandy to wash her hands before helping Ellie go potty. She hands Sandy a sterile urine specimen cup and says, "Allow Ellie to start urinating, and then place the cup in her urine stream to collect a sample midstream. When the cup is about half full or when Ellie's urine flow stops—whichever comes first—remove the cup and place the lid on the cup. The cup has already been labeled with Ellie's name and birthdate. Place the cup on the tray in the bathroom labeled 'specimens.' All clear?"

"Yes," Sandy says. She takes Ellie to the bathroom. Ellie is able to urinate and Sandy is able to collect the urine.

Liz runs a point-of-care test on Ellie's urine and reports the results as follows:

- Glucose: Negative
- Bilirubin: Negative
- Ketones: Negative
- Specific gravity: 1.023
- Blood: Small
- pH: 6
- Protein: None
- Urobilinogen: 0.4
- Nitrite: Positive
- Leukocytes: Positive

Dr. Engle returns to the exam room to talk with Sandy about the results. He shares the urine analysis results and explains that a urine test with positive nitrites and positive leukocytes is concerning for a UTI (Box 4.3). Ellie's urine will be sent to the laboratory for a culture to confirm the presence of bacteria and to determine which type of bacteria is present. If the culture comes back sensitive to a different antibiotic, Dr. Engle explains, he will change her to an antibiotic that the bacteria is most sensitive to. For now, he will prescribe trimethoprim/sulfamethoxazole (10 mg/kg/d divided every 12 hours). He explains that children treated with trimethoprim/sulfamethoxazole have shown higher cure rates than those treated with amoxicillin, which used to be the first-line antibiotic for UTIs, due to the rise in *Escherichia coli*, which is highly resistant to treatment with amoxicillin (White, 2011).

Box 4.3 Urinary Tract Infections in Young Children

- Annually, there are ~1.5 million ambulatory visits for urinary tract infections (UTIs) in children in the United States (Paintsil, 2013).
- UTIs are quite common in children.
  - By the age of 7 y, 8% of girls and 2% of boys will have had at least one UTI.
  - Moreover, 30%–50% of children will have at least one recurrence.
- Common uropathogens include: *Escherichia coli, Klebsiella, Enterobacter, Citrobacter, Staphylococcus saprophyticus*, and *Enterococcus*.
- *E. coli* (the most common bacteria found in a positive urine culture) has become increasingly resistant to treatment with antibiotics (White, 2011).

"She already takes that medicine," Sandy says (Analyze the Evidence 4.1). "Although I've not been giving Ellie her dose every night because she has been spitting it out."

"How many times a week does Ellie actually receive the dose?"

"Maybe 3 or 4 times a week."

"The dose I'm prescribing is much higher than the dose Ellie takes every night to help prevent a UTI. Ellie will need to take the medicine once in the morning and once in the evening for 7 days. If Ellie is not better within 48 hours or if she develops a high fever, vomiting, or more painful urination, call the office. Ellie is at high risk for pyelonephritis, considering her diagnosis of grade 3 vesicoureteral reflux. Pyelonephritis is a bacterial infection of the kidneys. If she develops it, she may need to be hospitalized for intravenous (IV) antibiotics or given different oral antibiotics."

"How do I get Ellie to take all this medication? She just spits it out and it becomes a big struggle," Sandy tearfully says to the doctor.

"Tell me how you currently try to give Ellie the medication."

"I tell her it is time for her medication and then she runs and hides. When I find her, I try to hold her down and squirt it in her mouth in the front. The nurse once told me I should put it in the back corner of her cheek but I do not want to make her choke. Some nights, I just don't feel like fighting with her and I give up."

"First, start with making the medication a 'must do' for Ellie. Have her sit in an upright position. Place the syringe behind the teeth or gum line or in the pocket of her cheek. Slowly trickle the medication in her mouth. If this does not work, you will need two people. One person holds Ellie on his or her lap and holds her head and hands down. The other person opens Ellie's mouth by pushing down on her chin or putting the finger inside her mouth along her gum line and opening the jaw. Then this person places the syringe on the back of the tongue, slowly dripping the medication in. It is fine to offer a reward if she takes the medication without a struggle."

"I don't understand—how could Ellie have gotten this infection?" Sandy says, trying to stay calm. "I'm so careful to wipe Ellie each time she uses the potty, from front to back, exactly the way I've been taught at previous visits, and I never allow her to soak in the bath tub or use bubble bath. I only use a fragrance-free soap for sensitive skin to wash Ellie during bath time. What more could have I done?"

"I'm sure you were doing everything possible," Dr. Engle replies. "Unfortunately, these infections can occur even when we're doing everything right. Has Ellie been constipated lately or had any episodes of diarrhea?"

Sandy, puzzled, says, "What does that have to do with a UTI?"

Analyze the Evidence 4.1 Prophylactic Antibiotics for Prevention of Urinary Tract Infections in Children With Vesicoureteral Reflux

For many years, prophylactic antibiotics have been used to prevent recurrent urinary tract infections (UTIs) and thus renal scarring and renal damage in young children, particularly with those diagnosed with vesicoureteral reflux. Children without vesicoureteral reflux also received prophylactic antibiotics if frequent UTIs were occurring on the assumption that they could help avoid recurrent UTIs and renal damage.

However, several studies have discredited this assumption. Islek et al. (2011) followed up on infants with ureteropelvic junction obstruction who were not prescribed antibiotic prophylaxis. During the 12–24 mo of follow-up, none of the 84 patients in the study had a UTI or renal scarring. Montini et al. (2008) found that children with or without nonsevere primary vesicoureteral reflux, who were followed up for 12 mo, had no difference in recurrence rates of febrile UTIs following their first episode. Prophylactic antibiotics did not reduce recurrence rates.

Therefore, the American Academy of Pediatrics currently does not recommend prophylactic antibiotics after first UTI in children aged 2–24 mo (Roberts, 2012).

"Constipation can cause a voiding dysfunction and an unstable bladder," Dr. Engle replies. "The bladder does not empty effectively when constipation is present, which can lead to bacteria growth in the retained urine."

"Ellie has been constipated in the past, but not lately."

Dr. Engle finishes answering Sandy's questions and reminds her to call the office if she feels Ellie is not getting better or if she has questions or concerns.

At the Hospital

Two days later, Ellie wakes up and vomits in her bed before Sandy can get to her room. She also has a temperature of 104.2°F (40.1°C). Sandy gives her a dose of ibuprofen, but her temperature remains at 101.8°F. Sandy phones the pediatrician's office at 8:00 a.m., when they open, and speaks with Dr. Engle. He suspects Ellie has pyelonephritis because her symptoms have worsened despite antibiotic therapy for almost 48 hours and her fever is greater than 102°F (38.9°C) (Morello, La Scola, Alberici & Montini, 2016). He instructs Sandy to bring Ellie to the hospital to be admitted.

Ellie is directly admitted to A3 North, a short-stay unit at the pediatric hospital about 30 minutes from the Raymore's home. Ellie has been admitted once before to this same unit for dehydration resulting from a gastrointestinal virus with severe vomiting and diarrhea. Upon arrival to the unit about 10:00 a.m., Ellie and her mother are greeted by the patient care assistant and the nurse, Sonya, who will be taking care of her today. Sonya walks with them to room A322.

Ellie is crying as they enter the room and tells her mom, "I want to go home!"

"I know, sweetie," Sonya says. "But I need to measure your weight. Can you help me with that?" Sonya points to a platform scale. Ellie shakes her head and keeps crying.

"Can we weigh her later," Sandy asks, "Once she's calmed down a bit?"

"I'm sorry," Sonya says, "But it really is important that we weigh her now. You see, the dosage of the medication she needs is based on her weight, and to safely and accurately administer it, we need to obtain a current weight. If you'd like, though, we can weigh you both together, while you're holding her, then weigh you separately, and find the difference."

Sandy agrees and steps onto the scale while holding Ellie. Sandy then sets Ellie down and weighs herself. The difference in the two weights is Ellie's current weight: 31.8 lb (14.5 kg).

"That sounds right," Sandy says, "because Ellie weighed 32 lb at her recent 3-year checkup." Sonya also confirms Ellie's full name and birthdate with Sandy and places an identification bracelet on her. Sonya tells Sandy it is okay to sit on the bed with Ellie since she is being very clingy and shy.

Sonya performs an initial assessment, explaining to Sandy, who is curious, that she is paying particular attention to what she calls "the priorities of care," which in this case include hydration status, pain, genitourinary assessment, and signs of

Priority Care Concepts 4.1

Monitoring a Patient With Pyelonephritis

Signs and Symptoms of Dehydration: Red Flags

- Decreased urinary output (<1 mL/kg/h for a 3-y-old)
- Dry mucous membranes
- Tachycardia
- Tachypnea
- Altered level of consciousness
- Sunken eyes
- Decreased skin turgor

Signs and Symptoms of Pain

- Inconsolable crying
- Agitation
- Refusing to urinate
- Crying when urinating
- Identifying pain in the back or flank area

Genitourinary Assessment

- Refusing to urinate
- Redness or irritation in the urethral area
- Discolored urine: cloudy or bloody
- Foul-smelling urine

Signs and Symptoms of Urosepsis

- Tachypnea
- Labored or irregular breathing
- Extreme tachycardia
- Fever > 100.4°F (38°C)
- Lethargy, difficult to arouse
- Change in mental status
- Vomiting
- Pale skin
- Urine output < 0.5 mL/kg/h

impending urosepsis (Priority Care Concepts 4.1). Sonya obtains Ellie's vital signs and reports them as follows:

- Temperature: 101.9°F (38.8°C)
- Apical pulse: 155 bpm
- Respiratory rate: 36 breaths/min
- Blood pressure: 89/48 mm Hg (taken on the right arm when Ellie is quiet, sitting on her mother's lap)
- O₂ saturation: 95% on room air

"When was the last time Ellie urinated?" Sonya asks.

"I think it was last night before bed," Sandy replies.

"I'm concerned Ellie may be dehydrated, particularly if she has had an ongoing fever," Sonya says. "About how much has Ellie had to drink since yesterday?"

How Much Does It Hurt? 4.1 FLACC Scale

The face, legs, activity, cry, consolability (FLACC) scale is a behavioral scale for measuring the intensity of pain in young children from 2 mo to 7 y old. The FLACC scale contains five indicators: face, legs, activity, cry, and consolability. Each item is ranked on a 3-point scale (0–2) for severity, with 0 representing no pain and 2 representing severe pain. A total score can range from 0 to 10.

Preschool children, like Ellie, are in the preoperational stage of cognitive development and have developed symbolic representation. However, they are not yet able to understand the concepts of greater and less and thus are not able to rate their pain on a scale. They can often tell where it hurts and when it hurts but cannot describe the severity. Therefore, preschool children do not understand when asked to rate their pain on a scale of 1–10. The FLACC scale is an ideal pain scale for this age group. A total score of 1–3 indicates mild pain, 4–6 is moderate pain, and 7–10 indicates severe pain.

	Scoring		
Categories	**0**	**1**	**2**
Face	No particular expression or smile	Occasional grimace or frown, withdrawn, uninterested	Frequent or constant frown, quivering chin, clenched jaw
Legs	Normal position or relaxed	Uneasy, restless, tense	Kicking or legs drawn up
Activity	Lying quietly, normal position, moves easily	Squirming, shifting back and forth, tense	Arched, rigid, or jerking
Cry	No crying, awake or asleep	Moans or whimpers, occasional complaint	Crying steadily, screams or sobs, frequent complaints
Consolability	Content, relaxed	Reassured by occasional hugging, touching or being talked to; distractible	Difficult to console or comfort

Adapted with permission from Merkel, S., Voepel-Lewis, T., Shayevitz, J. R., & Malviya, S. (1997). The FLACC: A behavioral scale for scoring postoperative pain in young children. *Pediatric Nursing, 23*(3), 293–297.

"She's been refusing to drink from her cup," Sandy says. "She may take a few sips at a time but has not drunk a whole cup of water or milk since yesterday morning."

"Has Ellie had any pain?"

"Yes," Sandy says. "She cries and complains of her back hurting and cries when she tries to urinate; she says it hurts." Sandy glances down at Ellie, who is sitting on her lap. "I don't think she's in pain now. She's just tired and weak."

"We'll keep Ellie as comfortable as possible and assess her frequently for pain, using this tool called the FLACC scale.

Please let me or the other nursing staff know if you think Ellie is in pain" (How Much Does It Hurt? 4.1).

Sonya orients Sandy and Ellie to the room and to the unit and explains the admission orders and plan of care for Ellie (Box 4.4). She says that Ellie will be receiving IV fluids to help rehydrate her and make sure she does not become further dehydrated. A urine sample will be sent for an analysis and culture, and blood will be drawn to determine whether Ellie's UTI has spread to her bloodstream. Also, antibiotics will be given via an IV line to help fight the infection.

Box 4.4 Admission Orders for Ellie Raymore

1. Start a peripheral intravenous (IV) line.
2. Dosing weight: 14.5 kg
3. Normal saline (NS; 0.9%) bolus of 290 mL IV over 1 h
4. Maintenance IV fluids: NS infused at 74 mL/h for 24 h
5. Obtain a clean-catch urine sample for urinalysis and culture.
6. Obtain blood for the following laboratory tests: basic metabolic panel, complete blood count, and peripheral blood cultures.
7. Diet: regular toddler diet
8. Take vital signs every 4 h: heart rate, respiratory rate, temperature, and blood pressure.
9. Ceftriaxone (Rocephin) 725 mg IV every 24 h, to start immediately after urinalysis/urine culture and blood cultures are obtained
10. Encourage the patient to drink fluids.
11. Out of bed as tolerated
12. Daily weight
13. Strict intake and output
14. Call the provider if urine output is <1 mL/kg/h.
15. Acetaminophen 477 mg by mouth every 6 h as needed for temperature >100.5°F (38°C) or mild-to-moderate pain
16. Ibuprofen 145 mg by mouth every 8 h for severe pain

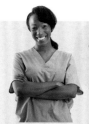

The Nurse's Point of View

Sonya: I call the phlebotomy team (also known as the vascular access team, at this hospital) to come and start an IV on Ellie and obtain blood cultures and the ordered laboratory tests. A child life specialist comes with the team to help with distraction and comfort during the IV start procedure. The team is successful in starting an IV line on the second attempt, and enough blood is obtained for the blood cultures and ordered laboratory tests. I start the normal saline bolus over 1 hour after checking to make sure the ordered volume is appropriate for Ellie's weight. I calculate the bolus to be 20 mL/kg, which I recall is an appropriate bolus when there is concern for a fluid deficit. I double-check the IV fluid rate to make sure it is appropriate for Ellie's weight. I realize that it is higher than it should be and contact the physician to clarify the order. (See Table 4.1 for a review of how to calculate maintenance fluids for pediatric patients.) The physician states he would like to infuse Ellie's IV fluids at a rate one-and-a-half times that of maintenance to keep her hydrated and help flush out the kidneys. Once the normal saline bolus is finished infusing, I will start the maintenance intravenous fluids (MIVF) at the ordered rate.

Table 4.1 Maintenance Fluid Intravenous Infusion Rate Calculation

Body Weight	Daily Infusion Rate (mL/kg/d)	Hourly Infusion Rate (mL/kg/h)
First 10 kg	100	~4
Second 10 kg	50	~2
Each additional kg	20	~1

Reprinted with permission from Kahl, L. K., & Hughes, H. K. (2018). *The Harriet lane handbook* (21st ed.). Philadelphia, PA: Elsevier.

Sonya returns to the room and says, "I have an order for a urinalysis and culture, so I'll need to collect a urine specimen from Ellie."

"But they just collected urine at the pediatrician's office 2 days ago," Sandy says. "Why do you need another sample?"

"The physician is concerned that the bacteria in Ellie's urine may be different from what was in the previous sample or may be resistant to the antibiotic Ellie was prescribed."

"Okay," Sandy says. "I can do it. I learned how at the pediatrician's office. I wipe Ellie first, then allow her to start urinating, and then, in the middle of her urine stream, put the specimen cup under her to collect urine, right?"

"You got it," Sonya says, handing Sandy the cup. "Let me know if you need any assistance."

Just then, Ellie starts crying and says, "My sides hurt!"

Sonya watches Ellie for a minute and says, "I'd call that a FLACC score of 4. That means I can give her a dose of acetaminophen."

"Yes, please do," Sandy says. "Anything that will help relieve her pain."

"Does Ellie normally take medication from a cup or a syringe at home? I've found that following home routines and practices makes taking medications much easier, especially for kids."

"She likes to take it from a cup," Sandy says.

"Great," Sonya says. "I'll be back in a minute." She disappears. A moment later, she returns and says, "I'm sorry—I forgot to ask whether Ellie has had acetaminophen or any other medications within the last 4 hours?"

"Let's see," Sandy says. "I last gave Ellie acetaminophen 6 or 7 hours ago."

Sonya soon returns with the medicine and says to Sandy, "You're welcome to give her the medicine, yourself, if you would like."

Ellie looks at Sandy and says, "Only my mom can give me medicine."

"Okay," Sonya says. "Let me just check the medication order against the label on the medication again to make sure we're giving her the right dose, by the right route, and for the right reason. Everything looks good. Now, I just need to check your armband, Miss Ellie, to make sure you are the right patient. Yes, you are. Okay, mom—here you go." She hands Sandy the medicine and Ellie takes it like a champ for her mom.

"Why is Ellie having pain with this infection?" Sandy asks. "And what exactly is pyelonephritis?"

Sonya explains that pyelonephritis is an infection of the kidneys where inflammation is present (Fig. 4.2). The pain can be from the inflammation as well as from the spasms. When a person has repeated episodes of pyelonephritis, scarring of the kidney and atrophy of the renal cortex can occur leading to long-term kidney damage.

About an hour after the normal saline bolus was finished and the IV fluids were started, Ellie is able to urinate. Sandy is successful in getting a clean-catch specimen when Ellie uses the bathroom. When Sonya comes in to get the specimen, she assesses what is in the cup for color, clarity, and odor, she explains. She says that Ellie's urine is dark amber and very cloudy and that some white casts are at the bottom of the cup. When she takes the lid off the cup, she says she notices a foul smell. Sandy sees Sonya enter her assessment of the urine

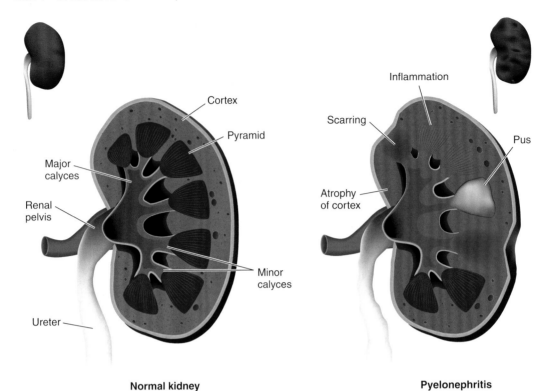

Normal kidney

Pyelonephritis

Figure 4.2. Changes in the kidney due to pyelonephritis. Changes in the kidney when pyelonephritis occurs include the following: inflammation, scarring, accumulation of pus (white cells), and atrophy of the renal cortex.

into Ellie's chart on her tablet, checking to make sure the specimen container is labeled with the correct patient label. She says she will send the specimen to the laboratory. Sonya also explains that she is documenting the 30 mL in the cup and 20 mL in the hat that she placed in the toilet so Ellie's output could be measured.

"I'm ready to start the first dose of ceftriaxone now," Sonya says to Sandy (The Pharmacy 4.1). She explains that it is an antibiotic and how the care team will determine whether it is working.

"Does Ellie have any allergies to medications? Whenever I give a medication, I like to ask about any medication allergies."

"No," Sandy says. "Ellie's not allergic to any medicine that I know of."

Sonya explains that nurses will monitor Ellie's temperature, heart rate, and blood pressure, assess her urine each time she urinates, monitor her pain level and frequency of pain episodes, and assess her intake and output. Ellie falls asleep while Sonya is hanging the antibiotic.

The Pharmacy 4.1 | **Antibiotics Used to Treat Urinary Tract Infections and Pyelonephritis in Children**

Medication	Classification	Route	Action	Nursing Considerations
Ceftriaxone (Rocephin)	Third-generation cephalosporin	• IM • IV	Inhibits bacterial cell wall synthesis	• May cause diarrhea • Monitor renal function
Cephalexin (Keflex)	First-generation cephalosporin	• PO	Inhibits bacterial cell wall synthesis	• May cause nausea, vomiting, or diarrhea
Sulfamethoxazole and trimethoprim (Bactrim)	Sulfonamide derivative	• PO • IV	• Kills bacteria • Inhibits sequential enzymes of the folic acid synthesis pathway	• Do not give if the patient has an allergy to sulfa • May cause nausea, vomiting, diarrhea, or loss of appetite • May be taken with or without food

IM, intramuscular; IV, intravenous; PO, oral.
Adapted from Taketomo, C. K., Hodding, J. H., & Kraus, D. M. (2018). Pediatric & neonatal dosage handbook (25th ed.). Hudson, OH: Lexicomp.

The Nurse's Point of View

Sonya: Evening has come, and it's near the end of my shift. I walk into Ellie Raymore's room and find both Sandy and Ellie sound asleep. There's a knock on the half-open door, and Kevin, the oncoming nurse, peers in. I step out into the hall with him and shut the door behind me. We greet each other, and I begin to give him my handoff report.

"The laboratory called several hours ago to report that Ellie's urine was positive for leukocytes and nitrites," I mention during the report. "I phoned the results to the nurse practitioner caring for her. She's been asleep now for over 5 hours."

Kevin nods and jots down some notes. "I'll be sure to assess her neurological status," he says.

"I think she's most likely tired from having a fever and being dehydrated when she arrived at the hospital. She was up at home last night with vomiting and a fever."

At the end of report, Kevin and I go in Ellie's room together to check the infusing IV fluids and the IV site and do a quick assessment of Ellie. Ellie is sleeping but easily arousable and asks for her cup of water. Sandy wakes up and helps Ellie get a drink and use the bathroom.

Throughout the night, the new nurse, Kevin, checks on Ellie every hour. At 11:30, he comes in and takes her temperature.

"What is it now?" Sandy says.

"It's up to a 103°F (39.4°C)," he tells her. He gives Ellie acetaminophen. "Has she urinated recently?" Kevin asks her.

"No," Sandy says. "Not in a while. Is that bad?"

"Since being admitted this morning, it looks like she has voided only 180 mL of urine," Kevin says. "I'm concerned that she may be dehydrated." He explains that Ellie has voided less than 1 mL/kg of body weight since admission. "I'll call the nurse practitioner who is covering the unit tonight and let her know."

The nurse practitioner arrives and assesses Ellie and looks at her heart rate trend and her urine output totals. She orders a normal saline bolus (0.9%) 290 mL IV over 1 hour. The nurse practitioner also asks Kevin to call if Ellie does not urinate within 2 hours of the bolus. Kevin starts the bolus.

About an hour after the normal saline bolus is finished, Kevin arrives to check on Ellie.

Ellie wakes up and says, "Mommy—I need to go potty." After she's done, Kevin inspects her urine.

"How is it?" Sandy says.

"Not as dark as before," he says, "which is a good sign." It's now yellow but is still a bit cloudy. Sandy puts her back in bed. "Could you drink some water for me, Ellie?" Kevin says. Ellie takes the cup from him and sips about 3 oz of water through the straw.

The rest of the night goes well. Ellie sleeps until almost 6:00 in the morning, when she wakes up to go potty. She is also crying and holding her sides. Kevin watches for a minute and reports her pain level as a 5 on the FLACC (face, legs, activity, cry, and consolability) scale. He checks the medication administration record to see when the last time Ellie had acetaminophen and says she can have another dose. He gives her a dose. Ellie falls back to sleep about 40 minutes after taking the medication.

On the second day of hospitalization, Ellie is starting to show improvement. Her urine output is now 2 to 3 mL/kg/h over the course of the day, and she has only had one fever, which was at noon. Her temperature was 101.8°F, for which she received a dose of acetaminophen. She did receive a dose of ibuprofen for severe pain about 9:30 a.m., but her FLACC score has been 0 to 1 the rest of the day. Ellie is also starting to drink more, but does not have much of an appetite. The physician has decreased her MIVF to 49 mL/h. Just as important, the laboratory results came back for the urine culture. Ellie's urine is positive for *E. coli*. Kevin explains that *E. coli* is the most common bacteria causing pyelonephritis, with a prevalence of about 80% to 90% (Morello et al., 2016).

On day 3 of her hospitalization, Ellie starts to feel better and the whole unit knows about it. Ellie is asking for puzzles to play with and wants to go outside. Sandy is happy to see Ellie feeling better. On morning rounds, the care team reviews the discharge goals for Ellie with Sandy and everyone agrees she is making progress. The first goal has been met, which is to achieve an adequate urine output for her weight and age. However, this is with MIVF infusing. The bedside nurse asks whether the MIVF can be stopped, because Ellie seems to be drinking enough fluids. The team agrees to stop the fluids and monitor her closely. The second goal, which is that her urine is free of bacteria, needs to be followed up with. Although the nurse reports that Ellie's urine looks clear yellow, a follow-up urinalysis and culture needs to be sent today. The nurse will ensure a urine sample is sent. The third goal, which is that Ellie is without fever for 24 hours, has almost been achieved. Ellie's temperature will be monitored closely today. And the final goal, that Ellie is drinking adequately and eating without nausea or vomiting, is progressing, as well.

At Discharge

Ellie has been fever-free for almost 2 days now. She is eating and drinking almost like she was before getting sick. Sandy tells Eric that Ellie "is back to her spunky self." On morning rounds, the nurse practitioner reports that Ellie is feeling better and has met all of her discharge criteria. The urine culture from

Box 4.5   Nursing Tasks Before Ellie's Discharge

- Provide teaching to Sandy regarding antibiotic therapy, prevention of urinary tract infections, and follow-up testing.
- Check Ellie's discharge orders.
- Ensure that prescriptions have been sent to the pharmacy the Raymores use.
- Remove Ellie's intravenous line.
- Ensure that follow-up appointments are listed on the discharge papers.

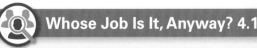

Whose Job Is It, Anyway? 4.1

Child Life Specialist

Child life specialists are trained to help children of all ages cope with the stressors of hospitalization, chronic illness, and grief. While children are in the hospital, child life specialists provide them with developmentally appropriate interventions through therapeutic play and distraction techniques to help children cope with hospitalization, prepare them for procedures, and help them deal with interventions that may provoke anxiety or fear. They provide education related to coping with pain, as well as dealing with fear and anxiety.

Adapted from Association of Child Life Professionals. (2017). *What is a certified child life specialist?* Retrieved from https://www.childlife .org/the-child-life-profession

yesterday came back negative. The team agrees that Ellie can go home today but will need to continue antibiotic therapy at home. The nurse practitioner will write a prescription for oral cephalexin as part of the discharge instructions.

Ellie's nurse, Kelly, tells Sandy she will have the paperwork ready within the hour and that it is okay for Ellie to get dressed in her own clothes so she can go home soon (Box 4.5). Ellie is eager to dress herself with the new clothes her dad brought yesterday in preparation for going home today.

Kelly and another woman arrive later with some papers and supplies. "Hi, Ellie!" Kelly says. "Are you ready to go home?"

"Yes!" Ellie shouts.

"Great, because we're here to help you get ready to go," Kelly says. "This is Anna, our child life specialist on the unit" (Whose Job Is It, Anyway? 4.1). While Anna is chatting with Ellie, Kelly turns and says to Sandy in a lowered voice, "First, I need to take out the IV."

Ellie overhears this and says, "I don't want it to hurt!"

Anna says, "Look, Ellie! I've brought some things for us to play with. Do you like to blow bubbles?" Ellie nods her head and squeals with delight. While they blow bubbles, Kelly comes to eye level with Ellie and is able to remove the tape and the IV without Ellie crying. When she's done, though, Ellie yells, "Go away now!" While Anna continues to play with Ellie, Kelly gives Sandy the discharge instructions.

Kelly reviews how to lessen the risk and possibly prevent a UTI in the future, beginning with reminders about hand washing. She also talks to Sandy about the importance of making sure Ellie does not become constipated, because this can contribute to the risk of UTIs.

"Yes," Sandy says, "We've had to deal with constipation before, so I know what to do to prevent it."

"What do you usually do?"

"We feed her a lot of fruits and high-fiber veggies and give her plenty of water throughout the day," Sandy says. "And if she doesn't have a bowel movement at least every other day, we give her prune juice. Occasionally we have to use polyethylene glycol, which our pediatrician recommends."

"Perfect," Kelly says. "You sound like a pro. You also probably already know to wipe Ellie from the front to the back after she uses the potty."

"Absolutely," Sandy says. "I've trained Ellie to do it, too."

"Great," Kelly says. "I also recommend that you encourage Ellie to use the bathroom every 2 to 4 hours throughout the day."

Kelly discusses the antibiotic regimen with Sandy and reviews the dosage, frequency, and importance of finishing the entire prescribed course of cephalexin to help ensure the infection is gone and to help prevent antibiotic resistance. Ellie will need to take the antibiotic for 14 days. Sandy nods her head in understanding. Kelly also reviews with Sandy the signs of a UTI and what signs and symptoms should prompt a visit to the pediatrician. When all the education is complete, Ellie is discharged from the hospital.

Think Critically

1. Why does vesicoureteral reflux make some children more susceptible to a urinary tract infection?
2. What suggestions can be given to Sandy to ensure that Ellie takes every dose of her medication and does not spit it out?
3. What should Sonya's priorities of care be in her initial assessment of Ellie on admission to the hospital?
4. What types of age-appropriate diversional activities can the nurse provide while Ellie is hospitalized?
5. Ellie has an intravenous (IV) line while hospitalized. Explain two ways the nurse can help reduce the risk of Ellie removing the IV.

References

American Academy of Pediatrics. (2017). *Developmental milestones: 3 to 4 year olds*. Retrieved from https://www.healthychildren.org/English/ages-stages/toddler/Pages/Developmental-Milestones-3-to-4-Years-Old.aspx

Centers for Disease Control and Prevention. (2017). *Preschoolers (3-5 years of age)*. Retrieved from https://www.cdc.gov/ncbddd/childdevelopment/positiveparenting/preschoolers.html

Foxman, B. (2014). Urinary tract infection syndromes: Occurrence, recurrence, bacteriology, risk factors, and disease burden. *Infectious Disease Clinics of North America, 28*(1), 1–13.

Islek, A., Güven, A. G., Koyun, M., Akman, S., & Alimoglu, E. (2011). Probability of urinary tract infection in infants with ureteropelvic junction obstruction: Is antibacterial prophylaxis really needed? *Pediatric Nephrology, 26*(10), 1837.

Montini, G., Rigon, L., Zucchetta, P., Fregonese, F., Toffolo, A., Gobber, D., & ... Zanchetta, S. (2008). Prophylaxis after first febrile urinary tract infection in children? A multicenter, randomized, controlled, noninferiority trial. *Pediatrics, 122*(5), 1064–1071.

Morello, W., La Scola, C., Alberici, I., & Montini, G. (2016). Acute pyelonephritis in children. *Pediatric Nephrology, 31*(8), 1253–1265.

National Institute of Diabetes and Digestive and Kidney Disorders. (2017). *Vesicoureteral reflux*. Retrieved from https://www.niddk.nih.gov/health-information/urologic-diseases/urine-blockage-newborns/vesicoureteral-reflux

Paintsil, E. (2013). Update on recent guidelines for the management of urinary tract infections in children: The shifting paradigm. *Current Opinion in Pediatrics, 25*(1), 88–94.

Roberts, K. (2012, November). Revised AAP guideline on UTI in febrile infants and young children. *American Family Physician, 86*(10), 940–946.

White, B. (2011). Diagnosis and treatment of urinary tract infections in children. *American Family Physician, 83*(4), 409–415.

Suggested Readings

American Academy of Pediatrics. (2017). *Preschool time*. Retrieved from https://www.aap.org/en-us/advocacy-and-policy/aap-health-initiatives/HALF-Implementation-Guide/Age-Specific-Content/Pages/Preschool-Timeline.aspx

National Institute of Diabetes and Digestive and Kidney Disorders. (2017). *Vesicoureteral reflux*. Retrieved from https://www.niddk.nih.gov/health-information/urologic-diseases/urine-blockage-newborns/vesicoureteral-reflux

Paintsil, E. (2013). Update on recent guidelines for the management of urinary tract infections in children: The shifting paradigm. *Current Opinion in Pediatrics, 25*(1), 88–94.

5 Maalik Abdella: Gastroenteritis, Fever, and Dehydration

Maalik Abdella, age 2 years

Objectives

After completing this chapter, you will be able to:
1. Describe normal growth and development of the 2-year-old.
2. Discuss an appropriate teaching plan for a healthy 2-year-old.
3. Compare the fluid distribution of infants and children with that of adults.
4. Identify signs and symptoms of dehydration in infants and young children.
5. Explain how to manage a fever and when a fever would not be treated.
6. Explain the use of oral rehydration therapy in the treatment of dehydration.
7. Recognize the signs and symptoms of hypovolemic shock.
8. Discuss aspects of culture to consider when providing health care to a Muslim patient.
9. Create a nursing plan of care for a toddler with severe dehydration.

Key Terms

Emesis
Hijab
Isotonic fluids

Lethargic
Parallel play
Regression

Background

Maalik Abdella is a healthy 2-year-old boy whose family immigrated from Mosul, Iraq, 3 years ago. Maalik's father, Kasim, brought his family to the United States when his city was in danger of attack. He wanted to seek a better and safer life for his family. At the time that Kasim and his wife, Farrah, left Iraq, they had a 4-year-old daughter, Sabeen. Sabeen is now 7 years old and, having grown up in the American culture, has assimilated well. On the other hand, neither Kasim nor Farrah spoke any English at the time they arrived in the United States. Their native language is Arabic, and they had a difficult time when they first arrived in the country.

The family moved to an area in which there is a large group of Muslim families who all practice the Islamic faith. This was comforting to both Kasim and Farrah initially because they had no family around to help them. In the Muslim culture, extended family is an important part of a child's life because of the belief that children are better off when they learn about life from more adults than just their parents (Hickey, 2013). The community to which they moved helped fill the role of the extended family that Kasim and Farrah had left behind in Iraq. In addition, the Abdellas joined the local mosque and were able to continue to practice their Islamic faith.

Within a few months of moving to their new community, Kasim began to work at the local butcher shop. The butcher shop is halal, meaning that it is one in which all meat is butchered according to Islamic principles and, practicing the food restrictions of Islam, no pork is sold (Johnson, 2019). About the time that Kasim began to work at the butcher shop, Farrah discovered that she was pregnant with her second child. Maalik was born without any complications, and the Abdella family began to acclimate to their new home and community.

Although the Abdella family has been living in the United States for 3 years, they continue to practice traditional customs of the Muslim culture and Islamic faith. Farrah wears a **hijab** when in public or when in the presence of other males. Both Kasim and Farrah play a role in deciding who their older daughter Sabeen's friends are. They wish her to have friends who are of the same faith as their family so as not to expose her to the excesses of American culture. In the Muslim culture, respect for others, delayed gratification, and self-discipline are of utmost importance (Hickey, 2013; Inhorn & Serour, 2011).

Both Kasim and Farrah have learned some English, although they still have difficulty with the language at times. Sabeen speaks Arabic at home but has learned to speak English through school and is able to help her parents when they struggle to find the correct wording. Maalik is learning to speak and is learning Arabic and English at the same time. His language skills are really starting to take off, and Farrah often hears him trying to say what his sister Sabeen says and sees him try to copy what Sabeen is doing, such as coloring pictures (Growth and Development Check 5.1).

Growth and Development Check 5.1

Two-Year-Old Milestones

Social/Emotional

- Likes to be around other children
- Tries to imitate both children and adults
- Engages in **parallel play**
- May have temper tantrums

Speech

- Speaks in two- to four-word sentences
- Is able to point to objects in a book
- Is able to point to body parts
- Follows simple instructions

Cognitive

- Identifies shapes and colors
- Builds a tower of at least four blocks
- Begins to show hand preference
- Can name items in a picture book

Gross Motor/Fine Motor

- Throws a ball overhand
- Stands on tiptoes
- Climbs on and off things
- Kicks a ball
- Starts to run

Adapted from the Centers for Disease Control and Prevention. (2016). *Learn the signs. Act early.* Retrieved from https://www.cdc .gov/ncbddd/actearly/milestones/milestones-3yr.html

Patient Teaching 5.1

Temper Tantrums

Temper tantrums occur as part of a normal stage of emotional development. Tantrums can begin as early as 12 mo of age but are typically seen between the ages of 2 and 3. Temper tantrums often occur when the child is frustrated and unable to verbalize what he or she wants. However, a toddler may also throw a temper tantrum as a way to get attention. Normal temper tantrums in toddlers consist of behaviors such as the following:

- Kicking and screaming
- Flailing of the arms
- Crying
- Throwing themselves on the floor

Dealing with temper tantrums can be frustrating. It is important for parents to understand that this is a normal developmental behavior. When a child is throwing a tantrum, parents should ignore the behavior as long as the child is safe. If the child is at risk of danger, the parent should hold the child tightly. If a child throws a tantrum in a public place, the parents may try to distract the child but may ultimately need to leave rather than giving in to the child.

The most important part of discipline with temper tantrums is to reward good behavior and ignore unwanted behavior. One exception to the rule is that biting and hitting should never be ignored and should be disciplined with a time out. Finally, make sure that parents understand their child's limits. Keeping a child out too long and missing a meal or a nap is the perfect setup for a tantrum.

Adapted from Daniels, Mandleco, and Luthy (2012); Swanson, W. S. (2018). *Top tips for surviving temper tantrums.* Retrieved from https://www.healthychildren.org/English/family-life/family-dynamics/ communication-discipline/pages/Temper-Tantrums.aspx.

Although Maalik is learning to speak well, he still throws temper tantrums (Patient Teaching 5.1). At times, when he doesn't get what he wants, he throws himself on the floor and cries for several minutes at a time. Farrah does not remember Sabeen throwing tantrums on a regular basis, but it seems as if Maalik is having a temper tantrum every day. It is getting very frustrating for the family, but luckily Maalik is not acting out in public places. Farrah remembers that Maalik has a checkup scheduled in a couple of days. She will ask the pediatrician how to help Maalik stop having temper tantrums.

Health Promotion

Farrah brings Maalik to the pediatrician's office for his 2-year-old checkup. She tells the nurse that she really has no concerns at this time other than the daily temper tantrums. The nurse reports that today Maalik's weight is 26 lb (11.8 kg), and he is 2.8 ft (34 in) tall (Growth and Development Check 5.2). The nurse plots his weight and height on the growth chart and calculates his body mass index (BMI). The nurse explains to Farrah

Growth and Development Check 5.2

Physical Growth

During the toddler years, physical growth is not as rapid as it was during infancy. Typically, the toddler gains 3–5 lb (1.36–2.27 kg) per year and grows about 3 in (7.62 cm) per year. A toddler will reach half of his or her adult height by 2 y old.

Adapted from American Academy of Pediatrics. (2015). *Physical appearance and growth: Your 2 year old.* Retrieved from https://www.healthychildren.org/English/ages-stages/toddler/Pages/Physical-Appearance-and-Growth-Your-2-Year-Od.aspx

that Maalik's weight is in the 25th percentile and his height is just above the 50th percentile. His BMI is 15.8, which is in the 27th percentile. These measurements indicate that Maalik is of a healthy weight, she says, adding that a healthy weight range for BMI is from the 5th percentile to the 85th percentile (Hughes & Kahl, 2018).

After Maalik is weighed, Dr. Peterman enters the room and greets them.

"Maalik's weight and BMI are healthy," Dr. Peterman says. "How is his walking?"

"Good," Farrah tells Dr. Peterman. "He can walk on his own. He is walking up and down the stairs on his own but still needs to hold on to the rail."

"That's good," Dr. Peterman says. "Holding on to the rail is fine at this age; there is no need to worry. Can he hold crayons, use them, and stack three or four blocks? Is he learning his colors?"

"Yes," Farrah says. "He is doing all of these things." Dr. Peterman charts that Maalik is meeting gross motor, fine motor, and cognitive milestones.

"How is his speaking?" Dr. Peterman asks.

"Good," Farrah says. "He is learning both English and Arabic. Kasim and I are learning English, but we speak Arabic at home. Maalik is speaking in short sentences in both languages and copies what his sister says and does. But he gets upset, falls down, and kicks and screams."

"Ah," Dr. Peterman says. "You mean he throws a temper tantrum?"

"Yes," Farrah says. "What should I do?"

"Temper tantrums are a normal part of development," he says. "Just make sure he is safe and then try to ignore the behavior. When Maalik realizes that you will not respond to the tantrum, he will stop."

Dr. Peterman makes some notes in Maalik's chart.

"Maalik does not need any immunizations at this checkup," Dr. Peterman says. "I would like to talk about nutrition, though. It's really important to limit the amount of sugary drinks and foods Maalik consumes in a day. Try to encourage him to eat and drink nutritious, high-quality foods and drinks, and don't worry as much about how much he

eats. Toddlers are picky eaters, and it's easy to worry that they are not getting enough to eat. However, they tend to eat the amount that they need. Maalik should be eating what the rest of the family eats, and you should offer healthy foods and not make separate meals for him. Also, at this time, Maalik can switch from whole milk to what the rest of the family drinks. He no longer needs the fat in the milk for brain development."

"I'd also like to talk with you about screen time," Dr. Peterman says. "Does Maalik watch television or spend time on a computer?"

"Yes," Farrah says. "He watches television some in the afternoon with his sister, Sabeen, when she gets home from school. He also plays games on a tablet often."

Dr. Peterman nods and says, "Children have a lot of access to devices now. It's important, though, to limit their screen time. The American Academy of Pediatrics recommends 1 hour of quality digital media per day and that parents watch the programming with their children" (Chassiakos, Radesky, Christakis, Moreno, & Cross, 2016). "Digital media can also interfere with a child's sleep patterns. Sleep is important for children, even toddlers. The recommended amount of sleep for a 2-year-old is 12 to 14 hours per day" (American Academy of Pediatrics [AAP], 2017). "Lack of adequate sleep can contribute to both obesity and behavioral problems" (Bathory & Tomopoulos, 2017).

Dr. Peterman ends the visit with safety tips for Farrah (Patient Teaching 5.2). "The most common cause of death in children from 2 to 4 years old is preventable injury, including burns, falls, poisoning, choking, drowning, and improper car seat use," he warns (AAP, 2015).

At Home

It is the beginning of summer vacation. Sabeen recently finished the school year with straight A's, so Farrah and Kasim decide to take their family to the community carnival. At the carnival, Maalik enjoys riding the smaller rides with his sister. In fact, he rides them over and over. Because it is the first warm weekend of summer vacation, the carnival is extremely crowded. After a few hours at the carnival, Farrah worries that, with so many people around, her children are being exposed to too many germs and decides it is time to go home.

Unfortunately, Farrah is correct. The next morning, Maalik wakes up with a fever of 101.3°F (38.5°C). Shortly after waking, he begins vomiting and has profuse watery diarrhea. Farrah knows that she needs to keep him hydrated. She wants to avoid giving him any medication if possible but is unsure whether she needs to give Maalik something to reduce his fever (Patient Teaching 5.3).

Three hours later, Maalik continues with vomiting episodes and diarrhea. He is unable to hold any liquids down. Farrah has not given him any medication, and his fever has gone up to 102.4°F (39.1°C). Maalik does not seem irritable; however, in fact, he seems more quiet than usual. This concerns Farrah, and she decides to call the pediatrician's office.

Patient Teaching 5.2

Safety

Preventing Burns
- Use the back burners when cooking on the stove.
- Keep the hot water heater no higher than 120°F (48.9°C).
- Keep toddlers away from hot objects such as grills, ovens, and irons.

Preventing Falls
- Do not allow children to climb on furniture.
- Supervise children when they are going up and down stairs.
- Supervise children when they are on playground equipment.
- Use gates at the top and bottom of stairs.

Preventing Poisoning
- Keep all cleaning products out of reach, and use cabinet locks if kept in low cabinets.
- Keep all medications out of reach.
- Have the number for poison control easily accessible.

Preventing Choking
- Avoid giving children foods that can cause choking, such as the following:
  - Nuts
  - Hard candies
  - Hot dogs
  - Whole grapes
  - Marshmallows
- Supervise children while they are eating.
- Cut food into small bites.

Preventing Drowning
- Have a fence around backyard pools.
- Supervise children when they are around water.
- Have locks on toilet seat lids.
- Do not leave buckets of water unattended.

Car Seats
- Children 2–4 y old who have outgrown the height or weight limit of their rear-facing car seats may ride facing forward in a seat with a five-point harness.
- Children must use this type of seat until they are at least 4 y old.

Adapted from American Academy of Pediatrics, Committee on Injury, Violence, and Poison Prevention. (2011). Policy statement—Child passenger safety. *AAP News*, 127, 4. doi:10.1542/peds.2011-0213. Retrieved from www.pediatrics.org/cgi/doi/10.1542/peds.2011-0213doi:10.1542/peds.2011-0213 and American Academy of Pediatrics. (2015). *Safety for your child: 2 to 4 years*. Retrieved from https://www.healthychildren.org/English/ages-stages/toddler/Pages/Safety-for-Your-Child-2-to-4-Years.aspx.

Call to the Pediatrician

Farrah calls the pediatrician's office and talks with the nurse, Amy. "My family was at the carnival yesterday," she explains. "And Maalik woke up sick this morning. He has vomited 4 times and had watery diarrhea 5 times since he woke 3 hours ago." Farrah continues,

Patient Teaching 5.3

Fever

- Fever is a way for the body to fight infection.
- Not every fever needs to be treated. If your child is eating and drinking, try to avoid giving antipyretics.
- If treating a fever with antipyretics, be sure you are giving the correct dose.
- Fever causes children to lose fluids at a rate higher than normal, increasing the risk for dehydration.
- Call your healthcare provider if any of the following occurs:
  - Your child is not eating or drinking
  - Your child is extremely fussy and irritable
  - Your child is lethargic or less responsive than usual
  - Your child seems to be getting worse
  - For children over 2 y old, the fever lasts >3 d.

Adapted from American Academy of Pediatrics. (2016). *Fever without fear: Information for parents*. Retrieved from https://www.healthychildren.org/English/health-issues/conditions/fever/Pages/Fever-Without-Fear.aspx

telling the nurse that Maalik's temperature is 102.4°F, he is unable to hold any food or liquids down, and he seems very tired. "I am afraid he will have a seizure because of his fever," she tells Amy.

"Has Maalik ever had a seizure related to fever before, or febrile seizure?" Amy asks.

"No," Farrah says.

"A febrile seizure usually only occurs when a child's temperature rises rapidly, so it is unlikely that Maalik is at risk," Amy explains. "Have you given Maalik any medicine to reduce his fever?"

"No," Farrah responds.

"Bringing his fever down may help Maalik become less **lethargic**, which may help with the eating and drinking," Amy says. "You may use either acetaminophen or ibuprofen, but I would advise you to use acetaminophen, because Maalik is at risk for dehydration" (The Pharmacy 5.1). After discussing the treatment for Maalik's fever, Amy begins to discuss treatment for the vomiting and diarrhea.

Oral Rehydration Therapy

"Maalik most likely has gastroenteritis," Amy tells Farrah over the phone. "That means he has an infection in his stomach and intestines. The most important thing to do is to give Maalik plenty of fluids and nutrition. You said that he seems very tired?"

"Yes," Farrah says.

"Does he respond to you when you talk to him?" Amy asks. "Does he seem awake?"

"Yes," Farrah says. "He is awake. He looks at me when I say his name. But he is not moving much."

"Does Maalik have any tears in his eyes?" Amy asks. "Does his mouth seem wet or dry?"

"He is not crying, so I don't know about the tears," Farrah says. "But his mouth seems sticky."

The Pharmacy 5.1   Analgesics

Medication	Classification	Route	Action	Nursing Considerations
Acetaminophen	• Analgesic • Antipyretic	• PO • Rectal • IM • IV	• Analgesic: inhibits CNS prosta-glandin synthesis and peripher-ally inhibits pain impulses • Antipyretic: inhibits the heat-regulating center of the hypothalamus	• Dosing: 10–15 mg/kg every 4–6 h • Do not exceed 4,000 mg/d • Metabolized by the liver • Can be hepatotoxic • Monitor LFT, ALT, and AST with long-term use • Monitor for s/s of liver toxicity
Ibuprofen	• Analgesic • Antipyretic • Anti-inflammatory	• PO • IM • IV	• Inhibits COX 1 and 2 • Decreases prostaglandin precursors	• Dosing is 5–10 mg/kg every 6–8 h • Do not exceed 1,200 mg/d unless directed by healthcare provider • Excreted by the kidneys • Can be nephrotoxic • Monitor intake and output • Monitor BUN and creatinine with long-term use • Do not give to infants under 6 mo of age due to immature renal system • Monitor for s/s of GI irritation and bleeding • Monitor for s/s of increased bruising/bleeding due to decreased platelet adhesion

ALT, alanine aminotransferase; AST, aspartate transaminase; CNS, central nervous system; COX, cyclooxygenase; GI, gastrointestinal; IM, intramuscular; IV, intravenous; LFT, liver function tests; PO, oral; s/s, signs and symptoms.
Adapted from Taketomo, C. K. (2018). *Pediatric & neonatal dosage handbook* (25th ed.). Hudson, OH: Lexicomp.

"I think Maalik is moderately dehydrated," Amy says. "You need to give him plenty of fluids to drink. We call this oral rehydration therapy, or ORT" (Analyze the Evidence 5.1). You can do this at home as long as he improves over the next 2 to 3 hours. If he does not improve or if he gets worse, you must take Maalik to the hospital. "If he feels like eating, you may feed him whatever you'd like; there are no restrictions on his diet" (Churgay & Aftab, 2012). "Maalik does not need to have any

laboratory work done at this time because ORT is his mainstay of treatment" (Box 5.1; Carson & Mudd, 2016).

"I recommend that you buy him a special drink at the store called an oral rehydration solution, or ORS, such as Pedialyte," Amy says. "Watch Maalik carefully to see if he is getting better or worse. Do you have an oral medicine syringe at home to measure the amount of fluid to give to Maalik?"

"No," Farrah says. "I don't think so."

Analyze the Evidence 5.1   Using Diluted Apple Juice for Rehydration

Traditionally, fluids high in sugar content have been discouraged for use in oral rehydration therapy. The thought has been that these types of fluids can induce osmotic diarrhea; therefore, only electrolyte solutions should be used for rehydration. However, parents indicate that children do not like the taste of electrolyte solution and often refuse to drink it. Therefore, they end up in the emergency department for intravenous rehydration.

Researchers performed a single-center randomized trial with 647 children. They found that, for mild dehydration,

parents who gave their children diluted apple juice actually experienced less treatment failure than those who used commercial electrolyte solutions. Furthermore, the children who received the diluted apple juice had no more diarrheal episodes than those who received the electrolyte solution. The greatest benefit was among children older than 24 mo.

The researchers concluded that for mild dehydration, promoting fluid consumption is more important than the amount of sugar in the fluid.

Adapted from Freedman, S. B., Willan, A. R., Boutis, K., & Schuh, S. (2016). Effect of dilute apple juice and preferred fluids vs electrolyte maintenance solution on treatment failure among children with mild gastroenteritis: A randomized clinical trial. *Journal of the American Medical Association, 315*(18), 1966–1974.

Box 5.1 Oral Rehydration Therapy: Types of Fluids

Current guidelines state that solutions used for oral rehydration should contain 75 mEq of sodium, 64 mEq of chloride, 20 mEq of potassium, and 75 mmol of glucose per liter, with total osmolarity of 245 mOsm/L. Examples are as follows:

- Commercial electrolyte solutions such as Pedialyte
- Homemade solutions
  - Chicken broth with 2 tablespoons of sugar
  - Four cups of low-calorie Gatorade (G2) with 1/2 teaspoon of salt

  Fluids high in sugar content should be avoided because of their osmotic properties, which may increase the severity of diarrhea.

Adapted from Bhutta, Z. A. (2016). Acute gastroenteritis in children. In R. M. Kliegman, B. F. Stanton, J. W. St. Geme III, N. F. Schor, & R. E. Behrman (Eds.), *Nelson's textbook of pediatrics* (20th ed.). Philadelphia, PA: Elsevier, Saunders; Carson, R. A., & Mudd, S. S. (2016). Clinical practice guideline for the treatment of pediatric acute gastroenteritis in the outpatient setting. *Journal of Pediatric Health Care, 30*(6), 610–616; University of Virginia Health System. (2016). Homemade oral rehydration solutions. Retrieved from https://med.virginia.edu/ginutrition/wp-content/uploads/sites/199/2018/09/Homemade-Oral-Rehydration-Solutions-9-2018.pdf; World Health Organization (2005).

"You may also use a measuring spoon—a teaspoon," Amy says. "Write down the instructions I'm about to give you." The instructions Amy gives Farrah are presented in Box 5.2. Amy explains that, based on Maalik's weight at his checkup, 11.8 kg, he will need about 15 mL of ORS every 5 minutes. She says that 5 mL is equal to 1 teaspoon, so 15 mL is equal to 3 teaspoons.

So, Amy instructs Farrah to give Maalik 3 teaspoons of ORS every 5 minutes, plus an additional 120 mL for each episode of diarrhea and an additional 24 mL for each episode of vomiting.

Box 5.2 Oral Rehydration Therapy: Fluid Replacement

Goals for fluid intake:

- 15 mL/kg/h
- Give small amounts every 5 min for 3–4 h

For every episode of diarrhea:

- Add 10 mL/kg

For every episode of vomiting:

- Add 2 mL/kg

Adapted from Carson, R. A., & Mudd, S. S. (2016). Clinical practice guideline for the treatment of pediatric acute gastroenteritis in the outpatient setting. *Journal of Pediatric Health Care, 30*(6), 610–616; Cincinnati Children's Hospital Medical Center (2011); Hughes, H. K., & Kahl, L. K. (Eds.). (2018). *The Harriet Lane handbook* (21st ed.). Philadelphia, PA: Elsevier.

Farrah writes this down while Kasim runs out to the store to get the ORS. When Kasim returns, Farrah begins the ORT regimen immediately. At first Maalik is responsive to the ORS. He takes the spoonfuls that Farrah gives him and seems to be perking up a little. However, after about 45 minutes, Maalik has several episodes of vomiting in a row. Farrah knows that she needs to give him the extra amount of fluid, but Maalik will not take it. After 30 minutes of back-to-back vomiting episodes with no fluid intake, Maalik becomes lethargic and Farrah and Kasim cannot get him to respond to them. Kasim hurries to get the car so they can take Maalik to the hospital.

At the Hospital

In the Emergency Room

By the time Farrah and Kasim arrive at the hospital emergency room, Maalik can barely open his eyes when stimulated. Kasim carries Maalik to the triage area, where they meet Sarah, a triage nurse.

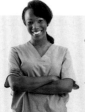

The Nurse's Point of View

Sarah: While I'm working triage, a man arrives carrying a young boy who appears to be nonresponsive. The man's name, I learn, is Kasim and the boy is Maalik. The boy's mother, Farrah, is also with them. I ask Kasim to lay Maalik on a bed so that I can assess him. Before he gets to the bed, however, Maalik vomits. The product of the **emesis** is mostly clear, with some mucus. I take a quick history on Maalik and realize that he is most likely very dehydrated.

In addition to obtaining his weight and vital signs, I also perform a focused assessment for circulation, fluid status, and neurological status. Maalik's vital signs and weight are as follows:

- Temperature: 102.3°F (39°C)
- Apical pulse: 140 beats/min (bpm)
- Respiratory rate: 40 breaths/min
- Blood pressure: 90/52 mm Hg
- O₂ saturation: 96% on room air
- Weight: 24 lb (10.9 kg)

I note that Maalik is slightly tachycardic and tachypneic, which could be related to his dehydration status. His blood pressure is within normal limits, so I know he is not exhibiting signs of shock.

I use the Clinical Dehydration Scale (Table 5.1; Analyze the Evidence 5.2) to assess Maalik's dehydration status. He is drowsy and limp, his eyes are slightly sunken, his mucous membranes are dry, and I cannot see any tears. I give Maalik a score of 7, indicating severe dehydration.

Table 5.1   Clinical Dehydration Scale for Children 1 to 36 Months of Age

	Score		
Characteristic	**0**	**1**	**2**
Description	No dehydration	Some dehydration (total score 1–4)	Moderate/severe dehydration (total score 5–8)
General appearance	Normal	Thirsty, restless, or lethargic but irritable when touched	Drowsy, limp, cold, sweaty, possibly comatose
Eyes	Normal	Slightly sunken	Very sunken
Mucous membranes (tongue)	Moist	Sticky	Dry
Tears	Present	Decreased	Absent

Adapted with permission from Goldman, R. D., Friedman, J. N., & Parkin, P. C. (2008). Validation of the clinical dehydration scale for children with acute gastroenteritis. *Pediatrics, 122*(3), 545–549.

Analyze the Evidence 5.2   Clinical Dehydration Scale

Dehydration secondary to gastroenteritis can be difficult to determine, especially if a preillness weight is not available. Researchers developed a simple four-item Clinical Dehydration Scale to assess the degree of dehydration in children with acute gastroenteritis and to evaluate the response to therapy. The scale takes a nurse ~2 min to complete.

Researchers validated the scale with the initial development and study of the Clinical Dehydration Scale. A study with a different sample of children indicated validity of the scale, as well. In the validity study, researchers concluded the scale is valuable in predicting a longer length of stay and need for intravenous fluids in children 1–36 mo with dehydration from acute gastroenteritis.

More recently, another group of researchers conducted **a meta-analysis** to determine the most accurate, non-invasive method for diagnosing dehydration in children with acute gastroenteritis. The researchers found that the Clinical Dehydration Scale consistently identifies severe dehydration with accuracy values of >80%. The researchers concluded that the Clinical Dehydration Scale provides overall improved diagnostic ability.

Adapted from Freedman, S. B., Vandermeer, B., Milne, A., & Hartling, L. (2015). Diagnosing clinically significant dehydration in children with acute gastroenteritis using noninvasive methods: A meta-analysis. *The Journal of Pediatrics, 166*, 908–916; Friedman, Goldman, Srivistana, and Parkin (2004); Goldman, R. D., Friedman, J. N., & Parkin, P. C. (2008). Validation of the clinical dehydration scale for children with acute gastroenteritis. Pediatrics, 122(3), 545–549.

When performing a circulatory assessment, I'm able to feel radial, brachial, femoral, and pedal pulses. However, his pedal pulses are weak and thready. I assess Maalik's capillary refill time and determine that it is greater than 3 seconds. I recall that a prolonged capillary refill time is another clinical sign of dehydration (Cincinnati Children's Hospital Medical Center, 2011).

Children are at greater risk of fluid loss than are adults, so I know that I must monitor Maalik's status very carefully (Let's Compare 5.1). As long as his sodium level is normal, he will need resuscitation fluids with **isotonic fluids** to improve his hydration status and prevent him from deteriorating to hypovolemic shock.

Maalik's weight in the emergency room is 10.9 kg.

"How much did Maalik weigh just before he became sick?" I ask Farrah.

Farrah does not answer, but Kasim does. Kasim says, "At the pediatrician's office recently, he weighed 11.8 kg."

It seems strange that Kasim answered the question and Farrah did not say anything. In fact, Kasim gives Maalik's history,

and it seems as if he is not letting Farrah take part in the conversation at all. I'm concerned about this interaction at first, but then I remember that in the Muslim culture men are the decision makers for the family (Hickey, 2013).

I know that to calculate fluid replacement volume, the physician needs to know Maalik's percentage of dehydration. So using an equation (Box 5.3), I determine that Maalik has 7% dehydration. I document this in his record.

I call the emergency physician and tell her Maalik's vital signs, weight, assessment, and dehydration percentage. The physician states that she will come to the emergency department soon, but that in the meantime I should start an intravenous (IV) normal saline bolus of 20 mL/kg over 1 hour. I write down the bolus order and repeat it back to the physician.

When I get off the phone, I explain to Kasim and Farrah that I am going to start an IV line to give Maalik some fluids that will help rehydrate him. I explain that initially fluids are given quickly to rehydrate and keep Maalik's condition from getting

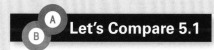

Let's Compare 5.1

Fluid Status

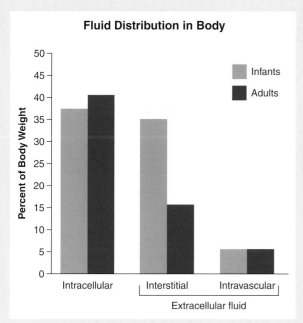

Fluid Distribution in Body

Infants and children have a relatively large amount of extracellular body fluids when compared with adults. To maintain fluid balance, infants and children require greater fluid intake. They also excrete a proportionately greater amount of fluid than do adults. These characteristics cause infants and young children to lose fluid at a faster rate than do adults and put them at greater risk for dehydration. Fluid loss occurs rapidly in infants and young children. Therefore, the fluid status of infants and young children should be closely monitored.

Fever increases the rate of fluid loss in infants and young children by increasing their metabolic rate and subsequently increasing insensible fluid loss.

Image adapted with permission from Hatfield, N. T., & Kincheloe, C. A. (2017). *Introductory maternity and pediatric nursing* (4th ed., Fig. 31-6). Philadelphia, PA: Wolters Kluwer.

Box 5.3 Calculating Dehydration

Equation for calculating dehydration:

$$\% \, dehydration = \frac{(preillness \; weight - illness \; weight)}{preillness \; weight} \times 100$$

Maalik's dehydration status:

$$\% \, dehydration = \frac{(11.8\,kg - 10.9\,kg)}{11.8\,kg} \times 100 = 7\% \, dehydration$$

worse. Once the initial bolus is given, then Maalik will be given IV fluids at a slower rate.

I start an IV line in Maalik's left arm. He continues to be drowsy and limp but does flinch and whine when the IV line is started. I calculate the bolus to be 220 mL. After priming the IV tubing, I hang the normal saline bolus. I set the pump to infuse 220 mL over 1 hour.

The emergency physician comes to the emergency department to check on Maalik. She reaches out to shake Kasim's hand, but I notice that he does not reciprocate but rather places his hand over his heart. I recall that in the Muslim culture, rather than shaking hands with the opposite sex, adults typically extend a greeting by placing their hand over their heart (Hickey, 2013). Once the physician assesses Maalik, she determines that he should be admitted for fluid replacement and observation. She enters orders (Box 5.4) and calls the unit to which Maalik is to be admitted.

I read the orders. I call a phlebotomist to arrange to have blood drawn for laboratory testing, including assessment of the complete blood count, serum electrolytes level, and blood glucose level. I tell Kasim and Farrah that the physician ordered a stool culture. Therefore, the next time Maalik has a bowel movement, they need to keep the diaper so I can collect a stool sample and send it to the laboratory.

Next, I give the ordered dose of ondansetron (The Pharmacy 5.2). I explain to Maalik's parents that the medication is to help with his vomiting. Shortly after I give him the medication, the unit calls and indicates that Maalik's room is ready. Meanwhile, I receive the results of Maalik's blood work and am glad to see that his serum electrolyte levels are all within normal limits. I call to the floor to give a report to Ann, the nurse who will be taking care of Maalik.

Box 5.4 Orders for Maalik Abdella

- Admit to unit B4 North
- Normal saline (NS; 0.9%) intravenous (IV) bolus of 220 mL over 1 h
- IV fluid replacement with NS, changing to dextrose 5% (D5) NS with 20 mEq of potassium after the first void:
  - 78 mL/h for the first 8 h
  - 61 mL/h for the next 16 h
- IV D5 NS with 20 mEq of potassium at 44 mL/h when fluid replacement is complete
- Ondansetron 3.3 mg IV × 1
- Acetaminophen 120 mg orally or parenterally every 4–6 h as needed for fever
- Laboratory tests
  - Serum electrolyte levels
  - Complete blood count
  - Blood glucose level
  - Stool culture
- Strict intake and output
- Daily weight
- Call for urine output less the 2 mg/kg/h
- Regular diet as tolerated

The Pharmacy 5.2			Ondansetron	
Medication	**Classification**	**Route**	**Action**	**Nursing Considerations**
Ondansetron	Antiemetic	• PO • IM • IV	• Selective 5-HT$_3$ receptor antagonist • Works in the chemoreceptor trigger zone	• Dosing depends on reason for use • For gastroenteritis in children 8–15 kg: • PO: 2 mg/dose × 1 • IV: 0.3 mg/kg/dose × 1, not to exceed 16 mg/dose • Monitor for agitation, anxiety with oral use • Monitor for sedation and drowsiness with IV use

IM, intramuscular; IV, intravenous; PO, oral.
Adapted from Taketomo, C. K. (2018). *Pediatric & neonatal dosage handbook* (25th ed.). Hudson, OH: Lexicomp.

On the Unit

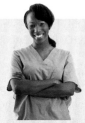

The Nurse's Point of View

Ann: I receive a report from Sarah in the emergency department about a 2-year-old patient named Maalik. I learn that a normal saline bolus is infusing and that about half of the ordered amount is left. Maalik has had blood drawn for his laboratory tests and received his ondansetron. The stool culture still needs to be collected, and he has not had any urine output. Sarah reports that Maalik remains limp and listless, his mucous membranes are dry, and his capillary refill time is greater than 3 seconds. His parents are with him.

I realize that although Maalik has a normal saline bolus infusing, he is still at risk for hypovolemic shock due to his dehydration status. I will have to monitor his status diligently for subtle changes. I will conduct a thorough assessment, paying close attention to Maalik's skin color and temperature, peripheral pulses, and blood pressure (Priority Care Concepts 5.1).

By the time Maalik arrives to the floor with his parents, there is about 15 minutes left of the normal saline bolus. I'm glad to see that the fluids seem to be helping Maalik. He is awake, although still lethargic. Upon further assessment, I find that his eyes still appear slightly sunken, his mucous membranes are still dry, and his capillary refill time is still greater than 3 seconds. Maalik's peripheral pulses are now 2+, and his skin is warm to the touch. I determine that Maalik has a score of 6 on the Clinical Dehydration Scale. His condition seems to be improving, but I know he still needs to be carefully monitored. He has had no urine output and no stool. On the unit, Maalik's vital signs are as follows:

- Temperature: 102.1°F (38.9°C)
- Apical pulse: 130 bpm
- Respiratory rate: 36 breaths/min
- Blood pressure: 98/56 mm Hg
- O$_2$ saturation: 96% on room air

Priority Care Concepts 5.1

Monitoring for Severe Dehydration and Shock

When a child is admitted for dehydration, it is imperative that the nurse monitor for changes in status to prevent the child from going into shock. Certain signs and symptoms of dehydration are red flags for possible progression to shock. Nursing intervention is necessary when a child exhibits any of these signs and symptoms.

Signs and Symptoms of Dehydration: Red Flags

- Altered responsiveness
- Decreased urinary output
- Sunken eyes
- Dry mucous membranes
- Decreased skin turgor
- Tachycardia
- Tachypnea

Signs and Symptoms of Shock

- Decreased level of consciousness
- Pale or mottled skin
- Cold extremities
- Tachycardia
- Tachypnea
- Weak peripheral pulses
- Decreased capillary refill
- Hypotension

I note Maalik's temperature. Sarah did not indicate whether he had received acetaminophen. I call the emergency room to double-check. Upon confirming that Maalik had not received acetaminophen, I give him a rectal dose of 120 mg.

After she assesses Maalik, the new nurse, Ann, shows Kasim and Farrah around the room and the unit. When she asks them whether they have any questions or concerns, Kasim says, "There are male nurses here?"

"Yes," Ann says. "Is that a concern for you?"

"In our culture, women should not be seen by men when they are not wearing the hijab" (Hickey, 2013). "My wife would like to remove her hijab while here in the room."

"Thank you for sharing your concern," Ann says. "I have two suggestions that I think will help Farrah be comfortable yet maintain her traditions. I can put a sign on the door requesting that all males please knock before entering. This will allow Farrah to dress properly before a male enters the room. I can also set up a folding screen in the room, so that Farrah can go behind it if she does not wish to put on her hijab when a male enters."

Ann also says, "You both speak English well. However, if at any time you have difficulty understanding what any of the healthcare providers say, I can call an interpreter to help" (Whose Job Is It, Anyway? 5.1).

Kasim and Farrah are both comfortable with this arrangement and settle into the room next to Maalik's bed. Once Maalik is stable, Kasim goes home to make sure that Maalik's sister, Sabeen, can be cared for by other members of their community.

Once things settle down, Ann asks Farrah, "Are you hungry? I can have food service bring you a tray of food, if you would like."

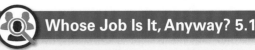

Whose Job Is It, Anyway? 5.1
Medical Interpreter

Most hospitals have access to interpreters for many different languages. These interpreters are trained in medical terminology and are often referred to as medical interpreters. Nurses are able to request an interpreter when families do not speak English or there is concern that a family may not understand instructions given to them. If there is any doubt whether a family fully understands their child's care and discharge instructions, enlist the help of an interpreter, if available, to prevent the child from harm.

"Thank you," Farrah says. "But it is the time of Ramadan now, when we Muslims fast. I may not eat from sunup to sunset" (Hickey, 2013). "Would it be permitted for Kasim to bring food after dark? We may only eat halal meat—meat from a special Muslim butcher—and may not have any pork."

"Yes," Ann says. "That would be fine. I am concerned for Maalik, though. Once he improves he will need to eat to get well."

"Young children and those who are ill do not have to fast," Farrah says (Hickey, 2013).

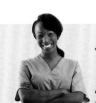

The Nurse's Point of View

Ann: Maalik's normal saline bolus is now complete. He has not had any urine output, so I hang normal saline at the ordered fluid replacement rate of 78 mL/h for 8 hours. About an hour after I hang the fluid replacement, Maalik has both urine and stool output. Although the stool is watery, I am able to scrape a sample from the diaper to send for culture. Next, I change the IV fluids to dextrose 5% in 0.45% normal saline (D5 1/2 NS) with 20 mEq of potassium, as ordered. I also recheck Maalik's temperature and find that it has gone down to 101°F.

I continue to monitor Maalik closely. He continues to improve each hour. Three hours into the replacement fluids, he is awake but irritable. His mucous membranes are sticky, and he is beginning to have tears. Maalik has some urine output, at a rate of 2 mg/kg/h. He has had one more watery stool. He has not had anything to eat or drink. I tell Farrah that my shift is over for the evening, but that I will be back in the morning.

The next day, Kasim arrives just in time for the morning rounds. The physicians assess Maalik and find that his condition has greatly improved. They explain to Kasim and Farrah that although he has improved, they would like to keep him overnight one more night to receive at least 24 hours of maintenance fluids. Kasim states that he understands and thanks the physicians.

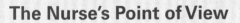

The Nurse's Point of View

Ann: This morning in report, I learn that Maalik had a few sips of diluted apple juice. He had no episodes of vomiting and one episode of watery stool. He currently is at hour 8 of the 16 hours of fluids at 61 mL/h. I enter Maalik's room to find him awake and in Farrah's lap. On assessment, I find that he is alert. His eyes no longer have a sunken appearance, his mucous membranes are moist, he has tears, and his capillary refill time is less than 3 seconds. His vital signs are as follows:

- Temperature: 99°F (37.2°C)
- Apical pulse: 102 bpm
- Respiratory rate: 30 breaths/min
- Blood pressure: 95/56 mm Hg
- O$_2$ saturation: 98% on room air
- Weight: 24.9 lb (11.3 kg)

I'm happy to find that Maalik's vital signs are within normal limits and that his weight is up. I offer Maalik some breakfast. He eats a few bites and drinks some milk. Thankfully, he holds it down.

Later in the day, when the 16 hours of fluid replacement at 61 mL/h is complete, I prepare to change the fluid to a maintenance rate. However, I realize that Maalik has gained some weight since the maintenance fluids were calculated yesterday (see Table 4.1). I decide to recalculate Maalik's maintenance rate to make sure he receives the correct amount of fluid (Box 5.5). I determine that the 44 mL/h rate is still correct and change the rate on the IV pump.

Box 5.5 Calculating Maalik's Maintenance Fluids

Maalik's current weight: 24.9 lb (11.3 kg)
First 10 kg: 100 mL/kg/d × 10 = 1,000 mL
Second 10 kg: 50 mL/kg/d × 1.3 = 65 mL
24-h fluid total = 1,065 mL
Hourly rate: 1,045/24 = 44 mL/h

That afternoon, the nurse, Ann, explains to Kasim and Farrah, "Maalik will receive fluids until he is discharged tomorrow. Encourage him to eat as he normally does."

Maalik continues to improve throughout the day.

Later, Farrah becomes frustrated with Maalik. She tells Ann, "I am trying to get Maalik to drink, but he won't drink from a cup and is asking for a bottle. He started drinking from a cup over a year ago. Why is he asking for a bottle now?"

"This type of behavior is normal for toddlers who have been very ill and in the hospital," Ann explains (Hospital Help 5.1). "It is called **regression** and is a defense mechanism usually due to some type of stress in the child's life. Once Maalik is home and back to his normal routine, these behaviors should disappear. I would let Maalik drink from a bottle, because at this point the priority is getting him to eat and drink and to make sure he can hold everything down."

Throughout the day Maalik eats small amounts and drinks well. He has no episodes of vomiting and only one episode of

watery stool. Ann reports that his urinary output is greater than 2 mg/kg/h. On evening rounds, the physician writes an order to stop the IV fluids and continue to monitor him overnight.

At Discharge

The next morning, after rounds, the physician writes discharge orders for Maalik. The stool culture results show that Maalik is infected with norovirus.

During the discharge instructions, Ann explains to the Abdella family, "Norovirus is a common cause for vomiting and diarrhea. Generally the infection does not last more than 3 days" (Payne et al., 2013). "Maalik could have a few more episodes of diarrhea over the next few days. As long as he is staying hydrated, acting like himself, and fever-free, there should be nothing to worry about. However, if Maalik stops drinking or becomes lethargic again, call his pediatrician."

Finally, Ann educates the Abdella family on how to prevent future episodes as this. "Proper hand washing is key to the prevention of norovirus, as well as many other infections," Ann tells them (Patient Teaching 5.4). "Washing your hands after changing diapers and before preparing food can help decrease the transmission of norovirus. Washing fruits and vegetables before you eat or prepare them is important, as well."

Maalik is awake, alert, and smiling. "Thank you for taking such good care of Maalik," Kasim says to Ann.

"Yes," Farrah says. "Thank you."

"You are welcome," Ann replies. "Do you have any further questions?"

"No," Kasim says. "We feel ready to take Maalik home." Kasim and Farrah sign the discharge papers and leave the hospital happy that Maalik is healthy again.

 Hospital Help 5.1

Building Toddler Autonomy and Managing Regression

Toddlers are in the Erikson stage of autonomy vs. shame and doubt. They are learning how to do things by themselves. Offering for the toddler to safely touch medical equipment, such as a stethoscope or penlight, may help gain cooperation when assessing a toddler. Also, allowing toddlers to have a comfort item in the hospital, such as a stuffed animal, can help alleviate fear and anxiety. Finally, allowing the parents to be present is important when the toddler is hospitalized.

While in the hospital, toddlers may experience regression. For example, they may begin to wet the bed after being potty-trained. Wanting a bottle or pacifier after having been weaned for a while is another common form of regression in toddlers. Explain to parents that this is normal behavior caused by the stress of illness and hospitalization. Although it may take a few weeks, the behavior will disappear when the toddler resumes a normal routine at home.

 Patient Teaching 5.4

Hand Washing

Hand washing is one of the best ways to prevent the spread of gastroenteritis. Be sure to wash your hands thoroughly with soap and water. Sing the song "Happy Birthday" twice to ensure you wash your hands for the proper amount of time. Always wash your hands after using the restroom, changing a diaper, before cooking, and before eating.

Think Critically

1. What are signs of developmental delay in a 2-year-old?
2. Discuss anticipatory guidance for a 2-year-old.
3. What are the differences between mild, moderate, and severe dehydration?
4. Why is it important that Farrah follow the directions for oral rehydration therapy?

5. What are important cultural considerations when caring for a Muslim family?
6. What would you expect Maalik's electrolyte levels to be if he were in metabolic alkalosis? Would this change the nursing care he needs?
7. What are the goals of nursing care for Maalik?

References

American Academy of Pediatrics. (2015). *Safety for your child: 2 to 4 years.* Retrieved from https://www.healthychildren.org/English/ages-stages/toddler/Pages/Safety-for-Your-Child-2-to-4-Years.aspx

American Academy of Pediatrics. (2017). *Toddler timeline.* Retrieved from https://www.aap.org/en-us/advocacy-and-policy/aap-health-initiatives/HALF-Implementation-Guide/Age-Specific-Content/Pages/Toddler-Timeline.aspx

Bathory, E., & Tomopoulos, S. (2017). Sleep regulation, physiology and development, sleep duration and patterns, and sleep hygiene in infants, toddlers, and preschool-age children. *Current Problems in Pediatric and Adolescent Health Care, 47,* 29–42. doi:10.1016/j.cppeds.2016.12.001

Chassiakos, Y. R., Radesky, J., Christakis, D., Moreno, M. A., & Cross, C. (2016). American Academy of pediatrics council on communications and media: Children and adolescents and digital media. *Pediatrics, 138*(5), e1–e18. doi:10.1542/peds.2016-2593

Churgay, C. A., & Aftab, Z. (2012). Gastroenteritis in children: Part II. Prevention and management. *American Family Physician, 85*(11), 1066–1070.

Cincinnati Children's Hospital. (2011). *Evidence-Based Care Guideline for Prevention and Management of Acute Gastroenteritis (AGE) in children age 2 mo to 18 yrs.* Retrieved from https://www.cincinnatichildrens.org/-/media/cincinnati%20childrens/home/service/j/anderson-center/evidence-based-care/recommendations/type/gastroenteritis-care-guideline

Daniels, E., Mandleco, B., & Luthy, K. E. (2012). Assessment, management, and prevention of childhood temper tantrums. *Journal of the American Academy of Nurse Practitioners, 24*(10), 569–573.

Friedman, J. N., Goldman, R. D., Srivastava, R., & Parkin, P. C. (2004). Development of a clinical dehydration scale for use in children between 1 and 36 months of age. *Pediatrics, 145*(2), 201–207.

Hickey, M. G. (2013). Our children follow our rules: Family and child rearing in U.S. Muslim migration. *Journal of Interdisciplinary Studies in Education, 1*(2), 4–26.

Hughes, H. K., & Kahl, L. K. (Eds.). (2018). *The Harriet Lane handbook* (21st ed.). Philadelphia, PA: Elsevier.

Inhorn, M. C., & Serour, G. I. (2011). Islam, medicine, and Arab-Muslim refugee health after 9/11. *The Lancet, 378,* 935–943.

Johnson, J. A. (2019). Islam. *Salem Press Encyclopedia, 7.*

Payne, D. C., Vinje, J., Szilagyi, P. G., Edwards, K. M., Staat, M. A., Weinberg, G. A., . . . Parashar, U. D. (2013). Norovirus and medically attended gastroenteritis in U.S. children. *The New England Journal of Medicine, 368*(12), 1121–1130.

World Health Organization. (2005). The treatment of diarrhoea: *A manual for physicians and other senior health workers.* Retrieved from http://apps.who.int/iris/bitstream/10665/43209/1/9241593180.pdf

Suggested Readings

Centers for Disease Control and Prevention. (2016). *Norovirus for healthcare workers.* Retrieved from https://www.cdc.gov/norovirus/hcp/index.html

Hickey, M. G. (2013). Our children follow our rules: Family and child rearing in U.S. Muslim migration. *Journal of Interdisciplinary Studies in Education, 1*(2), 4–26.

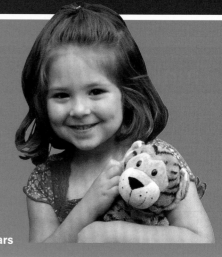

6 Abigail Hanson: Leukemia

Abigail Hanson, age 4 years

Objectives

After completing this chapter, you will be able to:
1. Describe normal growth and development of the 4-year-old.
2. Discuss an appropriate teaching plan for a healthy 4-year-old.
3. Identify presenting signs and symptoms of leukemia.
4. Apply principles of growth and development to the 4-year-old in the hospital.
5. Describe the psychological impact of a pediatric cancer diagnosis on the family.
6. Explain the progression from infection to sepsis.
7. Plan nursing interventions for the child undergoing chemotherapy treatment.

Key Terms

Absolute neutrophil count (ANC)
Alopecia
Central venous catheter (CVC)
Hepatosplenomegaly

Lymphadenopathy
Lymphoblast
Petechiae
Stomatitis

Background

Abigail Hanson is a 4-year-old girl who lives at home with her father, mother, and older sister. Abigail's father, Jack, is an investment banker who travels a great deal for work. When he is home, he is involved with his children and loves to take the girls to the zoo. Abigail's mother, Lucy, is a teacher but currently stays at home. She volunteers on two different community boards and plans on going back to work when both of the girls are in school full time. Isabelle, Abigail's sister, is almost 6 years old and is in half-day kindergarten. The family lives in the suburbs, about 30 minutes outside of a large metropolitan area.

Abigail is a typically developing 4-year-old (Growth and Development Check 6.1). She and Isabelle play well together most of the time but fight from time to time, as all siblings do. Abigail loves to play pretend. Her favorite game to play is "zoo." She has a stuffed animal for almost every animal that she has seen in the zoo with her dad. Abigail sets out the animals around her

playroom and has the animals act out different scenes. She can occupy herself for a couple of hours with her stuffed animals, and Isabelle often plays with her.

When she is not playing "zoo," Abigail likes to play outside with her friend next door. She plays on her swing set and loves to go down the slide. Abigail is a fast runner and loves to climb on things so much that Lucy is afraid that she is going to fall off of something and break a limb. Although Lucy wishes Jack were home more, she feels that she can't complain. She has healthy and happy girls, a nice house, and good friends.

Health Promotion

Lucy takes Abigail to the pediatrician's office for her 4-year-old checkup. Abigail actually turned 4 about 3 months ago.

"I feel guilty for not getting Abigail in sooner," Lucy tells the medical assistant in the office.

Growth and Development Check 6.1

Four-Year-Old Milestones

Social/Emotional

- Likes to do new things
- Engages in creative and imaginative play
- Likes to play with other children
- Is able to cooperate
- Talks about interests

Speech

- Uses "he" and "she" correctly
- Sings songs
- Tells stories

Cognitive

- Knows first and last names
- Is able to memorize address
- Can count to 10 or higher
- Knows at least four colors
- Begins to understand time, as in before and after
- Tells what happens next in a book

Gross Motor/Fine Motor

- Uses scissors
- Draws a person with two to four body parts
- Dresses and undresses without help
- Prints some capital letters
- Climbs and hops
- Stands on one foot
- Catches a bounced ball

Adapted from the Centers for Disease Control and Prevention. (2016). *Learn the signs. Act early.* Retrieved from https://www.cdc.gov/ncbddd/actearly/milestones/milestones-3yr.html

"No need to worry," the assistant tells Lucy. "It's good that you are getting her in for her check-up. Three months is not all that late."

The assistant weighs Abigail and takes her vital signs in a small room in the front of the office. She weighs 40 lb (18.1 kg) and is 3.5 ft (42 in) tall. Abigail's vital signs are as follows:

- Pulse: 102 beats/min (bpm)
- Respiratory rate: 25 breaths/min
- Blood pressure: 92/60 mm Hg
- Temperature: 98.2°F (36.8°C)

"Let's check how well you can see," the assistant tells Abigail, holding up a picture chart. "First, though, can you name the pictures you see on the chart? That will make it easier for me to know which pictures you are talking about." Abigail dutifully names the pictures on the chart. The assistant then has Abigail stand on a line and goes to another line 20 ft away. "Now, cover your left eye and call out the name of each picture I point to." The assistant points to pictures on different lines of the chart, and Abigail calls out the names. The assistant repeats this

procedure while having Abigail cover her right eye. Throughout the vision screening, Abigail has difficulty keeping one eye covered, Lucy notices. She keeps forgetting, and takes her hand off of her eye. The assistant estimates that her vision is 20/30.

The assistant shows Lucy and Abigail to an exam room. "Kevin is running a little behind schedule," the assistant says, "but the wait shouldn't be too long." Kevin is the nurse practitioner Abigail is scheduled to see. While they are waiting, Lucy notices that there are stickers on the wall that are different shapes and colors. She points them out and has Abigail practice naming the shapes and the colors. She is able to name red, green, blue, yellow, and black, but she cannot remember orange and purple. She gets all of the shapes correct. "Great job!" Lucy tells her daughter. At that moment, Kevin enters the room.

"Hi, Abigail!" Kevin says. "How are you today?" Abigail chatters for a moment in response. Kevin then turns to Lucy and says, "How are things going? Do you have any specific questions or concerns?"

"Actually, yes," Lucy says. "I'm a little concerned about Abigail's vision. Is 20/30 okay? Also, I noticed that Abigail did not seem to cooperate very well with keeping one eye covered during the screening. Could that have affected the result?"

"Although we check visual acuity with the picture chart at the 4-year-old checkup," Kevin says, "most children don't really understand how to follow the direction of keeping one eye covered until around the age of 5. I would not be concerned at this point. Children typically reach the visually acuity of 20/20 by the time they are 5 years old."

Kevin talks to Lucy about the measurements his assistant took at the beginning of the visit. He explains that Abigail's weight, 40 lb, puts her in about the 80th percentile for weight for all girls her age. Abigail's height, 3.5 ft, puts her in about the 90th percentile for height.

"Although these percentiles sound high," Kevin explains, "all they mean is that she is bigger than the average 4-year-old. Because her weight percentile is below her height percentile, I'm not concerned." He further explains that her body mass index (BMI) is 15.9, which is within the range of ideal weight. The range for ideal BMI is from the 5th to the 85th percentile, and Abigail is in the 69th percentile.

Kevin begins Abigail's physical exam. During the exam, he talks with both Abigail and Lucy.

"What do you like to do, Abigail?" he asks.

"I like to swing and ride my tricycle," Abigail tells Kevin.

"That's great!" he replies. "I'm so proud of you for being active and playing outside. That helps you stay healthy." He explains to Lucy how important activity is at this age and how it can prevent a sedentary lifestyle, which leads to obesity.

"What do you like to eat?" he asks Abigail.

"Pizza!" she shouts.

"Me, too," he says. "Do you know what fruits and vegetables are?"

"Yes."

"Can you name a fruit for me?"

"Apple," she says.

"That's right," he replies. "What about a vegetable?"

"Carrot," she says.

"We make sure that Abigail has at least one fruit or vegetable at every meal," Lucy says.

"It sounds like you are a good eater," Kevin tells Abigail. He explains to Lucy that most 4-year-olds eat three meals and two snacks per day and that it is important for parents to model healthy eating and offer healthy foods at each meal.

Kevin completes the physical exam and says, "Everything looks great, Abigail." He finishes up the appointment with some anticipatory guidance. "In general, when a child is 4 years old and 40 lb or more, he or she is able to use a booster seat with a back and a regular seat belt. But you should read the height and weight requirements for your specific car safety seat, as they can vary" (American Academy of Pediatrics [AAP], 2011, 2018).

"Sleep is another thing to consider," Kevin says. "It's so important for children. Not only does it help the child with cognitive development, adequate sleep can help prevent obesity beginning as early as infancy" (Taveras, Gillman, Pena, Redline, & Rifas-Shiman, 2014). "Preschool children typically need 11 to 12 hours per day. Does Abigail still take naps?"

"No," Lucy says. "She's more interested in playing with her older sister, Isabelle."

"That's fine," Kevin says. "Many children stop napping around the age of 4. However, no napping means that it is imperative that Abigail get 11 to 12 hours of sleep at night."

Continuing with his teaching, Kevin talks to both Lucy and Abigail about safety, especially stranger safety (Patient Teaching 6.1). "Preschoolers like to explore and meet new people," he says. "Sometimes they wander off in stores or parks. The good news is that by the age of 4, children have the cognitive ability to memorize their address and phone number. So, I encourage

you to work with Abigail to help her learn her address and phone number in case she ever gets separated from you."

Finally, Kevin explains to Lucy that with Abigail's increasing independence comes the need for new sets of rules (Patient Teaching 6.2). "Children tend to behave well when parents and other adults set rules and limits for them and follow them consistently," he says. "When children do not follow the rules, the consequences need to be logical and timely. Also, I

Patient Teaching 6.2

Discipline

Setting rules and limits can go a long way toward curtailing unwanted behavior in your child. When establishing household rules, be sure that your child is able to understand the rules and follow them. Similarly, be sure your child is able to accomplish the task he or she is asked to do. Children develop at different rates. Often children are not misbehaving, they simply are not at the developmental stage to accomplish what is being asked of them. Some tips for discipline in the 4-y-old include the following:

- Routines:
  - Establishing daily routines helps a child know what to expect each day.
  - Simple routines such as brushing teeth and reading a story before bed provide comfort and can help divert temper tantrums.
- Limits:
  - Setting limits lets children know what is expected, such as requiring them to always wear a helmet when riding a bike.
  - Explain the consequences of breaking the rules.
- Independence:
  - It is important to encourage independence within the set limits.
  - Independence within limits helps encourage self-confidence.
- Responsibility:
  - Encouraging responsibility with chores around the house fosters independence and self-confidence.
- Time-out:
  - When your child is not listening and a consequence must be enforced, time-out is a preferred method of discipline.
  - The goal of time-out is to separate your child from the situation.
  - Children should be warned that they are getting a time-out.
  - Choose a time-out spot.
  - Choose a time. A general rule of thumb is 1 min/y of age of your child.
  - If your child whines and fusses, then the time-out starts over.

Adapted from American Academy of Pediatrics. (2015). *Disciplining your child*. Retrieved from https://www.healthychildren.org/English/family-life/family-dynamics/ communication-discipline/Pages/Disciplining-Your-Child.aspx

Patient Teaching 6.1

Stranger Safety

At 4 y, children are becoming more independent. Children at this age are also very trusting. Therefore, it is very important to talk to children about safety with strangers. Parents should talk to their children about how to be careful when around strangers. Tell your child the following:

- Do not go with anyone you do not know.
- No one should touch you in the bathing suit areas unless the person is a doctor or a nurse, and then only if I say it is okay.
- If someone tells you to keep a secret from me, that is wrong; please tell me.
- If you get separated from me, try to find a security guard or police officer.

Parents can help their children learn tools to use when they are lost and in the presence of strangers. At this age, children are able to memorize their address and phone number. Help your child learn this information so that if your child gets lost, someone will be able to help him or her. In addition, in crowded places, point out safe areas and people who can help, such as police officers and security guards.

recommend that you encourage some independence in Abigail by having her dress and undress herself. Give her a chore to do such as picking up her dirty clothes. Daily routines will help her know what to expect and perhaps divert behavioral meltdowns."

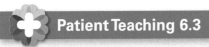

Patient Teaching 6.3

Immunizations for 4-Year-Olds

Immunizations

The immunizations that your child will get at his or her 4-y-old checkup are as follows:

- Diphtheria, tetanus, acellular pertussis (DTaP)
  - The DTaP vaccine protects against the following:
    - Diphtheria, a serious infection of the throat that can block the airway
    - Tetanus, otherwise known as lockjaw, a nerve disease
    - Pertussis, otherwise known as whooping cough, a respiratory infection that can have serious complications
- Inactivated poliovirus (IPV)
  - The IPV vaccine protects against polio, which can cause paralysis and death.
- Measles, mumps, rubella (MMR)
  - The MMR vaccine protects against the following:
    - Measles, a serious and highly contagious respiratory infection that causes rash and fever
    - Mumps, a highly contagious virus that causes fever, headache, and swollen glands under the jaw
    - Rubella, also known as "German measles," a virus that causes a rash and swollen glands
- Chickenpox (varicella)
  - The varicella vaccine protects against chickenpox, which is a disease that causes a rash that itches, forms blisters, and causes fever.
  - Chickenpox can be life-threatening in babies and children with weakened immune systems.

Common Side Effects

After your child gets immunizations, he or she may have the following:

- A fever of up to around 102°F
- Redness or a small amount of swelling at the injection site
- A mild rash 5–7 d after the MMR or varicella vaccine
- Fussier in the 24 h after immunizations
- More sleep in the 24 h after immunizations

When to Call the Healthcare Provider

- If your child has a fever and the temperature is 105°F (40.5°C) or higher
- If your child has a seizure
- If your child has uncontrollable crying for 3 h or longer

Adapted from the Centers for Disease Control and Prevention. (2017). *Diseases and the vaccines that prevent them.* Retrieved from http://www.cdc.gov/vaccines/hcp/conversations/prevent-diseases/provider-resources-factsheets-infants.html

After all of his teaching is complete, Kevin discusses Abigail's 4-year-old immunizations (Patient Teaching 6.3). "Abigail has had all of these immunizations before," he explains. "Each shot that she is getting today is a booster to her earlier immunizations. Two of the immunizations are live virus vaccines, meaning that Abigail receives a weakened form of the virus for which her body will form antibodies. The two live virus vaccines are the measles, mumps, and rubella, known as the MMR, and the chickenpox, or varicella, vaccines. Most 4-year-olds do not have reactions to the immunizations. However, if Abigail has side effects from the live virus vaccines, they are most likely to occur 5 to 7 days after the shots, so be aware. The most common side effects of the MMR and the chickenpox vaccines are fever and localized rash."

Abigail sits on the table like a big girl and gets her immunizations. She sits still and barely lets out a whimper. Lucy is so proud of her. On the way out of the office, Abigail picks out a sucker and a sticker and tells her mother that she is excited to get home and play with her stuffed animals.

At Home

A few days after her checkup, Abigail is not acting like herself, Lucy notices. She is grumpy and tired. She feels warm to the touch, so Lucy takes her temperature. It is 102.3°F (39°C). Lucy is not too concerned. She remembers that Kevin told her either the MMR or chickenpox vaccine could cause side effects 5 to 7 days later. She decides to keep an eye on Abigail over the next day or two to see what happens.

The next morning Abigail is worse. She wakes up, goes immediately to the couch, and lies back down. This is not like her at all. She usually bounces out of bed, eats breakfast, and is ready to play zoo with her stuffed animals. Abigail's dad, Jack, tries to entice her to eat breakfast, but she is just not interested. Abigail's temperature remains roughly the same, ranging from 101.8°F (38.8°C) to 102.3°F. Lucy gives Abigail some acetaminophen to help with the fever.

"Maybe we should call the pediatrician's office," Jack says.

"Not just yet," Lucy says, trying to stay calm. "I still think this is just a result of the immunizations."

Abigail stays on the couch and watches television most of the day. She cuddles with her blanket and her favorite stuffed tiger. Near bedtime, Abigail begins to complain that her legs hurt. Lucy gives her another dose of acetaminophen, rubs her legs to help her feel better, and lies down with Abigail until she falls asleep.

The next morning Abigail does not even want to get out of bed. She is now on day 3 of fever, and this morning her temperature is up to 102.9°F (39.4°C). Abigail is still complaining of her legs hurting. Lucy picks Abigail up to take her to the bathroom and notices small red spots on Abigail's arms (Fig. 6.1). She remembers that both the MMR and chickenpox vaccines can cause a rash, but these red spots concern Lucy. Lucy does not remember Isabelle having any trouble with her 4-year-old immunizations. She knows that every child can be different, but she also has a feeling that something is not right. She tells Jack that she is going to call the pediatrician's office.

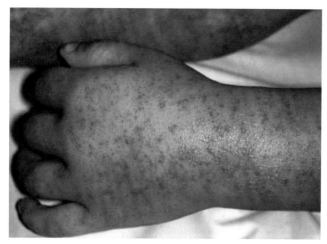

Figure 6.1. Petechiae. Petechiae are pinpoint, flat red spots that indicate bleeding under the skin. Reprinted with permission from Weber, J. R., & Kelley, J. H. (2017). *Health assessment in nursing* (6th ed., unnumbered figure in Abnormal Findings 14-4 in Chapter 14). Philadelphia, PA: Wolters Kluwer.

That morning Lucy calls the pediatrician's office and talks to the nurse. "Abigail received her immunizations 1 week ago, but her symptoms seem to be getting worse, not better. She has had a fever for 3 days that doesn't seem to be responding well to acetaminophen. She's been very sleepy, just not acting like herself, and this morning woke up with small red spots on her arms."

The nurse takes in this information and tells Lucy, "These symptoms do seem unusual for an immunization reaction. Bring Abigail into the office for a sick visit. An appointment is available at 11:30 a.m. We'll see her then."

At the Pediatrician's Office

Both Lucy and Jack bring Abigail to the pediatrician's office. The assistant takes Abigail's vital signs and reports them as follows:

- Pulse: 120 bpm
- Respiratory rate: 28 breaths/min
- Blood pressure: 90/58 mm Hg
- Temperature: 102.4°F (39.1°C)

Her weight is still at 40 lb. After completing the vital signs and measurements, the assistant takes Abigail and her parents to a room.

A few minutes later the nurse practitioner, Kevin, comes in. Lucy is glad that they are able to see him again since he just saw Abigail 1 week ago. Lucy tells Kevin the history of Abigail's present illness.

"You were right to bring Abigail in," Kevin says. "Although the immunizations that she received could cause fever, they would not cause fever of this intensity and duration."

Kevin completes a thorough physical exam. After he is finished, he tells Lucy and Jack, "I cannot find any overt signs that indicate what could be causing Abigail's fever. Her ears

are not infected, her lungs are clear, and her throat is not red or inflamed. Has she had any trouble urinating, complaints of burning, or foul-smelling urine?"

"No," Lucy says.

"I'm concerned because Abigail has mild **hepatosplenomegaly** and generalized **lymphadenopathy**," Kevin says, "meaning her liver, spleen, and lymph nodes are all enlarged. The red spots on her arms are called **petechiae**, which are caused by bleeding under the skin. All of Abigail's symptoms can be explained by a viral illness, but with the high fever, fatigue, and leg pain, the presentation is concerning. I'd like Abigail to have blood work done to help determine what is going on with her." Kevin explains that he is writing an order for a stat complete blood count (CBC) with differential and a comprehensive metabolic panel (CMP). He tells Abigail's parents that he will call them when he gets the results. Lucy and Jack take Abigail to the laboratory immediately to have blood drawn.

About an hour later, Lucy and Jack receive a call from Kevin. He tells them he has received the results of Abigail's blood work (Table 6.1) and asks them to come back to the office.

Back at the pediatrician's office, Kevin meets with Lucy and Jack and tells them that her blood work is concerning. "Her white blood cell (WBC) count is very high, higher than it should be for an infection. Her hemoglobin (Hgb) and hematocrit (Hct) levels are low, indicating that Abigail is anemic. Her platelet levels are slightly low, which could be the reason for the petechiae. The most concerning part of Abigail's blood work, however, is that she has 38% **lymphoblasts**. A lymphoblast is an immature WBC that does not work correctly." Kevin looks at Jack and Lucy with a somber expression and says, "The percentage of lymphoblasts in Abigail's blood along with the high WBC count and low Hgb, Hct, and platelet levels has me concerned that Abigail may have leukemia."

Jack and Lucy are absolutely stunned and cannot even speak. Lucy tears up but tries not to cry so as not to alarm Abigail.

"I'm going to have her admitted to the hospital with an oncology consult," Kevin continues. "The oncologists will want to conduct more tests for a definitive diagnosis. I know this is a terrible moment for you. I can assure you, though, that you will get the best care possible at the children's hospital. Go home, pack a bag for yourselves and Abigail, and go to the main welcome center at the hospital."

"How could this have happened?" cries Lucy. "Would her immunizations have caused this?" Suddenly, all Lucy can think about is that she did something to cause Abigail to develop this terrible illness.

Kevin looks at Jack and Lucy with compassion. "Abigail's immunizations in no way caused her to develop leukemia. We do not really know why children develop leukemia," he explains. "I can assure you that you have done nothing to cause this."

Jack and Lucy drive home and pack a bag for Abigail and Lucy. Jack will have to come home to stay with Isabelle. In the meantime, a neighbor is able to take care of Isabelle. Lucy is not sure what to tell Isabelle at this point, so she tells her that she and her daddy have to take Abigail to the hospital so the doctors can figure out what is making Abigail so sick and help

Table 6.1 Abigail's Initial Laboratory Results

Laboratory Test	Abigail's Results	Normal Range for a 4-Y-Old Female
Complete blood count with differential		
WBC, /µL	42,000	5,000–15,500
RBC, ×10⁶/µL	4	4.2–5.4
Hgb, g/dL	10	12.5
Hct, %	31	37
Platelets, ×10³/µL	90	150–350
Neutrophils—bands, %	50	3–5
Neutrophils—segmented, %	30	54–62
Lymphoblasts, %	38	N/A
Comprehensive metabolic panel		
Albumin, g/dL	4.3	3.6–5.2
Alkaline phosphatase, U/L	220	100–320
ALT, U/L	16	10–25
AST, U/L	22	13–35
BUN, mg/dL	7	5–18
Calcium, mg/dL	9.2	8.8–10.8
Chloride, mEq/L	99	99–107
Creatinine, U/L	32	20–180
Glucose, mg/dL	75	60–100
Potassium, mEq/L	4.1	3.4–4.7
Sodium, mEq/L	150	135–147
Total bilirubin, mg/dL	0.2	<1.5
Total protein, g/dL	7.2	6–8

ALT, alanine aminotransferase; AST, aspartate aminotransferase; BUN, blood urea nitrogen; Hct, hematocrit; Hgb, hemoglobin; RBC, red blood cell; WBC, white blood cell.
Adapted from Hughes, H. K., & Kahl, L. K. (Eds.). (2018). *The Harriet Lane handbook* (21st ed.). Philadelphia, PA: Elsevier.

her get better. Lucy and Jack kiss Isabelle goodbye and promise that daddy will be home to tuck her in tonight. They get in the car and drive to the hospital. Abigail is asleep in the backseat, clutching her stuffed tiger in her arms.

At the Hospital

Jack and Lucy do as Kevin instructed and stop at the main welcome desk of the hospital. The clerk looks up Abigail's name and finds her room number. The Hanson family is then escorted to a room in the hospital's oncology unit. Lucy is surprised; the unit almost looks like a hotel rather than a hospital.

The first person that Jack, Lucy, and Abigail meet is their nurse.

"Hi, I'm Norma," she says. "I'll be taking care of you all. I've been a nurse on the oncology unit for 20 years now. I like to work with children who are newly diagnosed because I feel it is my job to help families navigate through this difficult period." She takes Abigail's vital signs and weight. Abigail's weight is 39.8 lb (18 kg) on the hospital scale. Her vital signs are as follows:

- Pulse: 122 bpm
- Respiratory rate: 26 breaths/min
- Blood pressure: 91/56 mm Hg
- Temperature: 102.1°F (38.9°C)

Lucy watches Norma take Abigail's vital signs. She has been trying to stay strong but feeling extremely overwhelmed, Lucy breaks down and begins to cry. Jack sits next to Lucy and puts his arm around her.

The team of doctors comes in and Lucy brushes away her tears.

"Hi, I'm Dr. Redman, the attending physician," one says. She sits down in between the bed and the chair so that she can talk to Lucy, Jack, and Abigail at the same time. "We still need to do more blood work and some tests to be sure, but the initial blood work leads me to believe that Abigail has acute lymphoblastic leukemia (ALL)."

"When the percentage of lymphoblasts in a child's blood is greater than 20% and the WBC count is high, I suspect leukemia," Dr. Redman explains (National Comprehensive Cancer Network [NCCN], 2017).

"What are lymphoblasts?" Jack asks.

"Lymphoblasts are immature WBCs that do not function correctly, lowering the ability to fight infection, which is why Abigail has fever and lymphadenopathy," Dr. Redman says. "Furthermore, because the lymphoblasts are so proliferative, the bone marrow is not able to produce as many red blood cells (RBCs) and platelets. This explains why Abigail is anemic and has petechiae."

The entire time, Abigail listens to Dr. Redman and watches her mom and dad. Lucy can tell she is worried.

"What's wrong with me?" Abigail asks Dr. Redman.

"Well, sweetie, your body is making bad blood cells that are making you sick." She assures Abigail that she did nothing wrong to cause this to happen, explaining to Lucy and Jack that children at this age sometimes believe they caused their illness.

"Am I going to get better?" Abigail asks.

"I'm going to do my best to get the bad blood cells out of your body," Dr. Redman says.

"Can my tiger stay with me while I'm in the hospital?"

"Absolutely," Dr. Redman says. "He will help you feel safe while you are here."

Workup for All

"In addition to some more blood work," Dr. Redman tells Lucy and Jack, "Abigail will need to have a bone marrow biopsy and a lumbar puncture. The bone marrow biopsy will confirm the diagnosis and the lumbar puncture will determine whether the leukemia has spread to the central nervous system."

"Will these procedures hurt?" Lucy asks.

"They will be uncomfortable," Dr. Redman says, "But we will give Abigail some medicine to relax her and make her sleepy so she will not feel the discomfort during the procedure. However, she may be sore afterward. Norma, your nurse, is excellent and should be able to answer any questions you have." Dr. Redman explains that she must leave the room now to enter orders into the computer (Box 6.1).

Norma comes into the room and explains the tests and procedures that Dr. Redman ordered for Abigail. "The ECG, or electrocardiogram, and the echocardiogram are ordered as baseline tests of heart function because some of the chemotherapeutic agents can affect cardiac function," Norma tells Lucy and Jack. Turning to Abigail, she says, "These tests are just pictures, and they won't hurt."

Next, Norma talks about the bone marrow biopsy (Fig. 6.2) and lumbar puncture (Fig. 6.3). She tells Jack and Lucy, "Before the procedures, a child life specialist will show Abigail how the procedures are done on a doll. The child life specialist will also let Abigail play with some of the equipment the doctors and nurses will use for the procedures to help ease her anxiety."

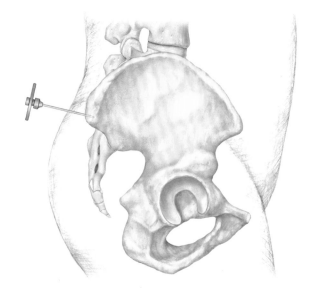

Figure 6.2. Bone marrow biopsy needle inserted in the right iliac crest. Reprinted with permission from Anatomical Chart Company.

A few hours later, Norma comes into the room and tells Jack, Lucy, and Abigail that the bone marrow biopsy and lumbar puncture could not be scheduled until the next day. She explains that nothing will happen this evening or overnight, so Jack should go home to be with Isabelle and come back in the morning.

The following day Abigail goes for the bone marrow biopsy and lumbar puncture. When she comes back to the room, she

Box 6.1   Orders for Abigail Hanson

- Admit to unit A6 West.
- Insert peripheral intravenous (IV) line.
- Dextrose 5% normal saline at 75 mL/h
- Nothing by mouth
- Acetaminophen 270 mg IV every 6 h as needed for fever
- Administer oxygen to keep saturation at 95% or higher.
- Complete blood count with differential
- Peripheral blood smear
- Blood type and screen
- Comprehensive metabolic panel
- Uric acid
- Prothrombin time
- Activated partial thromboplastin time
- Bone marrow biopsy
- Lumbar puncture
- Electrocardiogram
- Echocardiogram

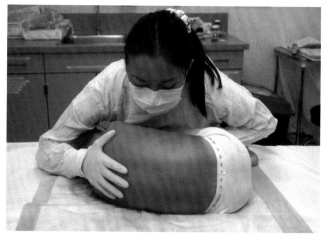

Figure 6.3. Positioning for a lumbar puncture. Reprinted with permission from Bowden, V., & Greenberg, C. S. (2013). *Children and their families* (3rd ed., Fig. 21-9B). Philadelphia, PA: Wolters Kluwer Health/Lippincott Williams & Wilkins.

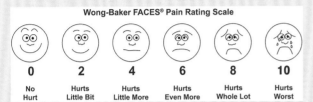

How Much Does It Hurt? 6.1

Wong-Baker FACES Pain Rating Scale

Preschool children are in the preoperational stage of cognitive development and have developed symbolic representation. However, they are not yet able to understand the concepts of "greater" and "less." Therefore, a preschool child does not understand when asked to rate his or her pain on a scale of 1–10.

Wong-Baker FACES® Pain Rating Scale

0	2	4	6	8	10
No Hurt	Hurts Little Bit	Hurts Little More	Hurts Even More	Hurts Whole Lot	Hurts Worst

The Wong-Baker FACES Pain Rating Scale shows a series of faces with different expressions. The faces range from a happy face at 0, or no pain, to a crying face at 10, or the very worst pain. These faces are the preschool child's symbolic representation of pain.

Image © 1983 Wong-Baker FACES Foundation. www.WongBakerFACES.org

Used with permission. Originally published in *Whaley & Wong's Nursing care of infants and children.* © Elsevier Inc.

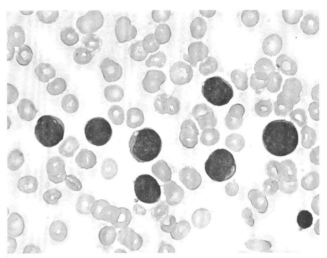

Figure 6.4. Peripheral blood smear. The dark purple cells without a nucleus are lymphoblasts. Reprinted with permission from Strayer, D. S., & Rubin, E. (2014). *Rubin's pathology* (7th ed., Fig. 26-56). Philadelphia, PA: Wolters Kluwer.

has a small bandage on her posterior left hip over the iliac crest. Abigail starts to cry. "Does it hurt where your boo boo is?" Norma says. Abigail nods her head yes. Norma uses something she calls the FACES scale to determine how much pain Abigail is experiencing (How Much Does It Hurt? 6.1).

Abigail points to the frowny face without tears, a number 8 on the scale. Norma checks the medication record and tells Lucy and Jack, "Abigail is due for some acetaminophen now." She administers the medicine and says, "If it does not relieve her pain, I will call Dr. Redman to get an order for a stronger pain medication."

Diagnosis

A while after Abigail returns to her room, Dr. Redman comes to discuss the procedure and blood work results with Jack and Lucy. Dr. Redman takes Jack and Lucy to a conference room down the hall. Norma accompanies them.

Dr. Redman sits down at the table with Jack and Lucy. She looks at them empathetically, and Lucy can tell from her expression that the news is not good. "The procedures and blood work confirm that Abigail does indeed have ALL." She explains to them that the repeat WBC is 43,000 and the peripheral blood smear showed lymphoblasts (Fig. 6.4). The bone marrow

biopsy showed 35% lymphoblasts, which is diagnostic for ALL, she says.

At this point Lucy feels like collapsing, but she stays strong and asks Dr. Redmond, "What happens now?"

Dr. Redmond continues with the remainder of the results. She tells Jack and Lucy that there is some positive news. Abigail's cerebral spinal fluid (CSF) is negative for leukemic cells. Abigail's age, WBC count, and negative CSF put her in the standard risk category, she explains. Children from 1 to 10 years old with a WBC count of less than 50,000 and negative central nervous system involvement have the highest cure rate, up to as high as 98% (Cooper & Brown, 2015).

Dr. Redman explains that while there is good news even in the face of this terrible diagnosis, it will still be a hard road for Abigail to get to remission. She finishes discussing the test results. The echocardiogram and ECG are normal. Abigail's bleeding times are normal, so she is not currently at risk for any serious bleed. Her uric acid level is a little high, indicating cell breakdown. Dr. Redman concludes the conversation by stating that the team would like to get chemotherapy started as soon as possible.

Norma takes Jack and Lucy back to Abigail's room. Norma asks them, "What questions do you have?"

Lucy feels overwhelmed, and Jack looks stunned. "What now?" Lucy asks.

"I know this is a lot of information, a lot to absorb," Norma says. "Please know that I am here to help you, and as you process things and questions come to mind, I'll be happy to answer them. I'll be off tomorrow, but for the rest of my shift today and when I come back the day after tomorrow, I'll be available to sit down with you and go over Abigail's treatment, as you feel ready."

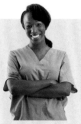

The Nurse's Point of View

Norma: When a child, like Abigail, is diagnosed with cancer, the parents are usually so over- whelmed they cannot process much of the in- formation they hear. And they are hearing a lot of information, including new terms and medical language they are unfamiliar with, which produces anxiety. It's a lot to absorb. That's why I like to sit in on meetings with the family and the physician and listen closely to all that is said. I'm like another set of ears for the par- ents. Later, once the initial shock of the diagnosis is over and the parents are ready, I can go over the information again with them a little at a time. I've learned over the years that providing infor- mation in small chunks allows the parents to think about the in- formation and ask questions. Psychological support is extremely important at the time of diagnosis, and I try to make sure the family has the necessary tools, resources, and support during this time (Cerqueira, Pereria, & Barbieri-Fegueiredo, 2016).

Initiation of Treatment

The next morning a surgeon comes to Abigail's room to discuss the placement of a **central venous catheter (CVC)** (Fig. 6.5). "The CVC allows chemotherapy to be delivered safely," the sur- geon explains to Lucy and Jack. "Also, all of Abigail's blood work will be drawn from the CVC, so she will no longer have to be stuck with a needle. Abigail is scheduled to have the CVC placed later this morning, so she will not be able to eat any breakfast."

Before Abigail leaves for surgery, the child life specialist, Meg, comes to show her a doll with a CVC so that Abigail will not be scared of the lines when she wakes up from surgery.

"That's brilliant," Lucy tells Jack. They watch as Abigail touches the lines, fascinated.

"It's like a straw coming out of her body," Abigail says.

"That's right," Meg tells her. "You will have special straws, too, so your body can drink in the medicine." Turning to Lucy and Jack, Meg says, "Some children even name their CVC. It helps them cope with their illness." Abigail decides to name her CVC "Sippy."

The CVC placement (Fig. 6.5) goes smoothly. When Abigail is back in her room, Dr. Redman stops by.

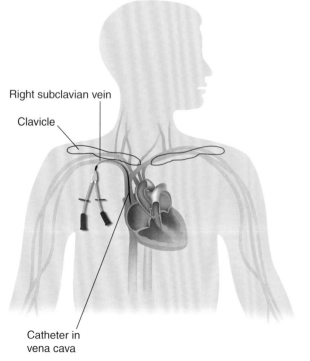

Right subclavian vein

Clavicle

Catheter in vena cava

Figure 6.5. The insertion site for a central venous catheter.

"I'll be writing orders for the chemotherapy to be started tomorrow," she says. Lucy is glad because she knows Norma will be back tomorrow, and she feels comfortable asking her questions about Abigail's treatment.

"The first phase of chemotherapy is the induction phase," Dr. Redman explains. "This phase lasts 4 to 6 weeks. Abigail's response to this phase will be a good indication of her potential for cure. A child who enters complete remission after the induc- tion phase is predicted to have a better chance of being cured" (Cooper & Brown, 2015).

"You mean she'll have to be in the hospital for the next 4 to 6 weeks?" Lucy asks.

"Not the entire time, no," Dr. Redman clarifies. "If she does not have any complications and is stable, she will be discharged in a week to 10 days and the remainder of the treatments can be conducted in the outpatient setting with close follow-up."

"Then what?" Lucy asks, trying to not panic.

"After the induction phase is the consolidation phase, which lasts approximately 6 to 9 months," Dr. Redman says. "The last stage of treatment is the maintenance phase. This phase lasts up to 2 years."

"Two years!" Jack says, distraught at this news. "So, alto- gether, Abigail's treatment will last around 3 years?"

Dr. Redman nods. "I'm sorry. I know this is a lot to take in. Why don't we stop here for now? We can discuss the details about the consolidation and maintenance phases later, when you're ready."

At this moment, Lucy realizes the full impact of Abigail's leuke- mia and treatment. This will be a new way of life for their family.

"Aren't there some natural therapies for the treatment of leuke- mia," Lucy asks, trying to think of any alternative to the news she has just heard. "A friend who practices alternative medicine told me there might be some herbs that could help Abigail" (Box 6.2).

"Many people ask about complementary therapies for cancer treatment," Dr. Redman says. "I do know of some, but I do not recommend any of them during the induction phase. I would be open to discussing them during the consolidation phase, however."

The following morning, Lucy and Jack are glad to see Norma return. "We have many questions about Abigail's chemother- apy," Lucy tells her. "Our biggest concern is about the side effects. She's been through so much in the last few days—a lum- bar puncture, a bone marrow biopsy, and a CVC placement. We just hate to see her go through more."

"I understand how overwhelming everything is right now," Norma says. "One thing I can do that might help is to tell you the names of the medicines before I give them and so that you can write them down and remember them. That way you can

Box 6.2 Complementary Therapy: *Astragalus membranaceus*

In a Taiwanese study conducted by Wang, Liao, Chen, Hsieh, and Li (2016), the researchers found evidence of prolonged overall survival when traditional Chinese medicine (TCM) was added to Western medicine in the treatment of patients with leukemia. The researchers also found that the addition of TCM may help with adverse effects of chemotherapy and provide an improved quality of life.

The most common herb used in pediatric patients diagnosed with leukemia is *A. membranaceus*. This herb increases the white blood cell (WBC) count. The pathophysiology of acute lymphoblastic leukemia involves an increased WBC count, and therefore physicians may be hesitant to have patients take these herbs, fearing they may worsen the leukemia. However, other researchers have determined that *A. membranaceus* increases the number of healthy WBCs and increases the breakdown of the tumor cells. Therefore, *A. membranaceus* should not exacerbate leukemia.

Box 6.3 Side Effects of Chemotherapy

Not all children on chemotherapy experience the same side effects. Similarly, side effects of chemotherapy may be experienced at different levels of severity among different children. The most common side effects are as follows:

- Nausea and vomiting
- Alopecia
- Stomatitis
- Fatigue
- Loss of appetite
- Immunosuppression
- Diarrhea
- Easy bruising

learn what side effects are typically associated with each drug and have some idea of what to expect. The chemotherapy that is ordered for Abigail is strong, because Dr. Redman wants Abigail to be in full remission after the induction phase."

"Every child experiences different side effects of chemotherapy," Norma continues, "and those side effects can range from mild to severe" (Box 6.3). "However, you should be prepared and prepare Abigail for her to lose her hair—a condition called **alopecia**. In addition, Abigail will most likely experience nausea and vomiting. Pediatric patients typically display delayed nausea and vomiting, occurring 24 hours or later after receiving chemotherapy" (Wood, Hall, Hockenberry, & Borinstein, 2015). "She may also develop **stomatitis**, or painful mouth sores that can affect eating. The most concerning side effect, though, is immunosuppression. The chemotherapy works on the immune system to suppress the cancer but in doing so also kills the working components of the bone marrow, WBCs, RBCs, and platelets. Suppression of the immune system could cause Abigail to develop a serious infection, anemia, and problems clotting due to low platelets."

"As for all children on chemotherapy," Norma says, "I'll be carefully monitoring Abigail to detect any complications

early. The effects of the chemotherapy, other than nausea and vomiting, may not appear for several days to weeks later. Also, Dr. Redman will not discharge Abigail until she is stable and you are comfortable with her care."

"I've heard that there are medications that can help with the side effects of chemotherapy," Lucy says. "Could you tell me what they are and whether Abigail will be allowed to have any?"

"Before each treatment with chemotherapy, I will give Abigail medication to help with nausea and vomiting," Norma replies. "She can continue to receive this medication every 8 hours. In addition, Abigail will need to do mouth care every 4 hours to prevent any sores that develop from becoming infected. This involves two medications, one that is swished around the mouth and spat out and one that is swished around the mouth and swallowed" (The Pharmacy 6.1).

"And we'll need your help, Abigail," Norma says after squatting to get on the child's eye level. "You have an important job to do. We'll give you a special sponge on a stick so you can rub the medicine around your mouth all by yourself. Do you think you can handle that?"

Abigail nods eagerly.

"I thought you could," Norma says. "And you know what else? Every time you do your mouth care on time, you will get a sticker. When you have 10 stickers, you may pick a prize out of the prize box in the playroom."

Abigail smiles for the first time all day.

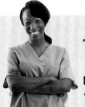

The Nurse's Point of View

Norma: A diagnosis of cancer introduces a "new normal" into a family's life. This new normal includes lengthy hospital stays, multiple outpatient visits, and often overwhelmingly stressful times when the child is very ill. I explain to Jack and Lucy that right now it may not seem possible to get some normalcy and routine back to their life, but for Abigail's and Isabelle's sake that they must try.

Although I encourage parents to participate in their child's care, I also encourage them to remain in the protector role while

collaborating in care (Darcy, Knuttson, Huus, & Inskar, 2014). I tell Jack and Lucy to remain Abigail's parents while learning how to care for her during her treatment. It is important that Abigail be treated like their 4-year-old daughter and not like a patient, especially once the family is discharged home. I encourage them to bring Abigail's sister, Isabelle, for a visit today. Sometimes siblings of children diagnosed with cancer make up what is happening in their heads because they cannot see their sick siblings. Sibling visits can help alleviate fears. I tell them that after Abigail's treatment begins, Isabelle may not be able to visit her if her immune system is suppressed. However, Abigail and Isabelle can communicate over the phone or through video calls.

The Pharmacy 6.1 — Ondansetron, Dexamethasone, Nystatin, and Chlorhexidine Gluconate

Medication	Classification	Route	Action	Nursing Considerations
Ondansetron	• Antiemetic	• PO • IM • IV	• Selective 5-HT$_3$ receptor antagonist • Works in the chemoreceptor trigger zone	• Dosing depends on reason for use • For chemotherapy-induced nausea: 0.15 mg/kg/dose 30 min before treatment, and then every 8 h • Monitor for agitation, anxiety with oral use • Monitor for sedation and drowsiness with IV use
Dexamethasone	• Corticosteroid • Antiemetic • Anti-inflammatory	• PO • IM • IV	• Decreases inflammatory mediators • Long-acting corticosteroid • Suppresses normal immune response • Antiemetic activity is unknown	• For chemotherapy-induced nausea: 10–20 mg 15–30 min before treatment • Prophylaxis for nausea, vomiting 4 mg every 4–6 h
Nystatin	• Antifungal	• PO	• Binds to fungal cell membrane • Changes cell wall permeability	• 400,000–600,000 U 4 times/d • Swish and hold in the mouth for as long as possible before swallowing • May use a mouth sponge to paint the inside of the mouth
Chlorhexidine gluconate	• Antibacterial dental rinse • Prophylactic dental rinse	• PO	• Activity against gram-positive and gram-negative organisms • Bonds to bacterial cell wall • At high concentrations, causes cell death	• Used to prevent oral infections in immunocompromised patients • For immunocompromised patients, use 10–15 mL 2–3 times/d • May cause mouth and teeth discoloration

HT, hydroxytryptamine; IM, intramuscular; IV, intravenous; PO, oral.
Adapted from Taketomo, C. K., Hodding, J. H., & Kraus, D. M. (2018). *Pediatric & neonatal dosage handbook* (25th ed.). Hudson, OH: Lexicomp.

Psychosocial Implications

"Continuing to foster Abigail's development while she is in the hospital is also important," Norma says (Hospital Help 6.1). "Encourage her to continue her play as she would at home, to the extent possible" (Silva & Cabral, 2014). "When Abigail feels like it, and as long as her WBC count is okay, she can go to the playroom to play. When her WBC count is low, a child life specialist can come to Abigail's room, provide toys and books, and engage in play."

"Will Abigail be allowed to have her stuffed animals?" Jack asks. "Abigail likes to play zoo with them. She only has her tiger with her now, which is her favorite, but I think it would cheer her up if she had more of her animals here."

"Absolutely," Norma says. "Feel free to bring her stuffed animals from home. The goal is to keep things as normal as possible and encourage her to play as she would at home."

Complications

One week later, Abigail has finished her first doses of chemotherapy in the induction phase. She is surrounded by her stuffed animals in her room, but her tiger always stays with her in her bed.

Hospital Help 6.1

Gaining Trust

Preschool children are active in imaginative play. This is the time of tea parties and superheroes. Preschool children are also very concrete thinkers, which, coupled with an active imagination, can make hospitalization a very scary time. The nurse should choose words carefully when discussing any tests or procedures with children. For example, telling a 4-y-old, "I am going to take your blood," might lead the child to think that the nurse is literally going to take all of the child's blood.

Gaining trust is important while a preschool child is in the hospital. Allowing the child to have a comfort item helps increase trust in the healthcare team and aids with cooperation from the child. It is important to let the child play with safe medical equipment. Any procedures can be explained using medical equipment and dolls. If the child has his or her own doll or stuffed animal, performing a "procedure" on the stuffed animal first, such as a dressing change, can help alleviate fear in the child.

It is now 2 days after her last dose of chemotherapy, and she is still having trouble with nausea and vomiting and unable to keep much food down. Later that evening Lucy notices that Abigail feels warm and appears flushed. Abigail's nurse today is Tom. He comes in to take her vital signs and reports them as follows:

- Pulse: 124 bpm
- Respiratory rate: 32 breaths/min
- Blood pressure: 94/56 mm Hg
- Temperature: 102.5°F (39.2°C)

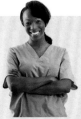

The Nurse's Point of View

Tom: I have a new patient today, Abigail Hanson. I conduct a quick assessment of her before calling Dr. Redman. I want to make sure I have all of the information so I can recommend a plan of action. When I changed her CVC dressing this morning, there was no redness or drainage at the site. Abigail's lungs are clear to auscultation, although she is tachypneic. Her skin is flushed and warm to the touch (Priority Care Concepts 6.1). Her mucous membranes are pink and moist. Her abdomen is soft and nontender. Her lower extremity pulses are weak and thready. Her capillary refill time in the upper extremities is <3 s, but in the lower extremities it is about 4 seconds.

I know I need to intervene quickly so that Abigail's status does not get worse (Vedi et al., 2015). I explain to Abigail's mother, Lucy, that I am going to call Dr. Redman to get some orders for blood work and antibiotics. I tell her that the blood work is to see if Abigail has an infection and the antibiotics are to treat any infection that may be there. She looks anxious, which is understandable.

I call Dr. Redman to get these orders (Box 6.4). She gives me orders for a blood culture and sensitivity, a CBC with differential, and a CMP. She also orders a broad-spectrum antibiotic to be started after the blood cultures are drawn. I carefully read back the orders to make sure they are correct.

Priority Care Concepts 6.1

Preventing Septic Shock

When a child with neutropenia develops fever, it puts him or her at risk of sepsis and septic shock. The nurse is responsible for monitoring the child closely and noticing small changes in status. Timely intervention can prevent progression from infection to shock.

When assessing a child with neutropenia, look for the following changes:

- Flushed skin progressing to mottled and blue skin, indicative of poor capillary refill and poor perfusion
- Warm extremities progressing to cooler and very cool extremities
- Tachycardia progressing to decreased blood pressure
- Tachypnea progressing to shallow breathing
- A sense of not feeling well progressing to tiredness and then severe lethargy

Box 6.4 Using ISBARR

Introduction: "Hi, Dr. Redman. This is Tom on unit A6W."
Situation: "I am taking care of Abigail Hanson. She has developed a fever. Her temperature is 102.5°F."
Background: "Abigail is a 4-y-old recently diagnosed with acute lymphoblastic leukemia. She finished her first round of treatment 2 d ago."
Assessment: "Abigail has a fever and is tachypneic and tachycardic. Her lungs are clear to auscultation bilaterally. Her abdomen is soft and nontender. Her skin is flushed and warm. Her lower extremity pulses are weak and thready, with a capillary refill time >3 s. Her central venous catheter site is without redness or drainage. I believe that Abigail has an infection and is at risk for sepsis."
Recommendation: "I would like to draw blood for cultures, a complete blood count with differential, and a comprehensive metabolic panel. Could I also have an order to begin broad-spectrum intravenous antibiotics after the blood for cultures is drawn?"
Read Back: Tom waits for Dr. Redman's orders. He will repeat them back to her once she is finished.

Tom returns to the room and explains the plan to Lucy. "I'd like to get the antibiotics started as soon as possible so that Abigail does not get sicker." Turning to Abigail, he says, "I'm going to give you some medicines now through your straw to help you feel better, okay?"

"His name is Sippy," Abigail says.

"Oh, okay," Tom says. "Sippy is going to help give you some medicine, then."

"Does my tiger need medicine too?"

"Yes, I think he needs medicine too," Tom replies. "I will make sure he gets some." Although weak, Abigail smiles at Tom.

About an hour later, Tom gets the results of Abigail's blood work and is looking over them intently (Table 6.2). Lucy asks him about the results. He tells her something about calculating Abigail's ANC based on her CBC (Box 6.5).

"What does that mean?" Lucy asks.

Table 6.2 Abigail's CBC Results After the First Round of Treatment

WBC, /µL	1,200
RBC, ×10⁶/µL	4
Hgb, g/dL	9.8
Hct, %	30
Platelets, ×10³/µL	88
Neutrophils—bands, %	4
Neutrophils—segmented, %	20

Hct, hematocrit; Hgb, hemoglobin; RBC, red blood cell; WBC, white blood cell.

Box 6.5 Calculating Absolute Neutrophil Count

$$ANC = \frac{(segs\% + bands\%) \times WBC}{100}$$

$$Abigail's\ ANC = \frac{(20 + 4) \times 1,200}{100} = 288$$

ANC, absolute neutrophil count; bands, neutrophils—bands; segs, neutrophils—segmented; WBC, white blood cell.

"Sorry," Tom says. "Let me try to put that into English for you. ANC stands for **absolute neutrophil count**. Neutrophils are a type of white blood cell. The ANC should be 1,500 or more. Anything less than that is considered neutropenia, meaning not enough neutrophils. An ANC <500 poses a severe risk for bacteremia, or a bacterial infection of the blood" (Hughes & Kahl, 2018).

"So," Lucy says, her voice quavering a bit. "What is Abigail's?"

"It's 288," Tom says.

"What do we do, then?" Lucy says, fighting back tears.

"Abigail should have limited visitors," Tom says. "You and Jack can still be in the room, but Isabelle cannot come to visit. Also, Abigail is not able to have any fresh fruit, vegetables, or flowers in the room. I'll monitor Abigail closely and will get the antibiotics started as soon as they come from pharmacy."

Lucy begins to cry and asks Tom, "Is there anything else we can do?"

"There is a medication called granulocyte colony-stimulating factor, or G-CSF, that stimulates the production of WBCs,"

Tom explains. "Once I get the antibiotics started, I will talk with Dr. Redman about ordering G-CSF" (The Pharmacy 6.2).

After 3 very intense days, Abigail's fever dissipates. Her WBC count comes up to 4,500, with an ANC of 2,200. Norma is back taking care of Abigail. She explains to Jack and Lucy that, because Abigail had such a rough time with the initial round of chemotherapy, Dr. Redman wants to keep Abigail in the hospital at least through the next round of chemotherapy to closely monitor her status.

At Discharge

Abigail tolerates the second treatment much better than the first, which is a big relief to Lucy. After Abigail has spent 3 weeks in the hospital, Dr. Redman is finally ready to discharge her home. Norma arrives and goes over discharge instructions with Lucy and Jack.

"You all have gotten used to the routine of the hospital, so returning home will be very disruptive," Norma says. "Abigail will need to protect her CVC. You should make sure the dressing is dry and intact and cover the dressing when Abigail takes a bath. Unfortunately, she will not be able to swim. One of the most important things to remember is when to call the doctor" (Box 6.6).

The Pharmacy 6.2   Filgrastim

Classification	Route	Action	Nursing Considerations
Granulocyte colony-stimulating factor	• IV • SC	• Stimulates the production, maturation, and activation of neutrophils • Increases neutrophil migration and cytotoxicity • Decreases neutropenia	• IV, SC: 5 µg/d once daily, beginning at least 24 h after chemotherapy • Continue for 14 d or until ANC reaches 10,000 • Monitor CBC with differential, platelet count, and uric acid level • Monitor temperature • Monitor liver function due to increased serum alkaline phosphatase • Monitor for musculoskeletal pain

ANC, absolute neutrophil count; CBC, complete blood count; IV, intravenous; SC, subcutaneous.
Adapted from Taketomo, C. K., Hodding, J. H., & Kraus, D. M. (2018). *Pediatric & neonatal dosage handbook* (25th ed.). Hudson, OH: Lexicomp.

Box 6.6 When to Call the Doctor

Parents of children receiving treatment for acute lymphoblastic leukemia should call the physician when any of the following occurs:

- The child has a temperature of 100.5°F (38.05°C) or greater
- There is any redness, swelling, or drainage around the central venous catheter insertion site
- The child becomes pale, listless, or lethargic
- The child has episodes of vomiting that are not well controlled with medication
- Any time there is a concern

Analyze the Evidence 6.1

Benefits of Having a Home Health Nurse

Caring for a child newly diagnosed with cancer is stressful for parents and any other caregivers of the child. Once a child is discharged home, the family faces many daily challenges. Often families find that although they became familiar with hospital routines, once they are home they are completely overwhelmed and may have a hard time remembering even the simplest of discharge instructions.

Branowicki, Vessey, Temple, and Lulloff (2016) found that having a home health nurse visit shortly after discharge provides comfort to families and makes them "feel safe." A visit from the nurse allows time to review discharge instructions and answer any new questions or unanswered ones families may have had at the time of discharge.

Home health nurses can also participate in care coordination with other members of the child's healthcare team. Overall, visits from home health nurses can lead to better outcomes of children undergoing treatment for cancer.

"Remember to treat Abigail like a normal child," Norma reminds them. "Let her play when she feels like it. Encourage interaction between Abigail and Isabelle. When Abigail is not feeling well, encourage Isabelle to read to her or watch a movie with her."

"Finally," Norma says, "I've arranged for a home health nurse to visit you tomorrow" (Analyze the Evidence 6.1). "Having a nurse visit helps ease fears and address any concerns once you're home. In fact, you may have multiple visits from the home health nurse, if you feel you need it. Do you have any questions?"

"No," Lucy says. "I think we're good."

Jack and Lucy have everything packed up. Abigail is excited that she gets to ride in a wheelchair to her car, her stuffed tiger in her lap. Lucy and Norma, who is pushing Abigail in the wheelchair, go out the main hospital entrance, where Jack is waiting in the car. Abigail gives Norma a hug, and Norma says, I'll see you for your next treatment." Isabelle is in the backseat, anxious for Abigail to get in the car. Lucy buckles Abigail in her booster seat, and the Hanson family heads home.

Think Critically

1. Norma does not discuss the need for O_2 with Abigail's parents. Why would Abigail need O_2?
2. In addition to antiemetics, what can you do to help Abigail cope with the myriad of side effects of chemotherapy?
3. Why does Norma create a sticker chart for Abigail to ensure that she does her mouth care?
4. What would be the course of action if Abigail continues to have trouble with vomiting and nutrition?
5. Besides nurses, physicians, and child life specialists, who else would be a member of Abigail's healthcare team?
6. What are ways in which you can encourage parents to be involved in their child's care?
7. If Abigail were older, such as 8 years old or 15 years old, how could you involve her in her care?

References

American Academy of Pediatrics. (2018). *Car seats: Information for families.* Retrieved from https://www.healthychildren.org/English/safety-prevention/on-the-go/Pages/Car-Safety-Seats-Information-for-Families.aspx

American Academy of Pediatrics, Committee on Injury, Violence, and Poison Prevention. (2011). *Policy statement—Child passenger safety.* Retrieved from www.pediatrics.org/cgi/doi/10.1542/peds.2011-0213. doi:10.1542/peds.2011-0213

Branowicki, P.A., Vessey, J.A., Temple, K.L., & Lulloff, A.J. (2016). Building bridges from hospital to home: Understanding the transition experience for the newly diagnosed pediatric oncology patient. *Journal of Pediatric Oncology Nursing, 33*(5), 370–377.

Cerqueira, C., Pereria, F., & Barbieri-Fegueiredo, M. C. (2016). Patterns of response in parents of children with cancer: An integrative review. *Oncology Nursing Forum, 43*(2), E43–E55.

Cooper, S. L., & Brown, P. A. (2015). Treatment of pediatric acute lymphoblastic leukemia. *Pediatric Clinics of North America, 62*, 61–73.

Darcy, L., Knuttson, S., Huus, K., & Inskar, K. (2014). The everyday life of a young child shortly after receiving a cancer diagnosis, from both the children's and parent's perspective. *Cancer Nursing, 37*(6), 445–456.

Hughes, H. K., & Kahl, L. K. (Eds.). (2018). *The Harriet Lane handbook* (21st ed.). Philadelphia, PA: Elsevier.

National Comprehensive Cancer Network. (2017). *National Comprehensive Cancer Network Guidelines for Patients: Acute Lymphoblastic Leukemia.* Retrieved from https://www.nccn.org/patients/guidelines/content/PDF/all.pdf

Silva, L. F., & Cabral, I. E. (2014). Cancer repercussions on play in children: Implications for nursing care. *Text Context Nursing, Florianopolis, 23*(4), 935–943. doi:10.1590/0104-07072014002380013

Taveras, E. M., Gillman, M. W., Pena, M., Redline, S., & Rifas-Shiman, S. (2014). Chronic sleep curtailment and adiposity. *Pediatrics, 133*(6), 1013–1022.

Vedi, A., Pennington, V., O'Meara, M., Stark, K., Senner, A., Hunstead, P., . . . Cohn, R. J. (2015). Management of fever and neutropenia in children with cancer. *Support Cancer Care, 23*, 2079–2087.

Wang, Y., Liao, C., Chen, H., Hsieh, C., & Li, T. (2016). The effectiveness of traditional Chinese medicine in treating patients with leukemia. *Evidence-Based Complementary and Alternative Medicine*, 1–12. doi:10.1155/2016/8394850

Wood, M., Hall, L., Hockenberry, M., & Borinstein, S. (2015). Improving adherence to evidence-based guidelines for chemotherapy-induced nausea and vomiting. *Journal of Pediatric Oncology Nursing, 32*(4), 195–200.

Suggested Readings

Childhood Leukemia Foundation. (n.d.). *For families.* Retrieved from https://www.clf4kids.org/forfamilies.php

Darcy, L, Knuttson, S., Huus, K, & Inskar, K. (2014). The everyday life of a young child shortly after receiving a cancer diagnosis, from both the children's and parent's perspective. *Cancer Nursing, 37*(6), 445–456.

National Institutes of Health, National Cancer Institute. *Support for families when a child has cancer.* Retrieved from https://www.cancer.gov/about-cancer/coping/caregiver-support/parents

7 Caleb Yoder: Heart Failure

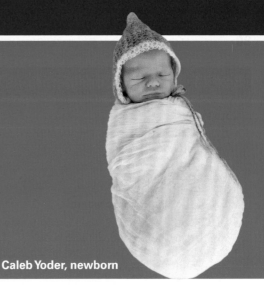

Caleb Yoder, newborn

Objectives

After completing this chapter, you will be able to:

1. Describe normal growth and development of an infant at 1 to 2 months of age.
2. Compare the anatomy and physiology of a normal infant heart with that of an infant heart with a ventricular septal defect.
3. Explain the anatomy and physiology of a ventricular septal defect.
4. Identify signs and symptoms of heart failure in an infant with a congenital heart anomaly.
5. Discuss nursing priorities for a 7-week-old with heart failure.
6. Explain nursing interventions for the care of an infant with a ventricular septal defect.
7. Describe the differences between the Amish culture and mainstream American culture and the impact these differences have on nursing care.

Key Terms

Cardiac output
Heart failure
Pulmonary vascular resistance

Ventricular septal defect (VSD)
Ventricular septum

Background

Caleb Yoder is a newborn boy born to Jacob and Sarah Yoder. The Yoders are Amish and live in a rural area in Pennsylvania. Jacob and Sarah have seven children: four boys and three girls. The oldest, Samuel, is 14 years old. Rebecca is 12 years old, Emma is 10, Elizabeth is 8, Roy is 6, and Eli is 3. The Yoders are part of an Old-Order Amish community of about 350 people. Amish communities are organized around church districts. Each district is governed by a set of rules specific to that particular district. This allows for some diversity and difference in the use of technology, use of modern medicine, dress, and degree of interaction with "the English" (non-Amish people). Typically, the Old-Order Amish do not use public electricity (tapping into public lines to power their homes), do not own computers, televisions, or modern farm equipment, and forbid owning automobiles (Amish Studies, 2019). Furthermore, the Amish forbid the following: education past the eighth grade, divorce, and joining the military (Amish Studies, 2019). The community the Yoders belong to follow these rules.

Caleb was born at home with a midwife present and was considered a full-term birth. Sarah did not have an ultrasound during her pregnancy, but the midwife did well-care visit pregnancy checks in the Yoders' home every 6 weeks. Sarah did not have any concerns or complications throughout her pregnancy. All of her other children were born without health problems. In the Amish community, the majority of families birth their children at home with a midwife or physician present

Box 7.1 Cultural Considerations When Caring for Amish People

Core Values

- Gelassenheit (Gay-la-sen-hite)—yielding oneself to higher authority
- Humility
- Obedience

View of the Healthcare System

- Use modern medical services to some extent; however, they believe God is the ultimate healer
- Do not subscribe to commercial health insurance; may have church aid plans or offerings collected for members who are hit with special or high-cost medical care
- Pay cash for medical expenses
- Are unlikely to seek medical attention for minor illness and injury
- Do not object to surgery and other advanced forms of treatment but rarely use heroic life-saving interventions

Nursing Considerations

- Use of modern technology may be okay but not when it disrupts family and community stability.
- Use home remedies
- Search for natural healing methods such as vitamins, homeopathic remedies, health foods, chiropractors, and natural antidotes rather than modern medicine as a first approach
- No dietary restrictions unless indicated by medical diagnosis
- Preventative health care, screenings, and immunizations are not routine.
- Modesty is part of the Amish culture; allow privacy when the patient is dressing or undressing.

Adapted from Heima, M., Harrison, M. A., & Milgrom, P. (2017). Oral health and medical conditions among Amish children. *Journal of Clinical and Experimental Dentistry, 9*(3), e338.

(Box 7.1; Weyer et al., 2003). Sometimes the first child is born at the hospital and subsequent births take place in the home.

Upon her initial assessment after birth, the midwife auscultated a heart murmur and noticed Caleb was breathing rather fast, oftentimes 80 to 90 times a minute. The midwife also noted Caleb had trouble nursing and seemed to breathe a bit faster when he nursed. Several hours after birth, Caleb continued to breathe 80 to 90 times a minute and was rather sleepy. The midwife began discussing the need for Caleb to be seen by a physician right away because she had concerns about Caleb's heart and lungs. Jacob and Sarah agreed for the doctor to come and see Caleb at their home.

The community to which the Yoders belong has a physician and a nurse practitioner who care for the entire community. The physician, Dr. Smith, makes home visits and also sees the families in his office, located in the next town over, when necessary. The Amish utilize modern medical services to some extent. Although the Amish cite no biblical decree against modern health care, they do believe that God is the ultimate healer (Amish Studies, 2019). Dr. Smith came, assessed Caleb, and explained to the Yoders that he believed Caleb may have a congenital heart defect. However, without the use of an echocardiogram (ECHO) and further evaluation of Caleb's heart, he could not be sure, he told them. Therefore, he recommended that the Yoders take Caleb to the hospital.

At the Hospital

After consulting with the elder community members, the Yoders agree to take Caleb to the nearest children's hospital, which is about 2 hours away. Often, the Amish do not make healthcare decisions on their own. They seek the counsel and advice of family and community (Garrett-Wright, Main, & Jones, 2016). Other barriers to seeking health care include cost of care, time

it takes to receive care, and negative provider attitudes toward the Amish way of life (Garrett-Wright et al., 2016). The Yoders have established trust with Dr. Smith and the providers in his office. Dr. Smith always seeks to understand the core values of the Amish and their use of home and natural remedies instead of more medically advanced forms of treatment. Most Amish prefer using natural and home remedies before seeking professional medical services and sometimes even afterward. In one study, 85% of Amish participants reported healthcare practices that included home remedies, supplements, and herbal products (Sharpnack, Griffin, Benders, & Fitzpatrick, 2010). The Yoders, however, are unsure and certainly not trusting of the hospital setting they are soon to encounter.

Jacob and Sarah seek an English person to drive them to the pediatric hospital. (English people are how Amish often refer to those non-Amish with whom they interact outside the Amish community.) They do not own a car and normally use a horse and buggy as transportation, so using a driver, which is expensive, is really their only option to get their infant to the pediatric hospital, which is so far away. Funds from the family, the community, and the church will pay for the transportation.

Upon arriving at the pediatric hospital, Jacob and Sarah go to the emergency room, as instructed by Dr. Smith, who spoke to the pediatric cardiologist earlier in the day. Jacob and Sarah have left their other children at home, under the care of Samuel and Rebecca (the Yoders' oldest children). Sarah's aunt will come and stay with the older children tonight. Sarah is worried about her children at home as well as about Caleb. She remains quiet during the initial triage, and Jacob does much of the talking. The triage nurse tells them that Caleb is breathing rapidly and that, because he is so young, she will assign him a room and a nurse right away.

The emergency room nurse, Olivia, and physician greet Jacob and Sarah within minutes of them arriving at the treatment room.

Olivia asks Sarah, "How much did Caleb weigh at birth?"

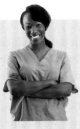

The Nurse's Point of View

Olivia: The Yoders, an Amish couple, just arrived with their newborn, Caleb, who has tachypnea. Their family physician, Dr. Smith, called us while the Yoders were en route to the hospital and told us of his concern about a possible congenital heart defect and of the cultural considerations related to this family. I know I will have to work a little harder than usual to win their trust, as they, like many Amish, tend to mistrust the American healthcare system, according to Dr. Smith. This trust is important for them to continue to bring Caleb for treatment. I take Caleb's vital signs and a brief history while the emergency room physician examines him. I also obtain four extremity blood pressures because a cardiac defect is suspected. Obtaining a blood pressure on all four extremities can provide important information about hemodynamic status as well as assist in ruling out certain cardiac anomalies such as coarctation of the aorta and interruption of the aortic arch (Patankar, Fernandes, Kumar, Manja, & Lakshminrusimha, 2016). Caleb's vital signs are as follows:

- Heart rate: 192 beats/min (bpm) (quiet and resting)
- Respiratory rate: 72 breaths/min
- Temperature: 97.2°F (36.2°C)
- O_2 saturation: 92% to 94% on room air
- Blood pressures:
  - Left arm: 66/32 mm Hg
  - Right arm: 65/28 mm Hg
  - Left leg: 72/40 mm Hg
  - Right leg: 74/42 mm Hg

Although at times his O_2 saturation levels are 92% to 94% and he looks like he is in respiratory distress, I don't give him O_2, because doing so on an infant with certain cardiac anomalies can worsen the infant's symptoms. O_2 dilates the pulmonary vasculature, which lowers **pulmonary vascular resistance**, thus creating pulmonary overcirculation or flooding of the lungs. I observe that Caleb has mild subcostal retractions that worsen when he is upset and crying.

"I don't know," Sarah says. "I'm not sure he was weighed then. He was born in our home, just as all of our other children were.

Olivia weighs Caleb on a special infant scale and measures his length with a length board. Olivia reports that Caleb weighs 5 lb 11 oz (2.58 kg) and is 1.6 ft (19 in) long.

"What did your other children weigh at birth?" Olivia asks.

"They all weighed about 6 or 7 lb (2.7 or 3.2 kg) at birth, as far as I can remember."

The physician comes in and explains the immediate plan of care for Caleb while he is in the emergency room, which includes a chest x-ray, an electrocardiogram (ECG), and an ECHO.

"For now," the physician says to Sarah, "You may nurse Caleb if he is interested in nursing."

"Are all these measures really necessary," asks Jacob. "They seem expensive."

"These are the most cost-effective ways to determine whether Caleb has a congenital anomaly," the physician explains. "And, if for some reason he does not, the exams will aid in determining what is causing his rapid breathing and heart murmur."

The pediatric cardiologist comes to the bedside to perform an ECHO. After a brief look at the heart, vessels, and chambers, the cardiologist explains that he believes Caleb has a **ventricular septal defect** (VSD; Fig. 7.1; Box 7.2). "The VSD appears moderate in size," he tells Jacob and Sarah, "which could explain Caleb's fast breathing, fast heart rate, pale color, and appearance of mild distress when he nurses. The chest x-ray and the ECG are normal at this time. I recommend that Caleb be admitted for further workup and diagnostic studies, as well as assessment of his ability to feed and gain weight."

By this time, Sarah's mother and father and Jacob's mother have arrived at the hospital to assist the Yoders in decision making and to provide support. The Amish family relies on support from family and community and often does not make healthcare decisions alone (Garrett-Wright et al., 2016). Sarah and Jacob look to their parents for advice on what treatment Caleb should have, whether he should be hospitalized, and what measures should be taken to care for Caleb.

After talking with their parents, Sarah and Jacob decide to have Caleb admitted to the cardiac stepdown unit at the pediatric hospital. Stephanie, an experienced pediatric cardiac nurse, admits Caleb to the stepdown unit.

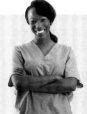

The Nurse's Point of View

Stephanie: I'm admitting Caleb Yoder today, a newborn with suspected VSD. After introducing myself to the parents, I verify his date of birth and his full name with them before placing an identification band on him. I note in the chart that Caleb was weighed in the emergency room and is 5.7 lb (2.58 kg).

Having an accurate weight is important in pediatrics because medications, intravenous fluids, and some treatments are based on weight. I orient Caleb's parents, Jacob and Sarah, to the room and unit. They remain very quiet the whole time and ask few questions while I explain the plan of care.

I inform them that while Caleb is in the hospital, we will be drawing blood to check his electrolyte levels, kidney function, and gas exchange. Also, I explain that the cardiologist will perform a more in-depth ECHO and an exam to determine the degree of Caleb's defect and to make sure his patent ductus arteriosus (PDA) is closing. Closing of the PDA may take a couple of days and is important to monitor when a VSD is present. The ductus arteriosus is the connection between the pulmonary artery and the aorta, which is necessary in utero for blood to bypass the lungs. When a baby is born, the ductus arteriosus closes over the first few days of life. Also, the cardiologist will check to make sure the foramen ovale is closed. If either the ductus arteriosus or the foramen ovale remains open, Caleb could experience decreased cardiac output.

Over the next several days, we monitor Caleb for signs of pulmonary overcirculation and decreased cardiac output.

Each shift, the other nurses and I perform in-depth assessments of his respiratory system and cardiovascular system and pay close attention to his intake and output as well as how well he is nursing. An essential piece of documentation is noting Caleb's tolerance and assessment before and after nursing. We also document whether he stays awake during feedings and what his respiratory rate and heart rate are before, during, and after nursing. This will help us determine whether the VSD is stabilizing and whether Caleb will be able to get enough calories without supplemental feedings, such as tube feedings. We also weigh Caleb daily. Any decrease in weight, other than an initial drop the first few days of life, may indicate Caleb is burning more calories than he is taking in.

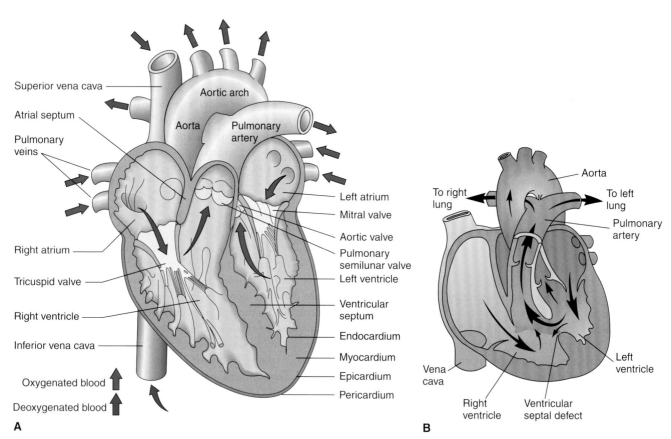

Figure 7.1. Comparison of blood flow in a normal heart and in a heart with a ventricular septal defect (VSD). (A) Blood flow in a normal heart. **(B)** Blood flow in a heart with a VSD. When a VSD is present, blood flows from the area of high pressure (left ventricle) to the area of low pressure (right ventricle), and thus is known as a left-to-right shunt. Oxygenated blood is mixed with unoxygenated blood and flows back through the pulmonary vasculature. (**A**, Reprinted with permission from Willis, M. C. (2002). *Medical terminology: A programmed learning approach to the language of health care*. Baltimore, MD: Lippincott Williams & Wilkins; **B**, Reprinted with permission from Pillitteri, A. (2014). *Maternal and child health nursing* (7th ed., Fig. 41.8). Philadelphia, PA: Lippincott Williams & Wilkins.)

Box 7.2 Ventricular Septal Defect

VSD is one of the most common congenital heart defects. It occurs in almost half of all patients with congenital heart disease (Fulton & Saleeb, 2016). A VSD occurs when there is a hole in the **ventricular septum** (the wall that separates the right and left ventricles). VSDs can occur in various locations on the ventricular septum and can be of varying degrees. The larger the hole, the greater physiological defect. A VSD allows O_2-rich blood to pass from the left ventricle to the right ventricle, where it mixes with O_2-poor blood. VSDs are anatomically defined as small, medium, or large, although there is no universally accepted definition of sizes. Generally, VSDs are considered small when the hole is <4 mm in diameter, moderate when the hole is 4–6 mm, and large when the hole is >6 mm (Fulton & Saleeb, 2016).

Initial goals of treatment while hospitalized for a newly diagnosed VSD include the following:
- Ensuring adequate cardiac output
  - Watch for patent ductus arteriosus to close.
  - Ensure that patent foramen ovale is closed.
  - Provide adequate but not overhydration.
- Reducing pulmonary overcirculation
  - Do not administer O_2 to a baby with normal O_2 saturation levels who is in respiratory distress. O_2 dilates the pulmonary vasculature, which causes lower resistance—therefore, there will be increased pulmonary circulation in an already overcirculated pulmonary system.
- Ensuring nutrition
  - Use high-calorie formula.
  - Provide frequent, small feedings.

After a week of being monitored and assessed and at 7 days of age, Caleb is cleared to be discharged home. Before discharge, Stephanie, who has cared for the Yoders 4 of the 7 days they've been in the hospital, provides discharge teaching to Sarah and Jacob, which includes how to assess Caleb before, during, and after feedings for tolerance to feedings; how to determine if he is getting enough intake (counting wet diapers and stools each day); when to contact the physician; and follow-up care for his diagnosis of a VSD.

"Caleb will need to be seen by the cardiologist to monitor his VSD, **cardiac output**, heart function, and growth," Stephanie explains.

"We are not sure what will happen with Caleb's care," Jacob says. "There will be a meeting of the elders and community to discuss medical costs and funding his care when we arrive back home."

Health Promotion

When Caleb is 4 weeks old, the nurse practitioner, Maria, visits the Yoders' home for Caleb's health checkup. Oftentimes in the Amish community, as long as children appear healthy, visits with the healthcare provider may not be as common as in non-Amish populations. However, since Caleb was discharged from the hospital at 7 days of life and diagnosed with a VSD, the Yoders' healthcare providers have strongly encouraged regular checkups and prompt attention to any health concerns they have with Caleb. Finally, after counsel with their community elders, Sarah and Jacob have reluctantly agreed to have Maria visit and assess Caleb. Maria is curious to assess Caleb's growth and development, particularly his weight gain. Infants with VSDs tire easily with feedings and have a high metabolic demand. Therefore, they may not be able to take in enough calories and may not adequately gain weight.

Maria arrives while Sarah is nursing Caleb. "Oh—I'm sorry to interrupt your feeding," Maria says when she sees that Maria is nursing. "I can wait if you'd like some time to finish."

"No problem," Sarah says. "Please come in and have a seat." Sarah drapes a baby blanket over Caleb as he nurses. She

appreciates Maria's sensitivity. Many Amish women, including some in Sarah's own community, are very modest and won't breastfeed while others are present. It doesn't bother Sarah so much, however, especially because it is a female nurse practitioner.

"What new things has Caleb been showing you?" Maria asks (Growth and Development Check 7.1).

"Caleb is a curious baby when he is feeling good," Sarah says. "Some days he is wide awake and alert, and other days he seems to be more sleepy and tires easily. He turns his head toward me when he hears my voice, as well as toward his siblings and dad when he hears their voices. He startles at loud noises. I've also noticed that his eyes cross at times."

Growth and Development Check 7.1

One-Month-Old Milestones

Gross Motor
- Brings hands within range of eyes and mouth
- Keeps hands in tight fists
- Requires head support; head will flop back if unsupported
- Moves the head side to side when lying on the stomach

Visual and Auditory
- Eyes wander and occasionally cross
- Prefers human face to all other patterns
- Recognizes some sounds
- May turn the head toward familiar sounds and voices
- Hearing is fully mature
- Crying is normal and may increase at 6–8 wk of age.

Smell and Touch
- Prefers sweet smells
- Recognizes smell of own mother's breast milk
- Prefers soft to coarse sensations

"That is normal for a baby at 1 month of age," Maria reassures Sarah. "How is Caleb nursing?"

"I feel like I spend much more time nursing Caleb than I did any of my other children," Sarah says. "In fact, I have barely been able to help with outside chores and gardening because it takes Caleb so long to nurse and he nurses so frequently. There are days when he wants to nurse every hour, and it may take 20 to 40 minutes for him to be finished."

"What concerns do you have regarding caring for Caleb since you have been home from the hospital?" Maria says.

"My only concern is about Caleb growing," Sarah replies. "I believe he is much behind in growth compared with his siblings at this age."

"At 1 month of age, a baby should be nursing or bottle feeding 8 to 12 times a day," Maria explains. "One way to tell whether Caleb is getting enough to eat is by how many wet diapers and bowel movements he is having each day. A typical 1-month-old has five to eight wet diapers a day and up to three to four stools per day."

"Caleb usually has five to six wet diapers per day and one bowel movement," Sarah tells Maria."

"I have a portable scale I bring with me when I make house calls," Maria says. "Would it be okay for me to weigh Caleb?"

"Sure," Sarah says.

As Maria sets up the scale, she asks Sarah, "How much did Caleb weigh when he was discharged from the hospital 3 weeks ago?"

"I think it was 6 lb 4 oz," Sarah replies (or 2.8 kg).

Maria weighs Caleb and measures his length. "Caleb now weighs 6 lb 6 oz," she tells Sarah (or 2.9 kg). "He measures 19.5 in (1.6 ft) in length." Maria looks at some notes she has from Caleb's hospital stay. "It looks like you are correct about Caleb's weight when he was at the hospital. Although Caleb has gained weight, he has not gained much and should be gaining 5 to 7 oz a week."

"I'd also like to talk about vaccinations," Maria says. "At 1 month of age, children who are following the recommended vaccination schedule should receive the second dose of the hepatitis B vaccine. However, Caleb did not receive the first dose at birth. Do you plan to vaccinate Caleb?"

"Most parents in the Amish community, including Jacob and I, have chosen not to vaccinate the children, for many reasons, including the costs and fees, lack of transportation to travel to vaccine clinics, fear of adverse reactions and effects, religious beliefs, and concern regarding the source of the vaccines. None of our other children have received any vaccines."

Maria drops the subject and moves on.

"Let's discuss safety concerns," Maria says (Patient Teaching 7.1). "What are your sleeping arrangements for Caleb?"

"He sleeps in a crib in the same room as Jacob and I," Sarah says.

"Remember to always put Caleb to sleep on his back," Maria says. "And keep any loose articles, including blankets and toys, in the crib or sleep area" (Moon, 2017). "This will help reduce the risk of sudden infant death syndrome, or SIDS" (Moon, 2017).

Patient Teaching 7.1

Safety

- Keep a hand on the baby during diaper changes and when changing the baby's clothes.
- Put the baby to sleep on his or her back.
- Keep soft objects out of the bed.
- Avoid crib bumpers.
- Do not use blankets in the baby's bed.
- Never shake the baby.
- Always check the temperature of bath water before placing the baby in the water.
- Wash your hands frequently.

Adapted from Bright Futures. *Bright futures parent handout: 1 month visit.* Retrieved from https://brightfutures.aap.org/Bright%20Futures%20Documents/A.Inf.PH.1month.pdf

"Hand washing is another important preventive measure," Maria says. "With so many siblings in the house and many community members coming to help out, Caleb is at risk for exposure to many germs and illnesses. Even catching a cold or virus could be especially difficult on Caleb, who already has periods of respiratory distress when feeding."

Maria ends the visit by discussing a plan with Sarah to monitor Caleb's weight gain and growth. "I'm concerned that Caleb is not gaining enough weight," Maria says, "perhaps because of the combination of feeding issues and the increased metabolic demand related to the VSD. One solution would be to supplement with a high-calorie formula."

"I would like to continue to just breastfeed," Sarah says. Sarah knows that formula is expensive and that she would have to discuss it with her husband first.

"I will discuss with Dr. Smith Caleb's current weight and his tachypnea, fatigue, and feeding issues," Maria says. If Dr. Smith needs any further information, he will get in touch with you. I suggest that you weigh Caleb at least twice a week. If he does not gain weight, you should schedule a visit with the pediatric cardiologist."

"I can't weigh him twice a week," Sarah tells Maria, "But I am okay with weighing him once a week, as long as you can make a home visit to weigh him."

"Yes," Maria says. "I can do that."

At Home

Since Caleb's initial hospitalization of 7 days when he was first born, Caleb has been home. However, despite Sarah's best efforts and patience with Caleb when trying to breastfeed, Caleb appears to be having a hard time nursing.

"Caleb just does not seem like he is able to eat," Sarah tells Jacob. "He gets tired easily and falls asleep when nursing. Each day, I hope Caleb will eat better but he just seems to be tired a lot. I've tried giving him a bottle with the high-calorie formula in it—using a sample I was given in the hospital—but he will not take a bottle and cries to nurse. I don't know what to do."

Jacob listens intently but says nothing.

Sarah's aunt visits daily to help the family with meals and home making. Today she says, "Caleb seems small, like he is not growing. I think he is not gaining weight."

"Caleb will be okay," Sarah replies. "I just need to continue to feed him frequently and pray that he will start growing soon."

Maria, the nurse practitioner, has visited once a week beginning when Caleb was 4 weeks of age. Sarah, who has been tracking Caleb's weight over the past few weeks, notices when reviewing her handwritten log that his weight has stayed essentially the same: Week 4, 2.83 kg; Week 5, 2.92 kg; and Week 6, 2.94 kg. Sarah has learned from Maria that, normally, a baby gains about 1 to 1½ lb (0.45–0.68 kg)/month or 5 to 7 oz/week. A healthy baby should grow 1 to 1½ in (2.54–3.81 cm) in length per month, as well. Although Caleb is gaining weight, he is well below an average infant in gaining weight and length. However, Sarah and Jacob insist on continuing to work on feeding and growing and do not want any further interventions or visits at this time.

Physician's Visit to the Yoders' Home

At about 6 weeks of age, Caleb begins having much more difficulty with nursing. Sarah notices that Caleb only sucks for a few seconds at a time and then pull his head away. But he always seems hungry. He also falls asleep very easily when nursing. Sarah also notices that Caleb is breathing really fast. As she was taught before Caleb was discharged from the hospital, she counts Caleb's respirations. He is breathing 90 times a minute. Sarah also notices that Caleb sounds very congested when he trying to nurse. She wonders whether this is the "wet" sound the nurse was describing during the teaching before being discharged from the hospital. Also, Sarah notices that Caleb sweats a lot, soaking through his clothes when he is feeding.

Sarah' aunt is over at their home helping with the other children. When she sees Caleb, she tells Sarah, "You need to call the physician. Caleb looks really pale and sick."

Sarah's aunt sends her teenaged son to the next town to ask Dr. Smith to visit. Dr. Smith agrees to come to the Yoders' home. After examining Caleb, he tells Sarah and Jacob, "You should take Caleb to the hospital now. I'm concerned that he has **heart failure**."

Later, Dr. Smith sends Sarah and Jacob word that he has called the children's hospital where Caleb was admitted at birth and spoken with the cardiologist who cared for Caleb, Dr. Stenson. He tells them that Dr. Stenson has requested that Caleb be admitted as soon as possible for further assessment.

Back to the Hospital

Hiring the same English driver who drove the Yoders to the hospital for the previous admission, Sarah and Jacob take Caleb back to the pediatric hospital, which is about 2 hours away from the Amish community where they live. Caleb is directly admitted to the cardiac stepdown unit. Dr. Smith has contacted Dr. Stenson directly regarding Caleb's current respiratory and cardiovascular status. Fortunately, one of the nurses who cared for Caleb during his first admission, Stephanie, is his nurse again.

Stephanie arrives at Caleb's room, greets Jacob and Sarah, and tells them she remembers them from their previous admission. This gives Sarah a bit of hope that someone knows Caleb.

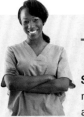

The Nurse's Point of View

Stephanie: Caleb Yoder has returned. I remember caring for him and his parents about a month ago, just after he was born. I learned a lot then about caring for Amish children and families and about their cultural practices. They are dressed today much like they were a month ago. Sarah is dressed in plain and simple clothes consisting of a three-piece dress, a cape, and an apron, and always wears a prayer cap. Jacob wears an Amish-style hat and vest. I learned last time that married Amish men are to grow a beard but not a mustache.

I weigh and measure Caleb upon arrival before getting his vital signs. Although he appears to be in mild respiratory distress, I quickly obtain a weight so the physician can begin writing orders. His weight is 6.39 lb (2.9 kg), and his length is 19.5 in. I explain to Sarah and Jacob that Caleb will need to be on continuous ECG and pulse oximetry monitoring. I attach the leads and look up to find that Caleb's rhythm is sinus tachycardia with a rate of 200 bpm. I auscultate his apical pulse and confirm that the rate is truly 200 bpm. His brachial pulses, while palpable, are not as strong as a normal infant's pulses. His capillary refill time is 2 to 3 seconds, and his hands and feet are cool to the touch. I notice that he is lethargic but can be aroused with gentle stimulation. Having cared for many infants with a VSD of moderate severity, I think Caleb may be in heart failure.

I anticipate that admission orders will include laboratory tests such as a basic metabolic panel (BMP), a brain natriuretic peptide (BNP) test, liver function tests, and, depending on the severity of his diagnosis, an arterial blood gas test. If Caleb's cardiac output is low, the blood gas test may reveal a state of acidosis. The BMP and liver function tests will help determine whether there is end-organ perfusion and even damage. When cardiac output falls, the kidneys and liver do not receive adequate blood flow and can become hypoxic and incur ischemic damage. The BNP test is usually used for determining the severity of heart failure. BNP is released in response to changes in pressure in the heart. BNP levels are high in patients with heart failure. I also anticipate orders for a diuretic such as furosemide and other cardiac medications such as digoxin to help control Caleb's heart rate and provide inotropy (The Pharmacy 7.1). I explain these laboratory tests and medications in simple terms to Sarah and Jacob without using medical jargon.

The Pharmacy 7.1			Cardiac Medications	
Medication	**Classification**	**Route**	**Action**	**Nursing Considerations**
Furosemide (Lasix)	Loop diuretic	• PO • IV	Inhibits reabsorption of sodium and chloride from the proximal and distal tubules and ascending loop of Henle, resulting in sodium-rich diuresis	• Monitor urine output following administration • Monitor potassium; may require potassium replacement • Perform daily weights • Monitor for orthostatic hypotension
Digoxin	Cardiac glycoside	• PO • IV	• Positive inotropic effect (increases force of myocardial contractions) • Increases renal perfusion • Negative chronotropic effect (decreases heart rate)	• Dosing in pediatrics is in µg/kg. • Monitor apical pulse for 1 min before administration; hold the dose if the pulse is <90 bpm in an infant • Avoid giving with meals
Enalapril	• ACE inhibitor • Anti-hypertensive	• PO • IV	• Blocks the conversion of angiotensin I to angiotensin II, which decreases blood pressure, decreases aldosterone secretion, slightly increases potassium, and causes sodium and fluid loss • In heart failure, also decreases peripheral resistance, afterload, preload, and heart size	• Monitor blood pressure for hypotension • May interact with OTC medications; have patient check with provider before taking any OTC medications • Adverse effects include cough, nausea, diarrhea, headache, and dizziness
Metoprolol (Lopressor) and carvedilol (Coreg)	Beta-1 selective adrenergic blocker	• PO • IV	• Blocks beta-adrenergic receptors in the heart and juxtaglomerular apparatus, which decreases the influence of the sympathetic nervous system on these tissues • Decreases the excitability of the heart, which decreases cardiac output and release of renin, which in turn lowers blood pressure	• Check apical pulse before administration; if <90 bpm, do not administer medication; consult the provider • Monitor blood pressure before administration • Be aware of the difference between the immediate- and extended-release forms of metoprolol; the extended-release form should not be crushed or chewed

ACE, angiotensin-converting enzyme; IV, intravenous; OTC, over-the-counter; PO, by mouth.

Adapted from Taketomo, C. K., Hodding, J. H., & Kraus, D. M. (2018). *Pediatric & neonatal dosage handbook* (25th ed.). Hudson, OH: Lexicomp.

Within an hour of Caleb being admitted, the cardiologist, Dr. Stenson, and the ECHO technician are at Caleb's bedside to perform an ECHO.

"An ECHO will show if Caleb is experiencing pulmonary overcirculation, right ventricle enlargement, and even if the right atrium has been affected," Dr. Stenson explains. "An in-depth look at the VSD will be obtained with the ECHO,

as well. Immediately before the ECHO, we'll obtain a portable chest x-ray to assess for pulmonary congestion." Dr. Stenson moves on without stopping to explain further.

While Caleb is undergoing the tests, Stephanie explains in simpler terms to Sarah and Jacob what is going on. She also explains about how heart failure can occur throughout the lifespan, but that the causes are different in children and adults (Let's Compare 7.1).

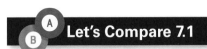

Let's Compare 7.1

Etiology of Heart Failure in Infants, Children, and Adults

Infants
- First week of life:
  - Coarctation of the aorta
  - Interrupted aortic arch
  - Total anomalous pulmonary venous connection
  - Adrenal insufficiency
  - Enzyme deficiency
  - Thyrotoxicosis
- From the 2nd week of life through infancy:
  - VSD (most common reason)
  - Atrial septal defect
  - Atrioventricular malformations
  - Patent ductus arteriosus

Children
- Endocarditis
- Myocarditis
- Kawasaki disease
- Rheumatic fever
- Anemia

Adults
- Myocardial infarction
- Hypertension
- Valve disorders
- Coronary artery disease
- Cardiomyopathy
- Infections
- Cardiac arrhythmias
- Other risk factors: thyroid disease, obesity, and diabetes

"Signs and symptoms of heart failure are a result of the heart attempting to compensate for the low cardiac output that ensues as the heart works harder and harder to pump," Stephanie says. "Caleb is experiencing many of these symptoms. His respiratory rate is often 70 to 80 breaths/min, and he occasionally coughs. At rest, his breathing is mildly labored with subcostal and suprasternal retractions. Although his heart rate is 190 to 200 bpm at rest, his blood pressure is within normal limits for his age. I'll be monitoring this closely, particularly if Caleb is given a diuretic."

Stephanie reviews the results of his chest x-ray with Sarah and Caleb and informs them that the radiologist has noted mild cardiomegaly. Stephanie says that Caleb has not gained an adequate amount of weight. Sarah tells Stephanie of Caleb's fatigue and sweating with feeding (Box 7.3).

As Jacob and Sarah are getting settled into the hospital, Dr. Stenson and a nurse practitioner come to explain the laboratory test, ECHO, and x-ray results to Jacob and Sarah as well as discuss a plan of care. For the immediate time period, interventions will be geared toward treating Caleb's heart failure. Once the heart failure is successfully treated, they explain, Caleb will need surgery to correct his VSD. Caleb will be hospitalized until he is stable enough for surgery. The surgery will consist of closing the VSD. Ultimately, closing the defect will redirect blood flow so that blood flows.

Sarah and Jacob remain quiet as they take in all the information. Sarah thinks about the decisions they will have to make regarding care for Caleb and how much they will rely on the community to come together to help them during this time.

Box 7.3 Signs and Symptoms of Heart Failure in an Infant

Respiratory
- Tachypnea
- Labored breathing
- Grunting
- Mild subcostal retractions
- Coughing
- Wheeze
- Crackles or rales in all fields (in severe heart failure)

Cardiac
- Tachycardia
- Hypotension
- Cardiomegaly
- Pulsus alternans (severe heart failure)
- Pulsus paradoxus (severe heart failure)

Neurologic
- Sleepy
- Fatigue

Gastrointestinal/Genitourinary
- Poor feeding
- Failure to gain weight
- Hepatomegaly

Skin
- Sweaty during feedings
- Pallor
- Cool hands and feet

Think Critically

1. What are some cultural considerations the nurse must incorporate when providing care for Caleb and his family?
2. Why is it so important to monitor Caleb's weight during the home visits and while Caleb is hospitalized?
3. What is the primary physiological problem associated with a VSD?
4. Discuss the two priority nursing assessments when monitoring a child with a VSD.
5. Differentiate the causes of heart failure in infants compared with adults.

References

Amish Studies. (2019). *The young center*. Retrieved from https://groups.etown.edu/amishstudies/

Fulton, D, & Saleeb, S. (2016). *Pathophysiology and clinical features of isolated ventricular septal defects in infants and children*. UpToDate. Retrieved from www.uptodate.com

Garrett-Wright, D., Main, M. E., & Jones, M. S. (2016). Anabaptist community members' perceptions and preferences related to healthcare. *Journal of Amish and Plain Anabaptist Studies, 4*(2), 187–200.

healthychildren.org. (2017). *Developmental milestones: 1 month*. Retrieved from: https://www.healthychildren.org/English/ages-stages/baby/Pages/Developmental-Milestones-1-Month.aspx

Heima, M., Harrison, M., & Milgrom, P. (2017). Oral health and medical conditions among Amish children. *Journal of Clinical and Experimental Dentistry, 9*(3), e338.

Moon, R. (2017). *How to keep your sleeping baby safe: AAP policy explained*. Retrieved from https://www.healthychildren.org/English/ages-stages/baby/sleep/Pages/A-Parents-Guide-to-Safe-Sleep.aspx

Nursing 322 Spring (2010). *The American Amish*. Retrieved from https://nursing322sp10.wordpress.com/the-american-amish/

Patankar, N., Fernandes, N., Kumar, K., Manja, V., & Lakshminrusimha, S. (2016). Does measurement of four limb blood pressures at birth improve detection of aortic arch anomalies? *Journal of Perinatology, 36*(5), 376–380. doi:10.1038/jp.2015.203

Sharpnack, P., Griffin, M., Benders, A., & Fitzpatrick, J. (2010). Spiritual and alternative healthcare practices of the Amish. *Holistic Nursing Practice, 24*(2), 64–72. doi:10.1097/HNP.0b013e3181d39ade

Weyer, S., Hustey, V., Rathbun, L., Armstrong, V., Anna, S., Ronyak, J., & Savrin, C. (2003). A look into the Amish culture: what should we learn? *Journal of Transcultural Nursing, 14*(139), 139–145. doi:10.1177/1043659602250639

Suggested Readings

Cincinnati Children's (2016). *Congestive heart failure*. Retrieved from https://www.cincinnatichildrens.org/health/c/chf

healthychildren.org. (2017). *Developmental milestones: 1 month*. Retrieved from https://www.healthychildren.org/English/ages-stages/baby/Pages/Developmental-Milestones-1-Month.aspx

Louden, M., Seroogy, C., Peterson, J., & Spicer, G. (2014). *Plain talk about providing health care to plain communities*. Retrieved from https://geneticsinwisc.wiscweb.wisc.edu/wp-content/uploads/sites/111/2017/03/ProvidingHealthCare_PlainCommunities.pdf

Madriago, E., & Silberbach, M. (2010). Heart failure in infants and children. *Pediatrics in Review, 1*(31), 4–10.

8 Andrew Hocktochee: Failure to Thrive

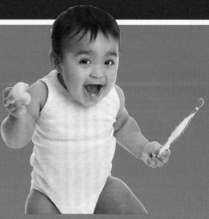

Andrew Hocktochee, age 6 months

Objectives

After completing this chapter, you will be able to:

1. Describe normal growth and development of the 6-month-old.
2. Discuss an appropriate teaching plan for a healthy 6-month-old.
3. Identify signs of developmental delay.
4. Explain the difference between organic and nonorganic failure to thrive.
5. Describe signs and symptoms of failure to thrive in infants.
6. Relate caloric needs to treatment of failure to thrive.
7. Discuss aspects of culture that are important to consider when providing health care to an American Indian patient.
8. Create a nursing plan of care for an infant with failure to thrive.

Key Terms

Galactagogues
Medicine Man
Navajo Nation

Nonorganic failure to thrive
Organic failure to thrive
Weight faltering

Background

Andrew Hocktochee is a 6-month-old American Indian male who lives on a reservation in the **Navajo Nation** with his family. His family consists of his mother, Dezba, his father, Sani, his three siblings, and his grandmother. Andrew's older brother, Caleb, is 5 years old and is starting kindergarten soon. He also has two sisters, Taylor, who is 4 years old, and Sarah, who is 2 years old. Andrew's maternal grandmother, Yanaha, has lived with the family for the past 4 years and ensures that the children are taught the ways of the Navajo tribe.

The Hocktochee family lives in a two-bedroom home on the same reservation the family has lived on for multiple generations. Although Andrew's parents have names that represent their Navajo heritage, both Dezba and Sani felt they wanted their children to be able to feel more comfortable around others

of a different culture. Besides, they will carry the Hocktochee name by which to remember their heritage.

Both Sani and Dezba have a high school diploma, but neither pursued higher education. Sani is currently unemployed, but has an interview with the Navajo City Transit for a position as a bus driver. He has had a difficult time keeping a job because of his lack of transportation. The family owns one vehicle, a small pickup truck that is unreliable. Fortunately, Sani's brother has a working vehicle and has offered for Sani to use it to get to both his interview and to work should he get the job. Sani's hope is that he will get the job and save money to buy a reliable vehicle for his family. Dezba stays at home with the children during the week. On weekends she works as a waitress at the local diner. Her mother, Yanaha, helps with the children when Dezba is working. Things have been difficult for the Hocktochee family with Sani out of work.

Andrew was born at 38 weeks of gestation at one of the hospitals run by the Navajo Area Indian Health Service. Labor and delivery was uncomplicated. Andrew weighed 7 lb, or 3.2 kg, at birth, which put him in the 25th percentile for his weight. Andrew's length, 1.9 ft (19 in), was also at the 25th percentile. He was the smallest of all of his siblings at birth, but the doctor reassured Dezba that Andrew's was a healthy weight. Dezba and Andrew stayed in the hospital overnight and were discharged 24 hours after delivery. Dezba is exclusively breastfeeding Andrew, as she did with all of her other children.

Although Andrew was born in a hospital, Dezba and Sani do not interact much with the traditional medical system. They have health insurance through the government because someone came to the reservation and encouraged them to sign up. However, the nearest clinic is 45 minutes away, which was not even addressed when the family was encouraged to sign up for the insurance. Without a reliable vehicle, it is very difficult for the family to go to any regular doctor's visits. Therefore, Dezba and Sani visit the tribe's **Medicine Man** when needed. He generally has an herbal remedy or tea that helps with any of the family's illnesses (Goss et al., 2017; Kessler, Hopkins, Torres, & Prasad, 2015; Portman & Garrett, 2006).

With regard to health, Yanaha insists that her family participate in the traditional ceremonies and healing rituals of the Navajo tribe. She imparts her wisdom regarding ancient beliefs that to live a balanced and healthy life, one must have a relationship with Mother Earth, the tribal community, the surrounding environment, and one's self. An unbalanced relationship with any of the four constructs leads to illness and distress (Goss et al., 2017; Kessler et al., 2015; Portman & Garrett, 2006). Yanaha does not trust traditional doctors. She feels that doctors practicing traditional medicine do not understand the healing practices of her tribe. When needed, Yanaha prefers to go to her tribe's Medicine Man for more traditional healing practices. She has instilled this practice of healing within her family, along with the distrust of traditional doctors.

Health Promotion

Despite Dezba's distrust of traditional medicine, she knows she needs to get her children to the clinic for a visit. She does get her children vaccinated, because she does not want to them to acquire a serious illness. She tells Sani, "I know that the doctors can help keep the kids healthy. I just wish they understood our culture more and would work with us to let us practice our ways along with theirs."

Sani nods his head in understanding. "I know what you are saying. If your mother had her way, the kids would never see a traditional doctor. I do agree, though, that we want to keep them healthy. Is it time for them to go for a visit? I can see if my brother's truck is available."

Dezba replies, "I know Andrew is overdue for a visit. I have only taken him to the clinic once since he was born. He seems to be doing okay but has been really fussy lately, and I don't know why. He is just so skinny, not like the others."

There are several barriers to actually getting to the clinic for the Hocktochee's. The closest clinic is 45 minutes away. In that clinic, pediatric care is only available on the fourth Monday of the month. Currently, that is 10 days away. If Sani gets his job and is working that day, Dezba will only be able to get the kids to the clinic if their truck decides to start. She could take them to another clinic, which offers pediatric care every day, but that clinic is almost 2 hours away.

Dezba decides to wait the 10 days to go to the closest clinic and hopes that transportation will be available on that day. In the meantime, Andrew continues to be fussy. Dezba is breastfeeding him multiple times a day and two or three times during the night. She has no idea why he is so fussy; she does not remember any of her other children being like this.

On the day before going to the clinic, Andrew is particularly inconsolable. Yanaha looks at Dezba and tells her, "He needs to eat more; feed him more often. Babies are supposed to be fat. He is too skinny."

Dezba listens to her mother and breastfeeds him more often that day. She thinks her mother is probably right, he needs to be fed more. However, it is difficult to breastfeed more often than she already is, with the three other children to take care of. Dezba does the best she can. In her culture, daughters listen to their mothers when it comes to child rearing and feeding practices (Eckhardt et al., 2014). In fact, she did not give her other children anything other than breast milk for the first 9 months of their lives based on her mother's advice. They are all happy and healthy, so her mother must be right.

The next day, Dezba gets all of the children ready to go to the clinic. Sani ended up getting the job with the Navajo Transit, so he has his brother's vehicle. Luckily, the pickup truck starts, and Dezba piles the four kids in the backseat, with Andrew on Caleb's lap. After the 45-minute drive, the family arrives at the clinic and discovers that the waiting room is extremely crowded. The receptionist explains to Dezba, "The nurses and doctors in the clinic are backed up. Have a seat. A nurse will come to get you when there is an opening. You will be seen today, but you may have to wait a while."

Dezba does as she is told and sits in the waiting room with her children. After about an hour, one of the nurses comes to the waiting room and calls for the Hocktochee family. Dezba, carrying Andrew, and the rest of the children follow the nurse to a room, where they are weighed. Andrew is starting to become agitated and fussy.

Dezba says, "May I feed him now?"

"Let me weigh him and get you into a room first; then you can nurse him," the nurse responds. In addition to Andrew being fussy, the 2-year-old, Sarah, is tired and extremely whiny because it is her nap time.

Dezba tells the nurse, "The children are getting fussy, and I don't want to be here very long. I should have left the older children at home with my mother."

The nurse reviews the charts and says, "Mrs. Hocktochee, it looks as if they are all due for a checkup. It might be best if they are all seen."

"Do any of them need shots besides Andrew?"

"Hmmm, let me see." The nurse refers to the charts. "It looks like Taylor needs her 4-year-old shots."

"I really am going to have to do that another time," says Dezba. "We have been here for a while, and the children are all getting irritable. I am mostly concerned about Andrew. He is so fussy lately. I will bring the others back another time."

The nurse glances at the other children. Dezba can tell she is concerned. She tells Dezba, "We will only see Andrew today, but the other children are behind on their checkups, so you will need to bring them back when we have the pediatric clinic again next month."

Dezba nods, but she is irritated. That nurse has no idea how difficult it is for her to get here.

The nurse takes Andrew's temperature, counts his pulse, and counts his respirations. "All of his vital signs are normal," the nurse indicates. Next, she weighs Andrew on an infant scale (Fig. 8.1). She has Dezba take off his clothes and diaper before she weighs him. Today Andrew weighs 13 lb 1 oz, or 5.9 kg. He is 25 in (63.5 cm) long. The nurse tells Dezba to put Andrew's diaper back on but leave his clothes off and escorts them to the clinic exam room.

A little while later, a young woman enters the room. "Hello, my name is Mary. I am the nurse practitioner seeing Andrew today." Noticing that the other children in the room seem unhappy to be there, especially the toddler, she pokes her head out the door and says to the medical assistant, "Would you please bring some blank paper and crayons to room three?"

The medical assistant returns with a few crayons, some paper, and even an old coloring book that still has some pages not colored. She hands these to Caleb, Taylor, and Sarah, and they seem satisfied to have something to do and somewhat calm down.

"Thank you," Dezba says to Mary. "They have been waiting a long time."

"I know, and I apologize for that. We had someone call in sick this morning, so we have been behind all day. What brings you to the clinic today?"

"I know that my children are behind on their visits. I have only brought Andrew once since he was born, so I thought it most important that he come to get his shots," explains Dezba.

Mary looks at the medical records for the other children and says, "It looks like the other children are due for checkups, as well. If you would like, I could examine them now, too."

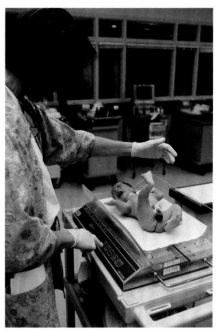

Figure 8.1. An infant being weighed lying down on an infant scale. Reprinted with permission from Jensen, S. (2018). *Nursing health assessment: A best practice approach* (3rd ed., Fig. 26.4). Philadelphia, PA: Wolters Kluwer.

Dezba responds, somewhat irritated, "I explained to the nurse that we have been here a long time today. I cannot handle having all four children here longer than need be today. I am not concerned about any of the children, other than Andrew. Please do his checkup and I will try to bring the other children back at another time."

"I understand," Mary says. "It's exhausting for both you and your children to have to wait so long. Normally, we are not this backed up. I apologize again for your wait." She looks over Andrew's chart again. "What are your concerns about Andrew?"

"Andrew is fussy all of the time lately. I don't know what to do. He is never happy; he won't smile or play with the other children. He is also so skinny. None of my other children were this way; they were all nice and fat, like babies are supposed to be."

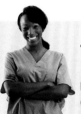

The Nurse's Point of View

Mary: I'm doing a well-care checkup for a 6-month-old, Andrew, today. His mother, Dezba, is concerned about his constant fussiness and lack of weight gain. I look him over as he sits in Dezba's lap. He is extremely thin. I look in his health record at his weight history. The last weight recorded for Andrew was at 3 months of age, the only time he has been seen at the clinic before today. At 3 months old, Andrew weighed 12 lb, or 5.4 kg. Today, Andrew weighs 13 lb 1 oz. Wow. Andrew has only gained 1 lb (0.4 kg) in 3 months (Growth and Development Check 8.1). This is not good. I try to maintain my composure in front of his mother, but I'm really concerned.

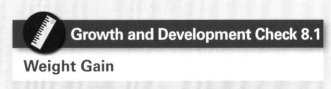

Growth and Development Check 8.1

Weight Gain

Age	Rate of Increase in Weight (oz/wk)
Newborn to 6 mo	5–7
6–12 mo	3–5

Note: Infants typically double their birth weight by 6 mo of age and triple their birth weight by 1 y of age.

Before I go any further, I plot Andrew's weights on a growth chart (Fig. 8.2). I pull out a paper chart, because this clinic does not have electronic medical records. There are three recorded weights for Andrew: his weights at birth, 3 months, and today. At birth he weighed 7 lb, which put him in the 25th percentile for weight. His weight at 3 months old (12 lb) put him in the 25th percentile again. His weight today (13 lb 1 oz) puts him below the 3rd percentile, which disturbs me. His length, however, still remains at the 25th percentile. What could be causing this lack of weight gain? I need to investigate further.

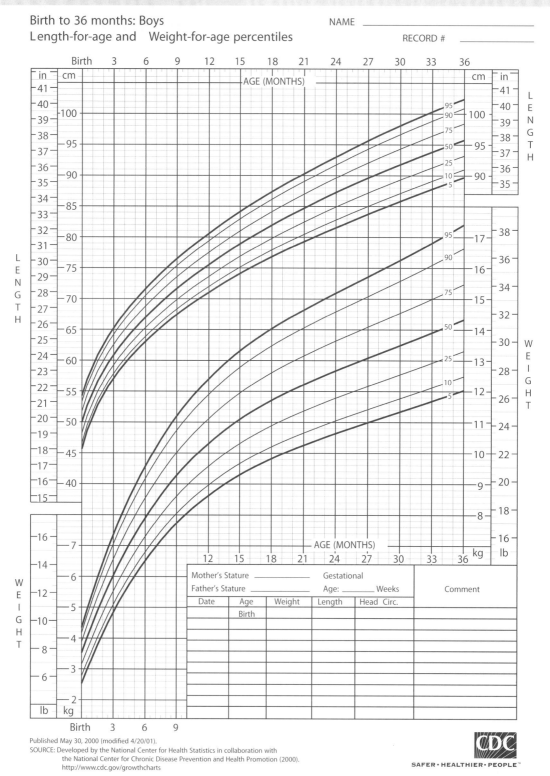

Birth to 36 months: Boys
Length-for-age and Weight-for-age percentiles

NAME _____

RECORD # _____

Published May 30, 2000 (modified 4/20/01).
SOURCE: Developed by the National Center for Health Statistics in collaboration with
the National Center for Chronic Disease Prevention and Health Promotion (2000).
http://www.cdc.gov/growthcharts

Figure 8.2. Growth chart for boys from birth to 36 months old, including length-for-age and weight-for-age percentiles.
Developed by the National Center for Health Statistics in collaboration with the National Center for Chronic Disease Prevention and Health Promotion (2000). Retrieved from http://www.cdc.gov/growthcharts

"What does Andrew usually eat?" Mary says.

"I'm breastfeeding him as much as I can," Dezba quickly explains. "My mother told me that he is too skinny, so I am trying to breastfeed him more, but it is hard with the other children to take care of."

"Is he eating any solid food?" Mary asks.

"Oh no, not yet. I don't feed my babies any food other than breast milk until they are 9 months old. This is what my mother taught me to do. My other children were fine with this," Dezba states emphatically.

"Okay," Mary responds. "Does he seem satisfied after he nurses, or does he seem hungry?"

"If he still seems hungry, I just let him nurse longer."

"Does Andrew ever seem to choke, or gag, when he is nursing?" Mary says.

"He doesn't seem to have any trouble at all. In fact, he nurses vigorously and he doesn't even spit up," Dezba replies.

Mary pauses, puts down her pen, and looks Dezba in the eye. "How are you doing having four children at home?" Mary asks.

"My mother is home to help me, although it is very busy. My husband, Sani, had been out of work for several months, so we had to start using food stamps."

"Are you getting enough to eat and drink?" Mary continues. "You need to make sure you are taking care of yourself so that you make enough breast milk for Andrew."

"I do my best," Dezba replies wearily. She is starting to feel like Mary is accusing her of not providing for her children. "Sometimes I do forget to eat, though, because I am so busy taking care of everyone else."

Mary picks up her pen again and says, "Let's talk about growth and development milestones (Growth and Development Check 8.2). What is Andrew able to do now? Is he laughing and cooing? Is he sitting up yet?"

"Andrew is rolling over both ways, but he is not sitting up yet; he really isn't able to sit long against pillows. Is he supposed to be? I don't remember." Dezba begins to get worried. Why is Mary asking all of these questions? She takes good care of her children. Maybe her mother is right. Maybe they can't trust traditional doctors.

"Andrew should be able to sit with support by now," Mary says, "meaning that he may not be able to sit completely by himself, but he should be sitting by supporting himself with his arms. This is called tripod sitting" (Fig. 8.3).

Mary continues, "Is Andrew laughing and smiling, reaching for toys, or babbling?"

Dezba, getting more and more irritated, states, "Andrew is fussy all of the time, he does not laugh, he only whines. I do not hear him making any other sounds. He doesn't seem interested in toys, either."

Growth and Development Check 8.2

Infant Milestones

Type of Development	Development Milestones at 6 Mo
Social and emotional	• Begins to differentiate strangers from people the infant recognizes • Enjoys looking at mirrors • Likes to play with others • Responds to own name • Is generally happy
Speech	• Babbles by stringing vowels together • Imitates sounds made by parents • Begins to say consonants such as "b" and "d"
Cognitive	• Explores with hands and mouth • Reaches for toys and other objects • Is interested in things around himself or herself
Gross and fine motor	• Is able to roll back and forth • Sits with the support of the hands (tripod sitting) • Supports the full weight on legs when held upright • Grasps food with the whole hand • Is able to move objects from one hand to the other

Adapted from the Centers for Disease Control and Prevention (2016, August 15). *Developmental milestones.* Retrieved from https://www.cdc.gov/ncbddd/actearly/milestones/milestones-6mo.html

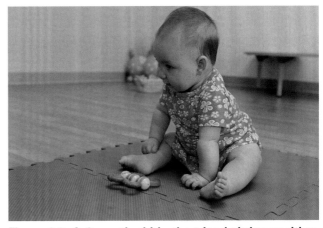

Figure 8.3. A 6-month-old in the tripod sitting position. Reprinted with permission from Kyle, T., & Carman, S. (2013). *Essentials of pediatric nursing* (2nd ed., Fig. 3.6B). Philadelphia, PA: Wolters Kluwer Health/Lippincott Williams & Wilkins.

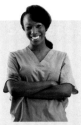

The Nurse's Point of View

Mary: In interviewing Andrew's mother, I was able to shed a little more light on possible causes of his lack of weight gain. He's not choking or gagging while nursing, which means he is not likely to have a swallowing disorder, something that can often lead to decreased weight gain (Romano, Hartman, Privitera, Cardile, & Shamir, 2015). I'm thinking that Andrew may not be getting enough nutrition. Breastfeeding exclusively at 6 months old is okay if the baby is getting enough milk. However, it appears that Dezba is tired and stressed, which can lead to a decreased milk supply. And, by her own admission, she is not eating enough herself, which also can decrease her milk supply.

I'm even more concerned because Andrew is not only behind on his weight, he is behind on his developmental milestones, as well. I believe that Andrew is suffering from failure to thrive, now often known as **weight faltering** (Homan, 2016). There are many reasons for failure to thrive, but the most common is inadequate intake (Homan, 2016; Romano et al., 2015). I will conduct a physical, but based on the history I've received, I think that Dezba is most likely not producing enough breast milk and, as a result, Andrew is malnourished.

I have Dezba keep Andrew on her lap while I conduct the physical exam. My findings are unremarkable. I can find no physical reason as to why Andrew is not gaining weight. I could order some blood work, but I don't really think it will show anything. I do not think that Andrew has an underlying medical problem causing **organic failure to thrive**, truly only a small proportion of infants with failure to thrive have a medical cause (Vachani, 2018). Besides, it seems most likely that Dezba is not picking up on Andrew's hunger cues because she is so tired and stressed. These factors, along with lack of weaning and complex social issues, are common in infants with **nonorganic failure to thrive** (Vachani, 2018).

Now, how do I convey this to the mother? I'll need to be clear but concise; the other children are getting restless, and once they start fussing, Dezba will not hear anything I say.

Following a physical, Mary tells Dezba, "I think that Andrew is fussy all of the time because he is not getting enough to eat. Most likely, because of everything you have going on with your family, your breast milk supply is drying up."

"What?" Dezba replies. She feels the anger in her rising.

"You have done nothing wrong," Mary quickly adds. "This is just something that happens. The best thing to do at this point is to begin supplementing your nursing with formula. I also recommend starting Andrew on solid foods" (Box 8.1).

Dezba replies angrily, "I did not start my other children on solid foods until they were 9 months old. Why should I start Andrew on solid foods now? I will talk with my mother. We will go see the Medicine Man. He can help me."

"It is really important that Andrew get the proper nutrition," Mary says quietly. "If his caloric intake is not enough, he will continue to fall behind in his developmental milestones. Lack of nutrition can also cause a delay in his cognitive development" (Analyze the Evidence 8.1; Homan, 2016). Mary continues, "I would like to have a nurse come to your home to discuss feeding Andrew and how to make the formula so that he will

Box 8.1 Starting Solid Foods

Most children are physically ready to start solid foods by the time they are around 4 mo old. Cues include disappearance of the tongue extrusion reflex, the ability to sit in a high chair, and that the birth weight is doubled. Most infants may begin eating pureed food between the ages of 4 and 6 mo. However, the American Academy of Pediatrics (AAP, 2018) recommends exclusively breastfeeding until infants are 6 mo old.

The traditional recommendation has been to start infants on a single-grain infant cereal. This recommendation is not necessary, and parents may start infants on fruits or vegetables first (AAP, 2018). Introduce a new food only every 5–7 d. By doing this, if an infant has an allergic reaction, it is easier to identify which food is the culprit. Call the healthcare provider if the infant develops a rash, has bloody stool, or has trouble breathing.

Under the current guidelines, there are minimal restrictions to solid foods. Avoid giving infants honey, because it may cause botulism. Infants should remain on breast milk or formula until 12 mo of age.

Analyze the Evidence 8.1

Effects of Nutrition on Cognitive Development

Black, Escamilla, and Rao (2015) underscore that poverty and malnutrition are prominent factors in developmental, cognitive, and physical delay. In their article, Black et al. (2015) discuss the need for programs that integrate nutrition and child development to maximize the growth and development potential of infants and children.

Despite much evidence of the need for integrated programs, there currently are no models for such programs. Black et al. (2015) indicate there are at least two essential components required for a successful program integrating nutrition with growth and development. First, a coordinated effort from policy makers is essential. Without governmental support, efforts will most likely be futile. Second, materials provided to families need to be culturally appropriate. Incorporating cultural differences into teaching and practice can make the difference in the developmental success of a child.

get enough calories. I am not trying to tell you how to raise your children, I am just trying to help you have Andrew be the healthiest that he can be."

"Fine," Dezba, says. She is done and just wants to get out of the clinic and go home. "But whoever you send out to our home is not going to understand our ways."

"I can tell you're frustrated," Mary says. "And I don't blame you. But there are a couple of other really important things I need to go over with you about Andrew's health. Can you hang in there with me just a few more minutes? I'll be as brief as I can."

Dezba nods, reluctantly.

Mary explains, "At 6 months old, Andrew should be happy and babbling, reaching for objects, and able to at least sit in the tripod position. The nurse I am sending to your home will help evaluate Andrew's development and, in addition to increased caloric intake, give you tools to help him meet his developmental milestones."

"In the next few months," Mary continues, "Andrew should become more mobile, scooting or crawling, so safety becomes extremely important. Make sure the low cabinets do not have any dangerous substances in them. Also make sure small objects are not on the floor. Babies Andrew's age like to put objects in their mouths, which may cause him to choke" (Patient Teaching 8.1).

"Andrew has only gotten one set of vaccines," Mary says. "He will need to get some immunizations today. Then, we should see him again in 1 month to get him on the catch-up immunization schedule" (Box 8.2).

Mary looks at an immunization schedule and explains to Dezba which immunizations Andrew will get today (Patient Teaching 8.2). "Do you have any questions?"

"No, I don't have any questions. I just really need to get home," Dezba replies.

"A nurse will call you to schedule a home visit," Mary says. "And remember to bring Andrew back in 1 month to catch up on his immunizations." Mary leaves the room.

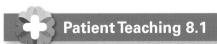

Patient Teaching 8.1

Anticipatory Guidance for 6-Month-Olds

Over the next 3 mo, you can expect your child to do the following:

- Become more mobile, either scooting or crawling
- Pick up small objects with the whole hand
- Begin to eat more table foods
- Begin to pull himself or herself up to a standing position holding onto a table or chair

Taking the following safety precautions is imperative as your child becomes more mobile:

- Store all cleaning materials and medicines in cabinets out of child's reach.
- Lock all guns in cabinets.
- Move cords out of the way or tape them to the floor.
- Remove any small objects or toys on the floor that are a choking hazard.

Box 8.2 Catching Up on Immunizations

The Centers for Disease Control and Prevention (CDC) produces the immunization schedules every year. For children who are >1 mo behind on their immunization schedule, the CDC has a catch-up immunization schedule. Healthcare providers must read and follow the instructions on this schedule carefully because the schedule and number of immunizations can vary greatly from the original schedule.

Patient Teaching 8.2

Typical 6-Month-Old Immunizations

Immunizations Given at the 6-Month Checkup

- Diphtheria, tetanus, acellular pertussis (DTaP)
  - The DTaP vaccine protects against the following:
    - Diphtheria, a serious infection of the throat that can block the airway
    - Tetanus, otherwise known as lockjaw, a nerve disease
    - Pertussis, otherwise known as whooping cough, a respiratory infection that can have serious complications
- *Haemophilus influenzae type b* (Hib)
  - The Hib vaccine protects against a type of bacteria that causes meningitis mostly in children under the age of 5 y.
- Hepatitis B (third dose)
  - Hepatitis B is a disease spread through contact with infected blood or other body fluids that can affect the liver.
- Pneumococcal conjugate vaccine (PCV13)
  - The PCV13 vaccine protects against 13 types of pneumococcal bacteria, which can cause pneumonia, meningitis, and certain types of blood infections.
- Inactivated poliovirus (IPV)
  - The IPV vaccine protects against polio, which can cause paralysis and death.
- Influenza
  - The influenza vaccine protects against the viral respiratory illness commonly known as "the flu."

Common Side Effects

After your baby gets immunizations, he or she may exhibit the following:

- Run a fever of up to around 102°F (38.9°C)
- Have redness or a small amount of swelling at the injection site
- Be fussier in the 24 h after immunizations
- Sleep more in the 24 h after immunizations

When to Call the Healthcare Provider

- If your child has a fever of 105°F (40.5°C) or higher
- If your child has a seizure
- If your child has uncontrollable crying for 3 h or longer

Adapted from the Centers for Disease Control and Prevention. (2017). *Diseases and the vaccines that prevent them.* Retrieved from http://www.cdc.gov/vaccines/hcp/conversations/prevent-diseases/provider-resources-factsheets-infants.html

After Andrew receives his immunizations, Dezba piles the four children into the truck and begins the 45-minute drive home.

At Home

When back at the house, Dezba tells Yanaha how upset she is. "That nurse just doesn't understand. She thinks that I am not a good mother!" She is almost in tears. "Mother, is there anything I can do to make sure Andrew is getting enough to eat without giving him formula?"

Yanaha looks thoughtfully at Dezba. "My dear, we can visit the Medicine Man. You are obviously out of balance in your mind, body, and spirit" (Goss et al., 2017; Kessler et al., 2015; Portman & Garrett, 2006). "I am sure that he will have an herbal remedy that can help with your milk supply. He can also help bring balance back to your life. There is no need to worry about what those nurses and doctors say. They do not understand our ways."

Yanaha takes Dezba and Andrew to see the Medicine Man. He says, "Dezba, you must bring balance back to your life. Are you giving thanks to the Creator each morning?"

"I try my best," says Dezba. "The kids keep me so busy that sometimes I forget."

"You must remember to give thanks to the Creator, Mother Earth, and the Four Directions each morning. Remember to start your prayers facing East to receive the blessings from the first rays of the sun" (Kessler et al., 2015; Portman & Garrett, 2006). "This practice is the first step to regaining harmony in your life."

"I will, I promise." Dezba makes a mental note to remember to set a time each morning to give thanks.

"When you bring balance into your life, you will reduce stress, which will help your situation." The Medicine Man continues, "In addition to practicing daily thanks, I will give you an herb that will increase your milk supply. The herb is called fenugreek. Take these leaves and steep them into a tea and drink it three times a day" (Box 8.3).

The Medicine Man gives Dezba an ample supply of fenugreek leaves to last her around 2 weeks. Dezba thanks him, and she and Yanaha make their way home.

Dezba makes sure that she gives thanks every morning to The Creator, Mother Earth, and the Four Directions. She faithfully drinks the fenugreek tea three times a day. However, it has been 4 days and Andrew still remains fussy. Dezba is frustrated. I am doing everything the Medicine Man told me to do, she thinks. Plus, Sani has a steady job now and we have money coming in. I don't feel as stressed, so why is Andrew still fussy? Am I a bad mother? Should I give him formula and food? If I do, I will feel like a failure.

A nurse has scheduled to come to the house tomorrow. Dezba wonders what the nurse will do. Dezba has heard of other families having their children taken away for many different reasons. Surely that won't happen to me, she thinks. I am only trying to do what I know is best for Andrew. I want him to be healthy. Dezba becomes anxious and has trouble sleeping that night, worried about what will happen when the nurse comes to visit.

Nurse's Home Visit

The next day Dezba hears a knock on the door. She gets the anxious feeling again. She really wishes Sani was here, but he is working today. Andrew is extra fussy but, thank goodness, Yanaha has Caleb, Taylor, and Sarah occupied.

Dezba, holding Andrew, opens the door to find a pleasant young woman standing in front of her. The woman appears to be of American Indian descent. Dezba even thinks that the woman looks as if she could be from the Navajo tribe. Instantly, Dezba relaxes.

The woman at the door introduces herself, "Hello, my name is Kai. I am a community health nurse with the Indian Health Service. We spoke yesterday on the phone."

Dezba knows by the nurse's name that she is a member of the Navajo tribe and feels comfortable letting Kai into her home. "Welcome, please come in."

Kai sets her bag down and gets out a scale. "How have things been going the last 4 days? I read in the chart that the nurse practitioner, Mary, instructed you to supplement Andrew's feedings with formula and to start some solid foods. Is he eating what you give him."

Upset, Dezba explains, "I have not done anything that Mary told me to do. I had lost balance in my life and was not doing

---

Box 8.3   Herbs to Increase Milk Supply

When women who are breastfeeding have trouble with milk supply, they often turn to supplements to increase milk supply. **Galactagogues** are dopamine antagonists that increase serum levels of the hormone prolactin. Although prolactin is important in the initial production of breast milk, once the milk supply is established, prolactin has very little role in maintaining it (Steyn & Decloedt, 2017). Galactagogues can be prescription medications; however, herbal galactagogues are the type most commonly used to increase breast milk supply.

Fenugreek is one of the most common herbs used by women to increase milk supply. Although the herb is widely used, no evidence shows that fenugreek actually has an effect on milk supply production (Steyn & Decloedt, 2017). However, Sim, Hattingh, Sherriff, and Tee (2014) found that women who used galactagogues felt empowered, which had an overall positive psychological impact. This feeling of self-empowerment is likely to have a positive impact on the breastfeeding experience.

my morning prayers on a regular basis. My mother took me to the Medicine Man. He told me to regain balance by resuming morning prayers and also gave me an herb to make into tea. It is supposed to help my breast milk supply."

"Okay, I understand that you wanted to approach this using traditional tribal ways. How does the herbal tea seem to be working?"

"I must admit, Andrew is still very fussy. I am not sure what to do. I am just trying to be a good mother the best way I know how." Tears come to Dezba's eyes.

"I believe that you are doing what you think is best. Let's weigh Andrew and see if he has gained any weight." Kai asks Mary to undress Andrew and set him on the scale. His weight is 13 lb, or 5.9 kg.

"Andrew's weight is down 1 oz," Kai says. "I am concerned that he has not gained any weight and that he is still fussy. I know it has only been 4 days, but I am not sure the herbal tea is going to work. We need to discuss ways to increase Andrew's caloric intake. We also need to talk about making sure he is doing well developmentally."

Dezba begins to cry. "I am scared that someone is going to take him away from me," she says. "I am not trying to do anything wrong."

Kai sits down next to Dezba, puts her arm around her, and says reassuringly, "Dezba, you have done nothing wrong and nobody is trying to take Andrew away from you. I am here to make sure that Andrew is healthy, and to help you make sure he is healthy, happy, and growing well. Isn't that what you want?"

Dezba's cry slows down to a sniffle. "Yes, it is. I guess it is time for me to do something else if the herb is not working."

"There is no reason you can't continue what you have been doing, we just need to add formula and solid food to the routine to get Andrew to the weight he should be at his age. Please continue your morning prayers; it is important to our culture. You may also continue the herbal tea if you would like, because it will not hurt anything." Kai pulls some sample cans of formula for Dezba out of her bag.

Kai tells Dezba that Andrew will need to have higher caloric intake than other infants his age until he reaches his target

---

Box 8.4 Increasing Caloric Intake

To determine how many calories an infant should consume to overcome failure to thrive, first determine the target weight.

Andrew's weight was at the 25th percentile at birth and at 3 mo of age. Therefore, the 25th percentile is a reasonable target weight. A 6-mo-old at the 25th percentile should weigh ~15 lb, or 6.8 kg.

A typically developing 6-mo-old should consume 98 kcal/kg/d (Homan, 2016). However, caloric intake for an infant with failure to thrive should be based on target weight.

Therefore, Andrew's caloric intake should be 6.8 kg × 98 kcal, or 668.2 kcal/d.

---

weight (Box 8.4). "To do this," explains Kai, "you will have to mix his formula differently than the directions on the can to increase the amount of calories Andrew gets with each bottle." Kai continues, "Normally, formula has 20 calories in an ounce. I want you to mix the formula so that there are 24 calories in an ounce. I have written the directions on how to do this on the can."

Dezba takes the can of formula and reads the directions Kai has written. "I don't have any bottles; I have never used bottles before."

Kai goes to her bag. "I brought three bottles with me. You will have to wash them often, but it should be enough to get you through."

Dezba takes the bottles and says, "Thank you."

"I would like you to make a bottle while I am here and feed it to Andrew. I want to see if he will take it or if he will need some convincing." Kai helps Dezba mix the formula in the bottle and watches patiently as Dezba offers the bottle to Andrew.

Andrew has no trouble taking the bottle and finishes it quickly. "He finished the bottle," says Dezba. "Is this a good sign?"

"Yes, it is."

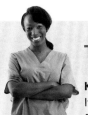

The Nurse's Point of View

Kai: I'm so glad that Andrew took the bottle. If he hadn't, I would've had to have arranged for an occupational therapist to come to the house to help him learn how to eat, and I'm not sure how Dezba would feel about that.

Andrew most likely just needs developmental surveillance and social work (Priority Care Concepts 8.1). If he has trouble with solid foods and textures, I will discuss with Dezba the need for occupational therapy.

Often, children who suffer from failure to thrive need a multidisciplinary team of healthcare workers to provide nutrition intervention and feeding behavior education (Romano et al., 2015; Vachani, 2018). However, because the Hocktochee family lives in a rural area and has difficulty with transportation, it is unlikely they would be able to make multiple visits to different specialists.

Now that Dezba has overcome the first hurdle by giving Andrew a bottle, I think I will take the visit one step further and see whether I can persuade her to take advantage of other resources to help Andrew with his development.

Priority Care Concepts 8.1   Monitoring Growth and Development

In the absence of underlying disease, the cause of failure to thrive is most likely decreased caloric intake (Romano et al., 2015; Vachani, 2018). Inadequate caloric intake affects not only an infant's weight but also his or her developmental milestones (Black et al., 2015). Therefore, it is essential that infants and children have adequate nutrition to meet developmental and cognitive milestones.

Goals

- Determine the infant's goal weight.
- Increase caloric intake on the basis of the goal weight.
- Reach developmental milestones appropriate for age

Nursing Interventions

- Assess developmental milestones.
- Monitor growth and development.
- Monitor weight.
- Teach caregivers a way to help infants achieve developmental milestones.
- Teach caregivers methods for increasing caloric intake.
- Make referrals as appropriate:
    - The Special Supplemental Nutrition Program for women, infants, and children
    - Early intervention programs
    - Social work
    - Occupational therapy
    - Physical therapy

"Dezba, I would like to talk to you about some services that are available to you to help Andrew be healthy and develop appropriately."

Dezba, overwhelmed with many different emotions at this moment, cautiously replies, "What do you mean?"

"I would like to refer Andrew to early intervention." Kai sees the confused look on Dezba's face. "Early intervention is a program that provides services such as nursing visits, social work visits, and many other services, if needed. The goal of early intervention is to support the development of Andrew."

"Why would I need a social worker? They will take my children!" Dezba becomes more anxious with each passing minute.

"Dezba, I understand that you believe social workers take children from their homes. This is not always the case. A social worker can help you get many services to allow Andrew to be happy and healthy." Kai tries to assure Dezba that a visit from a social worker does not mean she is at risk of losing her children (Whose Job Is It, Anyway? 8.1).

"If the social worker does not want to take my children, what is she going to do?" Dezba asks suspiciously.

Whose Job Is It, Anyway? 8.1
Social Worker

Social workers have a variety of tools to help children and families cope with the stressors of normal life. The goal of a social worker is to keep families intact. Social workers assess family situations, provide support, and coordinate resources to help families find solutions to their problems. Social workers are often the best advocates for families to receive the needed resources to have a better life.

"The social worker will help you access resources to meet your family's needs. The one resource that will help you tremendously is Women, Infants, and Children, or WIC. WIC will help you with nutrition education and will support Andrew until he is 5 years old" (United States Department of Agriculture, 2015). Kai continues to explain that early intervention services allow for her to continue to visit Andrew to monitor his weight and his development. "I want you to have all the support you need," emphasizes Kai.

"Okay," Dezba says to Kai after thinking about it for a few moments. "If you believe a social worker can help us, then I suppose it won't be all that bad."

"Great!" exclaims Kai. "Before I leave I want to know if you have any questions about making the formula for Andrew."

"How am I supposed to breastfeed and give him a bottle?" asks Dezba.

Kai explains, "You can breastfeed and then feed him a bottle, but that can be very time consuming. My advice would be to alternate every other feeding. If he continues to be fussy, you may need to stop breastfeeding altogether and only use formula. Remember, this is not because of anything you did wrong. It just happened."

"I understand," says Dezba.

Kai makes an appointment to visit Dezba next week. After Kai leaves, Dezba is torn. I am glad that Kai believes that I am a good mother, she thinks, but it is still difficult for me to accept that I can't provide nutrition for Andrew. I will do as Kai asks of me, though, because I love my son.

Nurse's Follow-Up Home Visit

Kai has visited the Hocktochee family every week for the past month. Andrew is now 7 months old. At the latest visit Kai is happy to see that Andrew has gained almost 3 lb, weighing 15 lb 14 oz, or 7.22 kg. She explains to Dezba that he is now close to the 10th percentile for weight.

"You are doing a great job!" Kai says. Andrew is no longer fussy. He is happy and smiling on this visit. He even giggles uncontrollably when Taylor and Sarah tickle him.

Dezba has been waiting for Kai to come today. "Look what Andrew can do," she says. She sits Andrew on the floor in a tripod position, she lets go, and he is able to support himself.

"How wonderful!" exclaims Kai.

"He is also eating rice cereal and bananas," Dezba says.

"You are doing an excellent job. I am so proud of you."

Dezba talks to Kai and tells her how helpful the social worker has been. The family has WIC, they have gotten car seats, and she has also helped find them some financial assistance. Until now, Dezba did not know that there were so many people willing to help. Even Yanaha has admitted that she was wrong to be so suspicious of traditional healthcare workers.

Dezba feels grateful to have Kai as their community health nurse. She understands the needs of the Navajo tribe. Although Dezba ended up having to stop breastfeeding altogether, she no longer feels guilty. She continues her morning prayer routine, and, although she realizes that Andrew still has a way to go, Dezba is thankful that her family is healthy.

Think Critically

1. Dezba piles her family into a pickup truck. What questions do you have surrounding this situation? What are the safety issues and how can nurses help with this?
2. What are other ways Mary could approach the subject of malnutrition with Dezba?
3. What are ways for caregivers to tell whether an infant is getting an adequate supply of breast milk?
4. Why might Dezba feel like a failure if she has to give Andrew formula? What can nurses do to alleviate this feeling?
5. Dezba relaxes when she senses the community health nurse is of American Indian Descent. Why is this?
6. How can nurses help ensure that Dezba and her family continue to have the resources they need to maintain health and wellness?

References

American Academy of Pediatrics. (2018). *Starting solid foods.* Retrieved from https://www.healthychildren.org/English/ages-stages/baby/feeding-nutrition/Pages/Switching-To-Solid-Foods.aspx

Black, M. M., Pérez-Escamilla, R., & Rao, S. F. (2015). Integrating nutrition and child development interventions: Scientific basis, evidence of impact, and implementation considerations. *Advances in Nutrition, 6,* 852–859.

Eckhardt, C. L., Lutz, T., Karanja, N., Jobe, J. B., Maupome, G., & Rittenbaugh, C. (2014). Knowledge, attitudes, and beliefs that can influence infant feeding practices in American Indian mothers. *Journal of the Academy of Nutrition and Dietetics, 114*(10), 1587–1593.

Goss, C. W., Daily, N., Bair, B., Manson, S. M., Richardson, W. J., Nagamoto, H., & Shore, J. H. (2017). Rural American Indian and Alaska native veterans' telemental health: A model of culturally centered care. *Psychological Services, 14*(3), 270–278.

Homan, G. J. (2016). Failure to thrive: A practical guide. *American Family Physician, 94*(4), 295–299.

Kessler, D. O., Hopkins, O., Torres, E., & Prasad, A. (2015). Assimilating traditional healing into preventive medicine residency curriculum. *American Journal of Preventive Medicine, 49*(5S3), S263–S269.

Portman, T. A., & Garrett, M. T. (2006). Native American healing traditions. *International Journal of Disability, Development, and Education, 53*(4), 453–469.

Romano, C., Hartman, C., Privitera, C., Cardile, S., & Shamir, R. (2015). Current topics in the diagnosis and management of the pediatric non-organic feeding disorders (NOFEDs). *Clinical Nutrition, 34,* 195–200.

Sim, T. F., Hattingh, H. L., Sherriff, J., & Tee, L. B. (2014). Perspectives and attitudes of breastfeeding women using herbal galactogues during breastfeeding: A qualitative study. *BMC Complementary and Alternative Medicine, 216*(14), 1–11.

Steyn, N., & Decloedt, E. H. (2017). Galactogogues: Prescriber points for use in breastfeeding mothers. *Obstetrics and Gynaecology Forum, 27*(1), 16–18.

United States Department of Agriculture. (2015, February). *About WIC—WIC at a glance.* Retrieved from https://www.fns.usda.gov/wic/about-wic-wic-glance

Vachani, J. G. (2018). Failure to thrive: Early intervention mitigates long-term defects. *Contemporary Pediatrics, 35*(4), 13–120.

Suggested Readings

Centers for Disease Control and Prevention. (2017, August 21). *A look inside food desserts.* Retrieved from: https://www.cdc.gov/features/fooddeserts/index.html

Portman, T. A., & Garrett, M. T. (2006). Native American healing traditions. *International Journal of Disability, Development, and Education, 53*(4), 453–469.

United States Department of Health and Human Services, Indian Health Service. (2017, September 3). *Navajo Nation.* Retrieved from: https://www.ihs.gov/navajo/navajonation/

9 Jessica Wang: Tonic-Clonic Seizures

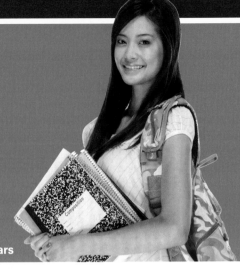

Jessica Wang, age 16 years

Objectives

After completing this chapter, you will be able to:

1. Describe normal growth and development of the 16-year-old.
2. Discuss an appropriate teaching plan for a healthy 16-year-old.
3. Identify the priorities of care for the child presenting with a seizure.
4. Apply principles of growth and development to the 16-year-old in the hospital.
5. Explain the psychological impact of a chronic illness such as epilepsy on a child.
6. Describe the progression of a seizure from an aura through the postictal phase.
7. Plan nursing interventions for the child diagnosed with a seizure disorder.

Key Terms

Absence
Atonic
Aura
Clonic
Epilepsy

Myoclonic
Postictal
Tonic
Tonic-clonic seizure

Background

Jessica Wang is a 16-year-old girl who loves playing tennis, hanging out with her friends, and volunteering at the local animal shelter. She is the oldest of three children in her family. Jacen, her brother, is 12 years old, and her little sister, Jennifer, is 8 years old. Jessica's parents are Lian and Mei Wang. Currently, Jessica is a sophomore in high school and is taking a driver's education course to gain experience and hours to get her driver's license by the time she turns 17. At school, she is enrolled in honors courses and is a member of several clubs and groups, including the school newspaper and drama club. Recently, although a quiet and reserved teen, Jessica has been hanging out more with friends and has even been invited to some weekend parties.

Jessica, along with her siblings, was born and has been raised in the United States. However, her parents, Lian and Mei, immigrated to the United States when they were in college. When Jessica was a baby, her paternal grandparents immigrated to the United States, as well. In their home, the Wangs speak both Mandarin, the official spoken language of China, and English. Jessica's grandparents, who live in the Wang home, do not speak much English. Many of the traditional customs of the Chinese culture are present in the Wang household, because her grandparents insist that the grandchildren are raised with the knowledge and awareness of their ancestors. Lian and Mei agree and are much appreciative of the grandparents' knowledge and willingness to teach the children the language and customs of their ancestors.

Box 9.1 Epilepsy

Epilepsy is a serious, common neurological disease and seizure disorder that affects males and females of all races, ethnicities, and ages. Most often, epilepsy presents in early childhood or older adulthood. Each year, approximately 460,000 children, from newborns to 17-y-olds, are treated in the United States for epilepsy (Centers for Disease Control, 2016). There are many types of seizures, but seizures can be separated into two categories, according to whether one or both sides of the brain are affected. Seizures that affect only one side of the brain are classified as focal seizures, whereas seizures that affect both sides of the brain are classified as generalized seizures. Box 9.2

defines each category and gives examples of the types of seizures that fall into each category. Recall that Jessica has a generalized seizure disorder and, specifically, has tonic-clonic seizures.

Epilepsy is diagnosed on the basis of one of the following:

- The occurrence of at least two unprovoked seizures more than 24 h apart
- The occurrence of one unprovoked seizure with a high probability of recurrence within the next 10 y
- A diagnosis of an electroclinical syndrome when evaluated by a neurologist (Fisher et al., 2014)

At the age of 4, Jessica had her first seizure. She had been ill with an upper respiratory virus and had been running a fever. Initially, she was treated for a febrile seizure and released from the hospital emergency department. Several months later, while playing on the playground, Jessica had another seizure. By the age of 5, she had had six seizures and was being seen by a pediatric neurologist for **epilepsy** (Box 9.1). Specifically, Jessica has **tonic-clonic seizures**, also known as convulsions (Box 9.2).

She began taking antiepileptic medications after her third seizure and has been on medications to prevent seizures since then. In the first year after diagnosis, Jessica's parents were reluctant to consistently give her the antiepileptic medications. Lian and Mei were torn between listening to Lian's parents and trusting the doctors who were caring for Jessica. In traditional

Chinese medicine (TCM), physical illness is an imbalance in yin and yang (hot and cold). Therefore, Jessica's grandparents often thought that Jessica was having an imbalance in harmony and yin and yang (Healthcare Chaplaincy, 2013). Also, those who practice TCM often stop taking medications when the symptoms disappear or are not obvious, or if side effects are present (Healthcare Chaplaincy, 2013). Jessica was sleepier at times when she first started her antiepileptic medications, and her grandparents did not believe that a child should suffer from the side effects of medications. They often persuaded Lian and Mei to not give Jessica her medication.

Adherence to antiepileptic medication therapy is essential and has been shown to have an impact on both short-term and long-term outcomes for children with epilepsy. According to a

Box 9.2 Seizures: Types and Definitions

Focal Seizures

Definition

Episodes of abnormal electrical brain activity in one or more areas on one side of the brain; also known as partial seizures

Types

- Simple focal: The patient is not likely to lose consciousness, may smell or taste something strange, and may see flashes of light or feel dizzy; fingers, arms, and legs may twitch briefly.
- Complex focal: It begins as a simple focal seizure and may include lip smacking, gagging, or rhythmic movements; it progresses to impairment in consciousness.

Generalized Seizures

Definition

Episodes of abnormal electrical brain activity in both sides of the brain with loss of consciousness and a **postictal** state afterward

Types

- **Absence:** The patient stares blankly, does not remember, and does not respond during the episode; the seizure lasts a few seconds.
- **Atonic:** The patient's muscles suddenly go limp; the patient is at high risk of injury from falling or dropping items.
- **Generalized tonic-clonic** (formerly known as grand mal): The patient's body shakes, stiffens, and jerks. The seizure may last 1–3 min or longer. The patient may lose consciousness or control of bowel or bladder.
- **Tonic:** The patient's muscles in the arms, legs, and trunk tense up; the seizure often occurs during sleep.
- **Clonic:** The patient's muscles spasm and jerk rhythmically in the arms, face, neck, or legs; the seizure may last several minutes.
- **Myoclonic:** The patient's muscles suddenly jerk.

Adapted from Beaumont Health. (n.d.). *Types of seizures in children*. Retrieved from https://www.beaumont.org/conditions/types-of-seizures-in-children

study by Modi, Rausch, and Glauser (2014), 31% of children who were nonadherent with antiepileptic medications after initial diagnosis continued to have seizures 4 years after diagnosis vs. only 12% of those with near-perfect adherence to their medication regimen. Jessica has had about one or two seizures a year since the age of 7. Most of these have been associated with missed doses of medication or additional stressors. Jessica has been on several antiepileptic medications since being diagnosed, including phenytoin, carbamazepine, and phenobarbital, all of which made her sleepy. For the past 5 years, Jessica has been taking levetiracetam and divalproex (The Pharmacy 9.1).

Health Promotion

Dr. Wong has learned many things about the Chinese culture over the course of taking care of the Wang children. For example, Dr. Wong respects the fact when the Wang children avoid eye contact, they are not ignoring the pediatrician; rather, they are showing respect for authority (Healthcare Chaplaincy, 2013). Dr. Wong also discovered, after teaching Jessica's parents about antiepileptic medications and learning that they did not understand the directions after all, that nodding politely does not mean the person understands the information being given and asking

The Pharmacy 9.1 — Anticonvulsants

Medication	Classification	Route	Action	Nursing Considerations
Carbamazepine (Tegretol)	Anticonvulsant	• PO	• Reduces polysynaptic responses; blocks posttetanic potentiation • Anticonvulsant	• Risk of TEN and SJS; discontinue administration at the first sign of a drug-related rash • Monitor laboratory test results for aplastic anemia and agranulocytosis • Increases in suicidal thoughts or behavior; monitor for signs of depression and changes in mood or behavior
Divalproex sodium (Depakote)	Anticonvulsant	• PO	• Blocks voltage-gated sodium channels and increases brain levels of GABA	• Monitor for hepatotoxicity • Risk for pancreatitis
Fosphenytoin (Cerebyx)	Anticonvulsant	• IV • IM	• Modulates sodium channels of neurons to stop seizure activity	• Rapid administration can lead to hypotension and cardiac arrhythmias
Levetiracetam (Keppra)	Anticonvulsant	• IV	• Inhibits presynaptic calcium channels, reducing neurotransmitter release	• Monitor for nonpsychotic behavior changes • Monitor for suicidal thoughts and behaviors
Phenobarbital	Anticonvulsant	• PO	• Acts on GABA receptors, increasing synaptic inhibition, which results in an elevated seizure threshold and reduction in the spread of seizure activity • Produces CNS depression	• May cause drowsiness • Monitor liver function • Monitor phenobarbital levels
Phenytoin (Dilantin)	Anticonvulsant	• PO • IV	• Slows impulses to the brain that lead to seizures	• Abrupt stopping of administration may precipitate status epilepticus • Increases in suicidal thoughts or behavior; monitor for signs of depression and changes in mood or behavior • Risk of TEN and SJS; discontinue administration at the first sign of a drug-related rash • Check with the provider before using OTC medications; many OTC drugs alter phenytoin levels

CNS, central nervous system; GABA, gamma-aminobutyric acid; IM, intramuscular; IV, intravenous; OTC, over-the-counter; PO, by mouth; SJS, Stevens–Johnson syndrome; TEN, toxic epidermal necrolysis.
Adapted from Taketomo, C. K. (2018). *Pediatric & neonatal dosage handbook* (25th ed.). Hudson, OH: Lexicomp.

questions may be disrespectful (Healthcare Chaplaincy, 2013). Health, in Eastern medicine, is seen as a balance between the physical, social, and supernatural environment (Carteret, 2011). Eastern medicine also assumes the body is whole and each individual part is closely connected with each organ, having both a physical and mental function (Carteret, 2011).

It's time for Jessica's annual well-care visit, so she and her mother drive to the office of her pediatrician, Dr. Mary Wong. Jessica has been a patient of Dr. Wong's since she was a newborn. Dr. Wong is also the primary provider for Jessica's brother and sister.

When her name is called, Jessica follows the medical assistant back to the exam room while her mother stays in the waiting room. Since the age of 14, Jessica has been seeing the pediatrician without her parents present in the exam room. Dr. Wong usually calls her mother back to the room at the end of the visit to address any questions or concerns her mother has. The medical assistant measures her vital signs, height, and weight and reviews Jessica's current medication list. The medical assistant reports her vital signs as follows:

- Heart rate: 65 beats/min (bpm)
- Respiratory rate: 14 breaths/min
- Blood pressure: 90/45 mm Hg
- O_2 saturation: 99% on room air

Her current weight is 122 lb (55.4 kg), and she is 64 in (5.3 ft). The medical assistant comments that Jessica has lost 1 lb (0.45 kg) since her well-care visit last year and that her body mass index is 20.9 (56th percentile), which is in the healthy range for her age and gender (Growth and Development Check 9.1).

Dr. Wong arrives and begins the exam like she usually does, by talking with Jessica about school, home, and friends. Jessica likes Dr. Wong and enjoys talking with her. Then, Dr. Wong asks, "What medications are you currently taking?"

"I'm taking divalproex and levetiracetam, both twice a day," Jessica tells Dr. Wong, trying hard to pronounce them correctly. At home, she just calls them her "meds."

"Have you missed any doses recently?" Dr. Wong asks, her eyebrows raised expectantly.

"Maybe one or two this past week," Jessica says sheepishly. She really tries to be good about taking them, but somehow still manages to forget. She braces herself for the lecture she knows is coming.

Dr. Wong's eyebrows drop and her forehead wrinkles. "What have we discussed before about your medications, Jessica?"

"That it's important that I follow the dosing schedule," Jessica says.

"*Strictly*," Dr. Wong says.

"Yes—that I *strictly* follow the dosing schedule," Jessica says.

"And why is it important?"

"Because if I don't, I'm more likely to have a seizure."

"And when is it particularly important to not forget to take your medications?"

"When there are extra stressors or seizure triggers in my life," Jessica says.

Dr. Wong reviews with Jessica some methods to help her remember to take her medicine, such as using a pill box, setting

Growth and Development Check 9.1

Adolescents (12–18 Years Old)

Physical

Early Adolescence (Aged 11–14 y)

- Continues to have growth spurts
- Experiences puberty changes, such as hair growth in the pubic area and breast enlargement in girls

Middle Adolescence (Aged 15–17 y)

- Is at or close to adult height and weight

Late Adolescence (Aged 18–21 y)

- Achieves adult height and weight

Emotional

- Distances self from parents
- Spends more time with friends
- Pushes the limits of authority
- Feels conflicted about leaving the safety of home

Intellectual

- Early and middle adolescence: views ideas as black and white, right or wrong
- Late adolescence: solves complex problems, appreciates subtleties of situations, and can look at future needs

Social

- Has friends of both the same and the opposite sex
- Has a circle of relationships that includes different ethnicities, social groups, and ages, including adults such as teachers, coaches, and mentors

Nutrition

- Requires about 2,200 calories/d (girls) or 2,800 calories/d (boys)
- May be deficient in vitamin D, calcium, zinc, or iron
- Requires 1,300 mg of calcium and 600 IU of vitamin D per day for proper bone health
- May drink either low-fat or nonfat milk
- May overconsume cholesterol and saturated fats (discuss at well-care visits)

Adapted from American Academy of Pediatrics. (2019). *Stages of adolescents.* Retrieved from: https://www.healthychildren.org/English/ages-stages/teen/Pages/Stages-of-Adolescence.aspx; American Academy of Pediatrics. (2016). *A teenager's nutritional needs.* Retrieved from https://www.healthychildren.org/English/ages-stages/teen/nutrition/Pages/A-Teenagers-Nutritional-Needs.aspx

reminders on her smartphone, and incorporating taking her medications into her daily routine. Jessica is already using a pill box, but she likes the idea of the smartphone app and promises to check into it.

"I know it's not easy living with epilepsy," Dr. Wong says, her tone softening. "How are you handling it lately?"

"Okay, I guess. I'm always a little scared that I will have another seizure. My biggest fear is that I'll have one at school, in front of everyone. That would be so humiliating. I feel relieved when I make it home every day and haven't had one."

"You told me that you've been spending some time with your friends lately," Dr. Wong says. "That's wonderful. It's important that you not let your fear of a seizure cause you to avoid people. Do your friends know what to do if you have a seizure when you're with them?"

"I don't know," Jessica says. "We haven't really talked about it. I feel a little weird bringing it up, you know. I can tell they already feel a little nervous being around me, like I'm a ticking bomb about to go off."

"Actually," Dr. Wong says, "They might be reassured if you were to give them some basic instructions on what to do if you should have a seizure. In fact, they would probably feel honored for you to trust them with that information and that they have an important role to play if something happens." As she usually does, Dr. Wong talks with Jessica about the additional stressors that people with epilepsy experience, such as decreased autonomy, stigma such as peer isolation and bullying, and socialization difficulties (Guilfoyle et al., 2017). Jessica can't relate to all of the things Dr. Wong mentions, but some of what she says is really helpful, and Jessica knows that Dr. Wong cares about her and is looking out for her.

"Have you missed any school in the past year?" Dr. Wong says. In the past, Dr. Wong has told Jessica and her mother that children with epilepsy are more likely to miss 11 or more days of school than children with other medical concerns (Centers for Disease Control, 2016).

"I only missed about 7 days of school in the past year," Jessica replies. "It was last fall, when I had a bad stomach virus. I forgot to take my seizure medications and then had a seizure." They discuss the seizure and then Jessica's current stressors and sleep habits. Dr. Wong reminds her that sleep deprivation can trigger seizures (Smith, Wagner, & Edwards, 2015a,b). Finally, Dr. Wong talks with Jessica about triggers of seizures that are common for her age group, which include poor nutrition and alcohol and drug use.

"What types of food do you eat on a typical day?" Dr. Wong asks.

"I'm pretty careful about what I eat," Jessica says. "Especially when I'm playing tennis. I eat cereal and fruit for breakfast, whatever is on the menu at school for lunch, and chips or fruit before tennis practice. For dinner, I eat whatever my mom makes, which usually includes meat, rice, vegetables, and fruit, along with tea."

"Have you tried any alcohol or tobacco products?"

"No, I don't drink and I've never tried tobacco." Jessica feels the weight of Dr. Wong's steady gaze and adds, "I mean, I did go to a party with friends last weekend where there was alcohol, but I didn't drink any."

"That's good," Dr. Wong says (Patient Safety 9.1). "Because, as you know, alcohol can trigger a seizure. Also, it can interact

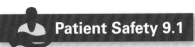

Patient Safety 9.1

Keeping Adolescents Safe

Parents should do the following to help keep their adolescents safe:

Driving

- Model good driving behaviors when behind the wheel.
- Offer as much practice time as possible before allowing licensure.
- Set rules for driving, such as no more than two friends in the car at once, no eating or drinking while driving, keeping music at low-to-moderate volume levels, no talking or texting while driving.

Helmet Safety

- Remember that adolescents have a greater tendency to not wear helmets, because of peer pressure and feeling invincible.
- Encourage helmet use when bicycle riding, roller skating, or riding an all-terrain vehicle or moped/scooter.

Substance Use

- Talk to children early and often about substance use.
- Note that 52% of teens admit to drinking alcohol, whereas only 10% of parents think their teens drink alcohol (Berchelmann, 2018).

Sex

- Openly address all of their children's concerns, questions, and comments about sex.
- Remain nonjudgmental of their teens' views or ideas regarding sex, sexuality, and related issues.

with your seizure medications and cause adverse effects. So don't even think about drinking. Are we clear?"

"Yes—completely clear, doctor."

"Do you have any health concerns or questions you would like to discuss?" Dr. Wong asks.

Jessica looks down at the ground and quietly says, "No, not today. Well, maybe. Can we talk about whether I will be able to get my driver's license soon? I have been reading and it sounds like some people with epilepsy cannot drive because of safety reasons. Is that true?"

"Actually, many people with epilepsy drive and do just fine," explains Dr. Wong. "There are some things you need to know in preparation for getting your license. Every state has different laws and requirements for obtaining a license if you have epilepsy. For example, our state requires you to be seizure-free for at least 3 months, taking your medications as prescribed, and you will need a statement from me or your healthcare provider stating your seizures are under control and you are under the care of a physician for your epilepsy.

Also, when you renew your license, a statement is required from your healthcare provider that you are taking your medications as prescribed and are safe to drive from a seizure-control standpoint."

"Thanks for explaining that," says Jessica. "So the chances of me getting my license are good as long as I take my seizure medications and I do not have any episodes, correct?"

"Yes, that is correct," replies Dr. Wong.

Jessica replies, "I think that was all I needed to talk about."

Dr. Wong asks Jessica's mother to join them and reviews pertinent health information with her, including reminders about medication adherence and balancing school, sports, and home life. Mei nods her head in agreement. Before the end of the visit, Jessica is given the second dose of MenACWY, the meningococcal vaccine. She received the first dose of the vaccine when she was 12 years old.

At Home and School

A month passes. Jessica has had a very busy few weeks at school and home. Tennis tryouts were last week, and Jessica had several difficult tests in math and English. She has also been having a difficult time getting along with her siblings. She feels that her mother is constantly blaming her for the squabbles and fights that ensue between Jessica, Jennifer, and Jacen. Furthermore, Jessica's dad just switched to working evenings and nights at his job, which has created some disruption in schedules at the Wang house. Jessica has not been sleeping well because of the extra stress. Jessica is aware that she is out of balance and harmony, but she is just not sure how to regain her balance with all this extra stress. In TCM, disharmony leads to disaster, disease, and bad luck (Carteret, 2011). She has tried talking to her grandmother and grandfather about her current stress levels. Her grandmother reminds her about balance and harmony and suggests that perhaps the increased stress is nature's way of telling her she is out of balance; her yin and yang need to be rebalanced. Her grandmother encourages her to reflect, meditate, and figure out how to find yin (the positive) and reduce yang (the negative) to restore harmony. In TCM, which her grandparents believe in and practice, yin–yang disharmony is the root cause of disease and illness. Jessica, her parents, and her siblings follow some TCM concepts but are also willing to use Western medicine, particularly when treating her seizures. Jessica has tried finding balance, but life just seems difficult right now.

While walking out to the tennis courts for practice after school one day, Jessica begins to feel funny and dizzy. She also hears buzzing in her ears. Jessica knows these signs (**auras**) happen before she has a seizure. She tells her friend, Nicole, that she doesn't feel well.

When she comes to, she hears voices around her talking and she finds herself lying on the ground. She feels very sleepy and disoriented. She opens her eyes a moment and sees bright, flashing lights. She slowly realizes that it is an ambulance. Then

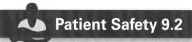

Patient Safety 9.2

Seizure Precautions and First Aid

1. Ensure that the patient's airway is clear and that breathing is not impaired.
2. Clear the area of any sharp or dangerous objects.
3. Do not hold the patient down; this may lead to injury.
4. Do not put anything in the patient's mouth.
5. Turn the patient's head to the side; this helps prevent saliva and mucus from blocking the airway and may help the patient breathe more easily.
6. If the seizure lasts more than 5 min, call 9-1-1.
7. In the hospital setting, prepare to give a rescue medication, such as lorazepam, midazolam, or diazepam in the event of a prolonged seizure.
8. In the hospital setting, pad the side rails of the bed, put all four side rails up, and have suction equipment readily available.
9. Offer supportive care.
10. Do not give the patient anything to eat or drink, including medications by mouth, until he or she is fully alert.

she sees Nicole and her tennis coach standing nearby. They are talking with some paramedics.

"Her body just went stiff, you know, and then she fell," Nicole says. "Then, her arms and legs began jerking around. I yelled for the coach, and he ran over."

"Fortunately, I've had training on how to respond to seizures," the coach says (Patient Safety 9.2), "So I knew to move her tennis racket and other things away from her, turn her on her side, and make sure she was adequately breathing. I had Nicole, here, call 9-1-1. She stopped convulsing about a minute before you all arrived."

"How long did the seizure last?" one of the paramedics asks.

"About 4 minutes," the coach replies.

"How was her breathing during the seizure?"

"It seemed fine. At no time did she appear to stop breathing."

Jessica opens her eyes again. One of the paramedics is crouched beside her. "Looks like she's coming to," he says. He takes her vital signs, and then they put her on a stretcher and load her onto the ambulance. En route, the paramedic checks her vital signs and reports them as follows:

- Heart rate: 72 bpm
- Respiratory rate: 12 breaths/min
- Blood pressure: 92/46 mm Hg
- O_2 saturation: 98% on room air

Jessica remains very sleepy but can still open her eyes when the paramedic taps her shoulders and calls out her name loudly, repeatedly.

At the Hospital

In the Emergency Room

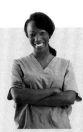

The Nurse's Point of View

Nicole: I'm working with a 16-year-old girl, Jessica Wang, who just arrived here at the emergency room (ER) by ambulance. She had a tonic-clonic seizure. She appears to have stopped seizing but is very sleepy and difficult to arouse. The paramedics report off to me and the ER physician, Dr. Beck, that the seizure activity lasted approximately 4 minutes, according to the tennis coach who witnessed the seizure. Her vital signs and breathing were stable throughout the transport. Jessica did not hit her head; she slumped down to the ground, according to her friend, who also witnessed the seizure.

Jessica's parents arrive shortly after the ambulance and are quiet but concerned about her. Jessica's dad appears to be the spokesperson while her mom remains quiet and avoids eye contact with the staff. Often, in TCM, the male is the spokesperson and makes decisions, I recall (Healthcare Chaplaincy, 2013). The chaplain is present to be with Lian and Wei while the staff get Jessica checked in and perform vital signs and an initial assessment (Whose Job Is It, Anyway? 9.1). The chaplain addresses Lian and Wei as Mr. and Mrs. Wang, which is wise, as calling a person by his or her first name can be disrespectful in the Chinese culture (Healthcare Chaplaincy, 2013).

Just after Jessica is placed on the stretcher in the exam room, she begins with tonic and then clonic motions of her arms and then her legs. Fortunately, the side rails of the stretcher are already padded. I watch her breathing closely and have suction equipment and oxygen set up and ready to use should Jessica aspirate, choke, or have apnea leading to oxygen desaturation during or after a seizure (Priority Care Concepts 9.1). This seizure lasts about 2 minutes. I record the start and stop times and document the types of movements and activity I noticed during the seizure. I monitor her for apnea.

The patient care assistant (PCA) and I remove Jessica's clothes, clean her perineal area and back, and place a hospital gown on her. Jessica was incontinent of urine during the seizure. During the clothes change, Dr. Beck and I examine Jessica from head to toe for bruises, cuts, scrapes, or any other injury she may have sustained during the first seizure. A bruise is present on her right knee, and her right elbow has several small abrasions. There are no other obvious deformities or open wounds. I make sure Jessica is lying on her side during the postictal period and observe her closely for signs of respiratory distress, apnea, or a change in her neurological status. I also place Jessica back on a continuous pulse oximeter and a heart rate monitor. During the seizure, before the leads came off, Jessica's heart rate was 142 bpm and her respiratory rate was 42 breaths/min.

Whose Job Is It, Anyway? 9.1

Hospital Chaplain

The chaplain is present when the Wangs arrive at the hospital. In many hospitals and ER settings, a chaplain is often available to offer spiritual and emotional care to patients and families.

Pastoral care services are a significant aspect in treating the whole patient in the hospital setting. Chaplains offer not only spiritual care but also emotional support to patients and families. Chaplains serve patients and families in many ways, including visiting and praying, offering encouragement and comfort, and discussing concerns about procedures or decisions. Furthermore, chaplains provide ministry services such as anointing of the sick, baptisms, communion, and worship services.

Providing spiritual and emotional care to patients and families in the ER and the hospital is essential to treating the patient in a holistic manner. Patients with illness or trauma and their families are complex humans who face unknown fears and demonstrate a variety of emotions. Chaplains can provide spiritual and emotional care, thus providing a more holistic approach during a health crisis, trauma, or illness.

Adapted from Best, M., Sarvaananda, S., Martin, J., White, P., & Martin, M. (2016). Spiritual care services in emergency medicine. In M. L. Martin, S. Heron, L. Moreno-Walton, & A. W. Jones (Eds.), *Diversity and inclusion in quality patient care* (pp. 83–100). Berlin, Germany: Springer International Publishing.

After the seizure, Jessica's heart rate is 72 bpm and her O_2 saturation is 98% on room air.

I perform a neurological examination. Jessica's pupils are 4 mm, briskly reactive, and equal in size, shape, and speed of reaction. Jessica arouses to gentle shaking and loud voice

Priority Care Concepts 9.1

Nursing Care During a Seizure

During a seizure, priorities of care include ensuring safety and maintaining a patent airway and adequate circulation. Positioning the patient on his or her side helps maintain a patent airway and prevent saliva and mucus from blocking the airway.

stimulation. She opens her eyes for a few seconds after I ask her several times. Jessica occasionally turns her head side to side on her own. She responds appropriately to painful stimuli by pulling her hand away and saying, "Stop that."

Dr. Beck orders a complete metabolic panel, a magnesium level, a urinalysis, a complete blood count, and a random drug level for divalproex sodium. Drug levels for levetiracetam are not routinely checked, so Dr. Beck does not order a test for this medication. Because Jessica is so sleepy, Dr. Beck has ordered a straight catheter to obtain the urine sample. Additional orders include the following:

1. Estimated dosing weight: 121.3 lb (55 kg)
2. Take seizure precautions.

3. Start a peripheral intravenous (IV) line with a saline lock.
4. Administer normal saline (NS) 3 to 5 mL every 8 hours and as needed to flush the peripheral IV.
5. Rescue medication: administer lorazepam 2 mg IV if seizure activity lasts more than 5 minutes. Notify the physician before administration of lorazepam (The Pharmacy 9.2).
6. Admit to A7 North for observation
7. NPO (nothing by mouth)
8. Dextrose 5% in half NS (D5 ½ NS) at 95 mL/h IV

The Pharmacy 9.2 Benzodiazepines

Medication	Classification	Route	Action	Nursing Considerations
Diazepam (Valium), lorazepam (Ativan), and midazolam (Versed)	Benzodiazepine	• IV • IM • PR[a]	Increases the action of GABA, a neuroinhibitory transmitter, thus depressing the CNS	• Monitor for respiratory depression • May cause bradycardia and hypotension • Dilute lorazepam with an equal amount of diluent

[a]Only diazepam may be administered rectally.
CNS, central nervous system; GABA, gamma-aminobutyric acid; IM, intramuscular; IV, intravenous; PR, rectal.
Adapted from Taketomo, C. K. (2018). *Pediatric & neonatal dosage handbook* (25th ed.). Hudson, OH: Lexicomp.

I gather supplies and ask the PCA to assist in holding Jessica's arm while I start the IV. Jessica is arousable to voice and touch but is delayed in following some commands. I'm not sure she will remain still during the IV start. To reduce the chance of getting an IV needle stick or losing an IV, I ask for the PCA's assistance. I arouse Jessica and explain what I'm about to do. Jessica nods her head slightly, but her eyes remain closed. I start a 20-gauge IV to the right forearm on the first attempt, secure the IV, and draw blood for laboratory tests. I flush the IV with 5 mL of NS. Jessica slightly pulls her arm back during the IV start and mumbles, "ouch," but then dozes off. Following the hospital policy for laboratory specimen safety, I check the laboratory labels against Jessica's identification band before labeling the blood tubes. The blood tubes are labeled at the bedside and sent to the laboratory. I start D5 ½ NS at 95 mL/h after calculating the correct IV fluid rate for Jessica's weight of 55 kg. Finally, I enlist the PCA to assist with the straight urine catheterization to obtain a urine sample. I am reassured about Jessica's neurological status during the catheter insertion when she wakes up and clearly states, "What are you doing?" I explain what I'm doing, and Jessica nods her head in agreement but remains quiet, with her eyes closed. Jessica's urine is dark yellow but appears clear in the sterile specimen cup.

Dr. Beck arrives in the room and examines Jessica. After ensuring that she is stable, Dr. Beck and I speak with Jessica's parents in the hall.

"Jessica is stable and in a postictal state," Dr. Beck informs Mr. and Mrs. Wang. "When was her last seizure?"

"It has been months since she has had a seizure," Lian replies.

"Do you know what might have triggered this one?"

Lian and Wei are quiet a moment, and then Lian explains Jessica's history of tonic-clonic seizures. "Jessica is currently taking divalproex and levetiracetam to control her seizures," Lian says.

"Has she been ill or exposed to anyone who is sick?" Dr. Beck asks.

"No," Lian answers.

"Has Jessica been taking her antiepileptic medications as directed?"

Lian replies, "Jessica is a very responsible young lady. We allow her to take her own medications. She would never miss a dose without telling us."

We walk with Jessica's parents back into her room. Jessica is asleep on the stretcher. The side rails are padded and up. I explain to Mr. and Mrs. Wang what has happened since Jessica arrived via ambulance to the ER. Lian tells Nicole that

Jessica usually sleeps for up to several hours after she has a seizure. Lian and Wei talk softly to Jessica and she moans hello and falls back to sleep.

About an hour after she arrived in the ER, we receive the results from Jessica's laboratory tests and learn that her antiepileptic drug levels are subtherapeutic (Table 9.1). Dr. Beck orders a loading dose of levetiracetam and then reassesses Jessica. He also informs Mr. and Mrs. Wang about the laboratory test results.

"Everything looks normal except for her divalproex level," Dr. Beck tells them. "Were her medication bottles brought to the hospital?"

"I will have to find them. Jessica keeps them on her often times because she is not at home when her medications are due," Mr. Wang tells Dr. Beck.

"I'm concerned that perhaps Jessica has not been taking her medications, because her levels are so low," Dr. Beck tells the Wangs.

Lian and Mei look to the ground and shake their heads.

"Jessica will be admitted for observation and medication adjustment to make sure her antiepileptic medication levels are therapeutic before discharge," Dr. Beck informs them.

Table 9.1 Jessica's Laboratory Test Results

Laboratory Test	Analyte	Result	Reference Range[a]	Unit of Measure
Complete blood count	RBC	4.5	3.9–5.5	$\times10^6/\mu L$
	WBC	7,000	4,500–11,000	$/\mu L$
	Hgb	12.3	14.0–17.5	g/dL
	Hct	38	41–50	%
	Platelets	230,000	150,000–350,000	$/\mu L$
Comprehensive metabolic panel	Sodium	145	136–142	mEq/L
	Potassium	4.1	3.5–5	mEq/L
	Chloride	100	96–106	mEq/L
	CO_2	24	22–28	mg/dL
	BUN	24	8–23	mg/dL
	Creatinine	0.7	0.6–1.2	mg/dL
	Glucose	85	70–110	mg/dL
	Phosphorus	1.1	0.74–1.52	mmol/L
Urinalysis	Color	Dark yellow	Light/pale to dark/ deep amber yellow	N/A
	Specific gravity	1.23	1.005–1.025	N/A
	pH	7.1	4.5–8.0	N/A
	Glucose	None	None	N/A
	Ketones	Negative	Negative	N/A
	Nitrates	Negative	Negative	N/A
	Leukocytes	Negative	Negative	N/A
Serum drug levels	Divalproex sodium	10	50–100	µg/mL

[a]Reference ranges for complete blood count and comprehensive metabolic panel adapted from the American Medical Association. (2007). *AMA manual of style: A guide for authors and editors* (10th ed.). New York, NY: Oxford University Press.
BUN, blood urea nitrogen; Hct, hematocrit; Hgb, hemoglobin; RBC, red blood cell; WBC, white blood cell.

On the Unit

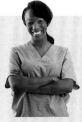

The Nurse's Point of View

Amy: A new patient, Jessica Wang, has just arrived on my unit, A7—the neuroscience unit at the pediatric hospital. She is being admitted for observation and seizure medication adjustment. I will be caring for Jessica until 7:30 tomorrow morning. The PCA and I greet Jessica and her parents at her room. Following safety procedures, I confirm Jessica's birth date and full name on her wrist band with Jessica's parents. Then the PCA and I assist the ER nurse in transferring Jessica to the hospital bed from the stretcher. Jessica is still sleepy and does not consistently follow several commands in sequence without falling asleep in between. However, she is opening her eyes when her mom or dad calls her name.

I ask Mr. and Mrs. Wang to step out so that I can examine Jessica from head to toe for any injuries and skin issues. I know that most 16-year-olds do not want their parents, particularly their fathers, present when being unclothed. I explain to Jessica what I am doing as I examine her. Jessica nods her head slightly and occasionally opens her eyes. To establish a baseline neurological status, I ask Jessica several questions.

"What is your full name?"

"Jessica."

"What is your last name?"

"Wang."

"Jessica, where are you?"

"I was at school."

"Where are you now?"

"Not sure."

"You are in the hospital because you had a seizure, and it is 9 o'clock at night," I tell her, reorienting her to place and time.

"I had a seizure?"

"Yes, on the tennis courts at school."

I continue my neurological exam and find Jessica's pupils to be 3 mm, equal, briskly reactive to light, and round.

Jessica follows some commands to follow the penlight to see whether she can track but dozes off before I am done with her examination. Jessica spontaneously moves her legs and arms but does not consistently grasp my hands or wiggle her toes yet. Jessica's vital signs are as follows:

- Heart rate: 76 bpm
- Respiratory rate: 12 breaths/min
- Blood pressure: 94/50 mm Hg
- O_2 saturation: 97% on room air

Jessica's O_2 saturation drops to 93% when she is deeply asleep, so I will keep oxygen close by. Thankfully, it does not go any lower.

I invite Jessica's parents back in and orient them to the room and to the unit rules.

"The hospital allows up to two people to stay the night with Jessica," I explain.

"We will not be staying," Mr. Wang replies. "We must go home because we have younger children there."

I discuss the plan of care for Jessica with them and then ask, "Do you have any questions or concerns at this time?"

Mrs. Wang is quietly tearful, looks at the floor, and shakes her head "no."

"Here is a unit resource pamphlet for parents that might be helpful," I tell them. "The phone number for the unit is printed on the front." I hand the pamphlet to Mr. Wang. "Please call at any time to check on Jessica or to let us know of any questions or concerns you have. Once Jessica is more awake, she will be able to be out of bed and resume her normal activities. For now, she will be allowed to sleep and rest and will receive IV fluids to make sure she stays hydrated."

Jessica sleeps throughout the night, except when I awaken her every 2 hours for a neurological exam. She does ask to use the bathroom once during an assessment. I realize it is unsafe to allow her to get out of bed, because she still seems sleepy and doesn't stay awake for more than 5 minutes at a time. So, the PCA and I help her use the bedpan. Jessica voids 800 mL of urine.

Jessica wakes up and realizes she is in the hospital. She is worried and a bit afraid, not remembering what happened. She realizes she is the only one in the room and presses the call light for the nurse. Jessica sits up in bed. She feels disoriented and upset.

A nurse comes in and says, "Jessica, what can I do to help? You put your call light on."

"I just realized I am in the hospital. I had a seizure, I think. Are my parents here? They are going to be so disappointed," says Jessica tearfully.

The nurse pulls up a chair and sits beside Jessica's bed. "Yes, you did have a seizure. You actually had two seizures. One at school on the tennis courts and one in the ER," explains the nurse. "My name is Amy. I've been caring for you since you arrived on the unit yesterday. How are you feeling now? Are you having any pain anywhere?"

"I feel okay. I am tired. My parents are going to be upset with me, I am sure. I have let them down again," replies Jessica.

"What makes you feel they are going to be upset?" asks Amy.

"I stopped taking my seizure medications. I have been so stressed lately. I forgot to take them one day and then just stopped taking them. I am tired of taking the medications. They make me feel different, and I don't like that. I thought maybe my grandparents were right. They told me I am just unbalanced and that is why I was so stressed. I thought if I stopped the seizure medications and tried to find harmony and balance, I would be okay and back to myself." Jessica cries harder and harder and stares downward.

"Jessica, I am sorry to hear you are so stressed and that things are so hard for you right now," Amy says. "We can talk about how to help you find ways of coping and dealing with stress. It is very, very important for you to take your seizure medications. The laboratory test results from the ER show that your levetiracetam and divalproex levels were low. It appears that not taking your medications led to your having the seizures."

"I know I need to take the medications, but I am just torn between my grandparents' thoughts about Western medicine and my parents' demands of taking my medication. Plus, I have so much stress with school, tennis, my brothers and sisters, and the demands of my parents and friends. I just don't make the medication a priority," says Jessica, sobbing.

At Discharge

By 2 days later, Jessica's antiepileptic medication levels are back within the therapeutic range. She has been taking her medications faithfully, and the neurologist informs her that she may now be discharged. Actually, several of the nurses have already been preparing Jessica for discharge, going over points about her epilepsy and how to manage it. Amy, one of the nurses who has been caring for her, comes in now to give her and her parents some final discharge teaching. First, Amy reviews triggers of seizures and strategies to lessen or avoid these triggers (Box 9.3). Next, she discusses the antiepileptic medications Jessica will be taking.

"You will be discharged on the same medications you were on before admission," Amy says. "The neurologist believes the seizures were a result of low drug levels, as evidenced by the laboratory test results on admission. You've done well with taking them the past couple of days, and I'm proud of you. But, as we've discussed, it is vital that you continue to take them

regularly. I believe by now you understand the consequences of not taking them, right Jessica?"

"Yes," Jessica replies. "I understand. I'm planning on taking them faithfully. I don't ever want to go through this again."

"I know how challenging it is to stick to your medication schedule," Amy says. She turns to Mr. and Mrs. Wang. "It's challenging for many teenagers—especially those who are on antiepileptic medications. Among adolescents with epilepsy, adherence to prescribed medication regimens has been consistently poor. Reports of nonadherence range from 35% to 79%" (Carbone, Zebrack, Plegue, Joshi, & Shellhaas, 2013).

Jessica's parents seem surprised to hear this information. "We will do whatever we can to help Jessica take her medications regularly," Mr. Wang says.

Amy discusses with Jessica and her parents the barriers to medication compliance and helps Jessica come up with solutions to avoid these barriers. Finally, Amy gives them a referral for adolescent behavioral health and counseling and encourages Jessica to follow up with the appointments to hopefully learn techniques to help with coping and stress management.

Box 9.3 Common Seizure Triggers

- Sleep deprivation
- Drugs
- Alcohol
- Increased stress
- Not eating well
- Flashing bright lights or patterns
- Illness or fever
- Use of certain medications
- Changes in menstrual cycle or hormones
- Specific time of day or night

Adapted from Schachter, S. C., Shafer, P. O., & Sirven, J. I. (2013). *Triggers of seizures.* Retrieved from http://www.epilepsy.com/learn/triggers-seizures

---

Think Critically

1. What other cultural implications should be considered while caring for Jessica, both in the hospital and as an outpatient?
2. What is the difference between Eastern medicine and Western medicine?
3. Why is it important for Jessica to have her blood levels of the antiepileptic medications checked on a regular basis? What factors may change Jessica's drug levels?
4. Why were Jessica's glucose and sodium levels checked as part of the initial diagnostic workup in the ER?
5. What factors could have precipitated Jessica's seizures?
6. What is a healthy weight range for a 16-year-old female?
7. What are the possible socioeconomic, health, and safety outcomes related to noncompliance with seizure medication?

References

Berchelmann, K. (2018). *Why to have the alcohol talk early: A pediatrician-mom's perspective.* Retrieved from: https://www.healthychildren.org/English/ages-stages/teen/substance-abuse/Pages/Why-to-Have-the-Alcohol-Talk-Early.aspx

Carbone, L., Zebrack, B., Plegue, M., Joshi, S., & Shellhaas, R. (2013). Treatment adherence among adolescents with epilepsy: What really matters? *Epilepsy & Behavior, 27*(1), 59–63.

Carteret, M. (2011). *Traditional Asian health beliefs & healing practices.* Retrieved from http://www.dimensionsofculture.com/2010/10/traditional-asian-health-beliefs-healing-practices

Centers for Disease Control. (2016). *Epilepsy in children.* Retrieved from https://www.cdc.gov/features/epilepsy-in-children

Fisher, R., Acevedo, C., Arzimanoglou, A., Bogacz, A., Cross, J., Elger, C., . . . Hesdorffer, D. (2014). ILAE official report: A practical clinical definition of epilepsy. *Epilepsia, 55*(4), 475–482.

Guilfoyle, S., Wagner, J., Modi, A., Junger, K., Barrett, L., Riisen, A., . . . Weyand, C. (2017). Pediatric epilepsy and behavioral health: The state of the literature and directions for evidence-based interprofessional care, training, and research. *Clinical Practice in Pediatric Psychology, 5*(1), 79–90.

Healthcare Chaplaincy. (2013). *Handbook of patients' spiritual and cultural values for healthcare professionals.* Retrieved from http://www.healthcarechaplaincy.org/userimages/Cultural%20Sensitivity%20handbook%20from%20HealthCare%20Chaplaincy%20%20(3-12%202013).pdf

Modi, A. C., Rausch, J. R., & Glauser, T. A. (2014). Early pediatric antiepileptic drug nonadherence is related to lower long-term seizure freedom. *Neurology, 82*(8), 671–673.

Smith, G., Wagner, J., & Edwards, J. (2015a). Epilepsy update part 1: Refining our understanding of a complex disease. *American Journal of Nursing, 115*(5), 40–47.

Smith, G., Wagner, J., & Edwards, J. (2015b). Epilepsy update part 2: Nursing care and evidence-based practice. *American Journal of Nursing, 115*(6), 40–47.

Suggested Readings

Epilepsy Foundation. (2017). *Tonic-clonic seizures.* Retrieved from http://www.epilepsy.com/learn/types-seizures/tonic-clonic-seizures

Victor, A. M. (2016). Caregiver's level of burden and coping strategies among patients with epilepsy: An exploratory study. *GSTF Journal of Nursing and Health Care (JNHC), 4*(1), 43–51.

10 Sophia Carter: Diabetes Mellitus Type 1

Sophia Carter, age 7 years

Objectives

After completing this chapter, you will be able to:
1. Describe normal growth and development of the 7-year-old.
2. Discuss an appropriate teaching plan for a healthy 7-year-old.
3. Identify signs of diabetes type 1.
4. Explain the pathophysiology of diabetes type 1.
5. Identify signs and symptoms of diabetic ketoacidosis and hypoglycemia.
6. Relate insulin therapy to the treatment of diabetes type 1.
7. Discuss the role of carbohydrates in the diet of a child diagnosed with diabetes type 1.
8. Create a nursing plan of care for a child newly diagnosed with diabetes type 1.

Key Terms

Basal insulin
Bolus insulin
Diabetes type 1
Glucometer
Glycated hemoglobin A1c (HgbA1c)
Insulin pump

Diabetic ketoacidosis
Ketones
Polydipsia
Polyphagia
Polyuria

Background

Sophia Carter is 7 years old and lives in an apartment in the city with her parents, Suzanne and Wayne. She is an only child. However, the Carter family has a small dog named Gus and a cat named Scout.

Sophia is in the second grade at a private school about three blocks from her apartment. Suzanne walks Sophia to school every morning before she goes to work, and most of the time Gus tags along, too. About 3 days a week, on their walk to school, Sophia and her mother stop at the cafe on the way to get drinks and pastries. Stopping at the cafe is one of Sophia's favorite things to do because it is special time with her mom. Suzanne is a high-powered business woman who works long hours. The morning walk to school is precious mother–daughter time.

Wayne, Sophia's dad, travels for business during the week but is home every weekend. He spends his time with Sophia going to the park, taking her to museums, or just walking with her around the city. After school, the babysitter, Megan, picks Sophia up and walks home with her. The Carters have no extended family near them. Both sets of grandparents, as well as aunts and uncles, live over 3 hours away. Megan is a sophomore at a nearby university studying to be a teacher. Most nights, Megan is at the Carters' apartment well into the evening. She is the one who usually fixes Sophia dinner and helps her with any homework. Although she arrives home late in the evening, Suzanne is always sure to be home to help Sophia get ready for bed. She reads a bedtime story to Sophia every night and cuddles with her until Sophia is almost asleep.

In the fall and spring, Sophia plays soccer on a local soccer team. She is passionate about soccer and has posters of the U.S. women's national soccer team in her room. During soccer season, Megan picks Sophia up from school and takes her on the subway to the soccer fields. The soccer fields are only two train stops from the school, but Sophia loves riding on the subway.

Sophia's health history is unremarkable. She suffered usual childhood illnesses such as strep throat, colds, and ear infections. She hasn't had any illnesses that have caused her to go to the doctor in over a year. Overall, Sophia is a happy 7-year-old who loves living in the city.

Health Promotion

While they are eating pastries on the way to school one morning, Suzanne says to Sophia, "You just had your seventh birthday. I guess that means it is time for your checkup with Dr. Hall."

"Mom, I don't want to go to the doctor. I haven't been sick. Why do I need to go?" protests Sophia.

Suzanne responds, "My dear, you are supposed to have a checkup every year to make sure you stay healthy. Dr. Hall has to check you out to make sure you are growing the way you should, although I can tell him you are growing like a weed. If you keep growing, I am going to have to put a brick on your head!"

Sophia giggles and says, "Mom, putting a brick on my head is not going to keep me from growing!"

"I know, but you are getting way too big way too fast. I will call Dr. Hall's office after I drop you off at school this morning." Suzanne and Sophia finish their pastries and drinks and head to school.

About 2 weeks later, Sophia has her appointment with Dr. Hall one morning before she goes to school. Dr. Hall has been Sophia's pediatrician since she was born. Suzanne feels lucky to have found such a great pediatrician; he is so good with Sophia. He makes her laugh, even if she feels terrible.

Sophia and her mom do not have to wait very long before her name is called. The assistant takes Sophia to a small room, where she measures her height, weight, and vital signs:
- Height: 49 in (4.1 ft)
- Weight: 52 lb (23.6 kg)
- Heart rate: 72 beats/min (bpm)
- Respiratory rate: 16 breaths/min
- Blood pressure: 102/65 mm Hg
- Temperature: 98.6°F (37°C)

The assistant takes Sophia and Suzanne to an examination room and tells them that Dr. Hall will be with them shortly.

While waiting for Dr. Hall, Sophia says, "Mom, do I have to get any shots today?"

"I don't think you need anything today," replies Suzanne. "Let's wait and see what Dr. Hall has to say."

A few minutes later, a monkey puppet on a hand appears through a crack in the door. "How's Miss Sophia today?" the monkey mouths in a silly voice. "I'm ready to do your checkup!"

Sophia starts giggling and says, "A monkey can't do my checkup!"

"Why not?" the monkey puppet replies. "Doctoring is part of my monkey business!" With that, Dr. Hall opens the door and comes in.

"Dr. Hall, you are so funny," says Sophia, still laughing. "It's not so bad coming here."

"How are you today?" Dr. Hall asks Sophia.

"I'm fine. I don't think I need to be here but my mom says I need to get a checkup every year, so that's why I'm here."

"Your mother is right; you do need a checkup every year. I need to make sure you are growing taller and gaining enough weight. I also need to make sure you are doing everything you are supposed to be doing in school."

"Thank you for explaining, Dr. Hall," states Suzanne. "I am not sure my daughter believed me!"

"I can tell you that I am doing everything I am supposed to in school. I get good grades and I never ever get in trouble. Right, mom?" Sophia declares proudly (Growth and Development Check 10.1).

"She is correct," replies Suzanne. "I have no trouble with her in school with either behavior or grades."

"That's good to know," says Dr. Hall. He looks at Sophia's chart. "I haven't seen you since your checkup last year." He continues asking questions of Sophia.

 Growth and Development Check 10.1

Early School-Aged Milestones

Type of Development	Development Milestones
Social and emotional	• Forms peer relationships • Establishes a best friend • Develops self-esteem • Is aware of body image
Speech	• Uses more complex grammar • Has the ability to think about language • Understands jokes and humor
Cognitive	• Likes to follow rules • Often likes to start collections • Begins to see things from another point of view • Develops a sense of self-worth through activities and accomplishments • Understands team sports
Gross and fine motor	• Improves in coordination and balance • Improves in rhythm • Improves in hand–eye coordination • Is able to participate in activities such as sewing, building models, or playing musical instruments

Adapted from the Centers for Disease Control and Prevention. (2017). *Child development: Middle childhood (6-8 years of age).* Retrieved from https://www.cdc.gov/ncbddd/childdevelopment/positiveparenting/middle.html

"What is your favorite thing to do when you are not in school?" asks Dr. Hall.

"That's easy. I love playing soccer. When it is soccer season, my babysitter, Megan, takes me to soccer practice after school. I just absolutely love it!" Sophia states emphatically. "I have posters of the U.S. women's soccer team on my bedroom wall. I want to play on that team someday. I know I can do it!"

"That sound like a nice goal. Do you wear all of your safety gear when you play?" asks Dr. Hall.

Sophia tells Dr. Hall, "I wear my shin guards and mouth guard every time I play because my mom and dad make me."

Dr. Hall tells Sophia and her mother that it is great she is so passionate about a sport, but Sophia needs to make sure she has time to do her homework and to get plenty of sleep.

"I make sure of that," Suzanne interjects (Patient Teaching 10.1). "Sophia is in bed by 8:30 every night. Megan is able to help her with homework if I have to stay at work late and Sophia's dad is out of town."

"Good, good," mumbles Dr. Hall as he is making notes in Sophia's chart. "What about friends?"

"Annie Sullivan is my very best friend. She plays soccer with me, and sometimes she gets to come to my house for a sleepover or I get to sleep over at her house."

"I am so glad you have a best friend, Sophia," continues Dr. Hall. "I'm going to change gears a little bit and talk about what you like to eat."

"Pastries and chicken nuggets," Sophia states matter-of-factly.

"This is an area we need to work on," Suzanne says. "Sophia is definitely not fond of vegetables. She will eat fruit, but veggies are an entirely different animal."

"How often do you eat pastries?" asks Dr. Hall.

Sophia replies, "Sometimes in the morning on the way to school. It is fun to have special time with mom. Sometimes our dog, Gus, comes too."

Dr. Hall looks at Sophia seriously and says, "Sweets like pastries are okay from time to time. I would like you to work on eating your vegetables, though. How about we make a plan that you will eat at least one serving of a vegetable a day? A serving

for you is the size of your palm. I will even let you put cheese on your broccoli or dip your carrots in ranch dressing!"

"How about it, Sophia," says Suzanne. "That plan doesn't sound too bad."

Sophia frowns and says, "I guess so."

Dr. Hall continues his conversation with Sophia and Suzanne. "Sophia, tell me about any chores you have at home."

"Well," Sophia starts. "I have to clean up all the stuff on my floor on Fridays, and I have to put my dishes in the dishwasher after I eat."

"That's good," Dr. Hall praises. "Those kinds of chores show me that you are responsible. Do you always do them?"

Sophia gets a sheepish grin on her face and her mother interjects, "Sometimes it takes a little prodding, but she is pretty good about getting things done."

Dr. Hall asks Sophia about her hygiene and oral health. Suzanne is proud of how Sophia responds and of how well she is doing.

"Sounds like you are doing great," Dr. Hall says. "You seem to be a happy, healthy, well-adjusted little girl."

Dr. Hall wraps up the health history by discussing safety (Patient Teaching 10.2). "We already talked about how important

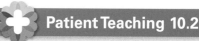

Patient Teaching 10.2

Safety for Early School Age

One of the greatest threats to children this age are injuries. However, most injuries are preventable by teaching children simple safety rules.

- Sports safety
  - Children should wear necessary sports equipment while playing.
- Water safety
  - Children should never swim alone.
  - Children should wear life jackets in bodies of water other than a swimming pool.
- Bike safety
  - Children should wear a helmet at all times when riding a bike.
  - Make sure the helmet fits securely and is buckled when worn.
- Car safety
  - Children under 4 ft 9 in tall should be in a booster seat with the regular car seatbelt.
  - Children may use a seat belt only when the lap belt fits on the hips and the shoulder belt is across the shoulder rather than the neck.
- Firearm safety
  - Store firearms in a locked cabinet.
  - Teach children the danger of firearms.

Adapted from the American Academy of Pediatrics. (2015). *Safety for your child: 8 years*. Retrieved from https://www.healthychildren.org/English/ages-stages/gradeschool/Pages/Safety-for-Your-Child-8-Years.aspx

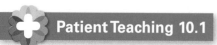

Patient Teaching 10.1

Parenting Tips for Early School Age

- Encourage physical activity daily.
- Help your child to make healthy food choices.
- Allow your child to help with meal choice and preparation.
- Help your child develop good homework habits.
- Continue reading to your child.
- Recognize your child's accomplishments.
- Set achievable goals.
- Have rules in place with consequences when the rules are broken.

it is for you to wear your safety gear when you are playing soccer. I want to check and make sure you are safe in other ways too." He looks at Suzanne and asks, "Do you have any firearms in the house?"

"No we don't," replies Suzanne. "I know that there is a firearm in Annie's house. That is Sophia's friend. Her dad has a gun, but I have talked with him and he assures me it is locked and out of reach of the girls."

Dr. Hall nods. "That's good. Adults should always make sure that firearms are locked away and out of reach of children. Unfortunately, there are too many avoidable accidents."

Next, Dr. Hall has Sophia hop up on the examination table. He completes her physical exam with complete cooperation from Sophia. "Sophia is perfectly healthy," Dr. Hall tells Suzanne after the exam. "I cannot even find anything on her physical exam to talk about."

Sophia smiles, but then a look of concern comes over her face. "Do I have to get any shots today?"

"The only shot you need this year is a flu shot. It is not quite time for that yet. You will need to come back in about a month. Your mom can schedule that visit when you leave," answers Dr. Hall.

"Yes!" Sophia shouts emphatically. "No shots today! Mom, let's go, I need to get to school."

Sophia and her mom thank Dr. Hall and make their way to the checkout counter. Sophia picks out a sticker and a sucker while her mom makes a flu shot appointment. They leave the office and make their way to school.

At Home

About a month after Sophia's visit to Dr. Hall, Suzanne notices that Sophia is more irritable and tired than usual. She figures it is because Sophia has been playing so much soccer and, unfortunately, getting to bed a little later at night. Sophia also seems to be hungry all of the time. This, too, Suzanne attributes to Sophia's playing soccer.

A few days after Suzanne notices changes in her daughter, Sophia comes to her mom and dad and says, "I don't feel good. My nose is all stuffy and I have to breathe through my mouth." Suzanne feels Sophia's forehead; she does not feel as if she has a fever.

"I think you are overdoing it, Sophia, and have gotten a cold," Suzanne says. "This weekend you should just stay at home and rest. We can watch movies and pop popcorn." Sophia goes back to bed and falls asleep.

Over the next few days, Sophia's cold symptoms neither worsen nor improve. In fact, Suzanne notices that Sophia is not only hungry all of the time but also seems to be drinking more. She assumes the increased thirst is because Sophia has been breathing through her mouth, which can cause a dry mouth.

Suzanne keeps Sophia home for a couple of days and watches her, hoping she will feel better after some much-needed rest. Wayne leaves town on business but tells Suzanne to keep him updated on how Sophia is doing.

The second morning Sophia stays home from school, Suzanne hears Sophia crying in her room. She goes to Sophia's room and finds Sophia lying on the floor, curled up in a ball, softly crying. "Honey, what's wrong?" Suzanne gently asks Sophia.

"Mommy, I had an accident—I wet the bed. I am so sorry!" Sophia begins to cry harder.

"It's okay, it's okay," assures Suzanne. "We will get you cleaned up and wash the sheets. Everything will be okay."

Suzanne helps Sophia get cleaned up. She tries not to let Sophia see that she is concerned. This is not like Sophia at all. She is tired, hungry, and thirsty all of the time lately and now she has wet the bed. Suzanne decides it is time to take Sophia back to see Dr. Hall.

At the Pediatrician's Office

Suzanne is able to get an appointment with Dr. Hall that afternoon. The assistant takes Sophia to get her weight and vital signs:

- Weight: 48 lb (21.8 kg)
- Heart rate: 100 bpm
- Respiratory rate: 16 breaths/min
- Blood pressure: 90/40 mm Hg
- Temperature: 100.8°F (38.2°C)

Suzanne notices Sophia's weight and is very concerned. Only about a month ago she weighed 52 lb. How could she have lost 4 lb, especially since she is eating all of the time? She begins to think that something is very wrong.

Sophia and her mother wait for Dr. Hall in one of the examination rooms. Suzanne can tell that Sophia is feeling worse today. She is even more tired than she has been over the past few days. Suzanne hopes Dr. Hall can figure out what is wrong. While they are waiting, Suzanne calls Wayne to let him know she is at the doctor's office with Sophia. She promises to call with an update after they see Dr. Hall.

Dr. Hall enters the room and frowns when he sees Sophia curled up in her mom's arms. "What's wrong with Miss Sophia today?"

"She has not felt well for a couple of weeks," Suzanne says. Suzanne recounts how she noticed Sophia was tired and eating more and how a few days ago she seemed to come down with a cold. "And a bedwetting incident this morning prompted me to schedule the visit."

Dr. Hall listens intently. He asks Sophia to sit on the table so he can conduct a quick exam. When he's done, he says, "Everything seems relatively normal, with the exception of decreased skin turgor. That means her skin doesn't return to its normal shape very quickly after I pinch it. It's often a sign of dehydration." He looks at her chart. "I'm also concerned that she has lost weight over the past month."

"What does this mean?" Suzanne asks.

"I have an idea," Dr. Hall says. "But I'd like check her blood glucose level, to make sure." Turning to Sophia, he says, "This test requires a quick prick of your finger. I need to check how much sugar is in your blood. The blood sugar level will help me determine what is making you feel so bad. The nurse will be in shortly to take care of you." Dr. Hall leaves the room.

Sophia is not happy that she has to have her finger pricked, but she is too tired to protest. She sits in Suzanne's lap while the nurse pricks her finger and puts a drop of blood on a small strip. "I will put the strip in a small machine that measures the amount of glucose in the blood," the nurse tells Suzanne and Sophia. "Dr. Hall will be back in shortly with the results." The nurse leaves.

A few minutes later, Dr. Hall enters the room and reports that Sophia's blood glucose level is 260 mg/dL. "Based on So-phia's symptoms—increased thirst, increased hunger, increased urination, weight loss, and fatigue—and now a high blood glu-cose level, I am afraid to say that Sophia meets the criteria for diabetes mellitus type 1" (Boxes 10.1 and 10.2).

Suzanne is stunned. She sits quietly for a moment collecting her thoughts. She is not sure where to even begin.

"What is diabetes?" Sophia asks quietly. "Am I going to die?"

Dr. Hall sits next to Sophia and says, "No, Sophia, you are not going to die. Diabetes is a disease where the cells in your body are not able to use a type of sugar, called glucose, for en-ergy. When the cells can't use glucose, the glucose stays in your blood and it makes you sick" (Box 10.3).

Dr. Hall continues to explain that insulin is what the body uses to absorb glucose into the cell. In diabetes mellitus type 1, the cells that make insulin have been destroyed and no insulin is produced. Therefore, the treatment for diabetes mellitus type

Box 10.1   Signs and Symptoms of Diabetes Mellitus Type 1

Children diagnosed with diabetes mellitus type 1 typically present with the following hallmark symptoms:
- **Polyphagia**
- **Polydipsia**
- **Polyuria**
- Fatigue
- Weight loss

Box 10.2   Criteria for the Diagnosis of Diabetes Mellitus Type 1

- **Glycated hemoglobin A1c** $\geq 6.5\%$
  or
- Fasting plasma glucose, defined as no calories for 8 h, ≥ 126 mg/dL
  or
- Two-hour plasma glucose ≥ 200 mg/dL during an oral glucose tolerance test
  or
- A random plasma glucose ≥ 200 mg/dL with classic symptoms of hyperglycemia

Adapted from American Diabetes Association. (2015). Classification and diagnosis of diabetes. *Diabetes Care, 38*(Suppl. 1), S8–S16; Mayo, P. (2016). An overview of diabetes. *Nursing Standard, 30*(46), 53–63.

Box 10.3   Pathophysiology of Diabetes Mellitus Type 1

Type 1 diabetes mellitus is the result of an autoimmune attack on the beta cells in the pancreas. Although there are many theories about what triggers this autoimmune re-sponse, the exact mechanisms are not well understood. Some predisposing factors for **diabetes type 1** include genetics, environ-mental factors, and other autoimmune condi-tions (Mayo, 2016).

Beta cells produce and regulate insulin to maintain a normal blood glucose level. When the beta cells are diminished or absent, little to no insulin is produced, causing a rise in blood glucose levels. Insulin signals cells to take in glucose to use for energy. Without insulin, glucose is not used by the cells and remains in the bloodstream. High blood glu-cose levels result in the symptoms associ-ated with diabetes type 1.

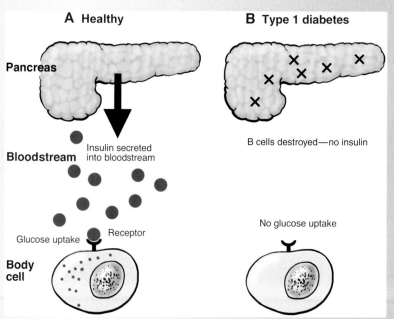

The pancreas and the action of insulin on the body cell in health and in type 1 diabetes mellitus. A. The healthy pancreas excretes insulin into the bloodstream, which enables glucose uptake by the body cell. **B.** In type 1 di-abetes mellitus, the pancreas produces no insulin and so the body cell can-not take up glucose. Reprinted with permission from Wilkins, E. M. (2016). *Clinical practice of the dental hygienist* (12th ed., Fig. 69.1). Philadelphia, PA: Lippincott Williams & Wilkins.

1 is to give insulin injections and control glucose levels in the blood.

After hearing the explanation, Suzanne asks, "Is there something I did wrong? Is it because we eat pastries on the way to school? Did I cause this to happen?"

"Absolutely not," assures Dr. Hall. "Sometimes, there is a genetic component to diabetes, meaning it runs in families, but most of the time we do not know why it happens."

"What now?" asks Suzanne.

"The next step is to get Sophia to the hospital and get her blood sugar under control. Her blood sugar is pretty high. If it gets higher, she could start having more severe symptoms. She is awake and alert but drowsy. I don't think she needs to be admitted to the ICU, or intensive care unit, but I will admit her to a unit where the nurses will be able to watch her closely."

Dr. Hall goes on to explain that the doctors that take care of children with diabetes mellitus type 1 are called endocrinologists. He tells Suzanne to go home, pack a bag, and then go to the emergency department at Children's Hospital. He will call to let them know they are coming.

Sophia starts crying. "I don't want to go to the hospital."

"Sophia, you have to go," Dr. Hall says. "Otherwise you will get worse instead of better. I promise you that after a day or two you will feel better and you will be able to go home." Dr. Hall tells Suzanne to go to the main desk in the emergency department and they should take Sophia up to the unit to be admitted.

Suzanne calls Wayne on her way back to the house. She tells him that Dr. Hall diagnosed Sophia with diabetes mellitus type 1 and she will be admitted to the hospital to start treatment. Wayne tells Suzanne that he will be on the next flight home.

At the Hospital

In the Emergency Department

Suzanne does as Dr. Hall instructed her and goes to the main desk in the emergency department. The receptionist does indeed have Sophia's name and indicates that she is to have some blood work drawn in the emergency department before she is taken up to the unit. The receptionist calls a nursing assistant to escort Sophia and Suzanne to a bed.

A few minutes later, a nurse comes to the bedside. "Hi, I'm Gina," she says. "I am going to take your vital signs and get some blood work."

"Why does she have to have her blood work done here?" inquires Suzanne.

"We can get the results of the tests quickly in the emergency department," explains Gina. "The doctors need some more test results before they know how much insulin Sophia needs."

Gina takes Sophia's vital signs. "I'm going to start an intravenous (IV) line and get the blood samples," she says. "That way, you only have to get stuck once." Gina starts the IV line and fills several tubes with samples of Sophia's blood. Gina also has Sophia give a urine sample. She tells Sophia and her mom, "You will probably be in the emergency department for about an hour or so. Do you need anything?"

Sophia says "I'm thirsty, can I have some juice?"

Table 10.1	Sophia's Laboratory Test Results		
Laboratory Test	**Result**	**Normal Range**	**Unit of Measure**
Blood glucose	260	70–100	mg/dL
Anion gap	14	8–12	mEq/L
Serum bicarbonate	17	18–25	mmol/L
Serum pH	7.29	7.35–7.45	N/A
Serum creatinine	1.2	0.8–1.4	mg/dL
Serum sodium	137	135–147	mEq/L
Serum potassium	4.6	3.4–4.7	mEq/L
Hemoglobin A1c	8.2	<7.5	%
White blood count	16,000	5,000–15,500	/mL
Urinalysis	Mild ketones	No ketones	N/A

Adapted from Harriet Lane Service (Johns Hopkins Hospital). In: Hughes, H. K., & Kahl, L. (2018). *The Harriet Lane handbook: A manual for pediatric house officers.* (21st ed.). Philadelphia, PA: Elsevier. Copyright © 2018 Elsevier. With permission.

"I don't think juice would be the best thing right now," Gina says. "How about I get you some water?" Gina gets Sophia some water and tells Suzanne she will check in on them soon.

About 45 minutes later, Gina returns and tells Suzanne that the results of Sophia's blood work are ready (Table 10.1). She also says, "I've called in the results to the endocrinologist, Dr. Price, who admitted Sophia. I've also arranged to transfer Sophia to the unit. She will need to be admitted to the ICU because she needs an insulin infusion. In the ICU, she can be closely monitored for unwanted side effects during the infusion. I talked with the nurse, Annie, who will be assuming care for Sophia and let her know that an assistant is bringing Sophia to the unit and that Dr. Price should be on the unit writing admission orders."

On the Unit

Sophia arrives at the ICU and is escorted to her room. A nurse who meets them says, "Hi, my name is Annie, and I am going to take care of you today."

"I'm scared," says Sophia. "There are so many lights and noises."

"I know it's scary, Sophia," Annie says. "The beeps and lights are nothing to be afraid of though. Would it be helpful to turn the TV on to try and forget about all of the other noises?"

"That would be good, I guess," Sophia says. She settles into the bed, with her mom sitting in the chair beside her. Annie does her best to distract Sophia and help her relax.

"I am going to check the doctor's orders and get some fluids and insulin started," explains Annie. "I will be right back" (Box 10.4).

Box 10.4   Orders for Sophia Carter

- Admit to A4 West.
- Start a peripheral IV line.
- Administer a normal saline bolus of 220 mL over 1 h.
- When the bolus is complete, start normal saline plus 40 mEq of potassium per liter at 97 mL/h (1½ × maintenance).
- Administer a continuous regular insulin drip at 2.3 U/h, with the goal of blood glucose level dropping by 80–100 mg/dL/h.
- Conduct blood glucose checks every 30 min during the insulin drip.

- Once the blood glucose level decreases by 80–100 mg/dL,
  - Change fluids to 5% dextrose in half normal saline plus 20 mEq of potassium per liter at 97 mL/h for 24 h.
  - Give insulin glargine 9 U subcutaneously and then stop the insulin drip.
- Insulin regimen
  - Administer insulin glargine 9 U daily.
  - Administer insulin lispro for carbohydrate coverage 1 U subcutaneously for every 25 g of carbohydrates.
- Check blood glucose level before meals and at 2 a.m.
- Refer the patient to a diabetes educator.
- Refer the patient to a dietitian.

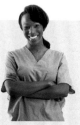

The Nurse's Point of View

Annie: I read Dr. Price's orders. Because Sophia's blood glucose level is over 250 mg/dL with positive **ketones** in her urine, a high anion gap, low serum bicarbonate, and low serum pH, I know that Sophia has **diabetic ketoacidosis (DKA)**. However, Sophia is awake and alert, although a little drowsy, and has no nausea, vomiting, or fruity breath, so her DKA is mild (Box 10.5). Sophia will need carefully monitoring over the next 24 hours. Because of the intensive insulin treatment for DKA, she is at risk for hypoglycemia (Box 10.5; Analyze the Evidence 10.1).

As I prepare to hang the insulin drip, I review the signs and symptoms of hypoglycemia in my head. Sophia's blood glucose level is high, but I've seen higher. It shouldn't take long for her blood glucose level to come down by 80 to 100 mg/dL. A blood glucose level <70 mg/dL is a warning value and means that insulin doses should be adjusted (American Diabetes Association [ADA], 2017). I will have to be vigilant in monitoring Sophia (Priority Care Concepts 10.1).

Box 10.5   Signs and Symptoms of Diabetic Ketoacidosis and Hypoglycemia

When taking care of patients with diabetes mellitus type 1, nurses should understand that the two critically acute complications are diabetic ketoacidosis and hypoglycemia. Recognizing small changes in status and intervening early can prevent either one of these life-threatening conditions.

Diabetic Ketoacidosis

- Blood glucose level > 250 mg/dL
- Venous pH < 7.3
- High levels of ketones in the urine
- Nausea
- Vomiting
- Tachypnea
- Fruity breath
- Dehydration
- Altered level of consciousness

Hypoglycemia

- Blood glucose level < 54 mg/dL
- Shakiness
- Sweating, chills, clamminess
- Irritability
- Altered level of consciousness
- Nausea
- Fatigue
- Seizures

Adapted from American Diabetes Association. (2017). Care of diabetes in the hospital. *Diabetes Care, 40*(Suppl. 1), S120–S127.

Analyze the Evidence 10.1

Diabetic Ketoacidosis at Diagnosis

Duca, Wang, Rewer, & Rewers (2017) conducted a 15-y longitudinal study to test the hypothesis that a child with diabetic ketoacidosis (DKA) at the time of diagnosis of diabetes mellitus type 1 is more likely to demonstrate poor long-term glycemic control. The study was a prospective cohort study that included 3,364 participants diagnosed with diabetes type 1 before the age of 18 y. The researchers measured each participant's hemoglobin A1c an average of 2.8 times/y. Controlling for race, gender, age, and socioeconomic status, the researchers found that mild, moderate, or severe DKA at diagnosis does predict poor glycemic control and increased complications of diabetes.

DKA causes severe hyperglycemia and inflammation, which leads to rapid destruction of the beta cells in the pancreatic islets. A decreased overall number of beta cells creates the need for higher amounts of insulin to achieve glycemic control. Thus, DKA at diagnosis is more than a complication. Children with DKA at diagnosis of diabetes mellitus type 1 have increased morbidity and mortality rates overall (Duca et al., 2017).

Priority Care Concepts 10.1   Monitoring for Hypoglycemia

Patients newly diagnosed with diabetes mellitus type 1 are at risk for moderate-to-severe hypoglycemia after the initiation of insulin therapy.

Goals
- Maintain blood glucose levels from 70 to 180 mg/dL.
- Maintain electrolyte levels within normal limits.
- Maintain adequate hydration.

Nursing Interventions
- Notify the healthcare provider of any blood glucose reading ≤70 mg/dL.
- Monitor for changes in cognitive status.
- Monitor for irritability, sweatiness, and slurred speech.
- Encourage the child to eat fast-acting carbohydrates such as juices, soft drinks, or a handful of candy.
- Retest the blood glucose level 15 min after carbohydrate ingestion.
- Adjust the insulin regimen as ordered.

As Annie is hanging the IV fluids and insulin drip, Dr. Price comes to assess Sophia.

"Hey there, young lady," begins Dr. Price. "My name is Dr. Price." He shakes hands with Suzanne and begins to explain Sophia's treatment.

"The insulin drip will get Sophia's blood glucose level under control quickly. We need to monitor Sophia very closely. If we don't, she could end up with a blood glucose level that is too low, and we don't want that, either. Once her blood glucose level comes down to around 160 mg/dL, we will stop the insulin drip and start her on a regimen of insulin shots."

"Shots!" shouts Sophia. "I hate shots! How many do I have to have?"

"I don't want to go into too much detail right now, but as part of the treatment for diabetes mellitus type 1, you will need to give yourself a few insulin shots every day."

"That sounds terrible," Sophia moans.

"Let's get you settled in and your symptoms taken care of before you think about anything else," interjects Dr. Price. "Once you are feeling a little better, our diabetes education team will come and talk with you and your mom about taking care of yourself at home."

"My dad will be here soon. He is coming home from a business trip," says Sophia.

"That's wonderful. You and your parents can all learn together, and we will be here to answer any questions." Dr. Price assures Suzanne that Sophia is in good hands and that he will be back in about an hour.

Insulin Therapy

It doesn't take long for Sophia's blood glucose level to decrease by 80 to 100 mg/dL, as ordered by Dr. Price. Annie discontinues the insulin drip. She explains to Sophia that she is going to give her the first insulin injection.

"Look at the needle, Sophia. The needle is very small. I am going to give you the shot in your belly. I will squeeze some skin and put the needle in the bunched up skin. I think you will hardly feel it at all," Annie does her best to reassure Sophia that the insulin injection is not so bad.

After the injection, Sophia exclaims, "You were right, Annie, that wasn't so bad!"

By this time, Wayne has arrived and is intently watching everything Annie does. Annie explains to Sophia and her parents that there are many different types of insulin and that they are classified depending on how long their effects last (The Pharmacy 10.1).

"How do we know which one to use?" asks Wayne.

Annie replies, "Dr. Price will prescribe an insulin regimen for Sophia. It will most likely need to be adjusted over the first few weeks until he finds what works best for Sophia."

Annie explains to Sophia and her parents that they will all have to learn how to draw up the correct amount of insulin in a syringe and give the injection (Hospital Help 10.1). "Ideally," says Annie, "Sophia will give the majority of injections herself. She is old enough. However, she will definitely need parental supervision for a while, until the treatment regimen is stable."

"I'll tell you what though," Annie continues, "When it is time for your next insulin injection, I am going to show you how, but you are going to do it yourself, Sophia" (Patient Teaching 10.3; Fig. 10.1).

"Really?" Sophia's eyes widen with both fear and excitement. "You mean I am going to give a shot to myself?"

"Yep," replies Annie. "You can do it."

As promised, Annie shows Sophia how to draw up insulin into the syringe and, with supervision, Sophia gives herself an insulin injection (Patient Teaching 10.4).

"Great job, sweetie," exclaims Sophia's dad. "I think you just jumped one of the biggest hurdles!"

"She did great," Annie agrees, "and, yes, this is a big hurdle. However, you all still have a lot to learn. You will need to make some lifestyle changes. Tomorrow, a diabetes education team will be in to teach you all how to manage diabetes at home.

The Pharmacy 10.1 Insulin Products

Rate of Onset	Insulin Product	Action	Nursing Considerations
Rapid	• Lispro (Humalog) • Aspart (Novo Log)	• Replacement of endogenous insulin in patients with type 1 diabetes • Onset: 5–15 min • Peak: 30–90 min • Effective duration: 5 h	• Administer via subcutaneous injection. • The dose is determined on the basis of age and blood glucose measurements. • Monitor blood glucose level regularly. • Monitor for hypoglycemia. • Store in a refrigerator until the expiration date. • Store at room temperature for 28 d.
Short	Regular U100	• Replacement of endogenous insulin in people with type 1 diabetes • Onset: 30–60 min • Peak: 2–3 h • Effective duration 5–8 h	• Administer via subcutaneous injection. • The dose is determined on the basis of age and blood glucose measurements. • Monitor blood glucose level regularly. • Monitor for hypoglycemia. • Store in a refrigerator until the expiration date. • Store at room temperature for 28 d.
Intermediate	Isophane (NPH, Humulin N)	• Replacement of endogenous insulin in people with type 1 diabetes • Onset: 2–4 h • Peak 4–10 h • Effective duration: 10–16 h	• Administer via subcutaneous injection. • Use as a supplement to a basal insulin injection. • The dose is determined on the basis of age and blood glucose measurements. • Monitor blood glucose level regularly. • Monitor for hypoglycemia. • Store in a refrigerator until the expiration date. • Once opened, this insulin is good for 31 d when stored in a refrigerator.
Long	Glargine (Lantus)	• Replacement of endogenous insulin in people with type 1 diabetes • Onset: 2–4 h • No peak • Effective duration: 20–24 h	• Administer via subcutaneous injection. • Use as a basal insulin dose. • Use with rapid- or short-acting insulin. • Monitor blood glucose level regularly. • Monitor for hypoglycemia. • Store in a refrigerator until the expiration date. • Store at room temperature for 28 d.
Long	Detemir (Levemir)	• Replacement of endogenous insulin in people with type 1 diabetes • Onset: 3–4 h • Peak: 6–8 h • Effective duration: 6–24 h, depending on the dose	• Administer via subcutaneous injection. • The usual maintenance range is 0.5–1.0 U/kg/d in divided doses. • Use as a basal insulin dose. • Use with rapid- or short-acting insulin. • Monitor blood glucose level regularly. • Monitor for hypoglycemia. • Store in a refrigerator until the expiration date. • Store at room temperature for 42 d.

Adapted from Hughes, H. K., & Kahl, L. K. (Eds.). (2018). *The Harriet Lane handbook* (21st ed.). Philadelphia, PA: Elsevier; Taketomo, C. K., Hodding, J. H., & Kraus, D. M. (2018). *Pediatric and neonatal dosage handbook* (25th ed.). Hudson, OH: Lexicomp.

I will not be back tomorrow, but I know that you will listen well and learn what you need to do to stay healthy, Sophia."

Diabetes Self-Management Education

The next morning, Dr. Price comes in to check on Sophia. "Looks like you had an uneventful night," he proclaims. "Today, you are going to learn a lot of information about how to manage diabetes. I want you to listen, but your mom and dad will be here to listen, too. When you have questions, be sure to ask

them. Maggie is our diabetes education nurse. She is a great teacher and loves to answer questions."

"How will we remember everything we are told?" Suzanne asks, feeling worried.

"Maggie will give you multiple handouts," Dr. Price says. "There is no way you will remember everything, and we don't expect you to. You will leave here knowing the most important things to get you through the next few days. We will monitor Sophia very closely in the first few weeks. If you have questions, we are only a phone call away."

Hospital Help 10.1

Encouraging Self-Care in School-Aged Children

School-aged children are able to participate in their care. Allow them to make choices when possible in the hospital. Give simple explanations for any procedures or medicines. Children at this age are able to tell time, so if a parent has to leave, letting them know a time of return can help alleviate anxiety.

School-aged children newly diagnosed with diabetes mellitus type 1 need to participate in administering insulin injections. To alleviate anxiety, children should practice drawing up insulin. Children can practice giving a "shot" with a needleless syringe to a doll. Practicing on a doll helps children become more comfortable with the procedure. Once children become comfortable with drawing up insulin and giving injections to a doll, they can then transition to giving their own insulin injections. Nurses are instrumental in the process of helping children and families become comfortable with insulin injections.

Suzanne looks at Wayne and relaxes a little. It is nice to know that she can call with questions. She hopes the diabetes nurse is just as reassuring as is Dr. Price.

As if on cue, Maggie walks into the room. Dr. Price smiles and says, "I'm leaving you in good hands. If all goes well, you

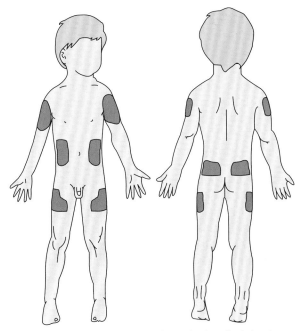

Figure 10.1. Insulin injection sites. An insulin injection may be given in any of the shaded areas. The same area should not be used each time; all sites should be included in rotation. Reprinted with permission from Silbert-Flagg, J., & Pillitteri, A. (2018). *Maternal and child health nursing: Care of the childbearing and childrearing family* (8th ed., Fig. 48.5). Philadelphia, PA: Wolters Kluwer.

 Patient Teaching 10.3

Drawing Up Insulin

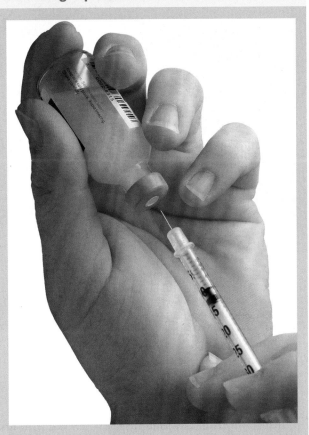

The nurse should first demonstrate how to draw insulin from the vial. The parents or caregivers should then perform a repeat demonstration of how to draw insulin from a vial. Return demonstrations should continue until there are no mistakes. School-age children and older should be involved in the procedure of drawing up insulin. Nurses should provide written material to families to reinforce learning.

Steps for drawing up insulin:
- Gather all equipment.
  - Syringe
  - Vial
  - Alcohol pad
- Clean the top of the insulin vial with an alcohol swab.
- Remove the syringe cap.
- Insert the syringe needle into the rubber stopper on the insulin vial.
- Measure the exact amount of insulin needed and remove the syringe from the vial.
- Tap the side of the syringe to remove air bubbles.

should be able to go home tomorrow. I will be by to check on you later this afternoon."

"Hi Sophia, I'm Maggie. I am going to teach you how to monitor your blood sugar and give your insulin at home."

Sophia grins widely, "I already gave myself a shot yesterday!"

Patient Teaching 10.4

How to Give an Insulin Injection

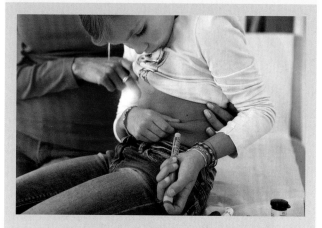

1. Pinch up some skin and quickly insert the needle at a 90° angle. Keep the skin pinched so the insulin does not go into the muscle.
2. Choose a site for the insulin injection (Fig. 10.1).
3. Push the plunger down all the way. Hold the syringe and needle in place for 5 s.
4. Let go of the pinched skin and remove the needle from the skin. If needed, press on the area for 5–8 s, but do not rub.
5. Discard the syringe in an appropriate sharps container.

Patient Teaching 10.5

Monitoring Blood Glucose

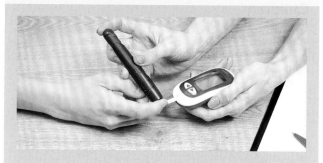

Monitoring blood glucose levels is the best way to determine whether the blood glucose is in a safe range. Blood glucose levels also help determine the amount of insulin needed. Common times to measure blood glucose levels include the following:
- First thing in the morning
- Before meals
- Before, during, and after exercise
- During times of illness
- As needed
   To measure blood glucose:
- Clean your hands with soap and water or alcohol wipes.
- Load the lancet device.
- Use the side of the fingertip to obtain a drop of blood with the lancet.
- Place a drop of blood on the test strip in the glucometer.
- Wait the appropriate amount of time and read the results.
- Record the results in a logbook or journal.

"That is wonderful!" exclaims Maggie. "That is a great first step, but there is a lot more to learn. The first thing I am going to do is teach you how to monitor your blood glucose level."

Suzanne smiles. She can tell that Maggie will be great with Sophia.

"I am going to tell you a lot of information this morning," Maggie says. "I will leave you with some things to read and come back later this afternoon. We will review information again later today and tomorrow morning. Before you go home, I will give you my cell phone number. I want you to text me your blood glucose level every time you check it for the first few days. It will help us get you on a stable regimen faster."

"Thank you so much," says Suzanne. "This is all so overwhelming."

"I know it is. That is why I am here. After I am done, a dietitian named Brett will come and talk to you about nutrition and diet as part of your treatment for diabetes."

"Caring for a child with diabetes is all about setting goals," Annie explains. "When monitoring blood glucose levels, you will need to consider two things. First, monitoring Sophia's blood glucose level at home with a **glucometer**; your goal is to have 80% of her blood glucose readings from 70 to 180 mg/dL." Maggie demonstrates how to use a glucometer for both Sophia and her parents (Patient Teaching 10.5).

After demonstrating the use of a glucometer, Maggie tells Sophia and her parents that the second number they will monitor is the hemoglobin A1c, or HgbA1c. This is a blood test that measures blood glucose control over time. Sophia's HgbA1c is currently 8.2%. Maggie explains that the HgbA1c should be less than 7.5%

for Sophia's age to indicate that the blood glucose levels have been well controlled over time (ADA, 2016). She tells Sophia's parents that they should see the number come down after a few months. The high HgbA1c is just another indication of new-onset diabetes.

"Now that we have talked about how to measure your blood glucose level, we need to talk about the insulin you are getting to help keep those numbers under control," Maggie tells Sophia.

Maggie begins her explanation of the different types of insulin and how the length of effect is different depending on the type of insulin. She tells the Carter family that Sophia will be on a basal bolus insulin regimen. This type of regimen requires multiple daily injections but is the most flexible, allowing for Sophia to eat more of the foods she likes. The **basal insulin** is given to steady Sophia's blood glucose levels, whereas the **bolus insulin** doses are given to correct for the amount of carbohydrates Sophia eats at any given meal.

"How will we know how much insulin to give Sophia when she eats?" asks Suzanne.

"You will have to count the number of carbohydrates that she eats. When Brett comes in, he will teach you how to do that," replies Maggie. "Also, we eventually hope to have Sophia on an **insulin pump**" (Fig. 10.2). "The pump gives a continuous

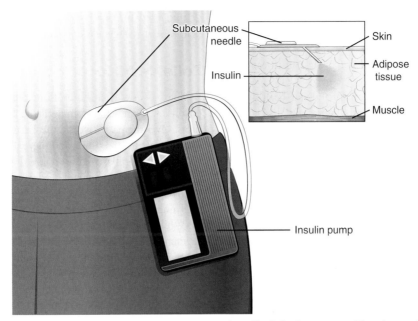

Figure 10.2. Continuous subcutaneous insulin infusion pump. The dose of continuous insulin is programmed into the pump and administered through a needle situated in the subcutaneous tissue. Reprinted with permission from Frandsen, G., & Pennington, S. S. (2018). *Abrams' clinical drug therapy* (11th ed., Fig. 41.3). Philadelphia, PA: Wolters Kluwer.

infusion of the basal insulin, reducing the number of insulin injections Sophia will need each day."

Maggie stresses to Sophia and her parents the importance of maintaining blood glucose levels within the recommended ranges, noting that multiple complications can occur if blood glucose levels are not maintained over time (Box 10.6). "If your blood glucose level is below 70 mg/dL or over 200 mg/dL, you need to call us right away, even if Sophia is acting okay. We will need to act on those numbers quickly so that she doesn't go into severe hypoglycemia, or into ketoacidosis. Either one of these is an emergency." Maggie continues by explaining the symptoms of both hypoglycemia and ketoacidosis.

"I know you have a lot of questions," says Maggie. "I am going to leave this information with you to read. As I said earlier, I will come back later this afternoon to review the information. In the meantime, write down any questions you may have."

"I have a question," Sophia says quietly. "Will I still be able to play soccer?"

"Absolutely, you will. However, we need to get this blood glucose level under control. Once you learn how to do that, then we will discuss what to do for exercise and sports. You will need to check your blood glucose levels more often when you are practicing or playing games." Maggie's answer makes Sophia smile.

"That's great, Sophia," says her dad. "We'll get you back to practice as soon as we can."

A few minutes later, Brett, the dietitian comes into Sophia's room (Whose Job Is It, Anyway? 10.1). "Hi there, Sophia. I'm here to teach you about eating healthy."

Box 10.6 Complications Associated With Diabetes Mellitus Type 1

Immediate Complications
- Hyperglycemia
- Diabetic ketoacidosis
- Hypoglycemia

Long-Term Complications
- Risk of other autoimmune diseases, especially hypothyroidism or celiac disease
- Nephropathy
- Retinopathy
- Cardiovascular disease
- Peripheral neuropathy
- Increased risk of infections

Adapted from Teuten, P., & Holt, S. (2016). Recognition and management of diabetes in children. *Emergency Nurse, 24*(8), 26–32.

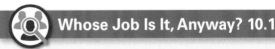 **Whose Job Is It, Anyway? 10.1**

Dietitian

Dietitians are experts in nutrition and can help children with diabetes mellitus type 1 and their families plan meals. They understand how food affects the body's blood glucose levels. A dietitian helps families learn to read food labels, determine the amount of carbohydrates in food eaten, and make adjustments to meal plans based on activities such as sports. A dietitian knowledgeable in diabetes mellitus type 1 is an essential member of the diabetes care team.

"I already told my doctor I will eat my vegetables. I don't need any more talking to about eating healthy." Sophia pouts and crosses her arms.

Brett laughs and says, "I'm glad you are going to eat your vegetables, but there are more things we need to talk about so you can keep your diabetes under control and stay healthy."

Brett explains that monitoring carbohydrate intake is a major part of maintaining blood glucose levels, along with insulin therapy.

"What is a carbohydrate?" asks Sophia.

"Carbohydrates are in foods and are turned into sugar in your digestive system. Too much sugar will make your blood glucose levels go too high."

"I can't have sugar!" cries Sophia. "Mom, what about our trips to the bakery before school? This isn't fair!"

"Calm down Sophia, let's hear what Brett has to say," Suzanne says soothingly.

"Sweets are okay every now and then, but you will need to adjust your insulin dose based on what you eat," says Brett.

Brett continues his teaching, talking about food labels. He tells Sophia and her parents that all packaged foods must have labels on them. They will need to know the total number of carbohydrates and serving size to correctly count how many carbohydrates Sophia eats. "Carbohydrate counting takes some getting used to, but it does allow flexibility in Sophia's diet. I promise it will get easier over time."

Follow-Up

Sophia has now been home from the hospital for 2 weeks. As promised, Maggie has been available for all of the family's questions. Over the past 2 weeks, the Carter family has met with the diabetes care team 3 times, and they still talk with Maggie at least once a day. Sophia is comfortable drawing up the insulin and giving her injections but still needs some help counting the number of carbohydrates she eats to determine her bolus insulin dose.

Things are slowly coming to a new normal in the Carter family. While Sophia and her family are learning about diabetes management, Wayne is not travelling and Suzanne is working from home in the afternoons after school. Megan, the babysitter, is learning how to take care of Sophia, as well. She plans on attending the next meeting with the diabetes care team so she is ready to go when Wayne and Suzanne resume their normal schedules.

Sophia remains a happy 7-year-old who likes to play soccer and play with her dog. Her parents know that they will worry at times, but Sophia seems to be settling into her treatment regimen fairly well. Suzanne even bought Sophia a pastry on the way to school this morning.

Think Critically

1. Why does Dr. Hall address most of his questions to Sophia rather than her mom, Suzanne?
2. Why does illness often precipitate the diagnosis of diabetes mellitus type 1?
3. What are some reasons insulin needs change over time in children with diabetes mellitus type 1?
4. When Sophia goes back to Dr. Hall's office, why is her weight down, her blood pressure down, and her heart rate up?
5. Potassium is added to Sophia's IV fluids after the normal saline bolus. How does potassium affect the transport of insulin?
6. Why is regular insulin used to treat diabetic ketoacidosis?
7. How does exercise affect insulin needs?
8. What are the advantages and disadvantages of an insulin pump over multiple daily injections?
9. What would a daily diet look like for Sophia?

References

American Diabetes Association. (2016). Children and adolescents. *Diabetes Care, 39*(Suppl. 1), S86–S93.

American Diabetes Association. (2017). Care of diabetes in the hospital. *Diabetes Care, 40*(Suppl. 1), S120–S127.

Duca, L. M., Wang, B., Rewer, M., & Rewers, A. (2017). Diabetic ketoacidosis at diagnosis of type 1 diabetes predicts poor long term glycemic control. *Diabetes Care, 40*, 1249–1255.

Mayo, P. (2016). An overview of diabetes. *Nursing Standard, 30*(46), 53–63.

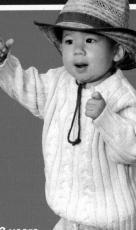

Chase McGovern, age 2 years

11 Chase McGovern: Second-Degree Burns

Objectives

After completing this chapter, you will be able to:
1. Describe normal growth and development of the 2-year-old.
2. Discuss an appropriate teaching plan for a healthy 2-year-old.
3. Identify immediate interventions for a patient with burns.
4. Apply principles of growth and development to the 2-year-old in the hospital.
5. Explain the psychological impact of pediatric burn trauma on the patient and family.
6. Distinguish between the varying degrees of thermal injury, from a superficial burn to a full-thickness burn.
7. Plan nursing interventions for the child being treated for second-degree burns.

Key Terms

Deep partial-thickness burn
Full-thickness burn
Parallel play

Superficial burn
Superficial partial-thickness burn

Background

Chase McGovern is a happy, healthy, active 2-year-old who is extremely curious about the world around him. Chase lives with his dad and mom, Gary and Liz, in a farmhouse in the country. The McGoverns raise pigs and goats and grow corn and soybeans. Gary also works full time at a factory making car parts, and Liz works part time as a waitress at a restaurant in a nearby town. Chase is the first child of Gary and Liz. Gary and Liz were full of joy when Chase was born and he has been the highlight of their lives ever since. Gary's parents live less than a mile down the road, and Liz's parents live about 20 minutes away. Often, Gary's parents babysit Chase while Gary and Liz are at work or taking care of their farm. Chase spends lots of time outside with his parents while they tend to the farm. He is an active boy, who climbs on everything and is like Houdini—he can disappear in the blink of an eye.

Liz had a normal pregnancy and Chase was born at 39 weeks of gestation via an uncomplicated vaginal birth. Chase has been relatively healthy other than a few bouts of mild respiratory viruses as an infant.

Health Promotion

It's time for Chase's 2-year-old checkup, so Liz drives him to the office of his pediatrician, Dr. Harper. The medical assistant leads Liz and Chase back to an examination room, where she measures his height and weight and takes his vital signs, which are as follows:

- Height: 35.5 in (90.2 cm)
- Weight: 29.5 lb (13.4 kg)
- Head circumference: 19.37 in (49.2 cm)
- Heart rate: 95 beats/min (bpm)
- Respiratory rate: 26 breaths/min
- Blood pressure: 90/55 mm Hg
- Temperature: 98.6°F (37°C)

Dr. Harper arrives soon. "Hi, Chase!" she says with a big smile. "How are you today?"

Chase grins back and says, "Hi!"

"Hi, Liz," Dr. Harper says. "Good to see you. How are things on your farm? I bet you and Gary are happy with all this rain we've been getting lately."

"Things are great," Liz responds. "Yes—we've loved having the rain. We're hoping for some bumper crops this season."

"Wonderful," Dr. Harper responds. "So it looks like you're in for Chase's 2-year-old checkup," she says, looking over Chase's paper chart. "Let's take a look at how he's growing."

After reviewing the most recent measurements taken by the medical assistant, Dr. Harper tells Liz that Chase is in the 76th percentile for weight and in the 78th percentile for height (Growth and Development Check 11.1). She explains that a 2-year-old boy in the 50th percentile weighs about 28 lb (12.7 kg) and is 34.5 in tall (87.6 cm). Chase's head circumference is in the 65th percentile for boys 2 years of age. She notes that Chase's weight and height have consistently ranged from the 70th to the 80th percentile since birth and his head circumference has ranged from the 55th to the 70th percentile since birth.

"So, Chase is growing well," Dr. Harper says.

"Now," Dr. Harper says to Chase. "It's time to check you out." Before starting the physical examination, she allows Chase to touch and play with her stethoscope, reflex hammer, and the light she is going to use to look in his eyes, ears and, throat. She also asks Liz if she would prefer Chase to sit on her lap or on the examination table. "I've found that toddlers generally cooperate and sit still for an exam better if they are held by the parent," she explains.

"I'll be happy to hold him," Liz says.

Dr. Harper completes Chase's physical exam and tells Liz that all of her findings are within normal limits.

"Let's talk about Chase's development," Dr. Parker says (Growth and Development Check 11.2). "How does he interact with kids his own age?"

"He likes to be around his cousins who are about his age and gets along with them well," Liz says. "They love to play with Legos. It's funny, though, because they'll sit right next to each

Growth and Development Check 11.1

Physical Growth

During the toddler years, physical growth is not as rapid as it is during infancy. Typically, the toddler gains 3–5 lb (1.4–2.3 kg) per year and grows about 3 in (7.62 cm) per year. A toddler reaches about one-half of his or her adult height by 2 y.

Adapted from American Academy of Pediatrics. (2015). *Physical appearance and growth: Your 2 year old.* Retrieved from https://www.healthychildren.org/English/ages-stages/toddler/Pages/Physical-Appearance-and-Growth-Your-2-Year-Od.aspx

Growth and Development Check 11.2

Two-Year-Old Milestones

Social and Emotional
- Likes to be around other children
- Tries to imitate both children and adults
- Engages in parallel play
- May have temper tantrums

Speech
- Speaks in two- to four-word sentences
- Is able to point to objects in a book
- Is able to point to body parts
- Follows simple instructions

Cognitive
- Identifies shapes and colors
- Builds a tower of at least four blocks
- Begins to show hand preference
- Can name items in a picture book

Gross and Fine Motor
- Throws a ball overhand
- Stands on tiptoes
- Climbs on and off things
- Kicks a ball
- Starts to run

Adapted from the Centers for Disease Control and Prevention. *Learn the signs. Act early. Important milestones: Your child by two years.* Retrieved from https://www.cdc.gov/ncbddd/actearly/milestones/milestones-2yr.html

other, but each one is doing his own thing, building his own tower of blocks. They enjoy being together while they play, but they don't actually play with each other, if that makes sense."

Dr. Harper is smiling. "Absolutely," she says. "That's called **parallel play** and is completely normal for 2-year-olds. So, Chase likes building with blocks?"

"Loves it," says Liz.

"What else does he like to do?"

"He likes for me to read to him, and he's so proud of himself when he can name the shapes and colors he sees in books. He has started to run and tries to kick every ball he sees."

"Perfect," Dr. Harper says. "How is his speech?"

"Coming along," Liz says. "His speech sounds very clear to me, but of course I'm his mom. Other friends and family seem to be able to understand him, though."

"Great. Is he speaking in sentences yet?"

"Yes," Liz says. "He can string together five to eight words when he speaks."

Dr. Parker jots down notes as Liz talks. Then she sets her pen down and says, "I'm really encouraged to hear all of this. It sounds like Chase is meeting all his growth and development milestones."

"Do you have any concerns about Chase that you'd like to discuss with me?" Dr. Harper says.

"Actually, I do," Liz says. "I'm concerned about what a picky eater Chase can be. I'm worried he is not taking in enough calories because he is so active and he only eats a few foods."

"I can understand your concern," Dr. Harper says (Patient Teaching 11.1). "Toddlers can be picky eaters at times. Part of this is because they are not growing as much as they were in their first year of life and so can be less interested in food. It is also common for toddlers to not try a new food until it has been served several times and to have different likes and dislikes in food from day to day. That's because they are becoming more independent and learning to make choices, and one way they assert this up-and-coming independence is by making their own food choices. Given Chase's healthy height and weight, though, I would not be too concerned about his eating. Just remain consistent with meal times and continue to offer a variety of foods with meals, introducing one new food at a time. How does he do with drinking?"

"He's a guzzler," Liz says. "He drinks up to 36 oz of milk a day several times a week."

"Wow," Dr. Harper says. "That is a lot. I'm glad to hear that Chase is getting plenty of calcium and vitamin D, but I recommend cutting back on the amount of milk he drinks, for a couple of reasons. First, if he drinks less milk, he will feel less full and may consume more solid food. Second, consuming too much milk can lead to an iron deficiency by hindering iron absorption."

"Do you have any other concerns about Chase?" Dr. Harper says.

"Yes," Liz responds. "Chase is so rambunctious, especially when he is at home. He climbs on everything and has no fear. He jumps off furniture, tries to run away when he is outside, and is impulsive."

Dr. Harper smiles and says, "He sounds like a handful! Yes, having a high activity level and a lack of fear is often normal for a 2-year old boy. How is his sleeping?"

"He goes to bed at 8 p.m. and wakes up at around 7 a.m. each day and sleeps soundly. He also takes a 1- to 2-hour nap each afternoon."

"Good," Dr. Harper replies. "Children 1 to 2 years of age should have about 11 to 14 hours of sleep a day, including naps" (Paruthi et al., 2016). "I'm happy to hear Chase is getting adequate sleep."

Next, Dr. Harper discusses safety issues such as burns, poisoning, drowning, and falls with Liz (Patient Teaching 11.2).

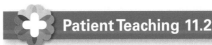

Patient Teaching 11.2

Toddler Safety

Burns
- Use the back burners when cooking on the stove.
- Keep the hot water heater set to no higher than 120°F.
- Keep toddlers away from hot objects such as grills, ovens, and irons.

Falls
- Do not allow children to climb on furniture.
- Supervise children when they are going up and down stairs.
- Supervise children when they are playing on playground equipment.
- Use gates at the top and bottom of stairs.

Poisoning
- Keep all cleaning products out of the reach of children; use cabinet locks if kept in low cabinets.
- Keep all medications out of the reach of children.
- Have the number for poison control easily accessible.

Choking
- Avoid giving children foods that can cause choking, such as the following:
  - Nuts
  - Hard candies
  - Hot dogs
  - Whole grapes
  - Marshmallows
- Supervise children while they are eating.
- Cut food into small bites.

Drowning
- Have a fence around backyard pools.
- Supervise children around water.
- Have locks on toilet seat lids.
- Do not leave buckets of water around.

Car Seats
- Have children ride facing forward in a seat with a five-point harness until they are 4 y old.

Adapted from American Academy of Pediatrics. (2015). *Safety for your child: 2 to 4 years*. Retrieved from https://www.healthychildren.org/English/ages-stages/toddler/Pages/Safety-for-Your-Child-2-to-4-Years.aspx

Patient Teaching 11.1

Toddler Nutrition

Healthy 2-y-olds should be eating three meals and one or two snacks a day. Also, a 2-y-old should be able to use a spoon, drink from a cup with one hand, and feed himself or herself a wide variety of finger foods. However, toddlers still may gulp food and are learning to chew and swallow efficiently. Parents should allow adequate time for toddlers to eat and little disruption at meal times to lessen the risk of choking.

At around the age 2 y, children should be offered low-fat or nonfat milk instead of whole milk. Intake of 16 oz of milk each day provides most of the needed calcium yet does not interfere with appetite.

Iron-deficiency anemia is a concern when a child eats very little meat, iron-rich cereals, or iron-rich vegetables, or drinks large quantities of milk (>32 oz a day), which can interfere with iron absorption.

Adapted from American Academy of Pediatric, 2017; Feeding and nutrition tips: Your 2-year-old. Retrieved from: https://www.healthychildren.org/English/ages-stages/toddler/nutrition/Pages/Feeding-and-Nutrition-Your-Two-Year-Old.aspx

"Yes," Liz says. "I'm concerned about his safety because he is so curious about the world and fearless and won't listen when I tell him 'no.'"

Dr. Harper discusses ways to help prevent burns such as keeping the hot water heater set no higher than 120°F (48.9°C) and using back burners when using the stove.

"I've found Chase turning the knobs on the stove on more than one occasion," Liz says. "Gary and I have even considered getting a new stove with the knobs above the burners, but we can't afford one right now."

"Actually, there's a much cheaper solution," Dr. Harper says. "Many stores sell child-proof stove knob covers, which are pretty effective. You also need to secure matches, lighters, and any other sources of fire. Another concern is poisoning. Where do you keep your cleaners, soaps, and medicines?"

"We keep all of that in a locked cabinet above the counters now, ever since the time Chase discovered toilet bowl cleaner in a lower cabinet and tried to open it."

"Great," Dr. Harper says. "You should also post the number to poison control in a prominent place, such as on your refrigerator, and enter the number in your cell phone. Drowning, of course, is another major danger for toddlers. Do you have any pools, ponds, or standing water on your farm?"

Liz smiles and says, "Oh yes. We have a pond and water tanks to feed the goats and pigs. Also, my in-laws, who live just down the street, have an in-ground swimming pool."

"Are those areas fenced off?"

"Yes, all except for the pond."

Dr. Harper instructs Liz on ways to prevent drowning, including not leaving buckets with water in them unattended, because toddlers can drown in as little as 6 in (15.2 cm) of water, and being sure that bodies of water are locked and secured, if possible. She also talks about falls and how to reduce the risk for Chase.

Liz sighs and says, "Yes, that's another problem. We gave up on using gates on stairs because Chase just climbs over them. At least when he does walk up the stairs, he uses both feet per step and holds on to the rail. Despite our best efforts, Chase climbs on everything, even the furniture."

"I'm sorry," Dr. Harper says. "I know that must be exasperating." She discusses the importance of a consistent, calm discipline and redirection when Chase chooses to act in an unsafe manner, such as jumping on furniture. "And just keep reminding yourself that this is just a phase. He will grow out of it."

"Well, I think that about covers it," Dr. Harper says. "Chase does not need any immunizations at this visit, as he is up to date on all his vaccines. I would encourage you, however, to bring him back in for an influenza vaccine in the fall. Do you have any more concerns or questions?"

"No," Liz says.

"Let's go, mommy," Chase says. "Let's go bye-bye."

"Goodbye, Chase!" Dr. Harper says. "I will see you again soon."

Chase leans into Liz's thigh and hides his head, acting shy for a moment. As Liz and Chase walk out, Chase shouts, "See you later alligators!"

At Home

A few days later, the McGoverns have family and friends over for a big summer celebration and to celebrate Chase's second birthday. The event is a success. It's now Sunday evening, and Liz and Gary decide to make spaghetti, something simple for dinner. Chase has just woken up from his nap. Surprisingly, he slept an extra hour today. He is playing with his cars on the play mat in the living room. Liz puts a pot of water on the stove to boil for the spaghetti and runs upstairs to put in a load of laundry, telling Gary, who is in the living room, to keep an eye on Chase so he does not get near the stove.

What seems like only a minute later, Liz returns to the living room on her way back to the kitchen. Chase is nowhere in sight. All of the sudden, Liz hears a loud thud and water spilling. Chase starts screaming, "Owie, owie." Liz and Gary run in to the kitchen and find Chase on the floor, soaked from the water in the pot. The pot is sitting beside Chase. Chase's right arm, right leg, and abdomen are bright red. Liz calls 911.

"My 2-year-old son just got burned with boiling water from the stove," Liz says to the 911 operator, trying to stay calm.

"I understand, ma'am," the operator says. "The first thing I want you to do is to check to see if his clothes are stuck to him; if not, I want you to remove them."

"He only has his diaper on because he just woke up from a nap," Liz says.

"Okay; then the next thing I want you to do is to cover the burned areas in cool, wet cloth or towels."

Liz relays this information to Gary, who is squatting next to Chase, trying to comfort him, and he jumps up and grabs some dish towels.

"Does your son appear to be breathing like he normally does?" the operator asks Liz.

"Yes," Liz says.

"Are there any burns to his face or neck?"

"No—just his right arm and leg and his belly," Liz responds. Liz begins to cry. The 911 operator stays on the line with her until the paramedics arrive.

At the Hospital

In the Emergency Room

The Nurse's Point of View

Cathy: Near the end of my shift, a 2-year-old boy, Chase McGovern, arrives by ambulance at the emergency room for a burn injury. As the paramedics bring him in on the stretcher, he is crying continuously and saying "Owie, owie, it hurts!" Each time anyone touches or moves him, he cries harder. Several nurses, including myself, a respiratory therapist, and the emergency room physician, Dr. Clark, are present to quickly assess Chase and implement life-saving interventions, if needed. As with any emergency, airway, breathing, and circulation are the priority of care. Chase does not appear to have any current airway or breathing issues, as he is crying constantly, his face and neck are not burned, and his pulse oximeter is reading 98% on room air. No chemicals or fire were involved with this burn, so inhalation injury is not likely to be a problem. I start two peripheral intravenous (IV) lines, one in the left forearm and one in the left antecubital area. Securing adequate IV access to administer fluids and resuscitation medications is essential in a burn patient. Furthermore, Chase will need medications for pain control. While I'm starting the IVs, another nurse obtains an initial set of vital signs, which are as follows:

- Heart rate: 156 bpm
- Respiratory rate: 48 breaths/min (he is crying continuously)
- Blood pressure: 86/52 mm Hg
- O₂ saturation: 98% on room air

Dr. Clark and I use a pediatric emergency resuscitation tape (commonly known as the Broselow tape) to estimate Chase's weight and height so we can give him the appropriate doses of medications and IV fluids. We estimate his weight to be 13 kg using the tape. Using the Faces Legs Activity Cry Consolability (FLACC) scale, I find Chase's pain rating to be 9, severe pain (How Much Does It Hurt? 11.1).

Dr. Clark orders 1.4 mg of IV morphine. I check the weight and appropriate dosing for pediatric patients and then administer the morphine. About 5 minutes after receiving the morphine, Chase has stopped crying continuously but still has a FLACC score of 5. Morphine can cause respiratory depression, so I place Chase on continuous pulse oximetry and an electrocardiogram (ECG) monitor. I will check his blood pressure every 15 minutes while monitoring for hypotension, both from the morphine and from the systemic effects of the burns.

Dr. Clark uses the Lund and Browder chart (Box 11.1) to calculate the percentage of body surface area burned. Chase's right arm, right leg, and abdomen appear to have **superficial partial-thickness** and **deep partial-thickness burns** (second-degree burns; Fig. 11.1). Approximately 37.5% of Chase's body has suffered second-degree thermal injury from the scalding water he poured over himself. His right hand has some white areas that do not blanch and delayed capillary refill, about 4 to 5 seconds; so, it appears to have a deeper injury. Dr. Clark tells me he is concerned that Chase may have a third-degree burn on that hand. However, his arm, leg, and abdomen are red, moist, and have blisters (some are broken) and most areas have a capillary refill of less than 2 to 3 seconds. (See Table 11.1 for a comparison of characteristics of burns.)

 How Much Does It Hurt? 11.1   **FLACC Scale**

The Faces Legs Activity Cry Consolability (FLACC) Scale is a behavioral scale for measuring the intensity of pain in children from 2 mo to 7 y old. FLACC contains five indicators: face, legs, activity, cry, and consolability. Each item ranks on a three-point scale (0–2) for severity. A total score can range from 0 to 10, with 0 representing no pain and 10 representing severe pain.

Toddlers, such as Chase, are in the preoperational stage of cognitive development and have developed symbolic representation. However, they are not yet able to understand the concepts of greater and less and thus cannot rate their pain on a scale. They can often tell where it hurts and when it hurts but cannot describe the severity. Therefore, the FLACC scale is an ideal pain scale for this age group. A total score of 1–3 indicates mild pain, 4–6 indicates moderate pain, and 7–10 indicates severe pain.

	Scoring		
Category	**0**	**1**	**2**
Faces	No particular expression or smile	Occasional grimace or frown, withdrawn, disinterested	Frequent to constant frown, quivering chin, clenched jaw
Legs	Normal position or relaxed	Uneasy, restless, tense	Kicking or legs drawn up
Activity	Lying quietly, normal position, moves easily	Squirming, shifting back and forth, tense	Arched, rigid, or jerking
Cry	No crying, awake or asleep	Moans or whimpers, occasional complaint	Crying steadily, screams or sobs, frequent complaints
Consolability	Content, relaxed	Reassured by occasional hugging, touching, or being talked to; distractible	Difficult to console or comfort

Adapted with permission from Merkel, S., Voepel-Lewis, T., Shayevitz, J. R., & Malviya, S. (1997). The FLACC: A behavioral scale for scoring postoperative pain in young children, *Pediatric Nursing, 23*(3), 293–297.

Box 11.1 Calculating Total Surface Area of Burn

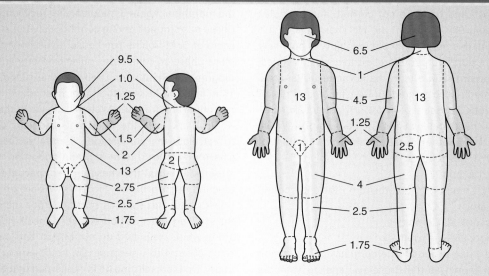

Infant   **Child (age 5)**

Area	Birth 1 y	1–4 y	5–9 y	10–14 y	15 y	Adult	2°	3°	Total
Head	19	17	13	11	9	7			
Neck	2	2	2	2	2	2			
Ant. Trunk	13	13	13	13	13	13			
Post. Trunk	13	13	13	13	13	13			
R. Buttock	2½	2½	2½	2½	2½	2½			
L. Buttock	2½	2½	2½	2½	2½	2½			
Genitalia	1	1	1	1	1	1			
R.U. Arm	4	4	4	4	4	4			
L.U. Arm	4	4	4	4	4	4			
R.L. Arm	3	3	3	3	3	3			
L.L. Arm	3	3	3	3	3	3			
R. Hand	2½	2½	2½	2½	2½	2½			
L. Hand	2½	2½	2½	2½	2½	2½			
R. Thigh	5½	6½	8	8½	9	9½			
L. Thigh	5½	6½	8	8½	9	9½			
R. Leg	5	5	5½	6	6½	7			
L. Leg	5	5	5½	6	6½	7			
R. Foot	3½	3½	3½	3½	3½	3½			
L. Foot	3½	3½	3½	3½	3½	3½			
						Total			

Lund and Browder chart. This chart, if used correctly, is the most accurate method for estimating the total body surface area burned. It compensates for the variation in body shape with age and therefore can give an accurate assessment of burns area in children. Reprinted with permission from Hatfield, N. T., & Kincheloe, C. A. (2017). *Introductory maternity and pediatric nursing* (4th ed., Fig. 41-10). Philadelphia, PA: Wolters Kluwer.

The Lund and Browder chart is a tool useful in estimating the total body surface area burned. The chart takes into consideration the patient's age and accounts for variations in body shape and percentage BSA with age.

Chase's burns:
Right arm = 9%
Right hand = 2.5%
Anterior abdomen and chest = 13%
Right leg = 13%
9% + 2.5% + 13% + 13% = 37.5%

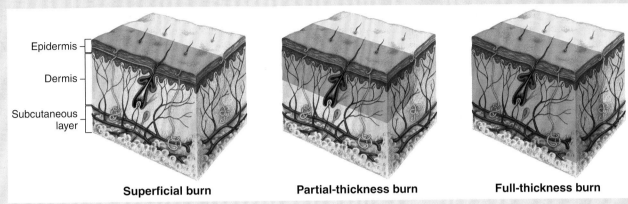

Epidermis —

Dermis —

Subcutaneous layer —

Superficial burn   **Partial-thickness burn**   **Full-thickness burn**

Figure 11.1. Degrees of burns. Superficial burns only affect the first layer of skin, the epidermis. Partial-thickness burns affect both the epidermis and some layers of the dermis. **Full-thickness burns** affect the epidermis, dermis, and the subcutaneous tissue. Reprinted with permission from Lippincott Williams & Wilkins. (2013). *Lippincott's nursing procedures* (6th ed., p. 99). Philadelphia, PA: Wolters Kluwer Health/Lippincott Williams & Wilkins.

Table 11.1 Comparison of Burn Characteristics

Burn Factor	Superficial Burns	Superficial Partial-Thickness Burns	Deep Partial-Thickness Burns	Full-Thickness Burns
Layers of skin involved	Epidermis	Epidermis and the papillary region (top layers) of the dermis	Deep into the dermis (the reticular region)	Beyond the dermis and into the subcutaneous tissue
Blisters	Absent	Present	Present and broken	Absent
Characteristics	Dry, red, sensation intact, no edema present	Moist, red, sensation intact	Moist, red, hemorrhagic	Dry, lack of sensation at the site, black or waxy-white appearance
Blanches (turns white when touched)	Yes	Yes	Yes, but delayed capillary refill	No
Pain	Mild to moderate	Extreme	May be extreme, but also may have reduced sensation	None
Treatment	Usually do not require medical treatment	• Application of cool, damp cloths to the area • Application of moisturizers such as aloe vera • Ibuprofen for pain	Depending on severity, may be treated like full-thickness burns	Surgical debridement and skin grafting
Healing time	7 d or less	14 d or less	21 d or more	Will not heal spontaneously

Adapted from Alquatani, S., Alzahrani, M., & Harvey, R. (2014). Burn management in orthopaedic trauma: A critical analysis review. *JBJS Reviews, 2*(10), 1–13.

Soon after our initial assessment of Chase, the decision is made to transfer him to the pediatric hospital, which is about a 2-hour drive away. Because he has burns over 37.5% of his body, Chase will need immediate and rapid transport to the pediatric facility for optimal care; therefore, he will be transported via a helicopter. Immediate and prompt resuscitation is critical because of a child's small circulating blood volume. Delays in resuscitation, even as little as 30 minutes, can result in increased rates of complications such as increased hospital stay, increased risk of renal failure, and even death (Romanowski & Palmieri, 2017). Dr. Clark consults with the pediatric hospital before transport. The pediatrician recommends starting IV lactated Ringer's solution at 100 mL/h. Because the total body surface area burned is greater than 20%, Chase is at risk for acute systemic responses, known as burn shock, and hypovolemia is likely to occur if adequate fluid resuscitation is not started in a timely manner (Rowan et al., 2015). Burn shock is characterized by several acute responses: (1) increased capillary permeability, (2) increased hydrostatic

pressure across the microvasculature, (3) fluids and proteins move from the intravascular space to the interstitial space, (4) increased systemic vascular resistance, (5) reduced cardiac output, and (6) hypovolemia (Rowan et al., 2015).

As soon as I've started the IV lactated Ringer's, the paramedics wheel Chase off to the helicopter pad. A moment later, I hear the helicopter take off.

Transfer to a Pediatric Hospital

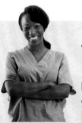

The Nurse's Point of View

Monica: Chase McGovern, a 2-year-old boy with pervasive second-degree burns, has just arrived by helicopter to the pediatric hospital where I work. It was a smart move to transfer him here. Our hospital has nurses, including myself, and pediatric providers trained in burn and wound care. Chase's parents, Gary and Liz, were not able to fly with him, but they are on their way by car. Our trauma team consists of two bedside nurses, a pediatrician specializing in pediatric

emergency care, a respiratory therapist, and a nurse team leader.

We see many cases each year of scalding burns, which, nationwide, account for about 65% of burn hospitalizations in young children under the age of 4 years (American Burn Association, n.d.). Mortality from burn injury is highest in children aged newborn to 2 years, due to the incompletely developed immune and organ systems in this population (Palmieri, 2016). Furthermore, because of the differences between a child's skin and an adult's skin, children are at higher risk for more severe injury when burned (Let's Compare 11.1).

Let's Compare 11.1 — Difficulties With Burn Injuries in Children vs. Adults

Difference in Children	Result
Shorter airway, with a smaller diameter	Greater risk for airway obstruction when inflammation or edema is present
More anterior pharynx, narrower cricoid area, and larger tonsils	More difficult to intubate (place a breathing tube) or secure an airway
Less-developed lungs (until about age 8 y) and a lack of pulmonary reserve	Compensation via increased work of breathing and increased respiratory rate; possible decompensation, often sudden, resulting in respiratory failure
Incompletely developed immune system	Increased risk of infection and sepsis
Greater ratio of body surface area to mass	More susceptible to hypothermia and increased need for fluid resuscitation
Body surface area distributed differently (head is larger, legs are smaller)	Require more intravenous fluids per kilogram than do adults
Limited cardiac contractility (in infants)	Only means of increasing cardiac output is by increasing heart rate; because tachycardia can also be related to pain, heart rate is not an adequate indicator of hypovolemia
Thinner skin	Deeper burns even with lower temperature of liquid, fire, or chemical; increased likelihood of third-degree burns; increased risk of hypothermia; avoid wet cloths and wet dressings
Less-developed communication skills	Greater difficulty assessing pain
Greater curiosity and use of concrete thinking; less aware of consequences of actions	More likely to suffer a burn injury

As a result of the greater body surface area, hypothermia is also a risk. So, I know I'll need to keep Chase covered with warm blankets and apply sterile, dry cloths to the burned areas. Because of the increased risk of hypothermia in the pediatric population, I know to avoid applying wet cloths to burned areas (Palmieri, 2016).

As soon as Chase arrives, the trauma team immediately assesses him for signs of burn shock. It has been about 90 minutes since the thermal injury occurred. Chase does not appear to be in shock at this time. I take his vital signs and find them to be as follows:

- Weight: 29.5 lbs. 13.4 kg
- Heart rate: 130 bpm (crying at times)
- Respiratory rate: 36 breaths/min
- Blood pressure: 88/48 mm Hg
- O_2 saturation: 99% on room air

The physician, Dr. Lee, uses the Parkland formula (Box 11.2) to calculate the total fluid volume Chase will need over the next 24 hours. Chase already has IV lactated Ringer's solution infusing at 100 mL/h from the outside hospital. On the basis of Chase's weight (13.4 kg), which I measure on his arrival, I adjust the IV pump to infuse at 125.6 mL/h and set the volume limit for 1,005 mL. Also, I start maintenance IV fluids, with 5% dextrose in normal saline infusing at 70 mL/h, to ensure Chase does not become hypoglycemic. The physician orders the placement of a urinary catheter. Monitoring hourly urine output is essential to determine whether adequate fluid replacement is being administered. We draw blood samples for a comprehensive metabolic panel and a complete blood count and send them to the laboratory stat. Knowing Chase's electrolyte

---

Box 11.2 Calculating Fluid Volume for Burn Resuscitation

1. Use the Parkland formula to calculate the total amount of fluid to replace over 24 h:
   4 mL × % of body surface area burned × mass in kg = total fluid to replace over 24 h
   Note that **superficial** (first-degree) **burns** should not be included in the percentage of body surface area burned in the calculation.
2. Give one-half of the total fluid volume in the first 8 h.
3. Give the remaining one-half over the next 16 h.

Example: Chase weighs 29.5 lb (13.4 kg). He has burns over 37.5% of his body.

4 mL × 37.5% × 13.4 kg = 2,010 mL over 24 h

2,010 mL/2 = 1,005 mL (This is half of the fluid, which should be administered in the first 8 h.)

Now calculate the hourly rate for the first 8 h:

1,005 mL/8 h = 125.6 mL/h

Next, calculate the hourly rate for the next 16 h:

1,005 mL/16 h = 62.8 mL/h

Thus, after the first 8 h, the rate should be changed from 125.6 to 62.8 mL/h.

---

values is essential to ensure that adequate fluid resuscitation is being administered.

Soon, I get word that they are ready to admit Chase to the pediatric intensive care unit (PICU).

On the Unit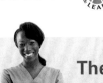

The Nurse's Point of View

Maria: Chase McGovern has just been admitted to the PICU, where I am on shift. I'm a certified wound and ostomy care nurse (CWOCN) and have specific training in burn care. My peers and I take classes annually on best practices for treatment of burns. On the basis of my training, I recognize that the priorities of wound care for Chase include the following: preventing wound infection, minimizing pain, promoting epithelialization, and minimizing scarring. I will be closely monitoring his fluid status, hemodynamic stability, and renal function and providing adequate pain control for dressing changes and ongoing pain (Box 11.3).

After Chase is settled in the PICU, I prepare to perform wound care on him. Before starting wound care, I consult with the care team and arrange for Chase to receive ketamine IV for analgesia and sedation. Once the ketamine is started, I begin cleaning the wound with soap and water to remove any debris and further evaluate the extent of the burns. During wound care, Brian, a PICU nurse, monitors Chase for pain, sedation, and procedure tolerance. Brian administers ordered medications such as ketamine and morphine for adequate pain control. I ask a fellow registered nurse, Sandy, to help me. Minimizing the time that skin is exposed to the air helps reduce fluid loss and heat loss. After we clean, assess, measure, and pat dry Chase's burns, I apply silver sulfadiazine cream, an antimicrobial agent, to the burned areas. Then I wrap the burns with nonadherent dressings and cover the dressings with gauze bandage rolls. I know the dressings need to be as toddler-proof as possible. Once Chase is stable, we will develop a wound care plan for him.

It is important to get Chase's parents back to see him as soon as possible after they arrive at the hospital. The unit secretary informs me that Chase's parents have been in the waiting room for 10 minutes. I ask her to allow the parents in. I meet Chase's parents at the door of his room and introduce myself.

"Hello. My name is Maria. I am the nurse caring for Chase. How was your drive here?"

"We couldn't get here fast enough," Liz says tearfully.

"Chase is stable right now. I have given him pain medication and some medicine to help him relax while I cleaned his burns, assessed them, and put dressings on them. He is still a little sleepy from the medications. If you would like to come on in the room and wash your hands, you can. Then you can talk to him and hold his hand. It is very important for everyone who comes to see Chase to wash their hands when they enter the room, before touching Chase," I explain.

"I just can't believe this happened. I just can't believe my baby is burned. I should have known better than to leave the pot of water on the stove without being in the kitchen. This is all my fault," Liz blurts out, sobbing.

I allow time for Liz and Gary to be with Chase while I do some charting on the computer in the room. I offer some tissues as Liz cries for a bit while holding Chase's hand. Gary is supportive of Liz, reassuring her that the accident is not her fault. He takes the blame for it and puts his arm around Liz. Sometimes, I do not know exactly what to say in these situations, but I have found that silence is okay. Just allowing parents to be present with their child is the appropriate thing to do. I will go over the plan of care with Liz and Gary, orient them to the room, and answer any questions they may have in a few minutes. I also page the doctor caring for Chase to come and speak with the parents. By having the doctor present during the initial meeting with the parents, I can gather essential information I may need to care for Chase and not

---

Box 11.3 Pathophysiological Changes in Burns

The first 24–72 h following a severe burn can result in critical care needs such as fluid and electrolyte challenges, volume redistribution resulting in hypovolemia, risk for shock and organ failure, and pain management issues. The edema and interstitial fluid shifts resulting in burn shock occur rapidly over the first 8 h after the burn and then continue to increase over the next 18 h but at a less rapid pace (Rowan et al., 2015). Fluid shifts can lead to decreased cardiac output, poor perfusion to organs, and, ultimately, hypoxemia to tissues and cellular and tissue death if adequate fluid resuscitation is not provided. Severe burns also send the body into a hypermetabolic and inflammatory response soon after the injury, which is associated with catabolism, protein and amino acid degradation, insulin resistance, hyperglycemia, and lipolysis.

These post-burn changes can contribute to organ failure. Prevention of organ failure is essential to reduce morbidity and mortality from a severe burn incident (Kraft, Herndon, Finnerty, Shahrokhi, & Jeschke, 2014). The hypermetabolic response begins immediately and may last for 6 mo. Nutrition, with increased calories, via the nasoenteral route, is often started as early as 12 h after the burn (Palmieri, 2016). Adequate caloric intake is necessary to reduce catabolism, thus reducing muscle and tissue breakdown, and for optimal wound healing.

have to ask the parents the same questions the doctor asked after he is finished talking to them. Dr. Sanders, the PICU attending physician, arrives soon after I page him.

"Hello, I am Dr. Sanders, the doctor who will be in charge of Chase's care while he is here in the pediatric intensive care unit. I am so sorry this has happened. We are going to take excellent care of Chase. Tell me what happened today."

"It's all my fault," Gary says. "I didn't keep a close enough eye on Chase, and he pulled a pot of boiling water off the stove on himself. I just can't believe this has happened. I knew he was a quick little Houdini, but I never imagined he would get near the stove. We tell him all the time how hot the stove it and that it will hurt him. But he is only 2 years old. It's not his fault. It's mine."

"Is Chase going to be okay? What is going to happen? Is he in pain? I just can't believe this is happening," Liz says.

"Chase is going to be okay," Dr. Sanders says. "The positive news is that children with second-degree burns like Chase's have a very good prognosis. If all goes well, Chase should be in the hospital for 7 to 10 days and then he will get to go home. He is currently sedated and sleepy from the medications we gave him when we assessed his burns, cleaned them, and put new dressings on them" (The Pharmacy 11.1). "We will monitor him closely for pain and give him medications to keep him comfortable. If at any time you feel he is in pain, please let your nurse know. We will do our best to control his pain. For the next few days, we will be monitoring the burns as the skin starts to heal. We will monitor for signs of infection, keep Chase hydrated with IV fluids, and keep a close eye on his electrolytes because, sometimes with burns like these, kids need their electrolytes replaced."

"I am so relieved to hear you say he will be okay. I am so worried and scared right now," Liz says.

The Pharmacy 11.1 — Medications for Patients With Burn Injuries

Medication	Classification	Route	Action	Nursing Considerations
Silver sulfadiazine or silver sulfadiazine and chlorhexidine-gluconate	Antimicrobial	Topical	Broad-spectrum antimicrobial with bactericidal effects for many gram-negative and gram-positive bacteria	• Apply under sterile conditions • Apply to a thickness of 1/16 of an inch • Assess the burned area for infection before administration
Morphine	Analgesic	• IV • IM • PO	Binds to opiate receptors in the CNS	• Monitor for respiratory depression • May cause hypotension • Constipation can occur; consider a bowel regimen
Ketamine (Ketalar)	• Sedative • Anesthetic	• IV • IM	Produces sedative, analgesic, and hypnotic effects while increasing sympathetic tone and maintaining airway tone and respiration	Monitor for emergent reactions, including the following: • Vivid imagery • Hallucinations • Dreamlike states • Confusion • Excitement • Irrational behavior These reactions can be counteracted with the simultaneous administration of a benzodiazepine.

CNS, central nervous system; IM, intramuscular; IV, intravenous; PO, by mouth.
Adapted from Taketomo, C. K., Hodding, J. H., & Kraus, D. M. (2018). *Pediatric and neonatal dosage handbook* (25th ed.). Philadelphia, PA: Lexicomp.

At Discharge

After Chase has been in the hospital for 7 days, the attending pediatrician, Dr. Simpson, clears him for discharge to home. Maria, one of the primary nurses providing care to Chase and his family during this time, enters Chase's room.

"Hi, Chase!" she says. "Are you ready to go home today?"

"Yes!" Chase shouts.

"And mom and dad?"

"Yes and no," Liz says. "I mean, of course we're happy he's coming home. But I'm also a little overwhelmed about the prospect of caring for his wounds."

"Me too," Gary says. "I'm afraid I'll do something wrong and hurt him even more."

"Well, I'm here to provide you with some final teaching and discharge instructions, which hopefully will help you feel more confident in taking care of him at home." As she has been doing for most of Chase's stay, she talks Gary and Liz through a burn dressing change and demonstrates how to care for Chase's skin so that they will be prepared to perform these tasks at home.

"One of the most critical goals in caring for Chase's burns is preventing infection, especially during dressing changes. Each time you change Chase's dressings, wash your hands properly before beginning, clean the wound with chlorhexidine solution,

and apply a fresh, sterile dressing to the wound, just as you've seen the nurses do here." Maria also instructs Liz and Gary on home cleaning routines to reduce the risk of infection while Chase continues healing at home.

"Another crucial goal is to prevent further burns," Maria continues, her voice softening.

Liz feels a knot forming in her stomach. "I should never have left that pot of water boiling on the stove," she says, beginning to get choked up. "I'm so sorry," she says, turning to Gary.

"No, you have no reason to be sorry," Gary says. "It was my fault. If I had just been watching him more closely, this never would have happened."

"Don't be so hard on yourselves," Maria says (Box 11.4). "Toddlers are incredibly accident-prone. You would have to be superhuman to protect them from every injury." She explains that approximately 91% of burn injuries in the pediatric population are accidental (Kramer, Rivara, & Klein, 2010) and that in children under the age of 5 years, scalding is the major cause (Kramer et al., 2010). "No one here is judging you. However, I would like to go over some prevention strategies with you. Would that be okay?"

"Sure," Liz says. "We'll do anything to keep this from happening again." Gary nods.

Box 11.4 Caring for the Psychosocial Needs of the Family of a Patient With Burn Trauma

Although the priorities of care for patients with significant burn trauma are certainly centered around their hemodynamic stability, pain control, and cardiorespiratory status, staff at the hospital know all too well about the importance of caring for the psychosocial needs of the families of these patients. A severe burn that requires hospitalization also requires a great deal of specialized care, including a significant inpatient hospital stay, pain, loss of control, and a need for the child and family to adjust their lives (Rimmer et al., 2015). The burn injury experience affects parents and caregivers in different ways. In fact, a childhood burn has been found to be one of the most stressful and overwhelming experiences a parent endures (Rimmer et al., 2015). Parents become stressed by the child's physical pain; uncertain outcomes; lengthy, tedious dressing change regimes; disfigurement; time away from home; and the need for multiple surgeries, therapies, and procedures (Rimmer et al., 2015). In one study, Rimmer et al. (2015) found that for parents the most difficult part of their child's burn injury was dealing with the pain the child endures, whereas the second-most difficult issue was the child's first hospital stay. In addition, parents of children with burn injuries often experience high rates of psychological trauma, such as depression, significant guilt, and post-traumatic stress syndrome (Bakker, Maertens, Van Son, & Van Loey, 2013).

How can nurses and hospital staff help parents with the stress of a burn-related hospitalization? Developing and using a pain medication plan with the parents' involvement is helpful for parents. Asking the parents for feedback about the current pain management regimen and using their feedback is also helpful. This also helps empower parents and give them some control over what is happening to their child (Rimmer et al., 2015). Involving the parents in dressing changes has been shown to have a significant impact on reducing the child's overall pain (Rimmer et al., 2015). Furthermore, discussion with parents about the anxiety, inability to sleep, pain control, and feelings of hopelessness can help them anticipate possible stressors and be more proactive and able to adjust to events as they occur. Using a social worker and psychologist in the early stages of burn injury can be helpful to parents and assist them in dealing with financial burdens, being away from home, and other stressors. Assisting parents to function in a positive manner by providing them with useful resources such as community support groups, using a child life specialist to help convey messages to siblings, encouraging them to schedule time with those at home, and helping them use their time most effectively may be helpful.

Box 11.5 Children and Burns: Prevalence and the Importance of Prevention

Fortunately, children with severe burns covering up to 90% of their body can survive today as a result of advances in burn care over the past 40 y (McDermott, Weiss, & Elixhauser, 2016). In 1970, burns covering only 20% of the body were almost always fatal. However, thermal injury continues to affect almost a million children each year in the United States (Gonzalez & Shanti, 2015). About 50,000 children are hospitalized each year for moderate and severe burns. Around 2,500 pediatric patients die each year from burns. Prevention is the key to reducing the incidence of burns in children.

"We like to talk about active and passive prevention strategies," Maria says (Box 11.5). "Active prevention strategies include making environmental changes, such as changing to a stove with knobs on the top, where they are harder to reach, not leaving the kitchen or area with heat and fire while Chase is present, and removing any climbing apparatuses near sources of thermal injury. Passive prevention strategies include locking and securing any source of heat or fire or burn mechanisms, such as matches and lighters, and installing safety devices such as gates and child-proof locks."

When Maria is done providing discharge instructions and answering Gary and Liz's questions, the McGovern family finally leaves the pediatric hospital. On the long drive home, Chase chatters excitedly and Liz is happy to have her boy back.

Think Critically

1. What factors led to Chase getting burned over 30% of his body? Use these to create a simple teaching plan for parents of a 2-year-old.
2. What are the priorities of care for a patient immediately following a thermal injury?
3. Why are young children at higher risk for more serious injury when a burn occurs?
4. Why is adequate nutrition a priority for a child with a thermal injury?
5. How is initial fluid resuscitation calculated for a child with burns?

References

American Burn Association. (n.d.). *Scald injury prevention educator's guide. A community fire and burn prevention program supported by the United States Fire Administration Federal Emergency Management Agency.* Retrieved from https://www.usfa.fema.gov/downloads/pdf/publications/burn_and_scald_prevention_flyer.pdf

Bakker, A., Maertens, K., Van Son, J., & Van Loey, N. (2013). Psychological consequences of pediatric burns from a child and family perspective: a review of the empirical literature. *Clinical Psychology Review, 33,* 361–371.

Gonzalez, R., & Shanti, C. (2015). Overview of current pediatric burn care. *Seminars in Pediatric Surgery, 24,* 47–49.

Kraft, R., Herndon, D., Finnerty, C., Shahrokhi, S., & Jeschke, M. (2014). Occurrence of multi-organ dysfunction in pediatric burn patients: Incidence and clinical outcome. *Annals of Surgery, 259*(2), 381–387.

Kramer, C., Rivara, F., & Klein, M. (2010). Variations in U.S. pediatric burn injury hospitalizations using the national burn repository data. *Journal of Burn Care and Research, 31,* 734–739.

McDermott, K., Weiss, A., & Elixhauser, A. (2016). *Burn-related hospital inpatient stays and emergency department visits, 2013. HCUP Statistical Brief #217.* Rockville, MD: Agency for Healthcare Research and Quality. Retrieved from http://www.hcup-us.ahrq.gov/reports/statbriefs/sb217-Burn-Hospital-Stays-ED-Visits-2013.pdf.

Palmieri, T. (2016). Pediatric burn resuscitation. *Critical Care Clinics, 32*(4), 547–559.

Paruthi, S., Brooks, L., D'Ambrosio, C., Hall, W., Kotagal, S., Lloyd, R, . . . Wise, M. S. (2016). Recommended amount of sleep for pediatric populations: A consensus statement of the American Academy of Sleep Medicine. *Journal of Clinical Sleep Medicine, 12*(6), 785–786.

Rimmer, R. B., Bay, R. C., Alam, N. B., Sadler, I. J., Richey, K. J., Foster, K. N., . . . & Rosenberg, D. (2015). Measuring the burden of pediatric burn injury for parents and caregivers: Informed burn center staff can help to lighten the load. *Journal of Burn Care and Research, 36*(3), 421–427.

Romanowski, K., & Palmieri, T. (2017). Pediatric burn resuscitation: Past, present and future. *Burns and Trauma, 5*(26), 1–9.

Rowan, M. P., Cancio, L. C., Elster, E. A., Burmeister, D. M., Rose, L. F., Natesan, S., . . . Chung, K. K. (2015). Burn wound healing and treatment: review and advancements. *Critical Care, 19*(1), 243.

Suggested Readings

American Burn Association. *Scald injury prevention educator's guide. A community fire and burn prevention program supported by the United States Fire Administration Federal Emergency Management Agency.* https://www.usfa.fema.gov/downloads/pdf/publications/burn_and_scald_prevention_flyer.pdf

Centers for Disease Control and Prevention. (n.d.). *Protect the ones you love: Childhood injuries are preventable. Burn prevention.* Retrieved from https://www.cdc.gov/safechild/burns/index.html

Healthy Children.org. (2017). *Burn treatment & prevention tips for families.* Retrieved from https://www.healthychildren.org/English/health-issues/injuries-emergencies/Pages/Treating-and-Preventing-Burns.aspx

12 Natasha Austin: Sickle Cell Anemia

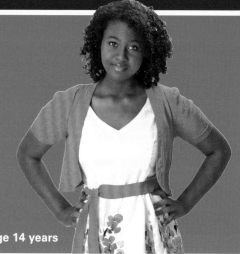

Natasha Austin, age 14 years

Objectives

After completing this chapter, you will be able to:
1. Describe normal growth and development of the 14-year-old.
2. Discuss an appropriate teaching plan for a healthy 14-year-old.
3. Identify triggers of a sickle cell crisis.
4. Identify signs and symptoms of impending sickle cell crisis in children.
5. Describe the treatment of acute chest syndrome in children and teenagers.
6. Create a nursing plan of care for a teenager with sickle cell anemia.

Key Terms

Acute chest syndrome (ACS)
Acute splenic sequestration
Atelectasis

Dactylitis
Vasoocclusive crisis

Background

Natasha Austin is a 14-year-old who loves listening to music, hanging out with her friends, and watching movies. She has one sibling, Madelyn, who is 10 years old and in the fourth grade. Her parents, Anita and Anthony, just celebrated their 20th wedding anniversary. Anita works full time as a social worker at the local community hospital. Anthony is the supervisor in the repair department at a local car dealership and often works 50 or more hours a week. Natasha is responsible for watching her sister after school until about 5 p.m., when her mom gets home from work. The Austins are actively involved in their church and spend Wednesday evenings and Sunday mornings participating in church activities.

Natasha just started her freshman year of high school about a month ago. She is a member of the drama club. Natasha likes school but has found it challenging to make new friends in high school. Many of her friends from junior high are attending a different, private high school. Her favorite classes are math and science. Natasha really wants to be an environmental engineer someday. One of her biggest challenges in school is keeping up with school work when she is absent because of symptoms and hospitalizations related to her sickle cell disease.

At birth, Natasha was identified as having sickle cell disease (Box 12.1) via the newborn screening process but was a healthy, full-term baby. At 6 weeks old, she had a second test to confirm she had sickle cell disease. Natasha's mother was aware she was a carrier, but her father was not sure whether he was or not. After Natasha was found to have sickle cell disease, Natasha's father did have genetic testing and was found to be a carrier of the sickle cell trait. Natasha remained symptom-free until about 6 months of age, when she developed an ear infection and cried inconsolably when she had a fever. At that time, she was found to be slightly anemic but did not require hospitalization for the ear infection, fever, and pain after being seen by the pediatrician.

Box 12.1 Sickle Cell Disease

Sickle cell disease is the most prevalent disease identified by newborn screenings. In the United States, where all states currently require testing for sickle cell disorders as part of newborn screening, sickle cell disease occurs in approximately 1 in every 2,500 births. A positive, or abnormal, screen indicates the need for further testing. More than 2 million people in the United States are either heterozygous or homozygous for the genetic disposition, with the majority of those being of African descent (National Institutes of Health, 2014). An estimated 70,000–100,000 Americans have the disease (Quinn, Rogers, McCavit, & Buchanan, 2010).

As seen in Figure 12.1, the red blood cells of a person with sickle cell anemia are of an irregular, sickle shape. A person with sickle cell anemia has a variant of hemoglobin, known as sickled hemoglobin (HbS), to which oxygen molecules are unable to attach, rather than a normal adult hemoglobin molecule, to which oxygen easily attaches and in which oxygen is carried to the tissues. Sickled cells cannot carry oxygen and can cause obstruction of blood flow and lead to multiple system failure, such as stroke, respiratory failure, and renal failure. Sickle cell disease is an autosomal recessive disorder. When both parents are carriers (as illustrated in the Punnett square, shown below), there is a 25% chance the child will develop the disease, a 50% chance the child will be a carrier of the disease but not develop it, and a 25% chance the child will not have the trait or the disease.

A Punnett square showing the genetic pattern for one who is homozygous for sickle cell anemia:

	S	s
S	SS	Ss
s	Ss	ss

Those who are sickle cell carriers may or may not have symptoms or complications from the disease. Those who are homozygous for sickle cell disease will demonstrate signs, symptoms, and complications of the disease.

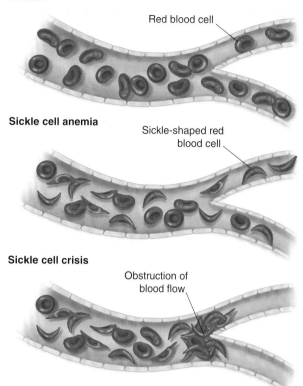

Figure 12.1. Sickle cell anemia. Sickle-shaped red blood cells are present in sickle cell anemia. Sickled cells are unable to carry oxygen and can cause obstruction of blood flow if present in large quantities, leading to sickle cell crisis. Reprinted with permission from Creason, C. (Ed.). (2011). *Stedman's medical terminology: Steps to success in medical language* (1st ed., Fig. 8-11B). Philadelphia, PA: Wolters Kluwer Health/ Lippincott Williams & Wilkins.

When Anita was pregnant with Madelyn, the obstetrician offered in utero DNA testing for the unborn child, but the Austins declined because the risks of chronic villus sampling and amniocentesis (the methods used to obtain DNA samples) outweighed the benefits (in the Austins' perspective) of knowing whether the baby had sickle cell disease before birth.

At 10 months of age, Natasha presented with her first episode of **vasoocclusive crisis** (Box 12.2). She had a severe case of **dactylitis**, with significant swelling and pain in both hands and feet, and was hospitalized for 5 days. Genetic testing confirmed that Natasha had homozygous sickle cell disease.

Anita remembers that time vividly. She was incredibly frightened and thought Natasha would always be sick and in pain. She had heard stories from several of her friends who have kids with sickle cell about the pain their children often had as a result of the disease. As any mother, she did not want to see her child be in pain. Anita remembers waking up in the middle of the night to Natasha crying uncontrollably and seeing that her fingers and feet were very swollen.

From the time she was an infant until the age of 5 years, Natasha received prophylactic penicillin and the conjugate pneumococcal and *Haemophilus influenzae* type B vaccine to reduce the risk of pneumonia and other infections that could lead to sepsis, as recommended (Brousse, Makani, & Rees, 2014). At the age of 4 years, Natasha had a splenectomy. In the year leading up to the splenectomy, Natasha had two **acute splenic sequestration** episodes. The hematologist caring for Natasha decided a splenectomy was necessary because of the severity of the episodes. The hematologist explained that acute splenic sequestration can be life-threatening. During an episode, blood becomes trapped in the spleen, causing enlargement of the spleen, a sudden drop in hematocrit, and a rise in the reticulocyte count. As a result of blood rapidly pooling in the spleen, circulatory compromise ensues. The spleen can trap enough blood volume that a patient can develop shock. The mortality rate for splenic sequestration has been reported as high as 12%.

Since being diagnosed at the age of 10 months, Natasha has been hospitalized too many times to count. On average,

Box 12.2 Vasoocclusive Crisis

Vasoocclusive crisis is the most common manifestation of sickle cell disease and occurs when the microcirculation becomes obstructed by sickled cells causing ischemia to tissues and organs, which results in pain. Pain associated with a vasoocclusive crisis can range from mild to severe. Pain begins suddenly and often lasts hours to days, ending just as abruptly as it started. Pain can affect any body part and most often affects the abdomen, joints, bones, and soft tissue. Dactylitis, acute abdomen pain, acute joint necrosis, and avascular necrosis are often how pain presents. During an episode, the patient may also have fever, malaise, and leukocytosis. Vascular injury also occurs, causing irreparable damage not only to the microcirculation but to larger vessels, as well. Repeated episodes can lead to end-organ failure. Sickle cell disease compromises spleen function which can lead bacteremia, sepsis, septic shock, and even death (Baskin, Goh, Heeney, & Harper, 2013).

Once a person is diagnosed with sickle cell anemia, it is imperative he or she understand the triggers of a vasoocclusive crisis and how to avoid them. Some common triggers are listed and described here:

- **Dehydration:** Acidosis results in a shift to the right of the oxygen dissociation curve, resulting in reduced hemoglobin (Hgb)-oxygen affinity.
- **Hyperthermia:** Fever results in a shift to the right of the oxygen dissociation curve, resulting in reduced Hgb-oxygen affinity.
- **Hypothermia:** A drop in body temperature causes peripheral vasoconstriction.
- **Hypoxia:** Deoxygenated sickled hemoglobin (HbS) becomes semisolid, enhancing adherence to endothelial cells.

until the age of 11 years, she was hospitalized 4 to 5 times a year for a vasoocclusive crisis or complications from sickle cell disease. At the age of 11, Natasha started taking hydroxyurea (The Pharmacy 12.1), which has seemed to lessen the number and severity of episodes of sickle cell crisis she has. Natasha has

also had to receive only one blood transfusion since the age of 11, compared with multiple transfusions each year before then. Anita is encouraged by Natasha's progress, but she also knows that Natasha still faces many long-term consequences of sickle cell disease (Box 12.3).

The Pharmacy 12.1   Medications Used in the Treatment of Sickle Cell Anemia

Medication	Classification	Route	Action	Nursing Considerations
Hydroxyurea (Hydrea)	• Antineoplastic • Antimetabolite	• PO	• Increases Hgb F, which inhibits the polymerization of Hgb S (McCavit, 2012) • Interferes with DNA synthesis • May alter characteristics of red blood cells • Reduces painful crisis and the incidence of acute chest syndrome (National Institutes of Health, 2014) • Reduces the need for blood transfusions • Lowers the number of leukocytes and reticulocytes, which contribute to vasoocclusion (Ware, 2010)	• Assess for signs of infection. • Monitor CBC with differential for anemia, thrombocytopenia, and neutropenia. • Assess for bleeding. • Monitor renal (BUN and creatinine) and liver function tests (AST, ALT, bilirubin, LDH).
Oxycodone	Opioid analgesic	• PO	• Binds to receptors in the CNS • Alters perception of and response to pain	• Do not confuse with hydrocodone. • Do not confuse short-acting oxycodone with long-acting Oxycontin. • Can cause respiratory depression; monitor respiratory status on initiation and when increasing dose. • Can cause drowsiness, confusion, and sedation • Can cause constipation; encourage the patient to drink plenty of fluids and increase fiber in diet.

ALT, alanine aminotransferase; AST, aspartate aminotransferase; BUN, blood urea nitrogen; CBC, complete blood count; CNS, central nervous system; Hgb, hemoglobin; Hgb F, fetal Hgb; Hgb S, sickle Hgb; LDH, lactase dehydrogenase; PO, by mouth.

Box 12.3 Long-Term Consequences of Sickle Cell Disease

Long-term consequences of sickle cell disease can affect every body system. As a result of obstructed blood flow to the microcirculation, cells become ischemic and die. The result of chronic sickling and vascular injury, as well as hemolysis, is silent but progressive organ failure. Also, acute infarcts (strokes) can occur in any organ, leading to sudden organ failure. Figure 12.2 shows how sickle cell anemia affects multiple body systems. Anemia and increased cardiac output can lead to cardiomegaly as a result of a constantly overworked heart. Eventually, heart failure can occur. Pulmonary infarcts and pneumonia can lead to ACS and respiratory failure. Renal infarcts and vascular injury to the kidney can cause acute or chronic renal failure. Retinopathy results from retinal infarcts, and, even in infancy and early childhood, infarcts to the cerebral vasculature can lead to neurologically devastating strokes. Sequelae of sickle cell disease are not always apparent, and undetected signs and symptoms can begin in early childhood. For example, children with silent central nervous system infarcts may present with developmental delays, learning difficulties, poor school performance, or social adjustment issues (National Institutes of Health, 2014).

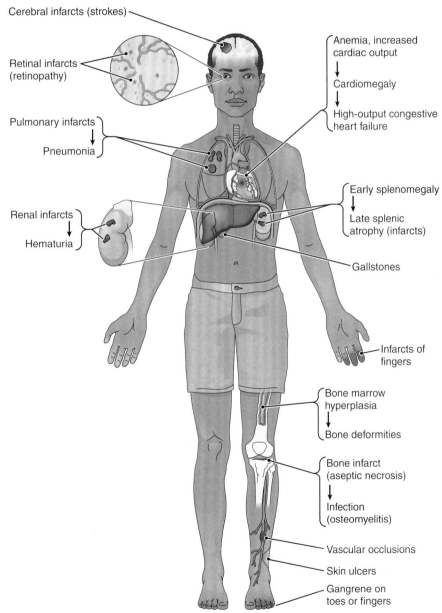

Figure 12.2. Systemic effects of sickle cell disease. Acute and chronic consequences of sickle cell disease affect every body system. Reprinted with permission from McConnell, T. H. (2014). *The nature of disease: Pathology for the health professions* (2nd ed., Fig. 7.6A). Philadelphia, PA: Wolters Kluwer Health/Lippincott Williams & Wilkins.

Health Promotion

Today, Anita takes Natasha to visit Janette, a pediatric nurse practitioner, for her annual well-care visit. Natasha sees one of her primary care providers, either Janette or Dr. Mallor, every 3 to 4 months as part of her sickle cell care plan. Her primary care providers collaborate with Dr. Anish, a pediatric hematologist, to provide comprehensive, collaborative care for Natasha.

The Nurse's Point of View

Janette: Natasha independently meets with me while her mother waits in the waiting room, as she's been doing since the age of 13 for well-care visits and some sick visits. Dr. Mallor and I believe children with sickle cell should play an active role in managing their disease, and meeting with them apart from their parents helps facilitate this. I will call her mother back to the room at the end of the visit, however, to address any questions or concerns her mother has.

"Hi, Natasha," I say as I enter the examination room. "How are you doing today?"

"I'm fine," she says.

"Great," I say. "Let me take a quick look at your chart, and then we'll get started." My registered nurse (RN) has already obtained and entered a set of vital signs for Natasha, along with her height and weight, and reviewed Natasha's current medication list with her. Her vital signs are as follows:

- Height: 5 ft 7 in (170.18 cm)
- Weight: 143 lb (65 kg)
- Heart rate: 74 beats/min (bpm)
- Respiratory rate: 16 breaths/min
- Blood pressure: 122/68 mm Hg
- O_2 saturation: 99% on room air

Natasha has gained 14 lb (6.3 kg) and grown 2 in (5 cm) since her well-care visit last year. Her body mass index is 22.4 (80th percentile), which is in the healthy range for her age and gender.

"It looks like you've had a relatively healthy year, Natasha," I tell her. "You only had to go to the hospital once for a sickle cell flare-up." In previous years, Natasha had been hospitalized on average 3 times a year for a vasoocclusive crisis. "You're doing a great job of taking care of yourself."

"Thanks," Natasha replies. "It's been really hard to take all the right steps to stay healthy. I'm getting really tired of taking my medications and having to be so careful about washing my hands, not getting infections, and drinking lots of water."

"I see in your chart that you had a scheduled visit with the hematologist last week that you didn't show up for. Can you tell me about that?"

Natasha looks down at the ground and says, "I forgot about it. My parents did, too."

"As we've talked about before, it's really important for you to make these appointments, Natasha. So, I want you to work extra hard this year on remembering to make them, okay?"

"Okay," she says.

I talk with Natasha about social things, such as school, home, and friends. She seems to be well adjusted socially.

"What medications are you currently taking?" I ask.

"I'm taking hydroxyurea for my sickle cell, ibuprofen for pain, and oxycodone when I have bad pain."

"Have you missed any doses of your hydroxyurea recently?"

"Maybe once this past week."

"I want you to work on taking your medication consistently," I tell her. "It's really important that you stick to the dosing schedule for the medication to help you the way it's supposed to." Natasha has been taking hydroxyurea for 3 years now, and I've noticed that she occasionally becomes nonchalant about her medication regimen. Hydroxyurea must be taken consistently for the most optimal effect (Analyze the Evidence 12.1). In fact, poor compliance is the biggest reason the drug is ineffective (Strouse & Heeney, 2012).

I also talk with Natasha about how her sickle cell disease is affecting her life, as I do at every visit. I'm acutely aware of how the diagnosis of sickle cell disease can affect both the teen and the family. Children with chronic sickle cell pain experience more symptoms of depression and anxiety, greater functional disability, and increased absences from school compared with their healthy peers (Sil, Cohen, & Dampier, 2016). Adolescents with sickle cell disease, in particular, may be at higher risk for depression, so I screen Natasha at every visit for depression (Graves, Hodge, & Jacob, 2016). On the basis of Natasha's responses this time and evidence of lack of self-care, I'm concerned that she might be displaying some signs of depression.

"Natasha, I am going to ask you a few questions about how you have been feeling lately," I say. "In the past few weeks, have you had trouble concentrating on things such as watching TV or reading?"

"No, not really," Natasha replies.

"Have you had any trouble falling asleep or staying asleep?"

"I am more tired than usual, but I sleep okay, I guess. Some nights better than others," answers Natasha, with her head down and looking at the floor.

"Do you feel sad or down in the dumps?"

"Not really. I just feel busy, like I have a lot going on sometimes and that gets to me. It makes me feel overwhelmed and then I feel down a bit," Natasha says.

"As you know, I am mindful of the fact that teens, particularly teens with chronic health concerns such as sickle cell

Analyze the Evidence 12.1 — Improving Medication Adherence in Patients Taking Hydroxyurea

Patients taking hydroxyurea for the management of sickle cell disease must take the medication regularly and as prescribed. The compliance rate for hydroxyurea in sickle cell patients was found to range from 49% to 94% (Walsh et al., 2014). For optimal effect, patients must take the drug regularly and not miss doses. Furthermore, Wang et al. (2013) found that among patients prescribed hydroxyurea for the management of sickle cell disease, those who adhered to their medication regimens experienced significant medical cost savings compared with those who did not.

Patients and parents who held negative beliefs about the drug were less likely to adhere to the medication regimen (Badawy et al., 2017). Oyeku et al. (2013) found that increased parent knowledge regarding hydroxyurea's therapeutic effects was significantly associated with more use of the medication. A study by Shahine, Kurdahi, Karam, and Abboud (2014) found that simply providing education materials in a simple language that is easily understood by fifth graders was beneficial in improving knowledge of sickle cell care, including medications, and reduced the

number of hospitalizations for complications from sickle cell disease. In a systematic review of medication adherence in sickle cell patients, Walsh et al. (2014) found that busy lifestyles, other competing demands, change in daily activities, and family stress all contribute to an increased number of skipped medication doses. Can adherence to a hydroxyurea dosing schedule be improved? One study suggests possible interventions to improve medication compliance in those taking hydroxyurea.

Interestingly, Estepp et al. (2014) studied the use of automated text message reminders to take hydroxyurea and found those who used automated text messaging had improved hematologic parameters, suggesting improved medication adherence. Patients were able to customize the text message timing, content, and frequency to deliver messages that were meaningful and specific to how and when they took their medication. Children using the text messaging system had higher mean corpuscular volumes, hemoglobin, and fetal hemoglobin percentages as well as lower reticulocyte counts and bilirubin levels, suggesting improved adherence to the medication regimen.

---

disease, are at risk for depression. What do you say we get you in touch with a counselor who can help you with some strategies to reduce your feelings of being overwhelmed and maybe talk about ways to cope with situations as they come up?"

"That sounds okay. Maybe talking with someone will help," responds Natasha.

Natasha appears to a typical teenager, meeting all the growth and development milestones expected for a 14-year-old, except for a delayed onset of puberty (Growth and Development Check 12.1). She did have a growth spurt this past year but remains in the normal range for height and weight. I notice that Natasha has had significant breast enlargement over the past year.

Growth and Development Check 12.1 — Adolescent Years 12 to 18 Years Old

Physical

Early Adolescence (Ages 11–14 y)
- Continues with growth spurts
- Experiences puberty changes, such as hair growth in the pubic area and breast enlargement in girls

Middle Adolescence (Ages 15–17 y)
- Is at or close to adult height and weight

Late Adolescence (Ages 18–21 y)
- Achieves adult height and weight

Emotional
- Distances self from parents
- Spends more time with friends
- Pushes the limits of authority
- Feels conflicted about leaving the safety of home

Cognitive
- Early and middle adolescence
  - Thinks in terms of black and white, right or wrong

- Late adolescence
  - Solves complex problems
  - Appreciates subtleties of situations
  - Can look at future needs

Social
- Has friends of the same and opposite sex
- Has relationships with people of different ethnicities and social groups and with adults such as teachers, coaches, and mentors

Nutrition
- Requires about 2,200 cal/d (girls) or 2,800 cal/d (boys)
- May be deficient in vitamin D, calcium, zinc, and iron
- Needs 1,300 mg calcium and 600 IU of vitamin D per day for proper bone health (girls)
- Should drink low-fat or nonfat milk
- Should discuss cholesterol and use of saturated fats at well-care checkups

Puberty in adolescents with sickle cell disease is often delayed, on average by 2.5 years (Serjeant, 2013). Despite the delay, there is no difference in menarche and time to first pregnancy compared with women without sickle cell disease (Serjeant, 2013).

"Have you started your period yet?"

Natasha nods. "About 2 months ago. I get these painful cramps when it starts."

"How have you been managing the cramps?"

"I usually use a heating pad on my lower abdomen, which my mom suggested, and I also try to exercise more which seems to help take my mind off of it," responds Natasha.

"I am glad heat and exercise help your cramps. Sometimes menstrual cramps can be quite painful. Let me know if you are not able to control the pain and we can talk about other possible ways to help."

I talk with her about sex, using contraception if she becomes sexually active, and the risks of pregnancy in women with sickle cell disease (Patient Teaching 12.1). Pregnancy in patients with sickle cell is associated with increased risk of acute chest syndrome (ACS), bone pain syndrome, and maternal death (Serjeant, 2013). In addition, I review the risks of getting pregnant while taking hydroxyurea. Hydroxyurea is a category D drug and may cause harm to the fetus. I inform Natasha that this is also a reason to use contraception if she does become sexually active.

Overall, the checkup goes well, and I have no concerns about Natasha's physical health after assessing her. When I call her mother back in, however, I go over the concerns I do have.

"As I told Natasha," I say, "It is critical that she make her appointments with the hematologist. Without adequate supervision and support during these teenage years, Natasha is

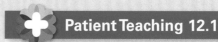

Patient Teaching 12.1

Keeping Early Adolescents Safe

Helmet Safety
- Greater tendency to not wear helmets, due to peer pressure and feeling invincible
- Encourage helmet use when bicycle riding, roller skating, or riding an all-terrain vehicle or moped/scooter.

Substance Use
- Talk to children early and often about the risks of substance use.
- Whereas only 10% of parents think their teens drink alcohol, 52% of teens admit to drinking alcohol.

Sex
- Openly address all concerns, questions, and comments with teens regarding sex.
- Remain nonjudgmental of the teen's views or ideas regarding sex and sexuality-related issues.

Adapted from American Academy of Pediatrics. Healthy Children. Org. (2015). *Stages of adolescents*. Retrieved from https://www .healthychildren.org/English/ages-stages/teen/Pages/Stages-of-Adolescence.aspx

at increased risk for complications and crisis episodes simply due to a lack of self-care and maintenance of the disease. I'd like you all to schedule a make-up appointment with Dr. Anish. I'll be following up with Dr. Anish to see how it goes."

"We understand and will work extra hard to make sure she doesn't miss any more appointments," Anita says.

At Home

It's now been a couple of months since Natasha's well-care visit, and Anita notices that Natasha has had a runny nose and sinus congestion for several days.

"How are you feeling, Natasha?" Anita asks.

"Fine, other than having to blow my nose constantly and being sleep-deprived," Natasha replies.

"You've been staying up too late. You need to go to bed earlier."

"I can't. I have all this homework and these projects that are due at school, and it takes me forever."

"Why don't you start on it as soon as you get home from school?"

"I have drama club right after school that I have to stay for."

"Maybe it's too much for you to do. We have to keep you healthy. Remember what they told us at the doctor's office?"

"But I landed the biggest role I've ever gotten for the winter play! The drama club is the one thing I care about at school. I am not giving that up."

Anita drops the matter but is still worried about Natasha.

The next morning at work, Anita gets a call on her cell phone from Natasha.

"I have a fever of 102.5," Natasha tells her. "I'm short of breath and there's this pain in my chest that's getting worse.

It started last night, but I didn't want to tell you. I'm sorry. I thought it would go away. I think I need to go the hospital, mom." She sounds scared.

"Take some ibuprofen and lie down," Anita says. "I'll be home to take you to the hospital as soon as I can get there. Okay?"

"Okay, mom. Thanks."

"It's going to be okay, Tash. Just hang tight."

Anita rushes home. On her way, she tries to stay positive. She's proud of Natasha for taking her own temperature and for calling her so quickly. Anita taught her to accurately take her temperature when she was 12 years old and staying home for short periods by herself. Also, Anita has tried to encourage Natasha to take an active role in her health and in managing her sickle cell disease. Anita picks Natasha up at home and takes her to the children's hospital, which is only about 10 minutes away.

At the Hospital

In the Emergency Room

Anita and Natasha arrive at the emergency room (ER) and are quickly taken back to a treatment room. They are met by a nurse,

Alexa, a respiratory therapist, Ryan, and a pediatric ER physician, Dr. Meyer. While Ryan places a continuous pulse oximeter on Natasha's index finger to check her O_2 saturation (SpO_2), Dr. Meyer asks Anita, "What brings Natasha to the ER?"

"She has sickle cell anemia and has had a cough, difficulty breathing, and a fever over the past 24 hours."

"And pain in my chest," Natasha adds.

"The monitor shows an oxygen saturation of 82%," Ryan says. "You need oxygen because your oxygen saturation is low."

He places an oxygen mask on her face and says he is setting it to a flow rate of 5 L/min. Her SpO_2 soon rises to 93% and remains steady at that level. Ryan listens to Natasha's chest with his stethoscope. "I'm finding decreased aeration and crackles to the right lower and middle lobes and left lower lobe," he reports to Dr. Meyer. "How is your breathing now, Natasha?" Ryan asks.

"A little better," she says. "The oxygen makes it a little easier to breathe."

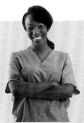

The Nurse's Point of View

Alexa: As soon as Natasha enters the examination room, I immediately begin my assessment by observing her breathing effort and mental status (Priority Care Concepts 12.1). I notice she is breathing faster than normal and is frequently lifting her shoulders to help her take each breath. Ryan's respiratory assessment reveals decreased aeration to the right lower and middle lobes and left lower lobe. I also auscultate coarse breath sounds in the upper lobes.

Although the oxygen is helping, Natasha still complains of difficulty breathing and chest pain. She tells me, "Sometimes it's hard to take a breath, my chest hurts, and when I cough, it really hurts."

Questions I have at this point are (1) What is her oxygenation status? (2) How long has she been breathing like this? (3) What is her mental status? Knowing her mental status/mentation can help me determine whether her oxygen and carbon dioxide levels are abnormal. Patients with high carbon dioxide levels and/or low oxygen levels often have an altered mental status: they are often lethargic, restless, or confused.

While I am speaking with Natasha about her complaints, another nurse is obtaining vital signs. Her vital signs are as follows:

- Heart rate: 128 bpm
- Respiratory rate: 28 breaths/min
- Blood pressure: 94/56 mm Hg
- Temperature: 101.5°F (38.6°C)

Priority Care Concepts 12.1

A Sickle Cell Crisis

1. Administer oxygen.
2. Hydrate the patient.
3. Control the patient's temperature. In this case, Natasha has a fever, so reducing fever is necessary. If Natasha were hypothermic, she would be warmed to a normal temperature.
4. Treat infection.
5. Control the patient's pain.

The patient's mother, Anita, tells me that Natasha's blood pressure is normally in the 120s for systolic and the 50s to 60s for diastolic. I note that her current systolic blood pressure of 94 mm Hg is lower than her baseline, possibly indicating volume depletion or onset of infection or sepsis.

"Did you take ibuprofen this morning?" I ask Natasha.

"Yes," she replies. "About an hour ago." I always ask patients I am caring for about medications they have taken recently so that I will not administer another dose (in this case, of ibuprofen) too soon.

I ask Natasha several questions, including ones about her full name and birthday, the current date, what grade she is in, and the names of her siblings. Natasha answers each question correctly, and, although she states she is sleepy, she remains awake and alert and a bit anxious in the examination room. This is reassuring to me, as her mental status appears to be within normal limits. Also, since Natasha has been on oxygen, she seems less anxious and is breathing more easily than when she arrived.

My next priorities, knowing that she has sickle cell anemia, are to treat her fever and pain and to begin hydrating her.

"How would you rate your pain on a scale from 0 to 10, 0 being no pain and 10 being the worst possible pain," I ask Natasha (How Much Does It Hurt? 12.1).

"My chest pain is an 8. My legs also hurt all the time; my leg pain is a 4."

"Tell me about your chest pain. What is it like?"

"I feel sharp pains whenever I take a deep breath, but I feel a gnawing pain all the time."

"What medication do you take for pain at home?"

"Oxycodone, 5 to 10 mg every 6 hours, when I need it. I took some this morning, but I don't know what time." I ask Dr. Meyer for pain medication orders after explaining what she takes at home.

Dr. Meyer, after examining Natasha, writes the following orders:

- Start a peripheral intravenous (IV) line.
- Draw the following labs: complete blood count (CBC), comprehensive metabolic panel, reticulocyte count, blood cultures, and a urinalysis (UA).
- After serum labs are drawn, give 1 L normal saline (0.9% NS) over 1 hour. Okay to give a normal saline (NS) bolus before obtaining the UA.

How Much Does It Hurt? 12.1

Assessing Natasha's Pain Using the Numeric Rating Scale

To adequately assess Natasha's pain, Alexa must perform an in-depth pain assessment and use an age- and developmentally appropriate pain scale. Because Natasha is of normal cognitive development, at the age of 14 y she should be able to describe, differentiate the characteristics of, and rate her pain. Alexa asks Natasha not only to rate the intensity of the pain but also to identify its location, acuity (acute or chronic), and quality (is it dull, sharp, stabbing, throbbing, gnawing, etc.).

For Natasha, a developmentally appropriate 14-y-old, the Numeric Rating Scale can be used to determine the severity of pain. The Numeric Rating Scale is a 0–10 scale, with a score of 0 indicating no pain and a score of 10 indicating the worst pain possible.

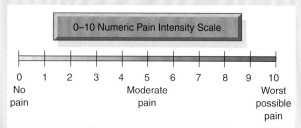

Numeric pain intensity scale. Reprinted with permission from Jensen, S. (2018). *Nursing health assessment: A best practice approach* (3rd ed., Fig. 6.4). Philadelphia, PA: Wolters Kluwer.

It is essential, because Natasha also has chronic pain related to her sickle cell disease, that Alexa differentiate her acute pain from her chronic pain. For example, a sickle cell patient could have chronic leg pain and rate it as a 4. However, the acute chest pain she is having may be a 10 on the Numeric Rating Scale. Patients with chronic and acute pain may have two separate pain scores.

- Hydromorphone (Dilaudid) 0.75 mg IV × 1 dose now (The Pharmacy 12.2)
- O_2 to maintain SpO_2 greater than 93%
- Ibuprofen 800 mg by mouth (PO) once for fever greater than 101.5°F
- Chest x-ray STAT
- Maintenance intravenous fluid (MIVF) to start after the NS bolus is complete: 5% dextrose (D5) in ½ NS at 105 mL/h

After reviewing the orders, I notice that there are no documented allergies for Natasha.

"Does Natasha have any allergies?" I ask her and her mother.

"No," they both reply.

"Have you ever had hydromorphone before for pain control?"

"Yes," Natasha replies. It is important for me to know whether patients have had medications before so that I can monitor them for reactions if it is the first time receiving a medication. I choose a 20-gauge IV because Natasha is a teenager and because she may need a blood transfusion or large-volume fluid boluses, both of which infuse better through a larger bore IV. I am also careful to not place the IV in her antecubital or wrist area, because she is a bit restless and moving around a lot, which could cause the IV to kink while fluids are infusing. To save time and to avoid an extra needlestick for Natasha, I draw the blood for labs when I start the IV, before I flush it.

After starting an IV in her right forearm, I gather supplies to give Natasha pain medication and start the fluid bolus. I do clarify with Dr. Meyer about the amount of fluid ordered. For some patients with ACS, caution should be taken to not overload them with fluid. Dr. Meyer and I discuss Natasha's fluid balance assessment and agree she probably needs the fluid. She has not urinated since last night, her mucous membranes appear a little dry, and her lips are dry. Natasha has rated her pain an 8 in her chest, so hydromorphone is appropriate, as it is for moderate-to-severe pain. I recheck Natasha's blood pressure and note her vital signs before giving her the pain medicine and starting the fluid bolus. I am monitoring for decreased

The Pharmacy 12.2 Medications Used in the Treatment of Sickle Cell Crisis

Medication	Classification	Route	Action	Nursing Considerations
Hydromorphone	• Opioid analgesic • Antitussive	• IV • IM • SC • PR	• Binds to opiate receptors • Alters response to painful stimuli; produces CNS depression • Suppresses cough reflex	• Can cause respiratory depression; monitor respiratory rate and effort after administration • Can cause hypotension; monitor BP before and after administration • Most common side effects: confusion, sedation, and constipation

	The Pharmacy 12.2		Medications Used in the Treatment of Sickle Cell Crisis (*continued*)		
Medication	**Classification**	**Route**	**Action**	**Nursing Considerations**	
Azithromycin	• Macrolide • Anti-infective	• PO • IV	• Bacteriostatic action against susceptible organisms	• Most common side effects: abdominal pain, nausea, and diarrhea • Assess for skin rash during therapy; may cause Stevens–Johnson syndrome, which can be life-threatening • May require dosage adjustment in patients with renal or liver impairment	
Ceftriaxone	• Third-generation cephalosporin • Anti-infective	• IV • IM	• Binds to bacterial cell wall membrane, causing cell death • Bactericidal action against susceptible bacteria	• Do not confuse with other cephalosporins such as cefazolin, cefoxitin, ceftazidime, or cefotetan. • Monitor IV site for phlebitis during and after administration. • Monitor for signs of pseudomembranous colitis (for up to several weeks after therapy ends): abdominal pain, bloody stools, diarrhea, and fever.	
Ketamine (Ketalar)	• Sedative • Anesthetic	• IV • IM	• Produces sedative, analgesic, and hypnotic effects • Increases sympathetic tone • Maintains airway tone and respiration	Monitor for emergent reactions, including the following: • Vivid imagery • Hallucinations • Dreamlike states • Confusion • Excitement • Irrational behavior These reactions can be counteracted with the simultaneous administration of a benzodiazepine.	

BP, blood pressure; CNS, central nervous system; IM, intramuscular; IV, intravenous; PO, by mouth; PR, by rectum; SC, subcutaneous.

respiratory rate and effort (related to the effects of hydromorphone) and want a baseline blood pressure and heart rate to assess what effect the fluid bolus has on her volume status.

Natasha is not the only patient I am caring for, so I let her and Anita know how long the fluid will infuse for and to utilize the call light if her pain worsens, her breathing becomes more difficult, or she needs anything else while I step out of the room for a few minutes. I tell her I will return in 10 to 15 minutes to reassess her pain and check on her. Because I gave her a narcotic, I want to make sure I frequently check her respiratory status and pain level. Also, with the fluids infusing at 999 mL/h, I need to assess the IV site frequently to watch for infiltration or extravasation.

While I am seeing my other patient, the radiology tech checks with me to see if she can do a portable chest x-ray on Natasha. I tell her yes and let her know, after stepping outside my patient's room so I do not violate the Health Insurance Portability and Accountability Act or confidentiality, that Natasha is having some significant chest pain, so if she needs assistance to position Natasha for the x-ray, to ask for the patient care assistant (PCA) to assist.

The laboratory calls about 30 minutes after I sent the blood samples to report critical laboratory values (Table 12.1). Natasha's red blood cell count and hemoglobin and hematocrit levels are reported as significantly lower than normal, whereas her white blood cell count is significantly elevated. I report these to Dr. Meyer and note in my charting that I have informed him of the results.

Natasha's chest x-ray results are also back. Natasha has evidence of right lower and middle lobe pneumonia and left lower lobe atelectasis. The x-ray is consistent with the physical findings of decreased aeration and crackles to those areas of Natasha's lungs. Dr. Meyer writes an order for a dose of ceftriaxone 1 g IV and a dose of azithromycin 500 mg IV.

Table 12.1 Natasha's Laboratory Test Results

Laboratory Test	Analyte	Result	Reference Range or Value[a]	Unit of Measure
Complete blood count	RBC	2.9	3.9–5.5	$\times 10^6/\mu L$
	WBC	19.5	4.5–11.0	$\times 10^9/L$
	Hemoglobin	6.2	14.0–17.5	g/dL
	Hematocrit	19.3	41–50	%
	Platelets	120,000	150,000–350,000	$/\mu L$
	Neutrophils—segmented	68.1	56	% of WBCs
	Neutrophils—bands	1.67	3	% of WBCs
	Lymphocytes	27	34	% of WBCs
	Reticulocytes	2.4	0.5–1.5	% of RBCs
Comprehensive metabolic panel	Sodium	146	136–142	mEq/L
	Potassium	3.5	3.5–5.0	mEq/L
	Chloride	101	96–106	mEq/L
	Carbon dioxide	24	22–28	mEq/L
	Blood urea nitrogen	35	8–23	mg/dL
	Creatinine	0.9	0.6–1.2	mg/dL
	Calcium	9.2	8.2–10.2	mg/dL
	Glucose	122	70–110	mg/dL
	Albumin	4.5	3.5–5.0	g/dL
	Alanine aminotransferase	60	10–40	U/L
	Alkaline phosphatase	120	30–120	U/L
	Aspartate aminotransferase	52	10–30	U/L

[a]Reference ranges and values adapted from the American Medical Association. (2007). *AMA manual of style: A guide for authors and editors* (10th ed.). New York, NY: Oxford University Press.
RBC, red blood cell; WBC, white blood cell.

Anita is a little overwhelmed by all of the people coming in and out of Natasha's examination room in the ER and all of the tests that are being done. It's hard for her to follow all that is happening.

Finally, Dr. Meyer returns to the room, looking like he has some news to share.

"Natasha has acute chest syndrome, or ACS, and needs to be admitted," he tells Anita and Natasha.

"Acute chest syndrome?" Anita asks. "Is that what's causing the pain in her chest?"

"Yes," Dr. Meyer replies. "ACS is an acute pulmonary illness that affects people with sickle cell disease. It is triggered by a vasoocclusion in the pulmonary vasculature. Signs and symptoms include chest pain, coughing, wheezing, fever, shortness of breath, and tachypnea. Lung auscultation often reveals crackles and diminished breath sounds."

"In other words, all the symptoms Natasha's had lately," Anita says.

"Exactly," Dr. Meyer says. "Clinically, ACS is described as a combination of fever, hypoxia, and a new infiltrate on a chest x-ray" (Kanter & Kruse-Jarres, 2013).

"So, what is the treatment for this condition?" Anita asks.

"We will continue to give her IV fluids for rehydration, along with other supportive care, and antibiotics to knock out the infection. We'll be monitoring her respiratory status closely using incentive spirometry and may need to give her bronchodilators if she continues to have trouble breathing. And she'll need a blood transfusion to maintain adequate hemoglobin levels and oxygen-carrying capacity."

Here we go again, Anita thinks. She calls Anthony to let him know.

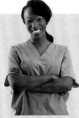

The Nurse's Point of View

Alexa: Once the fluid bolus is complete, I recheck Natasha' vital signs. They are as follows:

- Heart rate: 92 bpm
- Respiratory rate: 26 breaths/min
- Blood pressure: 102/62 mm Hg
- Temperature: 100°F
- O_2 saturation: 94% on 3 L of oxygen

I also auscultate her lungs to assess for crackles, a sign of fluid overloaded. Her lungs are unchanged from the initial assessment. When I reassess Natasha's pain 15 minutes after beginning the hydromorphone, she rates her pain a 3 in her chest and a 2 in her legs. She tells me that she is more comfortable since starting on the hydromorphone. She is sleepier now but easily arousable when I call her name and gently tap her shoulder. I let the physician know what her vital signs are after the bolus and he writes orders for MIVFs. It is important to ensure Natasha stays hydrated during a crisis to prevent further sickling of cells.

Natasha was not able to urinate before the fluid bolus, so I ask her if she thinks she can urinate now. She says she will try, so I grab some extension tubing for her oxygen so she can remain on oxygen while she is up and I assist her to the toilet. I am careful to use standby assistance and watch for dizziness because she received the hydromorphone. Natasha voids a small amount of dark-yellow urine. There is no odor and the urine is clear. I place a laboratory label on the specimen cup after I have verified that Natasha's name and birthdate are correct on the label and send the specimen to the laboratory. When Natasha gets back to the stretcher, she complains of shortness of breath. I stay with her and monitor her SpO_2 and respiratory rate until she feels better, which takes about 2 minutes in this instance. Her SpO_2 remains at 92% to 93% while she is short of breath. I make sure the side rails are up on her stretcher before stepping out of the room to get the antibiotics for administration.

I choose to give the ceftriaxone first because it can infuse over a shorter period of time (30 minutes). Once it has finished infusing, I can start the azithromycin, which is recommended to infuse over 1 hour. It is important to start the antibiotics as soon as they are available, particularly if Natasha has a respiratory infection or is becoming bacteremic, to prevent further decompensation and sepsis. I also make sure the blood cultures and urine specimen were received by the laboratory before giving the antibiotics. Cultures should ideally be drawn before antibiotic administration.

I call report to the nurse who will be caring for Natasha on the inpatient unit, Jill. Priority items I make sure to tell her include the following:

- Natasha's initial complaint
- A brief patient history
- Her initial and current vital signs
- Her respiratory assessment results and related interventions
- The current oxygen flow rate required to maintain her SpO_2 greater than 93%
- Her pain assessment results, related interventions, and response to interventions
- IV site and status
- Fluid bolus administration and response
- Labs drawn and abnormal results
- Chest x-ray findings
- Antibiotics given

It is important to communicate when the antibiotics were given so they are given at the appropriate time after admission. I also tell the nurse my concerns regarding Natasha's safety when she was out of bed to urinate.

On the Unit

Natasha is admitted to Unit A5 North, where the nurses and providers specialize in caring for children with hematologic disorders such as sickle cell disease. Jill, the RN, and Nicole, the PCA, meet Natasha, Anita, and the ER nurse in her room. Natasha has been hospitalized many times before and is usually on this unit, so many of the nurses and staff know her and her mom and dad.

"Hi, Natasha," Jill says. "I believe I've cared for you here before."

"Oh yeah!" Natasha says. "I remember." Anita is comforted by Jill's familiar face.

"Hey, Alexa. Before you go, I just wanted to confirm with you the IV infusion." Alexa verifies that D5 ½ NS is infusing at 105 mL/h, which corresponds with the order.

Jill then explains that she will assess the IV site for swelling, temperature to touch, color of surrounding skin, and dressing status. She reports that the IV site is within normal limits.

"Can you stand on the scale for me, Natasha, so I can get an accurate weight for you?"

"Sure," Natasha says. With Jill standing by ready to assist if needed, Natasha gets on the scale. Her weight is 145.5 lb (66 kg). Anita notices that Natasha is short of breath when she sits down in the bed. Jill switches Natasha's oxygen tubing from the portable tank used in transporting her to the floor to the wall unit in her room and then checks to make sure the oxygen flow is correct. It is set at 3 L/min.

Jill says, "It appears you are having some trouble breathing, Natasha. How do you feel?"

"I feel okay, but I do get a little short of breath when I stand up. It gets better once I lie back down," replies Natasha.

"Your oxygen is on. Do you feel it coming through the cannula?" asks Jill.

"Yes, I can feel it," says Natasha.

"I'm going to check your cannula by taking it out of your nose for a few seconds to see if oxygen is flowing. Yes—it's flowing just fine," Jill reports.

Next, Jill takes Natasha's vital signs. "Even though I've placed the electrocardiogram leads and a pulse oximeter on Natasha, it is important to confirm the monitor readings with an assessment," she explains. Jill reports Natasha's vital signs as follows:

- Heart rate: 130 bpm
- Respiratory rate: 28 breaths/min
- Blood pressure: 108/60 mm Hg
- Temperature: 98.8°F (37.1°C)
- O₂ saturation: 94% on 5 L of oxygen via face mask

When prompted by Jill, Natasha rates her pain a 5 in her chest and 3 in her legs.

"The physician has ordered that you can have two oxycodone tablets for moderate pain, Natasha," Jill says. "Would you like them now?"

"No," Natasha says.

"Natasha, I know generally you are pretty stoic and often do not want to take the pain medications when you are hurting. However, because you are already having some difficulty breathing, I am encouraging you to take the pain medication. It will help the pain in your chest and may help you breathe easier. It is okay to take the ordered doses for your sickle cell pain, particularly when your pain is worse than usual," explains Jill.

"I don't want to become addicted or be known as a drug addict," replies Natasha tearfully. Anita sits down on Natasha's bed and holds her hand. Jill pulls up a chair and remains quiet for a minute.

"Taking pain medication when you need it won't cause drug addiction," explains Jill in a calm, reassuring tone. "And, you have a disease that is painful at times. Part of managing your illness is managing your pain. Taking the pain medication actually helps you rest and heal during this sickle cell crisis."

"Okay, I will take it," Natasha says sniffling. After Jill leaves the room to get the oxycodone, Anita comforts Natasha and reassures her taking the pain medication is the right thing to do.

Jill returns with the oxycodone and, after verifying Natasha's name, birthdate, and allergies, she gives Natasha the medicine. "Natasha, as you may remember from previous admissions, I need to listen to your heart, lungs, and abdomen and check your skin. Do you want your mother to stay in the room while I complete my assessment, or would you like me to ask her to step out and she can come back in when I am finished?" Jill asks Natasha. Anita appreciates that Jill recognizes that adolescent girls can be modest and want privacy from their parents when body parts are exposed and that always she always gives Natasha a choice of having her mom present for assessments and toileting. Anita is prepared to leave, if Natasha wants her to, but she secretly hopes she can stay.

"My mom can stay. It's okay," Natasha responds.

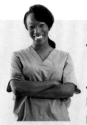

The Nurse's Point of View

Jill: I complete my assessment of Natasha's heart, lungs, and abdomen and check her pulses and skin. I note increased respiratory effort, coarse breath sounds bilaterally, and decreased aeration to the right middle and lower lobes and the left lower lobe of her lungs. I also see that although Natasha is not having to work as hard to breathe as she did after she stood on the scale, she still has some mild retractions suprasternally and is breathing 28 to 30 times a minute. Her other body systems are within normal limits, except that her lips and mucous membranes are slightly dry and noticeably pale, although her capillary refill is 2 seconds and her skin is warm to the touch.

I check the rest of the admission orders.

Admission orders include the following:

- Admit to Unit A5 North for ACS/sickle cell crisis.
- Maintain peripheral IV access; perform NS flushes 3 to 5 mL every 8 hours and prn.
- MIVF: D5 ½ NS at 105 mL/h
- Continuous pulse oximetry monitoring
- Cefotaxime 1 g IV every 12 hours
- Azithromycin 500 mg every 24 hours
- Oxygen to maintain O₂ saturation greater than 92%. Notify the physician if oxygen requirement exceeds 5 L/min.
- Obtain sputum culture.
- Ibuprofen 400 mg PO every 6 hours as needed for mild-to-moderate pain
- Oxycodone 5 mg PO every 4 hours as needed for moderate pain
- Morphine 4 mg every 4 hours as needed for severe pain
- Strict intake and output
- Notify the physician if urine output is less than 1 mL/kg/h.
- Diet: Clear liquids
- Activity: Bed rest. May use the bedside commode with assistance
- Incentive spirometer every hour while awake
- Packed red blood cells, leukocyte-reduced and negative 2 units to infuse over 4 hours
- Obtain CBC 1 hour after completion of packed red blood cells.

I get Natasha settled and perform an in-depth assessment on all systems. Then, after making sure that Natasha and Anita need no further assistance, I ask the health unit coordinator to call the vascular access team (VAT) to start a new peripheral IV on Natasha, because she will need a second IV to infuse blood through (Whose Job Is It, Anyway? 12.1). Natasha requested that the VAT team be called to start her IV because nurses have had trouble in the past getting an IV started on her.

Whose Job Is It, Anyway? 12.1   Vascular Access Team

Members of the vascular access team (VAT) play an important role, working in collaboration with providers and nurses to insert, help maintain, and care for all types of vascular access, from peripheral intravenous lines (PIVs) to peripherally inserted central catheters to central lines and dialysis catheters. VAT members help in assessing patients for the correct type of line and make recommendations to providers regarding which line would be the most appropriate for the patient's situation. Furthermore, VATs play an important role in central line care, including providing education and dressing care and monitoring for central line–associated bloodstream infections. The ability and authority to insert the different types of lines vary among hospitals. In some hospitals, the VAT is called for all line insertions, including PIVs. In other hospitals, nurses or phlebotomists insert PIVs and only call the VAT for central line needs.

In the hospital where Natasha is being treated, nurses are encouraged to call the VAT team for any patient who is a difficult IV stick or after a nurse has been unsuccessful after two attempts to start a PIV. The VAT team brings a special ultrasound machine that is used to find a peripheral vessel and assists the nurse in seeing where to guide the catheter to successfully place the IV line. Jill asks for the VAT team because Natasha and her mom requested them, because Natasha has required multiple attempts for PIVs in previous hospitalizations.

The doctor has ordered packed red blood cells to be administered over 4 hours. The blood bank calls the unit and informs me that the blood is ready to be administered. Following the hospital's policy for blood administration, I verify that Natasha has a patent IV, stable vital signs, and no fever before obtaining the blood from the blood bank. Knowing blood cannot be given through an IV that has anything but NS running, I flush Natasha's IV with saline well and find it patent. While in the room to check the IV and obtain vital signs, I also check the IV site with the MIVF infusing. The site is within normal limits and flushes easily. Natasha's vital signs are as follows:

- Heart rate: 105 bpm
- Respiratory rate: 30 breaths/min
- Blood pressure: 126/72 mm Hg
- O_2 saturation: 93% on 5 L of oxygen

The blood (packed red blood cells) arrives on the unit. I ask Terry, an RN, to check the blood with me. Together, we go into Natasha's room, confirm the blood order, check the blood compatibility and blood bank identification numbers, and check to ensure that the information on Natasha's identification band matches the information on the blood bag label. After performing the blood safety check, I spike the blood with special IV tubing that contains a blood filter and prepare to begin the infusion. I will need to stay in the room to observe Natasha for signs of transfusion reactions during the first 15 minutes of the transfusion and then monitor Natasha's vital signs and assess for reaction every hour until 1 hour after the infusion is complete (Table 12.2). Minimally, according to Maynard (2014), vital signs should be obtained and assessed immediately before, at 15 minutes after the start of, and at the end of the transfusion. However, transfusion reactions can occur anytime during or after the transfusion, so many blood transfusion policies mandate more frequent assessments of vital signs and assessments for transfusion reactions.

While observing Natasha following the start of the packed red blood cell infusion, I review in my mind the signs of the various reactions that can occur when a patient receives a blood transfusion. The most life-threatening reactions are an acute hemolytic transfusion reaction and allergic reactions causing anaphylaxis.

Table 12.2 Blood Transfusion Reactions: Signs and Symptoms

Type of Transfusion Reaction	What Happens	Signs and Symptoms	Interventions
Acute hemolytic	Rapid destruction of red blood cells (RBCs) when the patient is given incompatible blood; recipient antibodies react with donor RBCs	• Fever/chills • Chest pain • Hypotension • Back pain • Abdominal pain • Dyspnea • Vomiting • Diarrhea • Hemoglobinuria • Hematuria	• Stop the transfusion immediately • Provide supportive care, such as a fluid bolus, oxygen, and blood pressure support • Maintain urine output >100 mL/h • Draw blood for crossmatch and hematocrit

(continued)

Table 12.2 Blood Transfusion Reactions: Signs and Symptoms (*continued*)

Type of Transfusion Reaction	What Happens	Signs and Symptoms	Interventions
Delayed hemolytic	Recipient develops antibodies to an RBC antigen 24 h to 28 d after the transfusion	Same as for acute hemolytic but milder and may be absent; diagnosed with laboratory testing	• Supportive care
Febrile nonhemolytic	Most common reaction; no evidence of hemolysis	Fever/chills during or up to 4 h after the transfusion; generally mild and respond to treatment	• Acetaminophen • Diphenhydramine
Allergic	Patient has antibodies to donor proteins, leading to allergic reaction/anaphylaxis	• Itching • Hives • Respiratory distress • Flushing • Hypotension • Circulatory shock • Nausea	• Stop the transfusion • Administer supportive care • Normal saline bolus • Epinephrine (subcutaneous injection), if anaphylaxis • Epinephrine IV to support blood pressure • Diphenhydramine
Transfusion-associated circulatory overload	Volume overload from an excessively high infusion rate or too much volume	• Difficulty breathing • Cough • Fluid in the lungs • Pulmonary edema	• Oxygen; support respiratory symptoms • Diuretics • Elevate the head of the bed • Strict intake and output • Decrease total fluid intake
Transfusion-related acute lung injury	Fluid builds up in the lungs during or after a transfusion but is not related to volume; thought to be associated with antibodies in the blood	• Respiratory distress • Increased oxygen requirement • Dyspnea • Hypoxemia • Hypotension • Pulmonary infiltrates	• Supportive care • Oxygen; many need positive-pressure ventilation • Diuretics

Anita sits at Natasha's bedside, anxiously watching her. It's been 4 hours since they started the blood transfusion. An alarm sounds on the infusion pump, and Anita is concerned that something is wrong. She's about to pull the call light cord, but Jill walks in and checks the pump.

"Looks like the infusion is complete," Jill says, silencing the alarm. "Natasha has tolerated the infusion without any signs of reaction." Jill takes Natasha's vital signs and reports them as follows:

- Heart rate: 105 bpm
- Respiratory rate: 26 breaths/min
- Blood pressure: 118/74 mm Hg
- Temperature: 99°F (37.2°C)
- O$_2$ saturation: 95% on 5 L of oxygen

"Are those good numbers?" Anita asks.

"Definitely," Jill says. "Natasha's blood pressure has come up to what is more her baseline, and her heart rate is lower from when she was first admitted. These changes could be a result of her blood volume being replete, her no longer being febrile, or both."

Natasha is still sleepy but "easily arousable and appropriately oriented," as Jill puts it, before leaving.

About an hour later, Jill returns. "I'm going to draw some blood now to send to the laboratory for a CBC test," she says.

That evening, around 7:15 p.m., Jill enters the room with another nurse.

"Anita and Natasha, this is Adam," Jill says. "He will be Natasha's nurse for the night. Adam, this is Natasha and her mom, Anita."

Jill reports to Adam about Natasha. Following the report, Adam says to Natasha, "I'm just going to do a 1-minute assessment to make sure I have no further questions for Jill." Adam listens to Natasha's lungs, assesses her breathing, and asks her to rate and describe her pain. Adam has prioritized these assessments on the basis of Natasha's admitting diagnosis, he explains. Natasha rates her pain a 3 in her chest and a 2 in her legs.

"Do you need some pain medicine for the pain in your chest?" Adam asks.

"No thanks," Natasha says. "I'm okay. Maybe later, if it gets worse."

"Okay. I'll be back in a little bit to perform an in-depth assessment after I finish receiving reports on the two other patients I will be caring for."

Late in the afternoon on her second day of being in the hospital, Natasha is starting to feel better. Adam says that he turned down her oxygen rate to 4 L/min last night because her O$_2$ saturation levels were 96% to 97% on 5 L/min of oxygen and Natasha said she was breathing a little better. The respiratory therapist stops by to assess Natasha and reports that her O$_2$ saturation is 96% on 4 L/min.

"Natasha, I see that you are breathing mostly through your mouth," the therapist says. "Is that mainly how you've been breathing lately?"

"Yes, I guess so," Natasha replies. "I hadn't really thought about it."

"Okay, that's fine," the therapist says. "I'll leave you on the facemask for now. When we can wean your oxygen down to 3 L/min, I'll switch you to a nasal cannula."

The next morning, on day 3 of her hospital stay, Natasha tells the nurse she is feeling a bit better and would like to go for a walk. She has not been out of bed since she was admitted other than to sit in a chair or use the bedside commode. The nurse, Stephanie, agrees this is a good idea, but she must first obtain an order for Natasha to be up ambulating. The current order, she explains, is only for getting out of bed to sit in a chair or to use the commode. Stephanie takes some time to discuss discharge goals with Natasha and Anita, particularly since Natasha is feeling better and asking about ambulating.

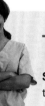

The Nurse's Point of View

Stephanie: I'm relieved to see how much better Natasha is doing today and to hear that she wants to get up to walk. Before I check on the order for that, though, I need to assess her lungs, breathing, and skin.

"How does your breathing feel compared to yesterday, Natasha?" I ask.

"I actually feel a little better. The pain in my chest is not as bad as yesterday and I do not feel short of breath as much when I turn myself in bed."

"I need to listen to your lungs. Is it okay that I do that with your mom and dad here in the room or would you like them to step out?"

Natasha's dad steps out, knowing Natasha does not like him in the room when nurses and doctors are examining her. I use this time to do a full assessment, including checking Natasha's skin on her back, buttocks, sacrum, and coccyx for pressure injury.

"Your lungs still have some coarse sounds in the lower lobes. Can you take some deep breaths and then cough for me, please?" Natasha coughs several times and I reassess her lung sounds. "Your lungs sound a bit better after you breathe deeply and cough. Have you been using your incentive spirometer?"

"Probably not as often as I should," responds Natasha.

It is imperative that patients with ACS begin using an incentive spirometer right away when they are hospitalized. These patients are at high risk for developing pneumonia and atelectasis, and an incentive spirometer aids in keeping the lungs open.

"Natasha, let me see you use the incentive spirometer. I would like to see what volumes you can maintain with the majority of your breaths." Natasha uses the incentive spirometer correctly, inhaling slowly and holding each breath for several seconds before she exhales. She is able to maintain a volume of 800 mL, which for her age and weight is below what I would expect, but she can reach that volume for all 10 breaths. I raise the volume to 1,000 mL and challenge her to try to reach that goal by tomorrow morning.

"Natasha, I would like to check your back and bottom for any skin issues. I know you have been in the hospital for only 3 days, but most of that time you have been in bed. Sometimes, pressure injuries can result when patients lie in bed for extended periods." Knowing that pressure injuries can occur after only a day of lying in bed, particularly if perfusion is compromised, I realize the importance of daily skin assessments. I also heard in report that previous nurses were concerned that Natasha was not moving enough in bed and was resistant at times to getting up to sit in the chair. These are also flags for me to thoroughly assess her skin.

"Yes, I know all about those pressure injuries. Last year when I was in the hospital for over a week, I had what the nurses kept calling a 'Stage I pressure injury' on my lower back, just above my bottom. It was sore and tender to touch but healed quickly once I started getting out of bed."

I check Natasha's back, buttocks, sacrum, coccyx, heels, ankles, and elbows for any signs of pressure injury. I also check the back of her head (occiput) because she has had her hair pulled tight and this is an area where patients can get pressure injury, as well. There are no areas of redness or tenderness.

"Everything looks great Natasha," I tell her.

After finishing my morning assessments and medication passes, I come back to help Natasha ambulate in the hallway.

"On morning rounds, the physician agreed Natasha should be out of bed walking at least 2 or 3 times a day unless she becomes short of breath or her oxygen saturation levels are not maintained on 5 L/min or less of oxygen," Stephanie reports to Anita and Natasha.

Stephanie connects Natasha's oxygen tubing to a portable oxygen tank and helps her get out of bed. Natasha actually walks to the end of the hall and back and only complains once of being slightly short of breath. Anita is proud of her and cheers her on. After a pause, she feels better and returns to her room.

"Even though it made me feel tired, I know I need to get out of bed and walk if I ever want to go home," Natasha tells Stephanie when she gets back to bed.

On day 4 in the hospital, Natasha continues to improve. The nurse tells Anita that Natasha's oxygen has been weaned down to 2 L/min via nasal cannula and that her O_2 saturation levels remain greater than 96% even when she is out of bed and walking. She still is not eating much but is drinking more, so they reduce her IV fluids to one half of the maintenance rate. Natasha also has not had a fever in over 24 hours.

By day 5, her oxygen is down to 1 L/min in the morning and she is on room air by the afternoon. The nurse reports that Natasha's lungs are clear but she still has a productive cough at times. She does not get short of breath when she gets out of bed but does still feel tired. Her O_2 saturation levels are greater than

97% on room air. By late evening on day 5, Natasha is able to eat almost all of her dinner and has drunk enough that her IV fluids are discontinued.

At Discharge

On day 6 of Natasha's hospital stay, Sandra, her nurse that morning, informs them that Natasha has met all the discharge criteria and is able to go home. Sandra goes over the discharge criteria for a patient admitted for ACS, which Natasha has now met; they include the following:

1. Respiratory status returns to baseline.
2. The patient maintains O_2 saturation levels greater than 96% on room air.
3. The patient is tolerating at least 50% of the required nutritional intake.
4. The patient is maintaining adequate hydration through PO intake.
5. The patient has been afebrile for at least 24 hours.
6. Pain is controlled with a home pain management regimen.

Before discharge, Sandra educates Natasha and her parents about ACS. She also reviews with them how to limit and avoid future episodes of sickle cell crisis, as well as signs of impending crisis (Patient Teaching 12.2). After a review of Natasha's

---

✚ Patient Teaching 12.2   Discharge Teaching Following a Sickle Cell Crisis

Topic	Information

Infection	1. Prevent or reduce the risk of infection
	  a. Wash your hands.
	  b. Avoid contact with sick people.
	  c. Avoid sharing cups and water bottles.
	2. Signs and symptoms of infection
	  a. Fever > 100.5°F
	  b. Shortness of breath or increased work to breathe
	  c. Increased phlegm or mucus
	  d. Redness, swelling, or warmth around open sores or cuts
	  e. Chills, muscle aches, malaise

Hydration	1. Maintain adequate hydration. 2. Signs and symptoms of dehydration
Pain	1. Maintain adequate pain control. 2. What to do if pain is not controlled by prescribed pain medication regimen?
Temperature control	1. Avoid extreme temperatures (too hot or too cold). 2. Wear extra layers and a hat and gloves when in cold temperatures. 3. Avoid prolonged exposure to heat on hot days; go outside in the early morning or late evening.
Sleep and rest	1. Get at least 8 h of sleep each night. 2. Consider a nap, when possible, if you do not feel well rested.
Signs of sickle cell crisis	1. Acute chest syndrome 2. Stroke 3. Vasoocclusive crisis

chart, Sandra reports that it appears that the staff have discussed most of the items on the discharge teaching plan but have not signed them off as complete. So, she says she will review all the items to ensure that Natasha and her parents understand the instructions. Other topics she covers include avoiding infections, maintaining hydration, managing pain, temperature control, and sleep.

As they pull out of the parking garage at the hospital, Anita feels relieved and grateful that Natasha is doing so much better. "I can't wait to sleep in my own bed tonight," Natasha says.

Think Critically

1. A parent asks, "What is sickle cell disease?" How would you respond?
2. What are the signs and symptoms of a vasoocclusive crisis?
3. What are three ways patients with sickle cell disease can lower their risk of a vasoocclusive crisis?
4. Why is it important for a patient with sickle cell disease to be seen early when a fever or signs of a respiratory infection are present?
5. What is the priority of care for a patient diagnosed with ACS?
6. What is the nurse observing for at the beginning and throughout administration of packed red blood cells to a patient?
7. What effect can dehydration have on a patient with sickle cell disease?

References

Badawy, S., Thompson, A., Penedo, F., Lai, J., Rychlik, K., & Liem, R. (2017). Barriers to hydroxyurea adherence and health-related quality of life in adolescents and young adults with sickle cell disease. *European Journal of Haematology, 98,* 608–614.

Baskin, M., Goh, X., Heeney, M., & Harper, M. (2013). Bacteremia risk and outpatient management of febrile patients with sickle cell disease. *Pediatrics, 131*(6), 1035–1041.

Brousse, V., Makani, J., & Rees, D. C. (2014). Management of sickle cell disease in the community. *British Medical Journal, 348,* g1765.

Crookston, K. P., Koenig, S. C., & Reyes, M. D. (2015). Transfusion reaction identification and management at the bedside. *Journal of Infusion Nursing, 38*(2), 104–113.

Estepp, J., Winter, B., Johnson, M., Smeltzer, M., Howard, S., & Hankins, J. (2014). Improved hydroxyurea effect with the use of text messaging in children with sickle cell anemia. *Pediatric Blood and Cancer, 61*(11), 2031–2036.

Graves, K., Hodge, C., & Jacob, E. (2016). Depression, anxiety and quality of life in children and adolescents with sickle cell disease. *Pediatric Nursing, 42*(3), 113–120.

Kanter, J., & Kruse-Jarres, R. (2013). Management of sickle cell disease from childhood through adulthood. *Blood Reviews, 27*(6), 279–287.

Maynard, K. (2014). Administration of blood components. In M. K. Fung, B. J. Grossman, C. D. Hillyer, & C. M. Westoff (Eds.), *AABB technical manual* (18th ed., pp. 545–559). Bethesda, MD: American Association of Blood Banks.

McCavit, T. (2012). Sickle cell disease. *Pediatrics in Review, 33,* 195–206.

National Institutes of Health. (2014). *Evidence-based management of sickle cell disease.* Retrieved from https://www.nhlbi.nih.gov/sites/www.nhlbi.nih.gov/files/sickle-cell-disease-report.pdf

Oyeku, S., Driscoll, M., Cohen, H., Trachtman, R., Pashankar, F., Mullen, C., . . . & Green, N. (2013). Parental and other factors associated with hydroxyurea use for pediatric sickle cell disease. *Pediatric Blood and Cancer, 60*(4), 653–658.

Quinn, T., Rogers, R., McCavit, L., & Buchanan, R. (2010). Improved survival of children and adolescents with sickle cell disease. *Blood, 115*(17), 3447–3452.

Serjeant, G. R. (2013). The natural history of sickle cell disease. *Cold Spring Harbor Perspectives in Medicine, 3*(10), a011783.

Shahine, R., Badr, L., Karam, D., & Abboud, M. (2015). Educational intervention to improve the health outcomes of children with sickle cell disease. *Journal of Pediatric Health Care, 29*(1), 54–60.

Sil, S., Cohen, L., & Dampier, C. (2016). Psychosocial and functional outcomes in youth with chronic sickle cell pain. *The Clinical Journal of Pain, 32*(6), 527–533.

Strouse, J., & Heeney, M. (2012). Hydroxyurea for the treatment of sickle cell disease: Efficacy, barriers, toxicity, and management in children. *Pediatric Blood and Cancer, 59*(2), 365–371.

Walsh, K., Cutrona, S., Kavanagh, P., Crosby, L., Malone, C., Lobner, K., & Bundy, D. (2014). Medication adherence among pediatric patients with sickle cell disease: A systematic review. *Pediatrics, 134*(6), 1175–1183.

Wang, W., Oyeku, S., Luo, Z., Boulet, S., Miller, S., Casella, J. F., . . . & Grosse, S. D. (2013). Hydroxyurea is associated with lower costs of care of young children with sickle cell anemia. *Pediatrics, 132*(4), 677–683.

Ware, R. (2010). How I use hydroxyurea to treat young patients with sickle cell anemia. *Blood, 115*(26), 5300–5311.

Suggested Readings

Centers for Disease Control and Prevention. *Sickle cell disease clinical guidelines.* Retrieved from https://www.cdc.gov/ncbddd/sicklecell/recommendations.html

Crookston, K. P., Koenig, S. C., & Reyes, M. D. (2015). Transfusion reaction identification and management at the bedside. *Journal of Infusion Nursing, 38*(2), 104–113.

Healthychildren.org. *Sickle cell disease: Information for parents.* Retrieved from https://www.healthychildren.org/English/health-issues/conditions/chronic/Pages/Sickle-Cell-Disease-in-Children.aspx

13 Jack Wray: Attention Deficit Hyperactivity Disorder

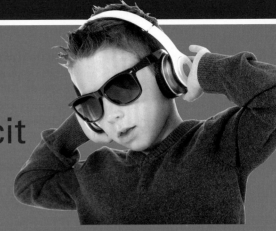

Jack Wray, age 8 years

Objectives

After completing this chapter, you will be able to:

1. Describe normal growth and development of the 8-year-old.
2. Discuss an appropriate teaching plan for a healthy 8-year-old.
3. Identify potential triggers and environmental stimuli that can worsen behaviors in a child with attention deficit hyperactivity disorder (ADHD).
4. Explain the use of behavioral therapy in the treatment of ADHD.
5. Identify the signs and symptoms of ADHD.
6. Discuss and differentiate the medications used in the treatment of ADHD.
7. Create a nursing plan of care for a school-aged child with ADHD.

Key Terms

Attention deficit hyperactivity disorder (ADHD)

Impulsivity

Background

Jack Wray is an 8-year-old boy who loves to ride his bike, wrestle with his brothers, and play with his superhero action figures. Jack is the youngest of three boys in the Wray family. Jeremy, who is 12 years old, is the oldest. Alex is the middle child and is 10 years old. Jack's parents, Kevin and Sherry, are always busy raising their three boys, who are active in sports and Boy Scouts. Kevin is an environmental engineer and the den leader for the boys' scout troop. Sherry is an accountant for a local accounting firm and also volunteers at the elementary school where Jack and Alex attend. The Wrays have a dog, Daisy. Daisy is a therapy dog for Jack. Daisy helps motivate Jack with different therapeutic interventions the Wrays use at home.

Shortly after Jack turned 5 years old, his parents became concerned about his inability to sit still and noticed that he was often very impulsive. At first, Kevin and Sherry thought this was just typical "boy" behavior, although they did not see the behaviors to this extreme in their older boys. Jack would often take risks, such as jumping off the top of the stairs, running away from his parents in a parking lot, and climbing on the counters and pretending to fly off of them. It seemed like no amount of time-outs, punishment, or removing privileges worked to lessen his impulsiveness. Sherry also thought that Jack was a bit more aggressive with his siblings than she thought was normal. It wasn't until Jack was enrolled in a prekindergarten program that the Wrays became really concerned about his behaviors. The teacher would often send a note home or even call with concerns regarding Jack's behavior. By the middle of Jack's kindergarten year, his parents and his pediatrician had begun to suspect that he had **attention deficit hyperactivity disorder (ADHD)**.

Sherry and Kevin quickly educated themselves about this disorder. They learned that ADHD is a chronic neurobehavioral disorder marked by a persistent pattern of inattention and/or hyperactivity and **impulsivity** that interferes with functioning and development (Felt, Biermann, Christner, Kochhar, & Harrison, 2014). They discovered that it is the most common behavioral disorder in children, and its prevalence is increasing. Recent national data that Sherry consulted revealed that approximately 11% of children aged 4 to 17 years (6.4 million children) are diagnosed with ADHD (Visser et al., 2014). More than two-thirds of these children take medication to control the symptoms of ADHD (Visser et al., 2014).

Sherry and Kevin also learned that diagnosis of ADHD is made by meeting criteria established by the American Psychiatric Association, which include symptoms characteristic of inattention and symptoms characteristic of hyperactivity and impulsivity. To be diagnosed, a person must meet six or more of the inattention behaviors or symptoms and/or six or more of the hyperactive/impulsive behaviors or symptoms. Furthermore, these symptoms of inattention and/or hyperactive/impulsivity must be present for at least 6 months, in two or more settings, such as home and school, and create a negative impact on social, academic, or occupational activities. Final diagnosis is based on the criteria delineated in the DSM-5 (APA, 2013); these are available at the following website of the Centers for Disease Control and Prevention (CDC): https://www.cdc.gov/ncbddd/adhd/diagnosis.html.

As part of the diagnostic process, Jack's pediatrician, Dr. Mario, asked his parents to fill out a screening questionnaire. A screening questionnaire was also submitted by his kindergarten teacher. Sherry still remembers when she and Kevin filled this out at home one night. They found it challenging to really be honest and open with all the behaviors Jack was displaying. Even though they knew it was in his best interest to be accurately diagnosed, the guilt they felt that their son was having difficulty was way more than they ever anticipated. Both their older boys are seemingly well-behaved, respectful, Straight-A students who have many friends and are very social. Jack is just the opposite.

Dr. Mario diagnosed Jack with ADHD soon afterward, on reviewing the questionnaires from his parents and teachers and the diagnostic criteria. In the inattention category, both his parents and teachers reported significant problems with listening to directions, keeping track of his belongings, not listening when spoken to directly, sustaining attention in play activities, and following through with even simple tasks such as putting his shoes on or getting dressed. Furthermore, Jack was very easily distracted by external stimuli; even the smallest noise, movement, or activity called his attention away. In the category of hyperactivity/impulsivity, Jack met all the criteria, and his parents and teachers provided multiple examples for each. For instance, anything that Jack had in his hand, he tapped or fidgeted with constantly, and he could not sit still for more than a minute. Even when interested in an activity, he was constantly moving. Jack's parents could not even begin to tell Dr. Mario how many times Jack had climbed and jumped off things, even after being told not to repeatedly or slightly injuring himself. His teacher reported that his behavior on the playground was quite daring and that he was often pulled aside to be reminded how to remain safe on the playground. These symptoms had persisted since he was in preschool and had seemingly gotten worse since entering kindergarten.

Health Promotion

Now, 3 years later, in late August, Sherry and Jack are going to see his primary care provider, Dr. Mario, for his 8-year-old well-care visit. They are late for their appointment by about 15 minutes because Jack had a meltdown when he had to leave school early. He could not find his book, lost his jacket, and was having difficulty following directions. Sherry attributes these things to the start of the new school year and transitioning to a new daily routine. When they arrive for the appointment, Sherry is worried about how Jack will behave while in the waiting room because they may have to wait longer. It has been a long day for Sherry, and sometimes she struggles to use any of the behavioral techniques she has learned to manage Jack's behavior by the end of the day. Luckily, they are seen quickly.

The medical assistant, Mandy, brings Jack and Sherry back to the examination room and measures his height, weight, and vital signs, including blood pressure. Mandy remembers Jack from a previous visit and has brought a small box of gadgets for him to play with while she asks Sherry the necessary questions for the visit. Mandy knows that Jack likes the surprise box and will follow directions to play with toys in the surprise box. All the toys in the box are age-appropriate, such as dinosaurs, cars, action figures, and Legos. Jack sits calmly and watches Mandy take his blood pressure and obtain pulse. Because Jack sits calmly, he is allowed to play with the surprise box. Mandy informs Sherry that Jack weighs 48 lb (21.8 kg) and is 49 in (4.1 ft) tall. She also tells Sherry that, based on the growth chart, the average weight for an 8-year-old boy is 57 lb (25.8 kg) and the average height is 50.5 in (4.2 ft). An 8-year-old boy in the 10th percentile for weight would weigh about 47 lb (21.3 kg), whereas one in the 95th percentile would weigh approximately 78 lb (35.4 kg).

"What medications is Jack currently taking?" Mandy asks Sherry.

"Jack takes a gummy multivitamin each day and takes dexmethylphenidate (Focalin) for his ADHD," Sherry replies.

"The dose for the dexmethylphenidate is 5 mg twice a day, correct?" Mandy asks.

"That's right," Sherry says. Mandy updates the information in Jack's record.

Dr. Mario comes in to see Jack. Jack is busy playing with some action figures, happy and content.

"Looks like you're having a tough day," Dr. Mario says as he enters the room. Sherry realizes how tired and frazzled she must look. "How are things going at home with the boys?"

"Some days are more challenging than others with these three boys," she replies. "Luckily, my older two boys are great kids, well-behaved, and helpful with Jack. It seems like some days Jack's ADHD symptoms are worse than other days, but I cannot put my finger on the pattern. It could also just be that I'm more stressed because I recently got promoted and am working longer hours some days. But, I think we are doing well, overall. It's just been a long day."

"I understand," Dr. Mario says. "Do you have any concerns or questions about Jack's development, growth, nutrition, or anything else?"

"I would like to talk about his weight and appetite," responds Sherry. "He is just not eating enough given how busy and active he is. Other than that, I think he is doing pretty well. School is just getting started and his teacher and guidance counselor have asked us to consider a meeting to discuss an IEP—you know, an individualized education program—so that he can perhaps get some accommodations for his tests and classwork, which he tends to take longer to complete. I have a phone meeting next week with the psychologist who sees Jack at the children's hospital to discuss what all that means. I just do not want him labeled or looked down upon because he has ADHD. He is a bright kid. I thought IEPs were for kids who have learning disabilities, hearing problems, or speech problems or who are developmentally delayed."

"Actually, IEPs are not a bad or negative thing and are used for children with many different types of developmental needs," Dr. Mario says. "Often parents find them helpful when their child has ADHD. Section 504 of the Rehabilitation Act and the Individuals with Disabilities Act were laws passed to help children who have many types of disabilities to have equal access to an education and can help children receive modifications and accommodations that will assist them in achieving educational goals," explains Dr. Mario. "If the school is requesting this, I would take advantage of these opportunities, because it may help him in the classroom setting. Accommodations can allow for more time to complete schoolwork, an aide to sit with Jack to help him stay focused, or even a nonstimulating environment to complete certain activities. Let me know if there is anything I can help you with after you speak with the nurse practitioner or psychologist."

Dr. Mario covers several areas during the well-care visit, including developmental milestones, safety, and anticipatory guidance (Growth and Development Check 13.1).

"Jack, are you riding your bike without training wheels?" asks Dr. Mario. Jack is playing with his dinosaurs and does not look up when Dr. Mario looks directly at him and speaks. Dr. Mario asks Jack a second time after moving closer to him and getting his attention.

"Oh yes I am!" responds Jack eagerly.

"He's actually pretty good at it," Sherry says.

"I also can beat my brothers in basketball. I make more baskets than they do," Jack adds. Sherry nods her head in agreement.

"What is your favorite activity or thing to do for fun?" asks Dr. Mario.

"I like to build things with play dough and clay. Mom lets me build animals with the clay and then we bake them and I paint them. I have a bunch in my room," Jack tells Dr. Mario.

"That seems to be Jack's main interest right now," Sherry confirms.

"How are you doing in school, Jack?" asks Dr. Mario.

"I sometimes don't like school because I can't find anyone to play with on the playground. And, I get in trouble sometimes for not staying in my seat," explains Jack.

"Does Jack have a best friend or any friends that he regularly talks about?" Dr. Mario asks Sherry. "At this age, kids typically

Growth and Development Check 13.1

Eight-Year-Old Milestones

Social and Emotional
- Develops hobbies such as model building and working with crafts and yarn
- Thinks about the future
- Gives attention to friendships
- Wants to be liked and accepted by friends
- Focuses less on self; has increased concern for others

Speech
- Is learning to talk through thoughts and feelings

Cognitive
- Reads
- Concentrates for increasingly longer periods of time
- Experiences rapid development of mental skills and use of judgment

Gross and Fine Motor
- Learns to ride a bicycle
- Shows increased coordination
- Is skilled in running, jumping, skipping, and hopping
- Throws objects with accurate aim and increased distance

want to develop friendships and want to be liked and accepted by friends."

"He does have a best friend who comes over to play after school often," Sherry says. "But he's a year older, so Jack doesn't see him at recess. Jack talks about a lot of different kids he plays with, but sometimes he would rather play alone or do his own thing."

"Are you concerned about friendships or Jack making friends at school, Sherry?" asks Dr. Mario.

"Not really. He seems pretty happy to go to school most days, and I believe he is having the normal friend-making challenge other kids his age have. I eat lunch with him occasionally, and he seems to always find kids to play with when I go outside for recess after lunch with him," explains Sherry.

"At times, kids with ADHD can have trouble making friends because of some of the behaviors they may exhibit, such as talking a lot, interrupting other children, not listening, and not waiting for their turn. I would keep an eye out and check in with Jack about friends and how he is feeling about his friends to make sure building friendships is happening. If he appears to be having difficulty, we may need to reassess how he is doing in other areas related to his ADHD and make sure his behaviors are under control," Dr. Mario tells Sherry.

"Okay. I will keep a watchful eye. I think it is okay for now," Sherry reassures Dr. Mario.

Dr. Mario goes over some anticipatory guidance topics for an 8-year-old, including the appropriate use of car seats, bicycle helmet use, firearm safety, and water safety (Patient Teaching 13.1). Dr. Mario reminds Sherry that around the age of 8 years, children develop a greater sense of independence and begin to give in to peer pressure; therefore, safety issues should be regularly addressed at home.

Safety is a particularly important concern for children with ADHD, Dr. Mario explains, because they have an increased incidence of accidents. In fact, he tells her, several studies have demonstrated that children are more likely to have higher rates of unintentional injuries, emergency room visits, smoking, drug use, and alcohol consumption (Bonander, Beckman, Janson, & Jernbro, 2016; Dalsgaard, Leckman, Mortensen, Nielsen, & Simonsen, 2015).

Dr. Mario reviews car safety with Sherry. He tells her that the American Academy of Pediatrics (AAP) recommends that children remain in an appropriate car seat or booster seat until they are between the ages of 8 and 12 years. Specifically, the AAP promotes the use of belt-positioning booster seats until the child has reached 57 in (4.75 ft) in height and is between the ages of 8 and 12 years. Motor vehicle accidents are the most common cause of death from unintentional injury in the school-aged population. Many of these deaths can be prevented when car seats and safety restraints are used appropriately, he tells her.

"As you know," Sherry says, "Jack was notorious for taking his seatbelt off while the car was moving. But ever since he turned five, we've been using a buckle guard on his seatbelt, just

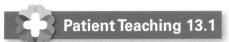

Patient Teaching 13.1

Eight-Year-Old Anticipatory Guidance

Safety

- Require the child wear protective gear when playing sports.
- Require the child to wear a helmet at all times when biking and skating.
- Have the child use a booster seat and remain in the back seat of the vehicle until he or she is at least 4 ft 9 in tall or 8 y old.
- Make sure that the child knows the family plan for exiting the house and meeting after a fire.
- Lock up guns and firearms.
- Supervise the child when he or she is near water, even if the child knows how to swim.
- Teach the child street safety: to avoid running after balls in the street and how to safely ride a bicycle and cross the street.

Social Development

- Meet and get to know the child's friends and their parents.
- Teach the child how to answer the phone and the door.
- Take time to talk with the child about his or her friends and relationships with peers.
- Monitor for signs of bullying.

as you recommended, and it's been great for keeping him from unbuckling his seatbelt. We're still using it, and probably will be until he turns 30," she says with a smile.

Dr. Mario examines Jack and tells Sherry he has no concerns related to his heart, lungs, abdomen, skin, and physical appearance.

"I'd like to talk now with you about the concerns you mentioned at the beginning of the visit," Dr. Mario says. "You're worried about his weight?"

"Yes," she replies. "Jack often has no appetite but is incredibly active."

"Let me look back at his record," Dr. Mario says, pulling up Jack's health record on a laptop computer. "It looks like Jack has only gained 1 pounds in the past year. On average, school-aged kids should gain about 4 to 7 pounds a year until puberty. I agree that his lack of appetite and less-than-average weight gain is a concern, particularly since he is on stimulant medications for his ADHD, which can cause a lack of appetite and weight loss in children."

"What type of foods does Jack like to eat, when he is hungry?" asks Dr. Mario.

"He generally eats a variety of foods, but over the past several months, he hasn't been interested in food at all, no matter what I put in front of him," Sherry tells the doctor. "And he is even calm and sits with us at breakfast and dinner, when we eat as a family. He just doesn't want anything and tells me he is not hungry."

"Have there been any changes in his medications, home routines, or meal times in the past several months?" asks Dr. Mario.

"No, but I have noticed that he goes through phases of not eating a lot and then eating way more than usual. But this most recent phase of not eating a lot has seemed to last a long time. We have tried adding high-calorie shakes and foods to just get the calories in, but he is not interested in them. I am wondering if it is the dexmethylphenidate. I understand that it can cause Jack not to be hungry," Sherry tells Dr. Mario.

"How is he sleeping? Does he seem more tired than usual?" asks Dr. Mario.

"He sleeps pretty well. He gets 9 to 10 hours of sleep most nights. He is a little more tired, but the school year just started, so all the boys are adjusting to earlier bedtimes and longer days. His activity level seems about the same, as well," explains Sherry.

"Well, let's do this. Can you keep a food log of what Jack eats each day for a week? Also write down how active he has been each day. I would like to see Jack back in a month for a weight and height check, and we will look at what his food intake has been. If he has lost weight, we will consult with the team at the children's hospital about possibly looking at his medication as the source of his lack of appetite. Does that sound reasonable?" Dr. Mario asks Sherry.

"Sure. We pack his lunch each day, so I can pay attention to what he brings home each day that he hasn't eaten. Should we keep trying the high-calorie shakes?" asks Sherry.

"I think that is fine, especially if you can find one that he likes. Just be sure those are not always taking the place of a meal. He needs a well-balanced diet with a variety of foods, too," Dr. Mario tells Sherry.

"I think this plan sounds fine," Sherry tells Dr. Mario.

Jack has already received all of his immunizations up to age 8 following the Centers for Disease Control and Prevention Guidelines; therefore, he does not receive any immunizations at the well-care visit. Dr. Mario reminds Sherry about the flu shot and recommends that Jack receive his flu shot today before he leaves. Sherry agrees but wishes she had thought about it before coming to the visit because she could have made sure Jack had his afternoon dose of dexmethylphenidate. Luckily, Jack sits still and gets the flu shot without any problems.

At Home

A month passes, and the Wray family is as much in chaos as ever, from Kevin and Sherry's perspective. With three active boys younger than age of 12, things get a little out of control when it comes to following rules, staying focused on necessary tasks, and doing chores. About the only calm times in the Wray house are breakfast and dinner. Last year, while meeting with a behavioral specialist to learn ways to help Jack focus and accomplish necessary tasks at home, the Wrays set a goal of finding methods to achieve a peaceful, calm dinner time. It took about 6 weeks of using the behavioral techniques, but at last, their goal was achieved.

In the morning, especially during the school year, it can be a challenge for everyone to get out the door on time. Kevin and Sherry have a very specific routine for Jack, which tends to work well most of the time. Jack gets up about 45 minutes before he must get on the bus for school. Sherry lays out his clothes the night before, and Jack is responsible for putting everything he needs for the next day in one spot by the door before he goes to bed. Kevin helps make sure he does it. Jack also takes a dose of his ADHD medication right before he gets on the bus. Kevin sets an alarm on his phone each night to remind him to help Jack take his medication before getting on the bus.

Recently, though, Sherry has noticed that Jack can't find his stuff at night and has trouble getting settled down for bed. In the mornings, he wakes up in time but loses track of what he is supposed to be doing. For instance, Sherry reminds him to brush his teeth and he goes to get the toothbrush but gets sidetracked and forgets to put the toothpaste on and goes to play with his dog. Sherry finds herself having to stay right beside Jack to keep him focused and on time. Kevin even notices Jack having a bit more difficulty in the evenings focusing on his school work. In fact, Kevin recently spent over an hour helping Jack complete an assignment that normally takes him 15 minutes. Kevin and Sherry discuss making an appointment with the nurse practitioner Jack sees at the children's hospital where they see a multidisciplinary team for ADHD.

At School

Jack is in the second grade. Generally, Jack likes school but has many challenges keeping up with school work and maintaining grade-level work. This year has already been exceptionally challenging, and they are only 6 weeks into the school year. Kevin has had to pick Jack up from school once because he became aggressive and was acting out at school, even after the counselor removed him from the classroom and worked with him. When called by

the counselor, Kevin was at a loss for what to do, so he picked Jack up from school. From that point, Jack has been having more good days than bad days behaviorally but is falling behind in his school work. He has had to stay in from recess at least once each day to complete assignments and often turns in work that is not completed. The classwork he does not get completed is sent home, and Sherry and Kevin are often spending well over an hour each night trying to help him stay focused and complete the work.

Kevin and Sherry meet with the teacher, guidance counselor, school psychologist, and principal to discuss the current issues and concerns Jack is having this year at school. Sherry always finds these meetings difficult because she really knows Jack cannot help his behavior at times and other times he can but chooses not to. This makes her feel like a bad mom at times because she cannot always "fix it" with the techniques she has been taught from the behavioral specialist and her mom instincts. At the meeting, the school staff brings up several concerns they have this year. Kevin and Sherry have had several meetings since Jack was diagnosed with ADHD, and at each meeting, Sherry has asked that concerns be categorized into behavioral concerns and academic/learning concerns. Here are the points of discussion the teacher brings to the meeting:

Academic performance:

- Jack's work is incomplete. He overlooks details when copying things from the board and makes careless mistakes on even simple assignments.
- Jack is intelligent but cannot sustain mental effort. He scores well on tests that last no more than 5 to 10 minutes but doesn't do well on longer tests.
- He forgets important instructions given by the teacher, his parents, and other authority figures at school.
- He does not concentrate in class. He often appears lost in his own little world.

Behavior:

- He is disorganized in the way he manages his belongings. He is always leaving his jacket somewhere, cannot find his books and art supplies, and forgets where he put his schoolwork.
- He cannot sit still. He often gets out of his seat and wanders around the classroom.
- Jack does not play in groups very well. He does not follow rules and often interrupts or intrudes on others while they are playing or talking.
- He talks a lot, often nonstop for several minutes at a time, and it is difficult for him to be redirected.
- Jack has difficulty waiting his turn.

After hearing the teacher discuss the list of concerns, Sherry says, "We're seeing some of these same behaviors at home, as well, and are concerned the current medication regimen may not be working for him. It's so hard for him to complete his homework—even just to read for 10 minutes a day."

"We're concerned about his safety, too," Kevin adds. "Just the other day, he just took off across a busy parking lot with no regard for vehicles coming and going."

"I know what you mean," Jack's teacher says. "Recently I had to bring him in from recess because he kept trying to jump off the top rung of the monkey bars with kids standing below. Once he did land on a kid."

Throughout the meeting, Sherry holds back tears. She feels like an incompetent mother when she hears some of the things the teacher says. Although she knows that these statements about his behavior are true and that Jack is having a hard time recently with ADHD, it is difficult to hear someone talk about her child when it is not positive. Also, Jack had been doing so well on the current medication regimen of dexmethylphenidate. At the end of the last school year, Jack was being praised for his behavior and his teacher said he was doing very well.

At the end of the meeting, Sherry says, "Kevin and I are planning to schedule an appointment with the team in the clinic at the children's hospital we have been working with. We're hoping they can help us put together a plan to address Jack's behaviors."

"I'll write up the academic and behavior challenges Jack has been having so you can take the list with you to the appointment," the counselor says.

As soon as they leave the school, Sherry calls the clinic and explains Jack's situation. Fortunately, there has been a cancellation for next week, and they are able to schedule Jack to see both the nurse practitioner and the behavioral medicine physician in back-to-back appointments.

In the Clinic

Last year, the pediatrician recommended that Jack see a behavioral medicine specialist to optimize his treatment for ADHD. Despite being prescribed dextroamphetamine/amphetamine (Adderall) by his primary pediatrician and taking it for 4 months, Jack was still having difficulty in school and at home with accomplishing necessary tasks (The Pharmacy 13.1). After a 6-month wait, they were able to see a multidisciplinary team, which includes a nurse practitioner, a behavioral medicine physician, and a clinical psychologist. The only downside is that the Wrays must travel about 2½ hours to get to the children's hospital where the multidisciplinary clinic is located. Together, the members of the multidisciplinary team provide and monitor treatment for Jack. At a previous visit, Jack was taken off the dextroamphetamine/amphetamine and placed on dexmethylphenidate. Sherry and Kevin saw much improvement in Jack after several weeks on the new medication, and, until recently, he had continued to do well on it.

The day of the appointments arrives, and both Kevin and Sherry have taken the day off work to take Jack to the clinic. Not long after Jack was diagnosed with ADHD, Kevin and Sherry agreed to attend Jack's appointments related to ADHD

The Pharmacy 13.1 ADHD Medications

Medication(s)	Classification	Route	Action	Nursing Considerations
Dextroamphetamine/amphetamine: short acting (Adderall) and long acting (Adderall XR) Dextroamphetamine: intermediate acting (Dexedrine)	Amphetamine	Oral	Stimulates the CNS	Monitor: • HR, RR, and BP before and periodically during use • Weight biweekly; report weight loss • Height; report growth inhibition Be aware of differences between the short-, intermediate-, and long-acting dosage forms
Methylphenidate: short acting (Ritalin), intermediate acting (Ritalin, Metadate ER), and long acting (Ritalin, Concerta, Metadate, Daytrana)	CNS stimulant	Oral	• Stimulates the CNS and respiration • Increases attention span in ADHD	Monitor: • HR and BP for tachycardia and hypertension • For common CNS side effects, including nervousness, insomnia, restlessness, and hyperactivity • Dietary intake and growth (height/weight), because it can cause anorexia Be aware of differences between the short-, intermediate-, and long-acting dosage forms
Dexmethylphenidate short acting (Focalin) Dexmethylphenidate long acting (Focalin XR)	CNS stimulant	Oral	• Stimulates the CNS and respiration • Increases attention span in ADHD	Monitor: • Weight biweekly and height periodically for signs of weight loss and growth suppression • HR, RR, and BP for tachycardia and tachypnea Be aware of differences between the short-, intermediate-, and long-acting dosage forms

ADHD, attention deficit hyperactivity disorder; BP, blood pressure; CNS, central nervous system; HR, heart rate; RR, respiratory rate.
Adapted from Taketomo, C. K. (2018). *Pediatric and neonatal dosage handbook* (25th ed). Hudson, OH: Lexicomp.

together so they could stay well informed regarding treatment and also to help relieve the burden of tackling this diagnosis alone. Jack's first appointment, with the nurse practitioner, is at 10:00 a.m., and then he is scheduled to see the behavioral medicine physician at noon. In addition to the list the school counselor gave her, Sherry brings with her a notebook of appointments, medications, and interventions that she has kept since Jack was diagnosed and a journal of his behaviors and triggers, which the nurse at the clinic suggested they keep. Kevin and Sherry have found journaling very helpful in communicating Jack's behavior and medication responses to his treatment team.

Karen, the nurse practitioner who sees Jack, greets him in the waiting room.

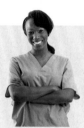

The Nurse's Point of View

Karen: I bring the family back to the examination room, along with a box of special toys for Jack. Another nurse takes Jack to weigh him and check his height, heart rate, and blood pressure while Sherry and Kevin sit down with me to open the dialogue about why they are here. The nurse takes a little extra time getting Jack back to the room by allowing him to pick a few things from the surprise box to play with during the visit. I always request that the nurse do this to give the parents a chance to communicate without Jack present. Sherry and Kevin are open with Jack, however, and usually do not have anything to say to me that they would not say in front of Jack.

The appointment goes well. I suggest increasing the dose of the dexmethylphenidate, monitoring Jack's caloric intake, and weighing him once a week at home. Jack has lost 2 lb since he saw his primary pediatrician for his yearly checkup a couple of months ago but has grown an inch. I would like to monitor his growth and, if he continues to lose weight, bring Jack back in for a change in medication or treatment plan. I believe the weight loss is the result of a combination of increased ADHD symptoms and the side effects of the medication. Kevin and Sherry agree to the plan.

During the behavioral medicine appointment, the physician listens to Sherry and Kevin's concerns regarding the increased ADHD behaviors and how they are affecting his academic performance and attention in school and at home. The psychologist is also at the appointment and, together, they teach Sherry, Kevin, and Jack some strategies and interventions to help with focus, getting things done on time, sustaining his mental effort, and staying organized in the classroom. Fortunately, there is now a satellite clinic closer to the Wrays' home, and Jack will attend therapy sessions there twice a week with Sherry and Kevin to work on these behaviors. Sherry and Kevin leave the appointments feeling reassured that Jack will improve but also recognizing that ADHD is challenging to deal with on a daily basis. They also realize it is hard for Jack and that he feels frustrated at times, as well.

Think Critically

1. Describe five behaviors a child may exhibit that lead to a diagnosis of ADHD.
2. Describe three stressors the Wray family encounters as a result of Jack being diagnosed with ADHD.
3. Why is it so important to monitor weight, height, and overall growth when a child is taking medication for ADHD?

4. Besides medication, what are two other interventions that may be helpful for a child with ADHD to improve behavior and focus?

References

American Psychiatric Association. (2013). *Diagnostic and statistical manual of mental disorders* (5th ed., pp. 59–60). Arlington, VA: Author.

Bonander, C., Beckman, L., Janson, S., & Jernbro, C. (2016). Injury risks in schoolchildren with attention-deficit/hyperactivity or autism spectrum disorder: results from two school-based health surveys of 6- to 17-year-old children in Sweden. *Journal of Safety Research, 58,* 49–56.

Dalsgaard, S., Leckman, J. F., Mortensen, P. B., Nielsen, H. S., & Simonsen, M. (2015). Effect of drugs on the risk of injuries in children with attention deficit hyperactivity disorder: A prospective cohort study. *The Lancet Psychiatry, 2*(8), 702–709.

Felt, B., Biermann, B., Christner, J., Kochhar, P., & Harrison, R. (2014). Diagnosis and management of ADHD in children. *American Family Physician, 90*(7), 456–464.

Visser, S., Danielson, M., Bitsko, R., Holbrook, J., Kogan, M., Ghandour, R., . . . Blumberg, S. (2014). Trends in the parent-report of health care provider-diagnosed and medicated attention-deficit/hyperactivity disorder: United States, 2003–2011. *Journal of the American Academy of Child & Adolescent Psychiatry, 53*(1), 34–46.

Suggested Readings

American Academy of Child and Adolescent Psychiatry. *ADHD resource center.* Retrieved from http://www.aacap.org/aacap/Families_and_Youth/Resource_Centers/ADHD_Resource_Center/Home.aspx

American Academy of Pediatrics, National Initiative for Children's Healthcare Quality. *Vanderbilt Assessment Scale (6 to 12 years of age; parent forms, teacher forms, and scoring instructions).* Retrieved from https://www.nichq.org/sites/default/files/resource-file/NICHQ_Vanderbilt_Assessment_Scales.pdf

Centers for Disease Control and Prevention. *Middle childhood (6–8-year-old).* Retrieved from https://www.cdc.gov/ncbddd/childdevelopment/positiveparenting/middle.html

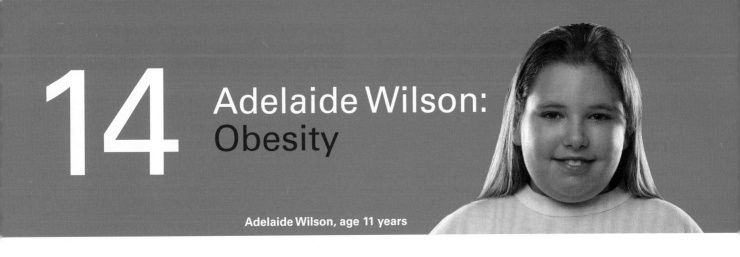

14 Adelaide Wilson: Obesity

Adelaide Wilson, age 11 years

Background

Adelaide Wilson is an 11-year-old girl of Irish descent who lives in a rural county of eastern Kentucky that is part of the cultural region known as Appalachia. Her county has been economically deprived for years owing to the failure of industries that were once a vital source of income for many of the families living in the area, including coal mining, timber, and oil. Unfortunately, owing to the economic collapse of her town, drug and alcohol use have become an epidemic (McGreal, 2015).

Adelaide resides with her mother, Nora, two older brothers, Ryan (age 13 years) and Sean (age 14 years), one younger sister, Shannon (age 9 years), and maternal grandparents. Adelaide's father has not been involved in her life for the past 2 years because of issues with drug and alcohol addiction. He lost his job 4 years ago and started using drugs and alcohol as a "way to make it through." Adelaide's mother works two part-time jobs to help support her family. Adelaide and her family live in government-subsidized housing and use government assistance for food and health care.

Adelaide is a shy girl who enjoys spending time with animals and attending church with her family. She has a dog and two cats. Sometimes, she walks to a nearby farm to help take care of the horses and goats. She has one close friend at school, Maddie, who also likes to play with animals. The other kids at school sometimes tease her for being chubby, which makes Adelaide feel sad. Adelaide often complains of having headaches and stomachaches, resulting in several unexcused absences from school. Nora is concerned about Adelaide's health and has decided to take her to the walk-in clinic at the local health department. Because Nora cannot get off work, Adelaide's grandmother, Barb, takes her to the clinic after school the next day. Her sister, Shannon, goes, as well, because no one is home to stay with her.

At the Clinic

Upon Adelaide's arrival at the clinic, the nurse, Sarah, begins the visit with a height, weight, and vital signs assessment. Adelaide is 60 in (5 ft) tall and weighs 175 lb (79.4 kg). Her vital signs are as follows:

- Temperature: 98.2°F (36.8°C)
- Heart rate: 98 beats/min (bpm)
- Respiratory rate: 16 breaths/min
- Blood pressure: 142/90 mm Hg

Sarah escorts Adelaide, Barb, and Shannon to the assessment room.

Sarah asks, "What brings you to the clinic today, Adelaide?"

Adelaide replies, "My mom wanted me to come today because I've been having a lot stomachaches and headaches and am missing a lot of school."

"Tell me a little more about the stomachaches and headaches," the nurse says.

"They usually start in the morning when I am getting ready for school," Adelaide says. "The only thing that makes them better is when I lie down or eat. They have been happening all school year."

"I'd like you to rate your pain using this tool called the visual analog scale, or VAS," Sarah says (Table 14.1; Fig. 19.1A). "Could you point to where your pain is on the scale?"

"Well, I don't really have any pain right now," Adelaide says. "But when I have a headache or stomachache, my pain is somewhere around there." She points to the middle of the VAS.

"The nurse practitioner, Jennifer, will be in soon to see you," Sarah tells Adelaide. Adelaide and Barb wait patiently for the nurse practitioner. However, Adelaide's sister, Shannon, is impatient and wants to leave. After 30 minutes of waiting in the assessment room, Shannon has annoyed Adelaide, causing her to become upset. She too wants to go home.

"Grandma, I'm tired and hungry," Adelaide says. "I'm only here because Mom made me come today."

Her grandmother tries to appease Adelaide by giving her a bag of Sour Patch Kids. As Adelaide eats her candy, Jennifer enters the room.

"Hi, I'm Jennifer, the nurse practitioner, and I will be managing your care today. I am very sorry for the long wait, but I am the only healthcare provider here today."

Jennifer begins her assessment by asking Adelaide what brought her to the clinic, and Adelaide tells her.

"They don't come to the clinic very often," Barb tells Jennifer. "However, her mom received a truancy notice from the school, so she decided to have Adelaide checked out."

Table 14.1 Common Pain Assessment Tools for Use in Early Adolescence

Visual analog scale	A self-report instrument used to measure pain intensity. The scale consists of a straight line with one end meaning "no pain" and the other end meaning "worst pain imaginable." The patient is asked to mark the point on the line that matches his or her pain (National Cancer Institute [NCI], 2016).
Numeric rating scale	A self-report instrument used to measure pain intensity. The patient is asked to rate his or her current pain on a scale from 0 to 10, with 0 meaning "no pain" and 10 meaning the "worst possible pain" (Pasero & McCaffery, 2011).
Adolescent pediatric pain tool	A self-report, multidimensional scale that evaluates the intensity, location, and quality of pain in children 8–17 y old (Jacob, Mack, Savedra, Van Cleve, & Wilkie, 2014).

Jennifer looks over Adelaide's medical record and then begins the exam.

"When do your headaches and stomachaches occur, Adelaide?" Jennifer asks.

"My stomach and head bother me most mornings before school, especially Mondays and Wednesdays."

"Tell me about your Mondays and Wednesdays," Jennifer says. "What are they like?"

"I go to school and have my normal classes, like math and science. I eat lunch, go to art, and then go to gym class."

"How do you feel about school?" Jennifer says.

"I like school okay, but I hate gym. Gym is really hard. Sometimes, the other kids laugh at me because I can't run fast and I have to stop and sit down when we play games."

Shannon interjects, "Adelaide gets made fun of because she is fat!"

"Shut up, Shannon!" Adelaide quickly responds. "You're just as bad as the kids at school!"

"That does sound hard, Adelaide," Jennifer says. "I understand how you could feel that way. Do you have any other issues or concerns, besides the headaches and stomachaches?"

"My knees hurt, and sometimes I feel like I can't catch my breath."

"Because it's been 2 years since your last visit to the clinic, I'm going to conduct a complete physical exam," Jennifer tells Adelaide (Table 14.2).

Table 14.2 Physical Examination for Preadolescents

System	Expected Findings	Adelaide's Findings
Integumentary	• Acne • Oily or dry skin	Striae distensae noted on hips and abdomen
Cardiac	• Normal S1 and S2 present • HR: 60–100 bpm	• Normal S1 and S2 present • HR: 98 bpm
Pulmonary	• No adventitious sounds • RR: 18–25 bpm • No dyspnea on exertion	• Lungs clear to auscultation • RR: 16 breaths/min
Reproductive	Tanner stages I–IV	Tanner stage II
Musculoskeletal	• No lateral curvature of spine (scoliosis screen) • Joint pain ("growing pains")	• No lateral curvature of spine • Complaint of "achy knees" with activity
Gastrointestinal	No dental caries or decay	Multiple dental caries

bpm, beats/min; HR, heart rate; RR, respiratory rate; S1, heart sound 1; S2, heart sound 2.
Adapted from American Academy of Pediatrics. (2010). *Performing preventive services: A bright futures handbook.* Retrieved from
https://brightfutures.aap.org/materials-and-tools/PerfPrevServ/Pages/default.aspx

Before Jennifer conducts the physical exam, she asks Barb about any significant family history.

Barb replies, "My husband and I both have high blood pressure and my husband has stents in his heart. Adelaide's dad has something wrong with his liver, but that is probably because he drinks a lot. Adelaide's mom suffers from depression from time to time, but who doesn't? Is that enough information?"

"Yes, thank you."

The Nurse's Point of View

Jennifer: I am sure glad her grandma brought Adelaide in today. I have several concerns about her health and well-being. I see in her medical record that her last visit was 2 years ago and that her weight at that time was only slightly above normal for her height. On the basis of her height and weight, Adelaide's **body mass index (BMI)** is 34.2, which is above the 99th percentile for girls of the same age (Growth and Development Check 14.1).

On assessment I find that she has a large, rounded, non-distended abdomen with bowel sounds active in all four quadrants. She denies pain upon palpation of the abdomen. Because Adelaide complains of headaches, I evaluate her visual acuity using the Snellen chart. Findings indicate no visual deficits. Her pupils are equal, round, reactive to light and accommodation, and her neurological exam is within defined limits. On the basis of Adelaide's age, I conduct a scoliosis screening. I note no evidence of lateral curvature of the spine or alteration in gait. However, I do notice that Adelaide has troubling reaching to her toes and complains of abdominal pressure when bending over. She shares with me that her knees "ache" when she is in gym class.

Unfortunately, Adelaide is obese and is likely to manifest additional health problems. I am fairly confident this is the reason that Adelaide has headaches and stomachaches on the days she has gym. I am sure she is self-conscious about her weight and her ability to keep up with the other kids at school. I am also concerned that Adelaide will develop additional health problems, such as type 2 diabetes mellitus, musculoskeletal issues, sleep apnea, and cardiovascular problems, such as **hypertension**, if she cannot get her BMI within a normal range. I really need to be open and honest with Adelaide and her grandma about my concerns so that we can develop a plan to help Adelaide obtain a healthy BMI. However, if I cannot get her entire family involved with the plan of care, outcomes may not be successful and Adelaide will continue to struggle emotionally and physically. On the basis of Adelaide's age, developing relationships with peers and gaining independence are so important. I really need to explore the psychosocial aspects of her development. I also fear that she may develop body image issues that will influence her normal growth and development.

Growth and Development Check 14.1

Middle Childhood

Physical

- Girls have rapid growth around age 11 ½ y
- Girls can gain nearly 10 in (25.4 cm) and 25 lb (11.3 kg) during puberty
- Boys lag behind in growth by 2 y

Social

- Grows more independent from family
- Gains a sense of responsibility
- Forms stronger, more complex relationships
- Experiences more peer pressure

Cognitive

- Has an increased attention span
- Finds academics more challenging

Emotional

- Becomes aware of body changes from puberty
- Is more likely to develop body image and eating problems

Adapted from American Academy of Pediatrics. (2018). *Physical development in girls: What to expect.* Retrieved from https://www .healthychildren.org/English/ages-stages/gradeschool/puberty/Pages/Physical-Development-Girls-What-to-Expect.aspx; Centers for Disease Control and Prevention. (2018). *Positive parenting tips: Middle childhood (9–11 years of age).* Retrieved from https://www.cdc.gov/ncbddd/ childdevelopment/positiveparenting/middle2.html

After completing the physical exam, Jennifer asks Adelaide, "What do you like to do for fun?"

Adelaide gets excited and tells Jennifer, "Me and my friend Maddie like to help take care of the animals on my neighbor's farm."

"That does sound like fun. What types of animals are on the farm?"

Adelaide responds, "Horses, pigs, and goats. The goats are always getting into trouble."

"What else do you do with your time?"

"I usually watch TV and help my grandma in the kitchen. She has been teaching me how to cook and bake."

"What foods do you like to make with your grandma?"

"Well, every Sunday after church, we have fried chicken, biscuits and gravy, macaroni and cheese, and sweet tea. I am learning how to fry the chicken so it tastes like my grandma's. We like to bake chess pie and peanut butter cookies, too. My brothers love the chess pie. My grandma also makes the best dried apple stack cake. My grandma is such a great cook!"

Barb tells Jennifer, "I love spending time with Adelaide in the kitchen. I want to share all my family recipes with her."

Jennifer responds, "It is great that you have such a good relationship; however, I am concerned about the amount of weight Adelaide has gained and its effect on her health."

Barb replies, "I would rather her have some meat on her bones than be too skinny."

Jennifer explains to Barb that Adelaide's BMI is 34.2, which is above the 99th percentile and indicates **obesity** (Box 14.1).

Jennifer explains that having a BMI in the obese range can lead to many health problems now and in the future.

"Adelaide will need some blood tests to further assess her health," Jennifer says.

Barb gets upset and states, "I brought her here because she has stomachaches and headaches and now you think she is fat and has all kinds of problems! I am going to talk to my daughter first before we do anything else."

Jennifer gives Barb information on obesity and nutrition. She includes a few free copies of *ChopChop*, a magazine of healthy recipes. Jennifer encourages Barb to schedule a follow-up appointment after she talks with her daughter. She also encourages Barb to have Adelaide's mother attend the appointment.

Box 14.1 Body Mass Index in Children and Teens

BMI for children and teens is age- and gender-specific. The BMI for age percentile growth charts are the most commonly used indicator to measure the size and growth pattern of children in the United States. Normal or healthy BMI is considered the 5th percentile to less than the 85th percentile. Obese is defined as equal to or greater than the 95th percentile.

Adapted from Centers for Disease Control and Prevention. (2015). *About child and teen BMI.* Retrieved from https://www.cdc.gov/ healthyweight/assessing/bmi/childrens_bmi/about_childrens_bmi.html

At Home

When Nora gets home from work, she asks Adelaide, "What did the doctor say about your stomachaches and headaches?"

Adelaide begins to cry and tells her mom, "The nurse said I was too heavy and I needed to have blood taken. Grandma got mad, and we left before I could have the tests done."

Nora finds her mom in the kitchen making dinner. "What happened at the appointment, Mom?" Nora asks.

"The nurse was more concerned about Adelaide's weight than her stomachaches or headaches. I don't see anything wrong with her weight. That nurse was being ridiculous. Adelaide just hasn't lost her baby fat yet." Barb hands Nora the paperwork from the appointment.

Nora reviews the paperwork and decides she should schedule a follow-up appointment for Adelaide. Nora has been concerned for a while about Adelaide's weight, but with her busy work schedule, she really has not had the time to deal with it. Besides, all of her children have some "meat on their bones," but Nora believes once they grow and get taller, they will be fine.

Follow-Up Appointment

A week later, Nora takes Adelaide back to the clinic. The nurse, Sarah, takes Adelaide's vital signs, height, and weight. Adelaide's weight remains the same and her blood pressure remains elevated at 138/88 mm Hg. Nora is shocked to see how much weight Adelaide has gained. Sarah tells Nora and Adelaide that Jennifer, the nurse practitioner from last week, will be in to see them soon.

Jennifer enters the room and says, "I'm so glad to see you back, Adelaide—and with your mom." Jennifer explains that she is concerned about Adelaide's BMI and blood pressure and recommends she have her cholesterol levels checked (Box 14.2). She explains that Adelaide has several modifiable behaviors, such as diet and activity level, that can be adjusted to manage her weight.

In addition, because Adelaide is 11 years old, she is due for some immunizations, Jennifer says (Patient Teaching 14.1). Nora anxiously agrees to the blood work and immunizations.

Box 14.2 Guidelines for Cholesterol Screening in Children

The American Academy of Pediatrics recommends universal cholesterol screening for children 9–11 y old and adolescents 17–21 y old.

Adapted from American Academy of Pediatrics. (2015a). *AAP releases summary of updated preventive health care screening and assessment schedule for children's checkups.* Retrieved from https://www.aap.org/en-us/about-the-aap/aap-press-room/Pages/AAP-Releases-Summary-of-Updated-Preventive-Health-Care-Screening-and-Assessment-Schedule-for-Children%27s-Checkups.aspx

---

Patient Teaching 14.1

Recommended Immunizations for 11- to 12-Year-Olds

- Diphtheria, tetanus, acellular pertussis (DTaP)
  - The DTaP vaccine protects against the following:
    - Diphtheria, a serious infection of the throat that can block the airway
    - Tetanus, otherwise known as lockjaw, a nerve disease
    - Pertussis, otherwise known as whooping cough, a respiratory infection that can have serious complications
- Influenza (Flu)
  - The influenza vaccine protects against the viral respiratory illness commonly known as "the flu."
- Meningococcal
  - The meningococcal vaccine protects against meningococcal disease, such as meningitis. Meningococcal disease can cause an infection of the lining of the brain, spinal cord, and blood.
  - The Centers for Disease Control and Prevention (CDC) recommends the meningococcal conjugate vaccine for children 11–12 y of age, with a booster at 16 y of age.
- Human papillomavirus (HPV)
  - The HPV vaccine protects against:
    - HPV is the genital virus contracted by skin-to-skin contact during sexual activity. There are about 40 types of HPV, some which cause cervical cancer and cancers of the anus, penis, vagina, vulva, and oropharynx. Other strains of HPV cause warts in the genital area.
  - The CDC recommends two doses of the vaccine for boys and girls 11–12 y old; the second dose is given 6–12 mo after the first dose.

Adapted from CDC (2017a). *2017 recommended immunizations for children 7–18 years old.* Retrieved from https://www.cdc.gov/vaccines/who/teens/downloads/parent-version-schedule-7-18yrs.pdf

---

"I'm not only concerned about Adelaide's physiological well-being but also about her psychological well-being," Jennifer delicately explains to Nora.

"During our last visit together, Adelaide talked with me about her headaches and stomach issues. It seems as though the pains occur on gym days. I would like Adelaide to keep a diary documenting her headaches and stomachaches over the next 2 weeks. This will help me to determine whether a pattern exists. In the meantime, I would like to discuss a plan for helping Adelaide lose some weight."

Nora replies, "I know Adelaide is heavy, but do you really think we need to make a big deal about this?"

"Obesity at her age can have significant health consequences in adulthood. It is important for Adelaide to work toward a healthy weight now."

Nora notices Adelaide is looking down at the floor and not saying anything. "Are you upset, honey?" Nora asks her.

Adelaide begins to cry. She says, "I hate being fat. I get made fun of at school and I am embarrassed when I go to gym class. I don't want to be fat, but I don't how to lose weight."

Jennifer sits beside Adelaide and places her arm on her shoulder. "You don't need to figure this out by yourself. We can make a plan together to help you lose weight and feel better. How does that sound?"

Adelaide sheepishly agrees.

Before leaving the appointment, Adelaide is given her recommended immunizations and has her blood work drawn. Nora schedules a follow-up appointment for 2 weeks.

At Home

When Nora and Adelaide return home, Barb is making supper.

"Why is Adelaide upset?" Barb asks Nora.

"She's gained a lot of weight over the past 2 years and is now considered obese," Nora tells her mom. "She had to have blood work taken and has to lose weight."

"I still think the nurse is overreacting," Barb says. She finishes making supper and then serves them fried fish sticks with macaroni and cheese.

Adelaide does not eat much. "My stomach hurts," she explains.

Adelaide talks to her friend Maddie the next day at school. She tells Maddie she went to the clinic and now she has to go on a "diet." Maddie tells Adelaide she would like to lose weight too and maybe they can do it together.

Two-Week Follow-Up Appointment

During the follow-up appointment, Jennifer reviews Adelaide's diary. It is apparent Adelaide's headaches and stomachaches correspond to gym days. Jennifer proceeds to review the laboratory work with Adelaide and Nora (Table 14.3). Her results indicate Adelaide has abnormal **high-density lipoprotein (HDL)**, **low-density lipoprotein (LDL)**, total cholesterol, and **triglycerides**.

"After reviewing your diary, Adelaide, it appears your headaches and stomachaches happen on gym days. I believe gym class causes you to feel stressed and upset and that is why your head and stomach hurt."

Jennifer also explains to Nora and Adelaide, "The laboratory work indicates that Adelaide's cholesterol and triglyceride levels are elevated. This means she will need to make changes to her diet and activity level."

Adelaide gets upset and whispers to her mom, "What does that mean?"

"Could you explain the test results to us a little more?" Nora asks Jennifer.

"**Cholesterol** is a type of fat found in your blood," Jennifer explains. "Cholesterol is helpful in the body, but too much can

Table 14.3 Adelaide's Laboratory Values

Laboratory Test	Normal Range in Ages 2–19 y (mg/dL)	Adelaide's Results (mg/dL)
Total cholesterol	<170	210
HDL	>35	35
LDL	<130	175
Triglycerides	<150	215

HDL, high-density lipoprotein; LDL, low-density lipoprotein.
Adapted from American Academy of Pediatrics. (2015). *Cholesterol levels in children and adolescents.* Retrieved from https://www.healthychildren.org/English/healthy-living/nutrition/Pages/Cholesterol-Levels-in-Children-and-Adolescents.aspx; Stanford Children's Health. (2018). *Cholesterol, LDL, HDL, and triglycerides in children and adolescents.* Retrieved from http://www.stanfordchildrens.org/en/topic/default?id=cholesterol-ldl-hdl-and-triglycerides-in-children-and-adolescents-90-P01593

cause health problems, such as damage to your heart and blood vessels. Your body makes cholesterol, and some cholesterol is found in certain foods. There are two types of cholesterol, HDL and LDL. Your HDL is the 'happy' cholesterol and your LDL is your 'lousy' cholesterol. The goal will be to increase your happy cholesterol and decrease your lousy cholesterol. We can achieve this goal by changing your diet and increasing your activity level. Your triglycerides are the most common fat in your body and store energy from your diet" (American Heart Association [AHA], 2018). "Changing your diet will also help lower your triglycerides."

"I don't know how to change my diet," Adelaide tells Jennifer, still upset, "because I eat whatever my grandma fixes for meals."

Jennifer responds, "We can start with some small changes to your diet. I will give your mom information on some better food options for you. I would also like you to pick out an activity you enjoy to increase the amount of exercise that you get each day. How does that sound?"

Adelaide begrudgingly replies, "That sounds really hard and I don't really like to exercise. I guess I can try."

"Adelaide, would you please step into the waiting room so I can talk to your mom for a minute?" Jennifer asks.

After Adelaide leaves the room, Nora begins to cry. "I feel like this is all my fault," Nora says. "I have to work two jobs and my mom does all the cooking. She is a great cook, but we do not eat very healthy. We have to eat what we get in our government boxes and what I can buy with my supplemental nutrition card. As you know, the 'healthy' foods are so expensive. I have four kids and my parents living with me, so I have to buy what will feed everyone. I know this is a problem, but what can I do?"

Jennifer puts her arm around Nora's shoulder and says, "I understand your concerns. We have many options, though, for improving Adelaide's health. Let me help you formulate a plan of care for Adelaide."

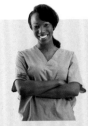

The Nurse's Point of View

Jennifer: I know Nora is trying her best given her situation. It is hard to focus on your health when you are just trying to survive. However, there are changes that are not expensive and actually not too difficult for Nora and Adelaide can make. The biggest challenge will be involving the entire family in the process. I will need to use a collaborative approach to help Adelaide manage her obesity (Priority Care Concepts 14.1). On the basis of Adelaide's age and developmental stage, it will be important to include her friends in the plan of care, as well. Because Adelaide is in Erikson's fourth developmental stage, Industry versus Inferiority, the peer group gains major significance and plays an important role in development of self-esteem (Erikson, 1963). In addition, the plan of care must include a physical therapist and registered dietician. I also need to find out what Adelaide eats at school, because that may be contributing to her weight gain. It is important for me to clearly establish a plan of care with the Wilson family to prevent the need for more complex weight management modalities, such as medication and bariatric surgery.

Priority Care Concepts 14.1

Obesity

Obesity Epidemic

Obesity affects approximately 12.7 million (17%) children and adolescents in the United States. Rates are higher for children and adolescents who receive federal assistance, such as the Special Supplemental Nutrition Program for Women, Infants, and Children or the Supplemental Nutrition Assistance Program (Centers for Disease Control and Prevention [CDC], 2017b).

Healthy People 2020 Goals

- Improve the healthy development, health, safety, and well-being of adolescents and young adults (annual yearly assessments).
- Promote health and reduce chronic disease risk through the consumption of healthful diets and achievement and maintenance of healthy body weights.

Office of Disease Prevention and Promotion, 2018. Nutrition and weight status. *HealthyPeople.gov*. Retrieved from https://www.healthy people.gov/2020/topics-objectives/topic/nutrition-and-weight-status

Goals for Adelaide

- Reduce caloric intake to reach a normal body mass index.
- Increase daily physical activity to 1 h each day.
- Encourage family involvement in healthy meal planning and exercise.

Nursing Interventions

- Monitor weight.
- Monitor blood pressure.
- Monitor laboratory values.
- Assess developmental milestones.
- Monitor growth and development.
- Teach the family how to incorporate healthy food options at mealtime.
- Make referrals as appropriate:
  - Registered dietician
  - Physical therapist

Later, when Adelaide has returned to the room, Jennifer explains that to begin Adelaide's weight loss program, they will need to meet with a registered dietician (Whose Job Is It, Anyway? 14.1). "We have one who works in several clinics in our region. Her name is Kathy, and she is great with kids. I will set up a time for you and your mom to meet with her. She will help you make better food choices so you can obtain a healthy BMI."

"I would also like to schedule a time for you to meet with a physical therapist," Jennifer continues (Whose Job Is It, Anyway? 14.2). "The physical therapist can help you develop an exercise plan so that you can lose weight and have less knee pain."

Nora comments, "Wow! This seems like a lot for Adelaide to do."

 Whose Job Is It, Anyway? 14.1

Registered Dietician

A registered dietician is an expert in food and nutrition for health promotion and disease management. Registered dieticians provide a variety of services, including meal planning with regard to budget, counseling on healthy eating habits, and evaluating effects of meal plans. Registered dietitians work in a myriad of settings, including hospitals, nursing homes, clinics, schools, cafeterias, and government institutions (Bureau of Labor Statistics [BLS], 2018).

Whose Job Is It, Anyway? 14.2

Physical Therapist

A physical therapist helps injured or ill people improve movement and manage pain. They are an important part of rehabilitation, treatment, and prevention of patients' chronic conditions. The physical therapist develops a plan of care that includes individualized exercises, stretches, hands-on therapy, and use of equipment to ease pain and improve mobility while facilitating health and wellness (BLS, 2018).

Physical therapists are trained to assist obese patients in weight management by helping them select exercises that are fun and help mitigate pain. By finding the right exercise, patients are able to better achieve their goals and make better choices (Avruskin, 2018).

Jennifer makes direct eye contact with Nora and states, "The best thing you can do to help Adelaide is to assist her with her nutrition and increase her activity level. If it will help, you can think of 'five-two-one-zero,' which stands for five fruits and vegetables a day, 2 hours or less of screen time a day, 1 hour of physical activity a day, and zero sugary drinks" (Maine Health, 2018). "The registered dietitian and physical therapist will provide the tools to assist you and Adelaide."

Nora responds, "I know that change needs to happen; I just feel overwhelmed."

"Understandably so, but you don't need to figure it out alone," Jennifer says. "We need to use other healthcare experts and connect with resources available in our community."

Nora and Adelaide agree to the plan. Jennifer tells Nora and Adelaide she will contact them when they can meet with the registered dietitian and physical therapist. Jennifer also states Adelaide will need to have laboratory work repeated in 3 months.

Meeting With the Dietician

A few weeks later, Adelaide, Nora, and Barb meet with Kathy, the registered dietician. The nurse, Sarah, sits in on the meeting with the Wilson family. Kathy begins by asking Adelaide to describe a typical breakfast, lunch, dinner, and snacks. Then Kathy provides the family with recommendations from *Bright Futures* (Patient Teaching 14.2). She also explains the importance of portion control. Kathy suggests Adelaide use the "MyPlate" method as a way to visualize proper portion control and food choices (Fig. 14.1; United States Department of Agriculture [USDA], 2017).

"What do you eat and drink while you're at school?" Kathy asks Adelaide.

Adelaide responds, "I love the school food, especially the cheese pizza and chicken patties. I also buy Mountain Dew from the machine when I have extra money."

"One simple but important change you can make to your diet is just to drink more water instead of sugary drinks," Kathy tells Adelaide. "Drinking Mountain Dew can cause cavities and

 Patient Teaching 14.2

Nutrition

General Recommendations from American Academy of Pediatrics Bright Futures Program
- Decrease daily sodium intake to <2,300 mg for healthy persons and to <1,500 mg for persons who have hypertension, diabetes, or chronic kidney disease. The 1,500 mg recommendation applies to about half of the U.S. population, including children and the majority of adults.
- Decrease daily intake of saturated fatty acids to <10% of total calories.
- Decrease daily intake of dietary cholesterol to <300 mg.
- Minimize intake of trans fatty acids, including foods that contain synthetic sources of trans fats.
- Decrease the intake of calories from solid fats and added sugars.
- Decrease the intake of foods that contain refined or milled grains, especially ones that also contain solid fats, added sugars, or sodium.
  Foods and Nutrients to Increase
- Increase vegetable and fruit intake.
- Consume a mix of vegetables, especially dark-green, red, and orange vegetables, and beans and peas.
- Eat at least half of all grains as whole grains.
- Increase consumption of fat-free or low-fat milk and milk products, such as yogurt and cheese.
- Select a mix of protein foods, which include seafood, lean meat and poultry, eggs, beans and peas, soy products, and unsalted nuts and seeds.
- Replace protein foods that are higher in solid fats with those that are lower in solid fats and calories.

Adapted from American Academy of Pediatrics. (2010). *Bright futures: Nutrition.* Retrieved from https://brightfutures.aap.org/Bright%20Futures%20Documents/BFNutrition3rdEdition_intro.pdf

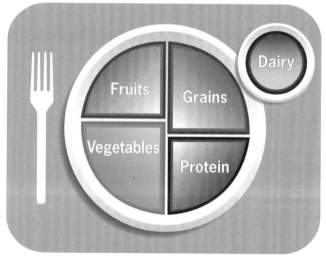

Figure 14.1. The MyPlate food portion size diagram. Reprinted from ChooseMyPlate.gov. https://www.choosemyplate.gov/

tooth decay." Turning to Nora and Barb, Kathy says, "Other changes would be to purchase whole grain bread instead of white bread and to grill or bake meats instead of frying them."

Adelaide sighs and looks discouraged.

"I know these dietary changes are difficult," Kathy says. "That's why I'm suggesting making small changes at first. You don't have to give up everything you like, but you do need to make better food choices."

Kathy also speaks to Nora and Barb about their access to healthy foods on a limited income. Kathy offers to provide Nora and Barb with examples of foods that can be purchased on a limited income. Also, she explains that, given that children consume up to half of their calories while at school (Kaiser Permanente, 2012), it is important to discuss what she eats while at school. Kathy tells them about government assistance programs and school interventions that help provide nutritious food to children, including the Supplemental Nutrition Assistance Program (SNAP) and SNAP-Ed, farm-to-school programs, self-serve salad bars, and better options for fruit and vegetables and whole grains (USDA, 2015).

At the end of their meeting, Kathy says, "I am going to send you home with some recommendations for a few basic changes that you can make over the next few months. We will follow up in 3 months to determine what type of progress you are making. I know Joe, the physical therapist, is waiting to meet with you. I will send him in."

Meeting With the Physical Therapist

Joe enters the room and greets Adelaide, her family, and the nurse, Sarah.

"Adelaide, I'm Joe. I am here to help you work on a plan to have fun while getting more physical activity."

"I don't like going to gym or exercising," Adelaide says.

Joe casually asks, "Well, what *do* you enjoy doing that's active?"

Adelaide replies, "I like to help out on my neighbor's farm. I usually go with my friend Maddie. My brothers are always playing ball in the yard and canoeing in the lake. Sometimes they let me play with them. They don't make fun of me like the kids at school."

"Working on the farm is great physical activity. How often do you go to the farm?"

Adelaide responds, "I usually go once or twice a week."

Joe states, "You need to do at least an hour of physical activity each day." Joe explains to Adelaide, Nora, and Barb that this activity should include aerobic, muscle-strengthening, and bone-strengthening activities (United States Department of Health and Human Services, 2019). "It would be great if you and Maddie could start exercising together" (Analyze the Evidence 14.1).

"I could talk to the Kramers about you spending more time on their farm," Nora says.

"That would be great," Joe says. "Also, Adelaide, is there any activity offered at your school that you might like?"

"I would really like to play softball. I play baseball with my brothers, and I can hit the ball far. But I'm embarrassed because

Analyze the Evidence 14.1

Influence of Peers on Diet and Exercise of Adolescents

A systematic review by Chung, Ersig, and McCarthy (2017) identified research studies that examined the influence of peers on diet and exercise. The review included 24 articles; 7 examined diet only, 14 examined exercise only, and 3 examined both. The results of the review indicated that the diet and exercise of adolescents were significantly associated with those of their peers. The association, however, depends on gender, type of exercise, and closeness of friends. The results of the review support the inclusion of peers in interventions that promote healthy diet and exercise.

I can't run fast. I'm not sure if I would make it to first base without being thrown out. I just don't think the other girls would want me to be on the team."

Adelaide begins to tear up. Joe leans in close to her, looks her in the eye, and says, "Adelaide, maybe you can't run fast today. Maybe you won't be able to run fast tomorrow. But if you let me help you, in time you will be able to do all the things you want to do."

During the rest of the meeting, Joe and Adelaide work together to establish activities to incorporate each day.

Sarah provides the Wilson family with a copy of the physical therapy plan. She reminds them to return in 3 months for blood work and health assessment.

Three-Month Follow-Up Appointment

Adelaide and Nora return to the clinic for a 3-month follow-up appointment. Sarah takes Adelaide's vital signs and her height and weight. Today, Adelaide's height is 60.25 in (5.02 ft) and she weighs 160 lb (72.6 kg). Her other vital signs are as follows:

- Temperature: 98.2°F (36.8°C)
- Heart rate: 88 bpm
- Respiratory rate: 18 breaths/min
- Blood pressure: 132/88 mm Hg

"Adelaide—you've lost 15 lb (6.8 kg), and your blood pressure is lower!" Sarah tells her. "That's wonderful!"

Adelaide gets a big smile on her face. "I've been working hard on the farm, and my grandma has been trying to make healthier dinners. Sometimes I have to remind her not to fry our food."

Nora interjects, "The changes have been hard, especially on my mom, but we are really trying and, believe it or not, my mom has already seen a drop in her blood pressure because of the diet changes!"

Jennifer soon enters the room and smiles when she sees Adelaide. "I can tell you've lost weight," she says. She explains that Adelaide's BMI has decreased from 34.2 to 31. Next, Jennifer reviews Adelaide's laboratory work with them (Table 14.4).

"I'm really pleased with the improvement in your laboratory tests," Jennifer says. "You've really been working hard." She gives Adelaide a hug.

"My brothers and sister have lost weight, too, because grandma is not making so many desserts," Adelaide tells Jennifer. "Now we only have chess pie on special occasions, like our birthdays."

"I'm so proud of you. You are making progress toward your goals. I would like you to keep with the plans we have established for you. How about the headaches and stomachaches?"

"I still get a headache on gym days sometimes, but I've been feeling a lot better," Adelaide shares with Jennifer.

"Jennifer, will you get a message to Joe for me?"
"Sure."

"I think I'm going to join the softball team next season. I believe I'll be ready to play by then."

Table 14.4 Adelaide's Follow-Up Laboratory Values

Laboratory Test	Normal Range in Ages 2–19 y (mg/dL)	Adelaide's Results (mg/dL)
Total cholesterol	<170	190
HDL	>35	40
LDL	<130	150
Triglycerides	<150	195

HDL, high-density lipoprotein; LDL, low-density lipoprotein.
Adapted from American Academy of Pediatrics. (2015). *Cholesterol levels in children and adolescents.* Retrieved from https://www.healthychildren.org/English/healthy-living/nutrition/Pages/Cholesterol-Levels-in-Children-and-Adolescents.aspx; Stanford Children's Health. (2018). *Cholesterol, LDL, HDL, and triglycerides in children and adolescents.* Retrieved from http://www.stanfordchildrens.org/en/topic/default?id=cholesterol-ldl-hdl-and-triglycerides-in-children-and-adolescents-90-P01593

Think Critically

1. How can the nurse and nurse practitioner help Adelaide continue to lose weight?
2. Identify other resources that should be incorporated into Adelaide's plan of care.
3. What other healthcare disciplines could be involved in the plan of care for an obese adolescent?
4. What cultural aspects should the nurse consider when developing a plan of care for Adelaide and her family?
5. What comorbid conditions are associated with obesity?
6. Discuss the impact of obesity on Adelaide's growth and development.

References

American Heart Association. (2018). *HDL (good), LDL (bad) cholesterol and triglycerides.* Retrieved from http://www.heart.org/HEARTORG/Conditions/Cholesterol/HDLLDLTriglycerides/HDL-Good-LDL-Bad-Cholesterol-and-Triglycerides_UCM_305561_Article.jsp#.WoL-GrGZNPM

Avruskin, A. (2018). *Physical therapist's guide to obesity.* Retrieved from https://www.moveforwardpt.com/SymptomsConditionsDetail.aspx?cid=df77f3aa-573b-4d1e-893b-18c88e6cedce

Bureau of Labor Statistics. (2018). *Dietitians and nutritionists.* Retrieved from https://www.bls.gov/ooh/healthcare/dietitians-and-nutritionists.htm#tab-2

Centers for Disease Control and Prevention. (2017a). *2017 recommended immunizations for children 7–18 years old.* Retrieved from https://www.cdc.gov/vaccines/who/teens/downloads/parent-version-schedule-7-18yrs.pdf

Centers for Disease Control and Prevention. (2017b). *Childhood obesity facts.* Retrieved from https://www.cdc.gov/obesity/data/childhood.html

Chung, S. J., Ersig, A. L., & McCarthy, A. M. (2017). The influence of peers on diet and exercise among adolescents: A systematic review. *Journal of Pediatric Nursing, 36,* 44–56.

Erikson, E. H. (1963). *Childhood and society.* New York, NY: W.W. Norton and Company.

Jacob, E., Mack, A. K., Savedra, M., Van Cleve, L., & Wilkie, D. J. (2014). Adolescent pediatric pain tool for multidimensional measurement of pain in children and adolescents. *Pain Management Nursing, 15*(3), 694–706.

Kaiser Permanente. (2012). *The weight of the nation.* Retrieved from https://share.kaiserpermanente.org/static/weightofthenation/docs/topics/WOTNCommActTopic_School%20Food_F.pdf

Maine Health. (2018). *Let's go.* Retrieved from https://mainehealth.org/lets-go/national-program

McGreal, C. (2015). America's poorest white town: Abandoned by coal, swallowed by drugs. *The Guardian.* Retrieved from https://www.theguardian.com/us-news/2015/nov/12/beattyville-kentucky-and-americas-poorest-towns

Medline Plus. (2018). *Cholesterol.* Retrieved from https://medlineplus.gov/cholesterol.html

Mosby's Medical Dictionary. (2008). *Human adipose tissue.* Retrieved from https://medical-dictionary.thefreedictionary.com/adipose+tissue

National Cancer Institute. (2016). *NCI dictionary of cancer terms.* Retrieved from https://www.cancer.gov/search/results

Office of Disease Prevention and Health Promotion. (2018). Nutrition and weight status. *HealthyPeople.gov.* Retrieved from https://www.healthypeople.gov/2020/topics-objectives/topic/nutrition-and-weight-status

Pasero, C., & McCaffery, M. (2011). *Pain assessment and pharmacologic management.* St. Louis, MO: Mosby.

United States Department of Agriculture. (2015). *The farm to school program 2012–2015: Four years in review.* Retrieved from https://fns-prod.azureedge.net/sites/default/files/f2s/Farm-to-School-at-USDA—4-Years-in-Review.pdf

United States Department of Agriculture. (2017). *Choose my plate.* Retrieved from https://www.choosemyplate.gov/what-healthy-eating-style

United States Department of Health and Human Services (2019). *Physical activity guidelines for Americans.* Retrieved from https://www.hhs.gov/fitness/be-active/physical-activity-guidelines-for-americans/index.html.

Wolters Kluwer Health. (2012). *Stedman's medical dictionary for the health professions and nursing.* Philadelphia, PA: Wolters Kluwer.

Suggested Readings

Centers for Disease Control and Prevention. (2016). *Childhood obesity causes and consequences.* Retrieved from https://www.cdc.gov/obesity/childhood/causes.html

Hagan, J., Shaw, J., & Duncan, P. (2017). *Bright futures: Guidelines for health supervision of infants, children and adolescents.* Elk Grove Village, IL: American Academy of Pediatrics.

Steele, R. G., Gayes, L. A., Dalton, W. I., Smith, C., Maphis, L., & Conway-Williams, E. (2016). Change in health-related quality of life in the context of pediatric obesity interventions: A meta-analytic review. *Health Psychology, 35*(10), 1097–1109.

Unit 2
Care of the Developing Child

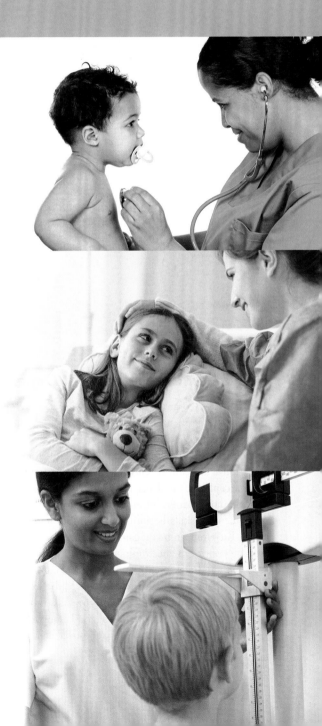

15 Care of the Newborn and Infant

Objectives

After completing this chapter, you will be able to:
1. Discuss normal growth and development in infants.
2. Describe the physical assessment of an infant.
3. Explain the development of gross and fine motor coordination and language milestones.
4. Explain the importance of nutrition in the first year of life.
5. Choose appropriate teaching topics for parents of infants.
6. Describe common developmental concerns in infants.
7. Identify common health problems in the first year of life.

Key Terms

Acrocyanosis
Cephalocaudal
Development
Fine motor
Gross motor
Growth

Meconium
Primitive reflexes
Proximodistal
Solitary play
Strabismus

Growth and Development Overview

Growth refers to an increase in size, whereas **development** denotes an attainment of different physical, psychosocial, and cognitive skills. The development of these skills takes place in a sequential order; one skill must be attained before a more complex skill is developed. Growth and development take place in both a **cephalocaudal** pattern and a **proximodistal** pattern. A cephalocaudal pattern of growth and development refers to the attainment of skills beginning at the head and moving downward. Therefore, an infant gains motor control of the head before gaining control of the trunk and legs. A proximodistal pattern of growth and development refers to the attainment of skills beginning at the trunk and moving out to the extremities. Consequently, an infant gains **gross motor** skills in the arms before gaining **fine motor** skills in the fingers. Throughout the first year of life, physical, cognitive, and psychosocial change is rapid. It is crucial for nurses to understand developmental milestones and recognize developmental red flags to promote optimum growth and development in the first year of life.

Nurses can monitor an infant's development by determining whether the infant meets milestones at appropriate ages, often simply through observation and physical assessment. Parental report is also a useful tool in determining whether an infant is meeting developmental milestones. In addition to history, observation, and assessment, different standardized developmental screening tools are available for nurses to use to gain an in-depth picture of an infant's developmental status, especially when there may be some developmental concerns. These tools include, but are not limited to, the Ages and Stages Questionnaire, the Parents' Evaluation of Developmental Status, and the Survey of Well-Being of Young Children (Hagan et al., 2017). These screening tools take anywhere from 10 to 15 minutes to administer and have strong psychometric properties, indicating high reliability.

Premature infants should be screened on the basis of their adjusted age. These infants reach typical developmental status by the time they are 2 years old.

Health Assessment

The infant stage of growth and development includes the newborn period through 12 months of age. Pediatric nurses should conduct routine health surveillance of children, including assessment of growth and development, at specified ages for well-child visits. These ages are designated by the American Academy of Pediatrics (Hagan et al., 2017) and include newborn, 1, 2, 4, 6, 9, and 12 months.

Conducting a thorough health assessment of a child in this age group requires significant involvement from the parents or caregivers. When obtaining a health history for an infant, ask the parents about prenatal care, growth and development, any recent illnesses, and social and living environments.

Involving parents or caregivers in the physical exam of an infant can also be beneficial. You may perform the physical exam on the exam table, but performing it while the infant is in the parent's lap (Fig. 15.1) calms the child, promotes a sense of safety, and often prevents crying, allowing for better inspection and auscultation. It also allows observation of the dynamics between the parent and child. Throughout the assessment, note the interaction between the parent and the infant. Do the parents respond to the infant's cues? Do the parents talk to the infant? Do they hold the infant? Do they appear interested in the infant's development? Reinforce positive parent–infant interactions and discuss any concerns.

Nurses may conduct a full head-to-toe exam on all infants at each well-child visit, depending on the setting in which the nurse is working. This requires flexibility, however, and you may not be able to conduct it literally from head to toe. For example,

if the infant is quiet, then auscultate the lungs first. In general, leave the most invasive procedures, such as looking in the mouth or ears, until the end of the physical exam. The infant needs to be undressed but can stay wrapped in a blanket, allowing you to uncover only the area you need to access at one time.

Head, Eyes, Ears, Nose, and Throat

Ask the parents or caregivers about their child's ability to see and hear. Questions to ask may include the following:

- "Do you think your baby focuses on your face when you are feeding him or her?"
- "Does your baby turn his or her head to the sound of your voice?"

If the parent answers no to either one of these questions, further investigation is warranted. Ask the parent or caregiver if the infant passed the newborn hearing screen in the hospital. If the infant did not pass the hospital hearing screen, then refer the infant for further testing.

In addition to seeing and hearing, ask the parents or caregivers about feeding. Ask questions such as the following:

- "Is the infant able to feed from the bottle or breast?"
- "Has the infant started any solid foods?"
- "Does the infant have any teeth?"

These questions help you determine the health status of the infant.

Head

Begin the assessment of the head by observing size and shape. The head is larger in proportion to the body in an infant than in an older child. Palpate the skull and neck for abnormalities such as enlarged lymph nodes. During palpation of the skull, note the anterior and posterior fontanelles (Fig. 15.2).

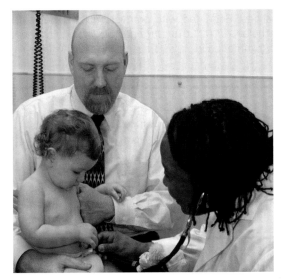

Figure 15.1. Infant assessment. Physical assessment of the infant can be completed while the infant is sitting on a parent's lap. Reprinted with permission from Jensen, S. (2015). *Nursing health assessment* (2nd ed., Fig. 8.6A). Philadelphia, PA: Wolters Kluwer.

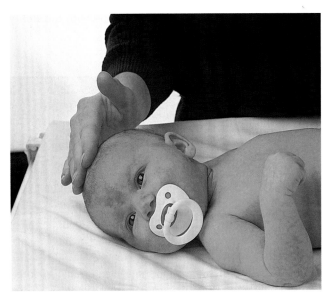

Figure 15.2. Anterior fontanelle. Palpating the anterior fontanelle. Photo by B. Proud.

The sutures of the skull are not fused at birth to allow for the rapid brain growth that occurs during the first year of life. The posterior fontanelle closes between 2 and 3 months of age. The anterior fontanelle, often called the "soft spot," closes between 12 and 18 months of age. The fontanelles should be flat and soft. Fontanelles that are bulging, sunken, or closed too early can indicate either a neurological abnormality or an alteration in fluid balance.

Eyes

The assessment of the eyes includes noting symmetry of the eyes on the face. Normal eye shape may vary, depending on the culture of the infant. **Strabismus**, or misalignment of the eyes, is common in the newborn up to 6 months of age (Burns, 2017; Fig. 15.3). Assess for a bilateral red reflex. It is difficult to assess ocular movement in a newborn. Visual fields are not tested until around 6 months of age, which is when infants begin to track objects.

Ears

Inspect the ears for symmetry and alignment. The top of the pinna of the ear should be in alignment with the outer canthus of the eye (Fig. 15.4). Inspect the ear for any drainage or redness. To inspect the tympanic membrane, pull the bottom of the pinna down and back to insert the otoscope, rather than up and back, as in an older child or adult.

Nose

The nose, as with other facial features, should be symmetrical. Some normal cultural variations include a flattened nose bridge in African American or Asian infants. Inspect the nares with either a penlight or an otoscope. To inspect the nares, gently tilt the infant's head back. The nares should be pink with no excoriation. Note any swelling of the turbinates. Nasal congestion in infants interferes with the ability to feed.

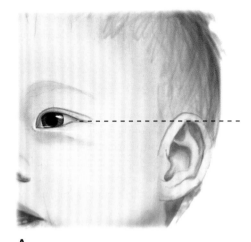

A

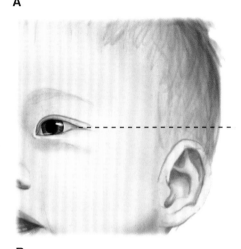

B

Figure 15.4. Infant ears. A. The top of the pinna should align along an imaginary line with the outer canthus of the eye. **B.** A pinna that sits below the imaginary line between the outer canthus of the eye could indicate chromosomal abnormalities. Reprinted with permission from Hatfield, N. T., & Kincheloe, C. A. (2018). *Introductory maternity & pediatric nursing* (4th ed., Fig. 13.7). Philadelphia, PA: Wolters Kluwer.

In Chapter 1, Chip Jones developed nasal congestion and had trouble breastfeeding. Why would a 4-month-old infant have difficulty breastfeeding with nasal congestion? What did the nurse at the pediatrician's office instruct Chip's mother, Diane, to do to assure adequate intake during his respiratory illness? How did Diane help to alleviate Chip's congestion before nursing him?

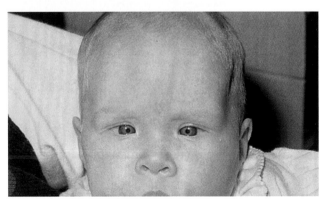

Figure 15.3. Strabismus. Strabismus in an infant. Reprinted with permission from Silbert-Flagg, J., & Pillitteri, A. (2018). *Maternal & child health nursing* (8th ed., Fig. 50.5). Philadelphia, PA: Wolters Kluwer.

Mouth and Throat

The lips should be symmetrical and free of lesions. The lips and oral mucosa should be pink and moist. An infant's tongue is large for the size of the mouth. The tongue extrusion reflex is present until about 6 months of age. This reflex causes the infant to push out any food placed on the tongue. The tonsils are not visible in infancy. The throat should appear pink and moist and without obstruction. With a gloved hand, palpate the hard palate. The palate should be solid, with no palpable opening.

Infants are typically born without teeth. Most infants have their first tooth eruption from 4 to 6 months of age. Teeth that are close to eruption can be felt and often seen. Palpate the gums to determine whether any teeth are close to eruption.

Neurological Assessment

During the first year of life, the neurological system changes rapidly. Assessment of the neurological system includes determining whether infants are achieving developmental milestones at expected ages, which often requires asking parents and caregivers about behaviors they have observed in the infant. Myelination of the nerves and spinal cord accounts for the rapid development in motor milestones and, throughout the first 2 years of life, allows for involuntary movements to come under voluntary control.

In addition, assessing to confirm that **primitive reflexes** disappear when expected is part of the neurological assessment in the first year. Primitive reflexes are those infants are born with and that disappear over the first year of the infant's life. The exception is the Babinski reflex, which is normally present until the age of 2 years. The primitive reflexes include the sucking, Moro (startle), stepping, palmar grasp, plantar grasp, and tonic neck reflexes (Table 15.1).

Table 15.1 Primitive Reflexes

Reflex	Photo	Description
Rooting		• **How to elicit:** Stroke the corner of the infant's mouth • **Infant's positive response:** Turns the head toward the stroking • **Purpose:** Allows the infant to find the breast or bottle • **Age it normally disappears:** Around 4 mo (AAP, 2009c)
Sucking		• **How to elicit:** Touch the roof of the infant's mouth • **Infant's positive response:** Initiates a sucking motion • **Purpose:** Allows for feeding • **Age it normally disappears:** Around 4 mo
Moro (startle)		• **How to elicit:** Startle the infant • **Infant's positive response:** Throws the head back and extends arms and legs • **Purpose:** Primitive fight-or-flight response • **Age it normally disappears:** Around 2 mo (AAP, 2009c)

(continued)

Table 15.1 Primitive Reflexes (*continued*)

Reflex	Photo	Description
Stepping	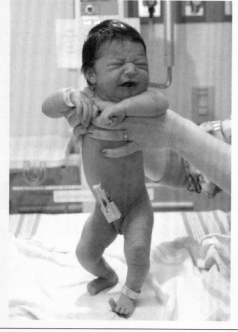	• **How to elicit:** Hold the infant upright on a flat surface • **Infant's positive response:** Makes a stepping motion • **Purpose:** Prepares the infant for walking • **Age it normally disappears:** Around 2 mo (AAP, 2009c)
Tonic neck (fencer)	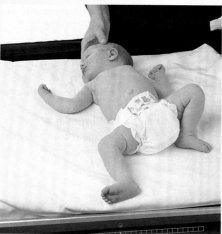	• **How to elicit:** Turn the infant's head to one side • **Infant's positive response:** Extends the extremities on the same side and flexes those on the opposite side • **Purpose:** Helps the infant transition from lying on the floor to crawling • **Age it normally disappears:** 5–7 mo
Palmar grasp	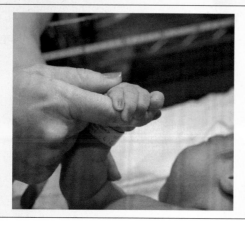	• **How to elicit:** Place an object in the infant's palm • **Infant's positive response:** Automatically grasps the object • **Purpose:** Prepares the infant for voluntarily grasping objects • **Age it normally disappears:** 5–6 mo (AAP, 2009c)

Table 15.1 Primitive Reflexes (*continued*)

Reflex	Photo	Description
Plantar grasp		• **How to elicit:** Stroke the bottom of the infant's foot • **Infant's positive response:** Flexes the toes • **Purpose:** Protects the sole of the foot • **Age it normally disappears:** 9–12 mo
Babinski		• **How to elicit:** Stroke the sole of the infant's foot from heel to toe • **Infant's positive response:** Extends the toes • **Purpose:** Protects the sole of the foot • **Age it normally disappears:** 2 years, although it may disappear as early as 12 mo

Images reprinted with permission from: Rooting and plantar grasp—Bickley, L. S. (2017). *Bates' guide to physical examination and history taking* (12th ed., first figure on p. 850 and Fig. 18.41). Philadelphia, PA: Wolters Kluwer. Sucking, Moro (startle), stepping, tonic neck (fencer), and palmar grasp—Reprinted with permission from Hatfield, N. T., & Kincheloe, C. A. (2018). *Introductory maternity & pediatric nursing* (4th ed., Fig. 13.10A–E). Philadelphia, PA: Wolters Kluwer. Babinski—Reprinted with permission from Kyle, T., & Carman, S. (2017). *Essentials of pediatric nursing* (3rd ed., p. 68, Table 3.1). Philadelphia, PA: Wolters Kluwer.

In addition to assessing reflexes, assess for attentiveness to visual and auditory stimuli. Elicit information from caregivers to determine whether further assessment is needed by asking questions such as, "Does your child turn to voices?"

Throughout the first year, the neurological assessment also includes evaluation of the infant's muscle tone, strength, and symmetry of movements. Assess for head lag by pulling the infant up to a sitting position. Head lag should be absent by 4 months of age. Figure 15.5 shows the progression of head control. Any head lag that persists beyond 4 months of age indicates tonal abnormality and could be related to a neurological deficit (Pineda et al., 2016).

Respiratory Assessment

The infant's respiratory system matures throughout the first year of life. The infant's lungs differ anatomically and physiologically from those of an adult. The infant's airways are smaller, the lungs have fewer alveoli, and the chest wall is more compliant. These anatomical differences account for the fact that infants are at risk for respiratory distress even with mild respiratory illnesses. Physiological differences in the infant, such as a poor hypoxic drive and decreased surface area for gas exchange, further increase the risk of respiratory distress (see Let's Compare 1.1).

Begin the respiratory assessment by asking the parents or caregivers whether they have any concerns regarding the infant's breathing. Inspect the thorax, assessing for symmetry with respiration. The infant normally appears barrel-chested, with a ratio of anteroposterior diameter to transverse diameter of 1:1. Infants are diaphragmatic breathers; therefore, their abdomens rise and fall with respiration. The respiratory rate is irregular and may have occasional pauses of a few seconds. Observe a respiratory rate for a full minute. The respiratory rate in infants ranges from 30 to 53 breaths/min. Observe for signs of respiratory distress such as retractions or nasal flaring.

Auscultate the lungs while the infant is quiet. If the infant is upset, the parents or caregivers may hold the infant to calm him or her down. Assess lung sounds with the diaphragm in all lung fields both anteriorly and posteriorly. Lung sounds should be clear and audible in all lung fields. Listen for adventitious lung sounds such as wheezing and crackles. If adventitious lung sounds are heard, further investigation is necessary. Note any

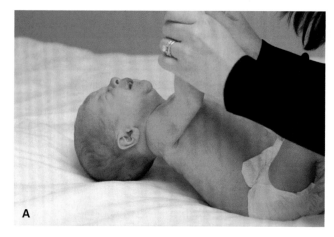

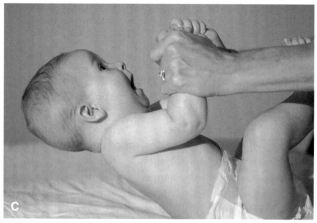

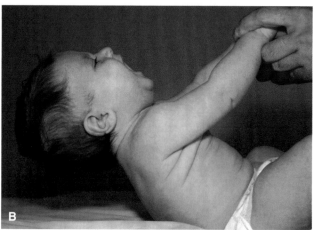

Figure 15.5. **Progression of head control in an infant. A.** Significant head lag. **B.** Improved head control. **C.** No head lag at 4 months of age. Reprinted with permission from Chow, J., Ateah, C. A., Scott, S. D., Ricci, S. S., & Kyle, T. (2012). *Canadian maternity and pediatric nursing* (1st ed., Fig. 25.4). Philadelphia, PA: Wolters Kluwer Health/Lippincott Williams & Wilkins.

adventitious sounds audible without a stethoscope, such as grunting. In addition to adventitious lung sounds, listen for nasal congestion. If adventitious lung sounds are heard in all lung fields, compare those sounds with the infant's nasotracheal sounds. The infant's lung walls are thin, and nasotracheal sounds can be transmitted throughout the lungs.

Think about Chip Jones from Chapter 1. Why did he experience respiratory distress with his illness? What signs and symptoms did he exhibit in his focused respiratory assessment? Why was the nurse practitioner, Laura, concerned about her findings on Chip's respiratory assessment?

Cardiovascular Assessment

While performing the cardiac assessment, ask the parents or caregivers whether the infant ever turns blue when crying, tires easily while feeding, or becomes diaphoretic while feeding. All of these can indicate congenital heart defects, which may or may not have been diagnosed at birth.

Throughout the assessment, observe the infant's color. The infant should be pink and warm. **Acrocyanosis** (Fig. 15.6), a condition of bluish hands and feet, may be present in newborns and can be a normal finding due to vasomotor instability (Cincinnati Children's Hospital Medical Center, 2015).

Assess the infant's pulses. In the infant, the point of maximal impulse (PMI) is in the fourth intercostal space and slightly right of the midclavicular line, as opposed to the fifth intercostal space, midclavicular line in older children and adults (Fig. 15.7). The heart rate in this age group is often irregular; therefore, assess the apical pulse (Fig. 15.8A) for one full minute to determine the heart rate. An infant's pulse can range from 80 to 160 beats/min. Also assess the brachial pulse (Fig. 15.8B) and femoral pulse (Fig. 15.8C). The brachial and femoral pulse rates should match the apical pulse rate. Abnormalities are often present in infants with congenital heart defects. In addition to the pulses, palpate the capillary refill time in both the fingers and toes. Compare the upper extremities with the lower extremities. The

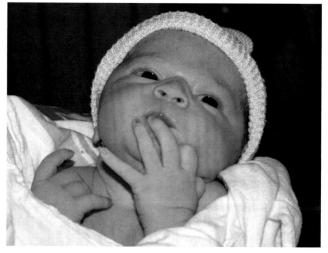

Figure 15.6. **Acrocyanosis.** Blue hands, indicating acrocyanosis. Reprinted with permission from Kyle, T., & Carman, S. (2017). *Essentials of pediatric nursing* (3rd ed., Fig. 3.3). Philadelphia, PA: Wolters Kluwer.

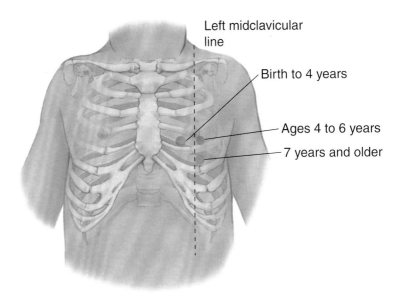

Figure 15.7. Point of maximal impulse (PMI).
Different locations of the PMI depending on age.
Reprinted with permission from Kyle, T., & Carman,
S. (2017). *Essentials of pediatric nursing* (3rd ed.,
Fig. 10.29). Philadelphia, PA: Wolters Kluwer.

capillary refill times in the upper and lower extremities should be equal and less than 3 seconds.

In the outpatient setting, blood pressure is not routinely assessed until the child is 3 years old (Hagan et al., 2017). If the infant has an underlying cardiac defect, however, assess blood pressure at routine visits during the first year of life. Systolic pressure ranges from 72 to 104 mm Hg and diastolic from 37 to 56 mm Hg in the first year.

When auscultating the heart, listen for murmurs and extra heart sounds. In addition to S1 and S2, S3 may be audible at the PMI and is often normal in infants (Bernstein, 2016). If you hear a murmur, listen for it in multiple positions. Place the infant supine, upright, left-side lying, and right-side lying. Note the location, associated body position, and intensity of the murmur. The intensity of murmurs is graded 1 to 6. A grade 1, the murmur is only slightly

audible with a stethoscope. A grade 6, it is audible with the diaphragm of the stethoscope held slightly away from the chest (Table 15.2; American Heart Association [AHA], 2015). Murmurs are often present and normal in asymptomatic infants. However, murmurs can also indicate congenital heart disease, especially at grade 3 or higher (Frank & Jacobe, 2011).

Think back to Caleb Yoder's history in Chapter 7. The nurse midwife auscultated a heart murmur shortly after birth. What additional information do you want to know? What should the nurse document? How did the nurse midwife determine that the murmur needed further investigation?

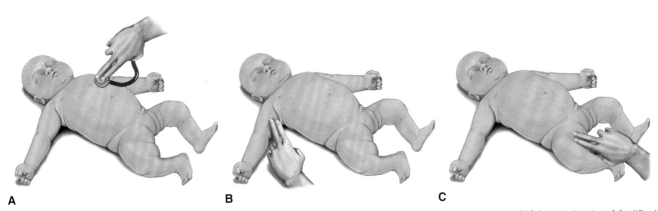

Figure 15.8. Techniques for assessing pulses in an infant. (A) Apical pulse, **(B)** brachial pulse, and **(C)** femoral pulse. Modified with permission from Kyle, T., & Carman, S. (2017). *Essentials of pediatric nursing* (3rd ed., Fig. 10.30). Philadelphia, PA: Wolters Kluwer.

Table 15.2 Classification of Murmurs

Grade	Description
1	Barely audible
2	Faint, but easily heard with a stethoscope
3	Moderately loud
4	Heard over a wide area; no palpable thrill
5	Loud, with a precordial thrill
6	Audible with the diaphragm of the stethoscope held slightly off the chest

Data from Frank, J.E., & Jacobe, K.M. (2011). Evaluation and management of heart murmurs in children. *American Family Physician, 84(7)*, 793–800.

Gastrointestinal Assessment

As part of the gastrointestinal assessment, ask the parents or caregivers about stool patterns. To understand the stool patterns, also enquire about what the infant is eating. Stool patterns and consistency change throughout the first year of life. The newborn's first stool, called **meconium**, is thick and green (Fig. 15.9). Infants who are breastfed generally have stools that are thinner in consistency and appear to be seedy and yellow. Infants who are bottle-fed have stools that are pastier in consistency and darker. Newborns and young infants may have up to 10 stools per day. As the infant gets older, stools become less frequent. It is not uncommon for infants to go several days without having a bowel movement. In addition, the color of the stool varies with the infant's diet.

Parents often worry that their infants are constipated if the infants do not have a bowel movement every day or appear to strain with bowel movements. Explain that it is normal for infants to appear to have difficulty with bowel movements because the gastrointestinal system is still immature (Patient Teaching 15.1). Teach parents that the consistency of the stool is what is important, not the frequency. Small, hard stools are of concern, whereas soft, although infrequent, stools are not.

The abdominal assessment is included as part of the gastrointestinal assessment. Inspect the abdomen, including the umbilicus. If the cord is present, there should be no redness or drainage. Note any umbilical or inguinal hernias. On palpation, the abdomen should be soft. The lower liver border is often felt in infants up to 2 to 3 cm below the costal margin. Bowel sounds should be audible in all four quadrants.

Genitourinary Assessment

At birth, the infant's total body water is 75% of the body weight; it decreases to 60% by the end of the first year of life Greenbaum, 2016). Premature infants have an even greater percentage of water per total body weight. In addition, the glomerular filtration rate (GFR) is lower in infants, which decreases the infant's ability to concentrate urine. Both the increased body weight and decreased GFR place the infant at greater risk for fluid imbalances.

To determine whether the infant is at further risk for fluid imbalances, ask the parents or caregivers whether the infant has a history of any genitourinary anomalies. Also ask about the number of wet diapers the infant has in a day, the color of the urine, the presence of any bad odors, and whether the infant cries when urinating.

As part of the genitourinary assessment in male infants, inspect the penis. Note whether the penis is circumcised.

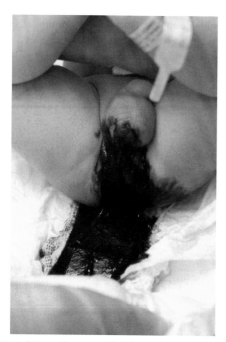

Figure 15.9. Meconium stool. Meconium stool is thick and green. Reprinted with permission from Ricci, S. S., Kyle, T., & Carman, S. (2017). *Maternity and pediatric nursing* (3rd ed., Fig. 25.2). Philadelphia, PA: Wolters Kluwer.

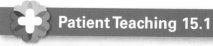

Patient Teaching 15.1

Abnormal Stools

Teach the parent the differences between normal and abnormal stools. If the infant is having infrequent stools, such as every third day, yet the stools are soft and either pasty brown or seedy yellow, there is no cause for concern. Instruct the parent to call the healthcare provider if stools are hard, red, mucousy, frothy, or extremely foul smelling.

If it is circumcised, assess for redness, swelling, or exudate. If it is not circumcised, you should be able to retract the foreskin over the glans and return the foreskin without difficulty. Note the location of the meatus, which should be directly at the tip of the glans. Also palpate for the position of the testicles.

For the female genitourinary assessment, inspect the labia. The labia may be swollen in the first few weeks of life due to maternal hormones. Inspect the vaginal and meatal openings. Note any abnormal findings such as labial adhesions.

Musculoskeletal Assessment

Ossification of bones occurs throughout childhood and until puberty. Because ossification is not complete, infants' bones are softer and made up of more cartilage than are those of older children and adults. The softer bones do not allow for infants to support their own weight. As ossification occurs, the infant develops and is able to meet gross motor milestones such as sitting, crawling, and walking.

During the musculoskeletal assessment, ask the parents or caregivers whether the infant is moving all four extremities equally. Also ask about any history of birth trauma, breech presentation, or congenital defects.

Assess range of motion in all four extremities. Assess the position of the feet. It can be normal for an infant to have metatarsus adductus from positioning in utero, a condition in which the foot is adducted but can be gently stretched into a normal position. In infants younger than 3 months old, assess for developmental dysplasia of the hip by performing Barlow and Ortolani maneuvers (see figures in Box 27.1). In infants 3 months of age or older, assess for hip dysplasia by examining for leg-length discrepancy, thigh-fold discrepancy, and appropriate abduction (Hagan et al., 2017).

Assess for muscular development by assessing for attainment of gross motor milestones at appropriate ages.

Integumentary Assessment

You may assess the skin throughout the entire time of the physical exam. The infant's skin should be pink. Look for signs of jaundice, such as a yellow undertone to the skin or yellowing of the sclera. Acrocyanosis may be present in the newborn. A newborn's skin may also appear mottled because of the instability of circulation at the surface of the skin (Fig. 15.10). Infants may have fine hair, called lanugo, on their face and torso. Lanugo is more common in premature infants and should disappear within the first few weeks of life.

Inspect the skin for normal variations and birthmarks. Normal variations include darker areolas in dark-skinned infants. Common birthmarks include salmon patches, strawberry hemangiomas, café-au-lait spots, and Mongolian spots (Table 15.3). Also inspect for abnormal findings in the infant, such as rashes, excoriation, cuts, and bruises. If any of these lesions are present, enquire as to what might be the

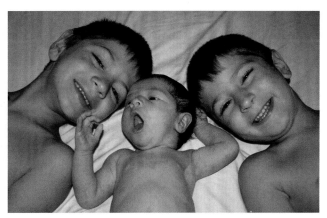

Figure 15.10. Mottling. Note the irregularity in color of the infant's skin. Reprinted with permission from Kyle, T., & Carman, S. (2017). *Essentials of pediatric nursing* (3rd ed., Fig. 3.3). Philadelphia, PA: Wolters Kluwer.

cause. If the parent's or caregiver's explanation for the abnormal findings does not seem plausible, suspect abuse and investigate further.

Palpate the skin with the back of the hand. The infant's skin should be warm and dry. It can be normal for an infant's skin to peel in the first few weeks of life. Peeling skin is more common in infants born post-term.

Immunological Assessment

For the first 3 to 6 months of life, infants rely on passive immunity received through the placenta. Maternal immunoglobulin G is passed to the fetus and protects the infant against infection early in life (Stoll & Shane, 2016). With exposure to pathogens and immunizations, the infant's active immune system becomes more developed (Analyze the Evidence 15.1).

To assess immune status, ask the parents about recurrent infections. Recurrent respiratory or candidal infections in infancy may indicate a weakened immune system. Assess the infant's immunization status.

Hematological Assessment

Infants are born with a high level of fetal hemoglobin (HgbF). HgbF constitutes 70% of the total hemoglobin when the infant is born (Christensen & Ohls, 2016). The production of HgbF decreases rapidly after birth and is replaced by the production of adult hemoglobin (HgbA). By 6 to 12 months of age, a normal pattern of HgbA is present.

In addition, fetal red blood cells are present at birth. Hematocrit levels at birth are higher than at any other time but fall quickly after birth (Christensen & Ohls, 2016). Fetal red blood cells have a lifespan of less than 120 days, precipitating the decrease in hematocrit. The decreased hematocrit may result in physiological anemia until HgbA is produced.

Table 15.3 Common Birthmarks

Birthmark	Photo	Description
Salmon patch		• A pink or light red area anywhere on the skin but most commonly seen on the back of the neck or the forehead • Commonly referred to as a "stork bite" or "angel's kiss" • Disappears as the infant gets older
Strawberry hemangioma		• A collection of widened blood vessels causing a raised red mark • Can appear anywhere on the skin • Typically disappears by 6 years of age without any treatment
Café-au-lait spot		• An area of skin with darker pigmentation • May become darker as the infant grows older • Usually not a concern
Mongolian spot		• Also known as congenital dermal melanocytosis • Bluish discoloration on the sacral area • More common in infants with darker skin, such as African American and Asian infants • Disappears over time

Images reprinted with permission from: Salmon patch, café-au-lait spot, and Mongolian spot—Bickley, L. S. (2017). *Bates' guide to physical examination and history taking* (12th ed., second figure on p. 820 and other unnumbered images). Philadelphia, PA: Wolters Kluwer. Strawberry hemangioma—Bowden, V. R., & Greenberg, C. S. (2014). *Children and their families* (3rd ed., Fig. 25.3). Philadelphia, PA: Wolters Kluwer Health/Lippincott Williams & Wilkins.

Analyze the Evidence 15.1   Maternal Immunizations

Eberhart et al. (2016) recently conducted a study to determine the optimal timing of maternal vaccination with the pertussis vaccine. The researchers considered the antibody levels present in newborns whose mothers were vaccinated after gestational week 13. After analyzing data from 335 women and their newborns, the researchers determined that the infants with the highest levels of antibodies for pertussis were born to mothers who had been vaccinated early in the second trimester of pregnancy. Therefore, the researchers concluded that the optimal timing for maternal vaccination with the pertussis vaccine is early in the second trimester of pregnancy.

During the physical exam, ask the parents or caregivers about any unusual bleeding or bruising. Assess for exposure to lead by asking about the age of housing and surrounding neighborhood conditions. Assess the infant for pallor, ecchymosis, and petechiae, all of which can indicate problems with platelets and red blood cell production.

Pain Assessment

Pain assessment in the infant requires an understanding of the infant's response to pain. The infant is unable to verbalize pain, and therefore it is important to assess changes in behavior and consolability. Use a developmentally appropriate pain scale to assess infant pain. The Neonatal Infant Pain Scale (NIPS) and the Face, Legs, Activity, Cry, and Consolability (FLACC) scale (see How Much Does It Hurt? 15.1) are two validated pain scales routinely used with infants.

NIPS is recommended for children younger than 1 year of age and is based on six domains. These domains are facial expression, cry, breathing pattern, arms, legs, and state of arousal. All of the domains are scored on a range of 0 to 1 based on the nurse's assessment, with the exception of cry, which is scored from 0 to 2. Presumed pain increases with a higher score (Lawrence, Alcock, McGrath, MacMurray, & Dulberg, 1993).

The FLACC scale was originally developed to assess postoperative pain in infants (Merkel, Voepel-Lewis, Shayevitz, & Malviya, 1997). However, the scale has recently been recommended for assessing procedural pain in infants (Shen et al., 2017). Using this scale, the nurse assesses infant expression, leg movement, activity, presence and quality of cry, and the ease of consolability. Each domain is scored from 0 to 2. A higher score indicates a higher level of pain experienced by the infant.

In addition to using validated pain scales, ask the parents or caregivers about the infant's pain level. Parents notice subtle changes in the infant that the nurse may not be aware of. During painful procedures such as heel sticks or immunizations, encourage nonpharmacological pain management such as swaddling and massage (Analyze the Evidence 15.2).

Physical Growth

Infants should have their weight, length, and head circumference measured at regular intervals to determine whether they are growing adequately. Nurses should understand the correct procedures for accurate measurements. Document the measurements appropriately and note any deviations in the growth pattern.

Weight

Infants lose up to 10% of their body weight in the first week of life. The weight is generally regained by the end of the second week. Average infant weight gain is 20 to 30 g/d for the first 1 to 3 months (Keane, 2016). On average, an infant's weight doubles by the age of 4 to 6 months and triples by the age of 12 months.

How Much Does It Hurt? 15.1

FLACC Scale

The FLACC scale is a behavioral scale for measuring the intensity of pain in young children from 2 months to 7 years old. The FLACC scale contains five indicators: face, legs, activity, cry, and consolability. Each item is ranked on a 3-point scale (0 to 2) for severity, with 0 representing no pain and 2 representing severe pain. A total score can range from 0 to 10.

| Categories | Scoring | | |
	0	1	2
Face	No particular expression or smile	Occasional grimace or frown, withdrawn, uninterested	Frequent or constant frown, quivering chin, clenched jaw
Legs	Normal position or relaxed	Uneasy, restless, tense	Kicking or legs drawn up
Activity	Lying quietly, normal position, moves easily	Squirming, shifting back and forth, tense	Arched, rigid, or jerking
Cry	No cry, awake or asleep	Moans or whimpers, occasional complaint	Crying steadily, screams or sobs, frequent complaints
Consolability	Content, relaxed	Reassured by occasional hugging, touching, or being talked to; distractible	Difficult to console or comfort

Adapted with permission from Merkel, S., Voepel-Lewis, T., Shayevitz, J. R., & Malviya, S. (1997). The FLACC: A behavioral scale for scoring postoperative pain in young children. *Pediatric Nurse 23*(3), 293–297.

Analyze the Evidence 15.2 | **Massage and Breastfeeding for Pain Relief**

A clinical trial of 75 infants was conducted to determine whether massage or breastfeeding during venipuncture had an effect on infant pain. The infants were randomized to three groups. The control group received no intervention before venipuncture. In another group, the infants breastfed before venipuncture. Venipuncture was done 2 minutes after breastfeeding. In the final group, the infants received a massage before venipuncture. Venipuncture was done 2 minutes after the massage. Using the NIPS 30 seconds after venipuncture, the researchers found that the lowest mean pain score was in the group of infants that experienced massage before venipuncture.

Data from Zargham-Boroujeni, A., Elsagh, A., Mohammadizadeh, M. (2017). The effects of massage and breastfeeding on response to venipuncture pain among hospitalized neonates. *Iranian Journal of Nursing and Midwifery Research, 22*(4), 308–312.

Weigh the infant with the infant naked and either lying or sitting on an infant scale. Plot the weight on the appropriate growth chart. There are separate growth charts for males and females (see https://www.cdc.gov/growthcharts). The infant's weight should generally fall in the same percentile throughout infancy. Note any drastic changes such as weight loss or weight gain.

In Chapter 8, Andrew Hocktochee was diagnosed with failure to thrive at 6 months old. Why was Mary, the nurse practitioner, concerned about Andrew's weight? What were some of the factors contributing to the diagnosis of failure to thrive? What are some other concerns with failure to thrive besides low weight? How did the home health nurse determine that Andrew's condition was improving?

Height

Length is most accurately measured with two people (Keane, 2016). The infant's length can be obtained using a measuring board or by making marks on the exam table paper. With the infant supine, straighten the infant's legs. Note the measurement on the board (Fig. 15.11). If no measurement board is available, mark the position of the head and the position of the heel and use a tape measure to measure the distance between the marks to determine the length. Plot the measurement on the appropriate growth chart. On average, infants grow 1.5 to 2.5 cm for the first 6 months of life and then 1 cm from 6 to 12 months of age. Generally, an infant's length increases by 50% in the first year (Feigelman, 2016).

Head Circumference

Head circumference is measured around the largest part of the skull. Place the tape measure at the forehead, around the occiput, and back to the forehead (Fig. 15.12). Record the measurement on the appropriate growth chart. Head

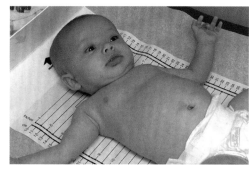

Figure 15.11. Measuring board. A measuring board is an accurate way to measure an infant's length. Reprinted with permission from Bickley, L. S. (2017). *Bates' guide to physical examination and history taking* (12th ed., Fig. 18.15). Philadelphia, PA: Wolters Kluwer.

circumference increases rapidly in the first 6 months of life and then slowly from 6 to 12 months of age. By 12 months of age, the head circumference has generally increased by 10 cm (Feigelman, 2016).

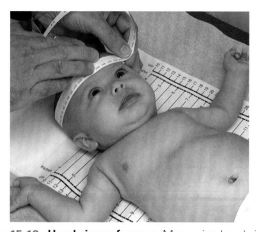

Figure 15.12. Head circumference. Measuring head circumference from the forehead around the occiput. Reprinted with permission from Bickley, L. S. (2017). *Bates' guide to physical examination and history taking* (12th ed., Fig. 18.16). Philadelphia, PA: Wolters Kluwer.

Developmental Theories

Theories of development are based in the psychoanalytic, cognitive, and moral domains. Psychosocial theories focus on behavior changes and ego development throughout the lifespan. Cognitive theories focus on the construction of knowledge. Moral theories are concerned with the development of moral perspectives through adulthood. Table 15.4 gives an overview of selected developmental theories.

Psychosocial

The establishment of trust is an important tenant of infant development. Through having needs met such as feeding, comforting, and diaper changing, infants learn to establish social trust (Erikson, 1963). Gradually, infants learn established patterns and become comfortable when parents or caregivers are out of sight for short periods of time. As the infant grows older, trust is further established through regular play and interaction (Hagan et al., 2017). If the infant's needs are not consistently met by parents or caregivers, then the infant develops mistrust, which has implications for problems in later developmental stages (Erikson, 1963).

Cognitive

According to Piaget (1930), the infant constructs reality through senses and motor skills. This stage is called the sensorimotor stage. In this stage, infants manipulate objects and begin to learn the idea of cause and effect. For example, an infant learns that shaking a rattle makes noise. Therefore, the infant begins to shake all objects to determine whether the object makes a noise. The infant learns which objects make noise and which ones do not and does not play with the silent toys.

During the sensorimotor stage, infants develop the concept of object permanence. This concept is fully developed by 8 months of age. With the development of object permanence, infants come to understand that just because an object cannot be seen does not mean the object is gone. At this stage, if the parent or caregiver hides a toy behind a table, the infant will try to find the toy. The development of object permanence also allows the infant to enjoy games such as "peek-a-boo" (Feigelman, 2016). By the end of the first year of life, infants also understand a sense of self, separate from parents and caregivers (Feigelman, 2016).

Motor Development

The acquisition of gross and fine motor skills is greater in infancy than in any other developmental stage. Assessment of motor development includes asking questions of the parents and caregivers, because the nurse is often not able to observe all of the gross and fine motor milestones the infant has reached. Parental report is acceptable to determine whether the infant is developmentally on target.

Gross Motor

Gross motor development occurs in a cephalocaudal manner. Infants gain control of their upper body before gaining control of muscles in the lower extremities. Attainment of gross motor skills occurs in a progressive manner. Each skill is developed sequentially. Therefore, sitting is not achieved until the infant has mastered rolling over. Table 15.5 describes the major gross motor development milestones of the first 12 months of life.

Fine Motor

Fine motor development occurs in a proximodistal manner, in which the infant develops skills from the center of the body (proximal) outward (distal). For example, an infant first picks up finger foods with the whole hand. As fine motor skills develop, the infant picks up finger foods using only the thumb and forefinger. By 12 months of age, the infant should be feeding him- or herself as well as holding and drinking from a cup (Hagan et al., 2017). Table 15.6 highlights some of the fine motor skills developed in the first year.

Communication and Language Development

Infants develop expressive and receptive communication skills throughout the first year of life. From the newborn period forward, infants are developing receptive language. Infants learn the meaning of different pitches in the voices they hear. Infants respond to an angry tone by crying. A soothing tone calms the infant because it is comforting (AAP, 2009a).

In early infancy, 0 to 3 months of age, the main method of expressive communication includes various intonations of

Table 15.4	Overview of Developmental Theories in Infancy		
Theorist	**Domain**	**Stage**	**Implications**
Erickson	Psychosocial	Trust vs. mistrust	Infants learn to rely on caregivers; their basic needs are met.
Piaget	Cognitive	Sensorimotor	Infants learn about the world around them through sensations.
Freud	Psychosexual	Oral motor	The infant is focused on oral sensations for pleasure, such as sucking and feeding.

Table 15.5   Gross Motor Development Milestones in Infancy

Age	Photo	Gross Motor Milestone
1 mo	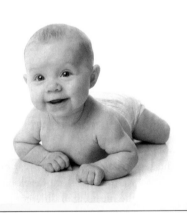	• Moves arms and legs together • Holds the chin up when lying on the stomach
2 mo		• Lifts the head and chest when lying on the stomach • Keeps the head steady when in a sitting position
4 mo		• Supports self on elbows and wrists when lying on the stomach • Rolls from the stomach to the back
6 mo	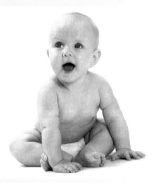	• Rolls from the back to the stomach • Sits in the tripod position • Sits briefly without support

Table 15.5 Gross Motor Development Milestones in Infancy (*continued*)

Age	Photo	Gross Motor Milestone
9 mo		• Sits well without support • Pulls to stand • Is able to go from a lying position to a sitting position • Crawls on hands and knees
12 mo		• Stands independently • May take first steps

Adapted from Hagan, J.F., Shaw, J.S., & Duncan, P. (Eds.). (2017). *Bright futures: Guidelines for health supervision of infants, children, and adolescents* (4th ed.). Elk Grove Village, IL: American Academy of Pediatrics; and Centers for Disease Control. (2017). *Learn the signs. Act early. Developmental milestones.* Retrieved from https://www.cdc.gov/ncbddd/actearly/milestones/index.html

Table 15.6 Fine Motor Development Milestones in Infancy

Age	Photo	Fine Motor Milestone
1 mo		• Opens fingers slightly at rest

(*continued*)

Table 15.6 Fine Motor Development Milestones in Infancy (*continued*)

Age	Photo	Fine Motor Milestone
2 mo	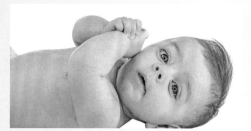	• Brings hands together • Opens and closes hands
4 mo	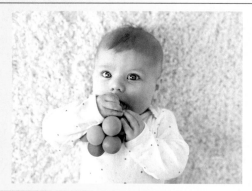	• Keeps hands relaxed • Grasps objects • Brings hands to the mouth
6 mo	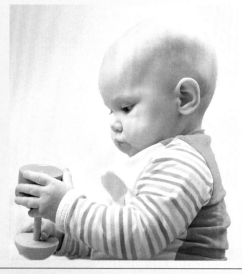	• Transfers objects from one hand to the other • Uses a raking grasp • Bangs objects on surfaces
9 mo	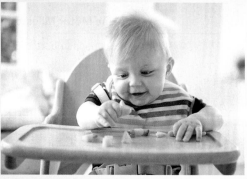	• Feeds self • Picks up small objects with three fingers and a thumb • Lets go of objects on purpose • Bangs objects together

Table 15.6 Fine Motor Development Milestones in Infancy *(continued)*

Age	Photo	Fine Motor Milestone
12 mo		• Uses a forefinger and a thumb to pick up small objects • Feeds self with a cup and spoon • Holds crayon with the whole hand

Adapted from Hagan, J. F., Shaw, J. S., & Duncan, P. (Eds.). (2017). *Bright futures: Guidelines for health supervision of infants, children, and adolescents* (4th ed.). Elk Grove Village, IL: American Academy of Pediatrics; and Centers for Disease Control. (2017). *Learn the signs. Act early. Developmental milestones.* Retrieved from https://www.cdc.gov/ncbddd/actearly/milestones/index.html

Growth and Development Check 15.1

Delayed Verbal Skills

If an infant is not imitating sounds or babbling by 7 mo old, the infant has a delay in language development and further investigation is warranted. Problems with hearing are often the cause of speech delay. Infants who have had recurrent ear infections often have speech delay due to fluid in the middle ear (AAP, 2009b).

crying. However, even as early as 2 months of age, infants begin to make a cooing sound. As infants begin to respond to parents' voices with sounds of their own, the relationship between parent and child changes, becoming more interactive (Growth and Development Check 15.1). Talking and reading to infants encourages language development and facilitates healthy interaction between parents and infants (Murray & Egan, 2014).

Infants who are born into bilingual families are often brought up learning the languages spoken in the home. However, not all infants brought up in a bilingual home end up learning both languages equally. The language best learned is influenced by the language spoken in the home and the characteristics of the child (Gathercole, 2014). Although infants may intermix words as they are learning to speak, the language development milestones are the same no matter the language (AAP, 2017a). Table 15.7 lists the major language development milestones in the first year.

Sensory Development

At birth, the infant's hearing is fully developed. Vision, taste, and touch continue to develop throughout the first year.

Vision

The infant's eyes are immature, resulting in 20/400 vision (Olitsky et al., 2016). Infants prefer to look at faces and recognize parents' and caregivers' faces early. Infants cannot see in full color until around

Table 15.7 Language Development Milestones in Infancy

Age	Language Milestone
1 mo	• Has different types of cries for hunger, discomfort, sleepiness
2 mo	• Coos • Makes gurgling noises
4 mo	• Turns to voices • Makes extended cooing sounds
6 mo	• Babbles by stringing vowels together • Begins to make consonant sounds • Has sounds for joy and displeasure
9 mo	• Copies sounds • Says "mama" and "dada" nonspecifically • Looks around when someone says, "Where's your toy?" • Understands "no"
12 mo	• Uses "mama" and "dada" specifically • Says one word other than "mama" and "dada" • Follows one-step directions • Uses simple gestures

Adapted from Hagan, J. F., Shaw, J. S., & Duncan, P. (Eds.). (2017). *Bright futures: Guidelines for health supervision of infants, children, and adolescents* (4th ed.). Elk Grove Village, IL: American Academy of Pediatrics; and Centers for Disease Control. (2017). *Learn the signs. Act early. Developmental milestones.* Retrieved from https://www.cdc.gov/ncbddd/actearly/milestones/index.html

7 months of age. Young infants, especially those 0 to 3 months of age, prefer black and white patterns. Until about 3 months of age, infants do not have full coordination of eye movement (Olitsky et al., 2016). Consequently, infants can appear cross-eyed.

Hearing

Newborns have hearing equal to that of an adult. From birth, infants are sensitive to the different vocal nuances present in any language (Langus & Nespor, 2013). Infants prefer voices of people, especially the high-pitched voices of women, rather than other sounds (AAP, 2009a). An infant who does not turn his or her head to sound should be evaluated.

Taste

Taste buds form during fetal development. Infants prefer sweet tastes over sour ones. If an infant has been breastfed, he or she will prefer breast milk over formula because of the sweet nature of the breast milk.

Touch

Touch is an important sense for parent–infant bonding (Carlo, 2016). Infants prefer soft, gentle touch. Cuddling, rocking, and swaddling are all forms of touch that can soothe and calm an infant. Rough sensations may elicit crying due to discomfort.

Social and Emotional Development

In the beginning, the infant spends most of the time sleeping. As the infant gets older, he or she becomes more social and interacts with parents and caregivers. Infants begin to mimic faces of caregivers and respond to singing and games such as "pat-a-cake." Social development of the infant depends on interactions between the infant and parents as well as other family members. Infants of mothers with postpartum depression often do not meet the appropriate social and emotional development milestones (Feigelman, 2016). An infant who is delayed in meeting these milestones warrants further assessment of the social situation at home (Growth and Development Check 15.2). Table 15.8 summarizes the pertinent social and emotional development milestones of infancy.

Growth and Development Check 15.2

Developmental Red Flags

If an infant is not reaching his or her development milestones, further investigation is needed into the reason. Is there a physical or medical reason the infant is delayed? Is there a social reason the infant is delayed? These are instances in which the nurse can play a major role in helping the parents foster appropriate growth and development in the infant through education and appropriate referrals.

Table 15.8   Social and Emotional Development Milestones in Infancy

Age	Social/Emotional Milestone
1 mo	• Looks at parent • Calms down when picked up or spoken to
2 mo	• Has a social smile • Has sounds that differentiate between happy and upset
4 mo	• Laughs out loud • Copies some facial expressions
6 mo	• Looks at self in a mirror • Knows familiar faces • Notices strangers
9 mo	• Plays games such as "peek-a-boo" and "pat-a-cake" • Has a favorite toy • Waves bye-bye • May be afraid of strangers
12 mo	• Imitates parents and caregivers • Cries when parents leave • Can put arms up to help with dressing

Adapted from Hagan, J. F., Shaw, J. S., & Duncan, P. (Eds.). (2017). *Bright futures: Guidelines for health supervision of infants, children, and adolescents* (4th ed.). Elk Grove Village, IL: American Academy of Pediatrics; and Centers for Disease Control. (2017). *Learn the signs. Act early. Developmental milestones.* Retrieved from https://www.cdc.gov/ncbddd/actearly/milestones/index.html

Think about Andrew Hocktochee from Chapter 8. He was mildly delayed in his gross motor development. What were some of the causes of the delay? How might the diagnosis of failure to thrive affect achievement of developmental milestones?

Stranger Anxiety

Around 8 months of age, infants begin to be wary of strangers. An infant may look from the stranger to the parent and become clingy with the parent. An infant who previously seemed easygoing may begin to cry when approached by a stranger (Feigelman, 2016). Reassure parents that this is a normal stage of development, and instruct them to have strangers approach the child slowly and calmly. Even with this approach, the infant may still cling to the parent.

Temperament

Temperament is an innate way of responding to the environment. Infant temperament is divided into three different types: easy, difficult, and slow to warm up. Understanding the infant's temperament allows the parents to predict how the infant will respond to certain situations. By understanding the infant's response, parents can tailor strategies to mitigate negative responses from the infant (Center for Child Development, 2015).

Easy

An infant with an easy temperament quickly establishes regular routines. The infant is generally happy and adapts easily to new situations.

Difficult

Infants with difficult personalities often require high levels of activity to keep calm. These infants are happiest in fast-moving infant swings or when being constantly walked around. Fussiness and crying are common in infants with a difficult temperament. Infants with this type of temperament have a hard time establishing routines and find it difficult to adapt to new situations.

Slow to Warm Up

Infants who are slow to warm up tend to be fussier than infants with an easy temperament but less fussy than infants with a difficult temperament. These infants have an initial negative reaction to new situations but adapt over time.

Health Promotion

Nurses play an important role in the health promotion of infants. Health promotion includes assessing the infant's environment and the parent's or caregiver's willingness to learn. Parental teaching is a large part of health promotion during the first year of life. Nurses are in a position to assist parents in giving their infant a healthy start in life. Anticipatory guidance is the portion of health promotion in which the nurse informs the parents of what their infant will be doing in the future. Anticipatory guidance includes information about growth and development, healthy sleep, safety concerns, immunizations, oral health, and nutrition, as well as common developmental concerns.

Promoting Healthy Growth and Development

Promoting healthy growth and development includes more than regular well-child visits (Priority Care Concepts 15.1). Seek to understand the infant's home environment. Questions to consider include the following:

- Is the infant living with family members who smoke?
- Is there mold in the home?
- Is the family housing secure and food secure?

Social and environmental factors can either positively or negatively affect an infant's growth and development. Nurses are in a position to refer families to appropriate resources when needed.

Priority Care Concepts 15.1

Promoting Healthy Growth and Development

Promoting optimum growth and development includes more than ensuring that infants meet the developmental milestones at the appropriate age. Nurses must consider the entire family to determine appropriate interventions to promote healthy growth and development. Cultural considerations, parental perspective, and social environment all play a role in the infant's health.

Social Determinants of Health

- Risks: Determine what risks are present in the home or family that could impede healthy growth and development, such as the following:
  - Tobacco exposure
  - Food insecurity
  - Housing insecurity
  - Parental substance abuse
- Protective factors: Determine what positive factors are present in the home or family that could promote healthy growth and development, such as the following:
  - Support networks
  - Positive family relationships
  - Adequate child care

Infant Behavior and Development

- Parent–infant relationships
  - Positive vs. negative interaction
  - Presence of maternal depression
- Daily routines
  - Feeding routines
  - Sleeping routines

Safety

- Home environment
- Parental knowledge

In addition to understanding the social and home environment, assess the parent's level of understanding regarding raising a child. Questions to consider are as follows:

- Is this the first child in the family?
- Does the family have support from other family members such as grandparents?

New parents of a firstborn child are often more nervous and lack knowledge about normal infant growth and development. Take every opportunity to reassure parents and provide them with appropriate education.

Safety

Providing teaching on safety in relation to an infant's developmental ability is essential for parents (Patient Teaching 15.2). Infants can wiggle off of elevated surfaces even if they are not

Patient Teaching 15.2

Safety Concerns in Infancy

Falls
- Never leave an infant alone on an elevated surface.
- Make sure infants are buckled in swings and bouncy seats.
- Once an infant is mobile, use safety gates at the top and bottom of stairs.
- Do not allow infants to use a baby walker.

Suffocation/Strangulation
- Make sure the infant's bed is free of any loose items.
- Keep the crib away from pull cords on curtains and blinds.
- Crib slats must be not more than 2⅜ in (6 cm) apart.
- Keep plastic bags away from infants.

Electrocution
- Mobile infants may stick objects in outlets.
- Cover electrical outlets.
- Keep infants away from electrical cords.

Choking
- Keep small objects away from infants.
- Make sure floors are clean once an infant is mobile.
- Cut food into small pieces.
- Foods with high choking risks:
  - Carrots
  - Popcorn
  - Hard candy
  - Grapes
  - Marshmallows
  - Hot dogs

Burns
- Do not carry hot liquids while carrying an infant.
- Make sure the hot water heater is set to no higher than 120°F (48.8°C; AAP, 2012).
- Never leave hot beverages on coffee tables

Poisoning
- Keep all cleaning products out of reach or in a locked cabinet.
- Keep all medications out of reach.
- Keep houseplants out of reach.
- Have the poison control number readily available.

Drowning
- Never leave an infant unattended in the bath.
- Do not leave any standing water such as in a bucket.

Motor Vehicle Safety
- Never leave an infant alone in a car for any amount of time.
- Infants up to 12 mo old *and* 20 lb should ride in a rear-facing car seat with a 5-point harness (AAP Committee on Injury, Violence, and Poison Prevention, 2011).
- Do not place an infant in a front seat with an airbag.

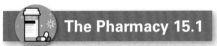

The Pharmacy 15.1

Medication Administration in Infants

Incorrect medication administration is a safety concern for infants. Over 7,000 children visit the emergency room every year because of incorrect medication administration and medication side effects (AAP, 2015). Safeguards to prevent medication errors and parental education can help mitigate this problem. Keep in mind and communicate to parents the following medication guidelines:

- Talk with the healthcare provider before administering medications to infants.
- Ensure that the medication is safe for infants.
- Use the infant's most current weight to determine the correct dose.
- Most medications are given in milligram per kilogram.
- Double-check that the medication is correct before administering it.
- Measure out the dose exactly using a medication syringe or dropper.
- Give medications at prescribed times.
- Place liquid medication in the side of the infant's mouth.
- Topical medications are quickly absorbed into the infant's skin, so use them sparingly.

rolling over yet. As infants become more mobile, falls become an even greater risk. Cabinets, cords, electrical outlets, and many other household items become safety hazards as infants grow and attain gross motor, fine motor, and cognitive skills. Teaching parents about hazards in the home, in the car, and around water, in addition to the importance of safe medication administration, is paramount to keep infants safe during the first year of life (The Pharmacy 15.1).

Oral Health

Oral health is crucial to the overall health of infants and thus should be considered in health promotion and disease prevention. There are large disparities in oral health among low-income ethnic groups and those living in medically underserved areas (Fischer, O'Hayre, Kusiak, Somerman, & Hill, 2017). Therefore, nurses should assess the sociodemographic status of families to determine risk of dental caries and other oral health problems.

Teeth erupt at different ages during the first year of life. Generally, the first tooth erupts around 4 months of age. From the time the first tooth erupts, infants are at risk for dental caries and tooth decay (Hagan et al., 2017). To promote healthy teeth and gums, parents should avoid giving infants any refined sugars. They should hold infants during feedings and not use something to prop up a bottle so that the infant can feed unattended. Parents or caregivers should not be put infants to bed with a bottle, because this contributes to dental caries.

Teach parents before tooth eruption to use a soft washcloth to wipe an infant's gums and after tooth eruption to use a very small amount of fluoridated toothpaste either with an infant toothbrush or with a washcloth to brush the infant's teeth twice a day. For families who do not have fluoridated water, infants should begin fluoride supplementation when 6 months old (Hagan et al, 2017).

Play

Play during infancy consists mostly of interacting with parents, family members, and other caregivers. Playtime consists of reading, singing, and playing with age-appropriate toys. Infants do not interact with other infants when playing with toys. This type of play is called **solitary play**. Appropriate toys for young infants include toys that can be batted with the hands and kicked with the feet, unbreakable mirrors, and toys with contrasting patterns. For older infants, toys that can be manipulated to make noise or light up, soft dolls, teething toys, board books, and large stackable blocks promote the development of both fine and gross motor skills.

Sleep

Around 3,500 infants die from sleep-related causes each year, including sudden infant death syndrome (SIDS) (AAP, 2016). Safe sleep habits can help prevent these unnecessary deaths (Patient Teaching 15.3; Fig. 15.13). Room sharing is recommended during the infant's first 6 months of life (Hagan et al., 2017). Infants should sleep in their own bed in the same room as the parents. Sleeping in the same bed increases the risk of sudden unexpected infant death (SUID) through suffocation.

Risk factors for SIDS and SUID include the following:

- Low-birthweight infant
- Maternal smoking
- Exposure to secondhand smoke
- Prone sleeping position
- Sleeping on soft surfaces
- Loose bedding
- Co-sleeping

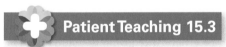

Patient Teaching 15.3

SIDS Prevention

Teaching parents and caregivers how to prevent SIDS and SUID is an important part of health promotion. SIDS and SUID prevention includes (AAP Task Force on Sudden Infant Death Syndrome, 2016) the following:

- Provide skin-to-skin care immediately after birth for 1 h.
- Place the infant on his or her back to sleep (Fig. 15.13).
- Use a tightly fitted crib sheet.
- Keep the crib bare, with no blankets, pillows, or bumper pads.
- Share your room, but not your bed, with your infant until the infant is 6 mo of age.
- Avoid exposing the infant to secondhand smoke.
- Offer a pacifier to the infant at naptime and nighttime.

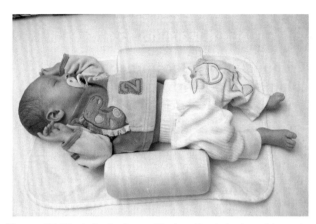

Figure 15.13. Infant sleep. Placing the infant on his or her back to sleep helps prevent SIDS. Reprinted with permission from Jensen, S. (2019). *Nursing health assessment* (3rd ed., Fig. 26.1). Philadelphia, PA: Wolters Kluwer.

Provide education to parents and other caregivers on safe sleep and SIDS prevention.

Healthy sleep is an important part of growth and development of infants. A consistent, predictable, and quiet place for sleep is important to establishing healthy sleep routines. A newborn sleeps around 16 hours a day, with nighttime sleep and daytime sleep evenly spaced through a 24-hour period. By 6 months of age, most infants sleep a 6- to 8-hour stretch at night with two naps during the day, for a total of 14 to 16 hours of sleep in a 24-hour period. By the end of the first year of life, infants sleep 10 to 12 hours at night with two naps during the day (Feigelman, 2016).

Discipline

During infancy, discipline involves teaching rather than punishment. Parents' understanding of infant behavior influences their reaction to the infant. Infant behavior is based on meeting needs, such as hunger and sleep. As infants grow and become more mobile, they become curious, which can place them in unsafe situations. At this time, infants should be redirected to safer places with safe toys. Distraction is appropriate discipline during the first year of life.

Immunizations

Immunizations protect against a variety of communicable diseases and are an important component of health promotion and disease prevention. Encourage routine immunizations at all well-child visits (Patient Teaching 15.4). In addition, assess parental knowledge, barriers to immunizations, and cultural and religious beliefs regarding immunizations.

Types of Vaccines

There are several different types of vaccines (Table 15.9).

Nursing Considerations

Nurses routinely give immunizations at well-child visits. The most up-to-date immunization chart is available at https://www.cdc.gov/vaccines/schedules/hcp/child-adolescent.html.

Patient Teaching 15.4

Immunizations Recommended for Infants, Along With Their Side Effects and Adverse Reactions

Immunizations

The immunizations that your baby will get during his or her first 12 mo are as follows:

- Diphtheria, tetanus, and acellular pertussis (DTaP)
  - The DTaP vaccine protects against:
    - Diphtheria, a serious infection of the throat that can block the airway
    - Tetanus, otherwise known as lockjaw, a nerve disease
    - Pertussis, otherwise known as whooping cough, a respiratory infection that can have serious complications
- *H. influenzae* type b (Hib)
  - The Hib vaccine protects against a type of bacteria that causes meningitis, mostly in children under the age of 5 y.
- Hepatitis B vaccine
  - The hepatitis B vaccine protects against the hepatitis B virus, which can cause chronic liver infection or liver failure.
- Pneumococcal conjugate vaccine (PCV13)
  - The pneumococcal conjugate vaccine (PCV13) protects against 13 types of pneumococcal bacteria, which can cause pneumonia, meningitis, and certain types of blood infections.
- Inactivated polio virus (IPV)
  - The inactivated polio virus (IPV) vaccine protects against polio, which can cause paralysis and death.
- Rotavirus (RV)
  - The rotavirus (RV) vaccine protects against a virus that causes severe diarrhea in infants and that can lead to dehydration and even hospitalization.
- Influenza
  - Protects against the influenza virus
  - Helps keep your child from spreading the flu virus
  - Cannot be given to a child under 6 mo of age

Common Side Effects

After your baby gets immunizations, he or she may exhibit one or more of the following:

- A fever of up to around 102°F (38.8°C)
- Redness or a small amount of swelling at the injection site
- Increased fussiness in the 24 h after immunizations
- Increased sleep in the 24 h after immunizations

When to Call the Healthcare Provider

- If your child has a fever of 105°F (40.5°C) or higher
- If your child has a seizure
- If your child has uncontrollable crying for 3 h or longer

Adapted from the Centers for Disease Control and Prevention. (2017). *Diseases and the vaccines that prevent them.* Retrieved from http://www.cdc.gov/vaccines/hcp/conversations/prevent-diseases/provider-resources-factsheets-infants.html

Table 15.9 Types of Vaccines

Type of Vaccine	Description
Live attenuated	• A weakened version of a virus • The immune system forms antibodies to the virus that is injected. • Examples: measles, mumps, rubella, and varicella (chickenpox)
Inactivated	• The virus is killed during the process of making the vaccine, but the vaccine is still capable of producing an immune response. • Example: inactivated polio vaccine
Toxoid	• Protects against bacteria that cause toxins • A weakened form of the toxin that does not produce illness but elicits an immune response • Example: diphtheria, tetanus, and acellular pertussis
Conjugate	• Protects against bacteria with a polysaccharide coating by allowing the immune system to recognize the bacteria and react • Example: *Haemophilus influenzae* type B

Adapted from Centers for Disease Control and Prevention. (2013). *Understanding how vaccines work.* Retrieved from: https://www.cdc.gov/vaccines/hcp/conversations/downloads/vacsafe-understand-bw-office.pdf

Discuss with the parents any side effects that are expected from the immunizations as well as any side effects for which the parent should call a healthcare provider. Provide vaccine information sheets to the parents and caregivers before administering immunizations. Ask the parents whether they have any questions. Parents must sign a consent form before any immunizations can be given. After giving the immunization, document the site, route, size of needle used, vaccine lot number, and expiration date.

Barriers

Assess any barriers to immunization. Common barriers include lack of transportation and financial concerns. Nurses are positioned to refer families to resources that can help them overcome these barriers. The Affordable Care Act ensures that vaccines are given free of cost as a measure to increase the vaccination rates in the United States. Another common barrier is concern regarding safety of the vaccines. Education is the best way to overcome these barriers. There is no evidence to support any claims that vaccines have detrimental effects such as autism. Providing education and encouraging parents, without judgment, to vaccinate their children can help prevent outbreaks of communicable disease.

Reporting Adverse Events

Nurses should understand the Vaccine Adverse Event Reporting System (VAERS). The Centers for Disease Control and Prevention closely monitors any concerns about adverse events through reports to VAERS (CDC, 2013). Adverse events reported after vaccination do not indicate that the immunization caused the adverse events but warrant further investigation. Examples of adverse events include seizures, fever not reduced with antipyretics, and uncontrollable crying for more than 3 hours.

Nutrition

Proper nutrition during infancy is necessary to promote physical growth, cognitive growth, and attainment of developmental milestones (Priority Care Concepts 15.2). In the first 6 weeks of life infants eat, sleep, and grow. Although growth is rapid throughout the first year of life, the greatest period of growth is in the first 6 months (Hagan et al., 2017).

This period of rapid growth requires a high intake of calories. Fat calories should not be restricted during the first 2 years of life, because fat is needed for the development of the nervous system (Hardy & Kleinman, 1994). Human milk and formula are both approximately 20 kcal/oz and have a fat content high enough to meet the infant's needs for the first 6 months. Caloric requirements in infants up to 6 months of age range from 110 to 120 kcal/kg/d. From 6 months to 1 year of age, the caloric requirements range from 95 to 100 kcal/kg/d (Consolini, 2017).

Breastfeeding

Breastfeeding not only provides optimal nutrition but promotes maternal–infant bonding, as well. The AAP (2017) recommends exclusive breastfeeding for the first 6 months and breastfeeding in addition to solid foods for the first year of life. Exclusively breastfed infants need vitamin D supplementation beginning at 2 months of age (AAP, 2017b). The World Health Organization (2017) recommends breastfeeding for the first 2 years of life and beyond. Benefits of breastfeeding include the following:

- Provides ideal nutrition for the infant
- Protects against certain infections
- Promotes healthy development of the neurological system
- May decrease the incidence of atopic diseases
- Facilitates an earlier return to prepregnancy weight for the mother
- Lowers the risk of maternal chronic disease
- Is free

Breastfeeding is not always easy and can be stressful for some women. Ensure that infants are latching on properly. The infant should have a large amount of the areola in his or her mouth and swallowing should be audible (Fig. 15.14). Refer to a lactation consultant as needed. Most women who breastfeed feed on demand rather than on a set schedule.

Ensuring that a breastfeeding infant is consuming enough milk is critical. Initially infants breastfeed every 2 to 3 hours or 8 to 12 times in a 24-hour period. As infants grow, they begin

Priority Care Concepts 15.2

Infant Nutrition

Feeding choices and guidance

- Breastfeeding vs. bottle-feeding
- Appropriate amount of intake
- Nonjudgmental guidance regarding feeding
- Assessment of cultural variation and perceptions

Hunger cues

- Rooting
- Moving hands to the mouth
- Sucking
- Crying
- Opening the mouth

Satiety cues

- Stopping sucking
- Pulling off the breast
- Pushing away
- Closing the mouth

Starting solid foods

- Infant readiness
- Parental understanding
- Education about food allergies

Starting table foods

- Knowledge of choking hazards
- Self-feeding

Weaning from the breast or bottle

- Infant readiness
- Parental readiness
- Transition to a cup

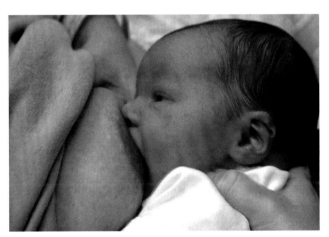

Figure 15.14. Breastfeeding technique. In proper breastfeeding technique, the infant should have most of the areola in his or her mouth. Reprinted with permission from Carter, P. J. (2016). *Lippincott textbook for nursing assistants* (4th ed., Fig. 44.6). Philadelphia, PA: Wolters Kluwer.

Analyze the Evidence 15.3   Breastfeeding in African American Women

African American women have lower rates of breastfeeding than do their Caucasian counterparts. Obeng, Emetu, and Curtis (2015) conducted a study regarding African American women's perceptions about and experiences with breastfeeding. The researchers found that although the women in the study understood the health benefits of breast milk, lack of information and lack of support from family and friends were the biggest barriers to the initiation of breastfeeding.

The researchers concluded that education of African American women's family support and community support circles is a primary intervention that may increase the likeliness to breastfeed.

to nurse for longer periods of time and less often. Weigh infants on a regular basis to determine whether their weight gain is adequate. Infants should have six to eight wet diapers per day.

Women may choose not to breastfeed, a decision that is often made in the prenatal period (Hagan et al., 2017). Educate women about the benefits of breastfeeding in a nonjudgmental manner. Assess barriers to breastfeeding and determine whether intervention is possible to promote breastfeeding (Analyze the Evidence 15.3). Barriers to breastfeeding include the following:

- Knowledge deficit
- Lack of family support
- Going back to work
- Lack of adequate private areas to pump while at work
- Inadequate break time to pump at work

Education regarding the benefits of breastfeeding goes beyond the family. Employers should understand that breastfeeding potentially reduces healthcare costs. Allowing women to pump while at work can reduce days missed because breastfeeding reduces the number of childhood illnesses.

Formula Feeding

Parents who choose to use formula should feed their infants iron-fortified formula. Newborns typically take 2 oz of formula every 2 to 3 hours. A newborn in the 50th percentile for weight consumes 16 to 24 oz of formula in a 24-hour period (Hagan et al, 2017). As infants begin to sleep for longer periods, their feeding patterns change, and they consume more formula at each feeding and feed fewer times during the day. At 4 months of age, infants need 26 to 36 oz of formula in a 24-hour period. By 1 year of age, infants consume about 30 oz/d, divided into four feedings.

Instruct parents on formula preparation according to directions. Parents may choose to use either tap water or bottled water for mixing formula. Instruct them to not heat formula in the microwave but rather to place the bottle in a pan of hot water on the stove. Teach parents to test the temperature of the formula before feeding the infant to prevent burns.

Starting Solid Foods

The AAP Committee on Nutrition recommends starting solid, or complementary, foods around 6 months of age (Hagan et al.,

2017). Cues that infants are developmentally ready for solid foods include the disappearance of the tongue extrusion reflex, increased formula intake or breastfeeding frequency, and the ability to sit in a high chair with good head control. Instruct parents to start with iron-fortified cereals mixed with either human milk or formula. Once the infant is comfortable eating from a spoon, parents or caregivers may introduce other pureed foods.

There is no evidence to support beginning with either pureed fruits or vegetables. Recommendations are to start with single-ingredient foods introduced one at a time. Parents should introduce new foods only as frequently as every 3 days. Once infants are able to sit independently, parents may introduce soft foods. When the pincer grasp develops, from 7 to 9 months of age, the infant is ready for table foods. As parents introduce table foods, remind them to cut the food into small pieces to reduce the risk of choking.

Infants should not have cow's milk during the first year of life (Patient Teaching 15.5). Cow's milk is difficult for infants to digest and does not contain the proper nutrients needed for healthy growth. Additionally, the high level of protein in cow's milk is difficult for the infant's immature kidneys to process.

Patient Teaching 15.5

Food Allergies

Food allergies can result in symptoms such as diarrhea, eczema, asthma, and anaphylaxis. However, true food allergies are not common. The most allergenic foods are cow's milk, eggs, wheat, peanuts, tree nuts, fish, and shellfish.

Current recommendations from the AAP and the American Academy of Allergy, Asthma and Immunology include introducing highly allergenic foods earlier rather than later. Introducing highly allergenic foods later than 6 months of age may actually increase the risk of food allergy (AAP, 2017b). The exception to this rule is with infants who have severe eczema, for whom allergy testing is recommended before starting allergenic foods (Togias et al., 2017)

Nuts, fish, eggs, and other allergenic foods should be introduced in the infant's diet per the normal guidelines for introduction of solid foods.

Other foods to avoid include honey, which can cause botulism in infants, and sugary foods. Parents should give fruit juices in moderation, no more than 4 oz/d.

Common Developmental Concerns

Parents are often concerned about many things during the infant's first year of life. Many concerns can be frustrating for parents but have no underlying medical concerns.

Teething

Typically, infants get their first tooth from 4 to 7 months of age. Once infants begin teething, they may become fussy and irritable and have increased salivation, low-grade fevers, and difficulty sleeping (Tinanoff, 2016). Some infants may not have any symptoms. Cold teething rings or washcloths to chew on can ease the discomfort associated with teething. Topical oral analgesics may be used sparingly. It is not recommended to give oral analgesics for mild teething symptoms.

Colic

Colic is a common concern in the first few months of life. The condition is self-limiting, with peak symptoms at 6 weeks and resolution of symptoms from 3 to 6 months of age. The etiology of colic is not well understood, and no underlying pathology has been identified. Symptoms include inconsolable crying lasting at least 3 hours at a time, usually in the evening, for 3 days a week for at least 1 week (Pace, 2017). Other symptoms include flatulence, clenched fists, and knees drawn to the chest. Instruct parents to contact the healthcare provider if the infant has bloody stools, fever, or persistent vomiting.

There is no treatment for colic, so parents need a great deal of support during this time. Alternative therapies have been shown to have mixed results in multiple studies, with some treatments having unwanted side effects (Pace, 2017).

Colicky babies can be very frustrating for parents. Reassure parents that they have done nothing wrong. Encourage parents when they are frustrated to either hand the infant to someone else or lay the infant down in the crib, even if he or she is still crying. It is important for parents of colicky infants to have a break during this time. Ensure that the parents have someone to care for the infant for short periods of time when needed. Remind parents that no matter how frustrated they become, it is never okay to shake the infant.

Spitting Up

Spitting up is a common concern of parents but can be perfectly normal in infants. In the first few months of life, spitting up, or wet burps, can occur with burping during feedings and up to 2 hours after feeding. In early infancy, the low tone of the lower esophageal sphincter is a cause of regurgitation. Additional causes are inadequate burping or overfeeding.

Reassure parents that spitting up is normal in the first few months of life. Spitting up may be improved with increased frequency of burping during feeds. Decreasing the amount of each feed and increasing the frequency of feedings may help, as well. Educate parents to contact the healthcare provider if the infant has projectile vomiting, is extremely irritable with spitting up, has bilious emesis, or is losing weight.

Media

Although parents may want to use digital devices to entertain infants for brief periods of time, the AAP (2016) recommends no screen time during the infant's first year. Evidence validates that infants cannot learn from screen time, even with those applications and shows that claim to teach infants (Hagan et al, 2017). Face-to-face interaction and being read to are the best activities for infant learning.

Health Problems of Infancy

Some health problems appear mostly during the first year of life. Many problems are common and easily treatable. However, some health problems of infancy often warrant further investigation.

Brief Resolved Unexplained Events

Brief resolved unexplained events (BRUEs), formerly known as apparent life-threatening events, are events in children younger than 1 year of age that are observed to include one or more of the following symptoms lasting less than 60 seconds (Tieder et al., 2016):

- Cyanosis or pallor
- Irregular, slowed, or absent breathing
- Hypertonia or hypotonia
- Altered level of responsiveness

These symptoms are frightening for parents and caregivers who observe them. Instruct parents and caregivers that any BRUE needs to be evaluated by a healthcare provider. Obtain a history of symptoms and previous illnesses. Most episodes of BRUE have no underlying cause and the physical exam is normal. Infants who exhibit other symptoms, such as nasal congestion, fever, or choking, should be evaluated further for illness.

Infants who have experienced BRUE should be evaluated to determine risk of having additional episodes. Infants at high risk of having another event may be admitted to the hospital for observation and monitoring. High-risk infants include those who are less than 2 months of age, have a history of prematurity, and have a history of more than one BRUE. Infants determined to be low-risk may be monitored at home (Tieder et al., 2016).

Diaper Dermatitis

Diaper dermatitis refers to any skin breakdown in the diaper region. Skin may be irritated by wet diapers, stools, diaper wipes, or even the diapers themselves. In this condition, the skin is erythematous and excoriated but the skin folds are not affected (Fig. 15.15; Dickey & Chiu, 2016).

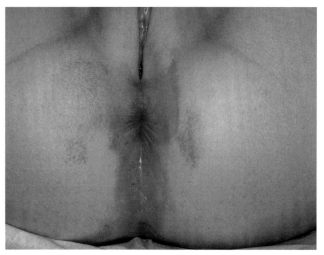

Figure 15.15. Diaper dermatitis. Diaper dermatitis with clearly demarcated borders. Note the skin folds are spared. Reprinted with permission from Edwards, L., & Lynch, P. J. (2018). *Genital dermatology atlas* (3rd ed., Fig. 14.5). Philadelphia, PA: Wolters Kluwer.

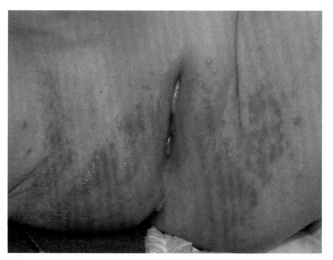

Figure 15.17. Candidal diaper rash. Diaper rash caused by a candidal infection. Note the pinpoint satellite lesions. Reprinted with permission from Edwards, L., & Lynch, P. J. (2018). *Genital dermatology atlas* (3rd ed., Fig. 14.9). Philadelphia, PA: Wolters Kluwer.

Diaper dermatitis is painful for infants. Treatment includes leaving the diapers off to allow the skin to dry as well as commercial barrier creams applied with each diaper change. Parents should consult their healthcare provider if they notice purulent drainage, odor, or fever.

Candidiasis

Candida is a common pathogen for fungal infections in infants. Candidal infections in the mouth are known as thrush. Symptoms of thrush include white patches on the tongue and buccal mucosa that cannot be scraped away (Fig. 15.16). Occasionally, thrush spreads to the esophagus, resulting in painful swallowing. Owing to the pain, infants may decrease intake until the infection is resolved.

Candida can also complicate diaper dermatitis. Candidal diaper infections are distinct. This type of diaper rash has a red raised border and often has pinpoint satellite lesions (Fig. 15.17). In addition, the erythema extends into the skin folds, unlike in diaper dermatitis.

Treatment for both thrush and candidal diaper infections is the antifungal nystatin (The Pharmacy 15.2). Oral liquid nystatin is used for thrush, whereas topical nystatin ointment is used in the diaper area.

Seborrhea

Seborrheic dermatitis, also known as cradle cap, is common in infants. The rash consists of scales and erythema, usually contained to the scalp (Fig. 15.18). Infantile seborrheic dermatitis typically resolves by the time an infant reaches 1 year of age. This type of dermatitis is not painful or itchy, as are other types of dermatitis.

Instruct parents to wash the infant's hair as normal. Using a soft brush can help gently remove the scales on the scalp. If seborrheic dermatitis extends from the scalp to behind the ears and in the creases of the neck, healthcare providers often instruct parents to apply 1% hydrocortisone cream to the affected areas.

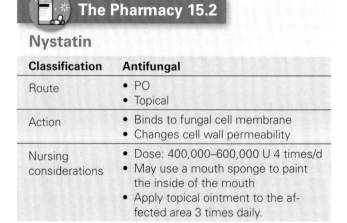

The Pharmacy 15.2

Nystatin

Classification	Antifungal
Route	• PO • Topical
Action	• Binds to fungal cell membrane • Changes cell wall permeability
Nursing considerations	• Dose: 400,000–600,000 U 4 times/d • May use a mouth sponge to paint the inside of the mouth • Apply topical ointment to the affected area 3 times daily.

PO, by mouth.
Adapted from Taketomo, C. K., Hodding, J. H., & Kraus, D. M. (2018). *Pediatric & neonatal dosage handbook* (25th ed.). Hudson, OH: Lexicomp.

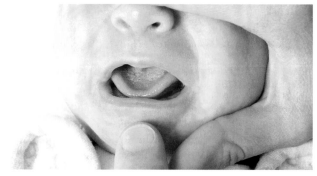

Figure 15.16. Thrush. An infant with the white plaques of thrush on the tongue.

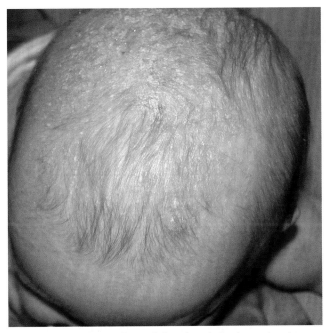

Figure 15.18. Seborrhea. Seborrhea infection, also known as cradle cap, on an infant's head. Reprinted with permission from Bachur, R. G., & Shaw, K. N. (2016). *Fleisher & Ludwig's textbook of pediatric emergency medicine* (7th ed., Fig. 65.10). Philadelphia, PA: Wolters Kluwer.

Acne Neonatorum

Acne neonatorum, or neonatal acne, is present in about 20% of newborns (Galbraith, 2016). In this condition, papules and pustules cover the forehead and cheeks (Fig. 15.19). The cause is unknown and treatment is generally not necessary. Reassure parents that the acne usually resolves within the first few months of life.

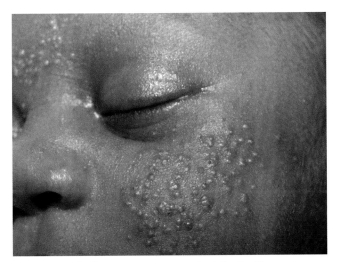

Figure 15.19. Acne neonatorum. An infant with papules on the forehead and cheeks. Reprinted with permission from Lugo-Somolinos, A., McKinley-Grant, L., Goldsmith, L. A., Papier, A., Adigun, C. G., Culton, D., . . . Lee, I. (2011). *VisualDx: Essential dermatology in pigmented skin.* Philadelphia, PA: Wolters Kluwer.

Roseola

Roseola infantum is a benign febrile exanthem in infancy caused by human herpesvirus 6 and human herpesvirus 7 (Caserta, 2016; Stone, Micali, & Schwartz, 2014). Transmission of the virus occurs through saliva.

Infants with this condition typically present with abrupt onset of high fever. The fever is usually 103.5°F (39.7°C) or higher and lasts approximately 72 hours. The characteristic rash of roseola appears after the fever is gone. The rash appears on the neck and trunk and consists of irregular rose-colored papules and macules that are about 2 to 3 cm in diameter (Fig. 15.20). Other clinical manifestations may include irritability, diarrhea, and upper respiratory symptoms (Stone et al., 2014).

Treatment for roseola is supportive. Ensure that the infant is appropriately hydrated. Antipyretics may be used to treat fever. Infants are contagious during the febrile stage of the illness.

Fever

Fever in infancy is defined as a rectal temperature greater than 100.4°F (38°C) (Harden, Kent, Pittman, & Roth, 2015). Infants are not developmentally able to hold a thermometer in their mouth for an oral temperature. Although temporal thermometers are useful, the rectal temperature is the most accurate for infants.

Fever indicates illness and is a sign that the infant is fighting the present infection. Fever initiates the activation of white blood cells to attack viruses. Moderate fever has no adverse effects on infants (Stone et al., 2014). Therefore, unless the infant is extremely irritable, administering an antipyretic is not recommended. Decreasing the fever may possibly prolong the illness.

Tachypnea and tachycardia are symptoms that are present during fever. Infants are generally more irritable while febrile. Often, infants sleep more when febrile. Educate parents on care for the infant during febrile illness, such as making sure the infant does not become overheated. Placing the infant in a cool bath is not recommended. Infants who appear toxic, lethargic, or cyanotic or who seem to have poor perfusion, hyperventilation, or hypoventilation should be evaluated immediately.

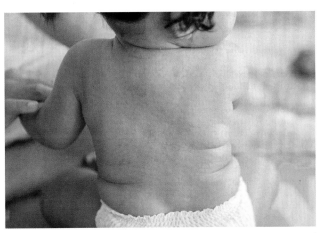

Figure 15.20. Roseola. An infant with the rash associated with roseola, which includes irregular rose-colored macules and papules 2 to 3 cm in diameter.

Think Critically

1. Why is it important to monitor growth and development in infants?
2. What are some developmental red flags in infancy? What can nurses do to help infants who are experiencing developmental delay to achieve optimal growth and development?
3. Develop a plan for optimal nutrition in the first year of life.

4. Why are solid foods introduced to infants one at a time every 3 to 4 days?
5. What are the most important components of anticipatory guidance during the first year of life?
6. What are the biggest safety concerns during infancy?

Unfolding Patient Stories: Jackson Webber • Part 1

Jackson Webber, age 3, is diagnosed with generalized seizures and started on phenobarbital. His mother is single and employed full time. The mother is concerned about his recent developmental regression and how that will affect his return to child care. What education can the nurse provide on normal growth and development for a 3-year-old and the relationship between developmental milestones and the new onset of an illness? What questions can the nurse ask to evaluate the adequacy and safety of the child care center that Jackson attends when considering his new diagnosis of seizures? (Jackson Webber's story continues in Unit 3.)

Care for Jackson and other patients in a realistic virtual environment: *vSim for Nursing* (thepoint.lww.com/vSimPediatric). Practice documenting these patients' care in DocuCare (thepoint.lww.com /DocuCareEHR).

Unfolding Patient Stories: Eva Madison • Part 2

Recall from Unit 1 Eva Madison, who had bacterial gastroenteritis. She is now at the clinic with her mother for a routine checkup. How can the nurse create an environment that is conducive to obtaining health information? How can the nurse prepare the child and the mother for the physical exam? What key areas of the health history and physical assessment should the nurse evaluate in this 5-year-old female?

Care for Eva and other patients in a realistic virtual environment: *vSim for Nursing* (thepoint.lww.com/vSimPediatric). Practice documenting these patients' care in DocuCare (thepoint.lww.com /DocuCareEHR).

References

American Academy of Pediatrics Task Force on Sudden Infant Death Syndrome. (2016). SIDS and other sleep-related infant deaths: Updated 2016 recommendations for a safe infant sleeping environment. *Pediatrics, 138*(5), e20162938

American Academy of Pediatrics, Committee on Injury, Violence, and Poison Prevention. (2011). *Child passenger safety.* Retrieved from www.pediatrics.org/cgi/doi/10.1542/peds.2011-0213

American Academy of Pediatrics. (2009a). *Hearing and making sounds.* Retrieved from https://www.healthychildren.org/English/ages-stages/baby/Pages/Hearing-and-Making-Sounds.aspx

American Academy of Pediatrics. (2009b). *Language development: 4–7 months.* Retrieved from https://www.healthychildren.org/English/ages-stages/baby/Pages/Language-Development-4-to-7-Months.aspx

American Academy of Pediatrics. (2009c). *Newborn reflexes.* Retrieved from https://www.healthychildren.org/English/ages-stages/baby/Pages/Newborn-Reflexes.aspx

American Academy of Pediatrics. (2012). *Safety for your child: Birth to 6 months.* Retrieved from https://www.healthychildren.org/English/ages-stages/baby/Pages/Safety-for-Your-Child-Birth-to-6-Months.aspx

American Academy of Pediatrics. (2015). *Medication safety tips.* Retrieved from https://www.healthychildren.org/English/safety-prevention/at-home/medication-safety/Pages/Medication-Safety-Tips.aspx

American Academy of Pediatrics. (2016). *Why to void TV in infants & toddlers.* Retrieved form https://www.healthychildren.org/English/family-life/Media/Pages/Why-to-Avoid-TV-Before-Age-2.aspx

American Academy of Pediatrics. (2017a). *7 Myths and facts about bilingual children learning language.* Retrieved from https://www.healthychildren.org/English/ages-stages/gradeschool/school/Pages/7-Myths-Facts-Bilingual-Children-Learning-Language.aspx

American Academy of Pediatrics. (2017b). *Starting solid foods.* Retrieved from https://www.healthychildren.org/English/ages-stages/baby/feeding-nutrition/Pages/Switching-To-Solid-Foods.aspx

American Heart Association. (2015). *Heart murmurs.* Retrieved from http://www.heart.org/HEARTORG/Conditions/More/CardiovascularConditionsofChildhood/Heart-Murmurs_UCM_314208_Article.jsp#.WgyEKLQ-e1t

Bernstein, D. (2016). Evaluation of the cardiovascular system: History and physical examination. In R. M. Kliegman, B. F. Stanton, J. W. St. Geme III, N. F. Schor, & R. E. Behrman (Eds.), *Nelson's textbook of pediatrics* (20th ed.). Philadelphia, PA: Elsevier, Saunders.

Burns, C., Dunn, A., Brady, M., Starr, N., Blosser, C., & Garzon, D. (2017). *Pediatric primary care* (6th ed.). St. Louis, MO: Elsevier.

Carlo, W. A. (2016). The newborn infant. In R. M. Kliegman, B. F. Stanton, J. W. St. Geme III, N. F. Schor, & R. E. Behrman (Eds.), *Nelson's textbook of pediatrics* (20th ed.). Philadelphia, PA: Elsevier, Saunders.

Caserta, M.T. (2016). Roseola (Human herpesviruses 6 and 7). In R. M. Kliegman, B. F. Stanton, J. W. St. Geme III, N. F. Schor, & R. E. Behrman (Eds.), *Nelson's textbook of pediatrics* (20th ed.). Philadelphia, PA: Elsevier, Saunders.

Center for Child Development. (2015). *Temperament and your child's personality.* Retrieved from https://childdevelopmentinfo.com/child-development/temperament_and_your_child/#.WhYpJrQ-e1s

Centers for Disease Control and Prevention. (2013). *Understanding how vaccines work.* Retrieved from https://www.cdc.gov/vaccines/hcp/conversations/downloads/vacsafe-understand-bw-office.pdf

Centers for Disease Control and Prevention. (2013). *Understanding the Vaccine Adverse Event Reporting System (VAERS).* Retrieved from https://www.cdc.gov/vaccines/hcp/conversations/downloads/vacsafe-vaers-bw-office.pdf

Christensen, R. D., & Ohls, R. K. (2016). Development of the hematopoietic system. In R. M. Kliegman, B. F. Stanton, J. W. St. Geme III, N. F. Schor, & R. E. Behrman (Eds.), *Nelson's textbook of pediatrics* (20th ed.). Philadelphia, PA: Elsevier, Saunders.

Cincinnati Children's Hospital Medical Center. (2015). *Cyanosis in infants and children.* Retrieved from https://www.cincinnatichildrens.org/health/c/cyanosis

Consolini, D. M. (2017). *Nutrition in infants*. Merck Manual. Kenilworth, NJ: Merck & Co. Retrieved from https://www.merckmanuals.com/professional/pediatrics/care-of-newborns-and-infants/nutrition-in-infants

Dickey, B. Z., & Chiu, Y. E. (2016). Contact dermatitis. In R. M. Kliegman, B. F. Stanton, J. W. St. Geme III, N. F. Schor, & R. E. Behrman (Eds.), *Nelson's textbook of pediatrics* (20th ed.). Philadelphia, PA: Elsevier, Saunders.

Eberhart, C. S., Blanchard-Rohner, G., Lemaitre, B., Boukrid, M., Combescure, C., Othenin-Gerard, V., . . . Siegrist, C. (2016). Maternal immunization earlier in pregnancy maximizes antibody transfer and expected infant seropositivity against pertussis. *Clinical Infectious Diseases, 62*(7), 829–836. doi:10.1093/cid/ciw027

Erikson, E. H. (1963). *Childhood and society*. New York, NY: W.W. Norton and Company.

Feigelman, S. (2016). The first year. In R. M. Kliegman, B. F. Stanton, J. W. St. Geme III, N. F. Schor, & R. E. Behrman (Eds.), *Nelson's textbook of pediatrics* (20th ed.). Philadelphia, PA: Elsevier, Saunders.

Fischer, D. J., O'Hayre, M. O., Kusiak, J. W., Somerman, M. J., & Hill, C. V. (2017). Oral health disparities: A perspective from the national institute of dental and craniofacial research. *American Journal of Public Health, 107*(S1), S36–S38.

Frank, J. E., & Jacobe, K. M. (2011). Evaluation and management of heart murmurs in children. *American Family Physician, 84*(7), 793–800.

Galbraith, S. S. (2016). Acne. In R. M. Kliegman, B. F. Stanton, J. W. St. Geme III, N. F. Schor, & R. E. Behrman (Eds.), *Nelson's textbook of pediatrics* (20th ed.). Philadelphia, PA: Elsevier, Saunders.

Gathercole, V. C. (2014). Bilingualism matters: One size does not fit all. *International Journal of Behavioral Development, 38*(4), 359–366.

Greenbaum, L.A. (2016). Composition of body fluids. In R. M. Kliegman, B. F. Stanton, J. W. St. Geme III, N. F. Schor, & R. E. Behrman (Eds.), *Nelson's textbook of pediatrics* (20th ed.). Philadelphia, PA: Elsevier, Saunders.

Hagan, J.F., Shaw, J.S., Duncan, P. (Eds.) (2017). *Bright futures: Guidelines for health supervision of infants, children, and adolescents* (4th ed.). Elk Grove Village, IL: American Academy of Pediatrics.

Harden, L. M., Kent, S., Pittman, Q. J., & Roth, J. (2015). Fever and sickness behavior: Friend or foe? *Brain, Behavior, and Immunity, 50*, 322–333.

Hardy, S. C., & Klingman, R. E. (1994). Fat and cholesterol in the diet of infants and young children: Implications for growth, development, and long-term health. *Journal of Pediatrics, 125*(5), S69–S77.

Keane, V. (2016). Assessment of growth. In R. M. Kliegman, B. F. Stanton, J. W. St. Geme III, N. F. Schor, & R. E. Behrman (Eds.), *Nelson's textbook of pediatrics* (20th ed.). Philadelphia, PA: Elsevier, Saunders.

Langus, A., & Nespor, M. (2013). Language development in infants: What do humans hear in the first months of life? *Hearing, Balance, and Communication, 11*, 121–129.

Lawrence, J., Alcock, D., McGrath, P., MacMurray, S. B., & Dulberg, C. (1993). The development of a tool to assess neonatal pain. *Neonatal Network, 12*(6), 59–66.

Merkel, S. I., Voepel-Lewis, T., Shayevitz, J. R., & Malviya, S. (1997). The FLACC: A behavioral scale for scoring postoperative pain in young children. *Pediatric Nursing, 23*(3), 293–297.

Murray, A., & Egan, S. M. (2014). Does reading to infants benefit their cognitive development at 9-months-old? An investigation using a large birth cohort survey. *Child Language and Teaching Therapy, 30*(3), 303–315. doi:10.1177/0265659013513813

Obeng, C. S., Emetu, R. E., & Curtis, T. J. (2015). African-American women's perceptions and experiences about breastfeeding. *Frontiers in Public Health, 3*, 273. doi:10.3389/fpubh.2015.00273

Olitsky, S. E., Hug, D., Plummer, L. S., Stahl, E. D., Ariss, M. M., & Lindquist, T. P. (2016). Disorders of the eye: Growth and development. In R. M. Kliegman, B. F. Stanton, J. W. St. Geme III, N. F. Schor, & R. E. Behrman (Eds.), *Nelson's textbook of pediatrics* (20th ed.). Philadelphia, PA: Elsevier, Saunders.

Pace, C. A. (2017). Infant colic: What to know for the primary care setting. *Clinical Pediatrics, 56*(7), 616–618.

Piaget, J. (1930). *The child's conception of physical causality*. London, England: Routledge & Kegan Paul Ltd.

Pineda, R. G., Reynolds, L. C., Seefeldt, K., Hilton, C. L., Rogers C. L., & Inder, T. E. (2016). Head lag in infancy: What is it telling us? *American Journal of Occupational Therapy, 70*(1), 1–8. doi:10.5014/ajot.2016.017558

Shen, J., Giles, S. A., Kurtovic, K., Fabia, R., Besner, G. E., Wheeler, K. K., . . . & Groner, J. L. (2017). Evaluation of nurse accuracy in rating procedural pain among pediatric burn patients using the Face, Legs, Activity, Cry, Consolability (FLACC) Scale. *Burns, 43*, 114–120.

Stoll, B. J., & Shane, A. L. (2016). Infections of the neonatal infant. In R. M. Kliegman, B. F. Stanton, J. W. St. Geme III, N. F. Schor, & R. E. Behrman (Eds.), *Nelson's textbook of pediatrics* (20th ed.). Philadelphia, PA: Elsevier, Saunders.

Stone, R. C., Micali, G. A., & Schwartz, R. A. (2014). Roseola infantum and its causal herpesviruses. *International Journal of Dermatology, 53*, 397–403.

Tieder, J. S., Bonkowsky, J. L., Etzel, R. A., Franklin W. H., Gremse, D. A., & Smith, M. (2016). Brief resolved unexplained events (formerly apparent life-threatening events) and evaluation of lower-risk infants. *Pediatrics, 137*(5), e20160590.

Tinanoff, N. (2016). Periodontal disease. In R. M. Kliegman, B. F. Stanton, J. W. St. Geme III, N. F. Schor, & R. E. Behrman (Eds.), *Nelson's textbook of pediatrics* (20th ed.). Philadelphia, PA: Elsevier, Saunders.

Togias, A., Cooper, S. F., Acebal, M. L., Assa'ad, A., Baker, J. R., Beck, L. A., . . . Boyce, J. A. (2017). Addendum guidelines for the prevention of peanut allergy in the United States: Report of the National Institute of Allergy and Infectious Diseases–sponsored expert panel. *Journal of Allergy and Clinical Immunology, 131*(1), 29–44.

World Health Organization. (2017). *Exclusive breastfeeding*. Retrieved from http://www.who.int/nutrition/topics/exclusive_breastfeeding/en/

Zargham-Boroujeni, A., Elsagh, A., & Mohammadizadeh, M. (2017). The effects of massage and breastfeeding on response to venipuncture pain among hospitalized neonates. *Iranian Journal of Nursing and Midwifery Research, 22*(4), 308–312.

Suggested Reading

Centers for Disease Control and Prevention. (2017). *For parents: Vaccines for your children*. Retrieved from https://www.cdc.gov/vaccines/parents/parent-questions.html

Murray, A., & Egan, S. M. (2014). Does reading to infants benefit their cognitive development at 9-months-old? An investigation using a large birth cohort survey. Child Language and Teaching Therapy, 30(3), 303–315. doi:10.1177/0265659013513813

Obeng, C. S., Emetu, R. E., & Curtis, T. J. (2015). African-American women's perceptions and experiences about breastfeeding. Frontiers in Public Health, 3, 273. doi:10.3389/fpubh.2015.00273

Shen, J., Giles, S. A., Kurtovic, K., Fabia, R., Besner, G. E., Wheeler, K. K., . . . & Groner, J. L. (2017). Evaluation of nurse accuracy in rating procedural pain among pediatric burn patients using the Face, Legs, Activity, Cry, Consolability (FLACC) Scale. Burns, 43, 114–120.

16 Care of the Toddler

Objectives

After completing this chapter, you will be able to:
1. Discuss normal growth and development in toddlers.
2. Describe the physical assessment of toddlers.
3. Explain the development of gross and fine motor coordination and language milestones during the toddler years.
4. Explain the importance of nutrition during the toddler years.

5. Choose appropriate teaching topics for parents of toddlers.
6. Describe common developmental concerns in toddlers.
7. Identify common health problems during the toddler years.

Key Terms

Animism
Echolalia
Effusion
Egocentrism
Expressive language
Food jag

Jargon
Parallel play
Physiological anorexia
Receptive language
Telegraphic speech

Growth and Development Overview

The toddler period is from 12 to 36 months of age. Although not as rapid as in the first year of life, growth and development during the toddler years contribute to developing independence. Gross motor, fine motor, language, and cognitive skills become more fine-tuned. Throughout the toddler period nurses continue to perform physical assessments, monitor growth and development milestones, and assess for developmental delay.

Health Assessment

Parents and caregivers remain an essential part of the toddler's health assessment. Parents can offer insight into any health problems or concerns regarding growth and development.

Allowing the toddler to sit on a parent's lap during the physical exam can elicit increased cooperation from the toddler.

During the physical assessment, note the interaction between the parent and the toddler. Does the parent act positively toward the child? Does the toddler interact with the parent? If siblings are in the room, how is the interaction between the toddler and the siblings? Lack of interaction between parent and toddler or negative interaction warrants further investigation.

When performing a physical assessment on a toddler, be flexible. Gather information about the toddler's health status through play. During the assessment, both the nurse and the parent can provide distraction to make the process easier. Toddlers respond to distractions such as singing, pictures, and toys. For example, singing to a toddler during abdominal palpation may help the toddler relax and allow the nurse to obtain more accurate assessment data. Allow the toddler to touch any safe medical equipment, such as a stethoscope or penlight (Fig. 16.1). Tell the toddler what you are going to do in simple terms. Do not ask the toddler for permission to perform any part of the exam. If asked, the toddler will most likely say "no." Praise the toddler for cooperating during the assessment. Use simple phrases such as, "you are doing a good job." If the toddler is not cooperative, move to a portion of the exam the toddler is likely to perceive as less scary. Complete the physical exam in the order that elicits the most cooperation. Always save the most invasive procedures for last.

Head, Eyes, Ears, Nose, and Throat

Ask the parents or caregivers whether they have any concerns about the toddler's vision or hearing. Does the child respond when you talk to him or her? Does the child turn his or her head toward loud noises? Has the toddler had a head injury? Are there any concerns about the shape of the toddler's head? Does the toddler have a history of eye or ear infections?

Head

Begin the assessment with observation of the shape and size of the toddler's head. The toddler's head is still large in proportion to the body, but the toddler should have full head control. The head should be round with no flattened areas. The midline of the head should align and be parallel with the midline of the neck. Note whether the toddler holds his or her head tilted to one side. Inspect for symmetry of facial features.

Palpate the anterior fontanelle. If the fontanelle is still open, it should be soft and flat. A sunken or bulging fontanelle is an abnormal finding. The anterior fontanelle should be closed by 18 months of age.

Eyes

Inspect the eyes for alignment. Strabismus at this age is considered an abnormal finding. Pupils should be equal, round, and reactive to light and accommodation (PERRLA; Fig. 16.2). Inspect the conjunctiva for redness and drainage. The sclera should be white. Any red, blue, or yellow of the sclera is an abnormal finding and needs to be documented.

Test extraocular motility by having a child track an object through the six visual fields. Depth perception continues to develop throughout the toddler years. Toddlers are still too young to use a Snellen eye chart for vision testing. Visual acuity during the toddler years is from 20/50 to 20/40.

Ears

Observe the ears for alignment with the outer canthus of the eye. Inspect the ears for redness or drainage. To inspect the inner ear, pull the pinna down and back (when the child reaches 3 years of age, a different technique is used; see Chapter 17).

Nose

Inspect the nose for symmetry and alignment on the face. Gently tilt the toddler's head back to inspect the nares. Note any redness or swelling of the turbinates as well as any drainage.

Mouth and Throat

The toddler's lips should be symmetrical on the face. Inspect the lips for lesions or excoriation. The buccal mucosa should be pink and moist. By 12 months of age, toddlers normally have several teeth. By 3 years of age, a child should have all 20 baby teeth. Inspect the teeth for color and cleanliness, determining the quality of oral hygiene.

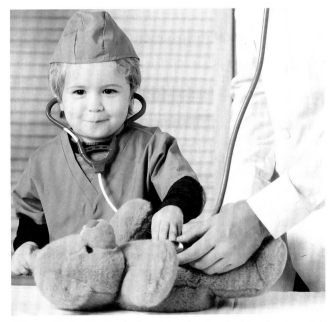

Figure 16.1. Medical play. Allowing the toddler to play with safe medical equipment can help elicit cooperation during the physical examination.

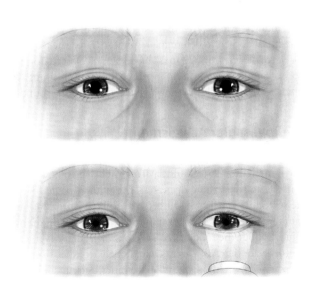

Figure 16.2. PERRLA. Pupils are equal, round, and reactive to light and accommodation. Reprinted with permission from Kyle, T., & Carman, S. (2016). *Essentials of pediatric nursing* (3rd ed., Fig. 10.19). Philadelphia, PA: Wolters Kluwer.

Observe the throat by asking the toddler to open his or her mouth. One way to gain cooperation is by playing a game with the toddler, such as telling the child, "Let's see if I can tell what you had for breakfast." Tonsils appear large throughout the toddler period and should appear pink. Ability to swallow indicates that the gag reflex is intact. However, should it be necessary to elicit a gag reflex, such as when assessing for suspected neurological injury, the uvula should be midline and rise smoothly.

Neurological Assessment

The toddler's brain continues to grow during the second year of life. Head circumference increases 2 cm from age 12 months to age 24 months (Feigelman, 2016). Head circumference is measured until the child is about 2 or 3 years of age. Myelination of the brain is complete around 24 months of age.

During the neurological assessment, ask the parents or caregivers whether they have any concerns about their child reaching growth and development milestones. Observe the toddler's gait both walking and running. Determine hand control by having the toddler scribble or stack blocks. Most children show a hand preference by 2 or 3 years of age.

Observe the interaction between the child and parent. Note eye contact, socialization, and the ability to follow commands. Assess the toddler's language ability and clarity of speech.

Respiratory Assessment

The respiratory system continues to develop during the toddler years. The alveoli increase in number but do not reach adult numbers. Therefore, the toddler is still at increased risk of impaired gas exchange. The trachea is narrower than that of an adult and the lower airways are smaller.

Ask the parents whether the child has a history of coughing, wheezing, or noisy breathing. Assess the toddler's respiratory effort. Toddlers still use the diaphragm to breathe; therefore, observe the abdomen to determine respiratory rate. The respiratory rate of toddlers is from 22 to 37 breaths/min. Observe for use of accessory muscles, indicating increased work of breathing. Auscultate in all lung fields, noting any adventitious lung sounds.

Cardiovascular Assessment

In the toddler, the point of maximal impulse remains at the fourth intercostal space, midclavicular line. The blood pressure increases and heart rate decreases. The normal range for heart rate in toddlers is 98 to 140 beats/min. Blood pressure ranges from 86 to 106 mm Hg systolic and 42 to 63 mm Hg diastolic. Enquire about the toddler's color. Does the toddler ever appear pale or cyanotic? Ask parents whether the toddler tires easily. Assess capillary refill in all four extremities. Auscultate for murmurs and document appropriately.

Gastrointestinal Assessment

The size of the stomach increases during the toddler years, allowing for longer times between meals. Intestinal length continues to increase. Stools may vary in color, depending on what the toddler eats. Stool frequency decreases, often to once daily. Toddlers are prone to constipation, especially during toilet training.

Assess the frequency and quality of stools. Stools should be soft and passed easily. A toddler who is straining with stools or whose stools are small and hard requires intervention. Determine whether the child has achieved bowel control. Toddlers generally have full bowel control by the time they are 3 years old.

Inspect the abdomen for shape, noting whether there is an umbilical hernia. Toddlers often appear to have a protruding abdomen. The abdomen should be soft and nontender on palpation. The lower liver border is normally palpable 2 to 3 cm below the intercostal margin. Palpate for hernias in the inguinal canal. Auscultate for bowel sounds in all four quadrants.

Genitourinary Assessment

Bladder capacity reaches adult volumes during the toddler years. By the end of the toddler period, the child should achieve daytime bladder control. The urethra remains shorter in toddlers, placing them at increased risk for urinary tract infection, especially females.

Determine whether the toddler has a history of dark or odorous urine. Does the toddler have pain with urination? Ask the parents about urine output, whether the toddler is still in diapers or is toilet trained. The normal urine output is 1 mL/kg/h. Assess for difficulty with toilet training.

In males, palpate the scrotum to determine whether the testes are descended. Note any swelling of the scrotum or penis. If the toddler is uncircumcised, retract the foreskin to inspect the glans. Inspect for discharge and foul odors. The foreskin should be able to be retracted.

In females, inspect the labia majora and minora. Observe for swelling, erythema, and discharge. Document any labial adhesions.

Musculoskeletal Assessment

During the toddler period, the musculoskeletal system continues to mature. During early ambulation, toddlers have a wide gait and tend to walk flat footed (Fig. 16.3A). By 3 years of age the gait narrows, and arms begin to swing with the gait (Baldwin, Wells, & Dorman, 2016). Toddlers walk with flat feet and bowed legs until the musculature is fully developed. A toddler's abdominal musculature is weak, giving the appearance of lordosis. Therefore, toddlers seem to have a potbelly (Fig. 16.3B). The abdomen should flatten out and the legs should straighten by the time the child is 3 years old.

As part of the musculoskeletal assessment, ask the parents or caregivers whether the toddler has altered gait, changes in coordination, or limited range of motion. Perform passive range of motion of all extremities. Observe the toddler's gait. Determine whether the child is meeting gross motor milestones.

Integumentary Assessment

Determine whether the child has had any recent injuries resulting in lacerations or bruising. Ask the parents or caregivers whether the child has a history of any rashes. Inspect the skin

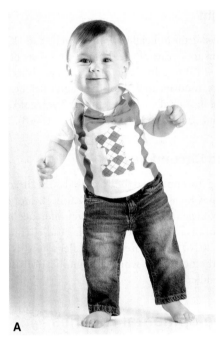
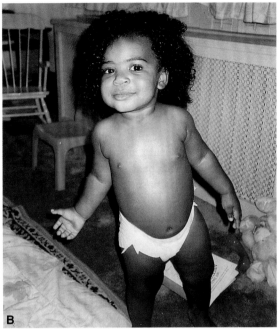

A **B**

Figure 16.3. Toddler stance. A. The toddler walks with a wide gait and flat feet to keep steady. **B.** The toddler's abdominal musculature is weak, giving the appearance of a potbelly. Part B reprinted with permission from Pillitteri, A. (2013). *Maternal and child health nursing* (7th ed., Fig. 30.1A). Philadelphia, PA: Wolters Kluwer Health/Lippincott Williams & Wilkins.

for lesions, abrasions, ecchymosis, and burns. If there are injuries, document whether the mechanism of injury matches what is seen on the toddler. If the injury does not match the parent's story, further investigation is warranted.

The skin should be pink. On palpation, the skin should be warm and dry. Note any discoloration of the palms or soles of the feet. Document any other abnormalities, such as petechiae, purpura, pallor, or yellowing of the skin.

Immunological Assessment

The immune system continues to develop during the toddler years. Most innate immunity is developed before school age but is not fully developed until the adolescent years (Ygberg & Nilson, 2017). Adaptive immunity continues to be immature during the toddler years, placing the child at increased risk of both viral and bacterial infections (Ygberg & Nilson, 2017).

Enquire whether the child has a history of frequent infections, specifically recurrent respiratory infections or fungal infections. Either of these may indicate a malfunctioning immune system.

Hematological Assessment

At 12 months of age, the toddler should have the hemoglobin ratio of a normal adult (Christensen & Ohls, 2016). The numbers of granulocytes and thrombocytes are equal to those of adults.

Determine whether the infant has a history of frequent infections or prolonged bleeding. Inspect for pallor, bruising, and petechiae, which may indicate dysfunction in the hematological system.

Pain Assessment

Toddlers are not developmentally able to provide a self-report of pain (Analyze the Evidence 16.1). Therefore, use of pain scales

Analyze the Evidence 16.1

Assessing Pain in Toddlers

Although there are several reliable and valid pain tools to assess pain in children, from the neonate to the adolescent, pediatric pain is still not well treated (Marrowen & Stinson, 2016). Part of the reason for inadequate pain treatment in children is due to their range of developmental and cognitive skills. The parent and patient report needs to be considered when developing a pain management plan for children.

For children with chronic pain, it is important to establish aggravating and relieving factors. There are currently no validated and reliable tools to measure these factors. Advances in technology, such as ePain diaries, make this easier for parents and children.

Genetics may play a role in pain management, explaining the fact that some children are more sensitive to pain than others. In addition, children whose parents experience chronic pain are more likely to experience pain themselves.

In conclusion, Marrowen and Stinson (2016) determined that pain assessment tools are used properly. However, the tools alone are insufficient for pain management. Self and parental report, assessing the impact of pain on the child's quality of life, and regularly assessing pain to determine the effectiveness of interventions are essential components of pain management.

requiring self-report are not appropriate during the toddler years (Manworren & Stinson, 2016). Ask the parents or caregivers about the child's experience with pain and painful procedures. As an objective measure of pain, the Faces, Legs, Activity, Cry, and Consolability (FLACC) scale is appropriate to use during the toddler years (Gomez et al., 2013; Merkel, Voepel-Lewis, Shayevitz, & Malviya, 1997).

Toddlers often react to painless procedures the same way in which they react to painful procedures. Crying, pushing away, kicking, screaming, and grimacing are all behaviors seen when a toddler experiences pain. Encourage the toddler to use his or her words for pain, such as "ouchie" or "boo boo."

Physical Growth

Toddlers should continue to have their height, weight, and head circumference measured routinely at well-child visits. Plot these measurements on growth charts to determine adequate growth, overweight, or underweight. When a child reaches 2 years of age, begin measuring his or her standing height.

Weight

In the early toddler years, children need to be weighed sitting on a scale (Fig. 16.4A). When a child reaches 3 years of age, begin obtaining his or her standing weight (Fig. 16.4B). During the toddler years, the child gains about 5 lb/y (2.3 kg). Once standing heights are measured, plot the toddler's body mass index on the growth chart to determine the risk of overweight or obesity.

Height

Toddlers gain in height approximately 5 in (12.7 cm) from 12 months to 2 years of age. From 2 to 3 years of age, the toddler grows 2 (5) to 3 in (7.6 cm) on average (Feigelman, 2016). By 2 years, toddlers are half of their adult height. Standing height can be measured when the child is 2 years old and understands to stand straight against the wall (Fig. 16.4B).

Head Circumference

Owing to continued head growth, the head circumference increases by about 2 cm from 12 to 18 months of age. By 2 years of age, the child's head circumference is approximately 85% of his or her expected adult head circumference (Feigelman, 2016). Therefore, the toddler's head is large compared with the body size, which has implications for safety during the toddler years.

Developmental Theories

During the toddler years, children move into different stages of psychosocial, cognitive, and moral development. Table 16.1 gives an overview of selected developmental theories for toddlers.

Psychosocial

Toddlers are developing the muscular maturity that allows them to explore their environment (Fig. 16.5). Erikson (1963) refers to this stage of development as autonomy vs. shame and doubt. This time of exploration can cause parents to become too restrictive for fear of the child injuring himself or herself. Alternatively, parents may not be firm enough, allowing children to become

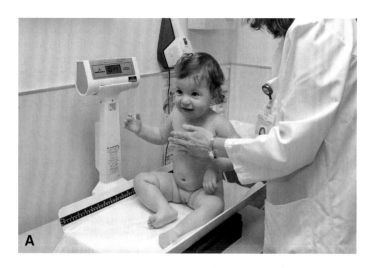

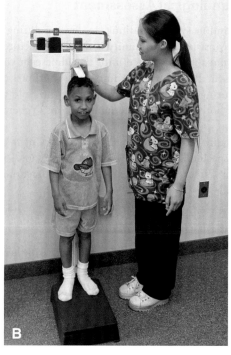

Figure 16.4. Toddler weight and height. A. Toddlers are weighed sitting on a scale until they are around 3 years old. **B.** Standing weight and height are obtained around 3 years old. Reprinted with permission from Hatfield, N. T., & Kincheloe, C. (2017). *Introductory maternity and pediatric nursing* (4th ed., Fig. 28.3B and C). Philadelphia, PA: Wolters Kluwer.

Table 16.1 Overview of Developmental Theories in Toddlers

Theorist/Type of Development	Stage	Implications
Erikson: Psychosocial	Autonomy vs. shame and doubt	Toddlers learn to do some things on their own and make choices.
Piaget: Cognitive	• Sensorimotor (up to age 2 y) • Preoperational (begins at age 2 y)	Toddlers manipulate objects to learn. They begin to imitate others.
Freud: Psychosexual	Anal	The toddler is focused on learning about when and where to defecate. Stool holding can be common during toilet training.
Kohlberg: Moral	Preconventional	The toddler is learning obedience.

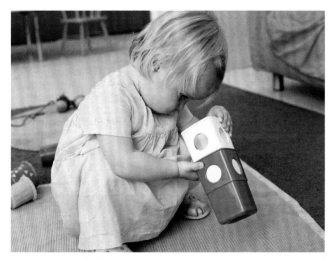

Figure 16.5. Toddler curiosity. As toddlers gain a sense of autonomy, they begin to explore their environment. Reprinted with permission from Kyle, T., & Carman, S. (2016). *Essentials of pediatric nursing* (3rd ed., Fig. 4.3). Philadelphia, PA: Wolters Kluwer.

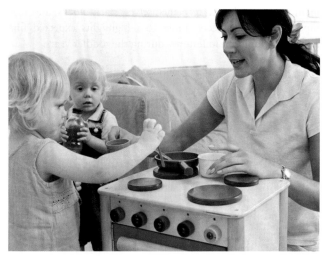

Figure 16.6. Appropriate use of objects. Toddlers begin to use toys appropriately, such as pretending to cook with pots and pans on a stove. Reprinted with permission from Kyle, T., & Carman, S. (2016). *Essentials of pediatric nursing* (3rd ed., Fig. 4.2A). Philadelphia, PA: Wolters Kluwer.

destructive. Either of these scenarios may lead to shame or doubt because the child is not given the proper direction to explore and to learn to perform tasks on his or her own. Establishing a sense of autonomy requires parents to allow the toddler to accomplish tasks independently yet establish firm rules to prevent harm. Giving toddlers choices, such as which book to read at bedtime or which shirt to wear, helps them achieve autonomy.

Cognitive

During the late sensorimotor stage, toddlers continue to explore the world through their senses. Using objects for their intended purpose becomes common (Fig. 16.6; Feigelman, 2016). Toddlers reach the early preoperational stage at 2 years of age. During this stage, the toddler begins to develop symbolic thinking. However, toddlers are egocentric in that they cannot think of life outside of their own body. A hallmark of the preconventional stage is the concept of **animism**, a state in which children believe

inanimate objects have a consciousness and other life-like properties (Piaget, 1930).

Moral

Kohlberg (1981) describes three levels of moral development, with each level divided into two stages. Toddlers are at the preconventional level of moral development. The first stage of this level is avoidance of punishment and obedience. The toddler is not focused on right and wrong, simply on avoiding punishment.

Motor Development

Both gross and fine motor development continue at a rapid pace during the toddler years. During the assessment, ask parents questions regarding their child's attainment of skills. If there are concerns, conduct a formal developmental evaluation using a validated assessment tool.

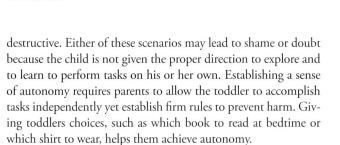

Gross Motor

Learning to walk is a hallmark accomplishment of the early toddler years. The toddler's gait is unsteady early on. The toddler walks with bowed legs and flat feet. By 3 years of age, the toddler is steadier and begins to walk in a heel-to-toe manner. As the toddler's large muscles develop, they acquire more gross motor skills, such as jumping and pushing toys (Fig. 16.7). Development of these skills contributes to the growing independence of the toddler, allowing the child to explore. Table 16.2 highlights expected gross motor skills during the toddler years.

Fine Motor

Fine motor skills continue to develop during the toddler years. Improved hand–eye coordination and small muscle development allow toddlers to feed themselves, stack blocks, and manipulate smaller objects. Table 16.3 highlights expected fine motor development milestones during the toddler years.

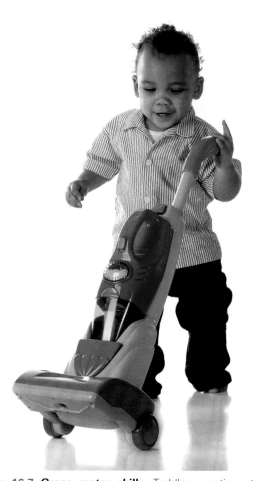

Figure 16.7. Gross motor skills. Toddlers continue to develop gross motor skills, making push–pull toys appropriate for this age. Reprinted with permission from Taylor, C., Lillis, C, & Lynn, P. (2014). *Fundamentals of nursing* (8th ed., Fig. 18.4A). Philadelphia, PA: Wolters Kluwer.

Table 16.2   Gross Motor Development Milestones in Toddlers

Age (mo)	Gross Motor Milestone
15	• Squats to pick up objects • Crawls up steps • Drinks from a cup
18	• Walks independently • Pushes and pulls toys when walking
24	• Runs • Kicks a ball • Jumps with two feet • Climbs on furniture
36	• Pedals a tricycle • Jumps forward • Walks up and down stairs with one foot on each step

Adapted from Hagan, J. F., Shaw, J. S., & Duncan, P. (Eds.). (2017). *Bright futures: Guidelines for health supervision of infants, children, and adolescents* (4th ed.). Elk Grove Village, IL: American Academy of Pediatrics; and Centers for Disease Control. (2017). *Learn the signs. Act early. Developmental milestones.* Retrieved from https://www.cdc.gov/ncbddd/actearly/milestones/index.html

Table 16.3   Fine Motor Development Milestones in Toddlers

Age (mo)	Fine Motor Milestone
15	• Marks with a crayon • Puts objects in and out of cups
18	• Scribbles spontaneously • Rolls a ball • Eats with a spoon • Helps undress self
24	• Copies straight lines and circles • Stacks objects • Turns pages • Throws a ball overhand
36	• Turns a door handle • Screws lids on and off • Copies a circle • Builds a tower of six or more blocks • Undresses self

Adapted from Hagan, J. F., Shaw, J. S., & Duncan, P. (Eds.). (2017). *Bright futures: Guidelines for health supervision of infants, children, and adolescents* (4th ed.). Elk Grove Village, IL: American Academy of Pediatrics; and Centers for Disease Control. (2017). *Learn the signs. Act early. Developmental milestones.* Retrieved from https://www.cdc.gov/ncbddd/actearly/milestones/index.html

Communication and Language Development

Receptive language develops at a more rapid pace than does **expressive language.** Toddlers are able to understand directions, follow commands, and point to pictures before they are able to put words together. However, during this developmental period, a toddler's vocabulary increases from one or two words to well over 200 (Feigelman, 2016). Table 16.4 highlights expected language milestones in toddlers.

As toddlers are learning to talk, they repeat words or phrases without knowing what they are saying. This is called **echolalia.** Echolalia is normal during the toddler years but can be a sign of autism if it persists beyond 3 years of age (Growth and Development Check 16.1; Stiegler, 2015).

By the time toddlers are 2 years of age, they are speaking in two-word sentences. These sentences contain only the necessary words for the toddler to get the point across. This type of speech is called **telegraphic speech.** Sentences such as "Want milk" or "Go bed" are examples of telegraphic speech. Stuttering can be a normal part of speech development and typically occurs from 2½ to 5 years of age. Normal stuttering includes repeating of

Growth and Development Check 16.1

Early Signs of Autism

Throughout the toddler years, nurses should monitor growth and development carefully to pick up on any motor, cognitive, or speech delays. In addition to general delays, the nurse should screen for autism during the toddler years. Signs of autism are typically evident in the second year of life. Screening should take place at 18 and 24 mo of age with a reliable and valid tool, such as the Modified Checklist for Autism in Toddlers (M-CHAT). (Refer to Chapter 33 for a more in-depth discussion about autism.) Behaviors associated with autism that are present during the second year of life include reduced response to name, abnormal communication, repetitive behaviors, abnormal visual attention, atypical emotional regulation, and reduced motor control (Zwaigenbaum et al., 2015). Early diagnosis and intervention lead to substantially improved growth and development outcomes. Nurses play a critical role in identifying signs of autism and helping families get the treatment needed to optimize their child's outcomes.

Table 16.4   Language Development Milestones in Toddlers

Age (mo)	Language Milestone
15	• Follows simple commands • Names a familiar object • Uses **jargon**
18	• Says single words • Shakes head no • Names two body parts • Names five objects
24	• Uses two-word sentences • Follows simple directions • Names five body parts • Points to pictures when named • Has a vocabulary of around 50 words
36	• Uses three-word sentences • Repeats a story from a book • Understands prepositions such as "over," "under," and "in" • Strangers can understand 75% of the child's speech. • Says name and age • Uses plurals

Adapted from Hagan, J. F., Shaw, J. S., & Duncan, P. (Eds.). (2017). *Bright futures: Guidelines for health supervision of infants, children, and adolescents* (4th ed.). Elk Grove Village, IL: American Academy of Pediatrics; and Centers for Disease Control. (2017). *Learn the signs. Act early. Developmental milestones.* Retrieved from https://www.cdc.gov/ncbddd/actearly/milestones/index.html

whole words rather than repetition of the first sound or syllable of the word (Coleman, 2016). If the child is exhibiting the latter form of stuttering, a speech evaluation is necessary.

During the toddler years, encourage parents to read to their child, as this can increase the child's vocabulary. Language development during this time helps set the child up for success in school (Norris, 2017). Toddlers exhibiting any speech delay should be further evaluated. Early identification of speech delay and referral to early intervention are crucial to maximizing communication skills.

Social and Emotional Development

During the toddler years, the child begins to understand the concept of self. Toddlers realize that they are separate from their parents. In the early period of this developmental stage, toddlers are not able to recognize emotions in others and do not understand the concept of sharing (American Academy of Pediatrics [AAP], 2015e). As a result of **egocentrism**, they may bite, hit, or poke a little too hard, not realizing they are hurting someone else. During this stage, encourage parents to tell the child "no" and redirect the child's behavior. By the time toddlers are 3 years of age, they begin to understand that their actions can hurt others and often show concern for others in distress.

Although toddlers are exerting newfound independence, they do not yet have many of the skills needed for safe exploration (AAP, 2015a). Common behaviors in toddlers that result from frustration include temper tantrums, biting, hitting, and sleeping issues (Hallas, Koslap-Petraco, & Fletcher, 2017).

Role modeling appropriate behaviors is important at this age. Toddlers imitate the behavior of others. They often feed a doll or a stuffed animal or give a doll a hug. When parents exhibit socially appropriate behavior, it sets an example for the toddler.

To help control some of these emotions and foster independence, encourage parents to give the toddler limited choices. For example, they should ask the child, "Do you want carrots or apples for snack?" Giving limited choices encourages independence while limiting frustration.

It is important to recognize the risk factors for emotional and behavioral problems. These risk factors include poverty, maternal depression, and exposure to toxic substances (Gleason, Goldman, & Yogman, 2016). Nurses should use systematic surveillance and screening to identify toddlers at risk for emotional and behavioral problems to start early treatment. Table 16.5 highlights expected social and emotional development milestones in toddlers.

Separation Anxiety

Toddlers may exhibit separation anxiety, although the anxiety does not typically last long after the parent is out of sight (AAP, 2015b). After infancy, separation anxiety may reemerge from 18 to 24 months of age (Hagan, Shaw, & Duncan, 2017). Keeping a consistent routine can help minimize separation anxiety for the toddler. If the toddler is in day care, dropping off and picking up at the same time each day can ease separation. Parents who are unable to have a consistent drop-off and pick-up time can create a goodbye ritual. This helps to comfort the toddler and convey that the parent is going to return. If the toddler is not in day care, it is important for the child to spend some time away from parents. Dropping the toddler off with grandparents or at a friend's house for a few hours helps the toddler become comfortable being away from his or her parents.

To help with anxiety, toddlers often have a security object, such as a blanket or toy (Fig. 16.8). These items are important for the child during times of separation, at bedtime, and during any unpleasant procedures such as immunizations. In addition, explaining to the toddler on his or her terms when the parent will return is important. Toddlers are not able to understand time. However, parents can explain to toddlers that they will return after naptime or after snack time. If the parent is going out of town, explaining to the toddler when he or she will return can be done in terms of the number of times the child goes to bed and wakes up, such as "mommy will be home after three sleeps" (AAP, 2015b). Younger toddlers will not be able to understand these terms, making the security object important. However, as the toddler nears the preschool years, he or she will understand these explanations. Similarly, if the toddler is in hospital, many of these techniques will work if the parent has to leave for a short period of time.

Age (mo)	Social or Emotional Milestone
15	• Hugs parents • Points to things he or she wants • May have a security object
18	• Looks at an adult if something new happens • May have temper tantrums • Begins to indicate when diapers are wet or soiled • Plays simple pretend games
24	• Imitates others • Likes to be with other children • Shows defiance • Shows more independence • Likes to talk about what is happening
36	• Eats independently • Begins to share • Separates easily from parents • Shows affection and concern

Table 16.5 Social and Emotional Development Milestones in Toddlers

Adapted from Hagan, J. F., Shaw, J. S., & Duncan, P. (Eds.). (2017). *Bright futures: Guidelines for health supervision of infants, children, and adolescents* (4th ed.). Elk Grove Village, IL: American Academy of Pediatrics; and Centers for Disease Control. (2017). *Learn the signs. Act early. Developmental milestones.* Retrieved from https://www.cdc.gov/ncbddd/actearly/milestones/index.html

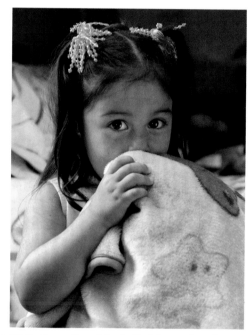

Figure 16.8. Security object. Toddlers often have a security object, such as a blanket, to help with separation anxiety. Reprinted with permission from Kyle, T., & Carman, S. (2016). *Essentials of pediatric nursing* (3rd ed., Fig. 4.5). Philadelphia, PA: Wolters Kluwer.

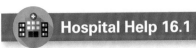

Hospital Help 16.1

Talking to Toddlers

Toddlers fear intrusive procedures and try to protect their bodies from being harmed. It is important for the nurse to understand how to talk to toddlers to help alleviate these fears. Before any procedures, allow the toddler to touch safe medical equipment to see that it is not harmful. Use positive words. When measuring blood pressure, tell the toddler you are "going to give his arm a hug." When inserting an intravenous catheter, tell the toddler you are "going to put a straw in her arm because she is too sick to drink." Although the child may still need to be held during some procedures, speaking in these terms may help elicit cooperation. Avoid phrases such as "take your blood" or "give you some dye" when explaining procedures, because these can frighten the toddler.

Fears

There is not a clear separation of self from body during the toddler period. As a result, the toddler may fear flushing stool down the toilet or fear bodily mutilation when undergoing intrusive procedures (Hospital Help 16.1). Other fears include new people and new places, such as day care centers. Helping the toddler ease into new situations a few hours at a time can help mitigate these fears. Toddlers may also be afraid of the dark. Having a nightlight in the toddler's room can help alleviate this fear and promote healthy sleep.

Temperament

The toddler's temperament determines how he or she reacts in different situations (refer to Chapter 15 for descriptions of different temperaments). The type of temperament exhibited during infancy continues during the toddler years. Some toddlers are easygoing, friendly, and do not seem to be overly anxious about new

situations. These types of toddlers easily regulate their eating and sleeping patterns. Some others may be passive and slow to warm up. These toddlers are quiet and more accepting of rules. However, they may take longer to mature because they tend to withdraw from social situations. The difficult toddler tends to be loud and fussy, pushing back against rules (Analyze the Evidence 16.2). These types of toddlers are generally highly reactive to changes in routine (Hagan et al., 2017). Toddlers with a difficult temperament respond well to structure. Deviation from the usual daily routines may result in temper tantrums.

Helping parents to understand their toddler's temperament allows the parents plan routines to minimize unwanted behaviors and promote positive ones. Explain to parents with a toddler who is slow to warm up that it will take a while for the child to become comfortable in new places and social situations. Encourage parents to keep exposing the toddler to novel places and to have patience when doing so. Parents of a child with a difficult temperament should pay particular attention to deviations in daily routines, especially in eating and nap times. Planning activities around routine eating and nap times may help minimize meltdowns.

Health Promotion

Nurses continue routine health promotion when children are seen for their well-child visits during the toddler years. Routine visits are conducted at 15 months, 18 months, 2 years, 2½ years, and 3 years of age (Hagan et al., 2017).

Promoting Healthy Growth and Development

Nurses play a critical role in promoting healthy growth and development of toddlers (Priority Care Concepts 16.1). Routine developmental surveillance allows for nurses to recognize developmental delays and refer toddlers for the interventions needed to promote optimal growth and development.

Nurses need to assess the growth and development of children with special healthcare needs as with any child. Determine where the child is developmentally and approach health promotion from the child's developmental stage, including such

Analyze the Evidence 16.2   Behavioral Problems in Children Living in Poverty

Holtz, Fox, and Meurer (2015) conducted a study investigating the frequency of behavior problems in children living below the federally identified poverty threshold. Children were from various ethnic groups, the primary caregivers were female, the amount of education of caregivers ranged from 8 to 18 y, and the family size ranged from one to eight children.

The researchers used two tools. The first was a demographic questionnaire. The second was the *Early Childhood Behavior Screen*. The screen is a 20-item self-report instrument developed for low-income toddlers and preschoolers.

The researchers concluded that there is a higher rate of challenging behavior in low-income families. This higher rate of behavioral problems is most likely due to a combination of family and environmental factors. Low-income children are not genetically predisposed to behavior problems. In addition, the researchers found differences in gender, with boys having a higher incidence of behavioral problems than girls.

This study reiterates the need to screen for and identify behavioral problems early to refer to treatment.

Priority Care Concepts 16.1

Promoting Growth and Development in Toddlers

Communication and Social Development
- Establishing daytime and nighttime routines
- Consistency in the toddler's environment
- Reading with the toddler

Sleep
- Bedtime routines
- Sleep through the night
- Daytime naps
- Parental knowledge

Oral Health
- Brushing teeth
- Dental visits

Safety
- Home environment
- Day care environment
- Parental knowledge

Nutrition
- Consistent meal times
- Healthy choices
- Limit sugars

The Pharmacy 16.1

Medications and Toddlers

Medications for toddlers usually come in a liquid form because toddlers are unable to swallow pills. It is important for parents to measure the correct amount of medication so as not to overdose or underdose the child. Regular silverware should not be used as a measuring device for liquid medications. Instruct parents to use a dropper, dosing spoon, or medicine cup.

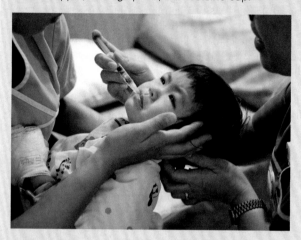

Many medicines have a palatable flavor for toddlers. However, some medications may have a bad taste. Having the child suck on a popsicle before and after taking the medication is one way to help relieve the unpleasant taste (AAP, 2015c).

Toddlers can be reluctant to take medications. Pretending to give medication to a doll or stuffed animal before the child can help elicit cooperation from the toddler.

activities as taking medicine (The Pharmacy 16.1). Help the parents understand how to promote growth and development based on the child's abilities, as well.

Be aware of and promote normal growth and development when interacting with toddlers in the hospital. Offer them books and toys when appropriate. Collaborate with child life specialists, who are often available as part of the healthcare team to provide developmentally appropriate activities to toddlers in the hospital.

No matter the developmental ability of the toddler or the healthcare environment, nurses need to evaluate the toddler's social determinants of health. What, if any, are the risk factors for the child? Understanding risk factors such as food insecurity, housing insecurity, or poor parental mental health allows the nurse to approach health promotion from the appropriate point of view and make referrals as necessary.

Safety

Understanding safety hazards for toddlers is imperative. As toddlers become more adept at exploring their environment, they are at greater risk for injury. Teaching parents about safety hazards can help them protect their toddlers and prevent unnecessary harm (Patient Teaching 16.1). Making sure electrical cords are out of the way, electrical outlets are covered, and windows are locked are important safety measures for the home. During

Patient Teaching 16.1

Safety in Toddlers

Burns
- Use the back burners when cooking on the stove.
- Keep the hot water heater set to no higher than 120°F (AAP, 2015f).
- Keep toddlers away from hot objects such as grills, ovens, and irons.

Falls
- Do not allow children to climb on furniture.
- Supervise children when they are going up and down stairs.
- Supervise children when they are on playground equipment.
- Have gates at the top and bottom of stairs.
- Have toddlers wear helmets as they learn to pedal a tricycle.

Poisoning (American Association of Poison Control Centers, n.d.)
- Keep all cleaning products out of reach; use cabinet locks if kept in low cabinets.
- Keep all medications out of reach.
- Have the number for poison control easily accessible.
- Keep plants off of the floor.
- Keep any alcohol or tobacco products out of reach.

Choking
- Avoid giving children foods that can cause choking:
  - Nuts
  - Hard candies
  - Hot dogs
  - Whole grapes
  - Marshmallows
- Supervise children while they are eating.
- Cut food into small bites.

Drowning
- Have a fence around backyard pools.
- Supervise children when they are around water.
- Have locks on toilet seat lids.
- Do not leave buckets of water around.

Firearm Safety
- Remove firearms from areas where children play and sleep.
- Lock all firearms in a cabinet.
- Make sure firearms are not loaded.

Motor Vehicle Safety
- Children can ride facing forward in a seat with a five-point harness (Fig. 16.9), but it is recommended to keep them rear facing until they are 2 y old (AAP, 2011).
- Children must remain in a forward-facing seat with a five-point harness until they are 4 y old.

the toddler years, parents should begin to teach their children to watch for cars as they are crossing the street and should place them in a forward-facing car seat when in the car (Fig. 16.9). Toddlers have impulsive behavior. Even the most watchful parents have toddlers who have accidents. Having safety measures in place helps minimize the risk of danger.

In Chapter 11, **Chase McGovern** was burned when he pulled a pot of boiling water off the stove. What was the situation that led to Chase's injury? Could anything have been done to prevent the injury? What teaching should nurses provide to help prevent this type of injury from happening?

Oral Health

Promoting oral health is important to healthy growth and development. Poor oral health leads to infections that can result in problems with speech, nutrition, and learning (Centers for Disease

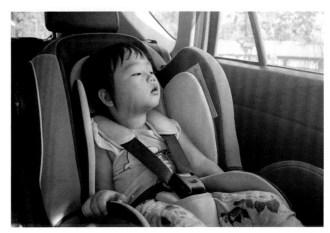

Figure 16.9. Car seat safety. Toddlers should be in a forward-facing car seat with a five-point harness.

Control [CDC], 2017). Teach parents how to prevent cavities and tooth decay. Parents should watch toddlers brush their teeth, helping as necessary (Fig. 16.10). Teach them to use a small, pea-sized amount of toothpaste on the toothbrush. Children younger than age 3 should only use a smear of fluoride containing toothpaste (CDC, 2017). Toddlers should have their first visit to the dentist around 1 year of age (Hagan et al., 2017).

Play

Play is an important part of the growth and development of children. At this age, toddlers engage in **parallel play**, playing alongside of one another but not playing with each other (Fig. 16.11).

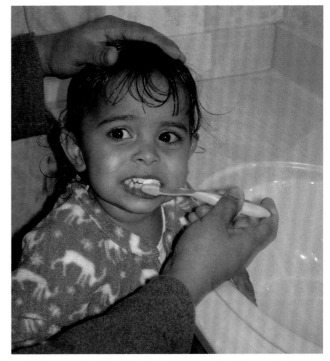

Figure 16.10. Brushing teeth. An adult should help the toddler brush his or her teeth to ensure a thorough cleaning. Reprinted with permission from Hatfield, N. T., & Kincheloe, C. (2017). *Introductory maternity and pediatric nursing* (4th ed., Fig. 24.5). Philadelphia, PA: Wolters Kluwer.

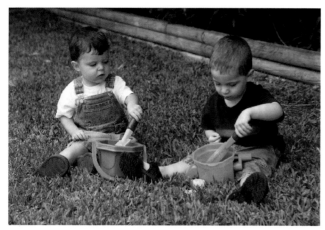

Figure 16.11. Parallel play. These toddlers are engaging in parallel play. They are playing with the same toys next to each other but not interacting with one another. Reprinted with permission from Hatfield, N. T., & Kincheloe, C. (2017). *Introductory maternity and pediatric nursing* (4th ed., Fig. 24.3). Philadelphia, PA: Wolters Kluwer.

Toddlers have a short attention span and frequently change the toy with which they are playing. Because toddlers are egocentric, they do not understand the concept of sharing (Piaget, 1930). In fact, toddlers often take a toy with which they wish to play from another child. By the end of the toddler period, children begin to understand the concept of sharing.

In Chapter 11, Chase McGovern's mother found it curious to see Chase engaging in parallel play with his cousins. What toy did they like to play with in this manner? What was Dr. Harper's comment about parallel play?

Playing with stacking blocks, push–pull toys, and dolls helps develop gross motor, fine motor, and social skills. In addition to playing with toys, toddlers like to listen to music and dance. Musical instruments are often favorite toys during this developmental stage. Teach parents about appropriate toys for toddlers, emphasizing that toys with small parts pose a risk of choking (Box 16.1). Active play is important as well. Playing outside promotes healthy growth and development and helps to prevent obesity (Fig. 16.12).

Encourage parents to participate in play with their toddlers, which encourages appropriate social interaction and promotes language skills, cognitive development, and school readiness (Manz & Bracaliello, 2016).

Sleep

Adequate sleep is necessary to promote growth, development, and cognitive functioning. Lack of sleep can lead to mood disturbances, poor behavior, irritability, and hyperactivity in the toddler (Owens, 2016). Toddlers need on average 11 to 13

Box 16.1   Age-Appropriate Toys for Toddlers

- Toys that can be pushed or pulled
- Tunnels to crawl through
- Household items such as wooden spoons and plastic containers
- Stackable blocks
- Large crayons or chalk
- Puzzles with large pieces
- Musical instruments
- Toys that can be manipulated, such as by putting the appropriate shape in the appropriate opening
- Dolls that have clothes with Velcro and large buttons that can be manipulated
- Bath toys such as rubber ducks

hours of sleep in a 24-hour period. On average, toddlers sleep around 9 hours at night and take two naps during the day until around 18 months of age. After 18 months, naps typically decrease to one 2- to 3-hour nap during the day, with nighttime sleep continuing to average 9 hours (Hagan et al., 2017).

Proper sleep hygiene encourages healthy sleep habits in toddlers. Bedtime routines help promote good sleep and decrease nighttime wakings (Bathory & Tomopoulos, 2017). Routines can include giving the child a warm bath and reading a bedtime story; watching television before bedtime, however, is not recommended. These daily routines signal to the toddler that it is time to transition from wakefulness to sleep. Toddlers should sleep in their own bed in a quiet, dark room. They should be adequately stimulated during the day to promote sleep. Naps should be spaced so that they are

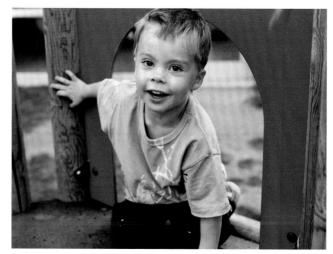

Figure 16.12. Outdoor play. Encourage toddlers to play outdoors to maintain a healthy weight and develop motor skills. Reprinted with permission from Ricci, S., Kyle, T., & Carman, S. (2016). *Maternity and pediatric nursing* (3rd ed., Fig. 26.8). Philadelphia, PA: Wolters Kluwer.

not too close to bedtime. Encourage parents to practice good sleep hygiene to avoid unwanted behaviors such as irritability and temper tantrums.

Discipline

A key to discipline is understanding the developmental age of the child. Toddlers are still unable to regularly incorporate rules into everyday life. Toddlers' inability to fully understand rules, coupled with their growing independence and propensity to explore, can often push parents to the edge. Often, what parents perceive as intentionally defiant behavior is really behavior resulting from the toddler's inability to understand what the parent is asking.

Discipline should be approached as teaching rather than as punishment. Rewarding good behavior and ignoring unwanted behaviors is an underlying principle of discipline for toddlers. Other recommendations for effective discipline include the following:

- Using developmentally appropriate approaches
- Emphasizing that the behavior is bad, not the child
- Being consistent
- Using nonphysical methods such as "time-out"

The toddler should never fear the parent as a result of discipline. In addition, physical forms of punishment such as spanking are not endorsed by the AAP (Hagan et al., 2017).

Parents should implement consistent discipline early. Once an unwanted behavior is allowed, it is difficult to reverse as the child grows older.

Immunizations

Immunizations continue to play an important role throughout the toddler years. The most up-to-date immunization chart is available at https://www.cdc.gov/vaccines/schedules/hcp/child-adolescent.html. Toddlers receive three vaccines that are not given to children younger than 12 months of age. These vaccines are measles, mumps, and rubella (MMR); varicella; and hepatitis A (Patient Teaching 16.2). Both the MMR and varicella vaccines are live attenuated vaccines (refer to Chapter 15). Side effects of these two vaccines include fever and rash. However, these side effects do not become apparent until 5 to 7 days after the vaccine is administered (Minor, 2015). Teach parents common side effects of the MMR, varicella, and hepatitis A vaccines, how to treat the side effects, and when to call the healthcare provider. Refer to Chapter 15 for nursing considerations, barriers, and reporting of adverse events associated with immunizations.

Nutrition

The eating habits of children change significantly during the toddler years. At 12 months of age, children are able to switch from formula or breast milk to cow's milk. The AAP recommends nonflavored whole milk until the age of 2 years (Hagan et al.,

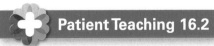

Patient Teaching 16.2

Immunizations for Toddlers

Immunizations

New immunizations that your child will receive during the toddler years include the following:

- MMR
  - The MMR vaccine protects against:
    - Measles, a respiratory disease that causes rash and fever with signs and symptoms of:
      - Cough, runny nose
      - Pinpoint red spots over the body
    - Mumps, a virus spread through coughing and sneezing with signs and symptoms of:
      - Headache
      - Muscle aches
      - Swollen glands in the neck and jaw
    - Rubella, a virus often referred to as "German measles" with signs and symptoms of:
      - Potentially, birth defects
      - Cough, runny nose
      - Rash over the body
  - Side effects of the vaccine may include the following:
    - Fever 5–7 d after administration
    - Rash resembling measles
    - Swelling at the injection site
    - Anaphylaxis (rare)
- Varicella
  - The varicella vaccine protects against the varicella virus, otherwise known as chickenpox, with signs and symptoms of:
    - Fever
    - Itchy rash with blisters
  - Side effects of the vaccine may include the following:
    - Soreness and swelling at the injection site
    - Fever 5–7 d after administration
    - Mild rash resembling chickenpox
- Hepatitis A
  - The hepatitis A vaccine protects against the liver disease hepatitis A with signs and symptoms of:
    - Stomach pain and vomiting
    - Fever
    - Yellow eyes
  - Side effects of the vaccine may include the following:
    - Soreness at the injection site
    - Fever
    - Headache

When to Call the Healthcare Provider

- If your child has a fever of 105°F (40.5°C) or higher
- If your child has a seizure
- If your child has uncontrollable crying for 3 h or longer
- If your child has an anaphylactic reaction

Adapted from the Centers for Disease Control and Prevention. (2017). *Disease and the vaccines that prevent them.* http://www.cdc.gov/vaccines/hcp/conversations/prevent-diseases/provider-resources-factsheets-infants.html

2017). If the child is overweight or there is a history of obesity in the family, 2% milk is recommended (AAP, 2018). Encourage parents to have the toddler drink milk from a cup rather than the bottle. Weaning from the bottle should be complete by the time the toddler is 15 months of age. Many mothers choose to breast-feed into the second year. Toddlers who are still breastfed should learn to drink from a cup by 15 months of age, as well.

After 2 years of age, both brain growth and physical growth slow down. Due to this slowdown in growth, toddlers have de-creased caloric requirements, leading to **physiological anorexia.** Older toddlers tend to become picky eaters, eating less than during infancy and the early toddler period. By the time a toddler reaches 3 years of age, **food jags** become common, which are times when the toddler only eats certain foods, such as apples and peanut butter. The toddler may be on a food jag for a few days and then suddenly refuse to eat the food anymore. Picky eating and food jags can be frustrating for parents. Teach parents that these are both normal phenomena during the toddler years and that it is important to continue to make mealtimes pleasant and offer a variety of healthy foods. Discourage parents from forcing children to finish their food. Toddlers typically eat what is neces-sary for their growth. If there is a concern about weight, either underweight or overweight, monitor the child's weight carefully.

Teach parents that early eating habits influence food choices, weight, and health later in life (Miles & Siega-Riz, 2017). Re-mind parents that, due to slowed growth, their child does not need a huge amount of intake. In general, the serving size for a toddler is about one-third that of an adult. Toddlers should have three meals and two snacks per day, totaling about 40 calories per inch of height (AAP, 2016). Snacks should include healthy foods such as fruit, vegetables, or yogurt. Educate parents on which foods to avoid in a healthy diet (Box 16.2). Caution par-ents on the amount of milk the child consumes. Sixteen to 24 oz of milk per day is adequate for toddlers. More than 24 oz of milk per day interferes with the toddler's appetite and increases the risk of iron-deficiency anemia (Hagan et al., 2017).

In Chapter 11, Chase McGovern's mother, Liz, indicated to Dr. Harper that Chase con-sumed an average of 36 oz of milk per day. Why was Dr. Harper concerned about the amount of milk? What teaching points did Dr. Harper give to Liz? Why does too much milk consump-tion place Chase at risk for iron-deficiency anemia?

Box 16.2 Foods to Avoid

- Candy
- Highly processed foods
- Fast food
- Sodas
- Other sugary drinks

Nurses play an important role, through education, in helping parents establish healthy eating patterns for toddlers. Nutrition education should focus on appropriate portion sizes, increas-ing vegetable consumption, and decreasing the consumption of sweetened beverages (Miles & Siega-Riz, 2017). To provide appropriate education, nurses should be aware of the barriers families may face in obtaining the appropriate healthy foods (Grossklaus & Marvicsin, 2014). In addition, understanding how culture influences food choices is important to providing proper education. Inquiring about staple foods in families of different cultures allows the nurse to incorporate these dietary preferences into an individualized nutrition plan.

Common Developmental Concerns

Parents often have concerns or questions about typical behaviors that occur during the toddler years. Toilet training and temper tantrums can be frustrating for parents. Regression is normal in new or stressful situations. Nurses play a role in educating parents about how to handle these behaviors.

Toilet Training

At around 2 years of age, many toddlers are ready to begin toilet training. This is the same time that myelination of the nerves in the brain is complete (Feigelman, 2016). However, the age at which children are cognitively ready to toilet train varies from 2 to 3 years. Signs that a toddler is ready to begin the process of toilet training include remaining dry for at least 2 hours at a time, having words for urine and stool, bringing a clean diaper to the parent to be changed (Fig. 16.13), and voicing discontent with having a soiled diaper (Hagan et al., 2017).

Positive reinforcement is the most effective way to teach a child to use the toilet. Toddlers generally feel more comfort-able using a potty chair (Fig. 16.14). Parents should reward

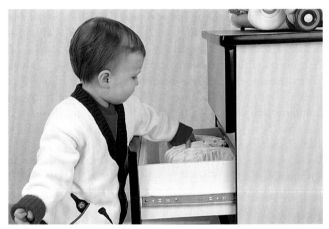

Figure 16.13. Toilet training readiness. Getting a diaper to be changed is one sign that a toddler is ready to begin the toilet training process. Reprinted with permission from Weber, J. R., & Kelley, J. H. (2017). *Health assessment in nursing* (6th ed., Fig. 31-5). Philadelphia, PA: Wolters Kluwer.

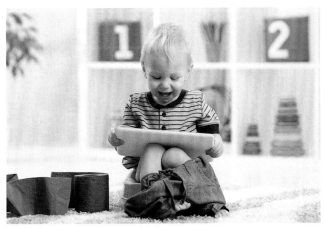

Figure 16.14. Toilet training. Toddlers feel more comfortable using a potty chair when toilet training.

their child for using the toilet with something such as a sticker chart. Toddlers may also enjoy the positive reinforcement of picking out "big kid" underwear. Punishing a child for having an accident is not effective and often deters the child from using the toilet.

Temper Tantrums

Because receptive language develops more rapidly than expressive language, toddlers have a hard time expressing their needs and wants. As a result, temper tantrums occur. Tantrums can begin as early as 12 months of age but typically occur from 2 to 3 years of age. Dealing with temper tantrums can be frustrating. Explain to parents that this is a normal developmental behavior.

The most effective way to address temper tantrums is to reward good behavior and ignore unwanted behavior. One exception to the rule is that biting and hitting should never be ignored but should be addressed by giving the child a time-out. Finally, remind parents of the importance of routine for toddlers. Disruption in routine, such as missing a nap, often leads to temper tantrums (Swanson, 2015; Daniels, Mandleco, & Luthy, 2012).

In Chapter 5, Maalik Abdella threw temper tantrums daily, which frustrated and concerned his mother. What behaviors did Maalik exhibit during his tantrums? What did Dr. Peterman tell his mother to do in response to these tantrums?

Regression

Regression is the loss of acquired developmental skills due to stress, change in routine, or major illness. Common causes of regression in toddlers include a new sibling, a new day care, a new home, or hospitalization (AAP, 2015). Regression can

manifest as different behaviors. Toddlers who are toilet trained may begin having accidents. Other behaviors include wanting a bottle or a pacifier after the toddler is weaned.

For toddlers exhibiting regressive behaviors, parents should determine the cause of the behavior. Encourage parents to sympathize with their child, telling the child that they understand that change is hard, and to maintain routines as much as possible with change or new situations. Parents should give the child clear expectations about behavior and use positive reinforcements to support toddlers through stressful situations (AAP, 2015).

In Chapter 5, Maalik Abdella exhibited regression while he was in the hospital. What behaviors did he exhibit? Why did he exhibit these behaviors? What advice did the nurse give Maalik's mother? Was this good advice? Should the nurse have done something different?

Media

Media use should continue to be limited during the toddler years. Children under 18 months of age should not watch television or digital media. For children 18 months or older, parents should limit screen time to 1 hour/day (Hagan et al., 2017). For these older toddlers, encourage parents to watch programming with the children to determine its quality. Video chats with family are a healthy way for parents to introduce digital media to toddlers. Educate parents about appropriate media use and remind them that toddlers learn best from interaction with parents and family members, such as being read to and being played with (Fig. 16.15).

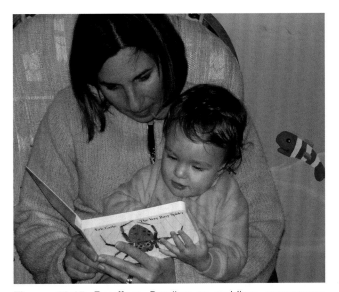

Figure 16.15. Reading. Reading to toddlers encourages learning and social interaction. Reprinted with permission from Kyle, T., & Carman, S. (2016). *Essentials of pediatric nursing* (3rd ed., Fig. 4.9). Philadelphia, PA: Wolters Kluwer.

Health Problems of Toddlers

A few illnesses are common mainly during the toddler years. Although older children may be prone to atopic dermatitis, common colds, and ear infections, these are generally first seen in toddlers.

Atopic Dermatitis

Atopic dermatitis, also known as eczema, is the most common chronic skin condition in children. Atopic dermatitis is one of several atopic diseases, including allergic rhinitis and asthma. Infants and toddlers with persistent atopic dermatitis are more likely to develop asthma later in childhood (Lowe et al., 2017). In addition, children diagnosed with eczema by 12 months of age are six times more likely to have egg allergy and 11 times more likely to have peanut allergy than children without eczema (Martin, Eckert, & Koplin, 2014).

Nursing Assessment

Atopic dermatitis is associated with immunoglobulin E sensitization (Leung & Sicherer, 2016). The hallmark symptom is severely dry skin. Other clinical manifestations include erythematous patches, with or without papules, and extreme pruritus (Fig. 16.16). Chronic atopic dermatitis leads to lichenification, or thickening of the skin, especially in skin folds (Fig. 16.17). Toddlers with chronic atopic dermatitis are at risk of infection in skin lesions due to skin breakdown from intense scratching.

Inspect for dry, scaly patches, especially in the skin folds of the elbows and the back of the knees. Document any erythematous papules or excoriated area. Assess for signs and symptoms of infection of lesions, such as purulent drainage, foul odor, or fever.

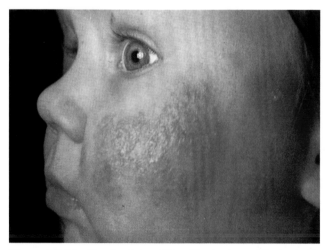

Figure 16.16. Atopic dermatitis. Atopic dermatitis typically manifests as dry erythematous patches that may or may not contain papules. Reprinted with permission from Kyle, T., & Carman, S. (2012). *Essentials of pediatric nursing* (2nd ed., Fig. 24.11). Philadelphia, PA: Wolters Kluwer Health/Lippincott Williams & Wilkins.

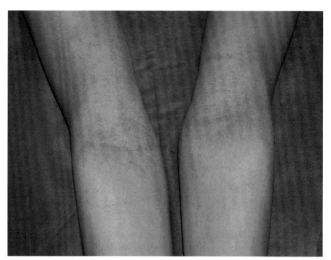

Figure 16.17. Lichenification. Thickening of the skin in the folds of the elbows from chronic atopic dermatitis. Reprinted with permission from Hall, J. C., & Hall, B. J. (2017). *Sauer's manual of skin diseases* (11th ed., Fig. 8.10). Philadelphia, PA: Wolters Kluwer.

Treatment

Prevention of atopic dermatitis begins with identifying the child's triggers and working to avoid them. Triggers may include foods, pets, soaps, dust mites, or extreme temperatures. Keeping the skin hydrated is also important in preventing outbreaks of atopic dermatitis. Applying a thick moisturizing cream or ointment after a warm bath helps the skin retain moisture. Caution parents to not make bath water too hot, as the heat may exacerbate the condition.

The main treatment for atopic dermatitis is topical corticosteroids (The Pharmacy 16.2), which are available in various strengths and as either creams or ointments (Leung & Sicherer, 2016). Although topical, these corticosteroids can have local and systemic effects. Thinning of the skin is a local adverse effect of chronic topical corticosteroid use. Adrenal suppression is a systemic effect and is generally only seen with chronic use

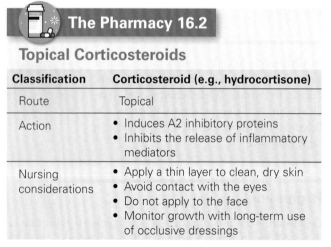

The Pharmacy 16.2

Topical Corticosteroids

Classification	Corticosteroid (e.g., hydrocortisone)
Route	Topical
Action	• Induces A2 inhibitory proteins • Inhibits the release of inflammatory mediators
Nursing considerations	• Apply a thin layer to clean, dry skin • Avoid contact with the eyes • Do not apply to the face • Monitor growth with long-term use of occlusive dressings

Adapted from Taketomo, C. K., Hodding, J. H., & Kraus, D. M. (2018). *Pediatric & neonatal dosage handbook* (25th ed.). Hudson, OH: Lexicomp.

of high-potency topical corticosteroids. High-potency topical corticosteroids should not be applied to the face. Educate parents on how to apply the creams and ointments safely to avoid adverse effects.

Common Cold

The common cold, or nasopharyngitis, is a common viral infection in childhood. Toddlers, especially those in day care, may have six to seven colds per year. The most common cause of the common cold is rhinovirus (Faschner, Ericson, & Werner, 2012). Other causes include parainfluenza virus, adenovirus, enterovirus, and human metapneumovirus. These viruses are concentrated in nasopharyngeal secretions. Viruses are spread via droplets through the process of sneezing and coughing. Colds are self-limiting and usually last 10 to 14 days.

Nursing Assessment

Symptoms of the common cold include rhinorrhea, cough, pharyngitis, nasal congestion, and fever. Assess for sore throat and enlarged turbinates. Any cough is generally nonproductive. Assess nasal drainage to determine whether it is clear or purulent, because either may be present with a cold. Although purulent nasal drainage does not necessarily indicate a bacterial infection, a toddler with purulent drainage that persists past 2 weeks should be evaluated for bacterial infection.

Treatment

Treatment of the common cold consists mainly of promoting comfort. Toddlers have a difficult time blowing their nose. Administration of saline nasal drops followed by suctioning with a bulb syringe can help alleviate nasal congestion. Use of cool mist humidifiers at night may also alleviate nasal congestion. Educate parents to clean humidifiers routinely to prevent the buildup of mold.

The efficacy of over-the-counter cough and cold medicines has not been adequately studied in children under the age of 6 years.

Therefore, the AAP recommends not giving these medications to children under this age (Lowry & Leeder, 2015). Furthermore, single-ingredient cough and cold formulations have the most reported overdoses in children younger than age 4 (Green et al., 2017). Educating parents of toddlers regarding the use of cough and cold medications is paramount to keeping toddlers safe. Because the common cold is a viral infection, antibiotics are not effective in treating it. Remind parents that the common cold is self-limiting and that comfort measures are the best modes of treatment. Finally, educate parents on preventing the spread of viruses that cause the common cold. Helping toddlers wash their hands thoroughly is the best way to prevent the spread.

Acute Otitis Media

Acute otitis media (AOM), otherwise known as an ear infection, is the most common reason for visits to healthcare providers in the first years of a child's life. Eighty percent of children have at least one episode of AOM by the time they are 3 years old (Kerschner & Preciado, 2016). The earlier the onset of the first episode of AOM, the higher the likelihood of a child having recurrent episodes.

Inflammation of the middle ear and middle ear **effusion** are the hallmark characteristics of AOM. With an acute infection, the fluid in the middle ear is purulent, causing the tympanic membrane to appear erythematous, bulging, and yellow (Fig. 16.18). Toddlers with recurrent AOM are at risk for speech delay because of the fluid in the middle ear. Fluid in the middle ear interferes with hearing, which, in turn, interferes with speech development.

Exposure to tobacco smoke correlates with an increased incidence of AOM (Csákányi, Czinner, Spangler, Rogers, & Katon, 2012; Kerschner & Preciado, 2016). Other risk factors for AOM include exposure to other children, such as in day cares, as well as congenital anomalies.

Protective factors against AOM, which are factors that decrease the incidence or risk of infection, include breastfeeding

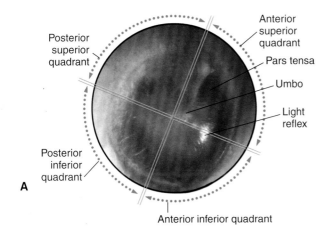
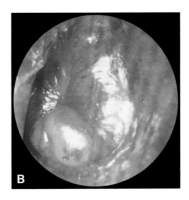

Figure 16.18. Acute otitis media. A. A normal tympanic membrane with light reflex visible. **B.** An erythematous, bulging tympanic membrane of AOM with no visible light reflex. Part A reprinted with permission from the Middle Ear Conditions ACC chart. Part B reprinted with permission from Moore, K. L., & Dalley, A. F., II. (1999). *Clinically oriented anatomy* (4th ed.). Baltimore, MD: Lippincott Williams & Wilkins.

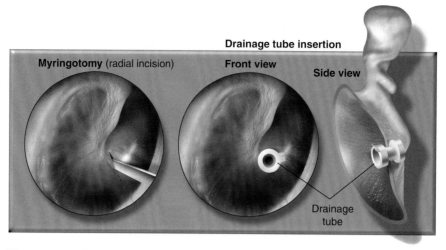

Figure 16.19. Myringotomy with pressure-equalizing tubes. Pressure-equalizing tubes inserted into the myringotomy incision to prevent buildup of fluid in the middle ear. Reprinted with permission from the Middle Ear Conditions ACC chart.

(Boone, Geraghty, & Keim, 2016) and vaccination with the pneumococcal vaccine (Wasserman & Gerber, 2017).

Nursing Assessment

AOM infections are generally accompanied by signs and symptoms of the common cold. Assess the toddler for rhinorrhea, fever, and irritability. Toddlers are not able to describe or quantify pain; therefore, symptoms such as irritability or decreased appetite may be the only indicators of pain.

If inspecting the tympanic membrane, pull the pinna down and back. Note the presence or absence of the light reflex. Assess the color of the tympanic membrane. Document whether the tympanic membrane is bulging.

Treatment

AOM is caused by several different strains of bacteria. Antibiotics are used to treat the infection. Educate parents that the toddler must finish the entire course of antibiotics, even if the child is feeling better. If there is no improvement after the course of antibiotics, the toddler should be reevaluated.

Comfort measures during an episode of AOM focus on pain relief. Acetaminophen or ibuprofen is given for fever reduction and pain relief. Warm olive oil drops in the affected ear may also help with pain relief.

For toddlers with recurrent AOM, a myringotomy may be performed. This is an outpatient procedure in which a small incision is made in the tympanic membrane to alleviate pressure and allow drainage of purulent fluid from the middle ear (Fig. 16.19). Small pressure-equalizing (PE) tubes are placed in the ear to help prevent future buildup of middle ear fluid.

Otitis Media With Effusion

After treatment for AOM, clear fluid may remain in the middle ear. Although otitis media with effusion (OME) is not an infection, it can have adverse effects for the toddler. Speech development is likely to be delayed in toddlers with OME. The persistent fluid in the ear interferes with the child's hearing, which then affects the child's speech development. Children with persistent OME are treated with a myringotomy and PE tubes.

Think Critically

1. Why is it important to monitor growth and development in toddlers?
2. What delays are of concern for autism? What is the nurse's role once these delays are discovered?
3. What are the most important components of anticipatory guidance during the toddler years?
4. Develop a plan for optimal nutrition during the toddler years. How does nutrition during these early years contribute to health later in life?
5. Create a teaching plan for a parent who is approaching toilet training a child for the first time.
6. Develop a nursing care plan for a toddler with severe atopic dermatitis whose triggers are house mites and cats.
7. What type of education is needed for a toddler with recurrent AOM?

References

American Academy of Pediatrics. (2011). Policy statement: Child passenger safety. *Pediatrics, 127*(4). Retrieved from www.pediatrics.org/cgi/doi/10.1542/peds.2011-0213

American Academy of Pediatrics. (2015a). *Emotional development: 2 year olds.* Retrieved from https://www.healthychildren.org/English/ages-stages/toddler/Pages/Emotional-Development-2-Year-Olds.aspx

American Academy of Pediatrics. (2015b). *How to ease your child's separation anxiety.* Retrieved from https://www.healthychildren.org/English/ages-stages/toddler/Pages/Soothing-Your-Childs-Separation-Anxiety.aspx

American Academy of Pediatrics. (2015c). *Medication safety tips.* Retrieved from https://www.healthychildren.org/English/safety-prevention/at-home/medication-safety/Pages/Medication-Safety-Tips.aspx

American Academy of Pediatrics. (2015d). *Regression.* Retrieved from https://www.healthychildren.org/English/ages-stages/toddler/toilet-training/Pages/Regression.aspx

American Academy of Pediatrics. (2015e). *Social development: 1 year olds.* Retrieved from https://www.healthychildren.org/English/ages-stages/toddler/Pages/Social-Development-1-Year-Olds.aspx

American Academy of Pediatrics. (2015f). *Safety for your child: 2 to 4 years.* Retrieved from https://www.healthychildren.org/English/ages-stages/toddler/Pages/Safety-for-Your-Child-2-to-4-Years.aspx

American Academy of Pediatrics. (2016). *Serving sizes for toddlers.* Retrieved from https://www.healthychildren.org/English/ages-stages/toddler/nutrition/Pages/Serving-Sizes-for-Toddlers.aspx

American Academy of Pediatrics. (2018). *Why formula instead of cow's milk?* Retrieved from https://www.healthychildren.org/English/ages-stages/baby/formula-feeding/Pages/Why-Formula-Instead-of-Cows-Milk.aspx

American Association of Poison Control Centers. (n.d.). *In the home.* Retrieved from http://www.aapcc.org/prevention/home

Baldwin, K. D., Wells, L., & Dorman, J. P. (2016). Bone and joint disorders: Growth and development. In R. M. Kliegman, B. F. Stanton, J. W. St. Geme III, N. F. Schor, & R. E. Behrman (Eds.), *Nelson's Textbook of Pediatrics* (20th ed.). Philadelphia, PA: Elsevier, Saunders.

Bathory, E., & Tomopoulos, S. (2017). Sleep regulation, physiology and development, sleep duration and patterns, and sleep hygiene in infants, toddlers, and preschool-age children. *Current Problems in Pediatric and Adolescent Health Care, 47*(2), 29–42.

Boone, K. M., Geraghty, S. R., & Keim, S. A. (2016). Feeding at the breast and expressed milk feeding: Associations with otitis media and diarrhea in infants. *The Journal of Pediatrics, 174,* 118–125.

Centers for Disease Control. (2017). *Learn the signs. Act early. Developmental milestones.* Retrieved from https://www.cdc.gov/ncbddd/actearly/milestones/index.html

Christensen, R. D., & Ohls, R. K. (2016). Development of the hematopoietic system. In R. M. Kliegman, B. F. Stanton, J. W. St. Geme III, N. F. Schor, & R. E. Behrman (Eds.), *Nelson's textbook of pediatrics* (20th ed.). Philadelphia, PA: Elsevier, Saunders.

Coleman, C. (2016). *Stuttering in toddlers and preschoolers: What's typical and what's not?* Retrieved from https://www.healthychildren.org/English/ages-stages/toddler/Pages/Stuttering-in-Toddlers-Preschoolers.aspx

Csákányi, Z., Czinner, A., Spangler, J., Rogers, T., & Katon, G. (2012). Relationship of environmental tobacco smoke to otitis media (OM) in children. *International Journal of Pediatric Otorhinolaryngology, 76*(7), 989–983.

Daniels, E., Mandleco, B., & Luthy, K. E. (2012). Assessment, management, and prevention of childhood temper tantrums. *Journal of the American Academy of Nurse Practitioners, 24*(10), 569–573.

Erikson, E. H. (1963). *Childhood and society.* New York, NY: W.W. Norton and Company.

Faschner, J., Ericson, K., & Werner, S. (2012). Treatment of the common cold in children and adults. *American Family Physician, 86*(2), 153–159.

Feigelman, S. (2016). The second year. In R. M. Kliegman, B. F. Stanton, J. W. St. Geme III, N. F. Schor, & R. E. Behrman (Eds.), *Nelson's textbook of pediatrics* (20th ed.). Philadelphia, PA: Elsevier, Saunders.

Gleason, M. M., Goldson, E., & Yogman, M. W.; Council on Early Childhood. (2016). Addressing early childhood emotional and behavioral problems. *Pediatrics, 138*(6), e20163025.

Gomez, R. J., Barrowmen, M., Elia, S., Manias, E., Royale, J., & Harrison, D. (2013). Establishing intra- and inter-rater agreement of the Face, Legs, Activity, Cry, Consolability scale for evaluating pain in toddlers during immunization. *Pain Research and Management, 18*(6), e124–e128.

Green, J. L., Wang, G. S., Reynolds, K. M., Banner, W., Bond, R., Kaufmann, R. E. ... Dart, R. C. (2017). Safety profile of cough and cold medication use in pediatrics. *Pediatrics, 139*(6), e20163070.

Grossklaus, H. & Marvicsin, D. (2014). Parenting efficacy and it's relationship to childhood obesity. *Pediatric Nursing, 40*(2), 69–86.

Hagan, J. F., Shaw, J. S., & Duncan, P. (Eds.). (2017). *Bright futures: Guidelines for health supervision of infants, children, and adolescents* (4th ed.). Elk Grove Village, IL: American Academy of Pediatrics.

Hallas, D., Koslap-Petraco, M., & Fletcher, J. (2017). Social-emotional development of toddlers: Randomized controlled trial of an office-based intervention. *Journal of Pediatric Nursing, 33,* 33–40.

Holtz, C. A., Fox, R. A., & Meurer, J. R. (2015). Incidence of behavior problems in toddlers and preschool children from families living in poverty. *The Journal of Psychology, 149*(2), 161–174.

Kerschner, J. E., & Preciado, D. (2016). Otitis media. In R. M. Kliegman, B. F. Stanton, J. W. St. Geme III, N. F. Schor, & R. E. Behrman (Eds.), *Nelson's textbook of pediatrics* (20th ed.). Philadelphia, PA: Elsevier, Saunders.

Kohlberg, L. (1981). *The philosophy of moral development.* New York, NY: Harper & Row.

Leung, D. Y. M., & Sicherer, S. H. (2016). Atopic dermatitis. In R. M. Kliegman, B. F. Stanton, J. W. St. Geme III, N. F. Schor, & R. E. Behrman (Eds.), *Nelson's textbook of pediatrics* (20th ed.). Philadelphia, PA: Elsevier, Saunders.

Lowe, A. J., Angelica, B., Su, J., Lodge, C. J., Hill, D. J., Erbas, B., ... Dharmage, S. C. (2017). Age at onset and persistence of eczema are related to subsequent risk of asthma and hay fever from birth to 18 years of age. *Pediatric Allergy and Immunology, 28,* 384–390.

Lowery, J. A., & Leeder, J. S. (2015). Over-the-counter medications: Update on cough and cold preparations. *Pediatrics in Review, 36*(7), 286–298.

Manz, P. H., & Bracaliello, C. B. (2016). Expanding home visiting outcomes: Collaborative measurement of parental play beliefs and examination of their association with parents' involvement in toddler's learning. *Early Childhood Research Quarterly, 36,* 157–167.

Marrowen, R. C., & Stinson, J. (2016). Pediatric pain measurement, assessment, and evaluation. *Seminars in Pediatric Neurology, 23,* 189–200.

Martin, P. E., Eckert, J. K., & Koplin, J. J. (2014). Which infants with eczema are at risk for food allergy? Results from a population-based cohort. *Clinical and Experimental Allergy, 45*(1), 255–265.

Merkel, S. I., Voepel-Lewis, T., Shayevitz, J. R., & Malviya, S. (1997). The FLACC: A behavioral scale for scoring postoperative pain in young children. *Pediatric Nursing, 23*(3), 293–297.

Miles, G., & Siega-Riz, A. M. (2017). Trends in food and beverage consumption among infants and toddlers: 2005–2012. *Pediatrics, 139*(6), e20163290.

Minor, P. D. (2015). Live attenuated vaccines: Historical successes and current challenges. *Virology, 479–480,* 379–392.

Norris, D. J. (2017). Comparing language and literacy environments in two types of infant-toddler childcare centers. *Journal of Early Childhood Education, 45,* 95–101.

Owens, J. A. (2016). Sleep medicine. In R. M. Kliegman, B. F. Stanton, J. W. St. Geme III, N. F. Schor, & R. E. Behrman (Eds.), *Nelson's textbook of pediatrics* (20th ed.). Philadelphia, PA: Elsevier, Saunders.

Piaget, J. (1930). *The child's conception of physical causality.* London, England: Routledge & Kegan Paul LTD.

Stiegler, L. N. (2015). Examining the echolalia literature: Where do speech-language pathologists stand? *American Journal of Speech-Language Pathology, 24,* 750–762.

Swanson, W. S. (2015). *Top tips for surviving temper tantrums.* Retrieved from https://www.healthychildren.org/English/family-life/family-dynamics/communication-discipline/pages/Temper-Tantrums.aspx

Wasserman, R. C., & Gerber, J. S. (2017). Acute otitis media in the 21st century: What now? *Pediatrics, 140*(3), e20171966.

Ygberg, S., & Nilson, A. (2017). The developing immune system: From foetus to toddler. *Acta Paediatrica, 101,* 120–127. doi:10.1111/j.1651-2227.2011.02494.x

Zwaigenbaum, L., Bauman, M. L., Fein, D., Pierce, K., Buie, T., Davis, P. A., ... Wagner, S. (2015). Early screening of autism spectrum disorder: Recommendations for practice and research. *Pediatrics, 136*(Suppl. 1), S41–S59.

Suggested Reading

American Academy of Pediatrics. (2016). *If autism is suspected, what's next?* Retrieved from https://www.healthychildren.org/English/health-issues/conditions/Autism/Pages/If-Autism-is-Suspected-Whats-Next.aspx

Green, J. L., Wang, G. S., Reynolds, K. M., Banner, W., Bond, R., Kaufmann, R. E., ... Dart, R. C. (2017). Safety profile of cough and cold medication use in pediatrics. *Pediatrics, 139*(6), e20163070.

Holtz, C. A., Fox, R. A., & Meurer, J. R. (2015). Incidence of behavior problems in toddlers and preschool children from families living in poverty. *The Journal of Psychology, 149*(2), 161–174.

17 Care of the Preschooler

Objectives

After completing this chapter, you will be able to:
1. Discuss normal growth and development in preschoolers.
2. Describe the physical assessment of preschoolers.
3. Explain the development of gross and fine motor coordination and language milestones during the preschool years.
4. Relate nutrition during the preschool years to obesity.
5. Choose appropriate teaching topics for parents of preschoolers.
6. Develop a health promotion plan for preschoolers.
7. Identify common health problems during the preschool years.

Key Terms

Intuitive thinking
Irreversibility
Magical thinking
Otoacoustic emissions

Preoperational thought
Prodromal
Transductive reasoning

Growth and Development Overview

The preschool period is from 3 to 6 years of age. During the preschool years, gross motor skills become more coordinated. The awkward gait and clumsiness of toddlerhood disappear as the preschooler becomes slenderer. Fine motor skills develop at an exponential pace during the preschool years, as preschoolers learn to use a pair of scissors, draw, and dress themselves. During this period, preschoolers are learning to take the initiative to try new things. This is also a time of magical thinking, imagination, and creative play.

Health Assessment

When assessing preschoolers, continue to involve the parents and caregivers in taking the health history. Parents give insight into the preschooler's growth and development. Ask parents whether they have any concerns about the child's motor skills, language development, or social development. The preschooler can be involved in the health history, as well. Asking simple questions or asking for a demonstration of the preschooler's skills encourages participation and cooperation in the health assessment.

Preschoolers begin to think of themselves as "big kids." Therefore, during the physical assessment, give the preschooler a choice of sitting on the parent's lap or sitting on the exam table. Continue to give choices throughout the exam, such as asking, "Do you want me to look in your ears first or your mouth first?" Presenting choices gives the preschooler some control, which helps illicit cooperation during the exam. Allow the preschooler to play with safe medical equipment, such as touching the light on an otoscope, to see that the equipment is not painful (Fig. 17.1). During the exam, discuss likes and dislikes with the child. This discussion not only helps distract the preschooler but makes him or her feel more comfortable. Perform the most invasive assessments last. These assessments include the ears, mouth, and genitalia.

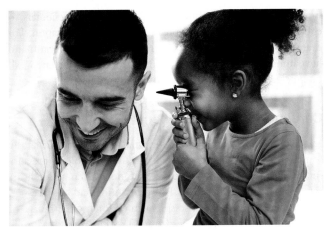

Figure 17.1. Preschool physical assessment. Allowing the preschooler to play with the medical equipment helps calm the child for the physical assessment.

Head, Eyes, Ears, Nose, and Throat

Ask the parents whether they have any concerns regarding the child's vision, hearing, or speech. Does the child have a history of recurrent ear infections? Does the child have pressure-equalizing tubes? Is there a history of eye infections? Does the child have a history of head injury? Has the child had any cavities? Has the child seen the dentist? Ask about recurrent pharyngitis, history of large tonsils, or difficulty swallowing.

Head

Inspect the head for shape and size. Test cranial nerve VII by asking the child to smile, stick out his or her tongue, and puff out his or her cheeks. Palpate the skull for symmetry. Palpate the lymph nodes of the head and neck, noting size, consistency, and mobility.

Eyes

Inspect the eyes for symmetry. Note the color of the sclera and conjunctiva. Assess that the pupils are equal, round, and reactive to light and assessment. Test cranial nerves III and IV by having the child perform extraocular movements. Preschoolers are more likely to cooperate with performing extraocular movements when asked to follow an interesting object such as a small toy. Older preschoolers, around age 5 years, are able to cooperate in the exam such as when asked to cover one eye in the cover/uncover test to assess for strabismus.

Preschoolers are able to cooperate with visual acuity testing between the ages of 4-5 years. Use a kindergarten test chart until the child is able to recognize letters (Fig. 17.2). Visual acuity reaches 20/20 between the ages of 4-5 years. (Feigelman, 2016).

In Chapter 6, Abigail Hanson had her vision assessed at her 4-year-old well-child visit. What tool did the medical assistant use to assess her visual acuity? What was the result of the assessment? Why was Abigail's mother, Lucy, concerned about the way the assessment proceeded? What did the nurse practitioner, Kevin, tell Lucy to address this concern?

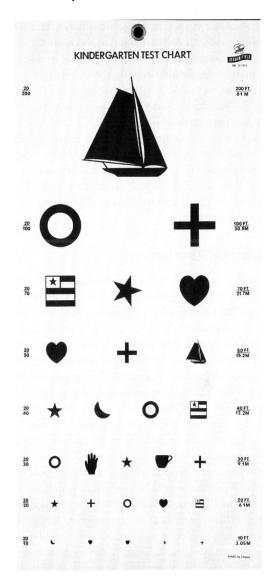

Figure 17.2. Snellen preschool chart. A Snellen chart appropriate for kindergarten children who are not yet able to read but can follow directions. Reprinted with permission from Kronenberger, J. (2016). *Lippincott Williams & Wilkins' clinical medical assisting* (5th ed., Fig. 15.7). Philadelphia, PA: Wolters Kluwer.

Ears

Assess the symmetry and placement of the ears. Note any redness or drainage. Palpate for swelling or tenderness. Assess hearing by performing an **otoacoustic emissions** test. If inner ear inspection is indicated, pull the pinna up and back, beginning at age 3 years.

Nose

Assess the nose for symmetry. Note any rhinorrhea or drainage. Inspect the turbinates by gently tilting the child's head back and inserting the otoscope into the nare. Note the color of the turbinates and the presence of any swelling.

Mouth and Throat

Inspect the lips for color, symmetry, and lesions. The buccal mucosa should be pink and moist, without lesions or swelling.

Assess cranial nerve XII, the hypoglossal nerve, by having the preschooler touch his or her tongue to the roof of the mouth and stick out the tongue and move it from side to side.

The preschooler should have 20 primary teeth by the age of 3 years. Assess for visible dental caries. Note any foul-smelling odor on the breath. The older preschooler, around age 6 years, may have lost one or two front teeth.

Inspect the throat, noting the size of the tonsils and the presence of exudate or erythema. Ask the preschooler to open his or her mouth and say "ahh." You do not need to use a tongue depressor if the child is cooperative. If the preschooler is not cooperating, ask the parents to hold the child during inspection of the mouth and throat.

Neurological Assessment

Brain growth slows during the preschool years. From 3 to 18 years of age, the head grows only 1.9 to 2.4 in (5 to 6 cm; Feigelman, 2016). However, preschoolers experience dramatic changes in the brain, including increased metabolic demand.

The neurological assessment during the preschool years includes assessment of sensory function, coordination, gait, balance, and development. Because of the increase in cognitive skills, more formal assessment tests can be performed. If there are any concerns about development, an in-depth developmental screening should be performed using a validated tool.

Ask the parents whether the child has had any trouble with balance or falling. Have they noticed any difficulties with speech? Is there any change in muscle strength or loss of motor skills?

Preschool children should be oriented to person. By the end of the preschool period, the child should be oriented to place. Ask the child his or her name and, if appropriate, where he or she is. Observe the preschooler walking, jumping, and hopping on one foot to assess gait and balance. To test for sensory function, have the child close his or her eyes. Touch the child in different places and have the child point to these places. The preschool child should also be able to perform the finger-to-finger test.

To further assess development, ask the child to draw a person. At 4 years of age, the child should be able to draw a person with three body parts. At 5 years of age, the child should be able to draw a person with six body parts. Preschoolers can also draw shapes such as circles, squares, and rectangles. Long-term memory develops at 4 years of age. Determine whether the preschooler knows his or her address or phone number.

Respiratory Assessment

The diaphragm remains the primary muscle for breathing until the age of 5 years, at which time the thoracic muscles take over. The number of alveoli is not yet at adult levels, keeping the preschooler at increased risk for respiratory distress.

Ask the parents whether the child has a history of coughing, wheezing, or noisy breathing. Assess the preschooler's respiratory effort. Until the age of 5 years, observe the abdomen for respiratory rate. The chest and abdomen should rise and fall simultaneously. The preschooler's respiratory rate ranges from 20 to 28 breaths/min. Observe for use of accessory muscles, indicating increased work of breathing. Play games with preschoolers to elicit cooperation with deep breathing during auscultation. For example, hold an index finger in front of the child's mouth and have him or her pretend to blow out a candle. Auscultate in all lung fields, noting any adventitious lung sounds.

Cardiovascular Assessment

In the preschooler, the point of maximal impulse remains at the fourth intercostal space, midclavicular line. The blood pressure increases and heart rate decreases. The normal range for heart rate in preschoolers is 80 to 120 beats/min. Radial pulses are acceptable for heart rate assessment in children over the age of 3 years. Blood pressure ranges from 89 to 112 mm Hg systolic and 46 to 72 mm Hg diastolic. At 3 years of age, begin routine measurement of blood pressure at well-child exams.

Inquire about the preschooler's color. Does the child ever appear pale or cyanotic? Ask parents whether the preschooler tires easily. Does the child have a history of a congenital heart defect? Assess pulses and note any difference between upper and lower extremities. Assess capillary refill in all four extremities. Auscultate for murmurs and document appropriately.

Gastrointestinal Assessment

The small intestine continues to grow in the early preschool years and reaches the adult length of 450 to 550 cm by 4 years of age (Liacouras, 2016). The child generally achieves bowel control by then. Preschoolers generally have one or two bowel movements a day.

For the gastrointestinal assessment, ask the parents whether the child has a history of diarrhea or constipation. Inquire about stool holding. As young preschoolers gain bowel control, they sometimes try to exhibit control over the toilet training process through stool holding. Signs include stool smears in the underwear, hard and dry stools, avoiding bowel movements on the toilet, and long periods between bowel movements.

Inspect the abdomen for symmetry and umbilical hernias. Auscultate for bowel sounds in all four quadrants. The abdomen should be soft and tender on palpation. Note the presence of inguinal hernias.

Genitourinary Assessment

Preschoolers typically achieve full daytime bladder control around 3 years of age. Nighttime bladder control takes longer and may not be achieved until 4 to 5 years of age. It is normal for children to still have occasional accidents. Inquire whether the child has achieved nighttime bladder control. If the preschooler continues to wet the bed beyond the age of 5 years, ask whether either parent has a history of bedwetting as a child, because sometimes the tendency runs in families. Determine whether the child has never achieved consistent nighttime dryness or achieved nighttime dryness but has regressed. The latter could indicate an underlying medical condition.

Ask the parents whether the child has a history of urinary tract infections. Pertinent questions include the following: Does the child complain of burning or hurting with urination? Does the child have urgency? Does the child urinate only small amounts at a time? Is there a foul odor to the urine? Preschoolers with a history of multiple urinary tract infections need further workup (see Chapter 24).

In Chapter 4, Ellie Raymore presented with signs and symptoms of a urinary tract infection. What were these signs and symptoms? Was her assessment normal or abnormal? Why was further testing warranted in Ellie's case?

When examining the genitalia, explain the assessment to the preschooler. Make sure the parents are present in the room. Explain that the assessment includes the private areas that are covered by underwear. Tell the preschooler, "Nobody should touch you in areas covered by your underwear unless mom and dad say it is okay." Have the parents reassure the child that the assessment is acceptable. In males, inspect the penis and scrotum. Note any drainage from the meatus. In females, assess the labia. Note any redness, swelling, or excoriation, which may be signs of abuse.

Musculoskeletal Assessment

The muscles continue to develop during the preschool years. At this time, the bones are still not fully ossified, leaving the preschooler vulnerable to injury. Preschoolers typically have genu valgum (knock-knees) in the early preschool period (Feigelman, 2016). As the legs straighten, the body becomes slenderer, losing the potbelly look of toddlerhood. Preschoolers are able to walk and run with ease.

Ask the parents about any concerns regarding muscle strength. Observe the preschooler's gait. Note persistent toe walking, which should be further investigated. Assess the spine, hips, and shoulders for symmetry, documenting unevenness. Assess lower muscle strength by having the preschooler press on the examiner's hands with his or her feet. Test upper extremity strength by having the preschooler squeeze the examiner's hand.

Integumentary Assessment

Inspect the skin for color, lesions, and rashes. The skin should be pink. Document pallor or cyanosis. Document any lesions, noting their size, color, and location. If rashes are present, document their appearance, color, and distribution. Palpate the skin, noting temperature and moisture. Assess for edema and skin turgor. The skin should feel soft, dry, and warm.

Assess for injuries such as burns or bruises. If either is present, inquire how the injuries occurred. Document the injuries, and if they seem suspicious, note that, as well.

Pain Assessment

Preschoolers are able to point to areas that hurt, but they are not able to describe their pain. For example, when asked, "Where

does it hurt?" the preschooler may point to the stomach. However, the preschooler will not be able to describe the quality of the pain. Cognitively, preschoolers understand the concepts of less and more. Therefore, children of preschool age are able to use self-report tools developed for this age group.

Two commonly used self-report pain scales for preschool-aged children are the Oucher scale and the FACES Pain Rating Scale (Analyze the Evidence 17.1). The Oucher scale consists of six points on a scale with corresponding color photographs of children's faces depicting different levels of pain. The faces have corresponding numbers of 0, 20, 40, 60, 80, and 100, with the higher number indicating a higher level of pain (Belter, McIntosh, Finch, & Saylor, 1988). The FACES Pain Rating Scale is a scale consisting of six cartoon faces with different expressions. The faces range from a happy face at 0, or no pain, to a crying face at 10, or the very worst pain. These faces are the preschool child's symbolic representation of pain (Wong & Baker, 1988).

Both the Oucher and the FACES Pain Rating Scale have been shown to be reliable for children 3 years and older (Belter et al., 1988). However, the studies reporting the validity and reliability of these two scales considered the children's ages in

Analyze the Evidence 17.1

Preschool Pain Scales

Standard self-report tools for preschoolers, such as the Oucher scale and the FACES Pain Rating Scale, include six different faces. Each face indicates a different level of distress and is associated with a corresponding number. During the early preschool years, children aged 3 and 4 y are able to describe concepts in terms of more or less but are unable to understand further differentiation.

Emmott et al. (2017) conducted a study to determine whether a simplified FACES Pain Rating Scale, using only three faces, is a valid tool for preschoolers under the age of 5 y undergoing procedural pain. The three faces were drawn in grayscale and represented mild, moderate, and severe pain.

Participants for the study were recruited from the Blood Collection Clinic of British Columbia Children's Hospital. The study was an observational study. Participants were randomized to either the standard scale or the simplified scale. There were a total of 180 participants: 60 each of 3-y-olds, 4-y-olds, and 5–6-y-olds.

The researchers found that children in the 4-y-old group distinguished pain from no pain more clearly when using the simplified FACES Pain Rating Scale. However, children in the 3-y-old group could not clearly distinguish pain from no pain even with the simplified scale. Therefore, it is recommended to continue using an observational tool, along with self-report, in 3-y-olds (Emmott et al., 2017).

aggregate. Preschoolers younger than age 5 do not yet have the cognitive ability to differentiate beyond no pain, a little pain, and a lot of pain. Therefore, to get an accurate view of pain in children younger than age 5, using a self-report tool as well as an observational tool, such as the Face, Legs, Activity, Cry, Consolability scale, gives the nurse the most accurate picture of the child's pain (Emmott et al., 2017).

In Chapter 4, Ellie Raymore experienced acute pain related to a urinary tract infection. Where did Ellie feel this pain? What tool did her nurse, Sonya, use to assess her pain? What was the result of the assessment? What intervention did Sonya use to address Ellie's pain?

Medications can be used to treat pain in preschoolers. However, nonpharmacological therapies, such as massage and acupuncture, can help decrease the preschooler's perception of pain. Distraction has been shown to work well in decreasing the preschooler's perception of pain, especially during procedures (Thrane, Wanless, Cohen, & Danford, 2016). Types of distraction include storytelling, cartoons, and toys.

In Chapter 6, Abigail Hanson experienced pain caused by an invasive procedure related to assessment for leukemia. What was this procedure? Where did Abigail have pain? What tool did her nurse, Norma, use to assess her pain?
What was the result of the assessment? What intervention did Norma use to address Abigail's pain?

Physical Growth

Continue to measure height and weight at each well-child visit during the preschool years. As muscle develops, preschoolers lose baby fat, giving them a slenderer appearance (Fig. 17.3).

Weight

From 3 to 6 years, preschoolers gain approximately 5 lb/y (2.3 kg). An average 4-year-old weighs 40 lb (18.1 kg). Measure the preschooler's body mass index (BMI) and plot the results on the appropriate chart (growth charts available at http://www.cdc.gov/growthcharts). Preschoolers with a high BMI are at increased risk for obesity in adulthood.

Height

Measure the child's standing height (Fig. 17.4). Preschoolers grow 2.5 to 3 in/y (6.1 to 7.6 cm). The average 4-year-old is 40 in (3.3 ft) tall.

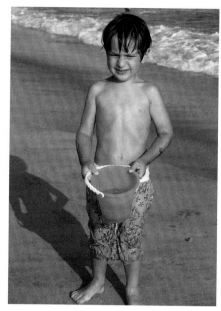

Figure 17.3. Preschool growth. Preschoolers take on a slenderer appearance. Reprinted with permission from Ateah, C. A., Scott, S. D., & Kyle, T. (2012). *Canadian essentials of pediatric nursing* (1st ed., Fig. 6.1). Philadelphia, PA: Lippincott Williams & Wilkins.

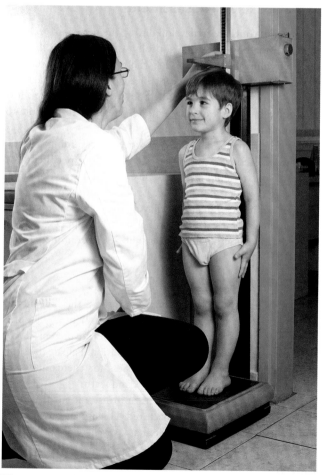

Figure 17.4. Measuring height. Measure a standing height in the preschooler.

Developmental Theories

Psychosocial, cognitive, and moral development continue. Table 17.1 gives an overview of selected developmental theories for preschoolers.

Psychosocial

The preschool period is characterized by the stage of initiative vs. guilt. According to Erikson (1963), the task of initiative builds on autonomy through undertaking new activities, planning games, and assertion of independence (Fig. 17.5). Preschoolers have a boundless amount of energy and learn through their successes and failures. However, when a child is not allowed to initiate new activities or engages in activities that are beyond the preschooler's capability, the result is a feeling of guilt. Initiative is a necessary skill for learning and positive interaction. Encourage parents to allow preschoolers to safely take initiative in daily activities.

Cognitive

Preschoolers are in the preoperational stage of cognitive development (Piaget, 1930). During the preoperational stage, the preschooler develops symbolic thinking. This process can be seen through the rapid development of language throughout the preschool years.

This stage is further divided into two substages. Children are in the preoperational stage until the age of 4 years. **Preoperational thought** is centered on egocentrism. Preschoolers cannot understand that others have a point of view that is different from their own. Furthermore, the preschooler's thinking is based on perception rather than logical thoughts. Therefore, the preschooler's perception is reality. **Transductive reasoning** is an example of thought during the preconceptional stage. The preschooler

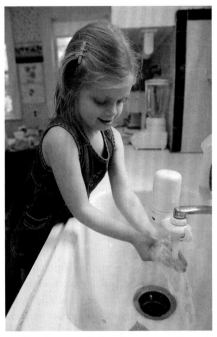

Figure 17.5. Psychosocial development. Preschoolers begin taking on tasks independently such as hand washing. Reprinted with permission from Kyle, T., & Carman, S. (2016). *Essentials of pediatric nursing* (3rd ed., Fig. 5.6). Philadelphia, PA: Wolters Kluwer.

connects seemingly related events that are not related at all. For example, the child may yell at a sibling and then the sibling comes down with a cold. The preschool child determines that the yelling caused the sibling's illness.

At 4 years of age, preschoolers move into the stage of **intuitive thinking**. During this stage, the preschooler begins to develop logical thought, although somewhat faulty. Logic continues to be based on perception. An example of this is the concept of

Table 17.1 Overview of Developmental Theories in Preschoolers

Theorist/Type of Development	Stage	Implications
Erikson: Psychosocial	Initiative vs. Guilt	• Plans and initiates activities • Wants to please parents • Asserts self more frequently • Makes up games
Piaget: Cognitive	Preoperational	• Focus on only one aspect of things • Imaginary play • Magical thinking • Knows right from wrong • Egocentrism lessens around 4 y of age • Animism lessens around 5 y of age • Uses transductive reasoning
Freud: Psychosexual	Phallic	• Genitals become an area of interest • Identifies more with the parents of the same sex
Kohlberg: Moral	Preconventional	• Learns good from bad based on punishment

irreversibility. The preschooler is unable to reverse the sequence of events. Animism, attributing lifelike qualities to inanimate objects, continues through the beginning of the intuitive phase. Transductive thinking lessens by the end of the preschool period.

Magical thinking is a hallmark of the preschool years. Preschoolers have a vivid imagination, and fantasy plays a role in thoughts and actions. The preschool child may think that the sun goes down in the evening because it is tired or that if fish stop swimming, the rivers will stop flowing (Piaget, 1930). Imaginary friends are often part of the child's magical thinking. These imaginary friends are often elaborate identities that are included in role play and help the child explore his or her world through make-believe (Mottweiler & Taylor, 2014).

Moral

Preschoolers continue in the preconventional stage of moral development. At this stage, preschoolers understand morality in terms of right and wrong or good and bad. Right and wrong is interpreted through consequences of actions such as punishments or rewards (Kohlberg, 1981). By the end of the preconventional stage, preschoolers conform to rules to avoid punishment and gain reward. Rules are seen as absolute. Preschoolers understand taking turns but complain if they feel their turn was shorter than that of others (Feigelman, 2016).

In addition, preschoolers value physical objects and desire to have the same objects as do their friends. They often do not understand the difference between make-believe and reality. Therefore, preschoolers, led by imagination, have a propensity to lie during the early preschool years. During this stage, preschoolers also learn how to deal with angry feelings. As the child is learning how to process these feelings, unwanted behavior, such as hitting and biting, may occur.

Motor Development

The preschooler's musculoskeletal system continues to mature, allowing for the refinement of skills and the development of new ones. Although the preschooler's gross motor skills continue to get stronger, fine motor skill development is the focus of the preschool period.

Gross Motor

The preschooler becomes adept at running, walking, and jumping. Walking up and down the stairs becomes more fluid, with the 3-year-old walking up and down the stairs with one foot on each step (Fig. 17.6). Preschoolers enjoy activities such as throwing and kicking balls, climbing, and riding tricycles. The preschool period is a time of constant physical activity. Table 17.2 gives examples of expected gross motor development milestones in preschoolers.

Fine Motor

During the preschool years, fine motor skills become more refined. By 3 years, the child has established whether he or she is

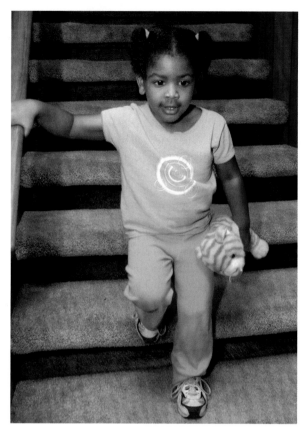

Figure 17.6. Gross motor development. Preschoolers walk down the stairs with one foot on each step. Reprinted with permission from Kyle, T., & Carman, S. (2016). *Essentials of pediatric nursing* (3rd ed., Fig. 5.4). Philadelphia, PA: Wolters Kluwer.

Table 17.2	Gross Motor Development Milestones in Preschoolers
Age (y)	**Gross Motor Milestone**
3	• Walks up and down stairs with one foot on each step • Pedals a tricycle • Runs well • Jumps forward
4	• Climbs and hops • Stands on one foot • Catches a bounced ball
5	• Swings • Climbs • Stands on one foot for 10 s • Somersaults

Adapted from Hagan, J. F., Shaw, J. S., & Duncan, P. (Eds.). (2017). *Bright futures: Guidelines for health supervision of infants, children, and adolescents* (4th ed.). Elk Grove Village, IL: American Academy of Pediatrics; and Centers for Disease Control. (2017). *Learn the signs. Act early. Developmental milestones.* Retrieved from https://www.cdc.gov/ncbddd/actearly/milestones/index.html

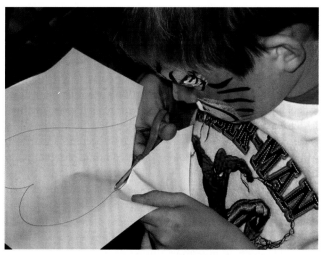

Figure 17.7. Fine motor development. Preschoolers are able to draw shapes. Reprinted with permission from Kyle, T., & Carman, S. (2016). *Essentials of pediatric nursing* (3rd ed., Fig. 5.5). Philadelphia, PA: Wolters Kluwer.

right or left handed. The child can hold a crayon like an adult, scribble, and begin to draw shapes and people (Fig. 17.7). Preschoolers are able to feed themselves and dress themselves. By the time the child is 5 years old, he or she is able to use a pair of scissors. Table 17.3 gives expected fine motor development milestones for preschoolers.

Table 17.3 Fine Motor Development Milestones in Preschoolers

Age (y)	Fine Motor Milestone
3	• Is able to put on a coat by self • Draws a single circle • Draws a person with a head and one body part • Does puzzles with three or four pieces • Builds a tower of more than six blocks • Turns pages one at a time • Holds a pencil with the whole hand
4	• Draws a person with three body parts • Draws a cross • Buttons and unbuttons large buttons • Grasps a pencil with the thumb and finger • Uses a pair of scissors
5	• Draws a person with at least six body parts • Prints some letters and numbers • Copies shapes • Uses a fork and spoon

Adapted from Hagan, J. F., Shaw, J. S., & Duncan, P. (Eds.). (2017). *Bright futures: Guidelines for health supervision of infants, children, and adolescents* (4th ed.). Elk Grove Village, IL: American Academy of Pediatrics; and Centers for Disease Control. (2017). *Learn the signs. Act early. Developmental milestones.* Retrieved from https://www.cdc.gov/ncbddd/actearly/milestones/index.html

Communication and Language Development

During the preschool years, language acquisition occurs at a rapid pace. Two-year-olds have a vocabulary of 50 to 100 words. By the time the child is 5 years, he or she uses up to 5,000 words (Feigelman, 2011). Not only does the preschooler's vocabulary increase, so does the ability to express thoughts and ideas. They speak in concrete language and are able to tell elaborate stories or recall recent experiences. However, preschool children are not able to understand abstract language and use the literal definition of words. Therefore, a preschool child will not understand commonly used phrases such as "stiff as a board" or "as thick as molasses." Table 17.4 gives expected language development milestones during the preschool period.

An important part of language development during preschool is exposure to the language and vocabulary of adults (McLeod, Hardy, & Kaiser, 2017). The more children are exposed to adults who read to them, ask questions, and encourage conversation, the more advanced their language skills become. These skills set the stage for reading and school readiness. Children living in poverty are more at risk for language delay than are other children (Growth and Development Check 17.1). Children living in poverty often live in a stressful home environment with less exposure to advanced vocabulary. Before entering kindergarten, language is learned through exposure to

Table 17.4 Language Development Milestones in Preschoolers

Age (y)	Language Milestone
3	• Speaks in three-word sentences • Strangers can understand 75% of the child's language. • Follows instructions with two or three steps • Names a friend
4	• Uses "he" and "she" correctly • Sings songs • Tells stories • Strangers can understand 100% of the child's language. • Uses four-word sentences • Knows some colors and numbers
5	• Counts to 10 • Names at least four colors • Uses full sentences • Knows name and address • Understands and uses the future tense

Adapted from Hagan, J. F., Shaw, J. S., & Duncan, P. (Eds.). (2017). *Bright futures: Guidelines for health supervision of infants, children, and adolescents* (4th ed.). Elk Grove Village, IL: American Academy of Pediatrics; and Centers for Disease Control. (2017). *Learn the signs. Act early. Developmental milestones.* Retrieved from https://www.cdc.gov/ncbddd/actearly/milestones/index.html

Growth and Development Check 17.1

Language Delay

Language delay in the preschooler may be a sign of one or more problems. Underlying causes of language delay may include the following:

- Autism
- Cognitive impairment
- Emotional delays
- Low socioeconomic status
- Neglect
- Underlying neurological disorders

It is important to assess the preschooler's language development. Any delays should be taken seriously, because language development is the foundation for school success (Feigelman, 2011). Nurses are able to develop interventions and educate parents on how to best help their child obtain optimal language development. Referrals to services such as Early Intervention and Head Start help place children in an environment for optimal development.

words and conversations with adults, which are typically decreased in lower socioeconomic households. As a result of these circumstances, children living in poverty may be behind in language acquisition when starting school. Stimulating language development through play and encouragement has been shown to be effective in at-risk children (McLeod et al., 2017).

Children growing up in a bilingual home may experience language development differently. Whichever language is predominantly spoken in the home will be the primary language learned by the child. In addition, who is speaking which language to the child will impact the child's language acquisition (Gathercole, 2014). Families from other cultures may speak the language of their culture at home while the child hears English at preschool or when with other families.

It is important to monitor language development. Language delay is often one of the first signs of either cognitive or emotional delays. Delay in communication could also indicate maltreatment or neglect (Feigelman, 2017).

Social and Emotional Development

Preschoolers experience and express a wide range of emotions, such as joy, happiness, fear, and anxiety. Learning how to cope with these emotions is part of the work of the preschool years. Imaginary play and imaginary friends are tools preschool children use to help them explore their emotions and different ways of communication. During this time, children often vacillate between fantasy and reality throughout the course of the day. It is important that parents not make fun of their child's imaginary play because it is a part of normal development.

Role play is important during the preschool years. Through role play, children learn about social interactions as well as

gender identity. By the time a child is 5 to 6 years old, he or she becomes interested in basic sexuality (American Academy of Pediatrics [AAP], 2015b). At the same time, interest in the opposite sex and in how boys and girls are different emerges.

Preschool is a time in which children begin to develop their own identity. As their skills develop, they want to exert more independence. It is important for parents to still maintain limits with preschoolers while giving them choices as much as possible.

During the preschool period, children become less selfish. Although cooperation becomes more common, parents often need to remind preschoolers to share and take turns. By the time children are 5 to 6 years old, they learn how to work out disagreements without much intervention from adults. Learning basic social skills in the early preschool period sets the child up for success in school. Table 17.5 highlights social and emotional development milestones during the preschool years.

In Chapter 4, Ellie Raymore's mother was concerned about some of her development. Why was she concerned? Were her concerns valid? What interactions could help Ellie with her development? How did Dr. Engle counsel Ellie's mother? What is the nurse's role in this situation?

Table 17.5 Social and Emotional Development Milestones in Preschoolers

Age (y)	Social or Emotional Milestone
3	• Goes to the bathroom by self • Cooperates and shares • Understands "mine" and "yours" • Separates easily from mom and dad • Copies adults • Shows concern
4	• Likes to do new things • Engages in creative and imaginative play • Likes to play with other children • Talks about interests • Follows simple rules • May not be able to differentiate "real" from "make-believe"
5	• Follows simple directions • Wants to please friends • Understands gender • Differentiates between "real" and "make-believe" • Is likely to follow rules

Adapted from Hagan, J. F., Shaw, J. S., & Duncan, P. (Eds.). (2017). *Bright futures: Guidelines for health supervision of infants, children, and adolescents* (4th ed.). Elk Grove Village, IL: American Academy of Pediatrics; and Centers for Disease Control. (2017). *Learn the signs. Act early. Developmental milestones.* Retrieved from https://www.cdc.gov/ncbddd/actearly/milestones/index.html

Friendships

Developing friendships is an important aspect of preschool development. Friendships help children develop social skills and understand appropriate social behavior. Through friendships, preschoolers learn to cooperate, share, and resolve disagreements. Friends are someone the child can play with, laugh with, sing and dance with, and pretend with (Fig. 17.8). First friendships are often formed through interactions that parents orchestrate. These interactions can be through the parents' friends, families in the neighborhood, scheduled playdates, or child care. Encourage the parents of children without siblings or with limited interaction with other children to seek out ways for their children to interact with others of preschool age to develop appropriate social skills.

Fears

Fears may grow out of the preschool child's overactive imagination. Children may be afraid of the dark or monsters they have created. They may fear new places and new people. Often, their fears may mimic those of older siblings or parents, such as fear of spiders or of big dogs. At this age, long-term memory begins to develop, allowing preschoolers to remember painful procedures, which may result in a fear of doctor's offices, hospitals, and healthcare workers. It is important for parents to work with their child to alleviate fears as best they can. For example, if a child is afraid of the dark, a night light might help.

Health Promotion

Nurses should continue to promote health with children and their families throughout the children's preschool years, scheduling annual routine health promotion visits from 3 to 6 years of age (Hagan, Shaw, & Duncan, 2017).

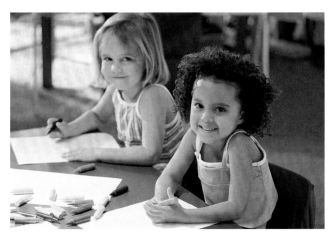

Figure 17.8. Social development. Preschoolers develop friendships and learn how to cooperate. Reprinted with permission from Jensen, S. (2010). *Nursing health assessment* (1st ed., Fig. 9.1C). Philadelphia, PA: Lippincott Williams & Wilkins.

Promoting Healthy Growth and Development

Helping families promote optimal growth and development is a key role for nurses (Priority Care Concepts 17.1). To provide appropriate teaching and anticipatory guidance, the nurse must understand the context in which the family lives. A family's culture influences its members' view of health and therefore should inform the approach the nurse takes with them in health promotion. For example, recommendations for ensuring adequate protein intake that a nurse makes for a preschooler from a Hindu family that practices strict vegetarianism would likely differ from those for a preschooler from a family that includes meat in the diet. Likewise, a family's culture influences the emphasis placed on education and social interaction, which in turn should inform the nurse's approach to these topics when working with the family.

Priority Care Concepts 17.1

Promoting Growth and Development in Preschoolers

Communication and Social Development

- Maintaining daytime and nighttime routines
- Consistency in the preschooler's environment
- Reading with the preschooler
- Providing social interaction

Sleep

- Bedtime routines
- Sleep through the night
- Nightmares vs. night terrors
- Parental knowledge

Oral Health

- Brushing teeth
- Dental visits

Safety

- Home environment
- Outside environment
- Preschool environment
- Parental knowledge

Nutrition

- Family meal times
- Allow the preschooler to make healthy choices
- Limit sugars

School Readiness

- Preschool
- Language development
- Experience in social situations

Social determinants of health should also influence teaching provided by nurses. Understanding the needs of families and the resources available to them helps the nurse tailor health promotion. Until basic needs are met, families have a hard time focusing on health. Assess the family's housing and food security, exposure to tobacco, and exposure to violence. In addition, assess the family's protective factors, such as social networks, family support, and community involvement.

During the hospitalization of preschoolers, nurses should continue to promote their healthy growth and development. Nurses must understand appropriate developmental milestones to recognize delays or signs of regression in the hospitalized child. Working with the family and other members of the healthcare team, such as the child life specialist, the nurse can help the child to maintain optimal development.

Early Learning and School Readiness

Early learning is important for preparing a child to begin school, and promoting early learning is a role of the nurse. The environment in which the child lives is a key aspect of early learning. Parents are their child's first teachers and serve as role models for all aspects of the preschooler's development. Encourage parents to read to their child (Fig. 17.9). Picture books and books with one or two words per page capture the preschooler's attention. Carrying on conversations and asking preschoolers open-ended questions help develop language skills, which are predictors of

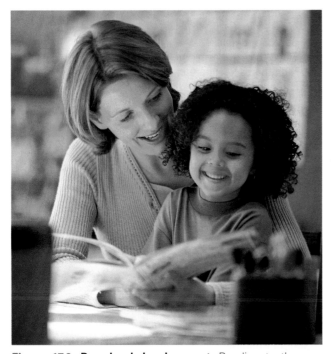

Figure 17.9. Preschool development. Reading to the preschooler promotes school readiness. Reprinted with permission from Taylor, C., Lillis, C., & Lynn, P. (2014). *Fundamentals of nursing* (8th ed., Fig. 18.5D). Philadelphia, PA: Lippincott Williams & Wilkins.

school readiness and academic success (Leech, Wei, Harring, & Rowe, 2018).

Providing structured environments with choices helps preschoolers learn how to act in social situations. Preschool programs help provide structure and allow children to interact with others their own age. Although it is not required that children go to preschool, it may help with the transition to kindergarten. Whether the child is starting preschool or kindergarten, the parent should prepare the child for the changes that will take place. Meeting the teacher and touring the school before the first day can alleviate some of the fear and anxiety of a new situation.

Children living in poverty often struggle with school readiness (Cavadel & Frye, 2017). Nurses can guide families to resources that can help their child with early learning and school readiness. Head Start services assist with school readiness of low-income families for children through the age of 5 years (U.S. Department of Health and Human Services, 2017). These services are provided through local communities and take place in various settings.

Safety

As preschoolers gain both cognitive and motor skills, they become more adept at exploring their environment. They often like new experiences and do not comprehend any risks involved. Teaching children the importance of safety is imperative at this age (Patient Teaching 17.1). Not playing close to the street, looking both ways before crossing the street, and wearing a helmet when riding a bike are all important safety lessons for preschoolers. Parents can help children learn to be safe by role modeling these behaviors.

Preschoolers tend to be very trusting. Therefore, stranger safety becomes a priority. Instruct and encourage parents to teach children not to go with anyone they do not know. Children should understand that no one should touch them in the areas covered by a bathing suit. In crowded situations, the parent should point out to the child safe areas and safe people, such as police officers, to go to in case the parent and child become separated. Having preschoolers learn their address and phone number is also helpful in case they are separated from their parents.

Firearm safety continues to be critical. Preschoolers' natural curiosity may cause them to get into things they should not. Make sure that firearms are out of sight and locked away. Instruct and encourage parents to teach children the danger of firearms and that they are not toys to be played with.

Oral Health

By this time, children should be seeing the dentist routinely every 6 months. Preschoolers should brush their teeth twice a day with a pea-sized amount of fluoridated toothpaste. Parents should have children spit the toothpaste out but not rinse their mouth. By doing this, the small amount of toothpaste left in the mouth is an additional protection against tooth decay (Hagan et al., 2017).

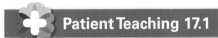

Patient Teaching 17.1

Safety in Preschoolers

Outdoor

- Check outdoor playground equipment for loose screws and sharp edges.
- Have preschoolers wear helmets when they ride a tricycle or bicycle.
- Teach children to look both ways before crossing the street.
- Have children wear sunscreen or clothing that protects them from the sun.

Strangers

- Teach children to say "no" to strangers.
- Have children memorize their address and phone number.
- Teach children about who are safe people to go to when in crowded places.

Falls

- Do not allow children to climb on furniture.
- Lock doors to dangerous areas.
- Supervise children when they are on playground equipment.

Poisoning

- Keep all cleaning products out of reach; use cabinet locks if kept in low cabinets.
- Keep all medications out of reach.
- Have the number for poison control easily accessible.

Water

- Have a fence around backyard pools.
- Supervise children when they are around water.
- Do not leave buckets of water around.

Car Seats

- Children can ride facing forward in a seat with a five-point harness until they are 4 y old.
- At 4 y old, children can move to a booster seat with a regular seat belt (Fig. 17.10).

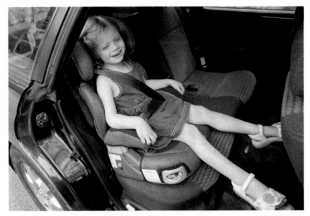

Figure 17.10. Preschool car seat safety. Preschool children can sit in a belt-positioning booster seat. Reprinted with permission from Kyle, T., & Carman, S. (2016). *Essentials of pediatric nursing* (3rd ed., Fig. 5.12). Philadelphia, PA: Wolters Kluwer.

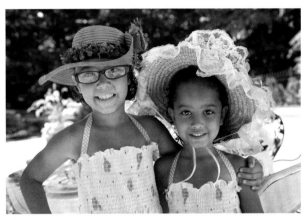

Figure 17.11. Imaginary play. Playing dress-up is an integral part of preschool growth and development.

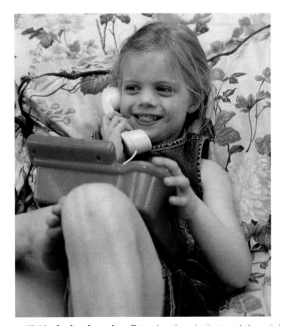

Figure 17.12. Imitative play. Preschoolers imitate adult activities such as talking on the phone. Reprinted with permission from Taylor, C., Lillis, C., & Lynn, P. (2014). *Fundamentals of nursing* (8th ed., Fig. 18.5E). Philadelphia, PA: Lippincott Williams & Wilkins.

Play

Preschool children engage in imaginary and creative play. Make-believe is often the activity of choice. Three-year-olds often have difficulty determining real from make-believe and often believe that the stories or characters they create are real. At 4 years of age, preschoolers understand the difference between imaginary and real characters but continue to engage in make-believe, creating characters and stories that involve dressing up, building forts, and other creative endeavors (Fig. 17.11). In addition, play at this age involves imitating adult activity (Fig. 17.12). As cognitive ability increases, the 5-year-old's imaginary play becomes more elaborate and detailed, often involving adults in the game.

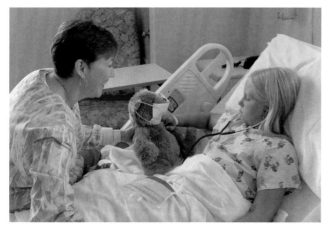

Figure 17.13. Hospitalization. Allowing the hospitalized preschooler to play with medical equipment can help alleviate anxiety. Reprinted with permission from Pillitteri, A. (2013). *Maternal and child health nursing* (7th ed., Fig. 35.2). Philadelphia, PA: Lippincott Williams & Wilkins.

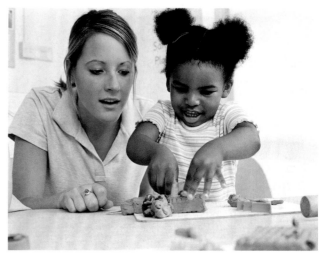

Figure 17.14. Creative play. Modeling clay helps preschoolers develop creativity. Reprinted with permission from Craven, R. F., Hirnle, C. J., & Henshaw, C. M. (2016). *Fundamentals of nursing* (8th ed., Fig. 37.1). Philadelphia, PA: Wolters Kluwer.

Play allows preschoolers to work through frustration and anxiety, as well. When a preschool child is hospitalized, providing opportunities for play allows the child some control. Having the child perform pretend procedures on dolls or stuffed animals gives him or her the opportunity to become familiar with medical equipment and can help alleviate fears of being in the hospital (Fig. 17.13).

In Chapter 6, Abigail Hanson enjoyed playing zoo with her stuffed animals. Is this appropriate developmentally for a 4-year-old? Did she have a favorite toy? How did this type of play help Abigail when she was in the hospital?

In addition to imaginary play, preschool children enjoy using their developing fine motor skills to color. Molding clay, building blocks, cars, trucks, and dolls are all toys that allow the preschool child to develop their creativity (Fig. 17.14). At this age, children are learning to share and take turns. Simple board games are appropriate during the preschool years.

Encouraging physical activity in preschoolers helps prevent obesity. Encourage families to participate in physical activity together. Preschoolers learn healthy habits from their adult role models. Teach parents that by increasing their own activity levels, they are encouraging children to live active and healthy lifestyles (Nerud & Samra, 2017). Playing outside, riding bikes, and playing on playgrounds are all appropriate activities (Fig. 17.15). Organized physical activities, such as sports, are not necessary at this time. If children are participating in sports, remind parents that preschoolers have a difficult time understanding the rules associated with different sports. Unstructured physical activity allows preschool children to be creative, use their imagination, and have fun.

Teach parents of preschoolers not only which types of toys promote growth and development but also which types of toys

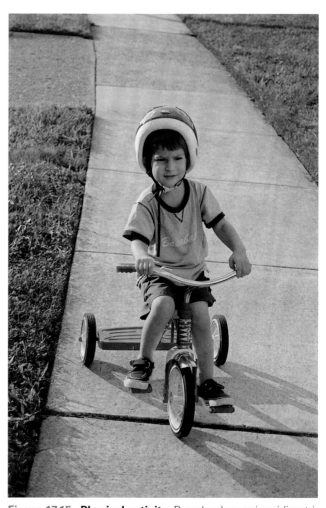

Figure 17.15. Physical activity. Preschoolers enjoy riding tricycles. Emphasize the importance of wearing a helmet for safety. Reprinted with permission from Weber, J. R., & Kelley, J. H. (2017). *Health assessment in nursing* (6th ed., Fig. 31.2). Philadelphia, PA: Wolters Kluwer.

Box 17.1 Appropriate Toys for Preschoolers

- Clothes for playing dress-up
- Art and craft supplies such as a pair of scissors, chalk, crayons, clay, paper, and pencils
- Blocks for building and stacking
- Dolls with clothes that can be taken on and off to practice dressing, undressing, and buttoning
- Puzzles with large pieces
- Simple board games
- Kitchen sets with pretend food and plastic plates, forks, and spoons
- Cars, trucks, and dolls
- Dollhouses
- Tricycles, bicycles, and other riding toys

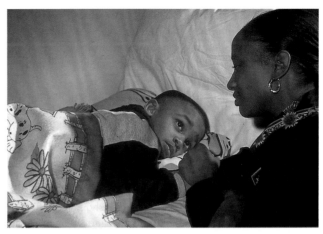

Figure 17.16. Nightmares. A parent comforts a preschooler after a nightmare. Reprinted with permission from Pillitteri, A. (2013). *Maternal and child health nursing* (7th ed., Fig. 31.4). Philadelphia, PA: Lippincott Williams & Wilkins.

to avoid (Box 17.1). Teach parents to not give preschool children toys with small parts. If the toy can fit into a toilet paper tube, then it is too small for the preschool child. Parents should also avoid toys that have paint containing lead and toys with small magnets, because accidental ingestion can cause serious harm to the gastrointestinal system (AAP, 2017).

Sleep

Sleep patterns during the preschool years change dramatically from those of infancy (Bathory & Tomopoulos, 2017). During the preschool years, the hours of sleep are consolidated into one long block. The average preschooler requires 10 to 13 hours of sleep per day (Hagan et al., 2017). At 3 years old, this total amount of sleep is typically divided between nighttime sleep and one daytime nap. The average preschooler stops taking naps around 4 years of age.

Promoting healthy sleep habits continues to be important. Establishing a time for bed with bedtime routines, such as a bath, brushing teeth, and story, helps the preschooler have a solid night of sleep. At this age, if children wake in the middle of the night, they should be able to get themselves back to sleep. Occasionally, due to an overactive imagination, preschoolers have nightmares. Nightmares often occur when the child is

overtired or under stress (AAP, 2013). If nightmares occur, parents should comfort their child as soon as possible (Fig. 17.16). They should try to determine what is scaring the child, reassure the child that he or she is safe, and stay with the child until he or she is ready to go back to sleep.

Night terrors can also occur during the preschool period. Night terrors differ from nightmares in that the child is not actually awake when they occur (Table 17.6). The child may scream and try to push the parent away before falling back asleep. Although night terrors can cause parents some concern, they are not harmful, and parents should not try to wake the child. Preschoolers do not remember night terrors.

Discipline

As children become more independent, parents need to develop a new set of expectations and new sets of rules. Preschoolers tend to behave better when they are allowed to explore their independence yet have set limits. In addition to having limits, daily routines can help avoid meltdowns.

Once parents have set rules, they should explain to the preschooler what the consequences are of breaking the rules. For example, riding a bike without a helmet might result in the

Table 17.6 Nightmares vs. Night Terrors

	Nightmares	Night Terrors (AAP, 2013)
Sleep/wake status	Wakes up scared	• Appears to be awake but is not • May appear glassy-eyed or confused
Crying status	May or may not cry	Cries uncontrollably
Behavior	Wants comfort from a parent	• Pushes the parent away • Kicks, screams, and thrashes
Response to event	• Can talk about it • Falls back asleep in a while	Does not remember it

child losing access to the bike for 3 days. Once the rules are established, it is important for parents to stick to them. If the child breaks the rules, the consequences must be logical and timely. Consistency is also paramount to establishing appropriate behaviors in preschoolers.

When preschoolers do not listen, it is important that parents not get frustrated. Remind parents that all children develop at different rates. Parents should make sure that the child is able to accomplish what he or she is asked to do. If the preschooler is misbehaving, implementing immediate forms of discipline, such as a time-out, is more effective than yelling. The goal of a time-out is to separate the child from the situation. When implementing this form of discipline, parents should tell children that they are getting a time-out and then direct them to the designated time-out spot. A general rule for a time-out is that it should last 1 min/y of age of the child. If the preschooler cries or fusses, then the time-out starts over (AAP, 2015a). The AAP does not recommend spanking, because it can lead to inconsistent discipline, aggression, or physical struggles.

Immunizations

Preschoolers need to have their immunizations before starting school (Patient Teaching 17.2). If the child is on schedule, the only immunizations needed are at the 4-year-old well-child visit. The immunizations the child receives at this visit are all boosters of vaccines they received at an earlier age. These immunizations include the following:

- Diphtheria, tetanus, acellular pertussis (DTaP)
- Inactivated poliovirus (IPV)
- Measles, mumps, rubella (MMR)
- Varicella

The most up-to-date immunization chart is available at https://www.cdc.gov/vaccines/schedules/hcp/child-adolescent.html. Remind parents of the side effects of these immunizations, how to treat them, and when to contact a healthcare provider. Refer to Chapter 15 for nursing considerations, barriers, and reporting of adverse events associated with immunizations.

Nutrition

Nutrition for preschoolers should be focused on a healthy, well-rounded diet. The AAP (2015c) recommends a nutrient-dense diet based on the food groups of whole grains, vegetables, fruits, milk and dairy, and lean protein (Box 17.2). Caloric requirements range from 1,200 to 1,400 calories/d depending on the gender of the child and his or her activity level (Parks et al., 2016). Teach parents to include healthy fats, such as omega 3 fatty acids, in their preschooler's diet, as they are needed for growth and brain development, but to avoid unhealthy fats, such as trans fats, which are found in highly processed food.

Parents should avoid giving their preschooler foods high in added sugar, such as soft drinks and sugary snacks. They should include milk in the diet, because it is an important source of protein, calcium, and vitamin D. Caution parents about including

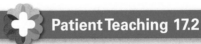

Patient Teaching 17.2

Immunizations for 4-Year-Olds

Immunizations
Immunizations that your child will receive at his or her 4-y-old checkup include the following:

- DTaP
  - The DTaP vaccine protects against:
    - Diphtheria, a serious infection of the throat that can block the airway
    - Tetanus, otherwise known as lockjaw, a nerve disease
    - Pertussis, otherwise known as whooping cough, a respiratory infection that can have serious complications
- IPV
  - The IPV vaccine protects against polio, which can cause paralysis and death.
- MMR
  - The MMR vaccine protects against:
    - Measles, a highly contagious respiratory infection that causes rash and fever
    - Mumps, a very contagious virus that causes fever, headache, and swollen glands under the jaw
    - Rubella, also known as "German measles," a virus that causes rash and swollen glands
- Chickenpox (varicella)
  - The varicella vaccine protects against chickenpox, which is a disease that causes a rash that itches, forms blisters, and causes fever.
  - Chickenpox can be life-threatening in babies and children with weakened immune systems.

Common Side Effects
After your child gets immunizations, he or she may have the following:

- Run a fever of up to around 102°F
- Have redness or a small amount of swelling at the injection site
- Have a mild rash 5–7 d after the MMR or varicella vaccine
- Be fussier in the 24 h after immunizations
- Sleep more in the 24 h after immunizations

When to Call the Healthcare Provider
- If your child has a fever of 105°F (40.5°C) or higher
- If your child has a seizure
- If your child has uncontrollable crying for 3 h or longer

Adapted from the Centers for Disease Control and Prevention. (2017). *Diseases and the vaccines that prevent them: For parents of infants and young children (birth through age 6)*. Retrieved from http://www.cdc.gov/vaccines/hcp/conversations/prevent-diseases/provider-resources-factsheets-infants.html

too much juice in the preschooler's diet. Even 100% fruit juice contains a high amount of sugar and should be limited.

Preschoolers typically eat three meals and one or two snacks per day. Parents should have the preschooler help prepare snacks

Box 17.2 Healthy Food Choices for Preschoolers

- Protein: 3–5 oz
  - Lean meat
  - Eggs
  - Fish
  - Beans
- Fruits: 1–2 cups
  - Fresh, whole fruits
  - Frozen or canned fruits with no sugar added
  - Dried fruits
- Vegetables: 1.5–2.5 cups
  - Whole, fresh vegetables
  - Canned vegetables
  - Provide a variety
- Grains: 4–6 oz
  - Whole grains
  - Limit refined grains such as white flour and pasta
- Dairy: 2.5 cups
  - Low-fat dairy products

Data from Mayo Clinic. (2018). *Nutrition for kids: Guidelines for a healthy diet.* Retrieved from https://www.mayoclinic.org/healthy-lifestyle/childrens-health/in-depth/nutrition-for-kids/art-20049335

when possible (Fig. 17.17). Teach parents to provide healthy snacks such as apples and peanut butter, cheese cubes, or yogurt. Snacks such as pretzels, fruit snacks, or snack crackers only provide empty calories. If the child is not hungry, the parent should not force him or her to eat, because this can lead to overeating. Allowing the child to determine when he or she is full can prevent overeating and potential obesity later in childhood. Preschoolers often remain picky eaters, which can be frustrating for parents. By the time preschoolers reach the age of 5 years, they are more willing to try new things. Encourage parents to keep offering healthy foods and snacks. Preschoolers should be expected to eat the same meal as the rest of the family. Teach parents that fixing preschoolers a separate meal only encourages picky eating.

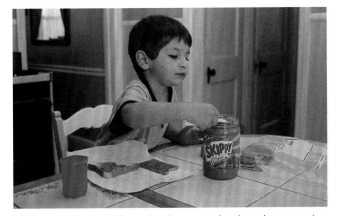

Figure 17.17. Nutrition. Involve preschoolers in preparing healthy snacks and meals. Reprinted with permission from Kyle, T., & Carman, S. (2016). *Essentials of pediatric nursing* (3rd ed., Fig. 5.2). Philadelphia, PA: Wolters Kluwer.

Nurses can educate parents on the benefits of a healthy diet for their preschooler. Healthy eating habits that begin during the preschool years help prevent obesity later in the school-age years, adolescence, and adulthood (Grossklaus & Marvicsin, 2014). Parental role modeling of healthy eating habits plays an important role in the preschooler's nutritional status. Help parents identify healthy food choices for their preschooler. Resources such as https://www.choosemyplate.gov/health-and-nutrition-information provide parents with ideas for healthy meals as well as ways to keep track of their preschooler's daily eating habits.

Common Developmental Concerns

Common developmental concerns during the preschool years include lying, masturbation, and media use. These are a normal part of preschool development. Educate parents on why these behaviors occur and how to manage them.

Lying

Lying occurs for different reasons during the preschool years. Sometimes preschoolers lie because of their overactive imagination and have a hard time distinguishing fantasy from reality. Other times, preschoolers lie to avoid punishment. Furthermore, the reason for lying changes as the preschooler gets older and cognitive abilities advance.

Young preschoolers, ages 3 to 4 years, tend to tell lies for themselves, trying to hide their own transgression (Talwar, Crossman, & Wyman, 2017). However, 5- to 6-year-olds tend to lie to prevent transgressions or harm to others (Harvey, Davoodi, & Blake, 2018; Talwar et al., 2017). At this age, preschoolers have the cognitive ability to understand that telling a lie can change the outcome for someone other than themselves (Harvey et al., 2018).

Although lying is common during the preschool years, encourage parents to teach children that lying is never okay. Before punishing the child for lying, the parent should find out the reason for the lie and then explain to the preschooler that telling the truth will get them in less trouble than lying. Punishment should be based on the severity of the transgression and the severity of the lie. Preschoolers should be praised for telling the truth. Remind parents that they are role models for their children and should tell the truth as well.

Masturbation

During the preschool years, children are discovering the differences between genders and exploring their own bodies. This exploration includes the genitals and takes place in the form of masturbation (Hagan et al., 2017). Parents are often appalled at this behavior. Reassure parents that this is normal behavior during the preschool years. Getting angry and punishing the behavior may result in the behavior occurring more frequently. Excessive or aggressive masturbation or acting out sexual intercourse should be further explored because it may be a sign of sexual abuse (Feigelman, 2016).

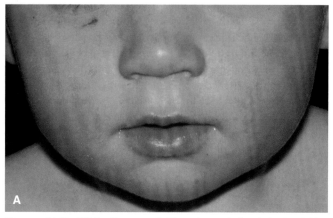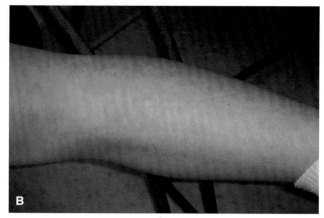

Figure 17.18. Fifth disease. A. The slapped-cheek look of fifth disease. **B.** The lacy rash of fifth disease on an extremity. Reprinted with permission from Bachur, R. G., & Shaw, K. N. (2015). *Fleisher & Ludwig's textbook of pediatric emergency medicine* (7th ed., Fig. 96.15). Philadelphia, PA: Wolters Kluwer.

Assess the parents' comfort with talking to their children about sexuality. Gain understanding of the influence of the family's culture on sexuality, which will determine how to address the topic. Teach children that this behavior only takes place in private. Furthermore, emphasize to preschoolers that no one should touch them in their private areas unless it is a doctor or nurse and then only with their parents' permission.

Media

During the preschool years, children can benefit from some educational media. Programs and applications designed to help children recognize letters and develop early math skills can be beneficial when used appropriately (Hagan et al., 2017). However, remind parents that these should not be the only educational opportunities for preschoolers. Encourage parents to read to their children and allow them to have unstructured play time both indoors and outdoors.

Parents should preview any programming and digital media with their preschooler to assure quality. Parents should avoid programs with violence or frightening content. Because of preschoolers' vivid imagination, this type of content could lead to behavioral problems or nightmares. No televisions or digital devices should be allowed in preschoolers' bedrooms. Excessive or inappropriate use of media can lead to aggressiveness, sleep disorders, and obesity (Hagan et al., 2017). Preschoolers should have no more than 1 hour of media exposure per day.

Health Problems of Preschool Years

A few illnesses are seen commonly during the preschool years, especially if children are in day care or preschool for the first time. Although these illnesses may be seen at other ages, they are commonly seen in the early preschool period.

Fifth Disease

Erythema infectiosum, more commonly known as fifth disease, is caused by the parvovirus B19. The virus is primarily spread through respiratory transmission, but it may also be spread through contact with blood (Koch, 2016). The virus peaks in late winter and spring.

Nursing Assessment

Fifth disease is often called the "slapped-cheek" disease because the child presents with bright red cheeks that look as if they have been slapped (Fig. 17.18A). The rash spreads to the trunk and upper extremities and takes on a lacy appearance (Fig. 17.18B). The child does not appear sick.

Inquire about **prodromal** symptoms such as mild fever, rhinitis, and headache. Generally, when the rash appears, the child no longer feels ill. Assess the cheeks and trunk. Document the appearance of the rash. Assess for pruritus, arthralgia, and lymphadenopathy, which can all accompany the rash.

Treatment

Fifth disease is a benign, self-limiting disease. Once the child presents with a rash, he or she is no longer contagious (Koch, 2016). Supportive treatment, such as maintaining hydration, is the main treatment for fifth disease. If arthralgia is present, acetaminophen or ibuprofen may be used for pain control. Pregnant women should try to avoid children with fifth disease because the virus may cause harm to the fetus.

Hand-Foot-and-Mouth Disease

Hand-foot-and-mouth disease is caused by the coxsackie virus. The coxsackie virus is spread through the fecal–oral route. Poor hand washing is the main cause of outbreaks in day cares and preschools.

Nursing Assessment

Coxsackie virus causes vesicular lesions in the oropharynx (Fig. 17.19) and vesicular or pustular lesions on the palms of the hands and the soles of the feet (Fig. 17.20), hence the name hand-foot-and-mouth disease (Abzug, 2016). The vesicles in the oropharynx may ulcerate.

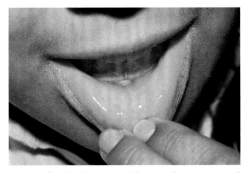

Figure 17.19. Oral ulcers with erythematous base of hand-foot-and-mouth disease. Reprinted with permission from Betts, R. F., Chapman, S. W., & Penn, R. L. (2002). *Reese and Betts' a practical approach to infectious diseases* (5th ed., Fig. 2). Philadelphia, PA: Lippincott Williams & Wilkins.

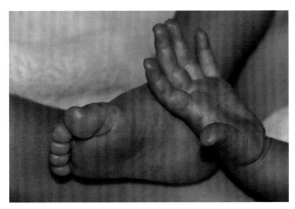

Figure 17.20. Pustular lesions of hand-foot-and-mouth disease on the palms of the hands and soles of the feet. Reprinted with permission from Salimpour, R. R. et al. (2013). *Photographic Atlas of Pediatric Disorders and Diagnosis* (category H, Fig. A, p. 105). Philadelphia, PA: Wolters Kluwer.

 How Much Does It Hurt? 17.1

Pain Assessment in Preschoolers

Maintaining pain control in the preschooler with hand-foot-and-mouth disease is imperative to promote hydration and nutrition. Preschoolers should be able to point to the area that hurts the most. Assess the preschooler's pain level using an age-appropriate self-report tool. Include parental report of the child's behavior to obtain an adequate picture of the child's pain.

Mild fever may or may not be present. Inspect the oropharynx for erythema, vesicles, and ulcerations. Inspect for vesicular and pustular lesions on the hands and feet. These lesions may also be present on the buttocks and groin. In children with eczema, inspect for excoriation in areas where coxsackie lesions are present. Assess pain level (How Much Does It Hurt? 17.1). Assess hydration status and ability to eat.

Treatment

Hand-foot-and-mouth is a self-limiting disease. Lesions generally resolve after 1 week. Supportive care is the mainstay of treatment. Make sure the child is maintaining adequate pain control. Pain control with acetaminophen or ibuprofen is imperative so that the child is able to eat and drink. Maintain hydration status.

Conjunctivitis

Inflammation of the conjunctiva is common in childhood. Conjunctivitis, more commonly known as "pink eye," may be caused by bacteria, viruses, or allergens (Table 17.7).

Table 17.7 Types of Conjunctivitis

Cause	Signs and Symptoms	
Bacterial	• Erythema of the conjunctiva • Purulent drainage • Crusting of the eyelids on wakening • Pruritus may or may not be present • Discomfort • Unilateral or bilateral manifestation	
Viral	• Erythema of the conjunctiva • Watery drainage • Pruritus may or may not be present • Unilateral manifestation • Occurs more in summer (Olitsky et al., 2016)	
Allergic	• Erythema of the conjunctiva • Edematous conjunctiva • Watery drainage • Pruritus almost always present • Usually bilateral	

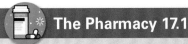

The Pharmacy 17.1   **Medications to Treat Conjunctivitis**

Classification	Route	Action	Nursing Considerations
Antibiotics	• Ophthalmic solution (e.g., ofloxacin 0.3%) • Ophthalmic ointment (e.g., gentamicin 0.3%)	Inhibit bacterial replication	• Solution: instill 2–4 drops in affected eye 4 times daily • Apply gentle pressure after installation • Ointment: apply ½ ribbon to affected eye 2–4 times daily
Mast cell stabilizers	Ophthalmic drops (e.g., nedocromil)	Inhibit inflammatory mechanisms by binding with mast cells	• Instill 1–2 drops daily while exposed to allergen • Avoid contact of bottle tip to cornea
Antihistamines	• Ophthalmic drops (e.g., azelastine) • Oral (e.g., cetirizine)	Inhibit the release of histamine by binding with the histamine receptor sites	• Ophthalmic: instill 1 drop to affected eye twice daily • Oral: monitor for dizziness, drowsiness, headache, bronchospasm, and pharyngitis

Adapted from Taketomo, C. K., Hodding, J. H., & Kraus, D. M. (2018). *Pediatric & neonatal dosage handbook* (25th ed.). Hudson, OH: Lexicomp

Nursing Assessment

Bilaterally inspect the conjunctiva and sclera. Note the amount and type of drainage. If purulent drainage is present, treat the condition as a bacterial conjunctivitis. Assess for upper respiratory symptoms, such as mild fever and rhinorrhea. These symptoms may precede conjunctivitis, especially during the preschool years. Assess for discomfort and pruritus. Determine whether the child has any known allergies.

Treatment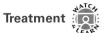

Bacterial conjunctivitis is treated with either antibiotic drops or antibiotic ointments (The Pharmacy 17.1). Warm compresses to the eye help alleviate discomfort (Olitsky et al., 2016). Teach parents to wipe the eyelid gently from the inner canthus to the outer canthus to clean drainage. Bacterial conjunctivitis is extremely contagious. Teach families that good hand washing is imperative to prevent spread.

Viral conjunctivitis is self-limiting. Warm compresses to the eye can help with discomfort in viral conjunctivitis. Allergic conjunctivitis is treated with antihistamines or mast cell stabilizers in either a topical or oral form.

Think Critically

1. Discuss pain assessment in preschoolers. How does pain assessment differ between the early and late preschool years?
2. How does the achievement of initiative affect the preschooler's development? How is development affected if initiative is not achieved?
3. What are some developmental red flags of the preschool years?
4. What are the most important components of anticipatory guidance during the preschool years?
5. Develop a teaching plan to promote early learning and school readiness in the preschool child.
6. Why is play important to development during the preschool years?
7. Develop a plan for optimal nutrition during the preschool years. How can preschoolers be involved in this plan?

References

Abzug, M. J. (2016). Nonpolio enteroviruses. In R. M. Kliegman, B. F. Stanton, J. W. St. Geme III, N. F. Schor, & R. E. Behrman (Eds.), *Nelson's textbook of pediatrics* (20th ed.). Philadelphia, PA: Elsevier, Saunders.

American Academy of Pediatrics. (2013). *Nightmares and night terrors in preschoolers.* Retrieved from https://www.healthychildren.org/English/ages-stages/preschool/Pages/Nightmares-and-Night-Terrors.aspx

American Academy of Pediatrics. (2015a). *Disciplining your child.* Retrieved from https://www.healthychildren.org/English/family-life/family-dynamics/communication-discipline/Pages/Disciplining-Your-Child.aspx

American Academy of Pediatrics. (2015b). *Emotional development in preschoolers.* Retrieved from https://www.healthychildren.org/English/ages-stages/preschool/Pages/Emotional-Development-in-Preschoolers.aspx

American Academy of Pediatrics. (2015c). *Sample menu for a preschooler.* Retrieved from https://www.healthychildren.org/English/ages-stages/preschool/nutrition-fitness/Pages/Sample-One-Day-Menu-for-a-Preschooler.aspx

American Academy of Pediatrics. (2017). *Dangers of magnetic toys.* Retrieved from https://www.healthychildren.org/English/safety-prevention/at-home/Pages/Dangers-of-Magnetic-Toys-and-Fake-Piercings.aspx

American Academy of Pediatrics Council on School Health, Committee on Nutrition. (2015). Snacks, sweetened beverages, added sugars, and schools. *Pediatrics, 135*(3), 1–9. doi:10.1542/peds.2014-3902

Bathory, E., & Tomopoulos, S. (2017). Sleep regulation, physiology and development, sleep duration and patterns, and sleep hygiene in infants, toddlers, and preschool-age children. *Current Problems in Pediatric and Adolescent Health Care, 47*(2), 29–42.

Belter, R. W., McIntosh, J. A., Finch, A. J., & Saylor, C. F. (1988). Preschoolers' ability to differentiate levels of pain: Relative efficacy of three self-report measures. *Journal of Clinical Child Psychology, 17*(4), 329–335.

Cavadel, E. W., & Frye, D. A. (2017). Not just numeracy and literacy: Theory of mind development and school readiness among low-income children. *Developmental Psychology, 53*(12), 2290–2303.

Emmott, A. S., West, N., Zhou, G., Montgomery, C. J., Lauder, G. R., & von Baeyer, C. L. (2017). Validity of simplified versus standard self-report measures of pain intensity in preschool-aged children undergoing venipuncture. *The Journal of Pain, 18*(5), 564–573.

Erikson, E. H. (1963). *Childhood and society.* New York, NY: W.W. Norton and Company.

Feigelman, S. (2016). The second year. In R. M. Kliegman, B. F. Stanton, J. W. St. Geme III, N. F. Schor, & R. E. Behrman (Eds.), *Nelson's textbook of pediatrics* (20th ed.). Philadelphia, PA: Elsevier, Saunders.

Gathercole, V. C. (2014). Bilingualism matters: One size does not fit all. *International Journal of Behavioral Development, 38*(4), 359–366.

Grossklaus, H., & Marvicsin, D. (2014). Parenting efficacy and its relationship to the prevention of childhood obesity. *Pediatric Nursing, 40*(2), 69–86.

Hagan, J. F., Shaw, J. S., & Duncan, P. (Eds.). (2017). *Bright futures: Guidelines for health supervision of infants, children, and adolescents* (4th ed.). Elk Grove Village, IL: American Academy of Pediatrics.

Harvey, T., Davoodi, T., & Blake, P. R. (2018). Young children will lie to prevent a moral transgression. *Journal of Experimental Child Psychology, 165*, 51–65.

Koch, W. C. (2016). Parvoviruses. In R. M. Kliegman, B. F. Stanton, J. W. St. Geme III, N. F. Schor, & R. E. Behrman (Eds.), *Nelson's textbook of pediatrics* (20th ed.). Philadelphia, PA: Elsevier, Saunders.

Kohlberg, L. (1981). *The philosophy of moral development.* New York, NY: Harper & Row.

Leech, K., Wei, R., Harring, J. R., & Rowe, M. L. (2018). A brief parent-focused intervention to improve preschoolers' conversational skills and school readiness. *Developmental Psychology, 54*(1), 15–28.

Liacouras, D. A. (2016). Stomach and intestines: Normal structure, development, and function. In R. M. Kliegman, B. F. Stanton, J. W. St. Geme III,

N. F. Schor, & R. E. Behrman (Eds.), *Nelson's textbook of pediatrics* (20th ed.). Philadelphia, PA: Elsevier, Saunders.

McLeod, R. H., Hardy, J. K., & Kaiser, A. P. (2017). The effects of play-based intervention on vocabulary acquisition by preschoolers at risk for reading and language delays. *Journal of Early Intervention, 39*(2), 147–160.

Mottweiler C. M., & Taylor, M. (2014). Elaborated role play and creativity in children. *Psychology of Aesthetics, Creativity, and the Arts, 8*(3), 277–286.

Nerud, K., & Samra, H. (2017). Make a move intervention to reduce childhood obesity. *The Journal of School Nursing, 33*(3), 205–213.

Olitsky, S., Hug, D., Plummer, L. S., Stahl, E. D., Ariss, M. M., & Lindquist, T. P. (2016). Disorders of the conjunctiva. In R. M. Kliegman, B. F. Stanton, J. W. St. Geme III, N. F. Schor, & R. E. Behrman (Eds.), *Nelson's textbook of pediatrics* (20th ed.). Philadelphia, PA: Elsevier, Saunders.

Parks, E. P., Maqbool, A., Shaikhkhalil, A., Groleau, V., Dougherty, K. A., & Stallings, V.A. (2016). Nutritional requirements. In R. M. Kliegman, B. F. Stanton, J. W. St. Geme III, N. F. Schor, & R. E. Behrman (Eds.), *Nelson's textbook of pediatrics* (20th ed.). Philadelphia, PA: Elsevier, Saunders.

Piaget, J. (1930). *The child's conception of physical causality.* London, England: Routledge & Kegan Paul Ltd.

Talwar, V., Crossman, A., & Wyman, J. (2017). The role of executive functioning and theory of mind in children's lies for another and for themselves. *Early Childhood Research Quarterly, 41*, 126–135.

Thrane, S. E., Wanless, S., Cohen, S. M., & Danford, C. A. (2016). The assessment and non-pharmacologic treatment of procedural pain from infancy to school age through a developmental lens: A synthesis of evidence with recommendations. *Journal of Pediatric Nursing, 31*, e23–e32.

Wong, D. L., & Baker, C. M. (1988). Pain in children: Comparison of assessment scales. *Pediatric Nursing, 14*(1), 9–17.

U.S. Department of Health and Human Services. (2017). *Office of head start.* Retrieved from https://www.acf.hhs.gov/ohs/about

Suggested Readings

American Academy of Pediatrics. (2015). *Energy in: Recommended food and drink amounts for children.* Retrieved from https://www.healthychildren.org/English/healthy-living/nutrition/Pages/Energy-In-Recommended-Food-Drink-Amounts-for-Children.aspx

Emmott, A. S., West, N., Zhou, G., Montgomery, C. J., Lauder, G. R., & von Baeyer, C. L. (2017). Validity of simplified versus standard self-report measures of pain intensity in preschool-aged children undergoing venipuncture. *The Journal of Pain, 18*(5), 564–573.

Healthy People 2020. (2014). *Early and middle childhood.* Retrieved from https://www.healthypeople.gov/2020/topics-objectives/topic/early-and-middle-childhood

18

Care of the School-Age Child

Growth and Development Overview

The school-age period of growth and development encompasses ages 6 through 12 years. During the school-age years, the child continues to mature in all aspects of growth and development. Coordination, balance, and strength improve, sparking an interest in sports, as well as in arts and crafts. The school-age child begins to think logically and see things from another's point of view. Friends become more important as children want to spend time with each other and learn to separate from their parents. Children develop self-confidence and learn how to deal with peer pressure. Starting school and academic preparedness are important aspects of the school-age years.

Health Assessment

Input from the child becomes an integral part of the health assessment in the school-age years. During the health history, direct questions at the child, especially with an older school-age child, but verify information with the parents and ask them questions to fill in gaps in information. Ask the younger school-age child simple and direct questions. With an older school-age child, ask more complex questions as needed to elicit more detailed information. Enquire of the child's health by asking him or her, "Do you think you are healthy?" and "What does being healthy mean to you?" Ask the parents whether they have any concerns about the child's development, school performance, or behavior. Finally, ask the parents about their child's abilities and what makes them proud.

School-age children should able to sit on an exam table during the health assessment. Perform the exam in a head-to-toe manner. If an exam of the genitalia is warranted, perform this exam last. Before performing each specific assessment, explain in concrete terms what will happen during it and why. For example, before auscultating the heart, tell the child, "I am going to listen to your heart to see how strong it is." Parents should remain in the room during the entirety of the exam during the school-age period.

Head, Eyes, Ears, Nose, and Throat

Enquire about the child's vision and hearing. Do the parents have any concerns? Ask the child whether he or she is able to see the board at school. Does the child have trouble seeing to read? Does the child have pressure-equalizing tubes? Is there a history of eye infections? Does the child have a history of head injury? Has the child had any cavities? Has the child seen the dentist? Ask about recurrent pharyngitis, history of large tonsils, or difficulty swallowing.

Head

Inspect the head and hair, noting any lesions or infestation with lice. Inspect the face for symmetry and the head for symmetry relative to the neck. Palpate the head for nodules. Palpate the lymph nodes, noting their size, shape, consistency, and movability. Frontal sinuses are fully developed by age 7 years. Palpate the sinuses for tenderness. Children at this age are old enough to follow directions and participate in cranial nerve testing.

Eyes

Inspect the eyes for symmetry. Note the color of the sclera and conjunctiva. Assess the pupils; they should be equal, round, and reactive to light and assessment. Perform all cranial nerve tests as for an adult.

School-age children are able to use the traditional Snellen chart (Fig. 18.1). All children should have a full eye exam by an ophthalmologist before entering school. Visual acuity other than 20/20 should be further evaluated.

Ears

Assess the symmetry and placement of the ears. Note any redness or drainage. Palpate for swelling or tenderness. Assess hearing using an otoacoustic emissions test. If it is not possible to conduct otoacoustic emissions, a simple whisper test will suffice. If inner ear inspection is indicated, pull the pinna up and back.

Nose

Assess the nose as previously described (see Chapter 17). Test for sense of smell in the school-age child by having the child close his or her eyes. Hold a familiar scent under the nose and have the child identify the scent.

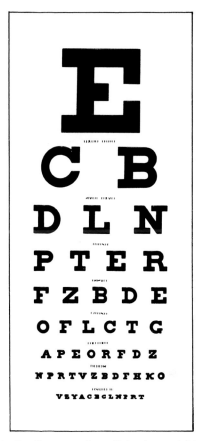

Figure 18.1. Snellen eye chart. School-age children can use the traditional Snellen eye chart to test their visual acuity. Reprinted with permission from Taylor, C., Lillis, C., & Lynn, P. (2014). *Fundamentals of nursing* (8th ed., Fig. 25.4). Philadelphia, PA: Lippincott Williams & Wilkins.

Mouth and Throat

Assess the mouth as previously described (see Chapter 17). Note the absence of primary teeth and presence of permanent teeth. Figure 18.2 indicates the ages at which the permanent teeth typically erupt.

Tonsils hypertrophy during the school-age years. Note the size and color of the tonsils and the presence of any exudate. Assess the uvula; it should be midline and rise with elicitation of the gag reflex.

Neurological Assessment

Brain growth slows during the school-age years. Between the ages of 6 and 12 years, the head grows only a total of 2 cm (0.7 in; Feigelman, 2016). Facial structure changes, becoming more elongated.

Ask the parents whether they have any concerns about their child's gait, balance, and coordination. Is the child oriented to person, place, and time? Is the child able to button and unbutton clothes, write with a pencil, and color with a crayon? Are there any concerns with speech? Have there been any changes in muscle strength?

The neurological assessment during the school-age years should include assessment of sensory function, coordination,

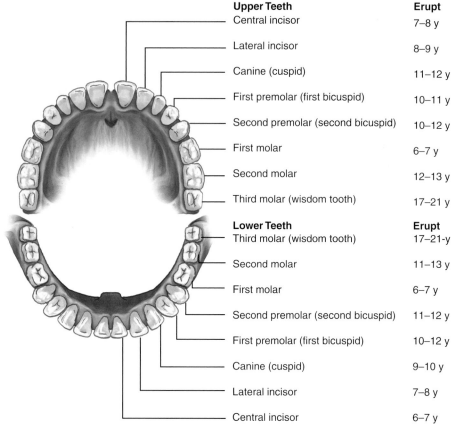

Upper Teeth	Erupt
Central incisor	7–8 y
Lateral incisor	8–9 y
Canine (cuspid)	11–12 y
First premolar (first bicuspid)	10–11 y
Second premolar (second bicuspid)	10–12 y
First molar	6–7 y
Second molar	12–13 y
Third molar (wisdom tooth)	17–21 y
Lower Teeth	**Erupt**
Third molar (wisdom tooth)	17–21-y
Second molar	11–13 y
First molar	6–7 y
Second premolar (second bicuspid)	11–12 y
First premolar (first bicuspid)	10–12 y
Canine (cuspid)	9–10 y
Lateral incisor	7–8 y
Central incisor	6–7 y

Figure 18.2. Normal pattern of tooth eruption. Reprinted with permission from Kyle, T., & Carman, S. (2016). *Essentials of pediatric nursing* (3rd ed., Fig. 10.23). Philadelphia, PA: Wolters Kluwer.

gait, balance, and development. Observe the child's gait. Ask the child to balance on each foot, jump up and down with both feet, and jump up and down on each foot. Have the child hop across the floor and skip back. Test the deep tendon reflexes, documenting the reflex response. Note whether the reflexes are equal bilaterally.

Conduct formal tests of cranial nerves and fine motor function on the school-age child. Test for sensation with sharp and dull touch. Test for coordination with the Romberg test, finger-to-finger test, finger-to-nose test, heel-to-shin test, and rapid, alternating hand movements.

The school-age child should be oriented to person, place, and time, at least to the day of the week. By the end of the school-age period, the child should also be oriented to today's date. School-age children should know their address and phone number.

Respiratory Assessment

School-age children may use their thoracic muscles to assist with breathing. Alveoli reach their adult-level numbers and function between 8 and 10 years of age. The maturation of the respiratory system results in fewer respiratory infections overall, although starting school exposes children to a myriad of infectious agents and may result in an increase in respiratory illnesses for a period of time.

Ask the parents whether the child has a history of asthma or other respiratory disorders. Assess respiratory effort. Normal respiratory rate in the school-age child is 16 to 22 breaths/min. Observe the rise and fall of the chest to measure respiratory rate. Note the use of any accessory muscles. Auscultate in all lung fields. Instruct the child to take deep breaths in and blow them out. Note if and where any adventitious lung sounds are heard.

Cardiovascular Assessment

Ask the parents whether the child has a history of congenital heart disease, cardiac surgery, or cardiac infection. If the child has a history of a congenital heart defect, determine the type of defect and the extent of the repair. Is the child still symptomatic? Does the child have activity intolerance?

During the school-age years, the point of maximal impulse moves to the fifth intercostal space at the midclavicular line (see Fig. 15.7). The heart rate ranges from 70 to 110 beats/min. Blood pressure ranges from 95 to 120 mm Hg systolic and 60 to 76 mm Hg diastolic. Assess pulses and note any difference between upper and lower extremities. Assess capillary refill in all four extremities. Auscultate for murmurs and document appropriately.

For children in the late school-age years, screen for hyperlipidemia. All children should have their total cholesterol and triglyceride levels checked at 11 years old. Children with a family history of high cholesterol should be screened earlier.

Gastrointestinal Assessment

Stomach size increases during the school-age years, allowing for increased time between bowel movements. Bowel movements become more regular, although constipation may still be an issue. At this age, bowel movements are greatly affected by diet and physical activity or lack thereof.

Determine whether the child has a history of gastrointestinal infections. Does he or she have frequent diarrhea or constipation? Does the child have a history of persistent nausea and/or vomiting? Inspect the abdomen. The abdomen should be flat, not sunken or protruding. Palpate the abdomen, noting any guarding, rigidity, tenderness, or hepatosplenomegaly.

Genitourinary Assessment

During the school-age years, bladder capacity increases, allowing for longer time between voidings. Children should achieve nighttime dryness by the beginning of the school-age period. If the child is still wetting the bed, determine whether there is a family history of bedwetting. If children have achieved nighttime dryness but begin wetting the bed again, further workup is warranted.

In Chapter 10, Sophia Carter wet the bed at 7 years. Had Sophia previously achieved nighttime dryness? What other symptoms was Sophia exhibiting? Why were her symptoms of concern? What are some other reasons children who have achieved nighttime dryness might begin wetting the bed?

Determine whether the child has a history of recurrent urinary tract infections. Is the child experiencing any discharge, dysuria, or foul-smelling urine? If the genitalia need to be examined, perform this exam last. Assure privacy for the child. Parents should remain in the room for the genitalia exam.

The end of the school-age years is characterized by a period known as prepubescence. Secondary sexual characteristics begin to develop in both males and females during this time. Development varies from child to child, depending on genetics, environment, and nutrition (Tanner, 1962). Obesity has an effect on the development of secondary sexual characteristics and on puberty. Obese females start puberty earlier than typical-weight females, whereas obese males start puberty later than typical-weight males (Reinehr, 2017). Assess for appropriate development of secondary sexual characteristics. Progression of secondary sexual characteristics is described and documented using **Tanner stages** (Holland-Hall & Burstein, 2016; Tanner, 1962).

Determine whether the child or parent has any questions about the development of secondary sexual characteristics or about puberty in general. Encourage parents to talk with their child about the upcoming changes in the child's body. Encourage the child to ask questions and emphasize that these changes are normal. Ask the parent and child whether they have any concerns about the child's development.

Males

Development of secondary sexual characteristics begins between 9 and 14 years of age in males, with an average of 12 years of age. The first sign of development is testicular enlargement to 3 mL or greater (Hendriks, Prentice, & Williams, 2017). Growth spurts in males tend to occur later in pubertal development.

Refer males showing signs of secondary sexual characteristics before the age of 9 years to an endocrinologist for evaluation for **precocious puberty**. See Figure 18.3 and Table 18.1 for information on the Tanner stages describing progression of secondary sexual characteristics for males.

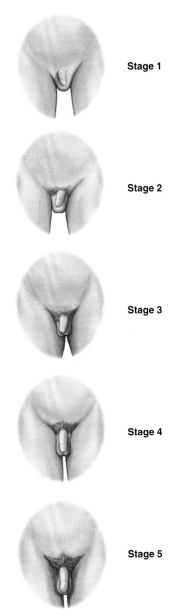

Figure 18.3. Male Tanner stages. Tanner sexual maturity stages for males depicting pubic hair and penile growth. Reprinted with permission from Kyle, T., & Carman, S. (2016). *Essentials of pediatric nursing* (3rd ed., Fig. 10.34). Philadelphia, PA: Wolters Kluwer; adapted from Tanner, J. M. (1962). *Growth at adolescence.* Oxford, England: Blackwell Scientific Publications.

Table 18.1 Tanner Sexual Maturity Rating for Males

Stage	Penis	Testes	Pubic Hair
1	No change	No change	None
2	No change	Enlarged scrotum	Scant, light in color
3	Increased length	Increased size	Darker, curls
4	Increased breadth	Scrotum darkens	Resembles adult but less quantity
5	Adult size	Adult size	Adult distribution

Data from Tanner, J. M. (1962). *Growth at adolescence.* Oxford, England: Blackwell Scientific Publications.

Females

Development of secondary sexual characteristics begins between the ages of 8 and 13 years in females, with an average of 11 years of age. The first sign of puberty is the development of breast buds, or **thelarche,** and a rapid growth spurt. The early growth spurt in girls results in them being taller, on average, than same-aged boys at the end of the school-age years (Hendriks et al., 2017).

Healthcare providers typically consider development of secondary sexual characteristics before the age of 8 years a sign of precocious puberty in females. However, new guidelines recommend that development not be considered precocious unless it is before the age of 7 years in Caucasian females and before the age of 6 years in African American females (Sultan, Gaspari, Maimoun, Kalfa, & Paris, 2018). **Menarche** generally occurs about 2 years after the development of breast buds. See Figures 18.4 and 18.5 and Table 18.2 for information on the Tanner stages describing progression of secondary sexual characteristics for females.

Musculoskeletal Assessment

Muscle strength and coordination increase throughout the school-age years. However, the bones are not fully ossified, and the child is still at risk for injury. Skeletal maturation is associated with staging of secondary sexual characteristics (Keane, 2016). The more the child progresses in the development of secondary sexual characteristics, the more progressive the skeletal development.

Enquire about any past musculoskeletal injuries. Do the parents or child have any concerns regarding the child's strength or coordination? Observe the child walk across the room normally and then walk back heel-to-toe. Test strength by having the child push his or her hands and feet against your hands. Assess the range of motion of all extremities.

Inspect for scoliosis by having the child lean over and touch his or her toes. Document any curvature in the spine. Have the child sit on the exam table, and observe for uneven shoulder height.

Integumentary Assessment

Acne often occurs with the development of secondary sexual characteristics. Inspect the child's face and back for **comedones,**

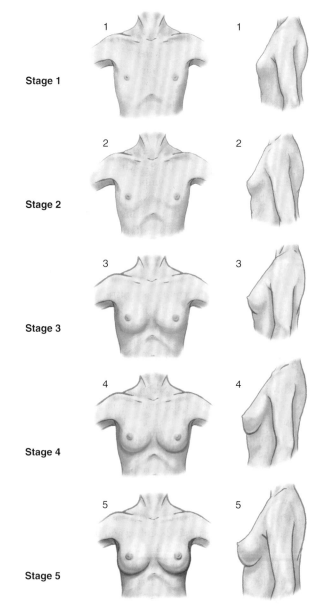

Figure 18.4. Female Tanner stages: Breast development. Adapted with permisison from Jensen, S. (2014). *Nursing health assessment* (2nd ed., Fig. 19.5). Philadelphia, PA: Wolters Kluwer.

Immunological Assessment

The immune system is fully developed by the end of the school-age years. Because of this, children may experience fewer infections during this time. Determine whether the child has a history of frequent illnesses and whether the parent or child has any concerns.

Pain Assessment

School-age children are able to locate, quantify, and describe pain. The descriptions of pain become more detailed as the child progresses through the school-age period. Continue to use the Oucher or FACES Pain Rating Scale for children younger than age 7 years (refer to Pain Assessment in Chapter 17). Children older than 7 years are able to use the Numerical Rating Scale (NRS; see How Much Does It Hurt? 3.1; Shields, Palermo, Powers, Grewe, & Smith, 2003). The NRS is a straight line with numbers spaced evenly along the line, generally labeled 0 through 10. The number 0 indicates no pain, and the number 10 indicates the worst pain ever felt by the child.

No matter which scale is used, ask the child to rate his or her pain (Analyze the Evidence 18.1). For younger school-age children, ask where the pain is. Ask questions such as, "Does it feel like someone is poking you with something sharp?" or "Does it feel like something is being twisted?" Older school-age children are able to understand when asked whether the pain is sharp, dull, or burning.

Nonpharmacological pain management such as distraction works well in the school-aged child. Music, television, video games, and guided imagery are all techniques that can be used effectively with this age group (Thrane, Wanless, Cohen, & Danford, 2016). For children who experience chronic pain, distraction can be important for maintaining activities of daily living. Conduct a thorough pain assessment, and do not assume that because a child is quiet and watching television that the child is not in pain.

When conducting a pain assessment, account for the child's cultural background. Some cultures look down upon expressions of pain. Therefore, nurses may not always be able to rely on visual and verbal cues, making self-report all the more important (Thrane et al., 2016).

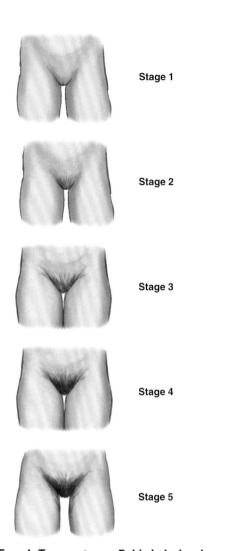

Stage 1

Stage 2

Stage 3

Stage 4

Stage 5

Figure 18.5. Female Tanner stages: Pubic hair development. Reprinted with permission from Kyle, T., & Carman, S. (2016). *Essentials of pediatric nursing* (3rd ed., Fig. 10.36). Philadelphia, PA: Wolters Kluwer; adapted from Tanner, J. M. (1962). *Growth at adolescence.* Oxford, England: Blackwell Scientific Publications.

pustules, and nodules. Inspect for any other rashes that may be present. Ask whether the parent or child has any concerns about the child's skin.

Table 18.2 Tanner Sexual Maturity Rating for Females

Stage	Breasts	Pubic Hair
1	No change	None
2	Breast elevated, areola enlarged	Scant, light in color
3	Breast and areola enlarged, no contour definition between breast and areola	Darker, curls
4	Areola forms mound separate from breast	Resembles that of adult but scant
5	Adult appearance, nipple projects	Adult distribution

Data from Tanner, J. M. (1962). *Growth at adolescence.* Oxford, England: Blackwell Scientific Publications.

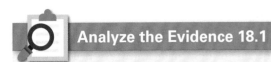

Analyze the Evidence 18.1

The Rainbow Pain Scale

In trying to develop a more valid self-report pain scale for preschoolers, researchers tested this new pain scale for validity in school-age children aged 5–10 y as a first step. The Rainbow Pain Scale (RPS) was originally developed by the mother of a young child. The scale allows the child to use colors to describe his or her pain. The child determines which color is associated with each level of pain. There are a total of five colors in the child's rainbow. Therefore, the pain scale is child-centered and individualized to each child.

Mahon et al. (2015) tested the validity of the RPS against the FACES Pain Rating Scale in children from 5 to 10 years old. Participants were 52 children in either an inpatient or outpatient setting at a tertiary medical center. The researchers found that the RPS showed high concurrent validity with the FACES scale. For future study, the researchers will test the validity of the RPS in the preschool-age group.

Physical Growth

During the school-age years, the child experiences changes in appearance. Some children have developed secondary sexual characteristics by the end of the school-age period, whereas others have not. Legs and arms grow faster at first than the rest of the body, giving older school-age children an awkward, gangly appearance. Body types and sizes vary depending on the onset of puberty, nutritional status, and physical activity. Physical maturity and cognitive maturity do not always correlate. Although a child may be more physically advanced for his or her age, he or she should be treated on the basis of cognitive maturity. The same goes for the child who develops late.

Weight

Weight gain averages 6.5 to 7.5 lb/y (2.9–3.4 kg; Feigelman, 2016) but varies depending on the child's diet and level of physical activity. Plot the child's body mass index (BMI) on the appropriate chart to determine whether the child is at risk for overweight or obesity (growth charts available at http://www.cdc.gov/growthcharts).

Height

Height increases about 2.5 to 3 in/ year (6.3–7.6 cm) during the school-age years (Feigelman, 2016). This growth occurs at discontinuous times throughout the year. There are months of no growth followed by months of rapid growth in height. Girls have a large growth spurt at the end of the school-age period, generally making girls taller than boys by the time they are 12 years old.

Developmental Theories

During the school-age years, children begin to understand points of view other than their own but are not yet able to think abstractly. Table 18.3 gives an overview of selected developmental theories for school-age children.

Psychosocial

Initiative is the psychosocial task of the school-age years. Children learn to master tasks and develop confidence that they can achieve their goals. The child learns to be productive and persevere to task completion (Erikson, 1963). If the child does not

Table 18.3	Overview of Developmental Theories in School-Age Children	
Theorist: Type of Development	**Stage**	**Implications**
Erikson: Psychosocial	Industry vs. inferiority	• Is learning to do more things on own • Develops confidence in ability to achieve goals • Develops competence • Likes to understand how things work
Piaget: Cognitive	Concrete operational	• Thinks about things in a logical and concrete manner • Can put items in a sequential order • Learns about objects through manipulation • Understands the concept of reversibility • Understands the concept of conservation • Understands the concept of time
Freud: Psychosexual	Latent	• Focuses more on relationships with same-sex peers
Kohlberg: Moral	Conventional	• Follows rules • Takes societal law into perspective • Begins to see things from different perspectives

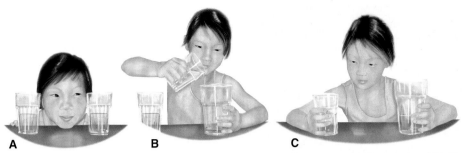

Figure 18.6. **Principle of conservation.** School-age children understand the theory of conservation **(A)**. If you pour an equal amount of liquid into two glasses of unequal shape **(B)**, the amount of water you have remains the same despite the unequal appearance in the two glasses **(C)**. Reprinted with permission from Kyle, T., & Carman, S. (2016). *Essentials of pediatric nursing* (3rd ed., Fig. 6.2). Philadelphia, PA: Wolters Kluwer.

achieve the task of industry, he or she risks feeling inferior. The feeling of inferiority comes from a sense of inadequacy from not achieving set goals.

To establish confidence, ensure that the child is able to master tasks and achieve goals set before them. Make sure that the child is involved in activities that match the child's abilities. Children at this age become involved in sports and other outside activities. Encourage parents to challenge their child but to set realistic, achievable goals, not ones that are so high that they are unachievable, particularly when it comes to academics, sports, and other activities. Teach parents to support and encourage the child when setbacks occur.

Giving school-age children chores around the house also helps them establish a sense of industry. Routine daily or weekly chores help instill responsibility and a sense of accomplishment in the school-age child.

Cognitive

The concrete operational stage is the beginning of logical and organized thought (Piaget, 1930). The school-age child understands the concepts of cause and effect. The school-age child also wants to understand how things such as an engine or a computer work. Therefore, the school-age child can often be seen building models or taking things apart to see how they work. Collecting objects and displaying them in some sort of sequential order or by classification occur during this stage, as well.

As part of logical thinking, school-age children develop an understanding of the concept of conservation (Fig. 18.6). **Conservation** allows the child to understand that when a liquid is poured from a tall, thin glass into a short, fat glass the amount of liquid stays the same. An additional hallmark concept of the concrete operational stage is **reversibility**. The school-age child understands that many sequences are reversible.

Moral

School-age children move to the conventional level of moral development, which is characterized by maintaining the expectations of the family and society (Kohlberg, 1981). Conformity to these expectations drives the school-age child's behaviors.

The conventional level is further divided into two stages. The first stage of the conventional level (the third stage, overall, in Kohlberg's theory of moral development), which occurs in the early school-age years, is the interpersonal concordance or "good boy, good girl" stage (Kohlberg, 1981). During this stage, the child's behavior is driven by wanting to be good. The 6- to 10-year-old is intent on following rules and conforming to the stereotypes of society. At this age, children want to please their parents, their teachers, and other authority figures. The second stage of the conventional level (the fourth stage, overall) is the "law and order" or "society" stage (Kohlberg, 1981). Older school-age children begin to understand that there is more than one point of view. Actions can be seen on the basis of intentions and judged less harshly if someone "means well." Behavior at this age is born out of respect for others.

Motor Development

The school-age period is a time of refinement of both gross and fine motor skills. Speed, accuracy, and coordination increase, allowing for participation in sports as well as in intricate activities such as sewing or building model cars. Asking what the child is involved in helps assess whether the child is meeting appropriate motor development milestones.

In Chapter 2, Mollie Sanders was seen for her well-child checkup when she was 8 years old. Was her motor development on target? What was she doing that led you to believe her development was or was not on target? Are there any other questions the healthcare provider could have asked Mollie about her activities, likes, and dislikes?

Gross Motor

Muscle coordination and balance improve during the school-age years. By the time a child is 7 to 8 years old, he or she may enjoy riding a bike, playing sports, or jumping rope (Fig. 18.7). Rhythm improves as well, allowing the school-age child to participate in dance or gymnastics. For the school-age child who enjoys sports, increased accuracy allows for a sense of confidence. If a growth spurt happens toward the end of the

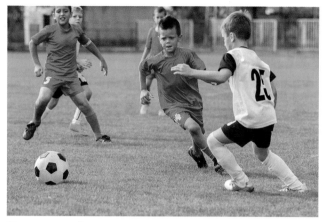

Figure 18.7. Gross motor development. School-age children enjoy participating in team sports.

school-age period, ages 10 to 12 years, the child may lose some coordination because of the awkwardness of the child's body. Assure both the child and the parent that the muscles will catch up with the skeletal growth and coordination will return.

Fine Motor

With the development of finger dexterity and hand–eye coordination, school-age children are able to participate in activities such as playing an instrument, braiding string for bracelets, and building models (Fig. 18.8). As these skills are developing, the

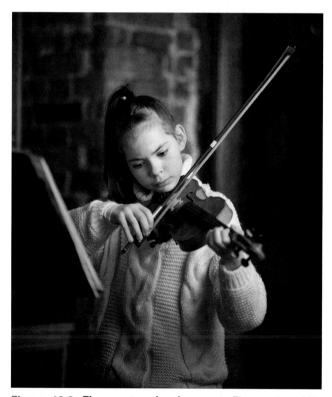

Figure 18.8. Fine motor development. Fine motor skills become fine-tuned, allowing school-age children to play instruments.

school-age child may become frustrated. Encouraging practice helps further develop fine motor skills. By the end of the school-age years, children have roughly the same manual dexterity as do adults.

Communication and Language Development

A child's understanding of language becomes more complex throughout the school-age period. The school-age child has the ability to think about language and how it is used. The use of jokes and humor is common during this period because at this age children understand play on words. Reading skills increase, and many children discover a love of reading at this age. The school-age child develops the ability to think about and talk through thoughts and feelings. Therefore, allow children time to express their feelings when they are upset, angry, or frustrated.

Social and Emotional Development

During this period children begin to separate from their parents. Peers and teachers have influence in the child's life in addition to the child's own family. Through interactions with others, children develop either a positive or negative self-esteem (Growth and Development Check 18.1). Encouraging parents to help their children develop a positive view of themselves will allow the children to deal with different pressures in social situations.

Friendships

Around the age of 7 years, children typically identify a best friend. Children at this age want to be accepted by their peers and must learn to deal with peer pressure. A child with positive self-esteem and good social skills will learn to not always give in to peer pressure. A child with poor social skills and a negative self-esteem may go to extreme measures to win acceptance by peers (Feigelman, 2016). Children who choose not to conform

Growth and Development Check 18.1

Signs of Low Self-Esteem

Children with low self-esteem feel they are not capable of completing tasks, developing talent, or having friends. These children tend to exhibit some of the following behaviors (AAP, 2015g):

- Gives up on tasks easily, fearing failure
- Cheats or lies to avoid failure
- Often says things such as "I'm stupid" or "I can't"
- Places blame on external forces
- Is strongly affected by negative peer comments
- Withdraws socially

to the norms of their peers may get made fun of or be a target for bullying. Parents should be aware of negative behavior changes in their child.

During the school-age years, peer groups tend to be same-sex. This helps children learn to work together and to see viewpoints different from their own. Parents should teach children that friends are people who don't ask them to do things that are harmful or scary. Knowing who their child's friends are helps parents keep their child safe and allows them to teach their child when there are problems among the peer group. Being part of a peer group helps with positive socialization of the school-age child.

School

Interactions in school have a profound influence on the child, second only to the child's individual family. Teachers can have a positive influence on school-age children. A teacher's support and positive attitude help the child to complete the task of industry and develop a positive self-esteem. Parents can assist in the transition to school by encouraging separation through positive reinforcement. Children who cling to their parents should not be allowed to continue the behavior, because it will hinder the transition to the classroom. When parents encourage their child to enter the classroom, they are allowing the child to develop independence, learn to follow rules, and develop the social skills needed to have a positive school experience (Fig. 18.9).

Body Image

A child's body image is often associated with the child's self-esteem. A child with a positive body image most likely will have a positive self-esteem, and a child with a negative body image most likely will have a negative self-esteem. It is important for the school-age child to be accepted by peers. Having the right clothes, shoes, and accessories becomes important to the child's self-image, especially during the late school-age years.

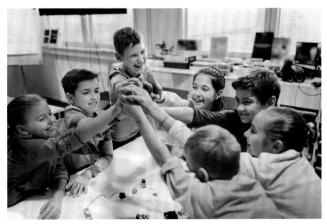

Figure 18.9. School-age development. It is important for school to be a positive experience for the school-age child.

The idea of body image is influenced by peers, adults, and media. Girls tend to be more concerned with appearance-related comparisons, whereas boys tend to be more concerned with sports-related comparisons (Tatangelo & Ricciardelli, 2017). As school-age children enter puberty, body types and shapes vary significantly. Girls who develop early may feel embarrassed, whereas boys who develop late may feel weaker than their peers. Remind school-age children that everyone develops at a different time and that their development is normal. Ask children whether they have any concerns about their body and encourage them to talk about it if they do.

Gender Identity and Gender Dysphoria

By school age, most children have fully identified with either the male or female gender. However, some children may identify with a gender that is different from their biological sex. **Gender dysphoria** occurs in the prepubescent child around the age of 9 or 10 years. For some children, gender dysphoria is long term, whereas for others it is not (American Academy of Pediatrics [AAP], 2015c). Gender dysphoria in the prepubescent period tends to resolve by the end of adolescence (American College of Pediatricians, 2017). However, children with gender dysphoria may grow up to identify with the opposite sex and/or to identify as gay, lesbian, or bisexual in orientation (AAP, 2015c).

Children who have gender dysphoria often have comorbid psychiatric disorders that worsen during puberty (Lopez, Stewart, & Jacobson-Dickman, 2016). Assure families that parenting did not cause gender dysphoria in their child. Although gender dysphoria is not well understood, members of the healthcare team must support families of children with gender dysphoria.

Nurses are in the position to assist families in adjusting to having a child with gender dysphoria. Remain nonjudgmental when caring for these families. Encourage parents to be open to the needs of their child and accept the child for who the child is. Teach parents behaviors to watch for that indicate bullying of their child. In addition, encourage parents to look for signs of anxiety, depression, and low self-esteem in their child. Social workers, psychiatrists, and adolescent medicine specialists should be involved in the care of a child with gender dysphoria to address all concerns.

Health Promotion

Throughout the school-age years, continue to promote health with children and their families. Help families through the changes that occur during this time, from starting school to entering puberty. Schedule routine health promotion visits yearly for children 6 to 12 years of age (Hagan, Shaw, & Duncan, 2017).

Promoting Healthy Growth and Development

Promoting healthy growth and development during the school-age years continues to involve assessing the family and social context in which the child lives (Priority Care Concepts 18.1). Assess social determinants of health and protective factors.

Priority Care Concepts 18.1

Promoting Growth and Development in School-Age Children

Communication and Social Development

- Self-esteem development
- Respectful communication
- Positive interactions between parents and child

Sleep

- Established bedtime
- No television, computer, or electronic devices in bedroom

Oral Health

- Brushing teeth and flossing
- Dental visits

Safety

- Home environment
- Outside environment
- School environment
- Internet safety

Nutrition

- Limit sugary beverages and snacks
- Appropriate portion sizes
- Importance of breakfast

School

- School attendance
- School performance

Physical Activity

- 60 min of physical activities daily
- Age-appropriate activities

Mental Health

- Dealing with anger and frustration
- Appropriate choices of friends

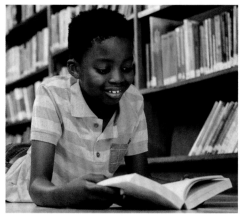

Figure 18.10. Promoting reading. Promoting reading during the school-age years fosters academic success. Reprinted with permission from Bickley, L. S. (2017). *Bates' guide to physical examination and history taking* (12th ed., Fig. 18.2). Philadelphia, PA: Wolters Kluwer.

school helps children learn to follow rules, adapt to new situations, and work with others.

Parents should continue to promote reading with their child (Fig. 18.10). Determine what types of books the child likes. The types of books children read become more complex throughout the school-age years. Allow the child to make choices in the types of books to read. Parents should determine the appropriateness of the books for their child and consult with teachers regarding appropriate reading level.

Children who struggle significantly in school should be evaluated for possible learning disabilities. If a child has an intellectual disability, parents, in conjunction with teachers and healthcare providers, should determine the best course of action for the child. An individualized education program (IEP) or 504 plan allows for accommodations so that the child can meet academic goals (Growth and Development Check 18.2).

In Chapter 13, Jack Wray's mother was concerned about Jack having an IEP. Why was she concerned about this? Why did Jack need an IEP? Was he a better candidate for an IEP or for a 504 plan? How could either of these help Jack with academic success?

Communication between the family and child allows for the child to be involved in making choices for a healthy lifestyle.

Learning

Formal schooling accounts for much of the learning throughout the school-age years. Parents and teachers must work together to ensure that the child is progressing appropriately. Parental support with homework helps the child with school success. A positive relationship with teachers allows the child to develop a positive self-esteem and master the task of industry. Being in

Safety

As school-age children gain more and more independence, parents need to be aware of the dangers their children face (Patient Teaching 18.1). Unintentional injury is the leading cause of death for children under the age of 19 years, overall, whereas motor vehicle accidents are the leading cause of death for children 5 to 19 years old (Centers for Disease Control and Prevention [CDC], 2016b). Parents play a major role in protecting their children from injury. Parents should address safety issues with their child and the importance of wearing safety equipment when riding

Growth and Development Check 18.2

Individualized Education Programs and 504 Plans

An IEP is a plan for children with disabilities that sets goals for the child. The plan outlines the services and supplemental aids that the school will provide for the child (AAP, 2015d). Many of the services can be provided in the regular classrooms. However, other services are too involved to be provided in the classroom. For more specialized services, children spend time in a resource room, often with other children having the same accommodations (KidsHealth, 2018b). Reasons for an IEP include, but are not limited to, the following:

- Physical disabilities
- Learning disabilities
- Autism
- Attention deficit hyperactivity disorder

   Students who need only mild accommodations in the classroom may qualify for a 504 plan. Such accommodations may include extra time on tests, verbal testing, visual aids, or modified textbooks (KidsHealth, 2018a). Whether a child has an IEP or a 504 plan, parents, teachers, and healthcare providers must work as a team to provide the best outcomes for the child.

bikes or playing sports (Fig. 18.11). Reminding children that they should never go with strangers and that nobody should touch them inappropriately continues to be important. For children who are home after school by themselves, parents should set rules and a safety plan for when a child is home alone. Remind parents that although their child may be getting older, the child still needs to be supervised for many activities.

Oral Health

By the school-age years, the child should have a dental home and be used to seeing a dentist twice a year for routine exams and cleanings. At this age, children are able to brush their own

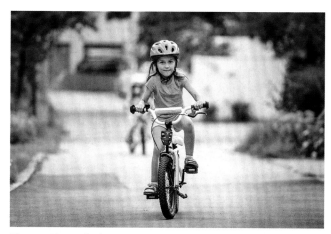

Figure 18.11. Safety. School-age children should wear appropriate safety equipment.

Patient Teaching 18.1

Safety for School-Age Children

Nurses are able to help promotion of safety through educating both parents and children on potential unintentional injuries and how to prevent them.

Sports
- Have children wear necessary sports equipment while playing.
- Learn to recognize signs of a concussion.
- Make sure children stay hydrated.
- Learn to recognize signs of dehydration and overheating.

Water
- Never allow children to swim alone.
- Have children learn how to swim.
- Have children wear life jackets in bodies of water other than a swimming pool.

Bike
- Have children wear a helmet at all times when riding a bike.
- Make sure the helmet fits securely and is buckled when worn.
- Teach children to watch for cars when riding on the road.

Car
- Children less than 4 ft 9 in tall should be in a booster seat with the regular car belt.
- Children may use a seat belt only when the lap belt fits on the hips and the shoulder belt is across the shoulder rather than the neck.
- Children under the age of 12 y should sit in the back seat.

Pedestrian
- Teach children to stop at the curb and look both ways before crossing a street.
- Have older children hold younger children's hands when walking on or near streets.

Firearm
- Store firearms in a locked cabinet.
- Teach children the danger of firearms.

Household
- Keep dangerous tools locked in a cabinet or shed.
- Warn children of harmful household products.

Fire
- Teach children how to be safe around campfires.
- Supervise children using matches.
- Have a fire escape plan for the home.
- Practice fire escape routes at home.

Data from AAP (2015e,f) and CDC (2017a,b)

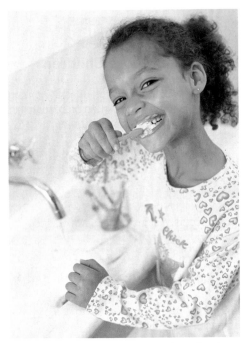

Figure 18.12. Oral health. Encourage the school-age child to brush his or her teeth in the morning and at bedtime as part of a routine. Reprinted with permission from Bowden, V., & Greenberg, C. S. (2013). *Children and their families* (3rd ed., Fig. 6-2). Philadelphia, PA: Lippincott Williams & Wilkins.

teeth (Fig. 18.12). Teach children to brush their teeth with fluoridated toothpaste twice daily for a full 2 minutes each time. Parents can set a timer near the sink so the child knows how long to brush. Another way the child can estimate 2 minutes of time is to sing the song "Happy Birthday" twice in a row. Flossing once a day is also important to prevent dental caries. Initially, children may need supervision with flossing. By the end of the school-age years, however, they should be flossing on their own.

Proper alignment of teeth is also important to oral health. Misalignment of teeth can affect both speech and appearance. During the school-age years, many children visit the orthodontist for the first time. Children with braces need to pay extra attention to brushing and flossing. Teach them to brush thoroughly around the brackets. Flossing is still possible with the use of a special tool to thread the floss, available from the orthodontist.

Nurses play an important role in promoting oral health. In addition to teaching children to practice good oral hygiene, teaching children to limit the number of sugary snacks and drinks they consume helps decrease the incidence of tooth decay. Children who do not have a fluoridated water supply should have fluoride supplements, as recommended by their dentist. Teaching children the importance of wearing mouth guards while playing any contact sports decreases the incidence of dental injury (Hagan et al., 2017).

Play

School-age children engage in cooperative play. They understand rules and are able to play team sports and participate in other organized activities. Increased coordination allows

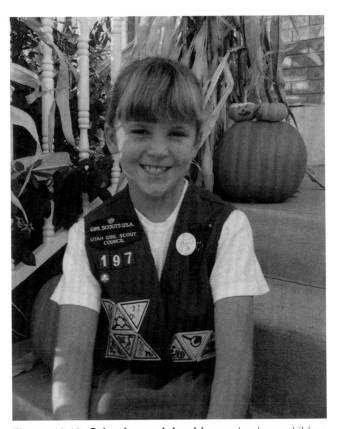

Figure 18.13. School-age clubs. Many school-age children enjoy participating in clubs with others of the same sex, such as Boy Scouts or Girl Scouts. Reprinted with permission from McGreer, M. A., & Carter, P. J. (2010). *Lippincott's textbook for personal support workers* (1st ed., Fig. 6.6). Philadelphia, PA: Lippincott Williams & Wilkins.

children to play team sports such as basketball or soccer. At this age, children understand the importance of working together as a team for a common goal and learn to value the rules associated with the team activity. Some children may enjoy participating in clubs such as Girl Scouts or Boys Scouts (Fig. 18.13).

In addition to team or group activities, school-age children also enjoy individual play (Fig. 18.14). This may take the form of individual sports such as cross-country or dance. Children

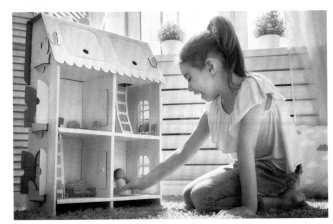

Figure 18.14. Individual play. School-age children enjoy individual play.

may also enjoy activities such as playing alone, reading, writing, or playing video games. Caution parents and children to monitor sedentary time. Remind families that children should continue to have at least 60 minutes of daily physical activity (Hagan et al., 2017). This activity can include team sports or individual activities such as walking or riding a bike.

Sleep

Healthy sleep habits are important for maintaining a healthy lifestyle. School-age children require 9 to 12 hours of sleep per night (AAP, 2017). Adequate sleep promotes a healthy immune system, better academic performance, and overall better mood. Sleep deprivation leads to behavior problems, poor academic performance, obesity, and depression (AAP, 2017).

Teach children about healthy bedtime routines. As much as possible, school-age children should go to sleep at the same time each night. The bed should only be used for sleep, not doing homework or watching television. No electronic devices should be kept in the child's room. Computers and televisions should be kept in family spaces. If the child has a mobile phone, the child should charge the phone outside the room at night. Daily physical activity promotes healthy sleep. However, overexertion may lead to sleep deprivation. Teach parents to recognize problems with sleep such as difficulty falling asleep, sleepiness during the day, poor academic performance, and moodiness.

Discipline

School-age children understand both rules and consequences. Parents should not only set family rules but also teach children societal rules. At this age, children still look to their parents for examples of appropriate behavior; therefore, parents should role model the behaviors they wish to see in their child. Children should learn to express emotions verbally and in a calm manner rather than by screaming, hitting, or acting out physical forms of anger in any other way. When children calmly express their feelings of being upset or frustrated, parents should praise them for it. However, if they break the rules, they should still receive consequences for their actions.

Although school-age children tend to want to follow rules, they often express their growing independence by pushing boundaries. Parents should establish clear consequences for breaking the rules up front. Consequences should be based on the age of the child and the severity of the discretion. Allowing children to have input into the consequences helps establish positive behavior. When the child breaks the rules, parents should listen calmly if the child wishes to explain his or her reasoning for breaking the rules. Unless there are extenuating circumstances, parents should then carry out the predetermined consequences. Consistency is important to disciplining the school-age child. If consequences are inconsistent, the child will not know what is expected of him or her and behavior may become erratic.

Drug and Alcohol Education

Drug use among eighth through 12th graders has continued to decline over the past several years (National Institute on Drug Abuse [NIDA], 2017). However, according to trends monitored

by NIDA, perception of risk with use of some substances, such as marijuana or over-the-counter cough and cold medicines, has declined among eighth graders. Starting education about the effects of drug and alcohol during the school-age years informs children of choices they may be facing in a few years. Teach parents to have open and honest conversations with their children about the subjects of drugs and alcohol. Education should be tailored to the child's age, being more simplistic for younger children and more in-depth for older children. Allow children to ask questions freely. Open communication may prevent children from trying illicit substances out of curiosity.

Immunizations

Immunizations are recommended for the school-age child at 11 to 12 years old (Patient Teaching 18.2). The recommended immunizations include the following:

- Influenza
- Diphtheria, tetanus, acellular pertussis
- Human papillomavirus (HPV)
- Meningococcal disease

Patient Teaching 18.2

Recommended Immunizations for 11–12-Y Olds

Immunizations

- Diphtheria, tetanus, acellular pertussis (DTaP)
  - Protects against the following:
    - Diphtheria, a serious infection of the throat that can block the airway
    - Tetanus, otherwise known as lockjaw, a nerve disease
    - Pertussis, otherwise known as whooping cough, a respiratory infection that can have serious complications
- Influenza (Flu)
  - Protects against the flu, a virus that spreads around the United States each year
  - Is spread by coughing, sneezing, and close contact
  - May make illness less severe if the child contracts the influenza virus
  - Prevents the spread of the flu to others
- Human papillomavirus (HPV)
  - Protects against HPV, a sexually transmitted infection, which is known to cause many types of cancers
    - Cervical cancer
    - Vaginal cancer
    - Throat cancer (in males and females)
    - Penile cancer
  - Protects against the strain of HPV that causes genital warts
  - Is administered as a two-dose series separated by 6–12 mo

- Meningococcal
  - Protects against meningococcal disease, a bacterial infection that can cause a severe form of meningitis
  - Meningococcal disease:
    - Spreads from person to person through close contact
    - Spreads quickly to people in close quarters, such as in locker rooms or dormitories
    - Kills about 15% of people infected
    - Causes lifelong disabilities in about 20% of survivors, such as the following:
      - Hearing loss
      - Brain damage
      - Amputation

Common Side Effects

After your child gets immunizations, he or she may have the following:

- Fever of up to around 102°F (38.8°C)
- Redness or a small amount of swelling at the injection site
- Soreness at the injection site
- Fainting spell

When to Call the Healthcare Provider

- If your child has a fever of 105°F (40.5°C) or higher
- If your child has a seizure
- If your child has trouble breathing

Adapted from the Centers for Disease Control and Prevention. (2017). *Diseases and the vaccines that prevent them: For parents of infants and young children (birth through age 6)*. Retrieved from http://www.cdc.gov/vaccines/hcp/conversations/prevent-diseases/provider-resources-factsheets-infants.html

Parents may have concerns about the HPV vaccine because HPV is a sexually transmitted infection. They may inquire as to why an 11- or a 12-year-old child needs a vaccine of this type. Teach parents that the two-dose series HPV vaccine protects their child from certain types of cancers. Although their child may not be sexually active at 11 or 12 years old, HPV infects 14 million Americans each year (CDC, 2016c). By vaccinating their child now, parents are protecting the child from contracting HPV once he or she does become sexually active.

The most up-to-date immunization chart is available at https://www.cdc.gov/vaccines/schedules/hcp/child-adolescent.html. Because these are immunizations the child has not received before, teach parents the reason for vaccine administration, as well as the side effects, how to treat them, and when to contact a healthcare provider. Refer to Chapter 15 for information on immunizations related to nursing considerations, barriers, and reporting adverse events.

Nutrition

Nutritional and caloric needs vary depending on gender and activity level (Table 18.4). Teaching children and families about specific caloric needs can help prevent children from becoming overweight. Involve school-age children in teaching so that they understand the importance of a healthy diet. Furthermore, allow children to assist in planning and making meals, which teaches them how to live and eat in a healthy way (Fig. 18.15).

Table 18.4 Nutritional Needs Based on Age, Gender, and Activity Level

Age (y)	Gender	Activity Level	Caloric Need per Day
6–8	Male	Sedentary	1,400
		Active	1,800–2,000
	Female	Sedentary	1,200–1,400
		Active	1,600–1,800
9–12	Male	Sedentary	1,600–1,800
		Active	2,000–2,400
	Female	Sedentary	1,400–1,600
		Active	1,800–2,200

Data from U.S. Department of Health and Human Services and U.S. Department of Agriculture. (2015). *2015–2020 Dietary guidelines for Americans* (8th ed.). Retrieved from https://health.gov/dietaryguidelines/2015/guidelines/appendix-2

In addition, encourage families to eat together; this allows the parents to role model healthy eating habits.

Healthy eating begins with a healthy breakfast. At this age, children may begin to skip breakfast before school to sleep later. Eating breakfast is correlated with improved academic performance and decreased BMI (Hagan et al., 2017). Ensure that there is an adequate intake of calcium and vitamin D. Because of the use of sunscreen and decreased outside activities, school-age children are at risk for vitamin D deficiency. Most milk is fortified with vitamin D and is a good source of calcium. Yogurt and cheese are also a source of calcium, protein, and other nutrients. If children consume other kinds of milk, such as soy or almond, they may need to take calcium and vitamin D supplements.

Teach children and families to choose foods from the five food groups (see Fig. 14.1). Nurses can direct families to

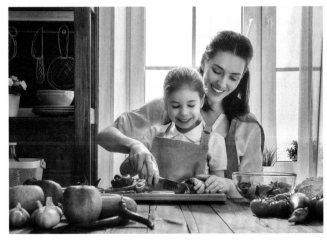

Figure 18.15. School-age nutrition. School-age children can be involved in meal preparation to promote healthy nutrition.

www.choosemyplate.gov for resources for both parents and children regarding healthy eating. Remind children to stay away from sugary snacks and drinks, including sports drinks. Sports drinks are often consumed after heavy physical activity, but they should not be used as a daily drink. Teach children that energy drinks are dangerous and may have life-threatening side effects. Children of any age should not consume any type of energy drink. Although sweet treats are acceptable occasionally in small amounts, these should be limited, as well.

Help families with limited resources or food insecurity find the necessary resources to promote healthy nutrition. The United States Department of Agriculture (USDA) has many resources to help provide children with the food they need. Programs provided by the USDA include the school lunch program, the school breakfast program, the summer food service program, and the fresh fruit and vegetable program (U.S. Department of Food and Agriculture: Food and Nutrition Service, 2018).

Common Developmental Concerns

Common developmental concerns during the school-age years include school refusal, bullying, obesity, cheating, lying, stealing, and excessive media use. Although common, these issues need to be addressed. If nurses and families do not address them during the school-age period, they may develop into more complex problems as the child reaches the adolescent years.

School Refusal

School refusal is not a diagnosis in and of itself, but it encompasses many factors. School refusal is characterized by the child's unwillingness to attend school and involves either multiple short absences or a prolonged absence. Parents are aware of their child's absences and, for the most part, have attempted to get their child to school without success. In general, school refusal is associated with severe emotional distress at the thought of attending school (Maynard et al., 2018). The most common ages for school refusal are from 5 to 7 years of age and 12 to 14 years of age, the typical times for school transitions (Nguyen, 2017).

Children with school refusal remain in bed, refuse to leave the car, or throw temper tantrums. In addition, they complain of many different vague somatic symptoms, including abdominal pain, nausea, headache, and sore throat (Nguyen, 2017). When children present with school refusal, conduct a thorough health history and physical assessment to rule out any underlying medical conditions. If you find no physical reason for the complaints, enquire about what is happening at school and why the child is avoiding the school environment. In the younger child, school refusal may be related to separation anxiety, whereas in the older school-age it may be related to fears, such as fear of failure or fear of not fitting in (Nguyen, 2017). Other possible causes for school refusal include a recent divorce in the family, a recent move, bullying, and low self-esteem (Maynard et al., 2018).

In Chapter 14, Adelaide Wilson did not like to go to school. What types of physical complaints did she have? What were the reasons she did not go to school? What interventions could the nurse discuss with both Adelaide and her mother to help Adelaide feel comfortable at school?

Treatment of school refusal begins with determining the underlying problem or problems deterring the child from going to school. Barring any safety issues for the child at school, the primary objective of treatment is to return the child to school as soon as possible (Maynard et al., 2018; Nguyen, 2017). Continuing treatment of school refusal involves anxiety management, cognitive behavioral therapy, social skills training, and, in some cases, pharmacotherapy. Treatment should be individualized to the child and family. Nurses can provide support to both the family and child to ensure a successful return to school.

Bullying

Bullying is a problem that typically begins during the school-age years and can continue into adolescence. With the increased use of digital and social media by children, bullying can take place in different ways. Children may experience bullying face-to-face at school or in friend groups. However, children may also be exposed to cyberbullying through the Internet. Regardless of the venue through which a child is bullied, the effects of bullying can be detrimental.

Bullying at School

Bullying during school is a common experience for many children. Although there is heightened awareness and anti-bullying campaigns, the behavior persists. An estimated 20% of children were bullied on school property in the past year (Stephens, Cook-Fasano, & Sibbaluca, 2018). The most common type of bullying in school is verbal and social bullying (U.S. Department of Health and Human Services, 2017b). Bullies can be either boys or girls and tend to pick on those who cry easily, get mad, give in, or are perceived as different (AAP, 2015a).

Assess for signs of bullying in children and teach parents to recognize these signs, as well. Children who are bullied experience changes in sleep and eating behaviors, depression, anxiety, social isolation, loss of interest in previously enjoyed activities, and vague health complaints (U.S. Department of Health and Human Services, 2017a). If a child is identified as being bullied, work with the parents and the healthcare team to alleviate the problem and prevent long-term psychosocial effects.

Cyberbullying

Bullying often extends beyond the school walls to digital and social media. Sending mean messages or embarrassing pictures or spreading rumors online are considered cyberbullying. Cyberbullying can take place at any time of the day, the bully is able to remain anonymous, and the mean messages can be forwarded on to others on social media (Moreno, 2018). As with face-to-face bullying, children who are bullied online are at risk for academic struggles, depression, and anxiety.

Teach parents to be alert to the signs of cyberbullying. Encourage children to talk about mean messages that are posted online. Parents should listen to and be supportive of their child. If possible, take a screenshot of the message or picture for evidence (Moreno, 2018). Report bad behavior through the reporting mechanisms on social media platforms. Talk with school counselors and refer children and families to resources available for bullying.

Obesity

Overweight is defined as having a BMI in the 85th to less than the 95th percentile for age. Obese is defined as having a BMI in the 95th percentile or greater for age. The prevalence of obesity in school-age children has increased from 6.5% in 1980 to 17.7 % in 2011 (Hagan et al., 2017). Obesity rates are higher in African American children, Hispanic children, and children living in poverty (Hagan et al., 2017). Obesity in childhood puts the child at risk for many diseases previously seen only in adults. These diseases include hypertension, type 2 diabetes, cardiovascular disease, and metabolic syndrome.

Overweight and obesity are caused by overconsumption of calories and lack of physical exercise. Nurses are able to identify those at risk for overweight and obesity at routine health promotion visits. In addition to monitoring weight and BMI, assess children for risk factors, including overweight or obese parents, overweight or obese siblings, low socioeconomic status, and maternal gestational diabetes (Hagan et al., 2017).

Treatment for overweight and obesity focuses on lifestyle changes and nutrition rather than on weight loss. Begin by encouraging basic healthy eating and increased physical activity, with the goal of decreasing BMI. Programs to help overweight and obese children achieve a healthier BMI are structured and require frequent monitoring by healthcare providers such as nurses. Often, overweight and obese children require the care of a multidisciplinary team that includes a dietitian and a counselor. For the most severe cases, children are referred to a pediatric weight management center.

In Chapter 14, Adelaide Wilson was identified as obese. What factors indicated that she was obese? What were her risk factors for additional health problems? What other disciplines were included in Adelaide's care? What interventions were implemented to help decrease Adelaide's BMI?

Cheating, Lying, and Stealing

Cheating, lying, and stealing are all common behaviors during the school-age years. Although these behaviors are common,

they should not be tolerated. Teach parents why these behaviors occur and how to stop them. In addition, remind parents to role model appropriate behavior. If children are exposed to cheating, lying, and stealing in the family, they are more likely to exhibit these behaviors.

Cheating

Cheating is common as children begin to play games with each other. Competitiveness among school-age children is often the reason for cheating. Early on, children learn that losing is bad, so they feel pressured to win and may cheat to do so. Children who have siblings, whether older or younger, are more likely to cheat than are only children, further underscoring competition as a basis for cheating (O'Connor & Evans, 2018). However, cheating at games when the child is past the school-age years is generally not tolerated by peers and has negative social consequences (AAP, 2015b).

School-age children may cheat at school because they are not in classes at the appropriate academic level. If school work is too difficult, children may feel the need to cheat and be successful rather than ask for help. If caught cheating at school, parents should discuss the matter with their child to help the child understand the seriousness of what has been done. Determine whether the child needs extra help in school, such as tutoring. If cheating persists, whether at games or at school, refer the family to a counselor to determine whether there are any underlying emotional issues (AAP, 2015b).

Lying

By 6 years of age, children understand what lying is. During the school-age years, children understand that lying is wrong but may continue to lie to push parental limits. Reasons children lie at this age include trying to protect themselves when they have done something wrong or when parental expectations have been set too high and to get attention (AAP, 2015h). Children with younger siblings have an increased propensity to lie (O'Connor & Evans, 2018). The larger the age gap, the more likely the older sibling is to lie. The younger the sibling, the more easily the sibling can be manipulated.

Teach parents when their child lies to let the child know he or she is lying. Strict punishment does not work in this situation. Have parents emphasize that the child will get in less trouble if he or she admits to lying and subsequently tells the truth. Educate parents on when to be concerned about their child's lying. Further evaluation is necessary if lying is in conjunction with other behavioral issues, if the child has low self-esteem or is depressed, or if the child shows no signs of regret about telling lies.

Stealing

Stealing during the school-age years may be a sign of peer pressure and a desire to fit in with a social group. By the age of 7 years, children understand the concept of property and that taking someone else's property is wrong. If a child is caught stealing, the transgression should be addressed immediately. If possible, the child should return the stolen item to the owner. Discuss with the child the reasons he or she stole. Further evaluation is necessary if the child shows no regret for stealing, if stealing is a consistent behavior, or if there are comorbid behavioral problems.

Media

During the school-age years, children become more interested in different types of media, such as video games and social media. Parents should monitor their child's Internet and media use. Younger children should not have any social media accounts, because they are not able to fully understand the dangers of disclosing personal information through social media. When children do start social media accounts, parents should monitor them. Parents should talk openly with their children about what are appropriate and inappropriate subjects to discuss on social media.

Teach parents and children about the adverse effects of media use. Overuse of media puts children at risk for obesity, poor school performance, Internet addiction, sleep problems, and cyberbullying (AAP, 2016). Encourage parents to have a family media use plan. This may include rules such as having a computer only in a common family space and not having digital devices in the bedroom or at the dinner table. The best way to teach children the appropriate use of digital media is role modeling. Parents can show children that it is not necessary to be connected all of the time by disconnecting from digital media themselves on a daily basis.

Health Problems of School Age

Certain illnesses and infections are more common during the school-age years, such as tinea infections. Others, such as influenza, pharyngitis, and tonsillitis, may occur at any age but are common during the school-age years due to greater exposure to children in school, clubs, and sports.

Influenza

Influenza viruses occur in many different strains and can cause a variety of respiratory symptoms. Every year there are three or four different types of influenza viruses in the United States. It is difficult to predict which strains will be prevalent. Every year the influenza vaccine contains three or four antigens to the strains of virus predicted to be most prominent (Havers & Campbell, 2016). The influenza vaccine is recommended for children over the age of 6 months who have no contraindications for the vaccine, such as a known allergy to the vaccine. The vaccine has been shown to reduce illness, prevent hospitalization, reduce deaths, and possibly reduce the severity of illness in those who do get infected with the influenza virus (CDC, 2017c).

Influenza viruses cause significant morbidity and mortality in children, with an estimated 20,000 children younger than age 5 being hospitalized during flu season in the United

States (Havers & Campbell, 2016). Children with the greatest risk of complications are those who are younger than 2, have underlying chronic medical conditions, or are immunosuppressed. Complications include worsening of the underlying condition, bacterial or viral pneumonia, co-infections such as myocarditis, respiratory failure, and multiorgan failure (CDC, 2016a).

Uncomplicated influenza begins with a sudden onset of fever, myalgia, chills, and malaise. Cough is often present. Younger children may appear toxic. Symptoms last 2 to 4 days. However, any cough can last for several weeks after the illness has resolved. Otitis media, pneumonia, and croup are common complications of the influenza virus in otherwise healthy children.

Nursing Assessment

Obtain a history of the present illness. Does the child have any underlying medical conditions? Has the child been around anyone else who is sick? When did the symptoms start? What symptoms is the child having? How high has the fever been at home? Is the child able to eat and drink? Is the child coughing? Has the child ever vomited from coughing?

Note the child's appearance. Is the child alert and talking or lethargic? Assess the child's vital signs. Inspect the child's throat. Palpate the child's skin for temperature. Note any clamminess. Auscultate the lungs in all lung fields, noting any adventitious lung sounds or decreased airflow. If the child has any underlying medical conditions, such as a congenital heart defect, note any changes from baseline.

Test for influenza with a rapid influenza test. Swab the child's nose and run the test as directed. Rapid influenza tests are only 50% to 70% sensitive but are 95% to 100% specific (Havers & Campbell, 2016). Therefore, false negatives may occur with the test. When the rapid flu test is negative, the healthcare provider must take into account the child's signs and symptoms when considering treatment.

Treatment

The antiviral agent oseltamivir is the most common treatment for influenza (The Pharmacy 18.1). The drug is approved for use in children as young as 2 weeks. When started within 48 hours of the onset of symptoms, oseltamivir reduces the severity and length of symptoms. Treatment is twice a day for 5 days. In addition to antivirals, adequate fluid intake and rest are important. Any concomitant bacterial infections should be treated with antibiotics. A child with uncomplicated influenza should begin to feel better in 48 to 72 hours. If the child's fever persists or symptoms are getting worse, the parents should bring the child to their healthcare provider.

Tinea Infections

Tinea infections are fungal infections that are further classified by where they occur on the body. Children with diabetes, cancer, or other forms of immunosuppression are at greater risk for developing these types of fungal infections.

Tinea Corporis

Tinea corporis, otherwise known as "ringworm," is a fungal infection that occurs on the body, excluding the palms, soles, and groin (Juern & Drolet, 2016). Lesions begin as dry scaly plaques and then become elevated and erythematous with a central clearing, giving the appearance of a ring (Fig. 18.16) Tinea corporis can be acquired by direct contact with infected persons or by contact with environmental surfaces with which infected persons have been in contact.

Nursing Assessment

Other than itching, no other symptoms are present with tinea corporis. Determine whether the child has been in contact with other infected children. Enquire as to whether the child plays sports, because sports mats and locker rooms may be a source of infection.

Treatment

Tinea corporis is treated with topical antifungal creams (The Pharmacy 18.2). Treatment lasts 2 to 4 weeks. Teach parents not to use combination antifungal/corticosteroid creams, because the corticosteroids could worsen the infection (Juern & Drolet, 2016).

Tinea Pedis

Tinea pedis, otherwise known as athlete's foot, is a fungal infection between the toes and on the soles of the feet. Excoriation and peeling of the skin surrounding the toes occurs with tinea pedis (Fig. 18.17) The area of infection itches and is tender to the touch. Occasionally, a foul odor may be present (Juern & Drolet, 2016). Warm weather and use of occlusive footwear, public showers, and swimming pools predispose children to tinea pedis.

Nursing Assessment

Ask the parent and child whether the child uses public showers or has been around any swimming pools. Inspect the child's feet for excoriation and erythema. Palpate the area for tenderness. Determine

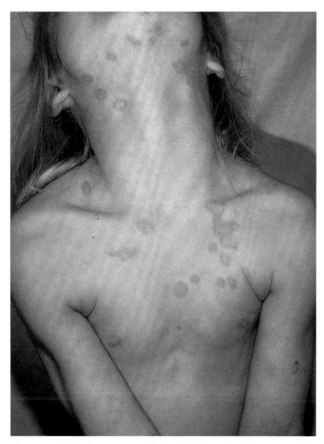

Figure 18.16. Tinea corporis. Multiple scaly plaques on the torso. Reprinted with permission from Burkhart, C., Morrell, D., Goldsmith, L. A., Papier, A., Green, B., Dasher, D., & Gomathy, S. (Eds.). (2009). *VisualDx: Essential pediatric dermatology* (1st ed., Fig. 4.206). Philadelphia, PA: Lippincott Williams & Wilkins.

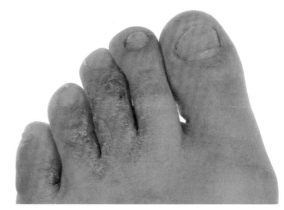

Figure 18.17. Tinea pedis. Tinea pedis commonly occurs between the toes.

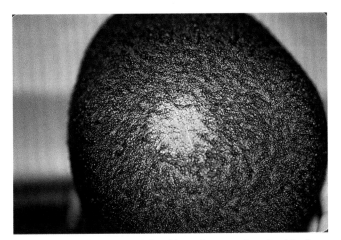

Figure 18.18. **Tinea capitis.** Alopecia associated with tinea capitis. Reprinted with permission from Kyle, T., & Carman, S. (2016). *Pediatric nursing clinical guide* (2nd ed., Fig. 2.16). Philadelphia, PA: Wolters Kluwer.

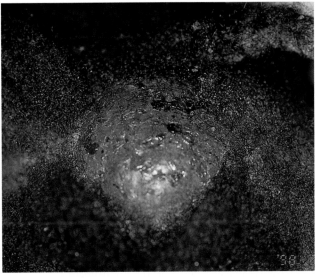

Figure 18.19. **Kerion.** A painful, swollen, boggy area associated with tinea capitis. Reprinted with permission from Fleisher, G. R., Ludwig, S., & Baskin, M. N. (2004). *Atlas of pediatric emergency medicine* (1st ed., Fig. 27.4). Philadelphia, PA: Lippincott Williams & Wilkins.

whether any foul odor is present. Assess for fever or inflammation of the infected area, which would suggest a more complex infection.

Treatment

Treatment of tinea pedis is with topical antifungals initially (The Pharmacy 18.2). Teach children to dry their feet thoroughly, including between the toes, before putting on socks and to wear flip-flops or sandals when using public showers or public swimming pools.

Tinea Capitis

Tinea capitis involves a fungal infection on the scalp (Fig. 18.18). This type of tinea infection is more common among African American children from 4 to 14 years old (Juern & Drolet, 2016). The infection typically starts as a black dot on the scalp with small areas of alopecia. Tinea capitis often resembles seborrheic dermatitis or psoriasis. In some cases, a severe inflammatory response occurs, resulting in one or more **kerions** (Fig. 18.19) on the child's scalp.

Nursing Assessment

Inspect the child's scalp for the black dots indicating tinea capitis. Inspect for scaliness, dry skin, and alopecia. Palpate the scalp to determine whether kerions are present. Palpate the cervical lymph nodes, noting any cervical lymphadenopathy. Determine whether the child has a fever. Culture the lesion for a definitive diagnosis.

Treatment

Treatment of tinea capitis consists of the antifungal griseofulvin (The Pharmacy 18.2). Treatment with griseofulvin is necessary for 8 to 12 weeks and, possibly, for up to 1 month after a negative scalp culture (Juern & Drolet, 2016). Teach parents that absorption of griseofulvin is improved with a fatty meal.

The Pharmacy 18.2   Medications to Treat Tinea Infections

Medication	Classification	Route	Action	Nursing Considerations
Griseofulvin	Antifungal	Oral	• Inhibits fungal cell mitosis • Treats tinea capitis	• Use for 6–8 wk • Concentrations increase with high-fat meals • May cause granulocytopenia or hepatotoxicity • Monitor CBC, LFTs
Terbinafine	Antifungal	Topical	• Inhibits an enzyme crucial to the development of the fungal cell wall, resulting in cell death • Treats tinea pedis and tinea corporis	• Apply to clean, dry, affected area • Apply once or twice daily for 7 d • Do not use occlusive dressings • Avoid contact with eyes

CBC, complete blood count; LFT, liver function test.
Adapted from Taketomo, C. K., Hodding, J. H., & Kraus, D. M. (2018). *Pediatric & neonatal dosage handbook* (25th ed.). Hudson, OH: Lexicomp.

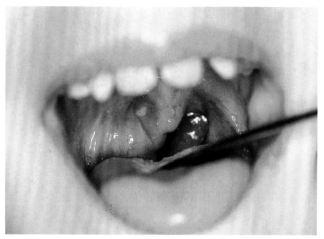

Figure 18.20. Streptococcal pharyngitis: Oral signs. Signs of streptococcal pharyngitis include erythematous tonsils with palatal petechiae and foul-smelling exudate.

Pharyngitis

Pharyngitis is inflammation of the pharynx, or a sore throat. Complaint of a sore throat is one of the most common reasons for a healthcare visit in children. Pharyngitis can be caused by both viruses and bacteria. The most common bacterial cause of acute pharyngitis is group A *Streptococcus* (GAS), commonly called strep throat. GAS causes 15% to 30% of cases of pharyngitis in school-age children (Tanz, 2016). It is important to determine whether the infection is viral or bacterial to determine the course of treatment. A thorough history of the illness and physical exam determine whether the child needs to be tested for GAS.

GAS pharyngitis presents with an extremely sore throat and purulent exudate on the tonsils (Fig. 18.20). Headache and abdominal pain can also accompany GAS pharyngitis. Sometimes a GAS infection produces a fine, papular, erythematous rash that feels like sandpaper, indicating scarlet fever (Fig. 18.21). GAS infections cause a higher fever and a more ill appearance in the child than do viral infections associated with pharyngitis. Symptoms such as otalgia and rhinorrhea are common with viral pharyngitis.

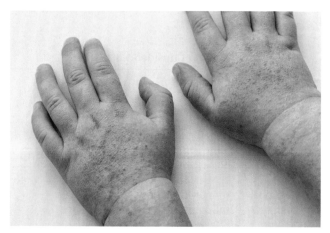

Figure 18.21. Streptococcal pharyngitis: Skin signs. The classic sandpaper rash associated with streptococcal pharyngitis.

Nursing Assessment

Obtain a history of the present illness. Determine the onset of illness. Document the appearance of the child. Assess the child's ability to swallow. Assess the temperature. Ask whether the child is having any other symptoms. Inspect the pharynx for erythema and the tonsils for exudate. Note any enlargement of the tonsils. Inspect the skin for rashes. Palpate the cervical lymph nodes, noting any enlargement and/or tenderness.

If you suspect a child of having GAS pharyngitis based on signs and symptoms, swab the child's throat and perform a rapid antigen-detection test for GAS.

Treatment

Viral pharyngitis is self-limiting and generally lasts about 7 days. Give ibuprofen or acetaminophen for pain and discomfort. Have the child gargle with warm salt water to alleviate discomfort, as well.

GAS pharyngitis is treated with a course of antibiotics. An intramuscular injection of penicillin is an option to treat GAS pharyngitis, but most healthcare providers choose to give a 10-day course of oral antibiotics. Amoxicillin or cefdinir are the most common antibiotics used in the treatment of GAS. As with viral pharyngitis, antipyretics and warm salt water gargles can be used for comfort. Teach parents that, although the child will most likely feel better 48 hours after starting the antibiotics, the child should complete the entire course of medicine. Untreated or partially treated GAS pharyngitis can lead to rheumatic fever. Children with recurrent GAS infections should be referred to an otolaryngologist to be evaluated for a tonsillectomy.

Tonsillitis

Acute tonsillitis is caused mostly by viral infections (Wetmore, 2016). Tonsils can become chronically infected with a variety of different microbes. Chronic infections are characterized by halitosis and chronic sore throats. Occasionally children experience tonsillar hypertrophy that leads to partial airway obstruction. Signs of airway obstruction include mouth breathing, snoring, and sleep apnea.

Nursing Assessment

Determine the history of the present illness. Ask whether this is a recurrent problem. Does the child have trouble breathing during the day? Does the child snore? Does the child have brief pauses in breathing while sleeping? Does the child appear tired during the day? Take vital signs to determine whether the child has a fever. Inspect the oropharynx, noting the size and color of the tonsils. Note any halitosis.

Treatment

Viral tonsillitis is self-limiting. Comfort measures are appropriate during the illness. For tonsillitis caused by bacteria, such as GAS, the child is treated with antibiotics. Children with recurrent or chronic tonsillitis are referred to an otolaryngologist to be evaluated for a tonsillectomy.

Think Critically

1. Discuss precocious puberty and the effects it can have on the school-age child.
2. How does the task of industry relate to self-esteem during the school-age years?
3. Develop a plan of care for a child with gender dysphoria.
4. What would you teach a parent who is concerned about the human papillomavirus vaccine?

5. Create a plan of care for the overweight or obese child. Is it important for the child to be involved in the development of the plan? Why or why not?
6. How can nurses help families who are concerned about their child's media use?
7. What are the most important teaching points regarding the influenza virus?

References

American Academy of Pediatrics. (2015a). *Bullying: It's not ok.* Retrieved from https://www.healthychildren.org/English/safety-prevention/at-play/Pages/Bullying-Its-Not-Ok.aspx

American Academy of Pediatrics. (2015b). *Competition and cheating.* Retrieved from https://www.healthychildren.org/English/family-life/family-dynamics/communication-discipline/Pages/Competition-and-Cheating.aspx

American Academy of Pediatrics. (2015c). *Gender non-conforming & transgender children.* https://www.healthychildren.org/English/ages-stages/gradeschool/Pages/Gender-Non-Conforming-Transgender-Children.aspx

American Academy of Pediatrics. (2015d). *Individualized education program.* Retrieved from https://www.healthychildren.org/English/health-issues/conditions/developmental-disabilities/Pages/Individualized-Education-Program.aspx

American Academy of Pediatrics. (2015e). *Safety for your child: 8 years.* Retrieved from https://www.healthychildren.org/English/ages-stages/gradeschool/Pages/Safety-for-Your-Child-8-Years.aspx

American Academy of Pediatrics. (2015f). *Safety for your child: 10 years.* Retrieved from https://www.healthychildren.org/English/ages-stages/gradeschool/Pages/Safety-for-Your-Child-10-Years.aspx

American Academy of Pediatrics. (2015g). *Signs of low self-esteem.* Retrieved from https://www.healthychildren.org/English/ages-stages/gradeschool/Pages/Signs-of-Low-Self-Esteem.aspx

American Academy of Pediatrics. (2015h). *Why children lie.* Retrieved from https://www.healthychildren.org/English/family-life/family-dynamics/communication-discipline/Pages/When-Children-Lie.aspx

American Academy of Pediatrics. (2016). *Constantly connected: Adverse effects of media on children & teens.* Retrieved from https://www.healthychildren.org/English/family-life/Media/Pages/Adverse-Effects-of-Television-Commercials.aspx

American Academy of Pediatrics. (2017). *Healthy sleep habits: How many hours does your child need?* Retrieved from https://www.healthychildren.org/English/healthy-living/sleep/Pages/Healthy-Sleep-Habits-How-Many-Hours-Does-Your-Child-Need.aspx

American College of Pediatricians. (2017). Gender dysphoria in children. *Issues in Law & Medicine, 32*(2), 287–304.

Centers for Disease Control and Prevention. (2016a). *Influenza signs and symptoms and the role of laboratory diagnostics.* Retrieved from https://www.cdc.gov/flu/professionals/diagnosis/labrolesprocedures.htm

Centers for Disease Control and Prevention. (2016b). *National action plan for child injury prevention.* Retrieved from https://www.cdc.gov/safechild/nap/index.html

Centers for Disease Control and Prevention. (2016c). *Vaccine information statements: HPV (human papillomavirus) VIS.* Retrieved from https://www.cdc.gov/vaccines/hcp/vis/vis-statements/hpv.html

Centers for Disease Control and Prevention. (2017a). *Child development: Middle childhood (6–8 years).* Retrieved from https://www.cdc.gov/ncbddd/childdevelopment/positiveparenting/middle.html

Centers for Disease Control and Prevention. (2017b). *Child development: Middle childhood (9–11 years).* Retrieved from https://www.cdc.gov/ncbddd/childdevelopment/positiveparenting/middle2.html

Centers for Disease Control and Prevention. (2017c). *Communications to healthcare providers.* Retrieved from https://www.cdc.gov/flu/pdf/professionals/Dear-Colleague-Letter-2017-2018.pdf

Erikson, E. H. (1963). *Childhood and society.* New York, NY: W.W. Norton and Company.

Feigelman, S. (2016). Middle childhood. In R. M. Kliegman, B. F. Stanton, J. W. St. Geme III, N. F. Schor, & R. E. Behrman (Eds.), *Nelson's textbook of pediatrics* (20th ed.). Philadelphia, PA: Elsevier, Saunders.

Hagan, J. F., Shaw, J. S., & Duncan, P. (Eds.). (2017). *Bright futures: Guidelines for health supervision of infants, children, and adolescents* (4th ed.). Elk Grove Village, IL: American Academy of Pediatrics.

Havers, F. P., & Campbell, A. J. P. (2016). Influenza viruses. In R. M. Kliegman, B. F. Stanton, J. W. St. Geme III, N. F. Schor, & R. E. Behrman (Eds.), *Nelson's textbook of pediatrics* (20th ed.). Philadelphia, PA: Elsevier, Saunders.

Hendriks, E., Prentice, P., & Williams, R. (2017). Disorders of puberty. *Medicine, 45*(9), 575–578.

Holland-Hall, C., & Burstein, G. R. (2016). Adolescent physical and social development. In R. M. Kliegman, B. F. Stanton, J. W. St. Geme III, N. F. Schor, & R. E. Behrman (Eds.), *Nelson's textbook of pediatrics* (20th ed.). Philadelphia, PA: Elsevier, Saunders.

Juern A. M., & Drolet, B. A. (2016). Cutaneous fungal infections. In R. M. Kliegman, B. F. Stanton, J. W. St. Geme III, N. F. Schor, & R. E. Behrman (Eds.), *Nelson's textbook of pediatrics* (20th ed.). Philadelphia, PA: Elsevier, Saunders.

Keane, V. (2016). Assessment of growth. In R. M. Kliegman, B. F. Stanton, J. W. St. Geme III, N. F. Schor, & R. E. Behrman (Eds.), *Nelson's textbook of pediatrics* (20th ed.). Philadelphia, PA: Elsevier, Saunders.

KidsHealth. (2018a). *504 education plans.* Retrieved from http://kidshealth.org/en/parents/504-plans.html

KidsHealth. (2018b). *What's and IEP?* Retrieved from https://kidshealth.org/en/parents/iep.html

Kohlberg, L. (1981). *The philosophy of moral development.* New York, NY: Harper & Row.

Lopez, X., Stewart, S., & Jacobson-Dickman, E. (2016). Approach to children and adolescents with gender dysphoria. *Pediatrics in Review, 37*(3), 89–96.

Mahon, P., Holsti, L., Siden, H., Strahlendorf, C., Turnham, L., & Guaschi, D. (2015). Using colors to assess pain in toddlers: Validation of "The Rainbow Pain Scale": A proof-of-principle study. *Journal of Pediatric Oncology Nursing, 32*(1), 40–46.

Maynard, B. R., Heyne, D., Brendel, K. E., Bulanda, J. J., Thompson, A. M., & Pigott, T. D. (2018). Treatment for school refusal among children: A systematic review and meta-analysis. *Research on Social work Practice, 28*(1), 56–67.

Moreno, M. (2018). *Cyberbullying.* Retrieved from https://www.healthychildren.org/English/family-life/Media/Pages/Cyberbullying.aspx

National Institute on Drug Abuse. (2017). *Trends and statistics.* Retrieved from https://www.drugabuse.gov/related-topics/trends-statistics

Nguyen, S. (2017). School refusal: Identification and management of a paediatric challenge. *Australian Medical Student Journal, 8*(1), 68–72.

O'Connor, A. M., & Evans, A. D. (2018). The relation between having siblings and children's cheating and lie-telling behaviors. *Journal of Experimental Child Psychology, 168,* 49–60.

Piaget, J. (1930). *The child's conception of physical causality.* London, England: Routledge & Kegan Paul LTD.

Reinehr, T., Bosse, C., Lass, N., Rothermal, J., Knop, C., & Ludwig, C. L. (2017). Effect of weight loss on puberty onset in overweight children. *The Journal of Pediatrics, 184,* 143–151.

Shields, B. J., Palermo, T. M., Powers, J. D., Grewe, S. D., & Smith, G. A. (2003). Predictors of a child's ability to use a visual analog scale. *Child: Care, Health, and Development, 29*(4), 281–290.

Stephens, M. M., Cook-Fasano, H. T., & Sibbaluca, K. (2018). Childhood bullying: Implications for physicians. *American Family Physician, 97*(3), 187–192.

Sultan, C., Gaspari, L., Maimoun, L., Kalfa, N., & Paris, F. (2018). Disorders of puberty. *Best Practice & Research Clinical Obstetrics and Gynaecology, 48*, 62–89. doi.org/10.1016/j.bpobgyn.2017.11.004

Tanner, J. M. (1962). *Growth at adolescence.* Oxford, England: Blackwell Scientific Publications.

Tanz, R. R. (2016). Acute pharyngitis. In R. M. Kliegman, B. F. Stanton, J. W. St. Geme III, N. F. Schor, & R. E. Behrman (Eds.), *Nelson's textbook of pediatrics* (20th ed.). Philadelphia, PA: Elsevier, Saunders.

Tatangelo, G. L., & Ricciardelli, L. A. (2017). Children's body image and social comparisons with peers and the media. *Journal of Health Psychology, 22*(6), 776–787.

Thrane, S. E., Wanless, S., Cohen, S. M., & Danford, C. A. (2016). The Assessment and non-pharmacologic treatment of procedural pain from infancy to school age through a developmental lens: A synthesis of evidence with recommendations. *Journal of Pediatric Nursing, 31*, e23–e32.

U.S. Department of Health and Human Services. (2017a). *Effects of bullying.* Retrieved from https://www.stopbullying.gov/at-risk/effects/index.html

U.S. Department of Health and Human Services. (2017b). *Facts about bullying.* Retrieved from https://www.stopbullying.gov/media/facts/index.html

U.S. Department of Food and Agriculture: Food and Nutrition Service. (2018). *School meals: Child nutrition programs.* Retrieved from https://www.fns.usda.gov/school-meals/child-nutrition-programs

Wetmore, R. F. (2016). Tonsils and adenoids. In R. M. Kliegman, B. F. Stanton, J. W. St. Geme III, N. F. Schor, & R. E. Behrman (Eds.), *Nelson's textbook of pediatrics* (20th ed.). Philadelphia, PA: Elsevier, Saunders.

Suggested Readings

American Academy of Pediatrics. (2016). *Constantly connected: Adverse effects of media on children & teens.* Retrieved from https://www.healthychildren.org/English/family-life/Media/Pages/Adverse-Effects-of-Television-Commercials.aspx

Centers for Disease Control and Prevention. (2018). *Influenza (Flu).* https://www.cdc.gov/flu/index.htm

Healthy People 2020. (2018). *Early and middle childhood.* Retrieved from https://www.healthypeople.gov/2020/topics-objectives/topic/early-and-middle-childhood

19 Care of the Adolescent

Growth and Development Overview

The adolescent period is one of many changes, as children become adults. These include changes in physical appearance and physiological processes, cognitive and neurological growth, and psychosocial development. The process of identity formation is ongoing throughout the adolescent period. As teens are discovering who they are, they are more likely to engage in risk-taking behaviors such as drinking, smoking, using illicit drugs, or engaging in sexual activities. Teach adolescents and parents about the dangers of these activities at all health promotion visits. Gain the trust of adolescents and help guide them, as well as their parents, through this often tenuous time.

The adolescent period is divided into three stages: early, middle, and late. Development varies by age, and teens have different needs depending on which stage they are in (Table 19.1). Although the stages of adolescence are defined by age, teenagers develop at different rates. Take into account an adolescent's

Table 19.1 Stages of Adolescence

Early adolescence	10–13 y
Middle adolescence	14–17 y
Late adolescence	18–21 y

physical, cognitive, emotional, and psychosocial development at each health promotion visit.

Health Assessment

Privacy during exams is important to the adolescent. Ensure the teen's privacy during the history and physical exam. Once adolescents begin to drive, they may be at health promotion appointments without a parent. Establish a good rapport with the adolescent, which helps to elicit accurate information about the adolescent's health and health-related behaviors.

While conducting the health history, address the adolescent directly. Confirm any information with the parent, if present, as needed. Ask the parent whether he or she has any concerns about the adolescent's health or behavior. To obtain an accurate history of substance use, smoking, or sexual activity, ask the parent, if present, to leave the room. Adolescents are not likely to be honest about these behaviors if a parent is in the room. In addition, ask the adolescent about social relationships, school, and any other areas of potential concern while the parent is not in the room. Assure adolescents that what they say is confidential unless they reveal an intention to hurt either themselves or someone else.

Conduct the physical assessment in a sequential, head-to-toe manner. Keep the adolescent's body covered as much as possible during the assessment to protect modesty. Explain to the adolescent what is happening during the assessment and why. As adolescents progress through the stages of adolescence, they may ask detailed questions about how the body works. Answer any questions they have.

Head, Eyes, Ears, Nose, Mouth, and Throat

Inquire about the adolescent's hearing and vision. Does he or she wear glasses or contacts? When was the last eye exam? If the adolescent does not wear glasses, ask whether he or she has difficulty seeing the board at school or reading road signs. If the adolescent plays contact sports, has he or she ever had a concussion?

Head

Inspect the scalp for lesions. Inspect the hair for lice. Palpate the head for nodules, noting their size, shape, and location if present. Palpate the lymph nodes and document their size, shape, consistency, and movability. Palpate the sinuses. Conduct cranial nerve testing as needed.

Eyes

Inspect the eyes for symmetry. Note the color of the sclera and conjunctiva. Assess the pupils; they should be equal, round, and reactive to light and assessment. Use the Snellen chart to assess visual acuity. Visual acuity greater than 20/20, not corrected with glasses, should be further investigated. Test cranial nerves III, IV, and VI by taking the adolescent through the cardinal fields of gaze.

Ears

Assess the symmetry and placement of the ears. Note any redness or drainage. Inspect for piercings, noting the number in each ear. Assess for signs of infection of any piercings, such as redness or drainage. Palpate for swelling or tenderness. Assess hearing by an otoacoustic emissions test. If inner ear inspection is indicated, pull the pinna up and back.

Nose

Assess the nose as previously described (see Chapter 17). Adolescents often have piercings other than ear piercings. Note any nose piercings and assess for signs of infection.

Mouth and Throat

Assess the mouth as previously described (see Chapter 17). Determine whether the adolescent has the last four molars, or wisdom teeth, and, if so, whether these teeth are affecting dentition. If the adolescent has braces, assess the buccal mucosa for lesions due to rubbing from the braces. Assess the gums for swelling, which, if present, may indicate poor oral hygiene in the adolescent with braces.

Neurological Assessment

The brain continues to develop throughout adolescence and into early adulthood. The frontal lobes, including the prefrontal cortex, are the last areas of the brain to fully develop (Holland-Hall & Burstein, 2016). The prefrontal cortex is responsible for impulse control, consideration of the consequences of various actions, and evaluation of risks vs. rewards. The later development of the frontal lobes explains the impulsive and risky behavior of many adolescents. Furthermore, adolescents tend to make impulsive decisions in the height of intense emotions, unlike mature adults, who are able to regulate these emotions.

Enquire about the adolescent's risk-taking behaviors, including experimentation with alcohol, tobacco, or any illicit drugs. Ask the parents about their child's impulse control, noting any issues with anger. Determine whether the adolescent has any trouble with muscle strength or coordination. Determine whether the adolescent is having frequent headaches. Conduct the neurological assessment as described in Chapter 18.

Respiratory Assessment

The lungs grow to adult size during adolescence. Lung volume and vital capacity increase. The respiratory rate decreases to that of an adult, or about 12 to 20 breaths/min. Growth of the larynx, pharynx, and pharyngeal cartilage is responsible for the deepening of both male and female voices.

Determine whether the adolescent has a history of chronic respiratory illness such as asthma or allergies. Ask about smoking, either tobacco or marijuana, as well as **vaping**. Observe the rise and fall of the chest to measure respiratory rate. Note the use of any accessory muscles. Auscultate in all lung fields. Instruct the adolescent to breathe deeply. Note whether and where any adventitious lung sounds are heard.

Cardiovascular Assessment

By the end of adolescence, the size and strength of the heart reach those of an adult. Blood pressure increases to 110 to 120 mm Hg systolic and 64 to 80 mm Hg diastolic. Normal heart rate in an adolescent is 60 to 100 beats/min (bpm). However, athletic adolescents may have a lower resting heart rate than 60 bpm.

Enquire about the adolescent's family history of heart disease. Determine whether the adolescent has a history of high levels of cholesterol or triglycerides. Continue to monitor cholesterol and triglyceride levels. Assess pulses and note any difference between upper and lower extremities. Assess capillary refill in all four extremities. Auscultate for murmurs and document appropriately.

Gastrointestinal Assessment

The gastrointestinal system reaches functional maturity during the school-age years. The spleen, liver, and gallbladder grow in size during the adolescent years, but their function does not change.

Enquire about a history of gastrointestinal problems such as recurrent or chronic diarrhea or chronic constipation. Inspect the abdomen. The abdomen should be flat, not sunken or protruding. Note any umbilical piercing and assess for signs of infection. Palpate the abdomen, noting any guarding, rigidity, tenderness, or hepatosplenomegaly. The spleen should not be palpable. Only the tip of the liver should be palpable in the adolescent.

Genitourinary Assessment

The urinary system has reached maturity by the time of adolescence. Determine whether the adolescent has a history of recurrent urinary tract infections (UTIs). If an adolescent female has frequent UTIs, find out whether she is sexually active, because sexual intercourse increases the risk of UTIs. Screen adolescent females who are sexually active for sexually transmitted infections (STIs).

Hormonal shifts, physical growth, and sexual maturity occur during adolescence. The onset of **puberty**, which is marked by the development of secondary sexual characteristics, is stimulated by gonadotropin-releasing hormone (GnRH). The release of GnRH stimulates the pituitary gland to release luteinizing hormone (LH) and follicle-stimulating hormone (FSH). Finally, LH and FSH stimulate the release of androgens and estrogens (Holland-Hall & Burstein, 2016).

Assess the stages of puberty using Tanner staging (see Figs. 18.3–18.5). Adolescents in whom the onset of puberty is delayed need further evaluation to determine the reason for delay. Adolescents with chronic illnesses often have delayed onset of puberty. If there is no previously known condition causing pubertal delay, refer the adolescent to an endocrinologist.

In Chapter 12, Natasha Austin had delayed onset of puberty. What about her development indicated that her onset of puberty was delayed? Why was the onset of puberty delayed in her case? How might the delayed onset of puberty have affected her emotional development and **body image?**

Males

After the onset of testicular enlargement, male adolescents experience penile growth. Table 19.2 describes the physical changes that males experience during puberty. Growth of pubic hair and axillary hair occurs as testosterone is released. Sometime in middle-to-late adolescence, male adolescents experience their first involuntary ejaculation, usually occurring at night, commonly referred to as a wet dream. Provide anticipatory guidance to the adolescent, letting him know that this is a normal part of development.

Females

Menarche occurs around 2 years after the development of breast buds, or thelarche. Table 19.3 describes the physical changes that females experience during puberty. After thelarche, pubic hair growth occurs. Anticipatory guidance for adolescent females includes preparing for monthly periods, menstrual cramps, and heavy bleeding. Explain what is normal and when the adolescent should see a healthcare provider.

Table 19.2 Male Physical Changes During Puberty

Stage of Adolescence	Physical Changes
Early (10–13 y)	• Tanner stages 1–2 • Testicular enlargement • Start of penile growth
Middle (14–17 y)	• Tanner stages 3–5 • Growth spurt • Nocturnal emissions • Body hair, facial hair
Late (18–21 y)	• Tanner stage 5 • Increased lean muscle mass

Table 19.3 Female Physical Changes During Puberty

Stage of Adolescence	Physical Changes
Early (10–13 y)	• Tanner stages 1–2 • Breast buds • Pubic hair, axillary hair • Growth spurt • Menarche
Middle (14–17 y)	• Tanner stages 3–5 • Peak growth velocity
Late (18–21 y)	• Tanner stage 5 • Increased muscle mass

Musculoskeletal Assessment

The skeletal system continues to mature during adolescence. In females, growth plates tend to close 2 to 2½ years after menarche. Growth slows after menarche and ceases when the growth plates close. In males, growth plates close later in adolescence. Full ossification occurs later in males than in females, as well. Inspect for scoliosis at each health promotion visit.

Muscle growth is affected by the release of hormones such as estrogen, progesterone, and testosterone. Muscle development in males is greater than in females. Lean muscle mass increases in both genders by the end of adolescence, with males having overall greater muscle mass.

Integumentary Assessment

Skin becomes thicker during adolescence. With the production of sex hormones, the sebaceous glands become more active, leading to acne on the face and back of many adolescents. Activity in the apocrine sweat glands increases, as well, to adult levels, leading to sweating during times of stress. These sweat glands are located around hair follicles, such as in the axillae and genital area and under the breasts.

Inspect the skin for both open and closed comedones. Inspect the face and the back. Determine the adolescent's cleansing routine. Enquire whether the adolescent is picking at his or her acne lesions. Inspect the skin for extreme dryness or oiliness. Inspect any moles, noting the size, shape, and color.

Pain Assessment

Adolescents are able to describe their pain in terms of intensity, type, location, and acuity (Growth and Development Check 19.1). The most common types of self-rating pain scales used with adolescents are the Visual Analog Scale (VAS) and the Numeric Rating Scale (NRS). The VAS is a 100-mm-long line with one end labeled "no pain" and the other end "pain as bad as it could possibly be" (Fig. 19.1A; Young, 2017). The NRS

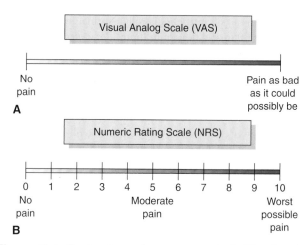

Figure 19.1. Scales for pain assessment. A. Visual analog scale. **B.** Numeric rating scale. Adapted with permission from Kyle, T., & Carman, S. (2016). *Essentials of pediatric nursing* (3rd ed., Fig. 14.6). Philadelphia, PA: Wolters Kluwer.

prompts adolescents to rate their pain from 0 to 10, with 0 indicating no pain and 10 indicating the worst possible pain (Fig. 19.1B; Young, 2017). A more recently developed pain scale is the clinically aligned pain assessment (CAPA) tool (Analyze the Evidence 19.1).

Be aware of the types of nonpharmacological pain management that are effective with adolescents. Behavioral interventions include preparation for procedures and positive reinforcement. Cognitive interventions include distraction and guided imagery. Music, acupuncture, and craniosacral therapy are complementary therapies that work well with adolescents. Additional interventions include deep breathing and hot or cold therapy to reduce pain (Short, Pace, & Birnbaum, 2017).

Physical Growth

Physical growth is genetically determined but is also affected by nutrition, environment, and physical activity. During adolescence, body fat increases in females in preparation for childbearing, whereas lean muscle mass increases in males (Fig. 19.2).

Growth and Development Check 19.1

Pain Assessment With Developmental Delay

When conducting a pain assessment, take into account the developmental level of the patient. Although the patient may be an adolescent by chronological age, his or her developmental age may be different. Adolescents who are developmentally delayed are not able to use either the Visual Analog Scale or the Numeric Rating Scale if the developmental age is below 7 y. For developmentally delayed adolescents, use a developmentally appropriate scale such as the Faces Pain Rating Scale. If the adolescent is nonverbal, use the Face, Legs, Activity, Cry, Consolability scale, along with parental report, to determine the patient's pain level.

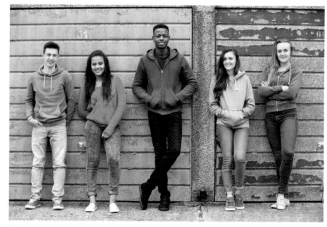

Figure 19.2. Physical growth in adolescents. Adolescents grow at different rates.

Analyze the Evidence 19.1 Clinically Aligned Pain Assessment Tool

The most commonly used pain scales are one-dimensional, only measuring pain intensity. However, pain encompasses so much more, and the experience of pain is individual to the patient. In 2012, the University of Utah piloted a multifaceted pain tool to assess the complexity of the patient's pain. This tool is called the clinically aligned pain assessment (CAPA) tool. In the pilot study, when the CAPA tool was implemented, patient pain satisfaction scores increased from the 18th percentile to the 95th percentile.

The CAPA tool engages the patient in a conversation about the pain experience. Sample questions include the following:

- How comfortable are you?
- Are you experiencing any pain?
- Is your discomfort improving or worsening?

- Has the medication/heating pad/ice helped manage your pain?
- Are you able to do what the staff is asking you to do (e.g., walking, coughing, physical therapy)?
- Have you been able to sleep? Is the pain waking you up?

On the basis of the results at the University of Utah, the University of Minnesota Medical Center adapted the CAPA as a tool for quality improvement. Researchers identified units on which the CAPA would be adopted. Nurses were then trained on the use of the tool. After implementation, units that fully embraced the CAPA tool saw patient pain satisfaction scores improve. In addition, patients indicated that they preferred the CAPA tool over the Numeric Rating Scale, indicating that assessing the entire experience of pain is important to the patient.

Data from Topham, D., & Drew, D. (2017). Quality improvement project: Replacing the numeric rating scale with a clinically aligned pain assessment (CAPA) tool. *Pain Management Nursing, 18*(6), 363–371.

Growth spurts start in the hands and feet and then move to the arms and legs, giving the adolescent an awkward appearance in the early adolescent years. Bone growth happens before bone ossification, which places the adolescent at risk for fractures. In addition, skeletal growth occurs before muscle growth, placing adolescents at risk for sprains and strains (Holland-Hall & Burstein, 2016).

Weight

Adolescence is a time of rapid increase in weight. A normal increase in weight is due to a change in hormonal regulation, increase in muscle mass, and bone growth. Poor diet and lack of exercise contribute to excessive weight gain during this time. Average weight gain varies throughout adolescence. Monitor the adolescent's weight relative to height, as quantified in the body mass index (BMI; growth charts available at http://www.cdc.gov/growthcharts). A healthy BMI is in the 5th to less than the 85th percentile.

Height

During adolescence, the greatest period of growth is during the growth spurt. For females, the peak growth rate is approximately 3 to 3.5 in/y (7.6–8.8 cm), which occurs about 6 months before menarche. Growth slows after menarche and continues for 2 to 2½ years, at which time the female adolescent has reached her adult height.

The peak growth rate for males is 3.5 to 4 in/y (8.8–10.2 cm), which occurs when the adolescent reaches Tanner stage 3 or 4, typically about 2 years after the female growth spurt. Males continue to grow 2 to 3 years after females stop growing.

Developmental Theories

The major tasks of adolescence are to develop an identity, a moral compass, and abstract thinking, all of which help the adolescent successfully transition to adulthood. Table 19.4 provides an overview of developmental theories in adolescence.

Psychosocial

The psychosocial task of adolescence is development of identity (Erikson, 1963). After a period of stability, adolescence is a time of rapid change both physiologically and in responsibilities. Erikson (1963) believed that, in their search for identity, adolescents must revisit all of the stages of childhood. Adolescents who did not successfully complete the tasks of previous stages could have difficulty with identity development. However, with the appropriate tools and support, adolescents can overcome the past and develop a secure identity by the end of adolescence (Erikson, 1963). In their search for identity, adolescents experiment with different styles, activities, and peer groups.

Adolescents discover identity through exploration of personal values and beliefs. The adolescent is caught between the ideology of a child and the ethics yet to be developed (Erikson, 1963). By the end of this stage, the adolescents should have a sense of what they want to do or be, as well as of their sexual identity. The adolescent who has trouble with identity development is at risk for role confusion. Adolescents experiencing role confusion may move frequently among peer groups or schools and often participate in risky behaviors. Those struggling with sexual identity are at risk for role confusion, as well. Adolescents require support from peers and family to successfully achieve identity development.

Table 19.4 Overview of Developmental Theories in Adolescence

Theorist: Type of Development	Stage or Level	Implications
Erikson: Psychosocial	Identity vs. role confusion	• Is self-conscious about the changing body in early adolescence • Is concerned with attractiveness in middle adolescence • Has a more stable body image in late adolescence • Is forming identity in late adolescence
Piaget: Cognitive	Formal operational	• Develops abstract thought in early-to-middle adolescence • Feels invulnerable during middle adolescence • Develops better impulse control by late adolescence • Can see others' perspectives
Freud: Psychosexual	Genital	• Experiments sexually • Settles into relationships
Kohlberg: Moral	Postconventional	• Understands that morally right and legally right are not always the same • Establishes own set of morals, which may be different from those of the family

In Chapter 9, Jessica Wang had a diagnosis of epilepsy. How did Jessica's epilepsy interfere with her development of identity? How did her family, including her grandmother, influence her development of identity? How did Jessica's pediatrician, Dr. Wong, assess and attempt to facilitate Jessica's psychosocial development?

Cognitive

The formal operational stage lasts from adolescence through adulthood. The adolescent develops the ability to think abstractly without having to manipulate a concrete object (Piaget, 1930). Logic and reasoning develop, and the adolescent is able to see things from many different points of view. Adolescents are able to hypothesize, debate different solutions to problems, and prioritize on the basis of the outcome desired.

In early and middle adolescence, teenagers are egocentric, thinking that everything revolves around them and assuming that everyone around them shares their same ideals and interests. This type of thinking can lead to risk-taking behavior, because adolescents think they are invincible. Adolescents also develop morals and viewpoints that are different from those of their families, which can cause family conflict.

Moral

Adolescents are in the postconventional level of moral development (Kohlberg, 1981). The first stage in this level (the fifth stage, overall, in Kohlberg's theory of moral development),

social contract, represents procedural democracy and is concerned with ensuring representation of all and understanding the establishment of laws (Kohlberg, 1981). The second stage of postconventional thought (the sixth and final stage, overall), universal principles, is reached in adulthood.

During this social contract stage of moral development, adolescents see the world from differing points of view and establish their own sets of morals and beliefs. These beliefs may be different from those of families and peers, causing some conflict among previously strong support networks. In addition, adolescents question the status quo and wonder why change doesn't occur when the status quo is no longer working. The adolescent discovers that morally right and legally right are not always the same but is able to reconcile these discrepancies.

Motor Development

During adolescence, both gross and fine motor skills continue to develop. Rather than continually developing new skills, adolescents refine the skills they already have. During growth spurts, both males and females may lose some coordination or flexibility. This loss may have an effect on activities, such as sports, during this time. Once the growth spurt is complete, any lost coordination or flexibility returns.

Gross Motor

Speed, coordination, and endurance increase throughout adolescence. By middle and late adolescence, teenagers tend to narrow their focus of interest in extracurricular activities (Fig. 19.3), which allows them to focus on skill and muscle development that benefit them in their chosen sport or activity.

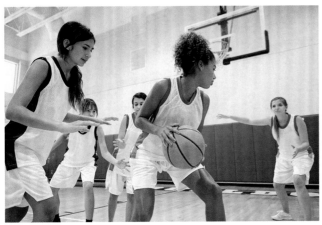

Figure 19.3. Gross motor development. Adolescents tend to narrow their focus, developing their gross motor skills for a desired sport.

Fine Motor

Dexterity continues to improve during adolescence. Whether playing a musical instrument, painting, drawing, sewing, or engaging in other hobbies, adolescents become steadier in their craft (Fig. 19.4). Improved hand–eye coordination also allows for advanced fine motor skills.

Communication and Language Development

During adolescence, one's vocabulary and use of language continue to increase in complexity. Abstract thought and the ability to understand the perspectives of others allow for communication at a deeper level. However, adolescents often use slang, making it difficult to communicate with adults. In addition, adolescents communicate through text using "text speak," further creating a divide in communication with adults. By the end of adolescence, language use is at the level of an adult.

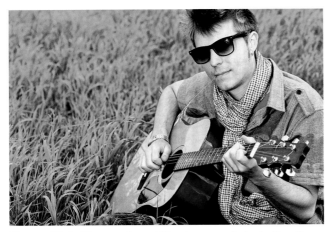

Figure 19.4. Fine motor skills. Increased dexterity allows adolescents to further develop their craft.

Social and Emotional Development

The majority of development in adolescence occurs in the areas of social and emotional development. Relationships change throughout adolescence as peers become more important and separation from parents occurs. Adolescents struggling with gender identity are at risk for anxiety and depression. Body image and self-esteem are affected either positively or negatively by relationships.

Relationships

The peer group becomes the most important source of information in early and middle adolescence. These relationships often cause conflict between adolescents and parents. By late adolescence, peer influence diminishes as identity is firmly established.

Parents

Although adolescents begin to separate from parents, the parents must maintain a relationship with their teenager. They need to continue to support the adolescent through communication. Adolescents are striving for independence, but parents still must enforce rules. Parents can set rules in conjunction with the adolescent, and the rules should not be too strict or too loose. Parents should be aware of who their adolescent's friends are and where they are when not at home.

As adolescents are spending more and more time on social media, it is crucial that parents maintain open and positive communication. Positive and supportive communication with parents seems to lessen the negative effects associated with excessive screen time in adolescence (Boniel-Nissim et al., 2015). Adolescents are moody and often shut themselves up in their rooms. Encourage parents to respect adolescents' space and privacy but to consistently communicate. Parents should be open and honest, not talk down to the adolescent, and admit when they make a mistake. Supportive and honest communication helps establish a positive relationship between the parents and the adolescent.

Peers

Peer influence during early and middle adolescence is higher than at any other point in development. Although peer influence is often associated with negative behaviors, evidence indicates that it also can foster positive social behaviors (Kilford, Garrett, & Blakemore, 2016). Peers can influence how adolescents dress, talk, and act and what activities they participate in. Peers have also been shown to influence an adolescent's diet and physical activity (Chung, Ersig, & McCarthy, 2017).

In early adolescence, same-sex peers have the most influence. In this stage, female groups tend to center around relationships, whereas male groups tend to focus on a particular sport or activity (Fig. 19.5; Holland-Hall & Burstein, 2016). As teenagers move into middle adolescence, both genders are included in peer groups (Fig. 19.6). During this stage, adolescents may

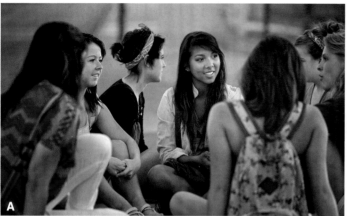
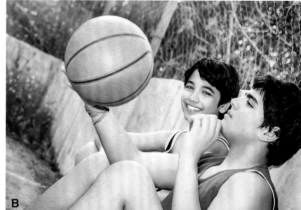

Figure 19.5. Peer relationships in early adolescence. A. Female relationships focus on social relationships. **B.** Male relationships tend to focus on sports or other activities.

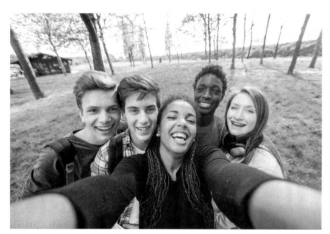

Figure 19.6. Peer relationships in middle adolescence. Peer groups in middle-to-late adolescence consist of both males and females.

Figure 19.7. Dating. One-on-one dating typically begins around the age of 16 years.

experiment with different peer groups to determine where they best fit in. During this time, some adolescents experiment with gang memberships.

Encourage parents to be aware of whom their adolescent is socializing with, both same-sex and opposite-sex peers. Remind parents to keep the lines of communication open with their adolescent to provide guidance, support, and role modeling. Adolescents without positive support and communication are more likely to become involved in risk-taking behaviors. Remind parents that adolescents are more likely to make positive choices if they are connected with family and positive peers and have clear rules (Hagan, Shaw, & Duncan, 2017).

Dating

Opposite-sex relationships may emerge by the end of early adolescence (Fig. 19.7). Dating begins around the age of 12½ years for girls and 13½ years for boys and initially occurs in groups rather than one-on-one (American Academy of Pediatrics [AAP], 2015c). Around the age of 16 years, adolescents begin dating one-on-one. Parents should talk with their adolescent

about healthy relationships. Both partners in the relationship should respect each other for who they are. There should be no bullying or threatening in any relationship. Parents should notice any change in their adolescent's behavior and encourage him or her to talk about any experiences, positive or negative, in the relationship. Dating can have either a positive or negative effect on self-esteem and academic performance, depending on the nature of the relationship.

Parents should begin talking with their adolescent about sex and dating early, optimally before the first date. Of adolescents surveyed in 2015, 41% had ever had sexual intercourse, 30% of those surveyed had had sexual intercourse in the past 3 months, and 43% of those adolescents surveyed did not use a condom (Centers for Disease Control and Prevention [CDC], 2017e). Early sexual behavior places adolescents at risk for STIs and teen pregnancy. Nearly half of the newly diagnosed STIs are in adolescents aged 15 years and older (CDC, 2017b).

Parents need to discuss with adolescents that "no means no" and that nobody should force them into any sexual act, including touching, oral sex, or sexual intercourse. Encourage adolescents to report any act of dating violence. Be honest and open with adolescents. Adolescents aged 12 to 19 years report that parents have a greater influence on sexual decision making than do peers (Hagan et al., 2017). Listen to what they have to say without being judgmental, and answer their questions. Talk to them about the dangers of STIs and how to prevent them. Explain pregnancy and how to prevent pregnancy, as well. Many parents do not feel comfortable talking to their adolescent about sex. Health promotion visits are ideal for nurses to talk with adolescents about sexual behavior and the risks associated with it.

Gender Identity

Gender identity is influenced by several factors beginning prenatally. Development of gender identity continues throughout childhood, adolescence, and adulthood. In addition to prenatal and hormonal factors, gender identity is influenced by sociocultural and psychological factors (Holland-Hall & Burstein, 2016). Gender identity and sexual orientation are two different constructs. Nurses should be aware of the differences. Gender identity refers to how adolescents see themselves, as male or female, regardless of their biological gender. Sexual orientation refers to attraction and whether the adolescent is attracted to males, females, or both (Bosse & Chiodo, 2016). Adolescents identifying as gay or lesbian may have expressed gender dysphoria during childhood. Nurses should be sensitive to the adolescent struggling with gender identity and sexual orientation that are different from the societal norms.

As adolescents move toward the task of identity formation, gender identity and sexual orientation are part of this process. Those adolescents who struggle with the integration of either one of these identities may face negative outcomes both physically and mentally (Bosse & Chiodo, 2016). Adolescents identifying as sexual minorities—as gay, lesbian, or transgender—are at greater risk of tobacco use, drug use, and violence-related behaviors (Kann et al., 2016). Be sensitive to the adolescent's identity formation process when discussing health promotion and risk-taking behaviors. If an adolescent identifies as a sexual minority, or a gender different from the adolescent's biological gender, note the interaction between the adolescent and the parent. Discuss counseling with families as needed. In addition, assess the prevalence of stigma and bullying that the adolescent experiences as a result of perceived nonconformity. In late adolescence, the adolescent may indicate the desire to pursue gender reassignment surgery. If this desire is expressed, refer the adolescent and family to a tertiary care center that specializes in this type of surgery for adolescents and can provide the psychosocial support services needed.

Body Image

Self-concept and **body image** are closely related. How an adolescent perceives himself or herself can lead to positive or negative self-esteem. There are a myriad of influences on body image perception. Females tend to be influenced by what their peers think about them. Media, specifically social media, also plays a role in a female adolescent's perception of herself. The higher the number of friends a female adolescent has on social media, the more likely she is to be concerned about her body image and, in particular, to desire to be thin (Tiggemann & Slater, 2017). Educate adolescents that what is posted on social media is not always a true depiction of reality.

Body image is also influenced by the development of secondary sexual characteristics. Early or late development of these characteristics can have a negative effect on body image and self-esteem. Males become concerned about muscle development, facial hair, and the size of their penis. Females become concerned about the size of their breasts and starting menstruation. Assess the adolescent's perception of his or her body. Refer those with obsessions about weight or appearance for counseling.

Health Promotion

Health promotion during the adolescent years focuses on the physiological, psychological, and social domains. During the adolescent period, parents and teenagers often have many questions. These questions center around the physiological changes of puberty, the adolescent's growing independence, and potential school or behavioral problems. Be sure to address the needs of both the parents and the adolescent. Ensure that the adolescent has the ability to talk privately with a healthcare provider if needed. Schedule routine health promotion visits yearly during adolescence (Hagan et al., 2017).

Promoting Healthy Growth and Development

When promoting healthy growth and development with adolescents, focus on their assets or strengths, rather than on potential problems (Priority Care Concepts 19.1). Considering assets, such as participation in extracurricular activities, allows parents and adolescents to set goals for healthy living (Hagan et al., 2017). Explain to parents that although adolescents are gaining independence, parental involvement is still important. Listening to the adolescent's wants and needs and involving the adolescent in mutual decision making fosters responsibility and self-reliance.

Continue to assess the social determinants of health, including both the risk factors and protective factors. Assess for interpersonal violence at home or in school, exposure to substance abuse, and food and housing security. In addition, assess for strengths, such as connections with family, peers, and other positive social groups.

Safety

Discuss with adolescents safety concerns and ways they can address them (Patient Teaching 19.1). The most common causes of injuries during the adolescent period are motor vehicle accidents, substance abuse, and firearms (Hagan et al., 2017).

Sports Safety

Many adolescents are involved in sports through school or the community. In addition to sprains, strains, and fractures, high

Priority Care Concepts 19.1

Promoting Growth and Development in Adolescents

Communication and Social Development
- Self-esteem development
- Respectful communication
- Positive interactions between parents and adolescent
- Supportive peer groups
- Developing independence

Sleep
- At least 7–8 h of sleep per night
- No television, computer, or electronic devices in bedroom

Oral Health
- Brushing teeth and flossing
- Dental visits

Safety
- Home environment
- Violence
- Internet safety
- Car safety
- Sports safety

Nutrition
- Limit sugary beverages and snacks
- Appropriate portion sizes
- Importance of breakfast

School
- School attendance
- School performance

Physical Activity
- 60 min of physical activities daily
- Extracurricular sports

Risk Reduction
- Pregnancy
- Sexually transmitted infections
- Substance abuse

Mental Health
- Dealing with anger and frustration
- Recognizing signs and symptoms of depression
- Recognizing signs and symptoms of eating disorders

Patient Teaching 19.1

Safety for Adolescents

Nurses are able to help promotion of safety through educating both parents and adolescents on potential unintentional injuries and how to prevent them. Involving adolescents in plans for injury prevention is more likely to result in compliance.

Sports
- Wear necessary sports equipment while playing.
- Learn to recognize signs of a concussion.
- Stay hydrated.
- Learn to recognize signs of dehydration and overheating.
- Learn to recognize signs of a concussion.

Water Sports
- Acquire proper licensure before driving a watercraft.
- Operate watercrafts safely.
- Wear a life jacket when in any body of water other than in a swimming pool.

Car
- Always wear a seatbelt.
- Avoid distracted driving.
- Follow the speed limit.
- Follow state driving laws.

Firearm
- Store firearms in a locked cabinet.
- Learn how to safely use firearms.

Fire
- Learn how to be safe around campfires.
- Use matches safely.
- Have a fire escape plan for the home.
- Practice fire escape routes at home.

Sun
- Use sunscreen when outdoors.
- Wear a wide-brimmed hat when in the sun.
- Do not use tanning beds.

Data from Centers for Disease Control and Prevention, 2018.

baseline cognitive functioning. If an adolescent sustains a head injury, healthcare providers can compare preinjury testing results with postinjury results to determine the effects of the injury (CDC, 2015). Knowing the difference between the baseline and postinjury test results also informs treatment decisions.

school athletes are at risk for concussions. It is imperative that adolescents wear all necessary safety equipment. However, some sports, such as soccer and basketball, do not require the use of a helmet, making adolescents more prone to concussion. Any high school athlete should participate in baseline concussion testing. This testing is done preseason and preinjury to establish

In Chapter 3, 12-year-old David Torres fractured his right ulna. What activity was David doing when he fractured his ulna? What type of fracture did he have? What treatment did receive for his fracture?

Motor Vehicle Safety

Although the legal age to begin driving and related laws vary from state to state, many adolescents begin driving independently during this period. Six teenagers are killed daily in motor vehicle crashes (CDC, 2017c). Injury and death from motor vehicle crashes are preventable. Teach adolescents and their parents about the principles of safe driving (Fig. 19.8). Distracted driving is a major cause of injury and death during the adolescent period. Nine percent of all drivers aged 15 to 19 years involved in fatal crashes reported driving distracted (National Center for Statistics and Analysis, 2017). Distractions while driving include texting, talking on the phone, and eating, among other things. Teach adolescents about the danger of being distracted on the road.

Other dangers associated with adolescent drivers include not wearing seatbelts, driving with other adolescents in the car, reckless driving, and driving at night. Parents play an important role in their adolescent's safe driving. Encourage parents to practice driving with their adolescents in different weather conditions, in heavy traffic, and at night. Both parents and adolescents should know the driving and curfew laws in their state.

Firearm Safety

Firearms should be kept in a locked cabinet and ammunition should be stored in a separate area. Households that have adolescents with a history of aggression, depression, or suicidal ideation should remove all firearms from the home (Hagan et al., 2017).

Adolescents who hunt should have a firearm safety class and understand that the firearm is only to be used when hunting.

Risk Reduction

Positive social development has been shown to be an effective means of reducing risks associated with adolescence (Hagan et al., 2017). Adolescents with positive social support are more likely to have higher self-esteem and emotional well-being.

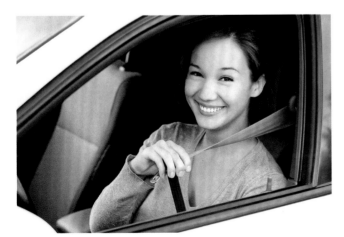

Figure 19.8. Motor vehicle safety. Teach adolescents the importance of wearing seatbelts.

When discussing risk reduction with adolescents, emphasize the importance of healthy relationships and activities that are meaningful to the adolescent. Encourage adolescents without positive family support to become involved in school or community groups.

For conversations involving sensitive topics such as sexual activity, pregnancy, STIs, and substance use, it is appropriate to ask the adolescent's parents to leave the room. Assure middle to older adolescents that anything they say is confidential unless they reveal they are going to hurt themselves or others. Early adolescents are generally not old enough to be deemed a mature minor, and, therefore, their parents must be involved. Know the laws for mature and emancipated minors in the state in which you practice.

Pregnancy and Sexually Transmitted Infections

Nurses should have open and honest conversations about sexual activity with adolescents. Determine whether the adolescent is engaging in sexual activity and therefore at risk for STIs or pregnancy (if female). Inform adolescent females that one in four have an STI such as chlamydia or the human papillomavirus (HPV) (CDC, 2017b). The incidence of STIs, such as chlamydia, gonorrhea, and syphilis, in adolescent males has increased in the past 4 years (CDC, 2017b). Although the incidence of STIs has increased, adolescent pregnancy rates have decreased over the years. The latest report, in 2015, showed a record low pregnancy rate of 22.3% in adolescent females aged 15 to 19 years (CDC, 2017d). Reasons for the decrease in adolescent pregnancies include increased age at initiation of sexual intercourse and more effective use of contraception (American College of Obstetricians and Gynecologists [ACOG], 2017).

Abstention is the best way to prevent STIs and pregnancy. However, if the adolescent admits to being sexually active, enquire whether he or she is using any kind of protection against STIs or any form of birth control. Adolescents are able to use any type of contraceptive approved by the Food and Drug Administration, including oral contraceptives and intrauterine devices. ACOG AAP (2017) recommends the use of long-acting reversible contraception (LARC), such as intrauterine devices, for adolescent females who are sexually active. Discuss sexual activity, reproductive plans, and contraceptive preferences with the adolescent before initiation of prescription contraception. Explain contraception failure rates and side effects of different types of contraception. Adolescent females desiring to start contraception such as LARC should be referred to a gynecologist.

Teach both male and female adolescents about the dangers of STIs and how they are passed from partner to partner, including through oral sex. Explain that abstaining from sexual activity is best practice, but also teach adolescents about safe sexual practices. Remind adolescents that contraception does not prevent STIs and that a form of barrier protection, such as a condom, should be used in addition to other forms of contraception. Ensure that the adolescent knows where he or she can obtain protection and screening for both STIs and pregnancy.

Substance Use

Substances, including alcohol, marijuana, and other illicit drugs, affect the development of the adolescent brain, specifically the prefrontal cortex. As a result, adolescents engaging in heavy substance use exhibit deficits in cognitive tasks such as recall, attention, spatial skills, and executive functioning (Silveri, Dager, Cohen-Gilbert, & Sneider, 2016; Squeglia, Jacobus, & Tapert, 2009). Executive functioning encompasses organizational skills, time management, planning, the ability to see different points of view, and emotional regulation. The earlier the age of onset of substance use, the poorer the cognitive outcomes (Jacobus et al., 2015). Furthermore, the age at onset of use inversely correlates with the likelihood of developing a **substance use disorder** (SUD; Levy & Williams, 2016). Because of this, it is imperative to not only provide intervention about abstaining from substances during the adolescent years but also intervene early with adolescents who are using substances to prevent neurocognitive deficits and future SUD.

Many adolescents experiment with substance use, including tobacco, alcohol, and other drugs. Discuss with adolescents the dangers of such use. Teach them how being under the influence of alcohol or drugs leads to poor decisions, such as driving while under the influence or engaging in unprotected sex. Educate adolescents about the dangers of tobacco use, and inform them that e-cigarettes are not necessarily safer than are traditional cigarettes. Provide education and materials on how they can resist peer pressure to engage in substance use.

When adolescents admit to substance use, determine their risk for SUD. Use validated screening tools, such as the CRAFFT (Car, Relax, Alone, Forget, Friends, and Trouble) and SBIRT (Screening, Brief Intervention, and Referral to Treatment) tools, to determine whether the adolescent is at low or high risk for substance abuse (Boxes 19.1 and 19.2; Substance Abuse and Mental Health Services Administration [SBIRT], n.d.). Discuss substance abuse further depending on the adolescent's answers to the CRAFFT screening tool.

Oral Health

Adolescents should continue to visit the dentist every 6 months. Ensure that the adolescent brushes his or her teeth twice daily. If the adolescent's home does not have fluoridated water, ensure that the adolescent takes fluoride until the age of 16 years to restore enamel and further prevent dental caries (Hagan et al., 2017). Discuss the importance of flossing to prevent gum disease.

Box 19.1   The Car, Relax, Alone, Forget, Friends, and Trouble Screening Tool

The CRAFFT screening tool is a six-item questionnaire recommended by the American Academy of Pediatrics to be used with all adolescents to identify those at risk for alcohol or other drug use disorders. The questions are as follows:

- **C**—Have you ever ridden in a **CAR** driven by someone (including yourself) who was "high" or had been using alcohol or drugs?
- **R**—Do you ever use alcohol or drugs to **RELAX**, feel better about yourself, or fit in?
- **A**—Do you ever use alcohol or drugs while you are by yourself, or **ALONE**?
- **F**—Do you ever **FORGET** things you did while using alcohol or drugs?
- **F**—Do your family or **FRIENDS** ever tell you that you should cut down on your drinking or drug use?
- **T**—Have you ever gotten into **TROUBLE** while you were using alcohol or drugs?

Healthcare providers should either give a brief intervention or refer adolescents for further evaluation and treatment depending on the adolescent's answers.

Data from D'Amico, E. J., Parast, L., Meredith, L. S., Ewing, B. A., Shadel, W. G., & Stein, B. D. (2016). Screening in primary care: What is the best way to identify at risk youth for substance use? *Pediatrics, 138*(6), e20161717. doi:10.1542/peds.2016-1717; Massachusetts Department of Public Health Bureau of Substance Abuse Services. (2009). *Adolescent screening, brief intervention, and referral to treatment for alcohol and other drug use using the CRAFFT screening tool.* Retrieved from https://www.integration.samhsa.gov/clinical-practice/sbirt/adolescent_screening,_brieft_intervention_and_referral_to_treatment_for_alcohol.pdf

---

Box 19.2   The Screening Brief Intervention and Referral to Treatment Screening Tool

The SBIRT tool is used to determine whether the adolescent is at low risk and can benefit from a brief intervention by the healthcare provider or at high risk and needs referral to treatment.

- **S**creening—Assess for risky substance use.
- **B**rief **I**ntervention—Have a short conversation with the patient in which you point out risky behaviors and offer advice.
- **R**eferral to **T**reatment—Refer the patient for additional services as needed.

Training is required before the healthcare provider can implement the SBIRT screening tool. Free online trainings are available at https://www.integration.samhsa.gov/clinical-practice/sbirt.

Personal Hygiene

Puberty requires meticulous personal hygiene. Discuss how to control body odor through daily showers and deodorant use. Teach the adolescent to brush and wash hair on a regular basis. Have adolescents wash their face twice daily. If the adolescent has acne, encourage him or her not to pick at the lesions.

When talking with an adolescent female, discuss hygiene related to menstruation. Whether using tampons or maxi pads, female adolescents need to understand how often to change them and how to keep the perineal area clean.

Screening for Reproductive Cancers

Although reproductive cancers do not typically occur in adolescents, breast, cervical, ovarian, and testicular cancer can occur in young adults (American Cancer Society, 2018). These cancers are often linked to environmental factors but, in young adults, may be related to DNA changes in cells. Teach adolescents about the different types of reproductive cancers and how to screen for them. Teach adolescent females to do breast self-exams and let their healthcare provider know of any changes, such as development of a lump. Although cervical cancer does not often occur in young adults, prevention begins in

adolescence. Cervical cancer is often caused by HPV and can be prevented with the HPV vaccine.

Testicular cancers often occur in younger males (American Cancer Society, 2018). Teach adolescent males how to do testicular self-exams. Teach males to contact a healthcare provider for further investigation if they notice a lump or scrotal swelling.

School

High school can be a time of high stress for adolescents (Fig. 19.9). Those who are struggling may experience stress because they are not doing well. High-achieving students may feel pressure to take advanced classes to get into college and get scholarships. Assess the adolescent's school performance. Perceived pressure in school can lead to negative outcomes. Discuss with parents whether the adolescent is in the correct level of classes. Inform adolescents and their families of school options after high school, including 4-year colleges, 2-year colleges, and trade schools. Some students may feel they are not ready for more schooling and plan to get a job and potentially pursue higher education at a later period in life. In any case, encourage the adolescent's participation in making choices about his or her future.

Sleep

Sleep deficit is common during the adolescent period due to a change in circadian rhythm. The typical adolescent sleep cycle is to go to bed around 11:00 p.m. and wake up around 9:00 a.m. (Hagan et al., 2017). This sleep cycle begins at the onset of puberty and lasts throughout adolescence. However, adolescents are generally unable to sleep on this circadian rhythm because of the early start time of school. Although they go to bed around 11:00 p.m., on average, they must get up for school earlier than 9:00 a.m., leading to a sleep deficit. The AAP (2014) has recommended that middle and high schools not start before 8:30 a.m. to combat the sleep deficits incurred by adolescents.

Sleep deficit can have significant effects on the adolescent. Adolescents who experience sleep deprivation may display negative mood and increased emotional reactivity (Tarokh, Saletin, & Carskadon, 2016). Lack of sleep leads to mood disorders such as depression and anxiety, behavioral disorders, eating disorders, substance use, and obesity (Analyze the Evidence 19.2; Zhang

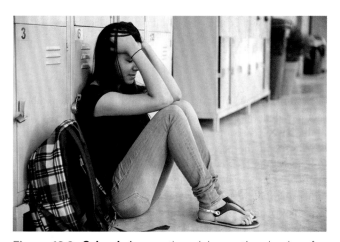

Figure 19.9. School. Assess the adolescent's school performance and stress level.

Analyze the Evidence 19.2 The Effects of Sleep on Food Choices

Asarnow, Greer, Walker, and Harvey (2017) conducted a study to determine whether the amount of sleep affected the intake of junk food in adolescents. The study was part of a National Institute of Child Health and Human Development–funded trial designed to improve sleep for 10- to 18-y-olds.

The study sample consisted of 42 adolescents. The participants were eligible if they scored in the lowest quartile of the Children's Morningness Eveningness

Preference Scale, meaning they preferred later bedtimes.

The study design consisted of the measurement of sleep through a sleep diary and the measurement of desire for weight-promoting foods in a laboratory. After a 6-wk intervention, sleep and desire for weight-promoting foods were measured again. The researchers found that in the adolescents with improved, or earlier, bedtimes, the desire to eat unhealthy foods decreased.

et al., 2017). Conversely, adolescents who get 8 to 10 hours of sleep per night have higher academic achievements, better nutritional status, and better overall quality of life (AAP, 2014).

Although adolescents are gaining independence, remind them about the importance of sleep and sleep hygiene. Bedtime should be the same each night. Adolescents should not have televisions or computers in their rooms or, at least, should turn them off 1 hour before going to sleep.

Discipline

Adolescence is a time of growing independence, and, as such, the adolescent is likely to break rules from time to time. Parents should establish a consistent set of rules for their child in early adolescence. The adolescent should have a clear understanding of the consequences of breaking the set rules.

As the child enters middle adolescence, parents can collaborate with him or her to establish rules and consequences for breaking those rules. This collaboration teaches the adolescent responsibility and fosters his or her growing independence in a healthy manner.

Immunizations

The adolescent needs to complete the HPV vaccine series if not already completed and needs the second dose of the meningococcal vaccine at age 16 years. In addition, the adolescent should receive the influenza vaccine yearly.

The most up-to-date immunization chart is available at https://www.cdc.gov/vaccines/schedules/hcp/child-adolescent.html. Remind parents and adolescents of the reason for vaccine administration as well as the side effects, how to treat them, and when to contact a healthcare provider. Refer to Chapter 15 for information on immunizations related to nursing considerations, barriers, and reporting adverse events. For patient teaching on immunizations, refer to Patient Teaching 18.2. Adolescents receive the same immunizations as do school-age children, with the exception that they do not receive the diphtheria, tetanus, and acellular pertussis immunization.

Nutrition

Talking to adolescents about nutrition continues to be important. Often, adolescents eat out with their friends and make food choices on their own. Educating them about making healthy nutritional choices, even when eating out, is crucial to preventing weight problems and other health problems later in life. Teach adolescents that high-quality diet alone, regardless of physical activity, is associated with less weight gain in the years between adolescence and young adulthood (Hu et al., 2017).

Discussing fad diets is also important. Fad diets often deprive the adolescent of vital nutrients needed for bone and muscle strength, immune system function, and cognitive function. Remind adolescents that energy drinks can have dangerous side effects. Discuss nutritional needs with the adolescent and determine whether the dietary intake is adequate. Adolescents often

Table 19.5 Nutritional Needs Based on Age, Gender, and Activity Level

Age (y)	Gender	Activity Level	Caloric Need Per Day
13–14	Male	Sedentary	2,000
		Active	2,600–2,800
	Female	Sedentary	1,600–1,800
		Active	2,200–2,400
15–16	Male	Sedentary	2,200–2,400
		Active	3,000–3,200
	Female	Sedentary	1,800
		Active	2,400
17–18	Male	Sedentary	2,400
		Active	3,200
	Female	Sedentary	1,800
		Active	2,400

From U.S. Department of Health and Human Services, & U.S. Department of Agriculture. (2015). *2015–2020 dietary guidelines for Americans*. 8th Edition. Retrieved from https://health.gov/dietaryguidelines/2015/guidelines/appendix-2/

overestimate how much food they need. Teach them about their needed caloric intake depending on their activity level (Table 19.5). Peers often have an influence on diet, depending on the sex of the peers and the closeness of the relationships (Chung, Ersig, & McCarthy, 2017).

Teaching about high-quality diets by targeting peer groups rather than individuals may be more effective. Resources are available for adolescents to plan their daily diet depending on the desired caloric intake. At https://www.choosemyplate.gov/MyPlate-Daily-Checklist, the adolescent can find the checklist appropriate for his or her age and the desired caloric intake (Fig. 19.10).

Common Developmental Concerns

Common concerns during the adolescent years include substance abuse, violence, eating disorders, depression, and incessant media use. The nurse may address any of these concerns. Educate parents on the signs and symptoms of these problems and when to seek help. Refer the adolescent to specialists as needed.

Substance Use Disorder

The terms substance use, substance abuse, and addiction are often used interchangeably. However, each condition affects the adolescent in a different way. Adolescents may use substances,

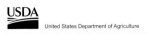 United States Department of Agriculture

MyPlate Daily Checklist
Find your Healthy Eating Style

Everything you eat and drink matters. Find your healthy eating style that reflects your preferences, culture, traditions, and budget—and maintain it for a lifetime! The right mix can help you be healthier now and into the future. The key is choosing a variety of foods and beverages from each food group—*and making sure that each choice is limited in saturated fat, sodium, and added sugars.* Start with small changes—**"MyWins"**—to make healthier choices you can enjoy.

Food Group Amounts for 2,000 Calories a Day

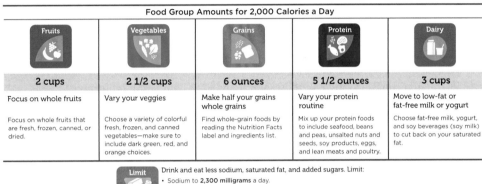

Fruits	Vegetables	Grains	Protein	Dairy
2 cups	**2 1/2 cups**	**6 ounces**	**5 1/2 ounces**	**3 cups**
Focus on whole fruits	Vary your veggies	Make half your grains whole grains	Vary your protein routine	Move to low-fat or fat-free milk or yogurt
Focus on whole fruits that are fresh, frozen, canned, or dried.	Choose a variety of colorful fresh, frozen, and canned vegetables—make sure to include dark green, red, and orange choices.	Find whole-grain foods by reading the Nutrition Facts label and ingredients list.	Mix up your protein foods to include seafood, beans and peas, unsalted nuts and seeds, soy products, eggs, and lean meats and poultry.	Choose fat-free milk, yogurt, and soy beverages (soy milk) to cut back on your saturated fat.

Limit Drink and eat less sodium, saturated fat, and added sugars. Limit:
- Sodium to **2,300 milligrams** a day.
- Saturated fat to **22 grams** a day.
- Added sugars to **50 grams** a day.

Be active your way: Children 6 to 17 years old should move **60 minutes** every day. Adults should be physically active at least **2 1/2 hours** per week.
Use SuperTracker to create a personal plan based on your age, sex, height, weight, and physical activity level.
SuperTracker.usda.gov

MyPlate Daily Checklist

Write down the foods you ate today and track your daily MyPlate, MyWins!

Food group targets for a 2,000 calorie* pattern are:

	Write your food choices for each food group	Did you reach your target?

Fruits — **2 cups**
1 cup of fruits counts as
- 1 cup raw or cooked fruit; or
- 1/2 cup dried fruit; or
- 1 cup 100% fruit juice.

Y / N

Vegetables — **2 1/2 cups**
1 cup vegetables counts as
- 1 cup raw or cooked vegetables; or
- 2 cups   salad greens; or
- 1 cup 100% vegetable juice.

Y / N

Grains — **6 ounce equivalents**
1 ounce of grains counts as
- 1 slice bread; or
- 1 ounce   cereal; or
- 1/2 cup cooked rice, pasta, or cereal.

Y / N

Protein — **5 1/2 ounce equivalents**
1 ounce of protein counts as
- 1 ounce lean meat, poultry, or seafood; or
- 1 egg; or
- 1 Tbsp peanut butter; or
- 1/4 cup cooked beans or peas; or
- 1/2 ounce nuts or seeds.

Y / N

Dairy — **3 cups**
1 cup of dairy counts as
- 1 cup milk; or
- 1 cup yogurt; or
- 1 cup fortified soy beverage; or
- 1 1/2 ounces natural cheese or 2 ounces processed cheese.

Y / N

Limit:
- Sodium to **2,300 milligrams** a day.
- Saturated fat to **22 grams** a day.
- Added sugars to **50 grams** a day.

Y / N

Activity — **Be active your way:**
Adults:
- Be physically active at least 2 1/2 hours per week.

Children 6 to 17 years old:
- Move at least **60 minutes** every day.

Y / N

* This 2,000 calorie pattern is only an estimate of your needs. Monitor your body weight and adjust your calories if needed.

MyWins Track your MyPlate, MyWins

Center for Nutrition Policy and Promotion
January 2016
USDA is an equal opportunity provider and employer.

Figure 19.10. Adolescent nutrition. Adolescents can use the MyPlate Daily Checklist as a healthy eating guide. From the U.S. Department of Agriculture. (2016). *MyPlate Plan.* Retrieved from https://www.choosemyplate.gov/MyPlatePlan.

such as tobacco, alcohol, and other drugs, as a result of social pressure from peer groups. Substance use refers to occasional use of substances, most likely in social situations. Often, adolescents use substances to cope with stress, anxiety, and depression, resulting in substance abuse. Substance abuse can cause damage to the body but does not interfere with daily life. Adolescents with substance abuse need intervention to understand the effect that their substance abuse has on their life and their future. Intervention could include outpatient or inpatient therapy.

One in four illicit drug users from age 12 to 17 years become addicted (AAP, 2015a). Addiction is related to biological and psychosocial factors and affects all areas of the adolescent's life. Addiction is determined by genetic conditions and comorbid psychiatric disorders. Relationships, academics, and self-esteem are all affected (Stager, 2016). Addiction and substance abuse are now commonly referred to as **substance use disorder (SUD)** and classified as mild, moderate, or severe. Adolescents with SUD find it hard to change their behavior regardless of the consequences.

Adolescents with low self-esteem, depression, eating disorders, and attention-deficit hyperactivity disorder (ADHD) are at risk for SUD (AAP, 2016a). Conversely, adolescents who have protective factors, such as positive social support, social connectedness, and parental involvement, are at lower risk for SUD (Hagan et al., 2017). In addition, adolescents should not have access to alcohol, tobacco, or drugs, especially in the home. Nurses can assess the risks and protective behaviors of adolescents. If the adolescent exhibits more risks than do protective behaviors, refer as needed for counseling, peer support, and community support.

Tobacco and Nicotine

Tobacco use in adolescents has decreased, yet 1 in 20 adolescents admits to being a daily smoker (U.S. Department of Health and Human Services, 2016a). Although smoking tobacco may be decreasing, the use of e-cigarettes is increasing, especially among children in early adolescence (U.S. Department of Health and Human Services, 2016a). E-cigarettes are thought to be harmful, but currently no long-term data support this belief. A popular type of e-cigarette is a small electronic vaping device known as a Juul. A Juul delivers a hit of nicotine similar to that of a cigarette. Inform adolescents that although Juuls may not contain cancer-causing tobacco, the high nicotine content may result in addiction.

Teach adolescents that tobacco use is the number-one cause of preventable deaths in the United States (U.S. Department of Health and Human Services, 2016). Provide the adolescent and parents with resources available to help them quit smoking. Refer adolescents to school- and community-based smoking cessation groups, because evidence has shown that these types of interventions have some success (U.S. Preventative Services Task Force, 2016).

Alcohol

Alcohol is the substance adolescents most widely use (SAMHSA, 2017). By the 10th grade, one in five adolescents admits to drinking alcohol, and the number increases to one in three by the 12th grade (U.S. Department of Health and Human Services [HHS],

2016b). Adolescents report drinking more often in a group than they do alone. Those at risk for alcohol abuse include adolescents with high levels of impulsiveness, aggressive behavior, conduct disorder, or other behavioral problems (SAMHSA, 2017). Risks associated with alcohol use in adolescence include risky sexual behavior, changes in brain development, increased incidence of violence, and long-term alcohol abuse.

Nurses can use screening tools such as the CRAFFT or SBIRT to determine the adolescent's risk for alcohol use and abuse. For adolescents who show binge-drinking behaviors, having five or more drinks at once for males and four or more drinks at once for females, referral to treatment may be necessary. Educate adolescents on the short- and long-term consequences of use of alcohol, including the risk of drunk driving and long-term health problems.

Illicit Drugs

Drug abuse in adolescence includes both the use of illicit drugs and the misuse of prescription drugs. Marijuana is the drug adolescents most commonly report using (HHS, 2017). The misuse of prescription medications, mainly opioids, is on the rise in adolescence (Stager, 2016). In a national survey, 3.6% of adolescents aged 12 to 17 years reported opioid misuse over the past year (HHS, 2017). Overdose and death are severe consequences of a opioid use disorder. The National Institute on Drug Abuse (2016) estimates that for every overdose death in adolescents there were 119 emergency room visits and 22 treatment admissions.

As with tobacco and alcohol abuse, adolescents with low self-esteem, poor parental support, and mental health disorders are at risk for drug abuse. Adolescents with ADHD are at increased risk for drug abuse due to impulsivity, poor judgment, and problems at school (AAP, 2016a). In addition, adolescents with ADHD may try to self-medicate. Other adolescents at risk for opioid abuse are those with chronic pain. Educate parents to look for changes in their adolescent that may indicate drug abuse. These behaviors include a change in mood or behavior, lack of interest in previously enjoyed activities, isolation, or hanging out with a new group of friends whom the parents do not know.

Nurses can use the CRAFFT or SBIRT screening tools to determine the extent of the adolescent's drug use. Treatment for drug abuse in adolescence is multidisciplinary and includes counselors, social workers, nurses, physicians, and mental health specialists.

Violence

Adolescents can be either the victims of violence or the ones inflicting violence. Violence can occur in the form of verbal abuse, physical abuse, sexual abuse, bullying, or cyber violence. Adolescents exposed to violence are at risk for anxiety and depression, posttraumatic stress disorder, antisocial behavior, and aggression (Heinze, Stoddard, Aiyer, Eisman, Zimmerman, 2017). Often, adolescents exposed to violence in one area of their life, such as at home, are exposed to violence in other areas, such as in the community. Adolescents exposed to continual violence are more likely to perpetrate acts of violence. Those most affected by and likely to commit acts of violence, excluding dating violence, are males, ethnic minorities, and those living in urban areas (Heinze et al., 2017).

The type of violence adolescents are most likely to experience is interpersonal violence at school, at home, or in the neighborhood. Neighborhood violence is often a result of gang violence. Adolescents experience cyber violence through video games, movies, or the posting of violent videos on social media (AAP, 2016b). Those who are perpetrators of violent acts may have behavior disorders, SUD, or other mental health disorders (Hagan et al., 2017). Furthermore, living in a single-parent home, low socioeconomic status, exposure to firearms, and poor family functioning are factors that increase violent behavior.

Nurses are able to assess the adolescent's exposure to violence. Determine whether the adolescent feels safe at home, at school, and in the neighborhood. Educate parents about violence in the media and online. Parents should routinely monitor their adolescent's exposure to violence through media, including social media. Encourage parents to know their adolescent's friends and note any behavioral changes. Engage adolescents and their parents in formulating and implementing solutions to create safe communities.

Eating Disorders

An eating disorder indicates that the adolescent is not satisfied with his or her weight or body image and involves dysfunctional weight control behaviors that can result in significant physical and psychosocial sequelae (Kreipe, 2016). Eating disorders in adolescence include anorexia nervosa, bulimia nervosa, and binge eating (see Chapter 33). More than 10 million adolescent females and over 1 million adolescent males have eating disorders (AAP, 2015b).

There is no single cause of eating disorders. They are a result of a complex interaction of psychosocial, cultural, family, peer, and genetic influences. Risk factors for development of eating disorders include a history of obesity, poor parental eating habits, perfectionism, low self-esteem, and participating in activities such as ballet or gymnastics (AAP, 2015b). The most common ethnic group affected is Caucasian females (Kreipe, 2016).

Adolescents with eating disorders such as anorexia nervosa demonstrate obsession diet, counting calories, and exercise. Those with bulimia nervosa may eat to relieve emotional distress and then purge to avoid weight gain. Regardless of the type, it is important to recognize and treat eating disorders early. Long-term problems result from eating disorders, including cardiac arrhythmias, electrolyte imbalances, oral health problems, gastrointestinal problems, endocrine disturbances, delayed growth and development, and early death (Hagan et al., 2017). Early referral to treatment is essential for the adolescent with an eating disorder. Encourage the family to be involved in the treatment plan. Family-based therapy has been shown to have the most positive outcomes for adolescents with eating disorders (Bryson, Lehman, Iriana, Lane-Loney, & Ornstein, 2018).

Depression

Depression is defined as a daily disruption of mood and loss of pleasure in activities that lasts 2 weeks or longer (Walter, Moseley, & DeMaso, 2016).

The incidence of depression in adolescents increases after the onset of puberty. Approximately 5% of adolescents exhibit depression at any point in time (Hagan et al., 2017). Depression risk doubles if the child has a parent with a depressive disorder. However, environmental influences appear to play a greater role than does genetics in the onset of depression after the age of 11 (Sallis et al., 2017). Environmental influences include stressful life events, such as the loss of a sibling or parent, community disasters, or chronic illness in a family member or the adolescent. Adolescents with depression often have comorbid mental health disorders such as anxiety or ADHD.

In adolescents, depression manifests not only as sadness but also as anger, aggression, problems with peer or family relationships, and substance use. Screen for depression at every visit. Ask questions of both the adolescent and the parents. Ask about things such as unusual sadness, tearfulness, withdrawal, and social isolation.

Unless there is an immediate threat, treatment begins with intensive psychotherapy. If there is no improvement after 4 to 8 weeks, pharmacotherapy is warranted. The most commonly used medications to treat depression in adolescents are selective serotonin reuptake inhibitors (The Pharmacy 19.1).

The Pharmacy 19.1 Fluoxetine

Classification	Route	Action	Nursing Considerations
Antidepressant	Oral	Inhibits serotonin reuptake in the central nervous system	• Assess for restlessness, hyperactivity, and agitation. • May cause nausea, vomiting, and diarrhea • Monitor for gastrointestinal bleeds. • Monitor for dizziness, headaches, and dry mouth. • Do not discontinue abruptly.

Adapted from Taketomo, C. K., Hodding, J. H., & Kraus, D. M. (2018). *Pediatric & neonatal dosage handbook* (25th ed.). Hudson, OH: Lexicomp.

Suicide

Suicide is the biggest concern in adolescents with depression. Suicide is the third-leading cause of death in adolescents (Hagan et al., 2017). It is imperative to determine the risk for suicide in an adolescent with depression. Tell parents to remove all firearms from the house, regardless of whether they are locked in a cabinet. Parents should remove all prescription medications with lethal potential from the home, as well. Educate parents to monitor their child's social media accounts for mention of suicidal ideation. Suicidal thoughts occur more commonly at the beginning of a major depressive episode. Recommendations are that adolescents exhibiting onset of depressive episodes with thought of suicide should be hospitalized immediately (Hagan et al., 2017).

Media

During the adolescent years, the use of media, especially social media, becomes more intense (Fig. 19.11). Parents must continue to monitor their adolescent's Internet and media use. Parents should openly talk with their children about what are appropriate and inappropriate subjects for social media. Be aware of any behavioral changes that may be associated with cyberbullying.

Teach adolescents the adverse effects of media use. Remind them to get at least an hour of daily activity per day. Overuse of media puts adolescents at risk for sleep disorders, anxiety, and depression (American Academy of Pediatrics Council on Communications and Media, 2016). Educate adolescents not to sleep with media devices in their room. Remind adolescents not to engage in unnecessary media use while doing homework. Encourage parents to have media-free time, such as at family dinners.

Health Problems of Adolescents

Health problems that are common in adolescence include infectious mononucleosis and acne vulgaris. **Dysmenorrhea** can occur in adolescent females.

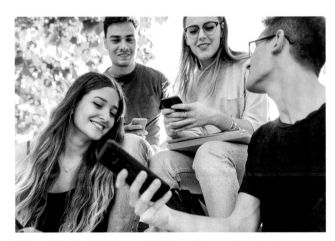

Figure 19.11. Media use. Talk to adolescents about appropriate social media use.

Infectious Mononucleosis

Infectious mononucleosis is a viral infection caused by the Epstein–Barr virus. The virus is spread through oral secretions and is therefore commonly referred to as the "kissing disease." The virus is shed in oral secretions up to 6 months after acute infection (Jensen, 2016). The common clinical manifestations include fever, pharyngitis, lymphadenopathy, and extreme fatigue. The sore throat, pharyngitis, and enlarged tonsils with exudate resemble the signs of strep throat (Fig. 19.12). Hepatomegaly and splenomegaly are often present at the time of diagnosis. Infection with the Epstein–Barr virus is common, with up to 83% of adolescents aged 18 to 19 years testing seropositive (Jensen, 2016).

Nursing Assessment

Obtain a history of present illness and determine whether the adolescent has been exposed to anyone with infectious mononucleosis. Ask the adolescent about the presence of fatigue and sore throat. Assess for fever. Inspect the adolescent's throat, noting erythema, tonsillar hypertrophy, and the presence of exudate. Inspect the skin for rashes. Palpate the cervical and submandibular lymph nodes for lymphadenopathy. Palpate the abdomen for hepatomegaly or splenomegaly.

Treatment

Treatment of mononucleosis includes supportive therapy such as rest and fluids. Treat symptoms such as headache, fever, and sore throat with antipyretics and analgesics. Instruct the adolescent to avoid participating in contact sports for 2 to 3 weeks because of the risk of splenic rupture. Acute symptoms last 2 to 4 weeks. Although full recovery occurs in most adolescents, fatigue may last up to 6 months.

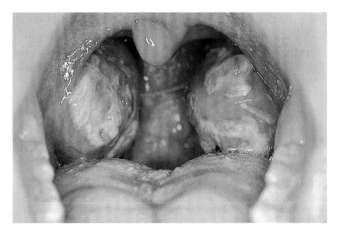

Figure 19.12. Infectious mononucleosis. Pharyngitis in infectious mononucleosis resembles streptococcal pharyngitis. Reprinted with permission from Hatfield, N. T. (2013). *Introductory maternity and pediatric nursing* (3rd ed., Fig. 41-12). Philadelphia, PA: Lippincott Williams & Wilkins.

Acne Vulgaris

Acne occurs in 80% of adolescents (Galbraith, 2016). Comedonal acne, which involves follicular sacs filled with keratinous material and bacteria, is the most common form of acne in adolescents and often the first sign of puberty. There are four types of lesions associated with acne vulgaris: open and closed comedones, papules, pustules, and nodular cysts (Fig. 19.13; Galbraith, 2016). Lesions can occur anywhere on the face, back, shoulders, and chest. Scarring may occur with chronic, unresolved acne. Acne flare-ups can be related to hormones and stress. Diet generally does not affect acne outbreaks.

Nursing Assessment

Ask the adolescent whether he or she is bothered by the acne. Determine the cleansing regimen used. Inquire whether the adolescent picks at the lesions. Inspect the skin for the presence of lesions. Note the distribution. Document the presence of open or closed comedones, papules, pustules, or nodules. Inspect for the presence of scabs and scarring.

Treatment

Treatment begins with a daily cleansing regimen. Adolescents may cleanse their face with over-the-counter products that contain salicylic acid or benzoyl peroxide. Warn adolescents not to scrub their face too hard or try to "pop" their acne. Instruct them to stop using any greasy cosmetic or hair products that may plug follicles on the forehead. Acne that is not controlled by over-the-counter products requires prescription treatments. The first line of treatment for comedonal acne is a topical retinoid and for inflammatory acne is a topical antibiotic (The Pharmacy 19.2). For acne that does not respond to topical treatments, systemic antibiotics may be used. Severe nodulocystic acne with the potential of scarring is treated with isotretinoin (Galbraith, 2016). Isotretinoin has serious side effects and must be used with caution. Educate adolescents and their parents on the side effects of the different treatments.

Dysmenorrhea

Dysmenorrhea, or painful uterine cramps before the onset of menses, occurs in 93% of adolescent females (Sucato & Burstein, 2016). The cramping is severe enough to interfere with school and other activities. Dysmenorrhea can be primary or secondary. Primary dysmenorrhea has no underlying cause and is the most common. Secondary dysmenorrhea has an underlying cause, such as endometriosis or pelvic inflammatory disease.

Primary dysmenorrhea presents as crampy lower back, pelvic, and upper thigh pain. Sometimes the pain is accompanied by nausea, diarrhea, and extreme fatigue. Symptoms occur before the onset of monthly menses and last 1 to 3 days (Sucato & Burstein, 2016). Pain that occurs between menstrual cycles or in a sexually active female should be further investigated for causes of secondary dysmenorrhea.

Nursing Assessment

Take a thorough history to determine possible underlying causes of pain. Determine whether the adolescent is sexually active. Ask about the timing, duration, and intensity of pain. Have the adolescent describe and rate the pain on an appropriate pain scale. Palpate the abdomen for any abnormalities.

Treatment

The treatment for primary dysmenorrhea is to decrease prostaglandin production. Start nonsteroidal anti-inflammatory medications (NSAIDs), such as ibuprofen, every 6 hours 1 day before the start of menses and continue for 5 days. Adolescents who have inadequate relief from NSAIDs are started on hormone therapy with oral contraceptives. Alternative forms of pain relief, such as heat, massage, acupuncture, and yoga, can also be effective in adolescents with dysmenorrhea.

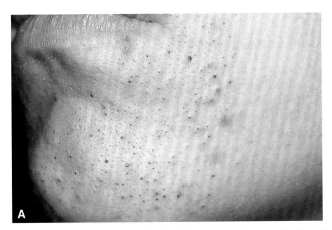
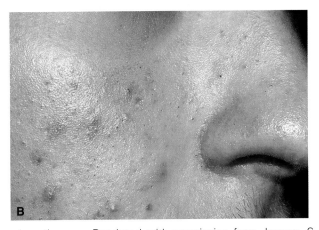

Figure 19.13. Acne vulgaris. A. Open comedones. **B.** Papular and cystic acne. Reprinted with permission from Jensen, S. (2018). *Nursing health assessment: A best practice approach* (3rd ed., Fig. 11.4). Philadelphia, PA: Lippincott Williams & Wilkins.

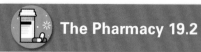

The Pharmacy 19.2 Medications to Treat Acne

Medication	Classification	Route	Action	Nursing Considerations
Tretinoin	Retinoid	Topical	• Vitamin A derivative • Modifies epithelial growth • Increases follicular turn-over, causing extrusion of comedones	• Apply once daily. • Educate that acne may get worse in the first 2 wk of use because of mechanism of action. • Improvement seen after 2 wk • Causes redness and dryness of skin with initial use; decrease application to every other day if severe • Increased photosensitivity; apply sunscreen to face daily.
Clindamycin	Antibiotic	Topical	• Inhibits bacterial protein synthesis • Bacteriostatic or bactericidal, depending on dose	• Apply once daily. • May cause a burning feeling in the skin • May cause facial redness
Minocycline	Antibiotic	Oral	Inhibits bacterial protein synthesis	• 100 mg once daily • Monitor BUN • Monitor LFTs • Increased photosensitivity; apply sunscreen daily. • Common side effects include diarrhea and dyspepsia. • Take with or without food
Isotretinoin	Retinoid	Oral	Reduces sebum production and sebaceous gland size in acne	• 0.5–1.0 mg/kg/d divided into two doses • Pregnancy category X • Patient must be part of the iPLEDGE program, which requires monthly pregnancy testing. • Female patient must start oral contraceptives concomitantly. • Monitor CBC. • Monitor LFTs. • Monitor for s/s of depression. • May cause arthralgia and back pain

BUN, blood urea nitrogen; CBC, complete blood count; LFT, liver function test; s/s, signs and symptoms.
Adapted from Taketomo, C. K., Hodding, J. H., & Kraus, D. M. (2018). *Pediatric & neonatal dosage handbook* (25th ed.). Hudson, OH: Lexicomp.

Think Critically

1. Discuss the effects of puberty on the physical and social aspects of adolescent development.
2. Discuss how relationships change during the adolescent years.
3. How does development of identity relate to self-esteem during the adolescent years?
4. How does sleep, or lack thereof, affect the adolescent?
5. Create a nutritional plan for the adolescent. What factors affect nutrition in adolescence?
6. What signs and symptoms are usually present with substance use or abuse?
7. Discuss how acne vulgaris affects social development in the adolescent. Create a plan of care for the adolescent with comedonal acne.

References

American Academy of Pediatrics. (2014). *Let them sleep: AAP recommends delaying start times of middle and high schools to combat teen sleep deprivation.* Retrieved from https://www.aap.org/en-us/about-the-aap/aap-press-room/pages/let-them-sleep-aap-recommends-delaying-start-times-of-middle-and-high-schools-to-combat-teen-sleep-deprivation.aspx

American Academy of Pediatrics. (2015a). *Is your child vulnerable to substance abuse?* Retrieved from https://www.healthychildren.org/English/ages-stages/teen/substance-abuse/Pages/Is-Your-Child-Vulnerable-to-Substance-Abuse.aspx

American Academy of Pediatrics. (2015b). *Is your teen at risk for developing an eating disorder?* Retrieved from https://www.healthychildren.org/English/health-issues/conditions/emotional-problems/Pages/Is-Your-Teen-at-Risk-for-Developing-an-Eating-Disorder.aspx

American Academy of Pediatrics. (2015c). *When to let your teenager start dating.* Retrieved from https://www.healthychildren.org/English/ages-stages/teen/dating-sex/Pages/When-To-Let-Your-Teenager-Start-Dating.aspx

American Academy of Pediatrics. (2016a). *ADHD and substance abuse: The link parents need to know.* Retrieved from https://www.healthychildren.org/English/health-issues/conditions/adhd/Pages/ADHD-and-Substance-Abuse-The-Link-Parents-Need-to-Know.aspx

American Academy of Pediatrics. (2016b). *Virtual violence impacts children on multiple levels.* Retrieved from https://www.healthychildren.org/English/news/Pages/Virtual-Violence-Impacts-Children-on-Multiple-Levels.aspx

American Academy of Pediatrics Council on Communications and Media. (2016). Media use in school age children and adolescents. *Pediatrics, 138*(5), e20162592.

American Cancer Society. (2018). *Cancers that develop in young adults.* Retrieved from https://www.cancer.org/cancer/cancer-in-young-adults/cancers-in-young-adults.html

American College of Obstetricians and Gynecology (2017). Committee opinion: Adolescent pregnancy, contraception, and sexual activity. *Obstetrics and Gynecology, 129*(5), e142–e149.

Asarnow, L. D., Greer, S. M., Walker, M. P., & Harvey, A. G. (2017). The impact of sleep improvement on food choices in adolescents with late bedtimes. *Journal of Adolescent Health, 60*, 570–576.

Boniel-Nissim, M., Tabak, I., Mazur, J., Borraccino, A., Brooks, F., Gommans, R., . . . Finne, E. (2015). Supportive communication with parents moderates the negative effects of electronic media use on life satisfaction during adolescence. *International Journal of Public Health, 60*(2), 189–198.

Bosse, J. D., & Chiodo, L. (2016). It is complicated: Gender and sexual orientation identity in LGBTQ youth. *Journal of Clinical Nursing, 25*, 3665–3675.

Bryson, A. E., Lehman, E. B., Iriana, S. M., Lane-Loney, S. E., & Ornstein, R. M. (2018). Assessment of parental knowledge and understanding of eating disorders. *Clinical Pediatrics, 57*(3), 259–265.

Centers for Disease Control and Prevention. (2015). *HEADS UP: FAQ's about baseline testing.* Retrieved from https://www.cdc.gov/headsup/basics/baseline_testing.html

Centers for Disease Control and Prevention. (2017a). *Diseases and the vaccines that prevent them.* Retrieved from http://www.cdc.gov/vaccines/hcp/conversations/prevent-diseases/provider-resources-factsheets-infants.html

Centers for Disease Control and Prevention. (2017b). *2016 sexually transmitted disease surveillance.* Retrieved from https://www.cdc.gov/std/stats16/adolescents.htm

Centers for Disease Control and Prevention. (2017c). *Parents are the key to safe teen drivers.* Retrieved from https://www.cdc.gov/parentsarethekey/danger/index.html

Centers for Disease Control and Prevention. (2017d). *Reproductive health: Teen pregnancy.* Retrieved from https://www.cdc.gov/teenpregnancy/about/index.htm

Centers for Disease Control and Prevention. (2017e). *Sexual risk behaviors: HIV, STD, and teen pregnancy prevention.* Retrieved from https://www.cdc.gov/healthyyouth/sexualbehaviors/

Centers for Disease Control (2018). *Information on Safety in the Home & Community for parents with teens (12-19).* Retrieved from https://www.cdc.gov/parents/teens/safety.html

Chung, S. J., Ersig, A. L., & McCarthy, A. M. (2017). The influence of peers on diet and exercise among adolescents: A systematic review. *Journal of Pediatric Nursing, 36*, 44–56.

Erikson, E. H. (1963). *Childhood and society.* New York, NY: W.W. Norton and Company.

Galbraith, S. S. (2016). Acne. In R. M. Kliegman, B. F. Stanton, J. W. St. Geme III, N. F. Schor, & R. E. Behrman (Eds.), *Nelson's textbook of pediatrics* (20th ed.). Philadelphia, PA: Elsevier, Saunders.

Hagan, J. F., Shaw, J. S., & Duncan, P. (Eds.). (2017). *Bright futures: Guidelines for health supervision of infants, children, and adolescents* (4th ed.). Elk Grove Village, IL: American Academy of Pediatrics.

Heinze, J. E., Stoddard, S. A., Aiyer, S. M., Eisman, A. B., & Zimmerman, M. A. (2017). Exposure to violence during adolescence as a predictor of perceived stress trajectories in emerging adulthood. *Journal of Applied Developmental Psychology, 49*, 31–38.

Holland-Hall, C., & Burstein, G. R. (2016). Adolescent physical and social development. In R. M. Kliegman, B. F. Stanton, J. W. St. Geme III, N. F. Schor, & R. E. Behrman (Eds.), *Nelson's textbook of pediatrics* (20th ed.). Philadelphia, PA: Elsevier, Saunders.

Hu, T., Jacobs, D. R., Jr., Larson, N. I., Cutler, G. C., Laska, M. N., & Neumark-Sztainer, D. (2016). Higher diet quality in adolescence and dietary improvements are related to less weight gain during the transition from adolescence to adulthood. *The Journal of Pediatrics, 178*, 188–193.

Jacobus, J., Squeglia, L. M., Infante, M. A., Castro, N., Brumback, T., Mereulo, A. D., & Tapert, S. F. (2015). Neuropsychological performance in adolescent marijuana users with co-occurring alcohol use: A three-year longitudinal study. *Neuropsychology, 29*(6), 829–843.

Jensen, H. B. (2016). Epstein-Barr virus. In R. M. Kliegman, B. F. Stanton, J. W. St. Geme III, N. F. Schor, & R. E. Behrman (Eds.), *Nelson's textbook of pediatrics* (20th ed.). Philadelphia, PA: Elsevier, Saunders.

Kann, E., Olsen, E., McManus, T., Harris, W. A., Shanklin, S. L., Flint, K. H., . . . & Zaza, S. (2016). Sexual identity, sex of sexual contacts, and health-related behaviors among students in grades 9–12—United States and selected sites, 2015. *Morbidity Mortality Weekly Report, 65*(9), 1–203.

Kilford, E.J., Garrett, E., & Blakemore, S. (2016). The development of social cognition in adolescence: An integrated perspective. *The Adolescent Brain, Neuroscience and Biobehavioral Reviews*, November 2016(7), 106-120.

Kohlberg, L. (1981). *The philosophy of moral development.* New York, NY: Harper & Row.

Kreipe, R. E. (2016). Eating disorders. In R. M. Kliegman, B. F. Stanton, J. W. St. Geme III, N. F. Schor, & R. E. Behrman (Eds.), *Nelson's textbook of pediatrics* (20th ed.). Philadelphia, PA: Elsevier, Saunders.

Levy, S. J., Williams, J. F.; Committee on Substance Use and Prevention. (2016). Substance use screening, brief intervention, and referral to treatment. *Pediatrics, 138*(1), e20161211.

National Center for Statistics and Analysis. (2017). *Traffic Safety Notes. Distracted Driving 2015.* Washington, D.C.: National Highway Traffic Safety Administration.

National Institute on Drug Abuse. (2016). *Abuse of prescription (Rx) drugs affects young adults most.* Retrieved from https://www.drugabuse.gov/related-topics/trends-statistics/infographics/abuse-prescription-rx-drugs-affects-young-adults-most?utm_source=external&utm_medium=api&utm_campaign=infographics-api

Piaget, J. (1930). *The child's conception of physical causality.* London, England: Routledge & Kegan Paul Ltd.

Sallis, H., Evans, J., Wooton, R., Krapoh, E., Oldehinke, A. J., Smith, G. D., & Paternoster, L. (2017). Genetics of depressive symptoms in adolescence. *BMC Psychiatry, 17*(321), 1–8.

Short, S., Pace, G., & Birnbaum, C. (2017). Nonpharmacologic techniques to assist in pediatric pain management. *Clinical Pediatric Emergency Medicine, 18*(4), 256–260.

Silveri, M. M., Dager, A. D., Cohen-Gilbert, J. E., & Sneider, J. T. (2016). Neurobiological signatures associated with alcohol and drug use in the human adolescent brain. *Neuroscience and Biobehavioral Reviews, 70*, 244–259.

Squeglia, L. M., Jacobus, J., & Tapert, S. F. (2009). The influence of substance use on adolescent brain development. *Clinical EEG and Neuroscience, 40*(1), 31–38.

Stager, M. M. (2016). Substance abuse. In R. M. Kliegman, B. F. Stanton, J. W. St. Geme III, N. F. Schor, & R. E. Behrman (Eds.), *Nelson's textbook of pediatrics* (20th ed.). Philadelphia, PA: Elsevier, Saunders.

Substance Abuse and Mental Health Services Administration. (n.d.). *SBIRT: Screening.* Retrieved from https://www.integration.samhsa.gov/clinical-practice/sbirt/screening

Substance Abuse and Mental Health Services Administration. (n.d.). *SBIRT: Screening, brief intervention, and referral to treatment.* Retrieved from https://www.integration.samhsa.gov/clinical-practice/sbirt

Substance Abuse and Mental Health Services Administration. (2017). *Underage drinking.* Retrieved from https://www.samhsa.gov/underage-drinking-topic

Sucato, G. S., & Burstein, G. R. (2016). Dysmenorrhea. In R. M. Kliegman, B. F. Stanton, J. W. St. Geme III, N. F. Schor, & R. E. Behrman (Eds.), *Nelson's textbook of pediatrics* (20th ed.). Philadelphia, PA: Elsevier, Saunders.

Tarokh, L., Saletin, J. M., & Carskadon, M. A. (2016). Sleep in adolescence: Physiology, cognition and mental health. *Neuroscience and Behavioral Reviews, 70*, 182–188.

Tiggemann, M., & Slater, A. (2017). Facebook and body image concern in adolescent girls: A prospective study. *International Journal of Eating Disorders, 50*(1), 80–83.

U.S. Department of Health and Human Services. (2016a). *Tobacco use in adolescence: preventing and reducing teen tobacco use.* Retrieved from https://www.hhs.gov/ash/oah/adolescent-development/substance-use/drugs/tobacco/index.html

U.S. Department of Health and Human Services. (2016b). *How common is adolescent alcohol use?* Retrieved from https://www.hhs.gov/ash/oah/adolescent-development/substance-use/alcohol/how-common/index.html

U.S. Department of Health and Human Services. (2017). *Opioids and adolescents.* Retrieved from https://www.hhs.gov/ash/oah/adolescent-development/substance-use/drugs/opioids/index.html#prevalence

U.S. Preventative Services Task Force. (2016). *Final recommendation statement: Tobacco use in children and adolescents: Primary care interventions.* Retrieved from https://www.uspreventiveservicestaskforce.org/Page/Document/RecommendationStatementFinal/tobacco-use-in-children-and-adolescents-primary-care-interventions#consider

Walter, H. J., Moseley, L. R., & DeMaso, D. R. (2016). Major and other depressive disorders. In R. M. Kliegman, B. F. Stanton, J. W. St. Geme III, N. F. Schor, & R. E. Behrman (Eds.), *Nelson's textbook of pediatrics* (20th ed.). Philadelphia, PA: Elsevier, Saunders.

Young, K. D. (2017). Assessment of acute pain in children. *Clinical Pediatric Emergency Medicine, 18*(4), 235–241.

Zhang, J., Paksarian, D., Lamers, F., Hickie, I. B., He, J., & Merikangas, K. R. (2017). Sleep patterns and mental health correlates in US adolescents. *The Journal of Pediatrics, 182*, 137–143.

Suggested Readings

Chung, S. J., Ersig, A. L., & McCarthy, A. M. (2017). The influence of peers on diet and exercise among adolescents: A systematic review. *Journal of Pediatric Nursing, 36*, 44–56.

Healthy People 2020. (2018). *Adolescent health.* Retrieved from https://www.healthypeople.gov/2020/topics-objectives/topic/Adolescent-Health

U.S. Department of Health and Human Services. (2017). *Opioids and adolescents.* Retrieved from https://www.hhs.gov/ash/oah/adolescent-development/substance-use/drugs/opioids/index.html#prevalence

Unit 3
Care of the Hospitalized Child

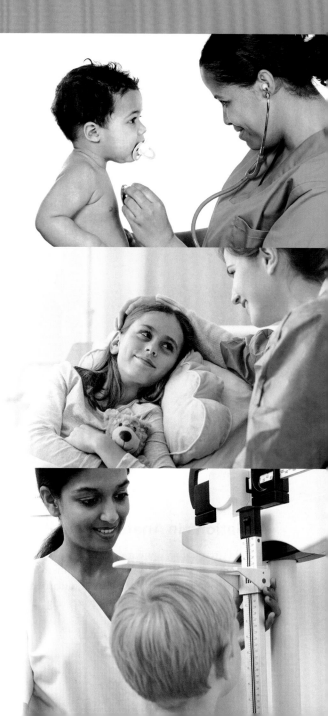

20 Alterations in Respiratory Function

Variations in Anatomy and Physiology

A child's respiratory system constantly changes and continues to grow until about 12 years of age. Differences between the pediatric and adult airways can be summarized by comparing the upper airways and the lower airways (Fig. 2.6).

Upper Airway

The upper airway comprises the nasopharynx and oropharynx and serves as the pathway for gas exchange during the process of **ventilation**. Recall that ventilation is the movement of oxygen into the lungs and the movement of carbon dioxide out of the lungs. A child's upper airway is much shorter and narrower than an adult's upper airway. A smaller nasopharynx can be more easily occluded when secretions, edema, or foreign bodies enter the upper airway. An infant's airway is approximately 4 mm, whereas that of an adult is about 20 mm. Imagine breathing through a small straw; this is about the size of a child's airway. During the first 5 years of life, the trachea grows in length but not as much in diameter.

Children have small oral cavities and large tongues in comparison to adults, which can lead to an obstructed oropharynx when a child is lethargic, has a swollen throat, or lacks head control. Children have long, floppy epiglottises, which can also lead to obstruction. A higher risk of aspiration is present in children as a result of a larynx and glottis that are higher in the neck in comparison to that of an adult. The cartilage supporting the neck and airways is much more flexible in children and a child's head is larger in proportion to the body, which may lead to airway compression if the head and neck are improperly supported. Narrower airways cause a greater increase in **airway resistance** (Fig. 2.5). Recall that airway resistance is the amount of force required to move air through the trachea into the lungs. Many conditions, such as croup, asthma, and epiglottitis, cause airway inflammation or edema, which can dramatically increase airway resistance.

Newborns are obligatory nose breathers. This means they only breathe through the mouth when they cry and do not automatically open the mouth to breathe when the nose is obstructed. Mouth breathing begins to occur when neurologic pathways mature, around 3 months of age. Infants up to 3 to 4 months of age can be obligatory nose breathers. As a result, it is vital to keep the nose of an infant open, patent, and free from any obstructions for adequate breathing and coordinated sucking to occur.

In Chapter 1, 4-month-old Chip had trouble nursing because of his nasal congestion. What effect did this nasal congestion have on him as his respiratory illness progressed? How did Chip's developmental level affect his risk for complications related to the congestion?

Lower Airway

The larynx (voice box) separates the upper airway from the lower airway. In a child, the right and left mainstem bronchi begin much higher and are at a steeper angle than those in an adult. The trachea divides into the right and left mainstem bronchi at the level of the T3 vertebra in children but at the level of the T6 vertebra in adults.

The number of **alveoli** in a full-term newborn is approximately 25 million, all of which may not be fully developed. By approximately 32 to 36 weeks of gestation, a fetus has enough functioning alveoli to maintain gas exchange. Adults, in comparison, have about 300 million alveoli. Not until 8 years of age do the size and complexity of the alveoli begin to increase. Also, the infant and the small child have narrower and fewer distal bronchioles, which may lead to less oxygen entering the alveoli. Table 20.1 summarizes the differences between the pediatric and adult airway anatomy.

Young children use different muscles to breathe than do older children and adults. Children younger than 6 years of age use the diaphragm as the principal muscle of inspiration. Before age 6, intercostal muscles are immature and much more flexible than those in older children and adults.

Table 20.1 Summary of Pediatric and Adult Airway Differences

Airway Structure or Factor	Infant or Child	Adult
Shape and size of the head	Larger in comparison to the body and neck; pronounced occiput	Flatter occiput
Tongue	Larger	Relatively smaller
Larynx	Level of the second and third cervical vertebrae	Level of the fourth and fifth cervical vertebrae
Epiglottis	U-shaped; floppy	Spade-shaped, flat, erect, more flexible
Hyoid/thyroid separation	Very close	Further apart
Glottis	Contains more cartilage	Only 1/4 cartilage
Cricoid	Narrowed area	No narrowing
Smallest diameter location	Cricoid ring	Vocal cords

Assessment of the Pediatric Respiratory System

Use the assessment guide in Table 20.2 to perform an in-depth nursing assessment of the pediatric respiratory system. Table 20.3 lists normal respiratory rates for pediatric age groups. Abnormal respiratory assessment findings are often compensatory in nature for the pediatric patient. For example, **grunting** helps keep the alveoli open at the end of expiration by maintaining pressure in the airways while the child exhales, and the use of accessory muscles in the chest and neck (retractions) is an attempt to assist with ventilation (Fig. 20.1). Table 20.4 lists abnormal assessment findings and their associated compensatory mechanisms.

Respiratory conditions are the most common cause of hospitalization in children aged 1 to 9 years. Respiratory problems in the pediatric population may occur as a primary problem or as a complication of a nonrespiratory problem. For example, children may have respiratory failure as a result of sepsis (a severe infection), trauma, such as a head injury, or severe dehydration as a result of excessive vomiting and diarrhea. It is important to remember the anatomical and physiological differences between children and adults and the changes pediatric patients undergo as they grow. The structure and function of the respiratory

Table 20.2 Assessment Guide: Pediatric Respiratory System

Element to Assess	Assessment Questions, Considerations, and Tips
Respirations	
Rate	Rate should be normal for age (see Table 20.3 for age-specific respiratory rates). Tachypnea? Bradypnea? Apnea?
Rhythm	Pattern should be regular. Newborns may have irregular respiratory rates.
Depth	Is the child taking deep enough breaths? Is the chest rising and falling adequately?
Symmetry	Chest rise should be equal and symmetrical bilaterally.
Effort	Is the child using accessory muscles to breathe? Does the child appear labored? How many words can the child say without taking a breath?
Cough	
Characteristics	• Dry—nonproductive • Wet—productive with mucus • Brassy—noisy, also known as musical • Croup-like—brassy or seal-like
When	Periodically? Only at night? Only when the child lies down? Only with eating or drinking?
Effort	Is the cough forceful or weak? Can the child bring up his or her own secretions?
Color	
Location	Mucus membranes, skin, and nail beds
Shade	Pink, pale, mottled, cyanotic
Cyanosis	A *late* sign of respiratory distress
When crying	Does color improve or worsen?
Adventitious Sounds	
Wheeze	• High-pitched whistling • Can be heard on inspiration, expiration (most common), or both
Stridor	Audible without a stethoscope; crow-like sounds
Crackles	• Fine: high-pitched, not continuous; heard at the end of inspiration ◦ Assessment Tip: Rub your hair together close to your ear. This is what fine crackles sound like. • Coarse

Table 20.2 Assessment Guide: Pediatric Respiratory System

Element to Assess	Assessment Questions, Considerations, and Tips
Pain	
Location	Throat? Chest?
Origin	On inspiration, expiration, or both? Only when coughing? When taking a deep breath?
Severity	Use an age-appropriate pain scale.
Odors	
Breath	Smells infectious? Improves after brushing teeth?
Mucus	Smells infectious?
Mucus	
Color	Clear, cloudy, white, yellow, green, brown?
Consistency	Thick, thin, chunky? Mucus plugs?
Position of Comfort	• Lying flat • Sitting up • Neck extended • Tripod position

Table 20.3 Normal Respiratory Rates for Pediatric Age Groups

Age	Respirations per Minute
Newborn	30–55
1 y	25–40
3 y	20–30
7 y	16–22
10 y	16–20
17 y	12–20

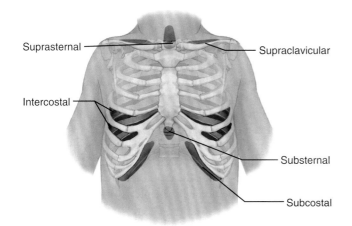

Figure 20.1. Location of retractions. Reprinted with permission from Kyle, T., & Carman, S. (2017). *Essentials of pediatric nursing* (3rd ed., Fig. 10.27). Philadelphia, PA: Wolters Kluwer.

system at various ages can impact the degree of alterations in gas exchange and ventilation.

Throughout the chapter, various infectious, noninfectious, and chronic respiratory disorders are explored. First, however, let's consider some general nursing interventions that apply to many of these conditions, as well as the difference between respiratory distress and respiratory failure in children.

General Nursing Interventions for Respiratory Disorders

Open and Maintain a Patent Airway

Perhaps no other nursing intervention is more critical to sustaining life than opening and maintaining a patent airway, no matter the age of the patient. It is the first priority of care in the ABCs of nursing priorities, which stands for airway, breathing,

Table 20.4 Abnormal Findings in Assessment of Pediatric Respiratory System

Finding	Cause
Head bobbing	Use of the sternocleidomastoid muscles to assist with ventilation
Nasal flaring	A physiologic attempt to increase the diameter of the air passages to decrease airway resistance and allow more air in
Grunting	A compensatory response to prevent end-expiratory alveolar collapse; helps keep alveoli open at the end of expiration
Hyperextension of head and neck	A form of accessory muscle use Child positions self in an attempt to open the airway.
Retractions	The chest wall is less compliant in children; the use of accessory muscles (chest and neck) is an attempt to assist with ventilation. • Mild distress: subcostal, substernal (Fig. 20.1) • Moderate distress: intercostal, supraclavicular • Severe distress: Suprasternal, sternal
Adventitious breath sounds	Accumulation of secretions (coarse crackles or rhonchi), obstructed airways (wheezing), accumulation of fluid, as in pulmonary edema (crackles)

and circulation. Moreover, given the narrower airway present in a child compared with that in an adult, this intervention is especially crucial in pediatric patients.

Respiratory disorders can lead to obstruction of the airway by secretions, such as mucus, tightened or swollen tissues of the airway, or a foreign object. Pneumonia, bronchiolitis, and cystic fibrosis (CF) all result in increased production of mucus and other secretions in the airway. Bronchopulmonary dysplasia (BPD) requires airway clearance of normal secretions to ease and improve ventilation and perfusion that have been compromised because of prematurity and damage to lung tissue as a result of mechanical ventilation. In epiglottitis, swollen tissues of the epiglottis resulting from a bacterial infection threaten obstruction of the airway. Asthma endangers airway patency in three different ways: increased mucus production, narrowing of the airways via bronchoconstriction, and inflammation of the airway tissues. A foreign body or object that a child inhales via the nostrils or mouth can also obstruct the airway.

Interventions to aid airway clearance vary depending on the cause, acuity, and severity of obstruction. In severe, acute cases of airway obstruction caused by excessive production of mucus and other secretions, such as in bronchiolitis, patients may require nasotracheal suction. More general interventions include chest percussion (chest physiotherapy) and postural drainage, which are used for CF and BPD. In milder cases, interventions may simply include encouraging the patient to cough with or without assistance, breathe deeply, and perform incentive spirometry. Encourage smaller children to breathe deeply and cough by having them blow bubbles or a pinwheel. Placing the patient in an upright, seated position and

encouraging frequent position changes also help move secretions and clear the airway.

Children with epiglottitis may require insertion of an endotracheal tube or even an emergency tracheostomy to open the airway. An acute asthma exacerbation requires treatment with bronchodilators and corticosteroids. Foreign body aspiration requires removal of the object, such as by back blows and chest thrusts in the case of complete obstruction of the airway.

Maintain Effective Ventilation

Like opening and maintaining a patent airway, maintaining effective ventilation is a critical intervention for patients—the second priority of care in the ABCs of nursing priorities (breathing). Respiratory disorders can make breathing difficult for children.

The ultimate intervention for respiratory dysfunction is mechanical ventilation, which may be required by premature neonates with underdeveloped respiratory systems and other children experiencing respiratory failure resulting from respiratory, cardiovascular, or other disorders. This intervention, however, poses its own risks to the patient, including the development of pneumonia, pneumothorax, or BPD.

An open pneumothorax, such as caused by penetrating trauma to the chest, requires covering the wound with an airtight seal; a gloved hand suffices until a dressing is available. Resuscitation may be needed for children with acute respiratory failure.

More commonly, children with respiratory disorders require supportive care to maintain effective ventilation, such as in

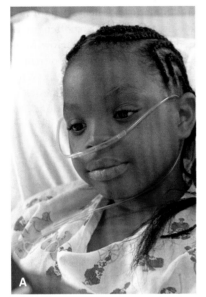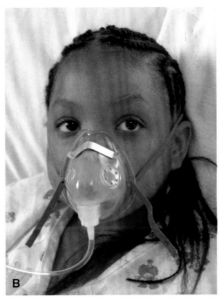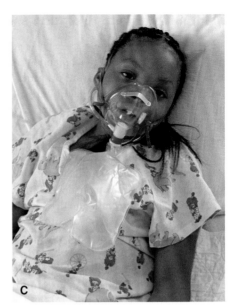

Figure 20.2. Oxygen delivery devices. A. A nasal cannula, which can deliver 24% to 35% oxygen (0.25–6 L/min of flow). **B.** A simple oxygen mask, which can deliver 35% to 50% oxygen (5–10 L/min of flow). **C.** A non-rebreather mask, which can deliver 70% to 100% oxygen (10–15 L/min of flow). Reprinted with permission from Chow, J., Ateah, C. A., Scott, S. D., Ricci, S. S., & Kyle, T. (2012). *Canadian maternity and pediatric nursing* (1st ed., Fig. 39.9). Philadelphia, PA: Lippincott Williams & Wilkins.

bronchitis and laryngotracheobronchitis (LTB). This care includes placing the child in a position of comfort, such as being held upright or over the parent's shoulder, which assists in achieving adequate lung expansion. Other supportive measures include humidification of air or oxygen to ease breathing, encouraging the child to breathe more slowly, and encouraging the child to rest.

Medications such as corticosteroids and racemic epinephrine may be ordered to help reduce airway inflammation.

Maintain Adequate Oxygenation

In addition to and, in part, as a result of compromising airway patency and ventilation, respiratory disorders can prevent adequate oxygen from entering the blood and being delivered to the cells of the body during respiration. Therefore, maintaining adequate oxygenation is another key nursing priority for children with respiratory disorders.

Whether poor oxygenation is a result of increased airway resistance, as in bronchiolitis and LTB, or impaired or damaged lung tissue, as in acute respiratory distress syndrome (ARDS), the needed interventions are the same: administration of supplemental oxygen and positioning of the child to promote optimal oxygenation. Oxygenation is measured by pulse oximetry, which determines the percentage of hemoglobin that is saturated with oxygen, or O_2 saturation. The appropriate oxygen delivery device to use with a child depends on how many liters of oxygen per minute are needed to maintain the infant's O_2 saturation. Many times, children only need oxygen via nasal cannula to maintain adequate O_2 saturation (Fig. 20.2A).

However, if children need higher concentrations of oxygen, they will require delivery via a facemask (Fig. 20.2B) or even a non-rebreather mask (Fig. 20.2C). Whatever the delivery device, the nurse should monitor the child's O_2 saturation level and adjust the oxygen flow rate to maintain saturation level at 90% or above or at the patient's baseline saturation if chronic respiratory disease is present (American Academy of Pediatrics [AAP], 2014). The nurse should also note the infant's color and monitor for mental status changes, both of which are indicators of oxygenation (Patient Safety 20.1).

Optimal positioning for oxygenation depends on the child's respiratory disorder. A more upright position, such as a semi-Fowler's or a high Fowler's position, helps clear the airway of secretions, which is appropriate for children with bronchiolitis and other respiratory infections. In ARDS, however, prone positioning may be more effective, because it allows previously nondependent air-filled alveoli to become dependent, thus increasing perfusion to air-filled alveoli and ultimately improving ventilation–perfusion matching.

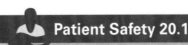

Cyanosis

Cyanosis is a LATE sign of respiratory distress. If you should find a child with cyanosis, prepare to intervene with stimulation, oxygen, and assisting with ventilation, if necessary.

Maintain Adequate Hydration and Nutrition

Because respiratory disorders can challenge fluid balance and food intake, interventions to maintain adequate hydration and nutrition are important nursing priorities. Several factors related to respiratory disorders contribute to dehydration in the child. Vomiting, such as may occur in bronchitis and other respiratory infections, results in increased insensible water loss. Fever, which increases evaporation of water from the skin and respiratory tract, and increased respiratory rate can lead to increased insensible fluid loss. The decreased ability and desire to drink fluids that accompany many respiratory disorders can reduce intake, also contributing to dehydration.

Because of this increased risk of dehydration, take care to assess for signs of dehydration, including poor skin turgor, sunken fontanel, low urine output, and dry mucus membranes. Closely monitor intake and output, as well as laboratory tests related to fluid, including blood urea nitrogen (BUN), creatinine, and urine specific gravity. Also, closely monitor serum electrolytes, such as potassium, particularly when diuretics are administered.

When dehydration is severe or the child is unable, such as in epiglottitis, or unwilling to take fluids by mouth, administration of intravenous (IV) fluids may be required, possibly with electrolytes. In other cases, encourage increased oral fluid intake via frequent sips of cool, noncarbonated, nonacidic fluids and favorite drinks or sucking on ice and other frozen items, such as popsicles, which, in addition to promoting hydration, may be soothing.

As with fluid intake, respiratory disorders can also disrupt food intake. In conditions in which children are unable to take in food by mouth, such as in ARDS, enteral feeding via a nasogastric tube is initiated. Early enteral feeding in critically ill children has been shown to improve outcomes and decrease mortality (Mikhailov et al., 2014). In other conditions, such as bronchiolitis, oral feeding may be possible but challenging due to nasal congestion, difficulty swallowing, or lack of appetite or desire to eat. In children with nasal congestion, suctioning before feeding may help increase oral intake. In other conditions, such as CF, children are likely to need a higher-than-normal caloric intake because of the increased work of breathing and higher metabolic demands. In general, offer children smaller, more frequent feedings, which they are more likely to tolerate.

Promote Pain Relief

Respiratory disorders can cause pain in a variety of ways. Frequent and forceful coughing, such as occurs in pneumonia and bronchitis, can cause children to experience chest pain, muscle pain and even pleuritic pain. Acute chest pain related to coughing can prevent the child from taking deep breaths. A child with a chest tube often has pain at the insertion site. Insertion of the chest tube requires the provider to go through the muscle layer of the lateral chest wall, resulting in incisional pain.

Analgesics and anti-inflammatories, such as ibuprofen, as well as nonpharmacological methods, are often useful in relieving pain associated with coughing (see How Much Does It Hurt? 20.1 for a discussion of assessment of pain in the child with pneumonia and pain relief strategies). When fever is present, antipyretics may be ordered. Analgesics are administered for pain related to chest tube insertion. Narcotics may be needed to control pain in some children with a chest tube.

How Much Does It Hurt? 20.1

Pain Assessment for a Child with Pleuritis

Pain associated with pleuritis and muscle pain from coughing can range from mild to severe. Assess pain using an age-appropriate pain scale.

Imagine you are caring for a 2-y-old boy admitted to the hospital with pneumonia. The mother repeatedly calls the nurse into the room stating that her child is in pain. The child is sitting in the crib and appears to be in mild respiratory distress. You notice mild intercostal retractions and intermittent nasal flaring. The child is on 2 L of oxygen via nasal cannula and appears sleepy but interacts appropriately when you present a toy to play with while assessing the patient. While you are in the room, the child begins to cough and then begins to cry. His mom states, "See—it hurts every time he coughs. Please help him."

How would you appropriately assess this child's pain? What are appropriate pain-relieving interventions for this child?

Appropriate pain scales to use for a 2-y-old include the FLACC scale (see How Much Does It Hurt? 11.1) and the Wong–Baker FACES Pain Rating Scale (see How Much Does It Hurt? 6.1).

Obtain a pain score while the child is coughing and when the child is not coughing. Include the mother in the evaluation of pain because the child is a toddler.

Interventions for mild pain may include the following: repositioning, assisting with splinting while the child coughs, and administration of prescribed analgesics, such as acetaminophen or ibuprofen. Teach the parent and child how to splint the chest wall using a pillow or favorite stuffed animal or doll. Recall that inflammation of the lining of the lungs as well as inflammation of the muscles used in coughing can be a primary source for the pain. Therefore, anti-inflammatory agents such as ibuprofen may be prescribed.

When a hospitalized child has moderate-to-severe pain that has not improved after other measures, administration of narcotics such as codeine, oxycodone, or stronger agents, such as morphine, may be prescribed.

Administer and Manage Medications

Medications used to treat respiratory disorders range from antibiotics (for CF, bacterial pneumonia, ARDS, epiglottitis, and tuberculosis), bronchodilators and corticosteroids (asthma), diuretics and vasodilators (ARDS), and mucolytics and pancreatic enzymes (CF). For details on specific medications, see the section Therapeutic Interventions for each condition throughout the chapter, as well as The Pharmacy features.

Prevent Infection

Hand washing is essential not just for clinicians but for anyone coming in contact with children who are vulnerable to respiratory infections, particularly those with respiratory disorders such as CF and BPD. Teach family and friends proper hand washing techniques. Limit and encourage parents to limit visitors both at home and in the hospital to those who are free from any respiratory symptoms. Children who have a peripherally inserted central catheter (PICC) line or central venous access are at increased risk for bloodstream infections. Provide proper care of the PICC line or central venous access line, as well as the IV site.

Provide Emotional and Psychosocial Support to the Child and Parents

Respiratory disorders and their potential complications can cause great anxiety in children and their parents. And often, this anxiety can further compromise respiratory status and contribute to respiratory distress in infants and children. During an acute asthma exacerbation, in particular, anxiety may be high because of the feeling of being unable to breathe. Use calming measures, such as guided imagery or distraction, with the child to try to reduce anxiety. Encourage the parents to participate in reducing the child's anxiety (and their own) by holding or talking to the child. Calm parents' anxieties by explaining the diagnosis, treatment, equipment, and procedures. Decrease anxiety by grouping nursing care to disturb the child as little as possible.

Respiratory Distress and Respiratory Failure

Respiratory distress, respiratory failure, and respiratory arrest occur on a continuum, with the milder respiratory distress progressing to respiratory failure and eventually to respiratory arrest. Respiratory distress occurs in many of the illnesses and diseases that affect the respiratory system. Signs and symptoms associated with respiratory distress result from the body's compensatory mechanisms used to avoid immediate respiratory failure (Patient Safety 20.2). Children can maintain a state of respiratory distress for a long time. However, signs of impending respiratory failure often occur suddenly, and the child may have a cardiopulmonary arrest if rapid assessment and intervention is

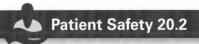

Patient Safety 20.2

Cardinal Signs of Respiratory Distress

The cardinal signs of respiratory distress are as follows:
- Restlessness
- Tachycardia
- Tachypnea
- Diaphoresis

Any child who appears with these signs should have an in-depth assessment of respiratory status and exam of the etiology of the signs.

not performed when a child appears with prolonged respiratory distress, worsening respiratory distress, or respiratory failure. Table 20.5 compares the clinical manifestations of respiratory distress and respiratory failure.

Respiratory failure occurs when a child's body can no longer maintain effective gas exchange, often when oxygen demand far outweighs oxygen supply and the child becomes extremely hypoxic. Other times, carbon dioxide levels rise as a result of hypoventilation to the point that the child becomes apneic. Serious acute or chronic respiratory or neuromuscular conditions can lead to respiratory failure. Acute lung injury, often caused by sepsis, pneumonia, aspiration, smoke inhalation, and near-drowning, can also lead to respiratory failure. Respiratory failure is the most common cause of cardiopulmonary arrest in children.

Hypoventilation of the alveoli precedes respiratory failure. What is hypoventilation and why does it occur? Hypoventilation occurs when the exchange of oxygen and carbon dioxide is disrupted in the alveoli due to oxygen demand far exceeding oxygen supply and/or carbon dioxide being inadequately cleared from the alveoli as a result of alveolar occlusion, damage, or injury. Etiologies for the disruption in gas exchange can be categorized as pulmonary or nonpulmonary.

Pulmonary causes of respiratory failure can be due to impaired integrity of lung tissue or increased airway resistance. Conditions that lead to impaired integrity of lung tissue include atelectasis, pneumonia, bronchiolitis, and ARDS, which can lead to ventilation–perfusion mismatch. Conditions that lead to increased airway resistance include foreign body aspiration, croup, and airway edema.

Nonpulmonary conditions that can lead to respiratory failure include respiratory muscle compromise, alterations in nervous system control of breathing, upper airway disorders, and cardiovascular and hematologic disorders. Recall that the chest wall of an infant or young child is extremely compliant, which compromises ventilation and leads to chest wall retractions. Respiratory muscle fatigue leads to hypoventilation because the child does not achieve adequate chest rise and thus adequate

Table 20.5 Comparing Respiratory Distress and Respiratory Failure

Factor to Assess	Respiratory Distress	Respiratory Failure
Respiratory rate	Increased	Increased, progressing to decreased (bradypnea)
Color	Pink, pale	Cyanotic, gray
Breath sounds	• Wheezing • Able to auscultate air movement	• Diminished significantly • Adventitious
Respiratory effort	• Nasal flaring • Retractions • Grunting	• Minimal chest expansion • Severe retractions • Apnea
Neurologic state/behavior	• Irritability • Increased restlessness • Confusion • Headache	• Difficult to arouse • Limp • Stupor • Coma
Cardiovascular	• Tachycardia • Diaphoresis • Hypertension	• Extreme tachycardia • Bradycardia (when hypoxia is present) • Hypotension
O_2 saturation	• May be normal or slightly lowered • May require oxygen to maintain level >93% • Mild hypoxia	• Unable to maintain level (often even with oxygen delivery) • Hypoxia worsens; oxygen deficit is beyond spontaneous recovery. • Cerebral oxygenation is severely affected.
Blood gas analysis	• pH: may be normal or alkalotic; mild acidosis may be present. • Pao_2: >60 mm Hg • $Paco_2$: <50 mm Hg	• pH: acidotic • Pao_2: <50 mm Hg • $Paco_2$: >50 mm Hg

lung volumes. Diaphragmatic hernia also leads to respiratory muscle compromise. Alterations in nervous system control of breathing that may lead to respiratory failure include the following: respiratory depression caused by narcotics, sedatives, or anesthesia; Guillain–Barre syndrome; head or spinal cord trauma; central nervous system infections; and central hypoventilation syndrome. Upper airway disorders leading to respiratory failure include choanal atresia and tracheoesophageal fistula. Finally, cardiovascular and hematologic disorders that can ultimately lead to respiratory failure include congenital heart disease, anemia, shock, and sepsis.

Acute Infectious Upper Airway Disorders

Pediatric respiratory infections can be described according to the location of the infection. The upper airway includes the oropharynx, nasopharynx, larynx (voice box), and the first part of the trachea. The lower airway includes the bottom of the trachea, left and right mainstem bronchus, bronchi, bronchioles, and alveoli. Remember that infections often spread from one respiratory structure to another.

Croup—which is the inflammation of the epiglottis, larynx, trachea, and possibly even the bronchi—is a very common pediatric disorder. Croup is the most common cause of cough, hoarseness, and stridor in children. Most children recover from croup without sequelae. However, because of the inflammatory nature of the croup syndromes, the small diameter of the child's airway, and other pediatric airway differences, croup can be life-threatening, particularly in very young children. Croup syndromes can be classified as viral or bacterial. Viral croup syndromes include spasmodic laryngitis and LTB. Bacterial croup syndromes include epiglottitis and bacterial tracheitis. Table 20.6 compares croup syndromes.

Laryngotracheobronchitis

LTB, which is the most common croup syndrome, is a viral infection of the upper airway, which includes the throat, larynx, and trachea. LTB is preceded by a recent upper respiratory infection. Although LTB is most likely to be diagnosed in infants and children aged 6 months to 3 years, it can occur in children up to 8 years of age. Boys are more likely than girls to be diagnosed with LTB.

Table 20.6 Comparing Croup Syndromes

Factor	Epiglottitis	Laryngotracheobronchitis (LTB)	Spasmodic Laryngitis	Tracheitis
Age	2–8 y	3 mo to 8 y	3 mo to 3 y	1 mo to 13 y
Etiology	Bacterial: *Haemophilus influenzae, Staphylococcus, Streptococcus*	• Viral: Parainfluenza, respiratory syncytial virus, influenza • Bacterial: *Mycoplasma pneumoniae*	Unknown; may be viral; may be brought on with allergic and/or emotional influences	Bacterial: *Staphylococcus, Haemophilus influenzae* (nontypeable)
Onset	Rapid progression; may progress to complete airway obstruction	Gradual; slowly progressive; initially appears as upper respiratory infection	Sudden; at night	Progresses from upper respiratory infection; usually in 1–2 d
Signs and symptoms	• Drooling • Dysphagia • Dysphonia • High fever • Extreme tachycardia • Tachypnea • Stridor that worsens when the child lies supine • Appears toxic	• Hoarseness • Brassy cough • Dyspnea • Restlessness • Irritability • Stridor • Low-grade fever • Rhinitis • Appears nontoxic	Afebrile, barking cough ("seal-like"), appears in mild respiratory distress	High fever, purulent secretions, croupy cough; Does not respond to interventions for LTB
Treatment and interventions	• Protect airway. • Antibiotics • Racemic epinephrine • Corticosteroids • Fluids for hydration	• Racemic epinephrine • Corticosteroids • Fluids for hydration	• Cool mist • Reassure parents of transient nature of episodes.	• Antibiotics • Fluids for hydration

Etiology and Pathophysiology

When viruses invade airway tissues, the tissues respond with inflammation and edema. Recall that the pediatric airway is most narrow in the subglottic and cricoid areas. The diameter of the airway significantly narrows as a result of the inflammation and edema caused by the virus. Narrowing of the airway obstructs air flow, which can lead to **stridor**, the hallmark sign of LTB.

Viruses causing croup are spread through direct contact with contaminated hands, which then touch the mucosa of the eyes, nose, or mouth, or through direct inhalation from an infected person's cough or sneeze. LTB is usually caused by a parainfluenza virus (75% of cases), influenza A or B, respiratory syncytial virus (RSV), or *Mycoplasma pneumoniae* (Wright & Bush, 2016).

Clinical Presentation

A child with LTB presents with a history of an upper respiratory infection or common cold. Parents may report that the child awakes at night with a low-grade fever, barking cough, and noisy breathing, as well as stridor. A child with LTB may appear agitated, restless, and frightened. A sore throat and rhinorrhea may be present.

Assessment and Diagnosis

Assessment of a child with LTB should focus on respiratory effort, severity of stridor, respiratory rate, use of accessory muscles, and O_2 saturation (Priority Care Concepts 20.1). Table 20.7 presents a tool for assessing children with stridor. Another helpful tool is a croup score, such as the Downes and Raphaely Croup Score, shown in Table 20.8. The higher the score, the more severe the croup symptoms and the more likely the child requires more intense treatment. Assessment of mental status is imperative to ascertain whether the child is suffering from **hypoxia** and potential respiratory failure. Diagnosis is often made by the clinical signs. However, radiographs of the chest and the upper airway may be taken to assess for airway narrowing in the subglottic area. This narrowing is often referred to as "**steeple sign**."

Assessment should include placing the child on a cardiorespiratory monitor and pulse oximeter and monitoring heart rate, respiratory rate, and O_2 saturation level. Place the child in an area that allows constant or frequent observation, which assists with identifying changes in respiratory effort, responsiveness, stridor, and preferred position. Note any behavior changes, and frequently reassess the child's respiratory ability, lethargy, and ease of arousal (Patient Safety 20.3).

Table 20.7 Assessing Children with Stridor

Sign	Rating					
	0	1	2	3	4	5
Stridor	None	Only with agitation or excitement	Mild at rest, heard with a stethoscope	At rest, heard without a stethoscope		
Retractions	None	Mild	Moderate	Severe		
Air entry	Normal	Decreased	Severely decreased			
Cyanosis	None				With agitation	At rest
Level of consciousness	Normal					Altered mental status

A score can range from 0 to 18. Mild respiratory distress = less than 3. Moderate respiratory distress = 3 to 6. Severe respiratory distress = greater than 6.
Reprinted with permission from Sobol, S., & Zapata, S. (2008). Epiglottitis and croup. *Otolaryngology Clinics of North America, 41*(3), 551–566.

Table 20.8 Downes and Raphaely Croup Score

Symptom	Score		
	0	1	2
Stridor	Normal	Inspiratory	Inspiratory and expiratory
Cough	None	Hoarse cry	Bark
Retractions and nasal flaring	None	Suprasternal	Suprasternal and intercostal
Cyanosis	None	In room air	In air with fraction of inspired oxygen of 40%
Inspiratory breath sounds	Normal	Harsh with rhonchi	Delayed

Reprinted with permission from Downes, J., Raphaely, R. (1975). Pediatric intensive care. *Anesthesiology, 43*, 238–250.

Priority Care Concepts 20.1 Patient With an Obstructed Airway

Priority Problem	Priority Interventions
Ineffective Airway Clearance • Inability to move air from the upper airway to the lower airway Goal: A. Maintain a patent airway.	1. Reposition the patient. Consider allowing parents to hold the child in a preferred position. 2. Open the airway using the jaw-thrust technique. 3. Administer medications such as bronchodilators and steroids. 4. Attach the patient to a cardiorespiratory monitor. 5. Auscultate breath sounds.
Impaired Gas Exchange • Oxygen deficit (inability to take in adequate oxygen) • Hypercarbia (inability to eliminate carbon dioxide) Goals: A. O_2 saturation levels are within normal limits for the patient. B. Carbon dioxide levels are within normal limits for the patient. C. There are no signs of respiratory distress.	1. Apply oxygen to maintain O_2 saturation levels >92%. 2. Reduce anxiety (anxiety can exacerbate dyspnea, leading to further compromise of gas exchange) (Bruera et al., 2000). 3. Place the patient in the semi-Fowler's position. 4. Position the patient prone (Patient Safety 20.4 and Analyze the Evidence 20.1). 5. Attach the patient to a cardiorespiratory monitor. 6. Auscultate breath sounds.

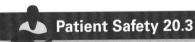

Patient Safety 20.3

A Child with Stridor Suddenly Becomes Quiet

Breath sounds and noisy breathing may actually diminish as the child uses remaining energy stores to maintain ventilation. Immediate assessment and intervention should occur when a stridulous or noisy breathing child suddenly becomes quiet. Reposition the child, open the airway, apply oxygen, and be prepared to assist with ventilation.

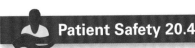

Patient Safety 20.4

Sudden Infant Death Syndrome

Prone positioning is associated with increased risk of sudden infant death syndrome. Therefore, prone positioning should only be used for children who are hospitalized and being continuously monitored.

Therapeutic Interventions

Children with LTB should be placed in a position of comfort, such as held upright over the parent's shoulder (see the section Maintain Effective Ventilation). Cool mist may be used for some children, although the evidence is not conclusive that

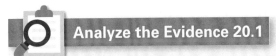

Analyze the Evidence 20.1

Prone Positioning

Clinical Question

Does prone positioning in the pediatric population improve oxygenation?

The Evidence

The effects of different body positions in hospitalized infants and children with acute respiratory distress were compared and analyzed. A review of 24 studies including 581 participants revealed prone positioning was significantly more beneficial than was supine positioning in terms of episodes of hypoxemia, oxygen saturation (SpO_2), and arterial oxygen (PaO_2). Also, respiratory rate associated with respiratory distress decreased. There were no adverse effects associated with prone positioning (Gillies, Wells, & Bhandari, 2012).

mist therapy is beneficial (Analyze the Evidence 20.2). Encourage rest, because an ineffective breathing pattern and poor respiratory effort can be worse when fatigue is present. Administer medications such as corticosteroids and racemic epinephrine as ordered to help reduce airway inflammation (The Pharmacy 20.1). Keep resuscitation equipment at the bedside. See the sections Maintain Adequate Oxygenation and Maintain Adequate Hydration and Nutrition.

Analyze the Evidence 20.2 Helpful Therapies for Croup

Clinical Questions

1. Does humidification improve respiratory status of a patient with croup?
2. Is the use of steroids, such as dexamethasone, beneficial for a patient with croup symptoms?

The Evidence

Johnson (2014) performed a systematic review to answer the clinical question, What are the effects of treatments in children with mild, moderate, or severe croup? In this systematic review, two of the specific areas examined were related to the outcomes when humidification was used in the treatment of croup and when dexamethasone was used as a therapy for treating croup.

The practice and treatment of delivering humidified air to patients with croup has been widely accepted since the 1800s. However, in the systematic review by Johnson (2014), the use of humidification was found unlikely to be effective in relieving symptoms. There were no randomized controlled trials (RCTs) with direct evidence supporting that humidification use decreases symptoms in children with mild croup. In relation to moderate-to-severe croup, Johnson (2014) found one systematic review and one RCT that examined the effects of humidified air and reduction of symptom severity in children with croup. The effects of humidified air were no more effective than nonhumidified or low-humidified air in reducing symptom severity at 30–60 min after initiation.

The use of dexamethasone has been shown to be beneficial in the treatment of mild, moderate, and severe croup in several RCTs. In studies examining the use of mild croup and use of dexamethasone, oral dexamethasone compared with a placebo was shown to reduce symptom severity in the first 24 h and reduce the need for additional medical attention in children with mild croup.

The Pharmacy 20.1   Medications Used to Treat Stridor

Medication	Classification	Route	Action	Nursing Considerations
Racemic epinephrine	Beta-agonist Beta-adrenergic	Nebulizer	• Rapid-acting bronchodilator • Decreases bronchial secretions • Decreases mucosal edema	Observe for: • Tachycardia • Hypertension • Headache • Dizziness • Nausea
Dexamethasone	Corticosteroid	Intravenous By mouth	• Anti-inflammatory • Decreases airway edema and inflammation	Observe for hypertension.

From Lexicomp. *Pediatric & Neonatal Dosage Handbook* (25th ed.), 2018.

Evaluation

Expected outcomes for a child with LTB include the following:
- The child has decreased respiratory distress.
- O₂ saturation levels are within normal limits for age and baseline health status.
- Administration of medications improves respiratory status and decreases stridor.
- The child has adequate fluid intake for age, as evidenced by adequate urine output for age (Growth and Development Check 20.1).

Discharge Planning and Teaching

Before discharge, assess parents for knowledge of symptoms of LTB and when to call the physician or to seek emergency treatment if symptoms recur or worsen. Parents should call the pediatric provider if any of the following occur:
- Mild symptoms do not improve with exposure to cool air or air-conditioning after 1 hour
- The child's breathing becomes more labored, respiratory rate increases, or the child becomes more lethargic
- The child does not take in adequate fluids for age and the urine output is reduced

Growth and Development Check 20.1

Age-Appropriate Intake and Output

Normal 24-h intake for an infant is as follows:
- 1 mo: 2–4 oz 6–8 times/d
- 2 mo: 5–6 oz 5–6 times/d
- 3–6 mo: 6–7 oz 5–6 times/d
- 6–8 mo: up to 24–32 oz/d
- 8–12 mo: 16–28 oz/d, depending on the amount of solid food eaten

Normal urine output for an infant is 1–3 mL/kg/h.
Normal 24-h intake for a toddler is 32–48 oz/d.
Normal urine output for a toddler is 1.5 mL/kg/h.

Epiglottitis

Epiglottitis, inflammation and swelling of the epiglottis, is a medical emergency. Recall that the epiglottis covers the larynx during swallowing to prevent food from entering the trachea. When the epiglottis becomes severely inflamed and swollen, the airway can become completely obstructed. Notice in Figure 20.3 the narrowing of the trachea caused by edema. An infant or child's airway is small, so even a little edema can result in a very narrowed or even obstructed airway.

Etiology and Pathophysiology

Acute epiglottitis is associated with significant morbidity and mortality if not diagnosed and treated promptly. *Haemophilus influenzae* type b (Hib) or *Streptococcus pneumoniae* (or other bacteria; see the list later) can colonize in the pharyngeal airway of children. The bacteria are spread through respiratory contact, often through close or intimate contact with another person. The bacteria then penetrate the oral mucosa and enter the bloodstream, leading to bacteremia. The bacteria then seed in the epiglottis. Other areas of the body where the bacteria may seed include the meninges, lungs, ears, and joints.

In the past, Hib was the predominant cause of epiglottitis, causing 90% of cases. Since the introduction of the Hib vaccine, the incidence of epiglottitis in children has dramatically declined to the current annual rate of 0.63 cases per 100,000 persons (Faden, 2006). Epiglottitis varies in prevalence according to the season and predominantly occurs in children aged 2 to 6 years. Other bacteria that can cause epiglottitis include the following: beta-hemolytic streptococci, *Staphylococcus aureus*, *Haemophilus parainfluenzae*, *Neisseria meningitides*, *Pseudomonas species*, and *Candida albicans* (more common in immunocompromised patients). Viral agents do not generally cause epiglottitis but can lead to a bacterial superinfection. Epiglottitis is more likely to affect males than females.

Clinical Presentation

Children with epiglottitis typically appear toxic or extremely ill. A high fever usually appears first; there are usually no prodromal signs of epiglottitis. The epiglottis is cherry red and swollen

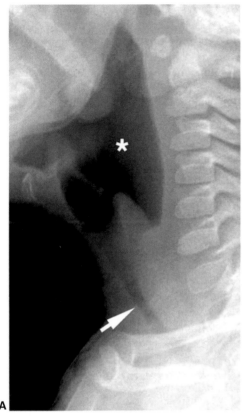 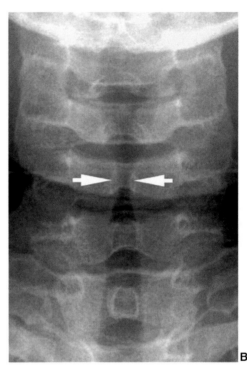

A B

Figure 20.3. **Steeple sign.** In the image on the **A**, there is a narrowing of the trachea where the arrow is pointed. Above the trachea, where the star is noted, there is a distended hypopharynx. In the image on the **B**, there is narrowing of the trachea between the two arrows. Reprinted with permission from Kline-Tilford, A. M., & Haut, C. (2015). *Lippincott certification review: Pediatric acute care nurse practitioner* (1st ed., Fig. 3.8). Philadelphia, PA: Lippincott Williams & Wilkins.

and obstructs the airway. Stridor may be heard. Secretions pool in the pharynx and larynx, above the epiglottis. Drooling is present in 80% of cases of epiglottitis. The child is unable to swallow and complains of a sore throat. Respiratory distress is common. Epiglottitis has a rapid onset; symptoms can appear and worsen to airway obstruction within 2 to 6 hours.

Assessment and Diagnosis

When assessing a child with suspected epiglottitis, try to keep the child calm and to avoid causing anxiety, which can lead to increased respiratory distress, crying, and ultimately to complete obstruction of the airway (Patient Safety 20.5). Crying stimulates the airway, which can precipitate **laryngospasm**, and increases oxygen consumption, which, given the limited oxygen supply due to the swollen airway, can lead to an imbalance in oxygen supply and demand and thus to hypoxia. Postpone invasive procedures, such as starting an IV line and obtaining a throat culture, until the airway is secure.

Examine the child for signs of an obstructed upper airway, which include **dysphagia**, **dysphonia**, drooling, the **tripod position** (or, in smaller children, the "sniffing position," in which the neck is extended). The tripod position, shown in Figure 20.4, involves the child sitting upright with hands on knees or supporting self with arms. The child often refuses to

Patient Safety 20.5

Epiglottitis

- Do not stick anything in the child's mouth.
- Allow the child to be in the position of comfort.
- Avoid procedures that are likely to upset the child or make the child cry; this can lead to an increase in the swelling in the airway.
- Observe the child continuously for inability to swallow, absence of voice, increased drooling, and increased respiratory distress. Increased drooling is an ominous sign of supraglottic obstruction.

lie down. Diagnosis is made on the basis of clinical symptoms and an X-ray of the lateral neck. The X-ray reveals soft-tissue edema, a narrowed airway (steeple sign), and a large, rounded epiglottis (Fig. 20.3).

Therapeutic Interventions

Children with epiglottitis often require immediate insertion of an endotracheal tube to maintain a patent airway. Placement of the endotracheal tube often takes place in the operating room,

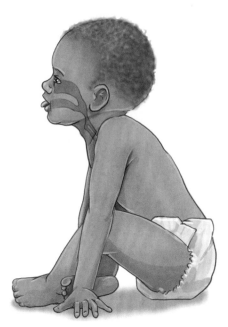

Figure 20.4. Tripod position. The child sits with head and neck extended upward to open the airway and supports self with arms. Reprinted with permission from Hatfield, N. T., & Kincheloe, C. A. (2017). *Introductory maternity and pediatric nursing* (4th ed., Fig. 36.3). Philadelphia, PA: Lippincott Williams & Wilkins.

in an environment where an emergent tracheostomy can be performed if the epiglottis completely obstructs the airway, making endotracheal intubation impossible. For children who are not immediately intubated, make readily available any equipment needed to assist with ventilation until an endotracheal tube can be placed.

As ordered, administer antibiotics in a timely manner once the airway is secured. Antibiotics should cover the most common organisms, such as *S. aureus* and group A streptococci (Faden, 2006). The child may also need antipyretics for fever and sedation to help maintain comfort.

Nothing should be administered by mouth. See the sections Maintain Adequate Hydration and Nutrition and Provide Emotional and Psychosocial Support to the Child and Parents.

Evaluation

Expected outcomes for a child with epiglottitis include the following:
- The child's airway remains unobstructed, breath sounds are equal bilaterally with adequate air entry auscultated, and stridor is absent.
- Oxygenation is within normal limits, with O_2 saturation levels greater than 92% and PaO_2 on an arterial blood gas test greater than 80 mm Hg.
- The child remains adequately hydrated.
- The child is afebrile.

Discharge Planning and Teaching

During the acute phase of care, parents may require much reassurance. The child may temporarily lose his or her voice;

reassure parents that the child's voice will return once the swelling decreases. Difficulty breathing can make even a calm child very anxious, thus producing much worry and concern for the parents. Explain the hospital environment, equipment, and monitors to parents. Endotracheal intubation often provokes anxiety in parents and the child, because the child cannot speak and communication is difficult. Provide age-appropriate alternative means of communication for the child, and reassure parents and the child that the inability to communicate is temporary.

Before discharge, instruct parents to make sure that the child completes the entire course of antibiotics. Also, teach the parents about signs and symptoms of respiratory distress and when to call the provider.

Tracheitis

Bacterial tracheitis is a secondary infection of the upper trachea. Viral laryngotracheitis leads to bacterial tracheitis. Tracheitis can be seen in any age group, with the mean age being 5 years. Tracheitis is also known as membranous LTB, bacterial LTB, and pseudomembranous croup.

Etiology and Pathophysiology

Fewer than 2% of cases of viral croup lead to tracheitis. Common bacteria that lead to tracheitis include the following: *S. aureus, S. pneumoniae,* and *Staphylococcus pyogenes*. However, *Moraxella catarrhalis* is a leading cause and is most likely to require endotracheal intubation. Tracheitis is more common in the fall and winter, when croup is more prevalent. Males are twice as likely to be diagnosed with tracheitis than are females. About 80% of children with tracheitis require intubation and 94% require intensive care (Kuo & Parikh, 2014). The potential for acute upper airway obstruction and hypoxia results in a mortality rate reported as high as 20% (Kuo & Parikh, 2014).

Clinical Presentation

The child with tracheitis appears ill or even toxic on presentation. A croupy cough is heard, a change in voice (dysphonia) or hoarseness is heard or reported by parents, and stridor is noted. The child is usually brought in because of a sudden decompensation characterized by noisy breathing, a much sicker appearance according to the parents, and presence of a high fever. Drooling is absent because the child is able to swallow secretions, unlike a child with epiglottitis.

Assessment and Diagnosis

Assessment of bacterial tracheitis is similar to that for LTB. However, left undiagnosed and untreated, tracheitis can lead to airway obstruction and respiratory arrest. The child presents with a history of upper respiratory infection. Clinical manifestations include the following: sore throat, dysphonia, croupy cough, stridor, high fever, and signs of respiratory distress. Characteristically specific to tracheitis, stridor usually does not improve with positioning. The child appears toxic or seriously ill. In contrast to epiglottitis, drooling is not present in cases of tracheitis. Thick, purulent secretions are common, which cause an increase in respiratory difficulties.

Tracheitis is diagnosed by culture and Gram stain of secretions. Specimens for culture and Gram stain are often obtained by a laryngotracheobronchoscopy or direct visualization of the trachea. Blood cultures are often obtained to monitor for bacteremia or spread of the organisms to the bloodstream. The child's white blood cell count is elevated.

Therapeutic Interventions

Nursing interventions for tracheitis are similar to those for epiglottitis. See the section Therapeutic Interventions for epiglottitis.

Evaluation

Expected outcomes for a child with tracheitis include the following:
- The child's airway remains unobstructed, breath sounds are equal bilaterally with adequate air entry auscultated, and stridor is absent.
- Oxygenation is within normal limits, with O_2 levels greater than 92% and PaO_2 on an arterial blood gas test greater than 80 mm Hg.
- The child remains adequately hydrated, and urine output is within normal limits for age.
- The child is afebrile.

Discharge Planning and Teaching

The section on Epiglottitis: Discharge Planning and Teaching, is appropriate also for the patient with bacterial tracheitis.

Acute Infectious Lower Airway Disorders

Pneumonia

Pneumonia, an inflammation or infection of the lower airways (the bronchioles and alveolar spaces of the lungs), occurs most commonly in infants and younger children. Pneumonia may be viral, bacterial, or mycoplasmal. Childhood immunizations have, fortunately, helped decrease the number of cases of pneumonia, particularly pneumonia caused by Hib and *S. pneumonia* infections. Worldwide, pneumonia is the leading infectious cause of death in children younger than age 5 years (Centers for Disease Control [CDC], 2017).

Community-acquired pneumonia is one of the most common serious infections in children. The annual incidence of community-acquired pneumonia requiring hospitalization among children younger than 18 years of age in the United States is 15.7 cases per 10,000 children (Jain et al., 2015). Children younger than age 2 years had the highest incidence, with 62.2 cases per 10,000 children (Jain et al., 2015). Approximately one-half of children younger than age 5 years who are diagnosed with community-acquired pneumonia require hospitalization. In the United States, hospitalization for pneumonia for children younger than age 5 years results in costs of about $1 billion/y (Pfuntner, Wier, & Steiner, 2011).

Etiology and Pathophysiology

Pneumonia is most commonly caused by viruses such as RSV, parainfluenza, influenza A and B, adenovirus, and human metapneumovirus. Bacterial pneumonia is more common in children older than age 5 years but can occur in any age group. Common bacterial organisms that cause pneumonia include *S. aureus*, *S. pneumoniae*, and *M. pneumoniae.*

Pneumonia can be acquired in the community or in a hospital (usually associated with mechanical ventilation). Children exposed to cigarette or woodstove smoke and those with chronic conditions such as asthma, CF, sickle cell disease, BPD, congenital heart disease, and immunodeficiency are at higher risk for community-acquired pneumonia.

Clinical Presentation

Although causative agents differ in cases of pediatric pneumonia, symptoms commonly include fever, **tachypnea**, and cough. The child may have decreased or poor oral intake, nausea, vomiting, and abdominal pain. Furthermore, the child may appear restless or even lethargic. Irritability is also common. Box 20.1 summarizes the clinical appearance of a child with pneumonia.

Assessment and Diagnosis

Assessment of the child with suspected pneumonia requires astute attention to respiratory changes, including changes in

---

Box 20.1 Clinical Presentation of a Child with Pneumonia

Behavior
- Irritability
- Lethargy
- Malaise
- Restlessness

Fever
- High (bacterial)
- Low or high (viral)

Respiratory
- Cough (productive or unproductive)
- Sputum (cloudy, white, yellow, tan)
- Tachypnea
- Retractions
- Nasal flaring
- Pallor
- Cyanosis (in moderate-to-severe cases)
- Breath sounds (crackles, decreased)
- Chest pain (worse with coughing)
- Dullness on percussion

Gastrointestinal
- Abdominal pain
- Anorexia
- Vomiting
- Diarrhea

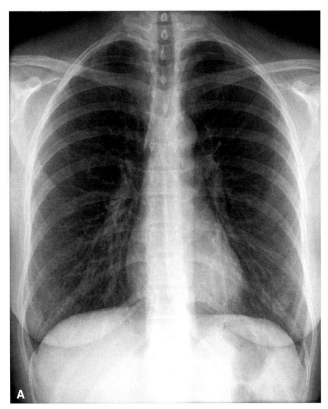

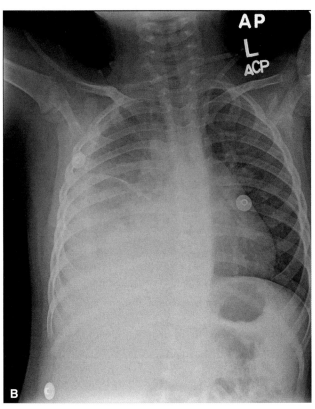

Figure 20.5. Comparison of a normal chest X-ray and an X-ray of a patient diagnosed with right-sided pneumonia. A. A normal chest X-ray: note the clear lung fields. **B.** Chest X-ray of a patient with right-sided pneumonia: notice that the right lung fields are dense and have areas of opacities. Part B reprinted with permission from Boyce, T. G. (2018). *Moffet's board review for pediatric infectious disease* (1st ed., Fig. 8.5). Philadelphia, PA: Wolters Kluwer.

respiratory rate, use of accessory muscles, respiratory effort, and level of consciousness. **Nasal flaring**, **dyspnea**, and grunting may be present. Auscultate and assess breath sounds for rhonchi, wheezes, and crackles, all of which may be signs of pneumonia. If cough is present, as it often is in pneumonia, assess it for sound, frequency, and associated findings. Consider the following questions during assessment:

- Does the cough sound wet, dry, hacking, or barky?
- Does the child become cyanotic with cough?
- Does the cough increase respiratory distress in the child?

Coughing episodes may result in cyanosis and vomiting of mucus. Children with pneumonia often complain of pain, particularly after coughing episodes and when asked to take a deep breath. Assess pain for timing, frequency, location, and severity (How Much Does It Hurt? 20.1).

Diagnosis is made by a chest radiograph. A chest radiograph consistent with pneumonia shows abnormal density of lung tissue, lobar consolidation, or patchy infiltrates (Fig. 20.5). Sputum cultures, if obtained, can be helpful in determining the causative agent. However, young children are not able to understand how to produce a sputum culture. Generally, children older than age 8 years can produce enough sputum for a culture. Respiratory viruses can be identified via a nasal swab or nasopharyngeal aspirate.

Therapeutic Interventions

Encourage the child with pneumonia to cough frequently and breathe deeply to help remove the thick, tenacious secretions in their bronchi, bronchioles, and lungs and maintain a patent airway (see the section Open and Maintain a Patent Airway, as well as Patient Safety 20.6).

For patients with bacterial pneumonia, administer antibiotics as ordered (The Pharmacy 20.2). Ensure that the child receives the appropriate weight-based dose and that the full course of antibiotic regimen is given. See the sections Promote Pain Relief and Maintain Adequate Hydration and Nutrition.

Patient Safety 20.6

Narcotic-Induced Respiratory Depression

If a narcotic is administered, pay close attention to the child's respiratory rate and effort, because narcotics can cause respiratory depression.

The Pharmacy 20.2 Medications Used to Treat Pneumonia

Medication	Classification	Route	Action	Nursing Considerations[a]
Penicillins (amoxicillin)	Antibiotic	• IV • PO	Kill or inhibit the growth of bacteria	• Monitor for allergic reactions. • Use with caution in patients with an allergy to cephalosporins. • Observe the child for at least 30 min after IV administration.
Cephalosporins (cefuroxime, cefdinir)	Antibiotic	• IV • IM • PO	Kill or inhibit the growth of bacteria	• Use with caution in patients allergic to penicillins. • Observe the child for at least 30 min after IV administration.
Macrolides (azithromycin)	Antibiotic	• IV • PO	Kill or inhibit the growth of bacteria	• Diarrhea and abdominal cramping should be reported to provider. • Monitor liver and renal labs.
Aminoglycosides (gentamicin)	Antibiotic	• IV • PO	Kill or inhibit the growth of bacteria	• Monitor drug levels: peak and trough. • Monitor for renal toxicity: BUN, creatinine, and I&O. • Monitor for ototoxicity: headache, dizziness, hearing loss, and tinnitus. • Monitor for superinfection.
Ibuprofen	• Analgesic • Anti-inflammatory	PO	Not completely understood; may be related to prostaglandin synthetase inhibition	Teach parents how to calculate and measure dose using an appropriate measuring device.

From Lexicomp. *Pediatric & Neonatal Dosage Handbook* (25th ed.), 2018.
[a]For all antibiotics, ensure that dosing is correct for the patient's weight, because antibiotic dosing in pediatrics is weight based.
BUN, blood urea nitrogen; IM, intramuscular; I&O, intake and output; IV, intravenous; PO, by mouth.

Evaluation

Expected outcomes for a child with pneumonia include the following:
• Optimal respiratory function is restored.
• Pain is adequately controlled; the pain score is within goals set by the parents and child.
• Medications, particularly antibiotics, are given as prescribed and for the duration prescribed.
• The child has adequate intake for age, as evidenced by adequate urine output for age.

Discharge Planning and Teaching

Before discharge, parents should be able to verbalize general care instructions for a child with pneumonia. Provide instructions to them on the following:
• Frequency and duration of antibiotic therapy and the importance of completing the entire prescription
• Proper and frequent hand washing to prevent the spread of infection
• When to call the physician:
  • Breathing is rapid or difficult
  • The child becomes lethargic or is difficult to arouse
  • Fever returns or is not controlled by antipyretics such as acetaminophen and ibuprofen.

Bronchiolitis and Respiratory Syncytial Virus

Bronchiolitis is a lower respiratory tract infection most commonly caused by RSV. Young infants are at greater risk for respiratory compromise from bronchiolitis because of their smaller airways. Although this infection is typically treated in the outpatient setting, approximately 5.2 of 1,000 children younger than age 24 months are hospitalized with bronchiolitis (Hall et al., 2013). The most common time for infants to develop bronchiolitis varies by region, but it is typically fall through early spring.

Etiology and Pathophysiology

RSV causes 50% to 80% of cases bronchiolitis. Other viruses known to cause bronchiolitis include human rhinovirus (5%–25%), parainfluenza virus (5%–25%), and human metapneumovirus (5%–10%) (Meissner, 2016). Regardless of the specific virus, the infection causes the cells in the lining of the small airways, the **bronchioles**, to die and accumulate in the lower airway, causing airway obstruction and leading to respiratory distress in the child. The obstruction compromises oxygen and carbon dioxide exchange through the alveoli, resulting in a lower O_2 saturation level (Casey, 2015; Meissner, 2016). Premature infants under 29 weeks of gestation and infants with underlying cardiopulmonary disease are at greater risk for complications from bronchiolitis, regardless of the causative agent.

Growth and Development Check 20.2

Obligatory Nose Breathing in Infants

Remember that infants are obligatory nose breathers until around 4 mo of age; therefore, any nasal congestion can cause difficulty with feeding.

Clinical Presentation

Bronchiolitis starts out with mild symptoms, such as nasal congestion, rhinorrhea, and "wet" sounding cough with or without fever. Parents and caregivers of infants 4 months and younger often indicate that the infant has difficulty feeding because of nasal congestion (Growth and Development Check 20.2).

After about 2 days, symptoms become more severe and infants begin to show signs of moderate respiratory distress, such as nasal flaring, grunting, and retractions. Tachypnea, tachycardia, and fever are common, along with adventitious lung sounds. In more severe disease, O_2 saturation levels fall below 90% and the infant appears lethargic. The decision to hospitalize the infant is based on the infant's respiratory status.

In Chapter 1, Chip was hospitalized because he exhibited signs of moderate-to-severe respiratory distress resulting from bronchiolitis. What were these signs? What was his O_2 saturation level? What additional risk did Chip's age pose?

Assessment and Diagnosis

Diagnosis of bronchiolitis is based on history and physical exam (Priority Care Concepts 20.2). Chest X-ray and laboratory studies are not recommended (AAP, 2014). Physical assessment is an important part of nursing care for the child hospitalized with

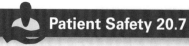

Patient Safety 20.7

Respiratory Decompensation

Note that a decreased respiratory rate in an infant who has been tachypneic does not necessarily indicate improvement; it could mean that the infant is decompensating. Be sure to take into account the full respiratory assessment of the infant to determine respiratory status.

bronchiolitis. Note adventitious lung sounds, the use of accessory muscles, and other symptoms of respiratory distress, such as tachypnea, pale or bluish skin color, and low O_2 saturation level. Closely monitor the work of breathing, because children can suddenly become unable to maintain it, which results in respiratory failure (Patient Safety 20.7). An increasing heart rate occurs as a compensatory effort to maintain effective perfusion to tissues. Monitor neurological status for increased irritability, increased lethargy, inconsolability, and arousability. When oxygen demand exceeds oxygen delivery or when carbon dioxide levels rise as a result of ineffective ventilation, a child's neurological status deteriorates. Communicate even minor changes to the healthcare provider in charge.

Therapeutic Interventions

Infants born at or before 29 weeks of gestation and those with underlying cardiopulmonary disease qualify for RSV prophylaxis. Prophylaxis with palivizumab occurs once a month for a maximum of 5 months during RSV season (The Pharmacy 20.3; AAP, 2014).

Perform nasotracheal suction to remove the copious amounts of mucus produced, maintain a patent airway, and alleviate respiratory distress (see the section Open and Maintain a Patent Airway). Suction the infant before feeding so that nasal

Priority Care Concepts 20.2   The Child with Bronchiolitis

Problem	Interventions
Ineffective Airway Clearance Goals: • Decreased adventitious lung sounds • Tolerate PO feedings	• Assess lung sounds every 4 h to determine the presence of adventitious lung sounds. • Suction before feedings to increase oxygenation and provide easier feeding.
Impaired Gas Exchange Goals: • Maintain oxygenation. • No signs of respiratory distress such as nasal flaring, grunting, or retractions • Respiratory rate and heart rate within normal limits	• Place in a position of comfort to maximize respiratory effort. • Monitor vital signs to determine improvement in status or to detect early decompensation. • Monitor O_2 saturation level every 2 h and adjust oxygen as needed to keep it at 92% to ensure adequate oxygenation.

The Pharmacy 20.3 Palivizumab

Medication	Classification	Route	Action	Nursing Considerations
Palivizumab (Synagis)	Monoclonal antibody	Intramuscular	• Exhibits neutralizing action against RSV • Inhibits RSV replication	• Given monthly throughout RSV season for 5 doses • Administer in the thigh

From Lexicomp. *Pediatric & Neonatal Dosage Handbook* (25th ed.), 2018.
RSV, respiratory syncytial virus.

congestion does not interfere with oral intake. Monitor lung sounds, noting any adventitious sounds and documenting the type of sound and where it is heard.

Chest physiotherapy is not recommended for infants with bronchiolitis because evidence has shown that this treatment does not decrease the length of hospitalization. Medications such as antimicrobials, corticosteroids, and bronchodilators are also not recommended because of lack of evidence showing any benefit from their use (AAP, 2014). See the sections Maintain Adequate Oxygenation and Provide Emotional and Psychosocial Support to the Child and Parents.

Evaluation

Expected outcomes for a child with bronchiolitis include the following:
- The child shows no signs of respiratory distress, such as nasal flaring, grunting, or retractions.
- The skin is appropriate in color for racial or ethnic background and dry to the touch.
- Vital signs are within normal limits for age.
- O_2 saturation level is maintained at or above 90% on room air.
- The child maintains adequate oral intake of fluids and food.

Discharge Planning and Teaching

Bronchiolitis is a self-limiting disease that should improve over about 2 weeks. Occasional adventitious lung sounds may still be present during the remainder of the illness. Cough may still be present for up to 2 weeks after discharge. Instruct parents that children should not be around secondhand smoke, because this increases the risk of repeat infections. Teach parents during the hospital stay how to bulb suction an infant. Having parents perform return demonstration before discharge is essential, because most patients with bronchiolitis are discharged home needing bulb suctioning before feeds or intermittently until secretions lessen.

Before discharge, parents should understand to call the healthcare provider if any of the following occur:
- The infant develops a fever of 101.5°F (38.6°C) or greater
- The infant begins to show signs of respiratory distress, such as listlessness, nasal flaring, grunting, or retractions
- The infant has decreased oral intake over 24 hours

Bronchitis

Bronchitis is an inflammation of the trachea, bronchi, and bronchioles, which generally, in children, occurs in conjunction with a viral respiratory tract infection. Acute bronchitis is characterized by cough due to the inflammation of the trachea, bronchi, and bronchioles (large airways) without evidence of pneumonia.

Etiology and Pathophysiology

Bronchitis is rarely a primary bacterial infection in children. The inflammatory response in the mucus membranes of the bronchial passages produces a hacking cough and thick phlegm. Viruses most often contribute to this inflammatory response (Brodzinski & Ruddy, 2009). Viral infections that cause bronchitis often include the following: adenovirus, influenza, parainfluenza, RSV, rhinovirus, coxsackie virus, and herpes simplex virus.

Males and females are equally likely to be diagnosed with bronchitis. Acute bronchitis occurs most commonly in children younger than age 2 years. However, children aged 9 to 15 years are more susceptible to bronchitis, as well. Throughout the world, bronchitis appears to be one of the top five reasons children visit the primary physician.

Clinical Presentation

Classic symptoms of bronchitis include the following: a coarse, hacking cough that worsens at night, chest pain as a result of frequent, deep coughing, and vomiting at night related to swallowing sputum. Excessive phlegm is also present. Some children may have fever. Symptoms are usually self-limiting, with the child returning to health in about 10 to 14 days.

Assessment and Diagnosis

Children often present to the care provider with symptoms of the common cold. Nasal discharge is present and may be purulent but without necessarily meaning that bacteria are present. Other symptoms include dyspnea, malaise, chills, fever, and pain in the chest and back. Assess cough for frequency, mucus production, and sound. Generally, cough is dry in the beginning of the course, becomes loose with mucus production, and worsens at night. The cough may sound dry, raspy, and harsh. When the cough loosens, parents often report a rattling sound in the chest. Children younger than age 5 years rarely cough up (expectorate) secretions. This leads to vomiting of thick mucus as a result of the child swallowing many of the secretions. Vomiting of pulmonary secretions is referred to as posttussive emesis. Breath sounds may be clear. However, wheezing, crackles, and rhonchi may be present throughout the period of illness.

Therapeutic Interventions

Support respiratory function by encouraging a comfortable position and rest and by providing humidification of air and oxygen if needed (see the sections Maintain Effective Ventilation and Maintain Adequate Hydration and Nutrition). Instruct parents to use a cool mist humidifier or vaporizer in the child's bedroom, particularly at night, when cough worsens. Children are often fatigued as a result of lessened periods of deep sleep at night related to coughing. However, antitussives and over-the-counter cough and cold medicines are not recommended for children younger than age 6 years because of a lack of research and potential risks, including a delay in seeking treatment, potential misuse and abuse, drug–drug interactions, and harmful side effects (Lowry & Leeder, 2015). See the section Promote Pain Relief.

Evaluation

Bronchitis is self-limiting. Resolution of symptoms indicates the end of the illness.

Expected outcomes for a child with bronchitis include the following:

- Pain is adequately controlled with pharmacological and nonpharmacological interventions.
- Fever is controlled with antipyretics, tepid baths, or cool cloths according to child and parent preference.
- The child is free from respiratory distress.

Discharge Planning and Teaching

Bronchitis often results in absenteeism from school related to coughing, fever, pain, and fatigue. Instruct parents that children may return to school when fever is no longer present, signs of infection have decreased, and alertness and strength have increased. Teach them pain management and use of analgesics, and if they smoke, advise them to quit or refrain around the child.

Tuberculosis

Pulmonary tuberculosis (TB) is a lung infection caused by the organism *Mycobacterium tuberculosis,* an acid-fast bacillus. In the past 25 years, the number of children with TB has greatly increased worldwide in the wake of the human immunodeficiency virus (HIV). Children are ineffective transmitters of the acid-fast bacillus and therefore do not get the attention of TB control programs. In the United States, there were approximately 9,582 cases of TB reported in 2013, of which 485 (5%) were among children younger than 15 years of age (https://www.cdc.gov/tb/topic/populations/tbinchildren/default.htm). Outside of the United States, children younger than 15 years of age account for 15% to 20% of TB cases. Infants and young children have higher morbidity and mortality rates related to TB than do older children and adults.

Risk factors for development of TB can fall into two categories: those pertaining to children recently infected with TB bacteria and those pertaining to children with medical conditions that weaken the immune system. Box 20.2 differentiates the risk factors for children with TB.

Box 20.2   Risk Factors for Tuberculosis in the Pediatric Population

Risk Factors Associated with Recent Infection with TB

- Close contact with a person infected with TB
- Immigration from or a visit to an area of the world with a high rate of TB (Mexico, the Philippines, Vietnam, China, India)
- Age younger than 5 y with a positive TB test result
- Homelessness
- IV drug use
- Close contact with someone exposed to those with high rates of TB: hospital, correctional facility, nursing home, and homeless shelter workers

Conditions that Weaken the Immune System

- Human immunodeficiency infection
- Substance abuse
- Head or neck cancer
- Low body weight
- Use of long-term corticosteroids
- Severe kidney disease
- Organ transplants
- Scoliosis
- Diabetes

Data from the Centers for Disease Control (CDC), (2016). *Tuberculosis: TB Risk Factors.* Retrieved from: https://www.cdc.gov/tb/topic/basics/risk.htm.

Etiology and Pathophysiology

TB is spread by airborne droplets. Infected droplet nuclei are generated when someone with pulmonary or laryngeal TB coughs, sneezes, or even talks and may be transmitted to a person in close proximity. These microscopic nuclei can remain airborne for minutes to hours after being expelled from the respiratory tract (Knechel, 2009). Once inhaled, the droplet nuclei enter the lungs and travel to the alveoli. Tubercle bacilli multiply in the alveoli. A small number of the tubercle bacilli enter the bloodstream and spread throughout the body, where TB disease is likely to develop. Within 2 to 8 weeks, macrophages ingest and surround the tubercle bacilli. These cells form a granuloma that acts as a barrier to keep the bacilli contained (latent TB disease). If the immune system cannot keep the bacilli under control, the bacilli rapidly multiply, resulting in TB disease.

There are two major patterns of TB: primary and secondary (Fig. 20.6). Primary TB, the initial infection, usually occurs in children, whereas secondary TB usually occurs in adults as a reactivation of infection. In primary TB, small subpleural granulomas and some lymph node infection occur, which form the Ghon's complex. These lesions usually heal, and the infection goes dormant. In secondary TB, the infection is reactivated as a result of a weakened immune system or a reinfection occurs.

Not every child who comes in contact with TB becomes ill. Two TB conditions exist: latent TB infection and TB disease. See Table 20.9 for a comparison the two conditions. Children with latent TB infection have the bacterium in their body but do not have TB disease and cannot spread the disease to others. Latent

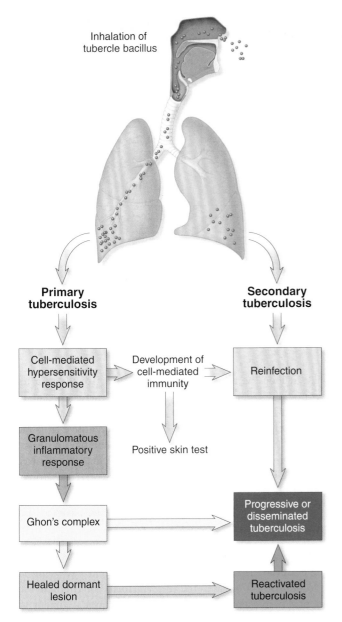

Figure 20.6. Pathogenesis of tuberculosis. Reprinted with permission from Braun, C. A., and Anderson, C. M. *Applied Physiology: A Conceptual Approach to the Mechanisms of Disease* (3rd ed., Fig. 5.16). Philadelphia, PA: Lippincott Williams & Wilkins; modified with permission from Porth, C. M. (2019). *Pathophysiology: Concepts of altered health states* (10th ed., Fig. 30.9). Philadelphia, PA: Lippincott Williams & Wilkins.

TB infection begins when bacilli are ingested by macrophages and presented to other white blood cells. This triggers an immune response in which white blood cells kill or encapsulate the bacilli. Granulomas then form and latent TB infection is established. Usually within several weeks, the body's immune system is able to halt the progression of the disease by stopping the multiplication of tubercle bacilli.

In some people, particularly those who are immunocompromised, tubercle bacilli overcome the immune system and TB disease develops.

Table 20.9 Comparison of Latent Tuberculosis Infection and Tuberculosis Disease

Factor to Consider	Latent TB Infection	TB Disease
Symptoms present?	No	Yes: severe cough, chest pain, bloody sputum, weakness, fatigue, weight loss, loss of appetite, chills, fever, night sweats
Feels ill?	No	Yes
Can spread disease?	No	Yes
Skin test result positive?	Yes	Yes
Chest X-ray?	Normal	Abnormal
Sputum?	Negative	Positive
Treatment?	Needs treatment to prevent TB disease	Needs treatment for TB disease
Isolation required?	No	Yes: airborne precautions

TB, tuberculosis.

Clinical Presentation

A child with latent TB disease is asymptomatic. A child with active TB disease presents with symptoms. Clinical features and symptoms vary according to the age of the child. Cough, lasting more than 3 weeks, is the common factor among all age groups. Infants often present with fever, persistent cough, decreased appetite or failure to thrive, and wheezing. School-age children often have mild symptoms, such as a dry cough. Adolescents present with a productive, persistent cough lasting longer than 3 weeks and systemic symptoms such as night sweats, fever, chills, and weight loss.

Assessment and Diagnosis

Multiple diagnostic tests are available to assist in identifying TB (Table 20.10). Among these tests are sputum smear, sputum culture, polymerase chain reaction, tuberculin skin test, QuantiFERON-TB test, and chest radiography.

Diagnostic testing for TB includes administering an intradermal tuberculin purified protein derivative (PPD) skin test when certain risk factors are present. A PPD should be administered if one or more risk factors are present. Risk factors for children for TB infection include exposure to high-risk adults,

Table 20.10 Diagnostic Tests for Tuberculosis

Diagnostic Test	Purpose	Time Required for Results
Sputum smear	• Detects presence of acid-fast bacilli • Does not confirm diagnosis; not all acid-fast bacilli are *Mycobacterium*	Rapid; usually within hours but up to 24 h
Sputum culture	Confirms active TB	Up to several weeks
Nasogastric tube aspirates (in early morning before feeding)	Confirms active TB for children under 12 y old who cannot produce sputum	Up to several weeks
TB skin test	Tests for *M. tuberculosis* infection; cannot confirm TB disease	48–72 h after intradermal injection
Blood test: interferon-gamma release assays	• Confirms diagnosis • Helps define drug sensitivity	Within 24 h
Chest X-ray	• Confirms presence of lesions • Can help rule out pulmonary TB for a child who tests positive on a TB skin test or blood test but is asymptomatic	Within hours

TB, tuberculosis.

being born in a country with a high prevalence of TB, and being homeless. Those who have had a severe allergic reaction to the TB skin test should not receive the test.

Skin tests are interpreted on the basis of two factors: the induration measurement (in millimeters) and the person's risk of being infected with TB and, if infected, of having it progress (Table 20.11). False-positive reactions may occur, in which the child does not have TB but reacts positively to the skin test. Causes of false positives may include the following: previous bacillus Calmette–Guérin vaccine, incorrect method of administering the test, incorrect interpretation of the results, incorrect bottle of antigen used, or infection with nontuberculous mycobacteria (CDC, 2016). False-negative reactions to the TB skin test may also occur, in which the child has TB but reacts negatively to the skin test. Causes of false negatives

may include the following: inability to react to the skin test because of weakened immunity (cutaneous anergy), recent TB infection (<8–10 weeks since exposure before the test), very old TB infection, age less than 6 months, recent live virus vaccination (i.e., measles or mumps), overwhelming TB disease, certain viral illnesses such as chickenpox or measles, incorrect method of administration of the test, or incorrect interpretation of the results.

Therapeutic Interventions

Nursing care and management of the child with TB differs in some aspects depending on whether the child has latent TB infection or TB disease. The primary focus for children with latent TB infection is to ensure that antibiotic regimens are

Table 20.11 Interpretation of the Tuberculin Skin Test Reaction: Populations Considered Positive at Various Indurations

Induration (mm)		
≥5	**≥10**	**≥15**
• HIV-infected persons • Persons with recent contact with a TB-infected person • Persons with a chest X-ray consistent with TB • Organ transplant patients • Immunosuppressed patients	• Recent immigrants (≥5 y) from countries with a high prevalence of TB • IV drug users • Laboratory personnel who work in mycobacteriology • Persons with clinical conditions placing them at high risk • Children <4 y of age • Residents and employees in high-risk settings • Infants, children, and adolescents exposed to adults at high risk	Anyone, including those with no known risk factors

HIV, human immunodeficiency virus; IV, intravenous; TB, tuberculosis.
Adapted from Centers for Disease Control and Prevention. (n.d.). *Fact sheets*. Retrieved from http://www.cdc.gov/tb/publications/factsheets/testing/skintesting.htm

The Pharmacy 20.4 — Medications Used to Treat Latent and Active Tuberculosis (Antitubercular)

Medication	Route	Action	Nursing Considerations
Isoniazid	• PO • IM	• Inhibits mycobacterial cell wall synthesis • Is bacteriostatic or bactericidal against *Mycobacterium*	• Monitor hepatic function before and during treatment, because it may cause drug-induced hepatitis. • Monitor the patient for signs of peripheral neuropathy.
Rifampin	• PO • IV	Inhibits RNA synthesis by blocking RNA transcription in susceptible organisms	• Administer 1 h before or 2 h after meals with a full glass of water. • The patient may take it with food if GI upset occurs. • Monitor hepatic and renal function throughout therapy. • Inform patient and family that saliva, sweat, tears, feces, and urine may become red-orange or red-brown. • It may discolor or permanently stain contact lenses. • It is teratogenic and decreases the effect of hormonal birth control; the patient should use alternative forms of contraception while taking rifampin.
Pyrazinamide	PO	• Is converted to pyrazinoic acid in susceptible strains of *Mycobacterium*; the pH is lowered in the environment. • Is bacteriostatic	Monitor hepatic function every 2–4 wk during therapy; elevation of AST and ALT may occur but is not predictive of drug-induced hepatitis.
Ethambutol	PO	• Inhibits growth of mycobacteria	• Administer with food or milk to reduce GI upset and irritation. • The patient should take it at the same time each day.

From Lexicomp. *Pediatric & Neonatal Dosage Handbook* (25th ed.), 2018.
ALT, alanine aminotransferase; AST, aspartate aminotransferase; GI, gastrointestinal; IM, intramuscular; IV, intravenous; PO, by mouth.

completed. Often, a child with latent TB infection is prescribed a course of isoniazid for up to 9 months. The primary focus for children with active TB disease is the administration of antibiotics, as well as supportive care for the symptoms, such as fever and cough (see the section Promote Pain Relief).

Initiation and completion of medication to treat TB is imperative to stop the spread of the disease and to prevent complications of the disease. Recommended medications for the treatment TB include isoniazid, rifampin, pyrazinamide, and ethambutol (The Pharmacy 20.4; Nahid et al., 2016). Less common medications for treating TB include amikacin, levofloxacin, moxifloxacin, streptomycin, capreomycin, cycloserine, and kanamycin.

Table 20.12 provides strategies for administering long-term antibiotics for children of specific age groups.

Evaluation

Expected outcomes for a child with TB include the following:
• The child completes the prescribed medication regimen.
• The child with latent TB does not develop active TB.
• Close contacts of the child are assessed and treated as deemed necessary by the provider.

Discharge Planning and Teaching

Teach the child and parents about infection control measures such as hand hygiene, coughing into tissues, and proper disposal of tissues into a closed bag. Also, review medication therapy before discharge, including adherence to the prescribed regimen (usually 6–12 months of daily medications) and side effects.

Acute Noninfectious Respiratory Disorders

Foreign Body Aspiration

Foreign body aspiration is the inhalation of an object into the respiratory tract. Objects can be solids, liquids, foods, or nonfoods. Small children explore their environment with their mouths and hands and are more prone to aspiration of foreign bodies. Children aged 1 to 3 years are most likely to aspirate a foreign object, either by sticking the object in their mouth or by sticking the object in their nose and then aspirating the object, such as a bead, into their trachea.

Etiology and Pathophysiology

Children are more susceptible to foreign body aspiration not only because of their need to explore with their mouths and hands but also because of the anatomy of the upper airway at a young age. The lack of molar teeth leaves the child incapable of chewing food sufficiently, and thus larger chunks are left to swallow. Also, chewing and swallowing are uncoordinated until

Table 20.12 Strategies for Administering Long-Term Antibiotics for Children at Various Ages

Age	Adherence Strategy
Infant (birth–1 y)	• Make sure parents and caregivers comprehend the need for treatment. • To promote compliance, offer medication when the baby is hungry. • Crush the pill, dissolve it in a small amount of warm water, and mix it with approximately 10 mL of breast milk or formula. • Avoid isoniazid liquid, which contains sorbitol and thus can cause diarrhea. • An isoniazid pill may be crushed and mixed with baby food, such as cereal or fruit, and given by spoon.
Toddler (1–3 y)	• Use distraction when administering. • Disguise the taste by mixing with a food of the child's choice. • Expect difficulty but be persistent. • Give simple explanations. • Use incentives for each daily dose if needed.
Preschooler (3–5 y)	• Give simple explanations. • Allow some negotiation for time of medication administration or method of administration. • Offer rewards and verbal praise, but be consistent and assertive.
School age (5–12 y)	• Discuss the treatment plan with the child. • Provide simple and accurate information. • Child may be able to swallow pills whole. • Have child receive the medication by DOT, if possible. • School DOT 2 or 3 times/wk may be an option and may be indicated to reduce dose-related side effects.
Adolescent (12–18 y)	• Use a calendar to document adherence. • Involve the adolescent in decision making. • There is potential for poor adherence. • School DOT is an excellent option, if available.

DOT, direct observation therapy.
Adapted with permission from New Jersey Medical School Global Tuberculosis Institute. (2009). *Management of latent tuberculosis infections in children and adolescents: A guide for primary care providers*. Retrieved from http://globaltb.njms.rutgers.edu/downloads/products/PediatricGuidelines.pdf

about the age of 5 years (Passali et al., 2010). Higher respiratory rates create increased likelihood of an open airway when objects are in the mouth. Children like to run, talk, laugh, and play while chewing. This increases the likelihood of a sudden aspiration of food that is in the mouth.

In the United States, foreign body aspiration accounts for approximately 17,000 emergency room visits per year in children aged 14 years or younger. Foreign body aspiration is the third-most common cause of unintentional injury leading to death in children younger than 1 year of age. An estimated 2,900 deaths occur annually in United States as a result of foreign body aspiration (National Safety Council, 2015).

Clinical Presentation

The child who has aspirated a foreign body often presents with a sudden episode of coughing. Dyspnea, stridor, and hoarseness may be present because of decreased air entry due to the obstructing object (Patient Safety 20.8).

Assessment and Diagnosis

Diagnostic studies include radiography of the upper airway and chest. However, thin, plastic materials often do not show up on an X-ray. Rigid bronchoscopy is also used to visualize the airway and remove the foreign body.

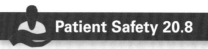

Patient Safety 20.8

Signs of Severe Respiratory Distress

A child who: (1) cannot speak, (2) is cyanotic, and (3) collapses is in severe respiratory distress and requires immediate attention. Without immediate airway intervention, the child can go into respiratory arrest and die within 4 min.

Therapeutic Interventions

For a child with a complete obstruction, perform back blows and chest thrusts to help remove the object (see the section Open and Maintain a Patent Airway). For a child with a partial obstruction, place in a position of comfort, usually sitting upright or in a semi-Fowler's position. Avoid any intervention that increases anxiety, because increased respiratory effort or sudden movements such as startling may cause the foreign body to move and cause further obstruction. Maintain a quiet environment and keep parents informed of any planned procedures or interventions. Following the removal of the foreign body, observe the child for respiratory complications such as stridor or increased work of breathing resulting from inflammation.

Evaluation

An expected outcome for a child with foreign body aspiration is as follows:

- Following removal of the foreign body or object, the child has spontaneous ventilations with bilateral breath sounds.
- Parents identify ways to prevent foreign body aspiration.

Discharge Planning and Teaching

Before discharge, teach parents how to prevent future incidences of foreign body aspiration. Encourage them to perform a detailed safety check of the home. Discuss with them common items associated with foreign body aspiration (Box 20.3). Primary care providers play a crucial role in helping parents prevent choking and foreign body aspiration through anticipatory guidance at each stage of development (Hayes & Chidekel, 2004).

Acute Respiratory Distress Syndrome

ARDS is an acute, diffuse inflammatory lung injury characterized by hypoxemia and stiff or noncompliant lungs. The hallmark sign of ARDS is hypoxemia that is unresponsive to increased oxygen delivery. Many children diagnosed with ARDS require care in the pediatric intensive care unit. Despite advances in modes of mechanical ventilation and a greater understanding of how to prevent lung damage in children receiving invasive ventilation, mortality rates remain high. The overall mortality rate in children from ARDS is approximately 24% (Wong et al., 2017).

Box 20.3 Common Items Associated with Foreign Body Aspiration

- Foods: nuts, seeds, popcorn, raw vegetables (e.g., carrots and celery), hot dogs, grapes, hard candy
- Household items: coins, safety pins, buttons, pieces of balloons, beads, disk batteries
- Toys: wheels, magnets, balls, marbles, caps off of markers or pens

Etiology and Pathophysiology

ARDS may be caused by direct injury to the lungs or indirect systemic insults that lead to lung injury. Direct causes of ARDS include pneumonia, aspiration of gastric contents, inhalation injury, pulmonary contusion, pulmonary vasculitis, and near-drowning events. Indirect causes include sepsis, major trauma, pancreatitis, severe burns, shock (noncardiogenic), drug overdose, multiple blood transfusions, and transfusion-related acute lung injury. Respiratory failure is a result of several common pathophysiologic changes that occur. In the early stages of ARDS, a proliferation of inflammatory mediators promotes neutrophil accumulation in the microcirculation of the lung. Neutrophils activate and then migrate in large numbers across the vascular endothelial and alveolar epithelial spaces. Proteases, cytokines, and reactive oxygen species are released. The migration of neutrophils and the release of mediators cause pathologic vascular permeability, open areas in the alveolar epithelial barrier, and necrosis of alveolar cells, all of which lead to pulmonary edema, hyaline membrane formation, loss of surfactant, and, ultimately, to decreased pulmonary compliance, making air exchange difficult. In later stages of ARDS, collagen deposition and fibrosis lead to worsening lung disease. Finally, as the lung recovers, multiple actions occur, including deactivation of neutrophils, reestablishment of the epithelial lining, and movement of fluid out of the alveoli and back into the pulmonary circulation (Fig. 20.7). Alveolar cells and macrophages remove protein compounds that block the alveoli, allowing oxygen to once again pass through the alveoli (Saguil & Fargo, 2012).

Clinical Presentation

Classic clinical signs of ARDS include hypoxemia, decreased lung compliance, and bilateral opacities on a chest radiograph. A child with ARDS initially appears tachypneic and tachycardic and has an increased work of breathing. O_2 saturation level is decreased, often despite an increase in oxygen delivery, and cyanosis may be present. Breath sounds are decreased bilaterally.

Assessment and Diagnosis

A complete and thorough respiratory assessment is warranted when caring for a child with ARDS, with particular focus on signs of hypoxia. Initially, the child is tachypneic and tachycardic with dyspnea, retractions, and use of accessory muscles. Auscultation of lung sounds may reveal normal lung sounds or fine, scattered crackles. Assess and monitor closely mental status and behavior for agitation and restlessness. As ARDS progresses and hypoxia worsens, the child may become lethargic and somnolent. The work of breathing increases, retractions worsen, color becomes pale or cyanotic, and, despite increased oxygen delivery, the child cannot maintain O_2 saturation levels above 90%.

Diagnostic studies and tests include assessment of arterial blood gases for decreased Pao_2, complete blood count (to assess white blood cell count, which may be elevated), and an electrolyte panel, as well as BUN and creatinine (for baseline

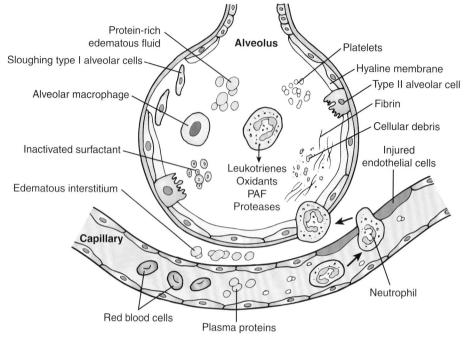

Figure 20.7. An alveolus injured by acute respiratory distress syndrome. PAF, platelet-activating factor. Reprinted with permission from Porth, C. M. (2015). *Essentials of pathophysiology: Concepts of altered health states* (4th ed., Fig. 22-11). Philadelphia, PA: Lippincott Williams & Wilkins.

renal function). Chest radiographs are essential in diagnosing ARDS. Findings may include atelectasis, infiltrates, and signs of pulmonary edema.

Therapeutic Interventions

Nursing management of the child with ARDS involves primarily supportive care. Children with ARDS are treated in the intensive care unit, because they are often intubated and mechanically ventilated as ARDS progresses. See the section Maintain Adequate Oxygenation, for interventions related to oxygenation.

Children with ARDS who are intubated and mechanically ventilated or who are receiving high levels of noninvasive positive pressure ventilation are at risk for decreased cardiac output and decreased perfusion. Administration of fluids to maintain cardiac output is often required in the care of a child with ARDS. Monitor heart rate and blood pressure frequently. Maintain blood pressure in the age-appropriate range. Monitor urine output, which is a key indicator of perfusion. This is because when perfusion to the kidney is decreased owing to decreased cardiac output, kidney function is decreased, reducing urine output. Mental status is also helpful in monitoring perfusion. A poorly perfused brain results in lethargy, alteration in mental status, and somnolence.

Medications often prescribed in the treatment of ARDS include antibiotics to treat infection, diuretics to reduce pulmonary fluid, and vasodilators to decrease pulmonary vascular resistance. Children who are diagnosed with ARDS are at high risk for kidney dysfunction and even kidney failure. Medications that affect kidney function should be adjusted accordingly. Gastric ulcer prophylaxis is initiated. Monitoring for side effects

of these medications is essential. See the section Maintain Adequate Hydration and Nutrition.

Evaluation

Expected outcomes for a child with ARDS include the following:
- The child is free from signs of respiratory distress.
- O_2 saturation levels are maintained at or above 92% throughout the illness.
- The child's oxygen requirement returns to baseline following resolution of ARDS.
- The child maintains adequate caloric intake throughout the illness.

Discharge Planning and Teaching

A child diagnosed with ARDS is often weak and may require oxygen at discharge. If oxygen is needed, educate the child and parents on oxygen safety and pulse oximetry monitoring. Encourage parents to provide opportunities for adequate rest, including naps, and to avoid activities that may overexert the child until activity levels return to baseline. Follow-up with the pediatrician or a pulmonary specialist is usually necessary to monitor pulmonary function. See the section Discharge Planning and Teaching for pneumonia for additional information related to discharge teaching.

Pneumothorax

A **pneumothorax** is an accumulation of air in the pleural space. Accumulating air between the visceral and parietal pleura increases intrapleural pressure, making it more difficult to expand the affected lung. Figure 20.8 shows a pneumothorax on the left side of the chest. As air accumulates in the pleural space, clinical

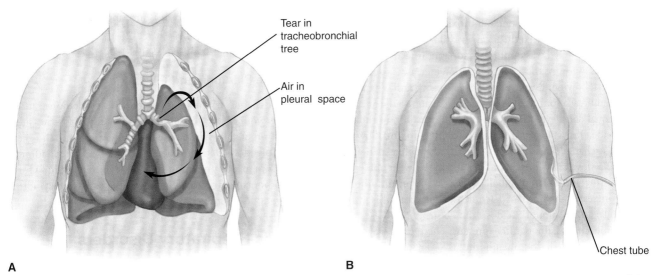

A   B

Figure 20.8. Pneumothorax on the left side of the chest. (A) Notice the air in the pleural space. **(B)** Note reinflation of the lung when the chest tube is present. Reprinted with permission from Kyle, T., & Carman, S. (2012). *Essentials of pediatric nursing* (2nd ed., Fig. 18.9). Philadelphia, PA: Wolters Kluwer.

manifestations appear. Notice that after the insertion of a chest tube to remove the air in the pleural space, the lung reexpands.

Etiology and Pathophysiology

The three major types of pneumothorax are spontaneous, traumatic, and tension. Primary spontaneous pneumothorax occurs in children with no history of lung disease, whereas secondary spontaneous pneumothorax occurs as a complication of chronic lung disease, such as BPD, CF, or asthma. Traumatic pneumothorax results from chest trauma. Penetrating chest trauma, such as a stabbing or gunshot wound, can lead to a pneumothorax. Blunt chest trauma, such as a fall or rib fractures, can also lead to a pneumothorax. A tension pneumothorax is a life-threatening emergency. Tension pneumothorax occurs when there is a rapid accumulation of air in the pleural space that results in severe hypoxia, difficulty in ventilation, and tracheal deviation, which may obstruct the airway. Furthermore, as pressure in the chest cavity increases, venous return to the heart decreases, ultimately leading to decreased cardiac output. A needle aspiration is the emergent treatment for a tension pneumothorax.

Pneumothorax, whether simple or complicated, is very common in pediatric blunt chest injuries (38% of injuries) and penetrating injuries (64% of injuries). The peak incidence in pneumothorax occurs in people aged 16 to 24 years. Even though the disorder is less common in children than in adults, newborns (both premature and full-term) have a relatively higher rate of pneumothorax, which declines during infancy. The highest risk group is premature newborns placed on mechanical ventilation.

Clinical Presentation

A child with a pneumothorax can present with a wide range of symptoms depending on the severity and origin of the air accumulation. Often, children with a small accumulation of air are asymptomatic, and the pneumothorax is only discovered as a result of an X-ray. Rapid breathing and short, shallow breaths

are classic signs in the initial phases of a pneumothorax. As air accumulates, children may become dyspneic, complain of chest and back pain, or have labored respirations, tachypnea, or tachycardia. O_2 saturation levels may be decreased, and hypotension can occur as the pneumothorax worsens. Figure 20.9 reveals a large pneumothorax on the right side.

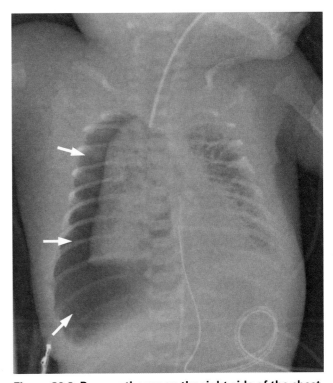

Figure 20.9. Pneumothorax on the right side of the chest. Notice that the lung is compressed by the accumulating air in the right pleural space (arrows). Reprinted with permission from Smith, W. L. (2013). *Radiology 101* (4th ed., Fig. 5.10). Philadelphia, PA: Wolters Kluwer.

Assessment and Diagnosis

Assessment of a child with pneumothorax varies depending on the severity of the air accumulation. A child with a small accumulation of air may be asymptomatic or appear tachypneic and have mild dyspnea. As the air accumulation increases, assessment reveals the following: dyspnea, tachypnea, tachycardia, hypoxia, diminished breath sounds, dullness on percussion to the affected side, unequal chest expansion, and tracheal deviation to the unaffected side. Tachypnea and shallow breathing do not allow for adequate exchange of gas to occur. Initially, the child experiences hypocarbia (low CO_2 levels), and if a blood gas were obtained, the analysis would reveal metabolic alkalosis. If a pneumothorax quickly increases in size or is left untreated, hypercarbia (high CO_2 levels) and respiratory acidosis can occur.

Pleuritic chest pain is often present; chest pain occurs in 95% of cases of pediatric pneumothorax (Gluckman & Forti, 2015). If the pneumothorax is a result of trauma, assessment should include exam of the chest wall for abrasions, bruises, and puncture wounds.

Diagnostic tools include a chest radiograph and an arterial blood gas test. A chest radiograph shows air accumulation and decreased lung volume on the affected side. An arterial blood gas test shows a decreased Pao_2.

Therapeutic Interventions

An immediate intervention for an open pneumothorax is covering the wound with an airtight seal, such as a gloved hand or a dressing (see the section Maintain Effective Ventilation). Place the child in a position of comfort. For children who are hyperventilating, encourage slow breathing, which helps optimize CO_2 levels.

Supplemental oxygen is often needed to maintain O_2 saturation levels within normal limits. The child initially has difficulty taking deep breaths, which prevents adequate air volume from entering the lungs, leading to hypoxia. After the insertion of a chest tube to remove the air in the pleural space, less supplemental oxygen may be needed as the lung reexpands (Fig. 20.8B). See the section Promote Pain Relief.

Make sure that safety equipment is readily available should the chest tube be accidently removed or become disconnected or dysfunctional. Place a pair of hemostats, a bottle of sterile water, petroleum jelly, gauze, and sterile gauze at the bedside. Position younger children in such a way they do not accidentally remove the chest tube. Use distraction, as well, to prevent them from removing the chest tube.

Explain to parents the purpose and function of equipment and monitoring devices used during hospitalization. Witnessing a child with a chest tube in place can increase anxiety in parents. Frequent reassurance and explanations regarding the chest tube can help alleviate anxiety.

Evaluation

Expected outcomes for a child with pneumothorax before the removal of the chest tube include the following:
- The child has equal breath sounds.
- O_2 saturation levels are within normal limits.
- The child is free of signs of respiratory distress.
- The child is without pain or is meeting the collaboratively established pain score goals.
- Safety equipment is at the bedside.

Discharge Planning and Teaching

Before discharge, parents should be able to demonstrate appropriate wound care for a chest wall incision (at the site of the chest tube). Instruct parents regarding the signs and symptoms of infection related to the incision. For a patient admitted with a spontaneous pneumothorax or who is at risk for a future pneumothorax, instruct parents regarding signs and symptoms that may appear if a pneumothorax should occur.

Chronic Respiratory Disorders

Asthma

Asthma is one of the most common chronic conditions of childhood. It is estimated that 8.7 million children aged 5 to 17 years have been diagnosed with asthma (American Lung Association, 2012). Asthma is characterized by chronic inflammation of the airways, intermittent bronchoconstriction, and increased mucus production. These three components of asthma contribute to remodeling of the airways, which is reversible with proper management and adherence to a treatment plan.

Etiology and Pathophysiology

Asthma is a multifaceted disease that can be characterized as a chronic inflammatory disorder of the airways. Bronchoconstriction, airway hyperresponsiveness, and airway edema are the pathophysiological processes that define asthma (Fig. 20.10). During bronchoconstriction, the bronchial smooth muscle contracts rapidly because of exposure to environmental triggers such as allergens or irritants, which narrows the airways and traps air in the lungs.

Airway hyperresponsiveness occurs as an exaggerated constriction of the bronchial smooth muscle in response to stimuli, further decreasing the diameter of the airways (Fig. 20.11). When a patient comes in contact with a trigger, the airways become inflamed, hypersecrete mucus, constrict, and develop bronchial edema, all leading to narrowed airways and obstruction of airflow.

As asthma becomes more persistent, the underlying inflammation causes edema of the airways and excess mucus production, further limiting airflow. This inflammatory process incorporates many different cell types and mediators within the airways. The inflammatory cells involved in asthma include the mast cells, eosinophils, neutrophils, lymphocytes, and macrophages. These cells have complex interactions with their mediators, leukotrienes, prostaglandins, interleukin, and platelet-activating factor to produce widespread and variable obstruction of airflow (Myers & Tomasio, 2011). This obstruction is often reversible with adherence to treatment.

Airway obstruction may not always fully reverse because of either disease severity or lack of compliance with treatment.

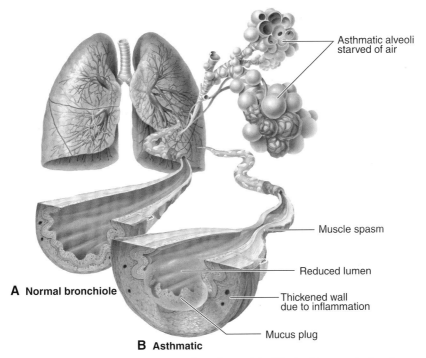

Asthmatic alveoli
starved of air

Muscle spasm

Reduced lumen

Thickened wall
due to inflammation

A Normal bronchiole

Mucus plug

B Asthmatic

Figure 20.10. **Pathophysiology of asthma.** Modified with permission from Anatomical Chart Company.

In this case, airway remodeling can occur. With remodeling, the epithelial lining of the airways becomes fibrotic, reducing lung compliance and further restricting air movement in the lungs. Hypersecretion of mucus, injury to the epithelial cells, and smooth muscle hypertrophy are other permanent changes that can occur (National Asthma Education and Prevention Program [NAEPP], 2007).

The causes of asthma appear to be the interaction of genetics and environment, and no one particular cause has yet been established. Current research in asthma pathophysiology and treatment is focusing on identifying asthma phenotypes. Focusing on phenotype characterization allows for more targeted and individualized treatment (Huffaker & Phipatanakul, 2015).

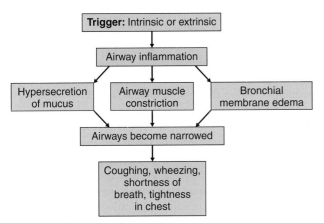

Figure 20.11. **The asthma pathway.**

Clinical Presentation

Remember Mollie in Chapter 2? Mollie was diagnosed with asthma at the age of 5 years after several episodes of wheezing and shortness of breath. What were her asthma triggers? What family history of asthma, if any, did Molly have? What event led her to be hospitalized for her asthma?

Asthma is a chronic condition that varies widely among children. The disease process can range from mild, with symptoms only appearing with certain triggers such as exercise, to severe, in which a child experiences daily symptoms. During an acute asthma exacerbation, the child experiences difficulty breathing, a tightness in the chest, and wheezing that is often audible without a stethoscope. The severity of asthma is determined on the basis of parameters such as frequency and severity of daytime symptoms, the frequency and severity of nighttime symptoms, and the frequency of use of short-acting beta-agonists. Figure 20.12 shows the classification of asthma severity and associated therapy levels. Figure 20.13 shows the different severity levels and the symptoms associated with each for children 12 years of age and older.

Asthma is most commonly treated in the ambulatory setting. A child being hospitalized with an acute asthma exacerbation indicates disease severity that requires a high level of assessment, monitoring, and care (Huffaker & Phipatanakul, 2015).

Components of Severity		Classifying Asthma Severity and Initiating Therapy in Children							
		Intermittent		Persistent					
				Mild		Moderate		Severe	
		Ages 0–4	Ages 5–11	Ages 0–4	Ages 5–11	Ages 0–4	Ages 5–11	Ages 0–4	Ages 5–11
Impairment	Symptoms	≤ 2 days/week		≤ 2 days/week but not daily		Daily		Throughout the day	
	Nighttime awakenings	0	< 2x/month	1-2x/month	3-4x/month	3-4x/month	>1x/week but not nightly	>1x/week	Often 7x/week
	Short-acting beta-agonist use for symptom control	≤ 2 days/week		≤ 2 days/week but not daily		Daily		Several times per day	
	Interference with normal activity	None		Minor limitation		Some limitation		Extremely limited	
	Lung Function • FEV₁ (predicted) or peak flow (personal best)	N/A	Normal FEV₁ between exacerbations > 80%	N/A	> 80%	N/A	60–80%	N/A	60%
	• FEV₁/FVC		> 85%		> 85%		75-80%		75%
Risk	Exacerbations requiring oral systemic corticosteroids (consider severity and interval since last exacerbation)	0-1/year (see notes)		≥ 2 exacerbations in 6 months requiring oral systemic corticosteroids, or ≥ 4 wheezing episodes/1 year lasting >1 day AND risk factors for persistent asthma	≥ 2x/year (see notes) Relative annual risk may be related to FEV₁				
Recommended Step for Initiating Therapy (See "Stepwise Approach for Managing Asthma" for treatment steps.) The stepwise approach is meant to assist, not replace, the clinical decision-making required to meet individual patient needs.		Step 1 (for both age groups)		Step 2 (for both age groups)		Step 3 and consider short course of oral systemic cortico steroids	Step 3: medium-dose ICS option and consider short course of oral systemic cortico-steroids	Step 3 and consider short course of oral systemic cortico steroids	Step 3: medium-dose ICS option OR step 4 and consider short course of oral systemic cortico-steroids

Key: FEV₁, forced expiratory volume in 1 second; FVC, forced vital capacity; ICS, inhaled corticosteroids; ICU, intensive care unit; N/A, not applicable

Notes:
• Level of severity is determined by both impairment and risk. Assess impairment domain by caregiver's recall of pervious 2–4 weeks. Assign severity to the most severe category in which any feature occurs.
• Frequency and severity of exacerbations may fluctuate over time for patients in any severity category. At present, there are inadequate data to correspond frequencies of exsacerbations with different levels of asthma severity. In general, more frequent and severe exacerbations (e.g., requiring urgent, unscheduled care, hospitalization, or ICU admission) indicate greater underlying disease severity. For treatment purposes, patients with ≥2 exacerbations described may be considered the same as patients who have persistent asthma, even in the absence of impairment levels consistent with persistent asthma.

In 2-6 weeks, depending on severity, evaluate level of asthma control that is achieved.
• Children 0-4 years old: If no clear benefit is observed in 4-6 weeks, stop treatment and consider alternative diagnoses or adjusting therapy.
• Children 5-11 years old: Adjust therapy accordingly.

Figure 20.12. Components of asthma severity: Impairment and risk. Asthma can be classified as intermittent or persistent. If persistent, a subclassification of mild, moderate, or severe is then determined. FEV, forced expiratory flow; FVC, forced vital capacity, ICS, inhaled corticosteroids; ICU, intensive care unit. Reprinted with permission from Arcangelo, V. P., & Peterson, A. M. (2011). *Pharmacotherapeutics for advanced practice* (3rd ed., Fig. 25.2). Philadelphia, PA: Wolters Kluwer.

Assessment and Diagnosis

The diagnosis of asthma is made on the basis of three key features: a detailed health history, physical assessment, and pulmonary function testing such as spirometry. The health history should include questions pertaining to the presence of wheezing and a history of cough or chest tightness. A health history that reveals symptoms that are worse in the presence of viral illness, exercise, change in weather, or environmental allergens or irritants or those that are worse at night is generally associated with the diagnosis of asthma (NAEPP, 2007). Spirometry is an objective measure of lung function that measures forced expiratory volume in 1 second, or the amount of air that can be forcefully exhaled in 1 second. This objective measure is essential to the diagnosis of asthma (NAEPP, 2007).

Assessment of the child with asthma should focus on respiratory effort, wheezing, use of accessory muscles, and oxygenation (Patient Safety 20.9). Pay attention to the child's mental status as an indication of oxygenation. Note the child's color and the condition of the skin. A child of any age hospitalized with an acute asthma exacerbation should be placed on a cardiorespiratory monitor with continuous pulse oximetry measurement. Position the child in a semi-Fowler's to a high Fowler's position to maximize respiratory effort.

Therapeutic Interventions

Patients hospitalized with acute asthma exacerbations are generally treated with a nebulized short-acting beta-agonist and an

IV corticosteroid such as methylprednisolone (The Pharmacy 20.5 and Whose Job Is It, Anyway? 20.1). Inhaled corticosteroids are not effective for acute exacerbations because of their delayed onset of action. In moderate asthma exacerbations, oral corticosteroids may be used (Myers & Tomasio, 2011).

Ensure that respiratory treatments and corticosteroids are administered as ordered. Monitor the child's respiratory status for improvements in lung sounds and respiratory effort. Monitor for tachypnea, chest pain, discomfort, and tachycardia not associated with medication use. Provide oxygen via nasal cannula or face mask to maintain O_2 saturation levels at 92% or above. See the section Maintain Adequate Hydration and Nutrition.

Patients with increased work of breathing have activity intolerance, as indicated by the need for frequent rest periods. Group nursing interventions should ensure adequate time for rest for the child. Provide activities that do not require much energy expenditure. Allow the child to increase activity as tolerated.

Asthma is a chronic condition that can have significant impact on the child and family (see the section Provide Emotional and Psychosocial Support to the Child and Parents). The child will need support in managing asthma care and understanding proper medication use. Assess whether the family needs help with eliminating environmental triggers in the home. Families may need support in obtaining medications and supplies such as a nebulizer machine or a peak flow meter. Refer families to a social worker as needed to help them find resources to care for their child's asthma (Whose Job Is It, Anyway? 20.2). Proper

Components of Severity		Classification of Asthma Severity ≥12 years of age			
			Persistent		
		Intermittent	Mild	Moderate	Severe
Impairment Normal FEV₁/FVC: 8–19 y 85% 20–39 y 80% 40–59 y 75% 60–80 y 70%	Symptoms	2 days/week	>2 days/week but not daily	Daily	Throughout the day
	Nighttime awakenings	2x/month	3–4x/month	>1x/week but not nightly	Often 7x/week
	Short-acting beta₂-agonist use for symptom control (not prevention of EIB)	2 days/week	>2 days/week but not daily, and not more than 1x on any day	Daily	Several times per day
	Interference with normal activity	None	Minor limitation	Some limitation	Extremely limited
	Lung function	• Normal FEV₁ between exacerbations • FEV₁ >80% predicted • FEV₁/FCC normal	• FEV₁ >80% predicted • FEV₁/FVC normal	• FEV₁, >60% but <80% predicted • FEV₁/FVC reduced 5%	• FEV₁ <60% predicted • FEV₁/FVC reduced >5%
Risk	Exacerbations requiring oral systemic corticosteroids	0–1/year (see note)	2/year (see note) ⟶		
		Consider severity and interval since last exacerbation. Frequency and severity may fluctuate over time for patients in any severity category. Relative annual risk of exacerbations may be related to FEV₁.			
Recommended Step for Initiating Treatment		Step 1	Step 2	Step 3 and consider short course of oral systemic corticosteroids	Step 4 or 5
(See figure 15-1 for treatment steps.)		In 2–6 weeks, evaluate level of asthma control that is achieved and adjust therapy accordingly.			

Figure 20.13. Classification of asthma severity in children 12 years or older. Note the similarity with that for younger children, except that here impairment includes specific peak flow values (forced expiratory flow/forced vital capacity [FEV₁/FVC]). EIB, exercise-induced bronchoconstriction. Reprinted with permission from Young, V., Kormos, W., & Chick, D. (2015). *Blueprints medicine* (6th ed., Fig. 15.2). Philadelphia, PA: Wolters Kluwer.

care at home with the proper resources helps reduce readmission for asthma exacerbations (Chung, Hathaway, & Lew, 2015).

Evaluation

Expected outcomes for a child hospitalized with an acute asthma exacerbation include the following:
- Lungs are clear to auscultation bilaterally.
- O₂ saturation level is 92% or above on room air.
- Vital signs are within normal limits for age.
- The child is able to maintain adequate respiratory function without repeated treatment with a short-acting beta-agonist.

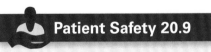

Patient Safety 20.9

Acute Asthma Exacerbation

In a child hospitalized with an acute asthma exacerbation, decreased wheezing does not necessarily indicate that the child's condition is improving. In fact, decreased wheezing may indicate lack of any air movement. Listen closely to determine whether the child has improved lung sounds or absent lung sounds. Perform a rapid focused respiratory assessment to fully determine the child's respiratory status.

- The family verbalizes understanding of medication use.
- The family verbalizes about being able to obtain proper medications and medical equipment.
- The family verbalizes that asthma is a chronic condition and that adherence to treatment is important in maintaining the child's lung function.

Discharge Planning and Teaching

The overarching goal of asthma treatment is to control asthma symptoms so that the child can go to school and participate in any activity he or she wants to. Asthma treatment involves medication, control of triggers, and education. All members of the family should be involved in education regarding the child's asthma treatment.

Begin discharge planning for the child hospitalized with an acute asthma exacerbation as soon as the child is stabilized. Education of the child and family is crucial to the child maintaining lung function and participating in desired activities. If thorough teaching cannot be completed in the inpatient setting, then it should be continued at the follow-up visit with either the primary care provider or the asthma specialist. A follow-up appointment should be made for 2 to 3 days after hospital discharge.

Topics to cover in discharge teaching include lifestyle factors affecting asthma outcomes, identification of asthma triggers, proper use of medications and medication devices, and use of a peak flow meter.

The Pharmacy 20.5 **Medications Used to Treat Asthma**

Medication Classification/Route	Action	Nursing Considerations
Bronchodilators: albuterol (Ventolin, ProAir, Proventil) Beta2-agonist—short acting Metered-dose inhaler Nebulizer	• Decreases airway resistance • Dilates the lower airways • Increases expiratory flow in the smaller airways	• Monitor heart rate for tachycardia. • May make patient shaky after use • Monitor for signs of toxicity.
Corticosteroids Methylprednisolone Prednisone Anti-inflammatory IV IM PO	• Reduces inflammation in the airways • Decreases obstruction in the airways • Enhances bronchodilating effects of beta2-agonists	• Monitor for increase in blood pressure. • Monitor weight with long-term use. • Monitor electrolytes. • Monitor serum glucose. • Monitor growth in long term use. • Monitor for signs/symptoms of infection with long-term use
Montelukast (Singulair) Leukotriene receptor antagonist PO (chewable, granules and tablets)	• Reduces inflammation process responsive for airway inflammation • Improves lung function • Decreases need for quick relief medications such as albuterol	• Administer in the evening. • May be given with or without food • Chewable tablets should be chewed, not swallowed whole. • Do not mix medication in liquid. • Granules may be mixed in applesauce or ice cream.
Salmeterol, formoterol Beta2-agonist—long acting Inhalation Nebulizer	• Relaxes smooth muscle in the airways • Prevents exercise-induced bronchospasm	• May be used to reduce nocturnal symptoms • Clinical data is for children ≥12 y old • Not studied in children < 4 y old
Beclomethasone, budesonide, flunisolide, fluticasone, mometasone, triamcinolone Anti-inflammatory Metered-dose inhaler Nebulizer Dry powder inhaler	• Decreased airway inflammation by inhibiting inflammatory mediators such as histamine, leukotriene and cytokines • Decreased inflammation reduces mucosal edema, secretions, and bronchoconstriction • Increases mucociliary action, promotes mobilization of mucus	• Do not abruptly stop taking medication. • Ineffective in acute bronchospasm; not used as a rescue inhaler
Theophylline Oral May be given IV in status asthmaticus	• Relaxes muscles that constrict airways • Dilates airways • Sustained release for prevention of nocturnal symptoms	• Do not crush or chew tablets. • Therapeutic level: 10–20 µg/L • Give at same time each day. • Avoid/limit caffeine intake. • Monitor for side effects: tachycardia, dysrhythmias, hypotension, tremors, restlessness, insomnia, severe headaches, vomiting diarrhea, seizures. • Serum levels must be monitored and dose adjusted for weight changes and therapeutic levels.

The Pharmacy 20.5 Medications Used to Treat Asthma (*continued*)

Medication Classification/Route	Action	Nursing Considerations
Omalizumab (Xolair) Monoclonal antibody Subcutaneous	• Used in moderate-to-severe allergic asthma not controlled with inhaled steroids • Inhibits immunoglobulin E from binding to the mast cells and basophils • Results in limited allergic response	• The injection is viscous and takes 5–10 s to administer. • Patients must be monitored for 2 h after each dose.
Mepolizumab (Nucala) Monoclonal antibody Subcutaneous	• Used in moderate-to-severe allergic asthma not controlled with inhaled steroids • Binds to and interferes with inter-leukin-5 cytokine • Reduces eosinophil production and survival	• Monitor for hypersensitivity reactions after injection. • Do not use for acute asthma exacerbation.

From Lexicomp. *Pediatric & Neonatal Dosage Handbook* (25th ed.), 2018.
IM, intramuscular; IV, intravenous; PO, by mouth.

 Whose Job Is It, Anyway? 20.1

Respiratory Therapist

In the hospital, patients with asthma receive respiratory treatments of nebulized short-acting beta-agonists. Patients in the intensive care unit may be on a continuous nebulizer. The respiratory therapist works with the healthcare team to provide these treatments and monitor the patient's overall respiratory status. The respiratory therapist assesses the patient before and after each treatment and monitors the response of each treatment.

 Whose Job Is It, Anyway? 20.2

Social Worker

Some families lack access to necessary resources to care for their child. Having a child with a chronic condition can put a significant burden on these already limited resources. Social workers are able to help families acquire medical equipment and medications. A medical home–based primary care provider would be ideal for many families of children with asthma. A social worker can help families explore options for a medical home. In addition, social workers may be able to help families reduce environmental asthma triggers in the home. A social worker can help reinforce asthma education and is an important member of the healthcare team, especially for families in need of resources such as assistance with obtaining medications and equipment due to the financial burden the costs often place on families.

Lifestyle Factors

Recent research has shown that poor control of asthma in childhood increases morbidity as the child transitions into adulthood (Bass, 2016). Many lifestyle factors can contribute to the severity of a child's asthma, including weight. Children who are overweight are more likely to have poor asthma control and increased risk for severe asthma exacerbations (Chen et al., 2014). Therefore, educating families about healthy lifestyles and healthy diets could have an impact on the child's morbidity. Counsel overweight children on healthy physical activity and need for weight loss as ways to control their asthma.

Identification of Asthma Triggers

Many different factors, both environmental and nonenvironmental, can trigger an asthma exacerbation. See Box 20.4 for a list of possible triggers.

Box 20.4 Examples of Asthma Triggers

Environmental Triggers
• Seasonal allergens
• Mold
• Pollen
• Tobacco smoke
• Pet dander
• Dust mites
• Cockroach droppings

Nonenvironmental Triggers
• Exercise
• Stress or anxiety
• Respiratory illness
• Gastroesophageal reflux

STEPWISE APPROACH FOR MANAGING ASTHMA LONG TERM

The stepwise approach tailors the selection of medication to the level of asthma severity (see page 5) or asthma control (see page 6). The stepwise approach is meant to help, not replace, the clinical decisionmaking needed to meet individual patient needs.

ASSESS CONTROL:

STEP UP IF NEEDED (first, check medication adherence, inhaler technique, environmental control, and comorbidities)

STEP DOWN IF POSSIBLE (and asthma is well controlled for at least 3 months)

		STEP 1	STEP 2	STEP 3	STEP 4	STEP 5	STEP 6
		**At each step:** Patient education, environmental control, and management of comorbidities						

0–4 years of age

	Intermittent Asthma	Persistent Asthma: Daily Medication — Consult with asthma specialist if step 3 care or higher is required. Consider consultation at step 2.				
Preferred Treatment[†]	SABA* as needed	low-dose ICS*	medium-dose ICS*	medium-dose ICS* + either LABA* or montelukast	high-dose ICS* + either LABA* or montelukast	high-dose ICS* + either LABA* or montelukast + oral corticosteroids
Alternative Treatment[†,‡]		cromolyn or montelukast				

If clear benefit is not observed in 4–6 weeks, and medication technique and adherence are satisfactory, consider adjusting therapy or alternate diagnoses.

Quick-Relief Medication	■ SABA* as needed for symptoms; intensity of treatment depends on severity of symptoms. ■ With viral respiratory symptoms: SABA every 4–6 hours up to 24 hours (longer with physician consult). Consider short course of oral systemic corticosteroids if asthma exacerbation is severe or patient has history of severe exacerbations. ■ Caution: Frequent use of SABA may indicate the need to step up treatment.

5–11 years of age

	Intermittent Asthma	Persistent Asthma: Daily Medication — Consult with asthma specialist if step 4 care or higher is required. Consider consultation at step 3.				
Preferred Treatment[†]	SABA* as needed	low-dose ICS*	low-dose ICS* + either LABA,* LTRA,* or theophylline(b) OR medium-dose ICS	medium-dose ICS* + LABA*	high-dose ICS* + LABA*	high-dose ICS* + LABA* + oral corticosteroids
Alternative Treatment[†,‡]		cromolyn, LTRA,* or theophylline[§]		medium-dose ICS* + either LTRA* or theophylline[§]	high-dose ICS* + either LTRA* or theophylline[§]	high-dose ICS* + either LTRA* or theophylline[§] + oral corticosteroids

Consider subcutaneous allergen immunotherapy for patients who have persistent, allergic asthma.**

Quick-Relief Medication	■ SABA* as needed for symptoms. The intensity of treatment depends on severity of symptoms: up to 3 treatments every 20 minutes as needed. Short course of oral systemic corticosteroids may be needed. ■ Caution: Increasing use of SABA or use >2 days/week for symptom relief (not to prevent EIB*) generally indicates inadequate control and the need to step up treatment.

≥12 years of age

	Intermittent Asthma	Persistent Asthma: Daily Medication — Consult with asthma specialist if step 4 care or higher is required. Consider consultation at step 3.				
Preferred Treatment[†]	SABA* as needed	low-dose ICS*	low-dose ICS* + LABA* OR medium-dose ICS*	medium-dose ICS* + LABA*	high-dose ICS* + LABA* AND consider omalizumab for patients who have allergies[††]	high-dose ICS* + LABA* + oral corticosteroid[§§] AND consider omalizumab for patients who have allergies[††]
Alternative Treatment[†,‡]		cromolyn, LTRA,* or theophylline[§]	low-dose ICS* + either LTRA,* theophylline,[§] or zileuton[‡‡]	medium-dose ICS* + either LTRA,* theophylline,[§] or zileuton[‡‡]		

Consider subcutaneous allergen immunotherapy for patients who have persistent, allergic asthma.**

Quick-Relief Medication	■ SABA* as needed for symptoms. The intensity of treatment depends on severity of symptoms: up to 3 treatments every 20 minutes as needed. Short course of oral systemic corticosteroids may be needed. ■ Caution: Use of SABA >2 days/week for symptom relief (not to prevent EIB*) generally indicates inadequate control and the need to step up treatment.

* **Abbreviations:** EIB, exercise-induced bronchospasm; ICS, inhaled corticosteroid; LABA, inhaled long-acting beta₂-agonist; LTRA, leukotriene receptor antagonist; SABA, inhaled short-acting beta₂-agonist.
[†] Treatment options are listed in alphabetical order, if more than one.
[‡] If alternative treatment is used and response is inadequate, discontinue and use preferred treatment before stepping up.
[§] Theophylline is a less desirable alternative because of the need to monitor serum concentration levels.
** Based on evidence for dust mites, animal dander, and pollen; evidence is weak or lacking for molds and cockroaches. Evidence is strongest for immunotherapy with single allergens. The role of allergy in asthma is greater in children than in adults.
[††] Clinicians who administer immunotherapy or omalizumab should be prepared to treat anaphylaxis that may occur.
[‡‡] Zileuton is less desirable because of limited studies as adjunctive therapy and the need to monitor liver function.
[§§] Before oral corticosteroids are introduced, a trial of high-dose ICS + LABA + either LTRA, theophylline, or zileuton, may be considered, although this approach has not been studied in clinical trials.

Figure 20.14. Stepwise approach for managing asthma long term. From the National Heart, Lung, and Blood Institute (NHLBI). (2012). *Asthma care quick reference: Diagnosing and managing asthma* (p. 7). Retrieved from https://www.nhlbi.nih.gov/files/docs/guidelines/asthma_qrg.pdf

Teach children and families to determine which triggers affect them and how to avoid or control these triggers, once identified. Common interventions include frequent vacuuming of carpet, covers for mattresses and pillows, avoidance of secondhand smoke, and avoidance of pets. Children who have seasonal allergies or pollen as a trigger may be prescribed antihistamines to help prevent asthma exacerbations. For those with exercise-induced asthma, treatment with a short-acting beta-agonist 30 minutes before exercise is required.

Proper Use of Medications, Inhalers, and Nebulizers

The types of medications used are determined by the severity of the child's asthma, using a stepwise approach (Fig. 20.14).

Educate children and their families on the different types of medications that they will be using in the management of asthma. Understanding when and why the medication is used can help both the child and family control asthma symptoms.

Short-acting beta-agonists are used as a "rescue" medication, when a child is experiencing signs and symptoms of respiratory distress such as wheezing and difficulty breathing. Ideally, the child should not use this medication more than twice in 1 week; more frequent use may indicate that the child's asthma is not well controlled.

Inhaled corticosteroids are "controller" or "maintenance" medications, meaning they are used on a daily basis even if the child is not experiencing any symptoms. Their purpose is to control the underlying inflammation associated with asthma. Emphasize to the child and family that the controller medication should be taken every day, even if the child feels fine.

Additional medications may be added to the child's therapeutic regimen if asthma is not well controlled with short-acting beta-agonists and inhaled corticosteroids. New medications, monoclonal antibodies, continue to be studied for children older than age 12 years with severe asthma (Bass, 2016). Refer to The Pharmacy 20.5 for additional medications that may be used.

In addition to the medications used in asthma treatment, teach children and families about various aerosol delivery devices, depending on the age. These delivery devices may include nebulizers, spacers, and metered-dose inhalers (Patient Teaching 20.1). Figures 20.15 and 20.16 show the different aerosol delivery devices used in asthma treatment. Aerosol delivery devices are selected on the basis of the child's age, and each has specific instructions for use. See Table 20.13 for instructions for use and the age range for each aerosol delivery device.

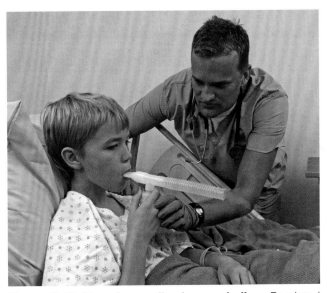

Figure 20.15. Use of a small-volume nebulizer. Reprinted with permission from Lynn, P. (2010). *Taylor's clinical nursing skills: A nursing process approach* (3rd ed., Fig. 3 in Skill 5-24). Philadelphia, PA: Lippincott Williams & Wilkins.

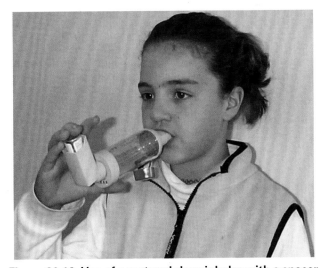

Figure 20.16. Use of a metered-dose inhaler with a spacer. Reprinted with permission from Pillitteri, A. (2013). *Maternal and child health nursing* (7th ed., Fig. 40.11B). Philadelphia, PA: Lippincott Williams & Wilkins.

Use of a Peak Flow Meter

A peak flow meter measures the amount of air forcefully exhaled in one breath. Figure 20.17 shows a peak flow meter. This device is useful for determining the degree to which a child's asthma is under control. Obtain a baseline reading while the child is not experiencing any symptoms, and then compare future readings with it to determine whether and to what degree the asthma is getting worse. A reading that is lower than a child's best indicates increased risk for an acute asthma exacerbation. Children on controller medications should ideally use the peak flow meter once a day to monitor their asthma (Patient Teaching 20.2).

✚ Patient Teaching 20.1

Use of a Nebulizer

Using a nebulizer can often be a struggle with a toddler or preschool child. Put stickers on the mask to make the experience more fun. Distract the child by reading, watching television, or playing a game.

Table 20.13   Aerosol Delivery Devices

Device/Drugs	Age for Use	Technique	Nursing Considerations
Metered-dose inhaler (MDI) • Beta-2 agonists • Corticosteroids • Cromolyn sodium • Anticholinergics	• ≥5 y • <5 y with a spacer	Actuate the MDI during a slow deep inhalation, followed by 10 s of holding breath.	Slow inhalation and coordination of actuation during inhalation may be difficult, particularly in young children. To ensure adequate delivery use a spacer with all ages.
Dry powder inhaler (DPI) • Beta-2 agonists • Corticosteroids • Anticholinergics	≥4 y	Rapid, deep inhalation. Most children <4 y of age do not generate sufficient inspiratory flow to activate the inhaler.	Dose is lost if patient exhales through device after actuating.
Spacer or valved holding chamber (VHC)	• ≥4 y • <4 y (VHC with a face mask)	• Slow deep inhalation, followed by holding breath for 10 s immediately following actuation • Actuate only once into spacer/VHC per inhalation. • If a face mask is used, it should have a tight fit and allow 3–5 inhalations per actuation.	• Indicated for patients who have difficulty performing adequate MDI technique • Spacers and/or VHCs decrease oropharyngeal deposition and thus decrease the risk of topical side effects (e.g., thrush). • It is as effective as a nebulizer for delivering short-acting beta-agonists (SABAs) and anticholinergics in mild-to-moderate exacerbations.
Nebulizer Beta-2 agonists • Corticosteroids • Cromolyn sodium • Anticholinergics	Patients of any age who cannot use an MDI with VHC and a face mask	• Slow tidal breathing with occasional deep breaths. Use a tightly fitting face mask for those unable to use a mouthpiece. • Using the "blow by" technique (i.e., holding the mask or open tube near the infant's nose and mouth) is not appropriate.	• Less dependent on patient's coordination and cooperation • May be expensive; time consuming; bulky • Potential for bacterial infections if not cleaned properly

Adapted from The National Asthma Education and Prevention Program. (2007). Expert panel report 3: Guidelines for the diagnosis and management of asthma (NIH Publication No. 07–4051). Bethesda, MD: National Institutes of Health, National Heart, Lung and Blood Institute.

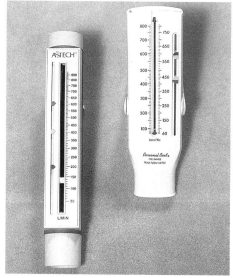

Figure 20.17. Peak flow meters. Reprinted with permission from Jones, R. M., & Rospond, R. M. (2008). *Patient assessment in pharmacy practice* (2nd ed., Fig. 11.12). Philadelphia, PA: Wolters Kluwer.

Each child diagnosed with asthma should have an asthma action plan (Box 20.5). The Asthma Action Plan form developed by the Asthma and Allergy Foundation of America (Fig. 2.2) is color coded such that the color of each specific action plan corresponds to a color on the peak flow meter markers. This form gives instructions as to how the child and parents should adjust the medications to try to prevent an acute asthma attack depending on whether the peak flow reading is in the red, yellow, or green zone (Fig. 2.2). Children not old enough to use a peak flow meter (younger than age 5 years) should have an asthma action plan, as well (Growth and Development Checks 20.3 and 20.4). However, the plan for younger children is based on symptoms alone.

Mollie in Chapter 2 had an asthma action plan. How did Mollie and her mother use the plan? How did the nurse at Mollie's school use the plan?

Patient Teaching 20.2

Using a Peak Flow Meter

A peak flow meter is used for baseline measurement when a child is symptom free. Instruct the child to do the following:

- Make sure the marker is at "0."
- Stand up straight.
- Take a deep breath.
- Close your mouth around the mouthpiece.
- Blow out as hard and quickly as possible.
- Note the number where the marker is and write it down.
- Repeat three times and record the highest number as the baseline reading.
- Use daily to determine asthma control.

Adapted from American Lung Association. (2016). *Measuring your peak flow rate.* Retrieved from http://www.lung.org/lung-health-and-diseases/lung-disease-lookup/asthma/living-with-asthma/managing-asthma/measuring-your-peak-flow-rate.html

Growth and Development Check 20.3

Peak Flow Measurement

Peak flow measurement is not used for children younger than 5 y of age because they have a hard time following the instructions for obtaining a reading owing to their stage of cognitive development. You may be instructing the child to blow as hard as the child can, but the child may actually inhale. One way to instruct children to exhale forcefully is to have them pretend they are blowing out candles on a birthday cake.

Box 20.5 Instructions Included with an Asthma Action Plan

- If the child's peak flow reading is in the GREEN zone or the child is not having symptoms, continue daily and/or as needed medications as prescribed.
- If the child's peak flow reading is in the YELLOW zone or the child has any of the symptoms listed on the action plan, increase or change medications as written by the healthcare provider. See the healthcare provider as instructed.
- If the child's peak flow reading or symptoms are in the RED zone, SEEK EMERGENCY TREATMENT IMMEDIATELY.

Cystic Fibrosis

Cystic fibrosis is a complex genetic disease affecting many organs. Simplistically, and often how the disease can be introduced to parents and children, CF is characterized by an abnormality in the body's salt, water, and mucus-making cells. It is an autosomal recessive disorder, meaning a person must have both copies of the abnormal gene to experience manifestations (Fig. 20.18). A person who only has one copy of the abnormal gene, known as a carrier, experiences no manifestations of the disease. An estimated 1 in 31 people in the United States are carriers of the CF gene. According to the Cystic Fibrosis Foundation 2015 Registry Report, the predicted median age of survival for patients with CF in the United States was 41.7 years. In 2015, approximately 65% of patients with CF in the United States who died, did so from respiratory and cardiorespiratory causes (Cystic Fibrosis Foundation, 2016).

Growth and Development Check 20.4 Developmental Stage and Asthma Care

It is important to remember the child's age when involving the child in asthma care. Think about Erikson's and Piaget's developmental stages when planning teaching.

Age	Developmental Stage	Teaching Strategies
Preschool	• Initiative vs. guilt • Preoperational	• Allow the child to play with empty aerosol delivery devices. • Include simple pictures in explanations. • Allow choices in when medication is taken.
School age	• Industry vs. inferiority • Concrete operational	• Provide a simple explanation of the disease process. • Explain how aerosol delivery devices work. • Involve the child in ways to avoid triggers. • Have the child breathe through a coffee straw and then a soda straw to demonstrate how the medications work.
Adolescence	• Identity vs. role confusion • Formal operational	• Involve the child in all aspects of care. • Provide detailed explanations of how asthma affects the lungs and long-term implications. • Explain how the medications work. • Have the child talk with other teenagers who have asthma. • Acknowledge that it is difficult to deal with a chronic illness but reiterate that with adherence to treatment the child can participate in all activities.

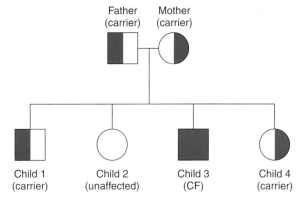

Figure 20.18. Family history genogram representing a mother and father who are both carriers of the cystic fibrosis (CF) defective gene. Child 1 and child 4 are carriers and asymptomatic. Child 2 is not a carrier and is unaffected. Child 3 has CF as a result of inheriting both copies of the defective gene from the parents.

CF affects the body from head to toe. The sinuses, lungs, skin, liver, pancreas, intestines, and reproductive organs can all be impacted by CF (Fig. 20.19). Thick, sticky mucus builds up in the sinuses and lungs. Salty sweat glands produce salty sweat. The pancreas and liver become blocked, leading to pancreas and liver dysfunction and obstructed bile ducts. Because the intestines cannot fully absorb nutrients, children with CF have constipation and abnormal stool patterns and stool composition. Infections are common, particularly in the sinuses and lungs.

Etiology and Pathophysiology

The gene associated with CF is the CF transmembrane conductance regulator protein, *CFTR*. Dysfunction of *CFTR*, the primary defect in CF, leads to a wide array of manifestations and complications. More than 1,000 changes can occur in *CFTR*, but the majority of people in North America with CF (70%) have the same defect: a gene mutation of delta F508. There are many less common mutations of the CF gene, which may cause milder symptoms. *CFTR* is commonly expressed in epithelial cells of the airways, the gastrointestinal tract (including the pancreas and biliary system), the sweat glands, and the genitourinary system.

Median age of diagnosis is 6 to 8 months, with most children being diagnosed by 1 year of age. CF occurs most frequently in white populations of North America, Northern Europe, Australia, and New Zealand. The prevalence is approximately 1 in 3,500 live births in these populations, compared with 1 in 9,200 of Hispanic descent and 1 in 15,000 of African American descent. In the United States, approximately 93% of those diagnosed with CF are white (Cystic Fibrosis Foundation, 2016).

As a result of the defective *CFTR* protein, chloride ion transport across exocrine and epithelial cell membranes is impaired and sodium absorption reduces water movement across cell membranes. Body secretions such as mucus in the airways and other secretions in the sweat ducts, pancreatic duct, intestine, biliary tree, cervix, vagina, and vas deferens become thickened. Lungs become obstructed with mucus, which leads to infection. The pancreas becomes obstructed and the flow of natural enzymes is stopped, leading to progressive pancreatic damage. Distal ileal bowel obstruction also occurs because of increased viscosity of intestinal mucus and prolonged intestinal transit time (Van der Doef, Kokke, van der Ent, & Houwen, 2011). Infertility results from thickening of secretions in the reproductive organs.

Insufficiency of the exocrine pancreas is present at birth in about two-thirds of patients with CF. By the age of 1 year, most

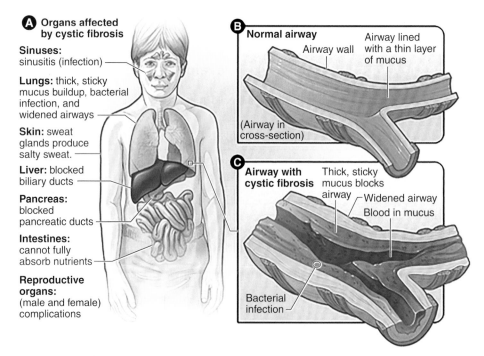

Figure 20.19. Effect of cystic fibrosis on body systems. Adapted from National Heart, Lung, and Blood Institute; National Institutes of Health; U.S. Department of Health and Human Services. (n.d.). *Cystic fibrosis.* Retrieved from https://www.nhlbi.nih.gov/health-topics/cystic-fibrosis

patients with CF have fat malabsorption. Recall that the function of the exocrine glands of the pancreas is to produce enzymes that help in the digestion of food. Patients with CF have fat malabsorption because the pancreas fails to make and release these necessary enzymes.

Clinical Presentation

The clinical presentation of a child with CF varies depending on the severity of the disease and which systems are affected. Initially, parents notice that their baby's skin tastes salty and that the infant does not pass stool normally soon after birth. The child presents with respiratory symptoms such as tachypnea, retractions, wheezing, recurrent pneumonia, dyspnea on exertion, and chest pain (in older children). Gastrointestinal complaints include abdominal distension, increased frequency of stools, meconium ileus, flatulence, foul-smelling bulky stools (**steatorrhea**), failure to thrive despite an increased appetite, jaundice, and gastrointestinal bleeding. Table 20.14 reviews by system the manifestations of CF.

Assessment and Diagnosis

Assessment involves identifying symptoms associated with CF, as described earlier. Also, young infants often present to the provider's office with symptoms of a respiratory virus or pneumonia one or more times before diagnosis. When caring for newborns and young infants, be astute to the clinical characteristics of CF, particularly in the first 6 months of life, when the majority of patients with CF are diagnosed. Newborn screenings for CF are mandatory in all 50 states and have led to an increased number of CF diagnoses before symptoms occur. In 2015, 59.6% of newly diagnosed CF patients were detected by newborn screening (Cystic Fibrosis Foundation, 2016). Diagnosis in the newborn period provides opportunities for children to begin treatment for CF early and can help parents learn ways to keep their child as healthy as possible during the early years.

Diagnosis is confirmed with several tests. The first, the sweat chloride test, involves collecting sweat and performing a chemical analysis of its chloride content. Sweat chloride tests are the standard approach to diagnosing CF. The presence of more than 60 mEq/L of chloride in sweat is diagnostic of CF when one or more other criteria are present. Exocrine pancreatic dysfunction, although clinically apparent in many children, can be assessed by measuring the fat balances in a 3-day stool collection. Another, simpler test, the quantification of elastase-1 activity in a fresh stool sample, can also indicate exocrine pancreatic dysfunction.

Table 20.14 Clinical Presentation of Cystic Fibrosis

System	Pathophysiology	Clinical Presentation
Respiratory	Upper respiratory tract: thickened mucus obstructs sinuses. Lower respiratory tract: thickened mucus obstructs the airways, reduces ciliary clearance; lungs become hyperinflated from air trapping which allows bacteria to remain in lungs and colonize. Long term: fibrotic changes occur in the lung tissue.	Cough; dry and hacking at first; then loose and productive Expectorated mucus is usually purulent. Extensive bronchiolitis with wheezing during the first few years of life Tachypnea Increased work of breathing Exercise intolerance Shortness of breath
Gastrointestinal	Thickened intestinal secretions result from failure to secrete enough chloride and fluid into intestines; decreased motility of the gut; obstruction of bile ducts. Long term: frequent small bowel obstructions	Frequent bulky, greasy stools (steatorrhea) Failure to gain weight despite excessive food intake Constipation Abdominal distension
Endocrine	Thickened mucus damages pancreatic ducts; enzymes necessary to digest fats and proteins are obstructed from entering digestive tract. Long term: buildup of enzymes damages pancreas; fibrosis leads to failure to produce enough insulin; cystic-fibrosis diabetes.	Stools contain visible droplets of fat. Excessive flatus Hyperglycemia Glucosuria, polyuria, weight loss
Reproductive	Females: decreased cervical secretions, thick vaginal discharge Males: vas deferens is absent; low levels of semen	Females: difficulty conceiving Males: infertility
Integument (sweat glands)	Excessive electrolyte loss via the sweat glands, particularly sodium and chloride	Very salty sweat Salt "frosting" on the skin Hyponatremia Hypochloremic alkalosis

Therapeutic Interventions

The plan of care for a patient with CF focuses on treating and managing the affected systems: respiratory, gastrointestinal, and endocrine. This care includes maintaining respiratory function, managing infections, optimizing nutrition, and maintaining adequate intestinal motility. A child with CF is often hospitalized multiple times throughout childhood for associated complications. When caring for children with CF, promote their normal growth and development and maintain a sense of routine for them throughout their lifespan. See Hospital Help 20.1 for strategies for maintaining growth and development for a hospitalized child.

As ordered, perform chest percussion, with or without high-frequency chest wall oscillation (Fig. 20.20), combined with postural drainage (see the section Open and Maintain a Patent Airway). This combination of therapy is useful because chest vibrations help move secretions from small airways, where expiratory flow rates are low, and cough clears mucus from larger airways. Airway clearance is often prescribed for 1 to 4 times a day, depending on the severity of lung dysfunction. Because secretions accumulate in small airways before symptoms are present, even patients with CF having mild lung involvement benefit from airway clearance and pulmonary hygiene. Immediate improvement of pulmonary function is not seen after chest physiotherapy. However, children with mild-to-moderate lung disease

---

🏥 Hospital Help 20.1   Maintaining Growth and Development

Children with chronic diseases are hospitalized often. When caring for a child with CF in the hospital, it is important to remember growth and development principles and apply them to nursing care. Maintain normal routines as much as possible and promote growth and development while the child is hospitalized.

Infants	Encourage parents and caregivers to stay with the child as much as possible. If they cannot stay, have them leave a familiar object or even a voice recording that the infant can listen to. Maintain home routines as much as possible.
Toddlers	Toddlers are in the stage of autonomy vs. shame and doubt. Do not ask whether they want to do something; give them a choice between two options or let them choose the order of interventions, if possible. When stating the duration of a treatment, do so in terms of shows and books. Example: "Your breathing treatment will be over after one show of Doc McStuffins."
	Explain to parents that children this age may show signs of regression during hospitalization. For instance, a child who was potty trained before hospitalization may begin wetting the bed.
Preschoolers	Preschool children are very literal. Explanations should be simple and concrete. Avoid using scary phrases such as "take your blood," because the preschooler may interpret this as taking all of the blood.
	Allow the child to touch and explore medical supplies and equipment when possible. Letting the child touch and examine a nebulizer, for example, may help elicit better cooperation with the treatment. Performing a pretend respiratory treatment on a doll or stuffed animal may help, as well, because preschool children love pretend play.
	If a parent or caregiver needs to leave, explain to the child when the person will be back in terms of something the child understands, such as a TV show. This will help relieve the anxiety of a parent being gone.
	As with toddlers, give choices when possible. Preschool children may also experience some regression while hospitalized.
School-age children	School-age children often try to be brave even though they may be anxious about hospitalization. Provide explanations of treatments and how they will help the child's condition. If the parents or caregivers need to leave, provide a time when they are expected to return.
	With prolonged hospitalizations, encourage the child to keep up with school work to the extent possible. Encourage communication with friends.
Adolescents	Adolescents do not like to be different; therefore, being in the hospital with a chronic condition may have impact on their psychosocial development. Assess for signs and symptoms of depression. Encourage the adolescent to talk with other teenagers who also have CF.
	Allow the adolescent to participate in the care process and help with decision making. With prolonged hospitalizations, encourage the adolescent to keep up with school work to the extent possible. Encourage communication with peers through social media, texting, FaceTime, etc.

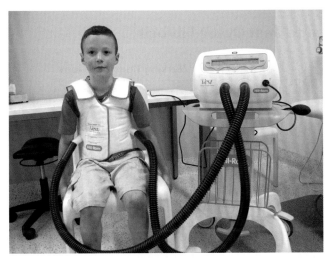

Figure 20.20. High-frequency chest wall oscillation. Reprinted with permission from Bronchiectasis Toolbox. *High Frequency Chest Wall Oscillation (HFCWO) in children.* Retrieved from http://bronchiectasis.com.au/paediatrics/airway-clearance/high-frequency-chest-wall-oscillation

who did not receive chest physiotherapy showed deterioration in lung function as early as 3 weeks without therapy. When therapy is resumed, lung function promptly improves (Egan, 2016).

A child with CF is likely to need a higher-than-normal caloric intake because of increased work of breathing and higher metabolic demands. A high-fat (Box 20.6), high-protein, high-calorie diet is recommended. Because pancreatic insufficiency results in malabsorption of the fat-soluble vitamins (A, D, E, and K), daily supplementation of these vitamins is necessary. Furthermore, children with CF need pancreatic enzyme replacement such as pancrelipase before snacks and meals.

Promote strict hand hygiene and avoid exposing the child to anyone with symptoms of respiratory infection (see the section Prevent Infection).

Medications used to treat patients with CF are numerous and can be overwhelming to the child and family, particularly upon initial diagnosis and when acute respiratory infections occur and the number of medications increases to treat infections

Box 20.6 Foods High in Fat

- Noodles with sauce (creamy sauces such as alfredo)
- Crackers with cheese or peanut butter
- Breaded fish or fish sticks
- Whole milk cheese
- Ice cream
- Pudding made with whole milk
- Mashed potatoes with butter, gravy, or sour cream
- Avocadoes
- Blueberry muffins
- Eggs scrambled with milk or cream added
- Pancakes
- French toast
- Thick creamy soups (cheese, potato, broccoli)
- Tuna or egg salad with mayonnaise added

and improve airway clearance. Children with CF need pancreatic enzyme replacements for the rest of their lives. Give pancreatic enzymes before every snack and meal and fat-soluble vitamins daily. Mucolytics and bronchodilators are also a daily regimen for CF patients. See The Pharmacy 20.6 for a complete list of medications, actions, and nursing considerations.

Evaluation

Expected outcomes for a child with CF include the following:
- Lung function is maintained as near to normal as possible with pulmonary hygiene and airway clearance measures.
- Incidences of respiratory infections are minimized and, when they do occur, are treated promptly and effectively with appropriate antibiotic therapy and respiratory clearance measures.
- The child receives adequate caloric intake and gains weight appropriately for age.

Discharge Planning and Teaching

Discharge from the hospital of a child with CF can be complex and a source of anxiety for parents, particularly in the early stages of diagnosis. Encourage parents to schedule and keep follow-up appointments. In the first year, infants are seen as often as every month during the first 6 months and every 1 to 2 months during the second 6 months of life. As the child grows, follow-up appointments are often every 3 to 4 months. Encourage parents and caregivers to keep a journal or log of current treatments, therapies, and medications, because interventions can change often as the child grows or encounters new complications as a result of CF. Instruct parents to call the healthcare provider if any of the following occur:
- Changes in bowel habits, including severe constipation or severe diarrhea
- Abdominal pain
- Vomiting
- Decreased appetite
- Being more tired than usual
- Difficulty taking part in daily activities
- Respiratory changes, including worsening shortness of breath or mucus becoming thicker or darker or containing blood
- Fever

Discharge teaching should cover infection prevention, immunizations, technique for airway clearance and postural drainage, nutrition, medications, exercise and physical activity, and genetic counseling. Each of these is discussed here.

Teach the child to help prevent infections by not touching his or her face with the hands. Teach the child and caregivers to wash their hands with soap and water and to vigorously rub their hands together for at least 20 seconds. Instruct them to keep hand sanitizer readily available in areas where soap and water are not. Teach children to not share water bottles and to avoid crowds, especially during the cold and flu season.

Recommend the influenza vaccine for all patients with CF who are 6 months and older. Children with CF should follow the current Centers for Disease Control and Prevention recommendations for standard immunizations, including the pneumococcal vaccine.

The Pharmacy 20.6 Medications Used to Treat Cystic Fibrosis

Medication	Classification	Route	Action	Nursing Considerations
Pancrelipase (Creon, Pancreaze, Ultresa, Zenpep)	Pancreatic enzyme replacement	PO	Aids in the digestion of nutrients; decreases fat in the intestines	• Swallow tablets whole; do not crush or chew. • Capsules may be opened and mixed with applesauce or pudding if difficult to swallow. • Take before or with meals. • Do not give with antacids or iron. • Monitor for steatorrhea.
Dornase alfa (Pulmozyme)	Mucolytic	Nebulized	• Thins secretions • Breaks down excess DNA in pulmonary secretions • May reduce risk of respiratory tract secretions	• Do not mix with other drugs in the nebulizer. • Keep refrigerated. • Monitor for improvement in sputum clearance.
Hypertonic saline 3% saline	Hypertonic solution	Nebulized	• Stimulates coughing • Hydrates airway secretion and mucus	• Give bronchodilator first.
Fat-Soluble Vitamins Vitamin A Vitamin D Vitamin E Vitamin K	Supplements	PO	Varies depending on the vitamin: A: important for growth and development, immune function and vision D: elevates plasma calcium and phosphate levels, which are required for bone mineralization E: antioxidant; protects cells against free radicals K: essential for blood clotting	• Absorption is improved when taken with pancreatic enzymes.
Ivacaftor (Kalydeco)	Cystic fibrosis transmembrane conductance regulator (CFTR)	PO	• Used only for patients with CF possessing a specific gene mutation • Increases chloride transport; reduces symptoms of CF	• Take with fat-containing foods such as eggs, whole milk products, cheese, peanut butter
Lumacaftor/ivacaftor (Orkambi)	Cystic fibrosis transmembrane conductance regulator (CFTR)	PO	• Used only for patients with CF possessing a specific gene mutation • Increases chloride transport; reduces symptoms of CF	• Take with fat-containing foods such as eggs, whole milk products, cheese, peanut butter.
Albuterol (Ventolin, ProAir, Proventil)	Bronchodilator Beta-agonist	MDI Nebulized	• Decreases airway resistance • Dilates the lower airways • Increases expiratory flow in the smaller airway	• Use before performing airway clearance. • Rinse mouth after administration.

From Lexicomp. *Pediatric & Neonatal Dosage Handbook* (25th ed.), 2018.

Give parents and caregivers ample opportunity to practice and demonstrate proper use of vests and airway clearance devices as well as techniques for postural drainage before discharge. Teach older children how to perform airway clearance and postural drainage independently.

Even when a child with CF is feeling well, a diet high in calories and protein is necessary to meet the metabolic demands CF creates on the body. Ensure that the caregiver and child are able to identify foods high in calories and protein. Teaching caregivers to read food labels will help them identify appropriate foods.

The child with CF is usually sent home with several different medications, including lung medications, pancreatic enzymes, fat-soluble vitamins, and, often, antibiotics. Review the medications at each discharge with parents and children who are school age and older. As the child grows, dosages change; therefore, make sure that the parents and the patient are familiar with the medications and understand the purpose, timing of administration, and dosages of all medications, which will help the child achieve optimal health.

Encourage children to exercise regularly and drink adequate liquids to replace water and salt losses during exercise.

For parents who have not had genetic testing and have a child diagnosed with CF, encourage follow-up with a genetic counselor and even having genetic testing done.

Bronchopulmonary Dysplasia

BPD, also called chronic lung disease, is a chronic obstructive pulmonary disorder occurring in infants as a sequela of prolonged use of supplemental oxygen and positive pressure ventilation after premature birth. More specifically, BPD is defined as the need for supplemental oxygen for greater than 28 days and/or the need for ventilatory support for greater than 28 days or beyond 36 weeks of postmenstrual age (Niedermaier & Hilgendorf, 2015).

Etiology and Pathophysiology

The pathophysiology of BPD is complex, and the exact pathogenesis remains unclear. As a result of prematurity, the alveoli do not develop correctly and alveolar simplification develops. Patients with BPD have a reduction in the overall surface area in which gas exchange can occur. Symptoms are a result of alveolar hypoventilation (insufficient ventilation that leads to increased carbon dioxide levels, or **hypercapnia**) and impaired gas exchange (Neidermaier & Hilgendorf, 2015). As hypoxia and hypercapnia develop, the child shows signs of respiratory distress, such as increased work of breathing and dyspnea. Also, as a result of prematurity, the microvasculature of the lungs is not well developed and capillary growth in and around the alveoli is reduced. Alveolar hypoventilation and vessel impairment lead to ventilation–perfusion mismatch in children with BPD. Chronic ventilation–perfusion mismatch, hypoxia, and hypercarbia may lead to pulmonary hypertension, interstitial fibrosis, and hypertrophy of the smooth muscles of the lungs (Niedermaier & Hilgendorff, 2015).

Although most likely to occur in premature, low–birth weight infants, BPD can develop in term or near-term infants, as well. Causes of BPD in term or near-term infants include the following: pneumonia, sepsis, lung hypoplasia, meconium aspiration, and diaphragmatic hernia (Baraldi & Filippone, 2007).

BPD most often occurs in infants of very low birth weight (VLBW; <1,250 g) who are born at 28 weeks of gestation or less (Islam et al., 2015). BPD is the most common morbidity seen in premature babies (Poindexter et al., 2015). In the United States, 5,000 to 10,000 cases of BPD are diagnosed each year in VLBW infants. VLBW is defined as a neonate weighing less than 1,500 g. Severity of BPD in infants born at a gestational age of less than 32 weeks and requiring at least 21% oxygen for at least 28 days can be categorized as mild, moderate, or severe (Askin & Diehl-Jones, 2009):

- Mild: The infant is breathing room air at 36 weeks of postmenstrual age or at the time of discharge from the hospital.
- Moderate: The infant requires supplemental oxygen of less than 30% at 36 weeks of postmenstrual age or at the time of discharge from the hospital.
- Severe: The infant requires supplemental oxygen of 30% or greater and/or positive pressure ventilation (via a tracheostomy) or nasal continuous positive airway pressure (CPAP) at 36 weeks of postmenstrual age or at the time of discharge from the hospital.

Clinical Presentation

Infants with BPD present with signs and symptoms of respiratory distress, including tachypnea, tachycardia, nasal flaring, grunting, and use of accessory muscles, resulting in retractions. Frequent oxygen desaturations are often seen in the patient with BPD. Wheezing and crackles may be audible and signs of pulmonary edema may be present. Irritability and restlessness are noticeable. Signs of failure to thrive, such as weight loss or inability to gain weight, poor intake, and fatigue, are present as a result of the increased oxygen demands of feeding that the child with BPD cannot meet. Episodes of sudden respiratory deterioration as a result of bronchospasms, mucus plugging, and increased air trapping can be frequent. Cyanosis may be seen in children with severe BPD.

Assessment and Diagnosis

The child with BPD requires meticulous and frequent assessment of airway patency and respiratory function. Place the child on a cardiorespiratory monitor and a pulse oximeter. Monitor heart rate and respiratory rate for tachycardia and tachypnea. Observe the child for paleness at baseline and behavior changes such as increased irritability and inconsolability, all of which can indicate worsening respiratory function. If the child has a tracheostomy, assess its patency and suction it as needed.

Laboratory tests and chest radiography can be used to evaluate and monitor the child with BPD. Arterial blood gas tests are used to assess for acidosis, hypoxia, and hypercarbia. Pulmonary function tests are used to monitor lung volumes (decreasing lung compliance leads to decreasing lung volumes). End-tidal carbon dioxide monitors can be used to monitor for hypercarbia. Chest X-rays may be obtained to determine the severity of BPD, assess for hyperinflation (as a result of air trapping), and rule out other causes of respiratory distress such as pneumonia, pneumothorax, pulmonary edema, or atelectasis.

Therapeutic Interventions

Position the child with BPD to facilitate breathing. Administer supplemental oxygen that is humidified. Perform chest physiotherapy to facilitate movement of secretions (see the section Open and Maintain a Patent Airway). Administer medications as prescribed (The Pharmacy 20.7). Bronchodilators decrease

The Pharmacy 20.7 Medications Used to Treat Bronchopulmonary Dysplasia

Medication	Classification	Route	Action	Nursing Considerations
Albuterol (Ventolin, ProAir, Proventil)	Bronchodilators Beta2-agonists, short acting	MDI Nebulizer	• Decreases airway resistance • Dilates the lower airways • Increases expiratory flow in the smaller airways	• Monitor heart rate for tachycardia. • May make patient shaky after use • Monitor for signs of toxicity.
Furosemide (Lasix), chloro-thiazide (Diuril), spironolactone (Aldactone)	Diuretic	PO IV during hospitalization	• Removes excess fluid from vascular space	• Monitor potassium levels. • Ensure adequate intake. • Teach patient and family about potassium- and sodium-containing foods.
Potassium chloride	Electrolyte replacement	PO (can also be given IV in the hospital setting)	• Prevents hypokalemia that may result from use of diuretics	• Monitor serum potassium level. • Teach patient and family about potassium-rich foods. Depending on which diuretic is prescribed, patient and family will need to add or avoid these foods.

From Lexicomp. *Pediatric & Neonatal Dosage Handbook* (25th ed.), 2018.
IV, intravenous; MDI, metered-dose inhaler; PO, by mouth.

airway resistance and stimulate mucus clearance. Suction as needed the tracheostomies of patients who have them.

Cluster and organize nursing care interventions to minimize the child's oxygen requirements and caloric expenditure. Excessive physical stimulation leads to increased respiratory effort and an increased oxygen demand.

The child with BPD is at risk for fluid overload, particularly in the lungs. Administer diuretics, as ordered, to remove excess fluid from lungs. Obtain daily weights to monitor fluid balance and weight gain. As ordered, provide a high-calorie formula (24–30 kcal/oz) to promote weight gain, because the increased work of breathing and feeding require extra calories. In some cases, a feeding tube may be used to ensure the child receives adequate calories. Nasogastric tubes are used as a short-term solution, whereas gastrostomy tubes may be placed as a long-term solution.

Promote strict hand hygiene and avoid exposing the child to anyone with symptoms of respiratory infection (see the section Prevent Infection). As ordered, administer palivizumab to infants monthly to prevent RSV infections.

Children with BPD often have repeated and prolonged hospitalizations, putting them at risk for delayed growth and development. Foster normal infant growth and development and parental bonding by promoting play with age-appropriate toys and objects of interest.

Evaluation

Expected outcomes for a child with BPD include the following:
• The child maintains a patent airway, and acute episodes of respiratory distress are managed without complications.
• The child maintains adequate hydration and receives adequate calories to sustain growth.

• The child remains free of infection.
• Growth and development are maintained, with age-appropriate milestones being met.

Discharge Planning and Teaching

Discharge of a patient with BPD from the hospital to home can range from simple (the child and family requiring few resources and referrals) to complex (requiring multiple resources). Infants with BPD may need supplemental oxygen, ventilation therapy (noninvasive ventilation such as CPAP or positive pressure ventilation requiring a ventilator attached to a tracheostomy), tracheostomy care, multiple medications, and specific nutrition regimens on discharge.

Community Referrals

As needed, refer the child for early intervention programs, including physical therapy, occupational therapy, speech therapy, and nutrition therapy. Early intervention for developmental care is often appropriate for children with chronic lung disease.

Home Care

Some families of children with BPD may need home health nursing assistance, particularly during the transition to home. They may also need assistance with home respiratory therapy, such as to set up home oxygen and deliver respiratory supplies.

Cardiopulmonary Resuscitation

Parents and those caring for a child outside the hospital setting should learn cardiopulmonary resuscitation. Children with moderate-to-severe BPD are at increased risk for respiratory distress, which may necessitate assisting the child to breathe with bag-valve

Patient Teaching 20.3   Home Care of a Child with a Tracheostomy

- Keep small toys, powders, plastic bibs, and any small particles away from child. These items place the child at an increased risk of aspiration or occlusion of the trachea.
- Wear loose bib over tracheostomy when eating to prevent food from entering tracheostomy.
- Use caution when bathing patient. Avoid getting water in tracheostomy.
- Observe skin around neck and stoma for redness, drainage, moisture and signs of infection.
- Always have assistance when changing tracheostomy ties in very young children. Change tracheostomy ties daily and as needed.
- Clean neck and area around stoma at least once daily with soap and water. Ensure skin is dried adequately.
- Suction tracheostomy when needed; suction only to end of tracheostomy; apply intermittent suction when removing suction catheter; limit suctioning to 5 s.

- Keep written instructions available at all times: size of tracheostomy tube, what to do in an emergency; how to suction tracheostomy and how to change the tracheostomy tube.
- An emergency bag with extra tracheostomies, suction catheters and a bag-valve mask should be available at all times.
- Notify utility companies and local emergency medical services of the child in the home who requires use of emergency equipment.
- No smoking in the home or around a child who uses oxygen
- Notify physician if:
  - Tracheal secretions increase
  - Tracheal secretions become purulent
  - Child develops respiratory distress or increased oxygen requirement
  - Child develops a fever

---

ventilation via the tracheostomy or giving rescue breaths to a child without a tracheostomy. Worsening hypoxia can lead to bradycardia, which may necessitate starting chest compressions.

Use of Home Monitoring Equipment

Train parents and caregivers to use home monitoring equipment such as a pulse oximeter and heart rate monitor. Discuss with them how to identify normal and abnormal O_2 saturation levels. Instruct them on appropriate assessments and steps to take when a monitor's alarm sounds and when the patient is desaturating.

Use of Oxygen

Instruct parents and caregivers on the proper use of oxygen and oxygen safety in the home. Teach them to keep oxygen tanks away from heat sources and to keep a fire extinguisher nearby. Smoking should not be allowed in the home of a child who is using oxygen therapy.

Tracheostomy Care and Safety

Instruct parents and caregivers regarding safety and care of the child with a tracheostomy, including emergency care, suctioning, stoma care, changing tracheostomy ties, changing the tracheostomy, and safety of the child and the environment. Patient Teaching 20.3 lists teaching points for the child with a tracheostomy. Have parents demonstrate proper care of their child with a tracheostomy many times before being discharged from the hospital (Fig. 20.21).

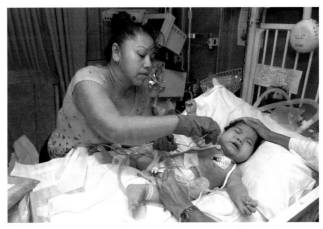

Figure 20.21. Child with a tracheostomy. Notice the caregiver suctioning and providing care for the child with a tracheostomy. Reprinted with permission from Bowden, V., & Greenberg, C. S. (2013). *Children and their families* (3rd ed., Fig. 16-11). Philadelphia, PA: Lippincott Williams & Wilkins.

Infection Control

Children with BPD are susceptible to frequent respiratory infections requiring hospitalization. Instruct parents and families on how to reduce the spread of infection and protect the child with BPD from potential infection. Teach proper hand washing. Anyone with respiratory symptoms should avoid contact with the child with BPD.

Think Critically

1. A 3-month-old presents to the clinic with a 2-day history of congestion and cough. The mother reports that the child is more sleepy than usual and barely took any of her bottle this morning. What signs and symptoms should the nurse look for to determine whether the infant is experiencing respiratory distress?

2. Liam, a 12-year-old boy who was diagnosed with asthma at the age of 5 years, has been hospitalized three times in the past 4 months for asthma exacerbations because he refuses to take his maintenance medications, montelukast and budesonide. What questions would you ask Liam to assist you in developing a teaching plan for Liam to increase his medication compliance?

3. The nurse is developing a teaching plan for a 4-year-old girl with pneumonia who is being discharged home later in the day. List and discuss three teaching points to review with the parents.

4. Why are infants more prone to developing respiratory distress from a respiratory virus than are school-age children?

5. The nurse enters the room of a 6-month-old admitted to the hospital 2 days ago with bronchiolitis, finds the infant head bobbing and grunting, and observes on the monitor a heart rate of 182 beats/min and a respiratory rate of 75 breaths/min. What other assessments should the nurse make? What immediate interventions should the nurse consider?

6. In a child with suspected epiglottitis, why should the nurse avoid sticking anything in the child's mouth?

7. The student nurse is reviewing causes of foreign body aspiration with her preceptor. What are contributing factors of foreign body aspiration in toddlers?

8. A 9-year-old is being treated in the emergency room for an asthma exacerbation. The nurse is preparing to administer a dose of IV methylprednisolone. How is methylprednisolone helpful in treating asthma?

Unfolding Patient Stories: Jackson Webber • Part 2

Think back to Jackson Weber, whom you met in Unit 2. He was diagnosed with generalized seizures 2 years ago at age 3. He had another seizure, and his mother brought him to the hospital. How would the nurse differentiate tonic-clonic seizures from other types of seizures? Compare and contrast the characteristics of each type of seizure.

Care for Jackson and other patients in a realistic virtual environment: *vSim for Nursing* (thepoint.lww.com/vSimPediatric). Practice documenting these patients' care in DocuCare (thepoint.lww.com /DocuCareEHR).

Unfolding Patient Stories: Brittany Long • Part 2

Recall from Unit 1 Brittany Long, a 5-year-old African American diagnosed with sickle cell anemia. She is having an acute pain crisis, and her mother brings her to the emergency department (ED). Her last visit to the ED was 1 year ago, when she was hospitalized for a vaso-occlusive crisis episode. How would the nurse prepare Brittany for insertion of an IV line and administration of IV fluids? How would the explanation differ for her mother? What nursing interventions safeguard the IV line and administration of fluids?

Care for Brittany and other patients in a realistic virtual environment: *vSim for Nursing* (thepoint.lww.com/vSimPediatric). Practice documenting these patients' care in DocuCare (thepoint.lww.com /DocuCareEHR).

References

American Academy of Pediatrics. (2014). Clinical practice guideline: The diagnosis, management, and prevention of bronchiolitis. *Pediatrics, 134*(5), e1474–e1502. doi:10.1542/peds.2014-2742

American Lung Association. (2012). *Trends in asthma morbidity and mortality.* Retrieved from http://www.lung.org/assets/documents/research/asthma-trend-report.pdf

Askin, D. F., & Diehl-Jones, W. (2009). Pathogenesis and prevention of chronic lung disease in the neonate. *Critical care nursing clinics of North America, 21*(1), 11–25.

Baraldi, E., & Filippone, M. (2007). Chronic lung disease after premature birth. *New England Journal of Medicine, 357*(19), 1946–1955.

Bass, P. (2016). Rethinking asthma: Prevention & management. *Contemporary Pediatrics,* 14–19. Retrieved from https://www.contemporarypediatrics.com/modern-medicine-feature-articles/rethinking-asthma-prevention-and-management

Brodzinski, H., & Ruddy, R. M. (2009). Review of new and newly discovered respiratory tract viruses in children. *Pediatric Emergency Care, 25*(5), 352–360; quiz 361–363.

Casey, G. (2015). Bronchiolitis: A virus of infancy. *Kai Tiaki Nursing New Zealand, 21*(7), 20–24.

Centers for Disease Control (CDC). (2016). *Tuberculosis: TB Risk Factors.* Retrieved from https://www.cdc.gov/tb/topic/basics/risk.htm.

Centers for Disease Control. (2017). *Pneumonia.* Retrieved from https://www.cdc.gov/pneumonia.

Chen, Y., Tu, Y., Huang, K., Chen, P., Chu, D., & Lee, Y. (2014). Pathway from central obesity to childhood asthma. Physical fitness and sedentary time are leading factors. *American Journal of Respiratory Critical Care Medicine, 189*(10), 1194–1203.

Chung, H., Hathaway, D., & Lew, D. (2015). Risk factors associated with hospital readmission in pediatric asthma. *Journal of Pediatric Nursing, 30,* 364–384.

Cystic Fibrosis Foundation. (2016). *Patient registry annual data report 2015.* Bethesda, MA: Cystic Fibrosis Foundation. Retrieved from https://www.cff.org/our-research/cf-patient-registry/2015-patient-registry-annual-data-report.pdf

Egan, M. (2016). Cystic fibrosis. In A. Nowak-Wegrzyn, H. A. Sampson, S. H. Sicherer, R. M. Kliegman, B. F. Stanton, J. W. St Geme, . . . R. E. Behrman (Eds.),. *Nelson textbook of pediatrics*. Philadelphia, PA: Elsevier.

Faden, H. (2006). The dramatic change in the epidemiology of pediatric epiglottitis. *Pediatric Emergency Care, 22*(6), 443–444.

Gillies, D., Wells, D., & Bhandari, A. P. (2012). Positioning for acute respiratory distress in hospitalized infants and children. *Cochrane Database of Systematic Reviews, (7)*, CD003645. doi:10.1002/14651858.CD003645.pub

Gluckman, W., & Forti, R. (2015). *Pediatric pneumothorax*. Retrieved from https://emedicine.medscape.com/article/1003552-overview

Hall, C. B., Weinberg, G. A., Blumkin, A. K., Edwards, K. M., Staat, M. A., Schultz, A. F., . . . Iwane, M. K. (2013). Respiratory syncytial virus-associated hospitalizations among children less than 24 months of age. *Pediatrics, 132*(2), e341–e348. doi:10.1542/peds.2013-0303

Hayes, N., & Chidekel, A. (2004). Pediatric choking. *Delaware Medical Journal, 76,* 335–340.

Huffaker, M. F., & Phipatanaku, W. (2015). Pediatric asthma: Guidelines-based care, omalizumab, and other potential biologic agents. *Immunology and Allergy Clinics of North America, 35*(1), 129–144. doi:10.1016/j.iac.2014.09.005

Jain, S., Williams, D., Arnold, S., Ampofo, K., Bramley, A., Reed, C., . . . Zhu, Y. (2015). Community-acquired pneumonia requiring hospitalization among US children. *New England Journal of Medicine, 372*(9), 835–845.

Johnson, D. W. (2014). Croup. *BMJ Clinical Evidence, 2014.*

Knechel, N. (2009). Tuberculosis: pathophysiology, clinical features, and diagnosis. *Critical care nurse, 29*(2), 34–43.

Kuo, C., & Parikh, S. (2014). Bacterial tracheitis. *Pediatrics in Review, 35*(11), 497–499.

Lowry, J., & Leeder, S. (2015). Over-the-counter medications: Update on cough and cold preparations. *Pediatrics in Review, 36*(7), 286–297.

Meissner, H. C. (2016). Viral bronchiolitis in children. *New England Journal of Medicine, 374,* 62–72.

Mikhailov, T., Kuhn, E., Manzi, J., Christensen, M., Collins, M., Brown, A., . . . & Goday, P. (2014). Early enteral nutrition is associated with lower mortality in critically ill children. *Journal of Parenteral Enteral Nutrition, 38*(4), 459–466.

Myers, T. R., & Tomasio, L. (2011). Asthma: 2015 and beyond. *Respiratory Care, 56*(9), 1389–1407.

Nahid, P., Dorman, S., Alipanah, N., Barry, P., Brozek, J., Cattamanchi, A., . . . & Higashi, J. (2016). Official American Thoracic Society/centers for disease control and prevention/infectious diseases society of America clinical practice guidelines: treatment of drug-susceptible tuberculosis. *Clinical Infectious Diseases, 63*(7), e147–e195.

National Safety Council. (2015). *Injury, death and fatality statistics*. Retrieved from http://www.nsc.org/news_resources/injury_and_death_statistics/Pages/InjuryDeathStatistics.aspx.

Niedermaier, S., & Hilgendorff, A. (2015). Bronchopulmonary dysplasia-an overview about pathophysiologic concepts. *Molecular and Cellular Pediatrics, 2*(1), 2.

Nierengarten, M. (2015). Diagnosis and management of croup in children. *Contemporary Pediatrics,* 31–33. Retrieved from https://www.contemporarypediatrics.com/contemporary-pediatrics/news/diagnosis-and-management-croup-children

Passàli, D., Lauriello, M., Bellussi, L., Passali, G. C., Passali, F. M., & Gregori, D. (2010). Foreign body aspiration in children: An update. *Acta Otorhinolaryngologica Italica, 30*(1), 27–32.

Pfuntner, A., Wier, L., & Steiner C. (2013, December). *Costs for hospital stays in the United States, 2011. HCUP statistical brief #168.* Rockville, MD: Agency for Healthcare Research and Quality. Retrieved from http://www.hcup-us.ahrq.gov/reports/statbriefs/sb168-Hospital-Costs-United-States-2011.pdf

Poindexter, B., Feng, R., Schmidt, B., Aschner, J., Ballard, R., Hamvas, A., . . . & Jobe, A. (2015). Comparisons and limitations of current definitions of bronchopulmonary dysplasia for the prematurity and respiratory outcomes program. *Annals of the American Thoracic Society, 12*(12), 1822–1830. doi:10.1513/AnnalsATS.201504-218OC

Saguil, A., & Fargo, M. (2012). Acute respiratory distress syndrome: Diagnosis and management. *American Family Physician, 85*(4), 352–358.

The National Asthma Education and Prevention Program. (2007). *Expert panel report 3: Guidelines for the diagnosis and management of asthma* (NIH Publication No. 07–4051). Bethesda, MD: National Institutes of Health, National Heart, Lung and Blood Institute.

Van der Doef, H., Kokke, F., van der Ent, C., & Houwen, R. (2011). Intestinal obstruction syndromes in cystic fibrosis: Meconium ileus, distal intestinal obstruction syndrome, and constipation. *Current Gastroenterology Reports, 13*(3), 265–270.

Wong, J., Jit, M., Sultana, R., Mok, Y., Yeo, J., Koh, J., . . . & Lee, J. H. (2017). Mortality in pediatric acute respiratory distress syndrome: A systematic review and meta-analysis. *Journal of Intensive Care Medicine.* doi: 10.1177/0885066617705109

Wright, M., & Bush, A. (2016). Assessment and management of viral croup in children. *Prescriber, 27*(8), 32–37.

Suggested Readings

American Academy of Pediatrics. (2014). Clinical practice guideline: The diagnosis, management, and prevention of bronchiolitis. *Pediatrics, 134*(5), e1474–e1502. doi:10.1542/peds.2014-2742

Asthma Center. *Pediatric asthma*. Retrieved from http://www.theasthmacenter.org/index.php/newsletter/pediatric_asthma

Cystic Fibrosis Foundation. Retrieved from https://www.cff.org

Wright, M., & Bush, A. (2016). Assessment and management of viral croup in children. *Prescriber, 27*(8), 32–37.

21 Alterations in Cardiac Function

Alterations in pediatric cardiovascular function may result from congenital heart defects, acquired infections, or injury to the heart or vascular system. Congenital heart defects, structural anomalies that are present at birth, occur in approximately 1% of live births (van der Linde et al., 2011). Approximately 40,000 babies are born annually with congenital heart defects. Congenital heart defects are also the leading cause of death related to birth defects during the first year of life (Mozaffarian et al., 2016).

Acquired infections such as Kawasaki disease, infectious endocarditis, cardiomyopathy, and rheumatic fever also cause alterations in cardiovascular function. Pediatric cardiology has grown rapidly in the past several decades because of new advances in diagnostic procedures and procurement of clinical data regarding both congenital heart disease and acquired heart disease. As a result, survival rates, both short term and long term, into adulthood, have increased dramatically (Shuler, Black, & Jerrell, 2013).

Variations in Anatomy and Physiology

The cardiovascular anatomy and physiology of infants and children, particularly of fetuses and newborns, are significantly different from those of adults. As the child grows, cardiovascular changes continue to occur until puberty. These differences relate to fetal circulation, transition to pulmonary circulation, and cardiovascular function. Understanding fetal and transitional circulation requires knowledge of a normal heart (Fig. 21.1).

Fetal Circulation

In the fetus, gas exchange occurs via the placenta, not in the lungs. A single umbilical vein delivers well-oxygenated blood to the fetus from the placenta. Most of this blood bypasses the liver via the ductus venosus. From the inferior vena cava, blood flows through the right atrium and, instead of going into the right ventricle, streams through the **foramen ovale**, an opening in the fetal heart between the right and left atria, into the left atrium. Deoxygenated blood returning from the head via the superior vena cava enters the right atrium and then flows into the right ventricle and out through the pulmonary artery. The fetus has a high pulmonary vascular resistance, which causes about 80% of blood from the pulmonary artery to flow across the ductus arteriosus and to the remainder of the body; the remaining 20% goes to the lungs (Fig. 21.2). The **ductus arteriosus** is a small blood vessel in the fetus that connects the pulmonary artery to the proximal descending aorta.

Transition to Pulmonary Circulation

At birth, the pulmonary vascular resistance drops significantly with the first few breaths. When the placenta is removed from circulation (the umbilical cord is cut), **systemic vascular resistance**, the resistance blood encounters in the vessels as blood travels throughout the body, increases and flow is reversed in the ductus arteriosus. Blood return to the left atrium from the lungs increases, and this increases left-sided heart pressures, functionally closing the foramen ovale. Within the first 24 to 48 hours of birth, the ductus arteriosus usually closes, due to two factors: increased O_2 saturation (the amount of oxygen being carried by hemoglobin in the blood) and removal of prostaglandins from circulation (Fig. 21.2). Table 21.1 compares fetal and neonatal circulation.

Cardiac Output and Total Blood Volume

Children also differ from adults in respect to cardiac output. **Cardiac output** is the volume of blood ejected from the left ventricle each minute and is the product of heart rate and stroke volume (CO = HR × SV). **Stroke volume** is the amount of blood ejected with each contraction of the heart. Contractility (the force with which the heart contracts), **preload** (the volume of blood in the ventricle at the end of diastole), and **afterload** (the resistance with which the ventricle must pump against to eject blood) are the three factors that determine stroke volume. Because children have a less developed heart muscle and thus less

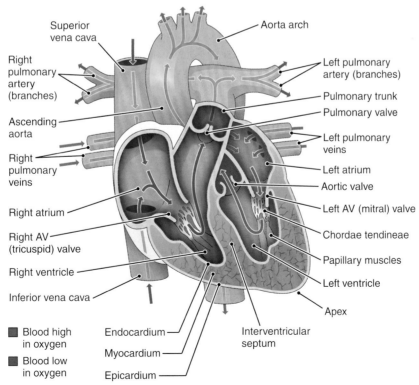

Figure 21.1. Normal heart anatomy. AV, atrioventricular. Reprinted with permission from Cohen, B. J., & Hull, K. L. (2015). *Memmler's structure and function of the human body* (11th ed., Fig. 13.4). Philadelphia: Lippincott Williams & Wilkins.

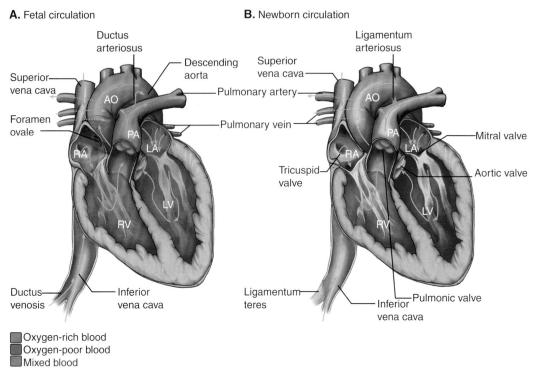

A. Fetal circulation

B. Newborn circulation

■ Oxygen-rich blood
■ Oxygen-poor blood
■ Mixed blood

Figure 21.2. Transition from fetal to newborn circulation. Reprinted with permission from Kyle, T., & Carman, S. (2016). *Essentials of pediatric nursing* (3rd ed., Fig. 19.1). Philadelphia, PA: Wolters Kluwer.

contractility than do adults, their hearts do not pump as forcefully and their stroke volume is less. Specifically, the neonatal myocardium has fewer contractile elements and a limited ability to change stroke volume. Therefore, cardiac output in children depends far more on heart rate than on stroke volume and the ventricle is less compliant than is the case in adults, which is why children have higher heart rates than adults. This situation

allows less time for diastolic filling and limits the child's ability to increase cardiac output by increasing the heart rate.

Another cardiovascular difference between children and adults is that children have lower total blood volume. Lower blood volume may present challenges when there is injury, surgery, or other sources of blood loss. A small amount of blood loss can lead to a large impact on a child's ability to maintain hemodynamic stability.

Table 21.1 Comparison of Fetal and Neonatal Circulation

Blood Vessels and Channels	Fetal Circulation	Neonatal Circulation
Pulmonary blood vessels	• Constricted • Low blood flow • Lungs not expanded	• Dilated • Increased blood flow • Lungs expanded
Systemic blood vessels	• Dilated • Low resistance • Blood mostly in placenta	• Arterial pressure increased because of loss of placenta • Increased systemic blood volume • Increased vascular resistance
Ductus arteriosus	• Large, no tone • Channels blood from pulmonary artery to aorta	• Constricts because of increased oxygen and body chemicals • Should close in 2–5 days
Foramen ovale	• Patent • Allows blood to flow from right atrium to left atrium	• Increased pressure in left atrium attempts to reverse blood flow • Flaps close on one-way valve
Ductus venosus	• Patent • Allows blood flow from placenta to liver and inferior vena cava	• Blood flow stops when umbilical cord is cut • Constricts and closes off

Assessment of the Pediatric Cardiovascular System

The nursing assessment of a child with potential or actual cardiovascular conditions involves the careful and in-depth review of many body systems and analysis of their relationship to cardiac function. Table 21.2 is a guideline for performing a comprehensive assessment of an infant or a child with an alteration in cardiac function, and Figure 21.3 shows anatomical locations of heart valves. Normal heart rate and blood pressure vary by age. Table 21.3 shows normal heart rates and blood pressures for various pediatric age groups. Many laboratory and diagnostic procedures are used to assist in the diagnosis of cardiovascular conditions. Box 21.1 lists these procedures and tests.

Table 21.2 Assessment Guide: Pediatric Cardiovascular System

Respirations	• Assess rate and depth. Tachypnea is a compensatory effect when oxygenation is poor or perfusion is inadequate.
Cough	• Present? Yes or no • Characteristics: Dry, wet, or productive? A wet-sounding cough can signal pulmonary venous congestion and heart failure. • When: Periodically? Only at night? Only when child lies down? Only with eating or drinking?
Color	• Pallor: A sign of anemia • Cyanosis (blue lips, nail beds, mucous membranes) or grayish/white color: A sign of hypoxemia • Mottled: A sign of poor perfusion • Does crying improve or worsen color? • Compare peripheral and central locations.
Adventitious breath sounds	• Rales/crackles: Signs of pulmonary congestion (heart failure) • Diminished: May be a sign of fluid in lungs (heart failure)
Heart rate/rhythm	• See Table 21.3 for normal heart rates. • Tachycardia • Bradycardia • Irregular or regular rhythm
Pulse characteristics	• Weak or absent? • Bounding? • Compare pulse sites for rate and strength (apical to brachial or radial, femoral, and pedal).
Capillary refill	• <2? • >4–5? • Compare upper extremities with lower extremities, as well as left side with right side.
Skin	• Diaphoretic • Warm, cool, or cold • Clammy?
Chest	• Palpate chest wall over heart. Are pulsations, heaves, or vibrations present? • Locate point of maximum intensity using topographic landmarks.
Heart sounds	• Auscultate heart sounds for quality: loud or weak, distinct or muffled. • Murmurs present? Murmurs may be innocent, functional, or pathologic. • Extra heart sounds? • Auscultate with child sitting and lying to detect differences in heart sounds (Fig. 21.3).
Fluid status	• Edema present? Periorbital, facial, or peripheral? • Signs of dehydration? Poor skin turgor or dry mucous membranes? Low urine output? • Weight increase or decrease? • Palpate for hepatosplenomegaly, which indicates possible fluid excess.
Activity	• Does child tire with feeding? • Is activity intolerance present? • Is child sleeping more than usual? • Have there been changes in child's activity level? • Does child become diaphoretic with activity?
Growth and development	• Assess growth patterns. • Is child gaining adequate weight for age?

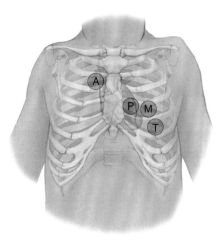

Figure 21.3. Areas where the sounds of heart valves radiate. A: Aortic valve—second intercostal space, just right of the sternum. P: Pulmonic valve—second intercostal space, just left of the sternum. T: Tricuspid valve—fourth intercostal space, just left of the sternum. M: Mitral valve—fourth intercostal space at the left midclavicular line. Reprinted with permission from Kyle, T., & Carman, S. (2016). *Essentials of pediatric nursing* (3rd ed., Fig. 10.32). Philadelphia, PA: Wolters Kluwer.

Table 21.3 Normal Heart Rate and Blood Pressure in Children

Age	Heart Rate (beats/min)	Blood Pressure, Systolic/Diastolic (mm Hg)
0–3 mo	100–150	65–85/45–55
3–6 mo	90–120	70–90/50–65
6–12 mo	80–120	80–100/55–65
1–3 y	70–110	90–105/55–70
3–6 y	65–110	95–110/60–75
6–12 y	60–95	100–120/60–75
>12 y	55–85	110–135/65–85

General Nursing Interventions for Cardiovascular Disorders

Caring for an infant, child, or adolescent with a cardiovascular disorder involves all aspects of the nursing process. Nurses care for children with cardiovascular disorders in schools, hospitals, clinics, pediatric offices, and homes. Although nursing care of the child with a heart condition is specific to the diagnosis, general nursing interventions that apply to many or most cardiovascular disorders are discussed later.

Maintain Adequate Oxygenation

Many hemodynamic changes accompany cardiovascular disorders, particularly underlying structural heart defects. Therefore,

adequate oxygenation is a key component in maintaining stability. Learn which conditions are likely to respond well to oxygen therapy, and provide humidified supplemental oxygen as ordered. Before and during oxygen administration, assess airway patency and respiratory effort. Position the child in a Fowler's or semi-Fowler's position to facilitate lung expansion. Monitor the child's heart rate, respiratory rates, lung sounds, color, and O_2 level. Be aware of the baseline or normal oxygenation saturation level for the child and the diagnosed defect. Some children may have a baseline O_2 level in the 70% to 85% range. This is considered normal for some defects, particularly those causing cyanosis (see Fig. 21.4), until surgical repair has been completed. Observe for signs of respiratory distress such as grunting, nasal flaring, retractions, and increasing tachypnea. Increased oxygen may be needed with exercise or increased activity or in the case of worsening heart failure.

Interventions for a child having a hypercyanotic spell are aimed at increasing systemic vascular resistance and promoting pulmonary blood flow. Oral propranolol may be prescribed to help prevent the episodes. When an episode occurs, it must be treated aggressively. Provide a calm, comforting approach to the child. Place the child in a knee-to-chest position or have older children squat down to increase systemic vascular resistance (Fig. 21.5). Reduce or remove any painful or noxious stimuli. Provide supplemental oxygen. Ensure that the patient is hydrated. Intravenous (IV) fluids may be necessary to increased central venous pressure and blood flow to the right heart and lungs. For patients experiencing pain or who are unable to be calmed, morphine may be given.

Maintain Adequate Cardiac Output and Tissue Perfusion

Many cardiovascular disorders, including congenital heart defect, heart failure, acute rheumatic fever (ARF), and infective

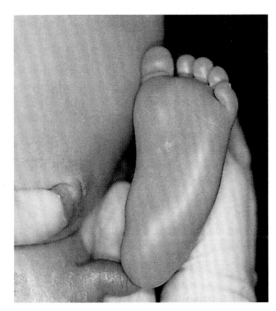

Figure 21.4 Cyanosis. A physical sign of poor perfusion or lack of oxygen in which the skin and mucous membranes turn a bluish color. (Reprinted with permission from Fletcher, M. (1998). *Physical Diagnosis in Neonatology*. Philadelphia, PA: Lippincott-Raven Publishers.

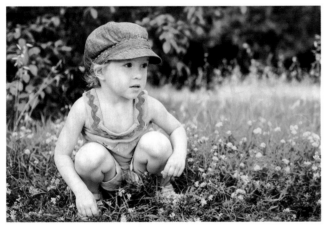

Figure 21.5. Knee-to-chest position during a hypercyanotic episode. Older children may squat to improve circulation during a hypercyanotic episode. Infants require being placed on their backs, with their hips and knees flexed, to assume this position.

carditis, pose a challenge to maintaining sufficient cardiac output to meet the body's metabolic demands. To counter this challenge, the nurse must work to optimize heart rate, preload, afterload, and contractility.

Assess the patient's vital signs and heart rhythm regularly for signs of decreased cardiac output (tachycardia, dysrhythmias, hypotension). Monitor heart rate by assessing the apical pulse in infants and children, and assess blood pressure using the right arm, preferably. Use a cardiac monitor to monitor for arrhythmias, which can lead to decreased perfusion. Children with heart failure, for instance, may require cardiac monitoring for bradycardia and arrhythmias. Note the child's heart rate and rhythm and changes in QRS, ST segments, and T wave. Monitor capillary refill and intensity of peripheral pulses.

Administer digoxin as ordered and according to heart rate parameters provided to increase contractility and regulate the heart rate. Elevate the legs if edema is present to promote venous return. Provide the child with rest periods, because rest decreases the need for higher cardiac output.

Monitor and maintain levels of electrolytes such as potassium, calcium, and magnesium according to provider orders. Potassium, in particular, plays a key role in contractility and heart rhythm stability, and hypokalemia can increase the risk of digoxin toxicity. Replace electrolytes as needed; potassium replacement, in particular, may be necessary for patients in heart failure.

Cardiac surgery is often necessary to correct a congenital heart defect or provide palliative symptom relief until corrective surgery can be performed. Surgery is most often planned but can be emergent in some cases. Open heart surgery involves opening the heart muscle to repair internal structures and may require cardiopulmonary bypass. Most surgeries to repair congenital heart defects require open heart surgery, but some can be done via cardiac catheterization.

Children are typically placed in the intensive care unit following surgery. Immediate postoperative care focuses on maintaining hemodynamic stability, ensuring adequate cardiac output, maintaining adequate oxygenation (as described earlier), maintaining thermoregulation, providing fluid and electrolytes, and managing pain (as described later). The child is often intubated and mechanically ventilated for one or more days. Chest tubes are in place to drain air, fluid, and blood from around the heart and lungs. **Inotropic** (altering the force or strength of a muscle contraction) medications may be necessary to maintain hemodynamic stability and blood pressure. Prophylactic antibiotics are usually administered. Heart arrhythmias are managed with antiarrhythmic medications.

Once the child is stable, care typically continues on a general nursing unit or a specialized cardiac unit. Priorities of care include pain management, promoting respiratory function, ensuring adequate fluids and nutrition, and preparing the patient and family for discharge home. The child may receive around-the-clock pain medication for several days. Avoid lifting a child who has just undergone heart surgery, particularly open heart surgery, by grasping under the arms, because this can put stress on the chest incision and cause pain. Encourage the child to take deep breaths and cough or provide age-appropriate activities such as bubbles or pinwheels to promote deep breathing, which promotes full lung expansion. Help the child splint under the chest using a pillow or stuffed animal to reduce the pain associated with deep breathing and coughing. Ensure that the child is maintaining adequate fluid and caloric intake, which is imperative to healing. Provide favorite foods and drinks. A bowel regimen may be needed, especially if opioids were used for pain management.

The patient with hypertrophic cardiomyopathy may need an implantable cardioverter-defibrillator, which has been proved effective for some children at risk for sudden death. For patients with severe or progressively worsening cardiomyopathy, despite treatment, a heart transplant may be needed.

Maintain Adequate Hydration and Nutrition

Patients with cardiovascular disorders, particularly heart failure and ARF with significant carditis, are at high risk for fluid imbalances, including hypervolemia and hypovolemia. Monitor intake and output carefully. With infants, weigh diapers to assess output. Obtain daily weights. Assess for peripheral edema and increasing abdominal girth. Administer diuretics as prescribed and monitor electrolytes (potassium and sodium). If fluid and/or salt restriction is ordered to decrease cardiac load, educate the patient and family regarding measuring fluids and maintaining fluid and/or salt restriction.

Conversely, following cardiac catheterization and for children with poor intake or experiencing vomiting and diarrhea, IV fluids may be ordered to help prevent dehydration. The contrast medium used during cardiac catheterization has a diuretic effect and can be harmful to the kidneys. Maintaining adequate hydration reduces the risk of hypovolemia and kidney dysfunction. Encourage the intake of small sips of clear liquids initially and then progress to other fluids and solid food as the child tolerates. Offering a favorite drink can be helpful in maintaining intake goals. Monitor the intake and output every 1 to 2 hours and notify the provider if the child's output exceeds the intake. Infants and children who are prescribed diuretics are at greater risk for dehydration. These patients may require additional IV fluids to maintain adequate intake.

Infants and children with congenital heart defects or heart failure often have imbalanced nutrition, particularly less than required, related to high metabolic demand and rapid tiring while feeding. Adequate nutrition is essential to foster growth and development and to reduce the risk of infection. Infants often require up to 150 kcal/kg or more per day to meet their metabolic demand and gain weight. Assist with providing these children with a balanced dietary intake of calories and fluids and refer to a dietitian when needed (Whose Job Is It, Anyway? 21.1).

For infants, a high-calorie formula (24–30 cal/oz) is used to provide sufficient calories. Hold infants at a 45° angle for feeding to promote breathing while eating and to help decrease venous return to the heart and reduce metabolic demand. Cutting a bigger hole in the bottle nipple decreases the work of feeding for some infants by causing the formula or breast milk to flow faster. Feedings are typically limited to 20 minutes or less because feeding for longer periods results in increased caloric expenditure. Rest periods during feeding, frequent small feedings, and using a slow-flow nipple can also be helpful. Frequent small feedings or meals require less energy for both intake and digestion. Provide older children with high-calorie snacks and a variety of foods, as well as frequent, small, high-calorie meals.

Enteral feeds via a nasogastric tube may be needed to meet caloric goals, especially for some children with heart failure who develop failure to thrive as a result of feeding difficulties. Tube feedings can provide calories without expending the child's energy to take in food. Some infants may take some formula or breast milk by bottle and then have the remaining amount gavage fed via a nasogastric tube.

Again, carefully record intake, including the amount and type of formula or food, to evaluate whether caloric and nutritional needs are being met. Weigh patients with heart failure daily. Weigh breastfed babies before and after feedings to assess volume intake.

Promote Pain Relief, Comfort, and Rest

Providing pain relief, comfort, and rest is important for children with cardiovascular disorders to help reduce metabolic demand or oxygen demand, especially those with heart failure, those recovering from surgery, and those with acute conditions, such as rheumatic fever, infective endocarditis, or Kawasaki disease.

Assess pain using an age-appropriate pain scale and provide analgesics as prescribed. High fever can lead to fluid loss, and pain and mouth discomfort can restrict a child's ability or desire to eat or drink. Provide children having fever with antipyretics as prescribed, offer them cool cloths, and keep their clothing and bed linens dry if diaphoresis is present. Keep their lips moist with a lubricant, particularly if cracks and fissures are present.

Provide infants and young children with frequent naps and rest periods every hour during the day, and establish a nighttime sleep routine. Space out activities that increase metabolic demand or oxygen demand. Plan age-appropriate activities, including those that can be done while in bed. Quiet activities such as watching a movie, coloring, reading a book, or listening to calm music provide necessary distraction to help keep the child still and calm. Offering the child a comfort item, such as a blanket, pacifier, or toy, can calm the child, as well. Talking with older children and engaging in conversation is often helpful to maintain a calm environment. Help the family set limits on visitors and activities that may overexpend the child's energy.

In children with ARF, joint pain is often present and can be difficult for children to understand. Administer anti-inflammatory medications as prescribed and place the child's joints in a neutral position. Handle the child carefully when turning, repositioning, or assisting with movement. Gradually increase activity as tolerated as soon as the child's C-reactive protein (CRP) and erythrocyte sedimentation rate (ESR) levels return to normal. Encourage quiet, developmentally appropriate activities at this time.

Administer and Manage Medications

A variety of medications are indicated for children with cardiovascular disorders (see The Pharmacy features throughout the chapter for details on these medications). Use careful aseptic technique

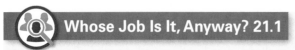

Whose Job Is It, Anyway? 21.1

Registered Dietitian

The registered dietitian plays an important role in caring for a child with a congenital heart defect. The dietitian determines the child's caloric needs and assists the provider in determining the appropriate prescription for feedings. Calories may need to be added to formula by mixing in supplements such as Polycose, oil, or protein powder. The dietitian monitors the child's caloric intake by evaluating recorded daily intake and calculating total calories received. For children receiving total parenteral nutrition, the dietitian calculates calorie, electrolyte, protein, fat, and dextrose goals and customizes a solution appropriate for the child.

when accessing IV lines and administering medications, and monitor the IV site for signs of infiltration or extravasation.

Common medications used in the treatment of heart failure, as well as ARF with significant carditis, include angiotensin-converting enzyme (ACE) inhibitors, diuretics, and digoxin.

Antibiotics are prescribed for ARF and infective endocarditis. Ensure the child is receiving the appropriate dose of antibiotics for age, weight, and organism identified. Antibiotics for ARF are prescribed to stop the group A streptococcal infection and most often include penicillin, amoxicillin, or cephalexin. Monitor for side effects of antibiotics, which often include nausea, upset stomach, diarrhea, and irritation to veins. Notify the provider of side effects.

Anti-inflammatory medications, such as aspirin or, if the child is allergic to aspirin, ibuprofen or naproxen, are prescribed for ARF and Kawasaki disease and should started as soon as the diagnosis is confirmed. Adjust doses to alleviate symptoms while avoiding toxicity and continue therapy until the patient has been asymptomatic for at least 2 weeks. During anti-inflammatory therapy, monitor for gastrointestinal upset, dyspepsia, bleeding around the gums, bruising, and signs of toxicity, which include tinnitus, headache, tachypnea, confusion, lethargy, agitation, and sweating. Assess the child's temperature every 4 hours while the child hospitalized.

Intravenous immunoglobulin (IVIG) therapy may be ordered for Kawasaki disease, because it has been shown to reduce the risk of coronary artery lesions if given within 10 days after onset of symptoms (McCrindle et al., 2017). The mechanism of action is unclear, but it is thought to neutralize microbial responses, decrease endothelial activation, and downregulate immune responses (Yim, Curtis, Cheyung, & Burgner, 2013). The infusion is often prescribed to run over 10 to 12 hours. During IVIG infusion, monitor the IV site for infiltration, obtain vital signs per hospital protocol, and monitor for side effects, including anaphylactic reactions.

Monitor for and Prevent Complications

Nursing care for children with cardiovascular disorders also includes monitoring for and helping prevent complications. Possible complications associated with cardiac catheterization include hematoma formation at the catheterization site, bleeding, arrhythmias, contrast-induced nephropathy, and clot formation. To help prevent these complications, maintain the child on bed rest for 4 to 6 hours after the procedure. Keep the head of the bed flat, because elevating it results in flexion of the hips, which is not permitted for 4 to 6 hours after the catheterization is complete. Limit the child's activity for up to 24 hours after the procedure. Maintain pressure on the catheterization site for 15 minutes after the catheter is removed and then apply a pressure dressing. Regularly check the dressing for bleeding and assess the site for formation of a hematoma. If the site begins to bleed, apply direct pressure over the site and notify the provider. Monitor the heart rate and rhythm, quality of peripheral pulses, and capillary refill in the distal extremities to assess perfusion. Decreased perfusion is a sign of possible clot formation in the affected vessel or bleeding internally. Monitor urine output for adequacy. Urine output should be greater than or equal to 1 to 3 mL/h in infants and 0.5 to 1 mL/h in children.

Patient Safety 21.1

Infection-Related Complications in Congenital Heart Defects

Children with congenital heart defects are at higher risks for compounding complications as a result of an infection.
- Fever increases metabolic rate and oxygen demand. The heart must work harder.
- Vomiting and diarrhea can lead to dehydration, particularly in the child taking diuretics.
- Dehydration puts the child with polycythemia at higher risk for thrombus formation.
- Respiratory infections worsen hypoxemia in children with a cyanotic heart defect.

Be astutely aware of how infection can impact the child with a congenital heart defect and provide interventions to prevent potential complications.

Complications of infectious endocarditis can include heart failure; thromboemboli in the heart, brain, bowel, arms or legs; aneurysms; and infections in other parts of the body (Patient Safety 21.1). Monitor for signs of complications and notify the provider promptly if signs of deep vein thrombosis (swelling, decreased pulses, redness, and pain) or change in neurological status or weakness occur, which could indicate an emboli in the brain. Monitor temperature every 4 hours for fever.

Promote Growth and Development

Bed rest, fatigue, multiple hospitalizations, and frequent procedures, interventions, and surgeries may lead to an environment of slowed growth and development for children with cardiovascular disorders, particularly those with congenital heart disease or heart failure. Encourage parents to play with their children, even when they are on bed rest or are hospitalized. Provide children with toys that stimulate hand–eye coordination and fine motor movements. Encourage sitting, standing, and walking when appropriate to foster development of large muscles. Provide adequate rest periods after physical activity. Collaborate with child life specialists to provide age-appropriate toys and activities for children. Occupational therapists (OTs) and physical therapists (PTs) play an important role in promoting growth and development. Collaborate with them to provide gross and fine motor development activities, promote muscle development, and prevent muscle loss from prolonged bed rest or inactivity. Help children develop cognitive and language skills by singing, playing music, and talking with them. Encourage interaction with peers.

Provide Emotional and Psychosocial Support to the Child and Parents

The parents and family of a child with a cardiovascular disease such as congenital heart disease or heart failure often feel overwhelmed and have increased anxiety related to the numerous exams, tests, and procedures the child must undergo. The parents may also fear long-term disability or even death. Serve as an advocate and liaison for parents, the child, and their family when interacting with them and with other healthcare providers who are involved in the child's care. Encourage parents to ask questions, explain all that is happening, and provide them with written materials and additional information when necessary. Allow time for the child and parents to voice their feelings, concerns, and questions. Learning about the child's diagnosis, setting goals, and working toward outcomes are often beneficial to children and families. Parents may tend to overprotect their child out of fear any activity will worsen his or her status. Encourage parents to stay with their child and continue parenting the child, even when the child requires extended hospital stays. Refer parents to support groups and offer resources related to the child's condition.

Congenital Heart Disease

Congenital heart disease occurs in approximately 1% of live births (van der Linde et al., 2011). Interestingly, congenital heart defects are one of the more common birth defects. The incidence is approximately 8 per 1,000 live births (Mozaffarian et al., 2016). Often, children are diagnosed either before birth as a result of ultrasound or immediately after birth at the initial assessment (Fig. 21.6). During the first week of life, 40% to 50% of patients with congenital heart disease are diagnosed as a result of symptoms. Within the first month of life, 50% to 60% are diagnosed. It is estimated that over 1 million children and 1.4 million adults were living with congenital heart disease in the United States in 2010 (Gilboa et al., 2016).

The fetal heart develops very early after conception, on day 18 of pregnancy. During the fourth and fifth weeks of fetal development, the atrial and ventricular septa form, as well as the blood vessels. Most cardiac defects form very early, during the first 8 weeks of gestation. Recall that this is also the time when the fetus is most susceptible to teratogens. Most heart defects

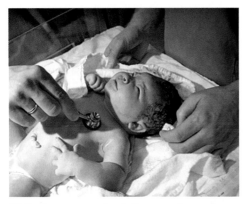

Figure 21.6. Assessment of the newborn for congenital heart defects immediately after birth. Reprinted with permission from Lippincott Professional Development September 2014.

> ### Box 21.2   Genetic Syndromes and Associated Congenital Heart Defects
>
> - Apert syndrome: VSD, ASD
> - Cri du chat syndrome: PDA, VSD, ASD, AV canal, tetralogy of Fallot
> - Duchenne muscular dystrophy: cardiomyopathy
> - Noonan syndrome: pulmonary stenosis, ASD, VSD, cardiomyopathy
> - Trisomy 21 (Down syndrome): VSD, ASD, AV canal

occur as a result of a combination of genetic and environmental factors. Some maternal medical conditions increase the risk of congenital heart disease, including type 1 diabetes, phenylketonuria, and rubella. Some medications taken by an expectant mother during pregnancy also increase the risk of congenital heart disease, including antiepileptics, lithium, and some acne medicines. Maternal alcohol and drug abuse have also been shown to cause heart defects.

Many syndromes and genetic conditions are associated with congenital heart disease. These include Apert syndrome, Cri du chat syndrome, DiGeorge syndrome, trisomy 21 (Down syndrome), Duchenne muscular dystrophy, Marfan syndrome, and Noonan syndrome. Box 21.2 lists the syndromes and their associated defects.

Congenital heart defects are often categorized by etiology or cyanosis status. In this chapter, heart defects are categorized primarily by etiology, although Figure 21.7 categorizes them according to whether cyanosis is present or not. In terms of etiology, most defects can be sorted into four categories: increased pulmonary blood flow, decreased pulmonary blood flow, obstruction to systemic blood flow, and mixed defects. Mixed defects can also fall into one of the previous three categories but have somewhat different approaches to repair and different prognoses, with survival being based on how the mixing of pulmonary and systemic blood flow occurs. See Table 21.4 for a breakdown of each category of congenital heart defects.

Increased Pulmonary Flow Disorders

The most common congenital heart defects are those that result in increased blood flow to the lungs. Recall that in a normal heart, the left side of the heart has higher pressures than does the right side of the heart. Defects with a connection between the right and left sides of the heart shunt blood from the area of higher pressure (left side) to the area of lower pressure (right side). This is referred to as a left-to-right shunt. Left-to-right shunting results in increased blood flow to the right side of the heart and to the lungs. Heart failure and right ventricular hypertrophy can result. In some cases, right ventricular hypertrophy can lead to a forcefully pumping right ventricle, which causes left-to-right shunting to reverse to right-to-left shunting. Overall blood O_2 is then lower as a result of deoxygenated blood mixing with oxygenated blood

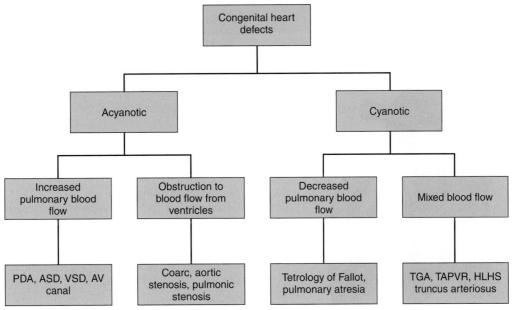

Figure 21.7. Acyanotic vs. cyanotic congenital heart disease. ASD, atrial septal defect; AV, atrioventricular; HLHS, hypoplastic left heart syndrome; PDA, patent ductus arteriosus; TAPVR, total anomalous pulmonary venous return; TGA, transposition of the great arteries; VSD, ventricular septal defect.

Table 21.4 Categorizing Congenital Heart Defects

Category	Defects	Clinical Presentation
Increased pulmonary blood flow	• Patent ductus arteriosus • Atrial septal defect • Ventricular septal defect • Atrioventricular canal	• Tachypnea • Frequent respiratory infections • Tachycardia • Murmur • Diaphoresis • Poor weight gain • Heart failure
Decreased pulmonary blood flow	• Pulmonic stenosis • Tetralogy of Fallot • Pulmonary atresia • Tricuspid atresia	• Cyanosis • Poor weight gain • Hypercyanotic episodes • Polycythemia
Obstruction to systemic blood flow	• Coarctation of the aorta • Hypoplastic left heart syndrome • Mitral stenosis • Interrupted aortic arch	• Diminished pulses • Delayed capillary refill • Poor color • Heart failure • Pulmonary edema
Mixed flow	• Transposition of the great arteries • Truncus arteriosus • Double-outlet right ventricle	• Cyanosis • Poor weight gain • Pulmonary congestion • Heart failure

during the right-to-left shunt. Congenital heart defects that lead to increased pulmonary blood flow include the following: patent ductus arteriosus (PDA), atrial septal defect (ASD), ventricular septal defect (VSD), and atrioventricular (AV) canal. Box 21.3 reviews the congenital heart defects that cause increased pulmonary blood flow. See The Pharmacy 21.1 for medications used to treat congenital heart disease. Refer to Table 21.5 for surgical procedures used to correct congenital heart defects.

Remember Caleb Yoder, the newborn who was diagnosed with a VSD in Chapter 7? What was Caleb's respiratory rate on assessment just after birth? What other sign of VSD did the midwife detect at this time? What effect did the VSD have on Caleb's ability to nurse?

Patent Ductus Arteriosus

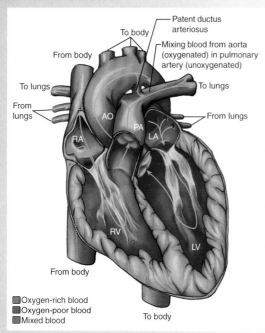

AO, aorta; LA, left atrium; LV, left ventricle; PA, pulmonary artery; RA, right atrium; RV, right ventricle. Figure reprinted with permission from Kyle, T., & Carman, S. (2016). *Essentials of pediatric nursing* (3rd ed., Fig. 19.7). Philadelphia, PA: Wolters Kluwer.

Pathophysiology

Abnormal blood flow occurs between the two major arteries that channel blood out of the right and left ventricles: the pulmonary artery and the aorta, respectively. Essentially, the ductus arteriosus fails to close. Recall that before birth, the pulmonary artery and aorta are connected by the ductus arteriosus, which during fetal circulation allows blood from the right ventricle to bypass the fetus's nonfunctioning fluid-filled lungs.

After birth, when pulmonary circulation begins and systemic vascular resistance increases, pressures in the aorta become greater than those in the pulmonary arteries, increasing circulation to the pulmonary system. Normally, the ductus closes by day 2 or 3 of life.

Facts

A common congenital heart defect, occurring in 5%–10% of infants with congenital heart disease (Elumalai & Thelma, 2016)

Clinical Presentation

- May be asymptomatic
- Respiratory: tachypnea, dyspnea, intercostal retractions; at risk for respiratory infections and pneumonia
- Cardiac: tachycardia; full, bounding pulses; widened pulse pressure; if low cardiac output, then hypotension, heart failure, hepatomegaly (if large defect), continuous murmur
- Growth: poor growth (if large)

Diagnosis

- Chest X-ray and ECG: show left ventricular hypertrophy
- ECHO: PDA visualized, left-to-right shunting measured

Therapeutic Interventions

Nonsurgical

Indomethacin IV or ibuprofen IV can stimulate closure of the ductus arteriosus in premature infants.

Surgical

Ligation of the PDA

Prognosis

- No long-term complications, as long as the PDA is closed before pulmonary hypertension or pulmonary vascular disease develops
- If left untreated, the child may develop pulmonary hypertension.

Atrial Septal Defect

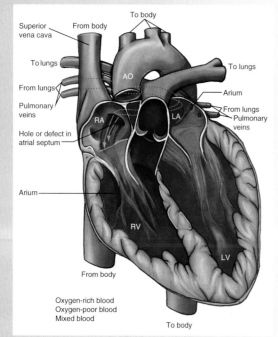

AO, aorta; LA, left atrium; LV, left ventricle; RA, right atrium; RV, right ventricle. Figure reprinted with permission from Kyle, T., & Carman, S. (2016). *Essentials of pediatric nursing* (3rd ed., Fig. 19.4). Philadelphia, PA: Wolters Kluwer.

Pathophysiology

There is a hole in the atrial wall. Oxygenated pulmonary venous return goes from the left atrium back into the right atrium (as a result of blood flow from higher to lower pressure; recall that the pressure in the left atrium is greater than that in the right atrium). The degree of left-to-right shunting depends on the size of the defect, vascular resistance in the pulmonary and systemic circulation, and the compliance of the ventricles. In large defects, a considerable amount of oxygenated blood is pumped back into the right atrium from the left atrium and then sent back in to the pulmonary vasculature.

Facts

Comprises 6%–10% of congenital heart defects

Clinical Presentation

- May be asymptomatic; often discovered inadvertently during a physical exam
- Large ASDs: may cause heart failure, failure to thrive (poor weight gain), and the child tiring easily
- Murmur may be present

Diagnosis

ECHO: dilated right ventricle (related to shunt size and blood overload)

Box 21.3 Pathophysiology, Clinical Presentation, and Therapies for Increased Pulmonary Flow Defects (*continued*)

Therapeutic Interventions

Nonsurgical

Small ASDs may close spontaneously. Heart failure can occur in untreated, larger ASDs or in patients who have an ASD and other heart defects.

Surgical

A patch is placed over the defect.

Prognosis

Children with repaired ASDs go on to lead normal, healthy lives. Unrepaired ASDs can cause cardiovascular and pulmonary problems in middle adulthood. The risk for stroke becomes more prevalent in adults with untreated ASDs because clots that are often filtered out by the lungs can pass directly to the left atrium via the ASD and into systemic circulation. Heart failure, atrial arrhythmias, and pulmonary hypertension can also develop in untreated adults.

Ventricular Septal Defect

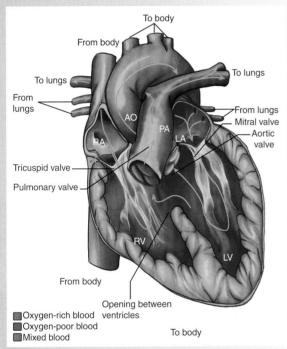

- Oxygen-rich blood
- Oxygen-poor blood
- Mixed blood

AO, aorta; LA, left atrium; LV, left ventricle; PA, pulmonary artery; RA, right atrium; RV, right ventricle. Figure reprinted with permission from Kyle, T., & Carman, S. (2016). *Essentials of pediatric nursing* (3rd ed., Fig. 19.5). Philadelphia, PA: Wolters Kluwer.

Pathophysiology

There is a hole in the ventricle wall between the left and right ventricles. The hole can range in size from very small to large. Oxygenated blood flows from the left ventricle (area of high pressure) to the right ventricle (area of lower pressure) and recirculates to the lungs.

Facts

About 20%–25% of all congenital heart defects are VSDs.

Clinical Presentation

- Respiratory: tachypnea, shortness of breath, increased pulmonary infections, pulmonary hypertension
- Cardiac: tachycardia, sweating while feeding, pale skin, systolic murmur
- Growth: failure to thrive (if large)

Diagnosis

- Chest X-ray: if large, may show enlarged heart and pulmonary vascular markings; if small, no signs
- ECG: may show signs of right and left ventricular hypertrophy
- ECHO: reveals shunting and establishes diagnosis

Therapeutic Interventions

Nonsurgical

- Aimed at preventing heart failure or treating it if it occurs
- Digoxin to control rate and rhythm
- Lasix for diuresis and to manage fluid balance
- ACE inhibitors to decrease aortic pressure, systemic vascular resistance, and left-to-right shunt

Surgical

- Palliative pulmonary banding to reduce blood flow to the lungs until a VSD patch can be placed
- VSD patch, placed at 3–12 mo of age

Prognosis

- For children who have VSDs that are completely surgically closed or that close on their own, no medications or restriction of activities are necessary.
- For children who have moderate-to-large VSDs or unrepaired VSDs, heart failure and/or pulmonary hypertension can develop over time.

Box 21.3   Pathophysiology, Clinical Presentation, and Therapies for Increased Pulmonary Flow Defects (*continued*)

Atrioventricular Canal

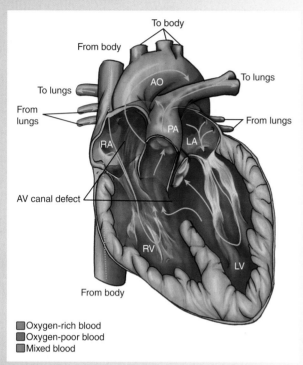

To body
From body
To lungs
From lungs
AO
To lungs
PA
From lungs
RA
LA
AV canal defect
RV
LV
From body

☐ Oxygen-rich blood
☐ Oxygen-poor blood
☐ Mixed blood

AO, aorta; LA, left atrium; LV, left ventricle; PA, pulmonary artery; RA, right atrium; RV, right ventricle. Figure reprinted with permission from Kyle, T., & Carman, S. (2016). *Essentials of pediatric nursing* (3rd ed., Fig. 19.6). Philadelphia, PA: Wolters Kluwer.

Pathophysiology

An AV canal is typically described as a large hole in the center of the heart with AV valve malformations. An AV canal can be partial or complete. A partial AV canal typically involves the right and left atria. An ASD is present with left-to-right shunting. Mitral valve regurgitation is common as a result of a cleft mitral valve. A cleft occurs when the valve has an extra leaflet. Volume overload occurs in the right ventricle and right atrium.

A complete AV canal involves all four chambers of the heart and both AV valves. A large VSD in the posterior portion of the interventricular septum is usually present as well as a large ASD in the anterior portion of the interatrial septum. The mitral and tricuspid valves are merged and form a single, multi-leaflet valve that crosses the ASD and VSD. Typically, left-to-right shunting is present, but bidirectional shunting is possible.

Facts

- Also known as an endocardial cushion defect
- Accounts for about 5% of all congenital heart defects
- Most common in infants with Down syndrome (about 15%–20% of infants with Down syndrome have an AV canal)
- Will need lifelong prophylaxis for infective endocarditis (before dental procedures, etc.)

Clinical Presentation

Symptoms depend on degree of left-to-right shunting.
- Respiratory: tachypnea, increased work of breathing, recurrent respiratory infections, respiratory failure
- Cardiac: weak pulses, ashen skin color, edema in legs, abdomen, holosystolic murmur
- Growth: lack of appetite, poor weight gain

Diagnosis

- Chest X-ray: **cardiomegaly**, or abnormal enlargement of the heart
- ECG: atrial enlargement, incomplete right bundle branch block, right ventricular hypertrophy
- ECHO: dilation of ventricles, septal defects, and valve malformation
- Cardiac catheterization: increased oxygen in right atrium and increased right ventricular and pulmonary artery pressure

Therapeutic Interventions

Surgical repair is required to correct AV canal, usually within the first year of life. The goal is to restore normal circulation by closing the septal defects and reconstructing the AV valves (mitral and tricuspid).

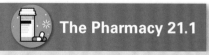

The Pharmacy 21.1   **Medications Used in the Treatment of Congenital Heart Disease**

Medication	Classification	Route	Action	Nursing Considerations
Alprostadil, prostaglandin E₁	Ductus arteriosus patency adjunct	IV	Directly relaxes smooth muscle of the ductus arteriosus	Monitor for side effects: • Apnea • Vasodilation • Bradycardia • Fever • Seizures

From Lexicomp. *Pediatric & Neonatal Dosage Handbook* (25th ed.), 2018.
IV, intravenous.

Table 21.5   Procedures Used to Repair Congenital Heart Defects

Procedure	Type of Defect	What Happens?
Arterial switch (Jatene procedure)	TGA	An arterial switch procedure is performed to connect the pulmonary artery to the right ventricle and the aorta to the left ventricle.
Balloon atrial septostomy	• TGA • Tricuspid atresia • Pulmonary atresia • TAPVR with restrictive ASD	An inflated balloon is passed across the interatrial septum through the PFO to create an ASD or make an ASD bigger to improve oxygenation of blood.
Balloon dilation or valvuloplasty	• Pulmonic stenosis • Aortic stenosis	An inflated balloon is used to relieve obstructions in stenosed valves.
Blalock–Taussig shunt	• Tricuspid atresia • Tetralogy of Fallot • Pulmonary atresia	A homograft tube or tube made of synthetic material is used to anastomose the right subclavian artery to the right pulmonary artery to direct blood flow from systemic circulation to the pulmonary circulation; increases pulmonary blood flow.
Fontan procedure	• Tricuspid atresia • HLHS	• A staged surgical repair. Stage 1 is palliative and involves pulmonary artery banding (to reduce pulmonary blood flow) or a Blalock–Taussig shunt (to increase pulmonary blood flow). • Stage 2 is a Glenn procedure. The main pulmonary artery trunk is removed and the distal end closed. The superior vena cava is anastomosed to the right pulmonary artery. • Stage 3 is Fontan completion. The inferior vena cava is connected to the right pulmonary artery either with a tunnel or a conduit.
Glenn procedure (Hemi-Fontan)	• Tricuspid atresia • HLHS	The second of three surgeries performed in which the ultimate goal is separation of the pulmonary and systemic circulations. The superior vena cava is anastomosed to the right pulmonary artery so that venous return from the upper body flows directly to the pulmonary artery.
Konno procedure	Aortic stenosis	Aortic root including valve and coronary arteries is removed. The left ventricular outflow tract is opened and enlarged. An aortic or pulmonary homograft is used to replace the aortic valve. The coronary arteries are then moved to the new aorta. The pulmonary valve is placed with a valved homograft.
Norwood procedure	HLHS	A three-stage procedure is used to convert the right ventricle from a pulmonary function to a systemic function and completely separate pulmonary and systemic circulations.
PDA ligation	PDA	The PDA is tied off at both ends and then cut in the middle.
Percutaneous balloon valvotomy	Aortic stenosis	An inflated balloon is used to relieve obstruction of a stenosed valve.
Pulmonary artery band	Pulmonary overcirculation	A band is placed around the pulmonary artery and adjusted to restrict flow to the branch pulmonary arteries and lungs.
Rastelli procedure	Cyanotic defects with a VSD and right ventricular outflow tract obstructions (tetralogy of Fallot, TGA, tricuspid atresia, truncus arteriosus, and some cases of DORV)	Several repairs are performed: patch repair of the VSD, excision of excess ventricular tissue, surgical closure of an abnormal or damaged pulmonary valve, and creation of an extracardiac conduit from the right ventricle to the bifurcation of the main pulmonary artery using an autograft or homograft.

(continued)

Table 21.5 Procedures Used to Repair Congenital Heart Defects (*continued*)

Procedure	Type of Defect	What Happens?
Ross procedure	Aortic stenosis	The stenosed aortic valve is removed and replaced with the child's pulmonic valve (autograft). The pulmonic valve is replaced with a human donor valve (homograft).
Synthetic patch aortoplasty	Coarctation of the aorta	Coarcted part of the aorta is resected and replaced with a synthetic patch or a homograft.
VSD repair	VSD	Procedure depends on the size of the VSD. For small VSDs, a direct suture and closing repair is performed. Patches using the pericardium or synthetic patches can also be placed to close a VSD.

ASD, atrial septal defect; DORV, double-outlet right ventricle; HLHS, hypoplastic left heart syndrome; PDA, patent ductus arteriosus; PFO, patent foramen ovale; TAPVR, total anomalous pulmonary venous return; TGA, transposition of the great arteries; VSD, ventricular septal defect.

Decreased Pulmonary Flow Disorders

Defects involving decreased pulmonary blood flow occur as a result of an obstruction of blood flow to the lungs. Because blood cannot adequately flow through the lungs, pressures in the right side of the heart increase and eventually become greater than pressures on the left side of the heart. Also, the lack of oxygenation in the lungs leads to an increased concentration of arterial deoxygenated hemoglobin, decreasing blood O_2 overall and causing cyanosis, a sign of hypoxemia (Patient Safety 21.2). Chronic hypoxemia can result in tissue and cell death. However, a child's bone marrow can respond to chronic hypoxemia by increasing production of red blood cells. This results in **polycythemia**, a greater-than-normal number of red blood cells (and hemoglobin), which are available to carry oxygen to the tissues. Although polycythemia can be beneficial, it can also cause complications such as thromboembolism resulting from platelet dysfunction.

Hypercyanotic spells may occur in children with cyanotic heart defects. Hypercyanotic spells occur when there is an abrupt or sudden increase in right-to-left shunting, which then decreases pulmonary blood flow. A **shunt** is a diversion of blood from one blood vessel to another through an abnormal anatomical or surgically created opening. An abrupt decrease in systemic vascular resistance or systemic perfusion, as occurs with hypovolemia, will leads to increased right-to-left shunting and may trigger a hypercyanotic episode. A sudden decrease or obstruction of pulmonary blood flow also results in increased right-to-left shunting via an intracardiac septal defect, triggering a hypercyanotic episode, also known as a "tet" spell. These episodes are characterized by rapid and deep breathing, worsening of cyanosis, decreased intensity of the heart murmur, and

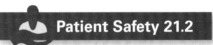

Patient Safety 21.2

Preventing Hypoxemia-Induced Cardiac Arrest

Children respond to hypoxemia initially with tachycardia. As hypoxemia worsens or goes untreated, bradycardia ensues. Cardiac arrest in children is most often the result of prolonged hypoxia related to respiratory failure or shock rather than a primary cardiac dysfunction. Bradycardia is therefore a significant warning sign in children that cardiac arrest is imminent. Respiratory interventions to improve hypoxemia often reverse bradycardia and prevent cardiac arrest.

periods of uncontrollable crying or panic. If prolonged, limpness, seizures, and death may result. Triggers of hypercyanotic spells are noxious stimuli such as phlebotomy, a bee sting, or an incident that leads to enhanced catecholamine output, such as prolonged crying and agitation on arising and early in the morning and or shortly after a nap when arising. Exercise, fever, and bathing (all of which can lead to decreased systemic vascular resistance) can potentiate right-to-left shunting and lead to hypoxemia as well.

Congenital heart defects that result in decreased pulmonary blood flow include pulmonic stenosis, pulmonary atresia, tricuspid atresia, and tetralogy of Fallot. These are covered in detail in Box 21.4.

Box 21.4   Pathophysiology, Clinical Presentation, and Therapies for Decreased Pulmonary Flow Defects

Pulmonic Stenosis

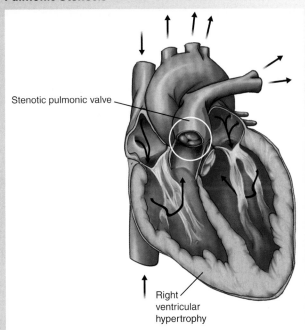

Figure reprinted with permission from Bowden, V. R., & Greenberg, C. S. (2013). *Children and their families* (3rd ed., Fig. 15.16). Philadelphia, PA: Wolters Kluwer Health/Lippincott Williams & Wilkins.

Pathophysiology

Pulmonic stenosis (pulmonary stenosis) is characterized by right ventricular outflow obstruction. There are three different types (subvalvular, valvular, and supravalvular), and each type can vary in terms of severity (mild, moderate, severe).

Flow from the right ventricle to the pulmonary artery is impeded as a result of excess tissue right below the pulmonic valve (subvalvular), narrowed pulmonic valve (valvular), or an obstruction in the pulmonary artery distal to the pulmonic valve (supravalvular).

Pulmonary Atresia

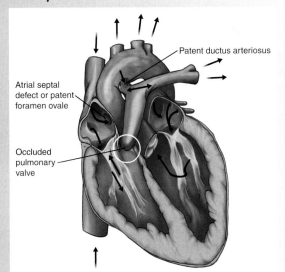

Figure reprinted with permission from Bowden, V. R., & Greenberg, C. S. (2013). *Children and their families* (3rd ed., Fig. 15.13). Philadelphia, PA: Wolters Kluwer Health/Lippincott Williams & Wilkins.

In some cases, there can also be narrowing and thus obstruction in the left and right branches of the pulmonary artery. This is known as branch stenosis.

Facts
- Second-most common congenital heart defect (5%–10% of all cases)
- Also referred to as right ventricular outflow tract obstruction
- Lifelong prophylaxis for infective endocarditis is needed.

Clinical Presentation
If mild, the child may have no symptoms.
- Respiratory: tachypnea, increased work of breathing, shortness of breath, cyanosis (if severe)
- Cardiac: tachycardia; edema in feet, ankles, face, eyelids, and abdomen; systolic ejection murmur

Diagnosis
- ECG: right atrial enlargement and right ventricular hypertrophy
- ECHO: information about pressure gradient across the valve
- Cardiac catheterization: used to determine right ventricular pressure (will be elevated) and pulmonary artery pressure (will be normal or low)

Therapeutic Interventions
Nonsurgical
Management of heart failure, if present

Surgical
For subvalvular stenosis, the excess tissue is removed just below the pulmonary artery. In valvular pulmonary stenosis, a balloon pulmonary valvuloplasty is performed during a catheterization procedure. For supravalvular pulmonary stenosis, surgery involves augmenting the pulmonary artery with patch angioplasty.

Prognosis
Children will lead normal lives if stenosis is treated. Regular follow-up is needed.

Pathophysiology
The pulmonic valve is underdeveloped or even completely closed by a layer of tissue. Therefore, blood cannot adequately flow to the lungs. This is a cyanotic defect, with cyanosis present shortly after birth. As the PDA closes, cyanosis becomes progressively worse. Therefore, the PDA must remain open to provide a source of pulmonary blood flow.

Typically, the right ventricle and the tricuspid valve are **hypoplastic** (small and dysfunctional).

Facts
- Unless very mild, must be managed at birth or the infant can become severely hypoxic
- In almost all cases there is an ASD with right-to-left shunting

Clinical Presentation
- Respiratory: cyanosis at birth, tachypnea, difficulty breathing
- Cardiac: pale, cool, clammy skin
- Growth: poor feeding

Diagnosis
- ECG: may show right atrial hypertrophy
- ECHO: there is no outflow tract or communication between the right ventricle and the pulmonary artery.

(continued)

Therapeutic Interventions

Nonsurgical

Prostaglandins are started immediately to keep ductus arteriosus open.

Surgical

Palliative repairs are done first, as described:
- A Blalock–Taussig shunt is used to establish a connection from the brachiocephalic artery or right subclavian artery to the right pulmonary artery through a homograft or synthetic graft.
- A pulmonary artery band may be placed in patients with pulmonary overcirculation.

Tricuspid Atresia

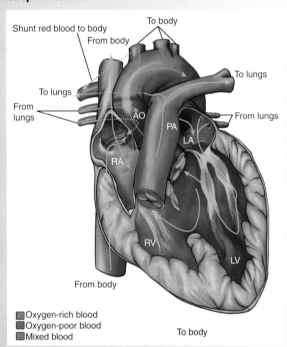

AO, aorta; LA, left atrium; LV, left ventricle; PA, pulmonary artery; RA, right atrium; RV, right ventricle. Figure reprinted with permission from Kyle, T., & Carman, S. (2016). *Essentials of pediatric nursing* (3rd ed., Fig. 19.3). Philadelphia, PA: Wolters Kluwer.

Pathophysiology

Tricuspid atresia is characterized by complete failure of the tricuspid valve (the valve from the right atrium to the right ventricle) to form. Therefore, there is no flow from the right atrium to the right ventricle because they are not connected. This is a cyanotic heart defect. An ASD is present with right-to-left shunting. This allows systemic venous blood to return to the left atrium, where it mixes with pulmonary (oxygenated) blood. The right ventricle is hypoplastic, and often the right atrium is enlarged and hypertrophic.

At a later date, the Fontan procedure is performed in stages to create passive pulmonary circulation that bypasses the right ventricle entirely.

Prognosis

Diagnosis and timely intervention are required for survival in a patient with pulmonary atresia.

Long-term outcomes vary depending on the corrective procedure and whether other defects are present. One study revealed 10-y survival rates ranging from 77% to 96% (Elias et al., 2018).

Because the left ventricle is volume overloaded (it receives both pulmonary blood and systemic blood from ASD), it is often enlarged and develops decreased function.

Facts
- One of every 10,000 babies born has tricuspid atresia (Mai et al., 2012).
- Prophylaxis for infective endocarditis is necessary after surgical correction.
- Long-term anticoagulant therapy may be necessary after surgical repair.

Clinical Presentation
- Respiratory: cyanosis present at birth, tachypnea, pulmonary edema, hypoxic episodes
- Cardiac: continuous murmur from the PDA, single S_2 heart sound in the aortic area, heart failure, hepatomegaly, polycythemia
- Growth: delayed

Diagnosis
- ECG: may reveal right atrial hypertrophy
- ECHO: reveals a hypoplastic (small and nonfunctional) ventricle and no flow from the right atrium to the right ventricle

Therapeutic Interventions

Nonsurgical
- Prostaglandins are started immediately to keep ductus arteriosus open. This provides the only blood flow to the lungs.
- Digoxin diuretics may be administered to control symptoms of heart failure.

Surgical

Surgical repair involves three separate surgeries to regulate pulmonary circulation: Blalock–Taussig shunt, Glenn procedure, and Fontan procedure. A Blalock–Taussig shunt is generally performed at 4–6 wk of age as a palliative measure. The Glenn procedure is performed at around 4–6 mo of age as a bridge to the final procedure, a Fontan procedure.

Box 21.4 Pathophysiology, Clinical Presentation, and Therapies for Decreased Pulmonary Flow Defects (*continued*)

Tetralogy of Fallot

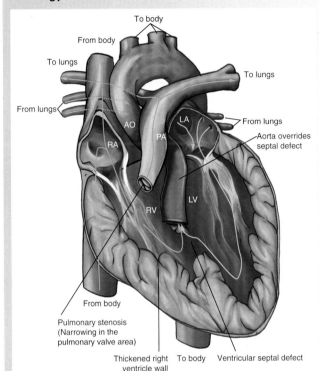

AO, aorta; LA, left atrium; LV, left ventricle; PA, pulmonary artery; RA, right atrium; RV, right ventricle. Figure reprinted with permission from Kyle, T., & Carman, S. (2016). *Essentials of pediatric nursing* (3rd ed., Fig. 19.2). Philadelphia, PA: Wolters Kluwer.

Pathophysiology

Four defects are present: pulmonic stenosis, right ventricular hypertrophy, VSD, and overriding aorta. The outflow portion of the right ventricle is undeveloped (hypoplasia) and not properly aligned, which leads to the four defects. Some children have a fifth defect, an open foramen ovale or an ASD. Elevated pressures on the right side of the heart (because of the increased blood volume and small right ventricle) cause a right-to-left shunt. The overriding aorta and VSD allow unoxygenated blood to enter the systemic circulation, hence cyanosis occurs.

The degree of right ventricular outflow tract obstruction determines the severity of the defect. When pulmonary stenosis is minimal, there may be little shunting across the VSD and thus very little unoxygenated blood enters the systemic circulation. This results in acyanosis. Conversely, a tetralogy of Fallot with severe pulmonary stenosis or even pulmonary atresia will be cyanotic.

Facts

- Most common cyanotic heart defect in infants
- Frequency among all cases of congenital heart disease of 10%
- Requires surgical repair
- Characterized by hypercyanotic episodes
- Squatting or a knee-to-chest position decreases return of systemic venous blood flow to the heart

Clinical Presentation

Symptoms depend on the severity of the right ventricular outflow tract obstruction and whether PDA is present.
- Respiratory: mild-to-severe cyanosis, tachypnea
- Cardiac: loud, harsh systolic ejection murmur, polycythemia, clubbing of fingers (over time), squatting in toddlers (if uncorrected)
- Growth: failure to gain weight

Diagnosis

- Chest X-ray: large right ventricle resulting in a boot-shaped heart, prominent aorta, decreased vascular markings
- ECG: right ventricular hypertrophy
- ECHO: obstructed pulmonary outflow, a VSD, an overriding aorta, and size of pulmonary arteries
- CBC: increased hematocrit, hemoglobin, prothrombin time, partial thromboplastin time (clotting time)

Therapeutic Interventions

Nonsurgical

Managing hypercyanotic episodes: monitor the child for prolonged unconsciousness and assess for metabolic acidosis.

Surgical

Palliative surgery is performed within the first few months of life for severe tetralogy of Fallot and a Blalock–Taussig shunt is performed.

Complete repair involves the following:
- Closing the VSD with a synthetic patch or autograft using the pericardium
- Closing the ASD, if present

Pulmonary stenosis is relieved by resecting the right ventricular outflow tract, a pulmonary valvotomy, or reconstruction using a patch.

Obstructive Disorders

Obstructive disorders involve **stenosis**, or narrowing of a major blood vessel, which interferes with blood flow through the vessel. Blood flow to systemic circulation is impaired; thus, peripheral circulation is decreased. Congenital heart defects that result in obstructed systemic blood flow include aortic stenosis, coarctation of the aorta, and hypoplastic left heart syndrome (Box 21.5).

Box 21.5   Pathophysiology, Clinical Presentation, and Therapies for Obstructive Defects

Aortic Stenosis

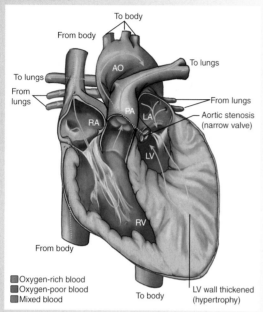

AO, aorta; LA, left atrium; LV, left ventricle; PA, pulmonary artery; RA, right atrium; RV, right ventricle. Figure reprinted with permission from Kyle, T., & Carman, S. (2016). *Essentials of pediatric nursing* (3rd ed., Fig. 19.9). Philadelphia, PA: Wolters Kluwer.

Pathophysiology

Aortic stenosis is an abnormal narrowing of the aortic valve. Blood flow from the left ventricle to the aorta is impeded. Therefore, systemic blood flow is compromised. Many times, the aortic valve has two leaflets instead of the usual three, and the leaflets may be stenotic (narrowed). There are three types of aortic stenosis: subvalvular, aortic, and supravalvular. Subvalvular is an obstruction below the aortic valve. Aortic stenosis involves the actual valve itself, and supravalvular involves obstruction of the ascending aorta just distal to the aortic valve.

Facts

- Requires bacterial endocarditis prophylaxis
- Exercise restrictions may be needed depending on the magnitude of the aortic valve dysfunction
- Chest pain, syncope (fainting), and sudden death may occur in symptomatic children, particularly during vigorous exercise

Clinical Presentation

- Respiratory: dyspnea on exertion or after exercise (uncommon)
- Cardiac: tachycardia, murmur, narrow pulse pressure (despite a normal blood pressure); in severe cases, low blood pressure and decreased peripheral pulses
- In neonates with severe aortic stenosis, closure of the PDA results in severe hypoperfusion, cardiogenic shock, profound metabolic acidosis.
- Growth: in severe cases, poor feeding, poor weight gain; most children grow and develop normally.

Diagnosis

- ECHO: increased left ventricular systolic pressure, size of valve opening, number of valve cusps present, size of aorta
- Exercise testing: in asymptomatic children to determine the amount of allowable exercise

Therapeutic Interventions

- Balloon valvuloplasty or surgical valvotomy
- Ross procedure (when severe)

Coarctation of the Aorta

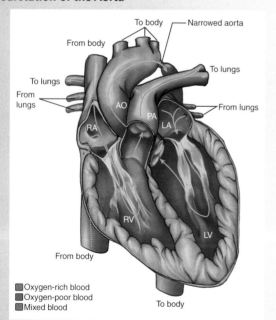

AO, aorta; LA, left atrium; LV, left ventricle; PA, pulmonary artery; RA, right atrium; RV, right ventricle. Figure reprinted with permission from Kyle, T., & Carman, S. (2016). *Essentials of pediatric nursing* (3rd ed., Fig. 19.8). Philadelphia, PA: Wolters Kluwer.

Pathophysiology

There is narrowing of the proximal portion of the descending aorta, usually just distal to the left subclavian artery. The narrowing may only involve a small segment of the aorta or may involve much larger segments. Typically, symptoms are not present at birth but can start developing as early as the first week of life. As long as the PDA remains open, perfusion to the lower extremities is adequate. Once the PDA closes, impaired perfusion to the lower extremities can occur.

Facts

- Blood pressures in the arms significantly higher than in the legs (10 mm Hg or greater)
- Relatively common, occurring in 5%–8% of all children with congenital heart disease; occurs in 4 out of every 10,000 babies born each year (Bjornard, Riehle-Colarusso, Gilboa, & Correa, 2013)

Clinical Presentation

- Respiration: tachypnea, increased work of breathing
- Cardiac: upper extremity hypertension, lower extremity blood pressures lower than upper extremities, weak/absent/delayed femoral pulses, pale and cold skin on legs/feet, sweating, loud S_2 on auscultation, systolic ejection murmur, palpable thrill in the suprasternal notch
- If severe, when ductus arteriosus closes at 8–10 d of life, development of shock, heart failure, metabolic acidosis,

Box 21.5 Pathophysiology, Clinical Presentation, and Therapies for Obstructive Defects (*continued*)

hypoglycemia, renal failure, necrotizing enterocolitis, and hypothermia
- Growth: poor feeding, poor weight gain
- Neurologic: irritability

Diagnosis
- Chest X-ray: cardiomegaly, pulmonary venous congestion
- ECG: left ventricular hypertrophy; in severe cases, right ventricular hypertrophy
- ECHO: size of aorta and actual coarctation, function of aortic valve and left ventricle

Therapeutic Interventions

Nonsurgical

- If severe in the newborn period, prostaglandin infusion required to keep ductus arteriosus open to perfuse the lower body and kidneys

- Treatment with diuretics, oxygen, and inotropic medications

Surgical

Several different surgical options are available depending on the severity of the defect and whether other heart defects are present:
- Synthetic patch aortoplasty
- Resection with end-to-end anastomosis (preferred because it preserves the left subclavian artery)
- Left subclavian artery patch (impairs blood flow to the left arm because of loss of the blood flow from the left subclavian artery)

Hypoplastic Left Heart Syndrome

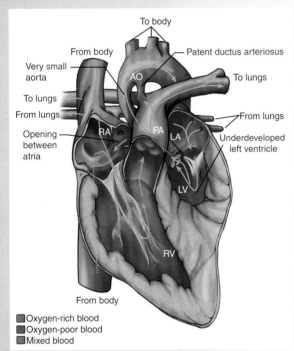

AO, aorta; LA, left atrium; LV, left ventricle; PA, pulmonary artery; RA, right atrium; RV, right ventricle. Figure reprinted with permission from Kyle, T., & Carman, S. (2016). *Essentials of pediatric nursing* (3rd ed., Fig. 19.14). Philadelphia, PA: Wolters Kluwer.

Pathophysiology

The left side of the heart is severely underdeveloped, including the left ventricle, the mitral and aortic valves, and the ascending aorta. The mitral valve is stenosed or there is mitral valve atresia. There is decreased blood flow to the left ventricle as a result.

The left ventricle is hypoplastic, reducing the force of contraction it can produce. Aortic stenosis or aortic atresia can be present, causing a narrowed tract for blood to leave the left

ventricle. Therefore, systemic blood flow is greatly reduced and the already hypoplastic ventricle must work harder.

In the right ventricle, mixing of oxygenated and unoxygenated blood occurs. The open PDA allows systemic circulation as it allows right-to-left shunting. In fact, in many cases, systemic circulation depends on the PDA remaining open.

Facts
- The most common cause of death among neonates with congenital heart disease
- Usually, the right ventricle becomes dilated and may be hypertrophic.

Clinical Presentation

The infant becomes symptomatic as ductus closes and systemic perfusion becomes increasingly compromised.
- Respiratory: tachypnea, increasing respiratory distress, cyanosis
- Cardiac: decreased pulses, signs of low cardiac output
- Growth: feeding difficulties
- Neurologic: irritable, not easily consoled, lethargy (late sign)

Diagnosis

During prenatal ultrasound, this defect can be diagnosed via ultrasound.
- Chest X-ray: pulmonary venous congestion and cardiomegaly
- ECHO: small size of left ventricle

Therapeutic Interventions

Nonsurgical

Prostaglandins are administered to keep ductus arteriosus open and maintain systemic perfusion.

Surgical

The Norwood procedure, which involves three stages of surgery, is used to repair the defect. Within the first few days of life, the procedure converts the right ventricle from pulmonary function to a systemic function. Later, the procedure allows complete separation of the pulmonary and systemic circulations.

Mixed Flow Disorders

Mixed defects involve the mixing of well-oxygenated blood with poorly oxygenated blood. Overall, the systemic blood flow contains a lower oxygen content as a result of the mixing. Cardiac output is also decreased, and heart failure occurs. Mixed flow disorders include transposition of the great arteries, truncus arteriosus, total anomalous pulmonary venous return, and double-outlet right ventricle (DORV; Box 21.6).

Cardiac Catheterization

Children with congenital heart disease, as well as some with acquired heart diseases, undergo cardiac catheterization to diagnose and, in some cases, treat their condition, and monitor their heart function. Cardiac catheterization can be performed on an outpatient basis or while the child is hospitalized. Before the procedure, laboratory studies, including a complete blood count (CBC) and electrolytes, and diagnostic

---

Box 21.6 Pathophysiology, Clinical Presentation, and Therapies for Mixed Flow Defects

Transposition of the Great Arteries

To body
From body
To lungs
To lungs
From lungs
AO   PA
From lungs
RA   LA
RV   LV
From body

■ Oxygen-rich blood
■ Oxygen-poor blood
■ Mixed blood
To body

AO, aorta; LA, left atrium; LV, left ventricle; PA, pulmonary artery; RA, right atrium; RV, right ventricle. Figure reprinted with permission from Ateah, C. A., Scott, S. D., & Kyle, T. (2012). *Canadian essentials of pediatric nursing* (1st ed., Fig. 20.11). Philadelphia, PA: Lippincott Williams & Wilkins.

Pathophysiology

The aorta and pulmonary arteries are connected to the wrong ventricles. The pulmonary artery is attached to the left ventricle and the aorta is attached to the right ventricle. Therefore, oxygenated blood from the left ventricle is recirculated to the lungs via the abnormally connected pulmonary artery. Also, deoxygenated blood returning to the right heart from the body recirculates to the body via the abnormally connected aorta.

Necessary blood flow occurs because one or more of the following defects is also present: PDA, ASD, and/or VSD. The PDA allows blood to shunt between the aorta

and the pulmonary artery. The ASD allows blood to flow from the right to the left atrium, and the VSD allows blood to flow between the right and left ventricles.

Facts

- Most common cyanotic heart defect; occurs in 5% of all newborns with congenital heart disease
- Twenty-five percent of children with this defect also have a VSD.
- If left untreated, 50% of children die within the first month of life.

Clinical Presentation

- Respiratory: cyanosis that does not improve with supplemental oxygen, hypoxia, tachypnea without signs of respiratory distress
- Cardiac: S_2 is loud, systolic murmur if VSD is present, signs of heart failure, polycythemia
- Growth: failure to gain weight

Diagnosis

- Chest X-ray: narrowed cardiac silhouette gives the heart a classic egg-shaped appearance, cardiomegaly
- ECG: right ventricular hypertrophy
- ECHO: abnormal position of the great arteries

Therapeutic Interventions

Nonsurgical

- IV prostaglandins are started soon after birth to keep the ductus arteriosus open.
- Monitor and treat heart failure.

Surgical

- Balloon atrial septostomy is performed palliatively to make a larger ASD (by enlarging the foramen ovale) to allow more mixing of oxygen-rich and oxygen-poor blood, thus increasing O_2 to approximately 80%.
- Surgical repair involves an arterial switch (the Jatene procedure). This procedure is usually performed within the first 2 wk of life.

Prognosis

Without treatment, 50% of infants die within the first month and 90% die within the first year of life. Following an arterial switch procedure, the 20-y survival rate is 97% (Van Velzen et al., 2015).

Box 21.6 Pathophysiology, Clinical Presentation, and Therapies for Mixed Flow Defects (*continued*)

Truncus Arteriosus

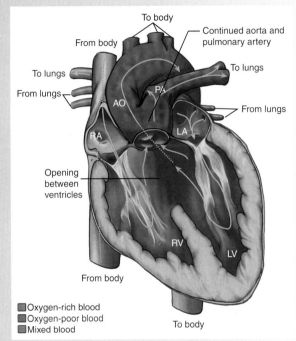

AO, aorta; LA, left atrium; LV, left ventricle; PA, pulmonary artery; RA, right atrium; RV, right ventricle. Figure reprinted with permission from Kyle, T., & Carman, S. (2016). *Essentials of pediatric nursing* (3rd ed., Fig. 19.13). Philadelphia, PA: Wolters Kluwer.

Pathophysiology

A single great artery with a common trunk overriding a large VSD is present. During fetal development, the truncus arteriosus (common trunk) fails to divide into the pulmonary artery and the aorta. Therefore, instead of a pulmonary artery arising from the right ventricle and an aorta arising from the left ventricle, there is one common great artery. Also, the aortic and pulmonic valves are fused together, forming one large semilunar valve with multiple leaflets. Cyanosis is common.

There is a large malaligned VSD. Left-to-right shunting or bidirectional shunting is always present. There is pulmonary overcirculation and systemic desaturation. The left atrium and left ventricle may be enlarged because of volume overload. Often, pulmonary hypertension and heart failure develop, particularly if surgical repair does not occur early.

Facts

- Can be associated with DiGeorge syndrome
- Child should not participate in competitive or strenuous sports.

Clinical Presentation

- Respiratory: cyanosis soon after birth, tachypnea, dyspnea, retractions, nasal flaring, frequent respiratory infections, pulmonary hypertension
- Cardiac: increased pulse pressure, irritability, bounding peripheral pulses, neck vein distension, facial swelling; over time, cardiomegaly, polycythemia, clubbing of fingers
- Growth: fatigue, poor feeding, poor growth

Diagnosis

- Chest X-ray: cardiomegaly, large aorta
- ECG: right and left ventricular hypertrophy
- ECHO: a VSD, a single great artery, and only one semilunar valve

Therapeutic Interventions

Nonsurgical

Treat heart failure with diuretics and digoxin.

Surgical

Corrective surgery involves the following three major components:
1. Separating the pulmonary arteries from the main truncus
2. Closing the VSD using a patch
3. Creating a connection between the right ventricle and the pulmonary arteries via a conduit (usually a homograft pulmonary artery)

(*continued*)

Box 21.6 Pathophysiology, Clinical Presentation, and Therapies for Mixed Flow Defects (*continued*)

Total Anomalous Pulmonary Venous Return

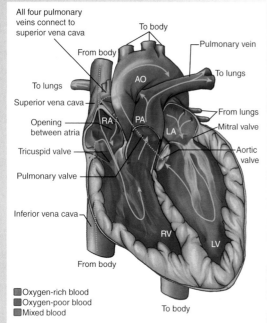

AO, aorta; LA, left atrium; LV, left ventricle; PA, pulmonary artery; RA, right atrium; RV, right ventricle. Figure reprinted with permission from Ateah, C. A., Scott, S. D., & Kyle, T. (2012). *Canadian essentials of pediatric nursing* (1st ed., Fig. 20.12). Philadelphia, PA: Lippincott Williams & Wilkins.

Pathophysiology

Instead of returning to the left atrium, the pulmonary veins empty into the right atrium or systemic circulation, which returns to the right atrium. The foramen ovale must remain open or an ASD must be present for mixed blood from the right atrium to pass to the systemic circulation for the body to be partially oxygenated. Cyanosis, in varying degrees, is present.

Facts

- Occurs in about 1% of congenital heart defects
- Survival without surgery is not possible

Clinical Presentation

If there is no obstruction of blood along abnormal course of the blood flow, infants and children can be asymptomatic. If any obstruction occurs, cyanosis occurs.

- Respiratory: tachypnea, mild cyanosis, increasing cyanosis with feedings as the esophagus compresses the common pulmonary vein
  - Note: when pulmonary veins are compressed, the following manifest: tachycardia, dyspnea, retractions, crackles, pulmonary edema, hepatomegaly, irritability, poor feeding
- Cardiac: tachycardia; heart failure; palpable precordial bulge; S_2 has a wide, fixed split, **gallop** rhythm (a third, typically abnormal, heart sound)
- Growth: failure to thrive

Diagnosis

- Chest X-ray: enlarged heart, pulmonary edema
- ECG: right atrial and ventricular hypertrophy
- ECHO: dilated right heart, smaller left heart, dilated pulmonary arteries, patent foramen ovale

Therapeutic Interventions

Nonsurgical

- Prostaglandins must be started to maintain a PDA.
- Heart failure is treated with digoxin and diuretics.

Surgical

- Palliative: balloon atrial septostomy to increase blood flow to the left side of the heart until patient is stable
- Corrective: reconnecting the pulmonary veins to the back of the left atrium

Double-Outlet Right Ventricle

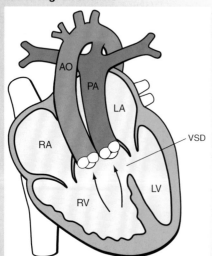

AO, aorta; LA, left atrium; LV, left ventricle; PA, pulmonary artery; RA, right atrium; RV, right ventricle; VSD, ventricular septal defect. Figure reprinted with permission from Abuhamad, A. Z., & Chaoui, R. (2015). *A practical guide to fetal echocardiography* (3rd ed., Fig. 27.1). Philadelphia, PA: Wolters Kluwer.

Pathophysiology

Both the aorta and the pulmonary artery exit from the right ventricle. This is a cyanotic heart defect, as unoxygenated blood leaves the right ventricle via the aorta and returns to the right heart without going through the lungs. The only outlet for oxygenated blood to enter systemic circulation is through a VSD (oxygenated blood flows from the left ventricle to the right ventricle and out the aorta). A VSD is always present in a patient with a DORV.

Facts

- A child with a DORV most likely has additional heart defects, including pulmonic stenosis, coarctation of the aorta, and transposition of the great arteries.
- Prophylaxis for infective endocarditis if often required for life.

Clinical Presentation

Symptoms depend on the position of the VSD and the degree of pulmonary valve stenosis.

- Respiratory: cyanosis, tachypnea at birth
- Cardiac: systolic murmur, loud S_2
- Growth: failure to thrive

Box 21.6 Pathophysiology, Clinical Presentation, and Therapies for Mixed Flow Defects (*continued*)

Diagnosis
- ECG: right bundle branch block, right ventricular hypertrophy, right atrial hypertrophy, first-degree atrioventricular block
- ECHO: both great arteries originating from the right ventricle, VSD, absence of left ventricular outflow

Therapeutic Interventions
Nonsurgical
Heart failure treatment is administered, including digoxin and diuretics.

Surgical
- If severe cyanosis: modified Blalock–Taussig shunt
- When VSD is too small: balloon atrial septostomy
- Corrective surgery: arterial switch, Rastelli or Fontan procedure depending on severity of defect and location of defects

tests, including an electrocardiogram (ECG), chest X-ray, and ECHO, may be ordered. The child should have nothing by mouth for several hours before the procedure. Administer medications, as ordered, up to the time of the procedure. Immediately before the procedure, have the child void. The child is sedated during the procedure. Infants and smaller children may need deeper sedation or anesthesia to keep them still during the procedure.

Care of the child undergoing a cardiac catheterization includes physical and psychosocial assessment of the child and family both before and after the procedure, as well as monitoring for complications and preparing the child for discharge home.

Assessment and Diagnosis

Before the procedure, assess the child using the assessment guidelines in Table 21.2. Be sure to note the heart rate, quality of peripheral and central pulses and capillary refill, and the temperature of the skin on all extremities. Ensure that the child has had nothing by mouth by questioning the parents regarding the time the child last had something to eat or drink. Obtain baseline hematocrit and hemoglobin levels before the procedure.

During the procedure, monitor the child's vital signs and assess for pain and anxiety. Immediately after the procedure, assess the catheter site for pulses or signs of bleeding or hematoma formation; distal to the site for pulses, heart rate, and blood pressure. If bleeding occurred during the procedure, obtain hemoglobin and hematocrit levels as ordered.

Therapeutic Interventions

Priorities of care for the child after a cardiac catheterization include monitoring and preventing complications, providing a restful, quiet environment, and maintaining hydration. See the section General Therapeutic Interventions for Cardiovascular Disorders for details on these interventions.

Evaluation

Expected outcomes for a child undergoing a cardiac catheterization include the following:
- Complications such as bleeding and clot formation are quickly identified and managed.
- The child maintains bed rest and avoids flexing the hips for 4 to 6 hours after catheterization.
- Intake and output are balanced after catheterization.

Discharge Planning and Teaching

Preparing a child and family for discharge after a cardiac catheterization includes teaching them the signs and symptoms of infection, signs of bleeding and clot formation, signs of dehydration, and when to call the provider. Teach parents the signs of infection, including fever, redness, warmth, increasing pain, and drainage or discharge from the catheter site. Instruct them that signs of bleeding and/or clot formation include the foot on the side of the catheterization being cooler than the other foot and having a loss of feeling. Teach parents how to apply pressure to the site if it begins to bleed.

Review signs of dehydration with parents, as well, and instruct them to notify the provider if they observe dry mucous membranes, an absence of tears, or a strong odor to the urine. Ask parents to note and report any decrease in wet diapers or frequency of voiding. Before discharge, parents should be able to state when to call the provider.

Discharge teaching following heart surgery should include information necessary for parents to continue to care for the child at home, such as the following topics:
- Congenital heart defect, surgical repair, and prognosis information
- Medication prescribed and the ordered schedule and dose
- Incision care and identification of signs of infection at the incision site
- Nutrition requirements and feeding strategies, especially for infants

- Follow-up appointments and laboratory testing
- Bacterial endocarditis prophylaxis, if ordered
- Activity restrictions until the chest is healed

Acquired Cardiovascular Disorders

Heart Failure

Heart failure is defined as a complex clinical and pathological syndrome resulting from structural or functional impairment of the heart ventricle. In children, heart failure is most commonly attributed to congenital heart disease. Specific heart malformations pose different risks of heart failure in the pediatric patient. Heart failure can also occur in the context of other diseases, such as sepsis, cancer, cardiomyopathy, myocarditis, and Kawasaki disease. In the United States, heart failure is estimated to affect 12,000 to 35,000 children each year, with more than 14,000 children being hospitalized annually for heart failure–related issues (Rossano et al., 2012).

Etiology and Pathophysiology

Heart failure in children can be divided into pathophysiological categories, which aids in the understanding of its underlying physiology and clinical manifestations. Three categories of heart failure are ventricular dysfunction, volume overload with normal ventricular contractility, and pressure overload with normal ventricular contractility. Ventricular dysfunction can be further divided into that which occurs in children with structurally normal hearts and that which occurs in those with congenital heart defects. Causes of ventricular dysfunction in children with structurally normal hearts include the following: cardiomyopathy, myocarditis, myocardial ischemia, arrhythmias (complete heart block and supraventricular tachycardia), drugs and toxins (children receiving chemotherapy or immunosuppressive therapy after organ transplant), and noncardiac issues, such as sepsis, chronic kidney disease, chronic lung disease, human immunodeficiency virus, and systemic lupus erythematous. Ventricular dysfunction in children with complex congenital heart disease can result from surgical repair or palliation early in childhood.

Heart failure resulting from volume overload with preserved ventricular contractility may be due to cardiac or noncardiac causes. When a moderate or large shunt occurs between the systemic and pulmonary circulations, volume overload can occur. Congenital heart defects that can lead to volume overload include the following: VSD, PDA, AV septal defect, aortic stenosis, and mitral valve regurgitation. A long-term complication following tetralogy of Fallot repair can be pulmonary regurgitation, which can lead to volume overload, as well. Noncardiac volume overload heart failure can occur in children diagnosed with oliguric renal failure.

Heart failure from pressure overload with preserved ventricular contractility often results from ventricular outflow obstruction. Mild outflow obstruction may be asymptomatic, whereas severe outflow obstruction often presents early in infancy because of low cardiac output. Aortic stenosis, coarctation of the aorta, and pulmonary stenosis can lead to heart failure as a result of pressure overload. Pulmonary hypertension can also result in pressure overload on the right ventricle and may lead to right-sided heart failure.

Regardless of the etiology, decreased cardiac output develops in heart failure. When cardiac output remains insufficient, the body's organs and tissues do not receive adequate perfusion and thus adequate oxygenation. Cytokine-induced inflammation also occurs. Decreased cardiac output leads to production of metabolites in organs, which results in vasodilation and decreased blood pressure. The renin–angiotensin system and the sympathetic nervous system are activated as compensatory mechanisms. As blood pressure falls, angiotensin and kidney mechanisms are stimulated (the renin–angiotensin aldosterone system), resulting in vasoconstriction to preserve end-organ function and water and sodium retention to increase preload and thus increase cardiac output. Systemic vascular resistance also increases to maintain mean arterial pressure and organ perfusion. The activation of the sympathetic nervous system and increased release of catecholamines result in tachycardia, increased myocardial contractility, and hypertrophy of the myocardium. Although these actions improve the child's cardiac output and maintain blood pressure, the continued increased work of the heart worsens symptoms (Masarone et al., 2017).

Clinical Presentation

In Chapter 7, Caleb Yoder, the newborn with a VSD, developed congestive heart failure. As his heart failure progressed, what signs did Caleb demonstrate? What was his heart rate and general appearance when he arrived at the hospital?

Clinically, the manifestations of heart failure in the pediatric patient vary according to the child's age, cardiac output, degree of volume overload, and degree of pulmonary or systemic venous congestion. Infants commonly appear with tachypnea and diaphoresis during feeds, irritability, decreased volume of feeds, and poor weight gain. Young children may have gastrointestinal symptoms such as abdominal pain, nausea, vomiting, and poor appetite, as well as easy fatigability and recurrent cough and wheezing. Older children may present with anorexia, abdominal pain, edema, palpitations, chest pain, and dizziness, as well as exercise intolerance and respiratory symptoms (wheezing and dyspnea).

Assessment and Diagnosis

Heart failure in children may be subtle initially and not immediately apparent. The diagnosis of heart failure primarily depends on physical symptoms, so astute nursing observations are important. Using a systems approach, the nurse recognizes that changes in respiratory, cardiovascular, neurological, gastrointestinal, and kidney function may indicate onset and worsening of heart failure. Respiratory changes to assess for include tachypnea, increased work of breathing, crackles upon auscultation, and decreasing O_2 levels. Respiratory findings are a result of pulmonary congestion. Cardiovascular assessment may reveal tachycardia, generalized edema, capillary refill time greater than 2 seconds, cool extremities, pallor, and diaphoresis. Tachycardia and signs of poor perfusion are a result of decreased cardiac output. Neurological changes include increased irritability, fussiness, or lethargy and sleepiness. Feedings may take longer in infants, and older children may demonstrate a loss of appetite. Urinary output may be less than usual or less than age-specific norms (infants: 1–3 mL/kg/h; older children: 0.5–1 mL/kg/h), and parents may report fewer wet diapers or trips to the bathroom for potty-trained children. Hepatomegaly and ascites may be present as a result of systemic congestions. Table 21.6 summarizes the clinical manifestations of heart failure according to the corresponding etiology.

The diagnosis of heart failure is based on a combination of clinical and laboratory findings, as well as radiographic, ECG, and ECHO. Laboratory studies for suspected heart failure include brain natriuretic peptide (BNP), troponin, CBC, and serum chemistries. Box 21.7 lists laboratory studies and the rationale for their use in patients with suspected heart failure. Chest X-ray may reveal cardiomegaly, pulmonary congestion, or pleural effusions. An ECG may demonstrate sinus tachycardia and can be helpful in determining the underlying cause of heart failure. ST-segment and T-wave abnormalities are common in cardiomyopathy, whereas changes in QRS voltage occur in ventricular hypertrophy, cardiomyopathy, and myocarditis. An ECHO is the most useful tool in diagnosing heart failure, because it reveals information regarding heart chamber size, ventricle function, ventricle size, wall thickness, and pulmonary pressures (Masarone et al., 2017).

Therapeutic Interventions

Care of the child with heart failure requires a collaborative approach and involves performing careful assessment, promoting oxygenation and cardiovascular function, supporting growth and development, supporting the child and family during hospitalization, and providing them with resources for care at home. The nurse not only provides direct intervention

---

Box 21.7 Laboratory Studies Observed in Heart Failure

BNP
- Used to assess severity of heart failure and monitor therapy
- Elevated BNP levels are seen in patients with left-to-right shunting defects.
- Elevated BNP levels are present in patients with low ejection fractions; the lower the ejection fraction, the higher the BNP (Sugimoto et al., 2010).

Troponin
- Elevated in myocarditis and myocardial ischemia

Complete blood count
- Anemia contributes to heart failure or exacerbates severity of symptoms.

Serum chemistries
- Sodium: hyponatremia may be seen in children with severe heart failure.
- Blood urea nitrogen and creatinine: elevated levels seen in renal failure; renal failure may be a contributing factor or worsen preexisting failure.
- Aspartate aminotransferase and alanine aminotransferase: liver enzymes may be elevated because of hepatic congestion.

---

but also functions as a liaison for teams involved in the child's care. Pediatric cardiologists, primary care providers, respiratory therapists, dietitians, social services professionals, home care nurses, PTs, and OTs are some of the team members involved in planning and implementing care for a child with heart failure.

Nursing care of the child with heart failure involves maintaining adequate oxygenation, maintaining cardiac output and myocardial function, monitoring fluid balance, administering medications (The Pharmacy 21.2), monitoring for effects and complications of medications, providing adequate nutrition, promoting rest, ensuring growth and development, and supporting the patient and family. See the section General Nursing Interventions for Cardiovascular Disorders earlier for details on these interventions.

Table 21.6 Clinical Manifestations of Heart Failure

Etiology	Clinical Manifestations
Pulmonary venous congestion	• Early: mild tachypnea, respiratory infections, labored breathing during feeding, cough • Progressive: increased tachypnea at rest, wheezing, crackles, grunting, cyanosis, increased diaphoresis and tachypnea during feedings
Systemic venous congestion	• Early: peripheral edema, periorbital edema, weight gain associated with fluid retention • Progressive: enlarged liver, ascites, abdominal distention, jugular venous distension
Impaired cardiac output	• Early: tachycardia, pallor, tiring with play, cool extremities • Progressive: weak pulses, hypotension, delayed capillary refill, oliguria, irritability
Increased metabolic demand	Diaphoresis, slow weight gain or weight loss, failure to thrive

The Pharmacy 21.2 Medications Used to Treat Heart Failure

Medication	Classification	Route	Action	Nursing Considerations
Furosemide (Lasix)	Loop diuretic	• PO • IV	Inhibits reabsorption of sodium and chloride from the proximal and distal tubules and ascending loop of Henle, resulting in sodium-rich diuresis	• Monitor urine output following administration. • Monitor potassium; may require potassium replacement. • Perform daily weights. • Monitor for orthostatic hypotension.
Digoxin	Cardiac glycoside	• PO • IV	• Positive inotropic effect (increases force of myocardial contractions) • Increases renal perfusion • Negative chronotropic effect (decreases heart rate)	• Dosing in pediatrics is in micrograms/kilogram. • Monitor apical pulse for 1 min before administration. Hold the dose if the pulse is <90 beats/min in an infant. • Avoid giving with meals.
Enalapril, captopril	• ACE inhibitors • Antihypertensive	• PO • IV	• Blocks the conversion of angiotensin I to angiotensin II, which decreases blood pressure, decreases aldosterone secretion, slightly increases potassium, and causes sodium and fluid loss • In heart failure, also decreases peripheral resistance, afterload, preload, and heart size	• Monitor blood pressure for hypotension. • May interact with OTC medications; have patient check with provider before taking any OTC medications. • Adverse effects include cough, nausea, diarrhea, headache, and dizziness.
Carvedilol (Coreg)	Beta-1-selective adrenergic blocker	• PO • IV	• Blocks beta-adrenergic receptors in the heart and juxtaglomerular apparatus, which decreases the influence of the sympathetic nervous system on these tissues • Decreases the excitability of the heart, which decreases cardiac output and release of renin, which in turn lowers blood pressure	• Check apical pulse before administration. If <90 bpm, do not administer medication; consult the provider. • Monitor blood pressure before administration.

From Lexicomp. *Pediatric & Neonatal Dosage Handbook* (25th ed.), 2018.
ACE, angiotensin-converting enzyme; IV, intravenous; OTC, over-the-counter; PO, by mouth.

Evaluation

Expected outcomes for a child with heart failure depend on the etiology and type of heart failure. Here, however, are some common expected outcomes:
- The child achieves adequate caloric intake.
- The child's weight gain is adequate for age.
- Symptoms of heart failure are controlled with medications, diet, and activity.
- The child's cardiac output is sufficient to meet the body's metabolic demands.
- Intake and output are balanced.
- Skin integrity remains intact.
- Parents have necessary information and support to care for their child with heart failure.

Discharge Planning and Teaching

Long-term health maintenance for a child with heart failure requires a multifaceted approach and collaboration between the child's primary care team and cardiologist. Health maintenance includes the following: immunizations, monitoring growth, monitoring cardiac symptoms, treating respiratory illnesses, exercise and physical activity, antibiotic prophylaxis, and careful planning of noncardiac surgeries, if needed. Children with heart failure should receive all routine childhood vaccinations, including pneumococcal and yearly influenza vaccines. Eligible infants should also receive immunoprophylaxis for respiratory syncytial virus. Teach parents to monitor their child's weight at home and to report any significant increase or decrease in weight to the provider, per the provider's orders. Make sure parents are aware of the signs of respiratory illness, and encourage them to seek early treatment for respiratory illnesses, which are associated with considerable morbidity and mortality in children with heart failure.

Antibiotic prophylaxis for the prevention of bacterial endocarditis is essential for many patients with heart failure, particularly those with cyanotic heart defects or heart failure caused by rheumatic fever. Educate parents on not just the importance of but also the specific indications for, and proper dosing, administration, and duration of prophylaxis.

Teach parents and older children how to recognize signs of worsening heart failure. Instruct parents to take the child's pulse and report significant changes to the provider. An increase in pulse can indicate worsening heart failure, whereas a decrease in pulse can indicate digoxin toxicity. Teach parents the signs of dehydration (fewer wet diapers, dry lips, decreased urine output), particularly for infants and children taking diuretics.

Before discharge, parents of infants should demonstrate how to properly feed an infant with heart failure and parents of older children should be able to identify appropriate high-calorie foods and snacks. If tube feedings are necessary after discharge, have parents demonstrate proper technique for this intervention. Ensure that parents know how to monitor and record the patient's intake and output if requested by the provider.

Keeping follow-up appointments with the cardiologist and other providers, obtaining and administering medications, and having blood drawn for laboratory tests as ordered are essential in the care of a child with heart failure. Teach parents the importance of follow-up care and laboratory studies. Refer families to a social worker for information regarding resources for medication assistance, transportation to appointments, and respite care.

Acute Rheumatic Fever

ARF is an autoimmune, inflammatory reaction affecting the heart, blood vessels, and joints that can develop as a result of being infected with group A streptococcus (GAS). ARF generally arises 2 to 4 weeks after an untreated infection with GAS. ARF can be prevented with the appropriate use of antibiotic treatment for GAS up to 9 days after the onset of pharyngitis (Watson, Jallow, Le Doare, Pushparaja, & Anderson, 2015).

Etiology and Pathophysiology

The pathophysiology of ARF remains unclear, but two theories of the pathogenesis have been seriously considered: the cytotoxic theory and the immunologic theory. The cytotoxic theory suggests that a GAS toxin is involved. GAS produces several enzymes that are cytotoxic, including streptolysin O, which has a direct cytotoxic effect on human cells. The immunologic theory suggests that some people have a specific immune response to repeated infections with GAS. This specific population develops a decrease in suppressor activity after repeated episodes of GAS throat infections. This leads to increased humoral and cellular immune response to the streptococcal antigen, which cross-reacts with specific human tissues such as the heart and joints. Autoantibodies against these tissues are then made, and the combination of these antibodies and the cellular response leads to the clinical manifestations seen in ARF (Carapetis et al., 2016).

The incidence of initial ARF is highest in children aged 5 to 15 years. Children who have had one attack of rheumatic fever are more susceptible to additional attacks. In some developing countries, the incidence exceeds 50 per 100,000 children. Most cases occur in low- and middle-income countries and among indigenous groups. Worldwide, rheumatic heart disease remains the most common form of acquired heart disease in all age groups. In the continental United States, however, the incidence is approximately 0.04 to 0.06 cases per 1,000 children (Stockmann et al., 2012).

Clinical Presentation

Children with rheumatic fever can present with subtle symptoms or very distinct symptoms. Many parents simply bring the child to the provider because of a low-grade fever that does not resolve. On questioning, the provider then learns that the child has had a recent sore throat and has not been treated or may have been treated for a strep throat. Other children present with obvious manifestations, such as severe joint pain and arthritis-like pain, a red rash over their trunk, or nodules on their elbows and knees (Fig. 21.8). The nurse should consider ARF if there is a history of a recent sore throat, particularly if it was not treated with antibiotics.

Assessment and Diagnosis

The diagnosis of ARF is made using the Jones criteria (Table 21.7). The Jones criteria consist of three groups of findings: five major manifestations, four minor manifestations, and

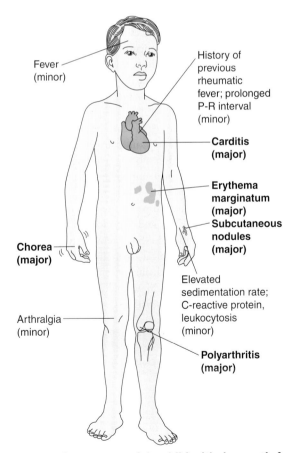

Figure 21.8. Assessment of the child with rheumatic fever. Reprinted with permission from Pillitteri, A. (2003). *Maternal and child health nursing* (4th ed., Fig. 41.3). Philadelphia, PA: Lippincott Williams & Wilkins.

Table 21.7 Jones Criteria Used in Diagnosing Acute Rheumatic Fever

Major Manifestations	Minor Manifestations	Evidence of Group A Streptococcal Infection
• Carditis • Polyarthritis • Sydenham chorea • Erythema marginatum • Subcutaneous nodules	• Fever • Polyarthralgia • Elevated C-reactive protein level or erythrocyte sedimentation rate • Prolonged PR interval	• Positive throat culture result • Positive antigen test result • Elevated or rising antistreptolysin-O titer

one essential criterion of evidence of preceding GAS infection. Diagnosis of ARF requires the presence of at least two major manifestations *or* one major and two minor manifestations *and* evidence of a GAS infection (Gewitz et al., 2015).

The major manifestations include carditis, polyarthritis, Sydenham chorea, erythema marginatum, and subcutaneous nodules. Carditis (inflammation of the heart) is seen in approximately 50% to 65% of patients who are diagnosed with ARF. Although the pericardium, epicardium, myocardium, and endocardium can all be affected, valvulitis is the most consistent feature of ARF (Gewitz et al., 2015). Detection of a murmur, cardiomegaly on a chest X-ray, or pericardial friction rub or effusion is often how carditis is diagnosed. Polyarthritis is often the earliest manifestation and is seen in 50% to 70% of patients diagnosed with ARF within 21 days of a GAS infection (Gewitz et al., 2015). Polyarthritis manifests as inflammation, erythema, heat, tenderness, edema, and pain in two or more joints, with the knees and ankles being the most frequently affected. Sydenham chorea, a neurologic sequela, manifests as myasthenia, emotional instability, and spontaneous involuntary movements that lack a consistent rhythm. Approximately 10% to 30% of patients with ARF have symptoms of chorea (Gewitz et al., 2015). Fewer than 6% of patients present with erythema marginatum, a nonpruritic, transient, macular erythematous rash that has folded-up borders and pale centers (Gewitz et al., 2015). In severe cases of ARF, subcutaneous nodules are found; they are firm, nontender, freely mobile nodules in the subcutaneous tissues, over bony prominences.

The minor manifestations include fever, polyarthralgia, an elevated CRP level or ESR, and a prolonged PR interval on an ECG. Fever is considered a body temperature greater than 38.5°C (101.3°F). Polyarthralgia—pain in multiple joints without signs of heat, edema, erythema, or tenderness—is a nonspecific minor manifestation. An abnormally elevated CRP level or ESR is almost always seen in patients with ARF. A prolonged

PR interval, after accounting for variability due to age, can be present, particularly if carditis is also present. Although not part of the Jones criteria, other clinical symptoms may occur in patients presenting with ARF, including abdominal pain, malaise, pallor, fatigue, epistaxis, tachycardia at rest, anorexia, and weight loss.

Therapeutic Interventions

Nursing management related to ARF includes prevention, treatment, and supportive care. The most important role of the nurse is prevention of rheumatic fever. Help prevent ARF by ensuring that all children with possible streptococcal infections seen in clinics, offices, and schools have a throat culture. If a throat culture returns a positive result, emphasize to the family the importance of completing the entire prescribed course of antibiotics. For the child diagnosed with ARF, nursing care focuses on assessing the child's condition, administering antibiotics and anti-inflammatory medications (The Pharmacy 21.3), promoting rest and recovery, relieving pain, providing supportive care, and ensuring the child and family adhere to the treatment regimen. See the section General Therapeutic Interventions for Cardiovascular Disorders earlier for details on these interventions.

Evaluation

Expected outcomes for a child with rheumatic fever include the following:
- No further episodes of GAS pharyngitis occur.
- The child achieves optimal cardiac function.
- Pain is controlled throughout the acute phase of rheumatic fever.

Discharge Planning and Teaching

Hospitalization for rheumatic fever can be for an extended period of time, particularly if severe carditis and heart failure

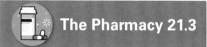

The Pharmacy 21.3 Medications Used in the Treatment of Acute Rheumatic Fever

Medication	Classification	Route	Action	Nursing Considerations
Naproxen	NSAID	PO	• Inhibits prostaglandin synthesis • Reduces inflammation • Reduces pain	• May cause dizziness or nausea • Monitor for GI bleeding

From Lexicomp. *Pediatric & Neonatal Dosage Handbook* (25th ed.), 2018.
GI, gastrointestinal; NSAID, nonsteroidal anti-inflammatory drug; PO, by mouth.

are present. When the child is ready to be discharged from the hospital, provide teaching on the following:

- Prevention of future GAS infections by the patient taking prophylactic antibiotics (a daily oral dose or monthly long-acting antibiotic injection) until the patient reaches his or her 20s or early 30s
- The importance of getting a throat culture if streptococcal infection is suspected and, if treated for GAS, the importance of finishing the entire 10-day course of antibiotics
- The signs of heart failure, including the following: shortness of breath, swelling of the legs, rapid heartbeat, fatigue and weakness, rapid weight gain, and reduced ability to exercise or participate in physical activity
- The need for prophylaxis with antibiotics to prevent infective endocarditis in children with heart valve damage
- The importance of follow-up care, particularly because patients with a history of ARF are at increased risk for developing rheumatic heart disease

Infective Endocarditis

Infective endocarditis is an infection of the endocardium (the heart's inner lining) and, possibly, the heart valves. Vegetations can grow in or around the affected endocardium or valves (Fig. 21.9). Infective endocarditis is also referred to as bacterial endocarditis, because most cases are caused by bacterial pathogens.

Etiology and Pathophysiology

Infective endocarditis is the result of complex interactions between bloodborne pathogens and a damaged endothelium. In children with congenital heart disease or indwelling central venous catheters, the endocardial surface is initially injured by

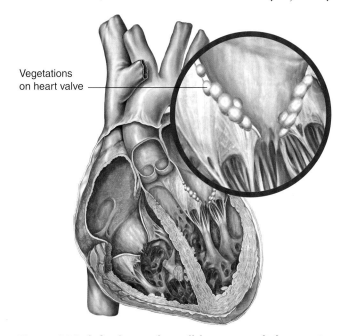

Vegetations on heart valve —

Figure 21.9. Infective endocarditis can result in vegetations in the heart tissue. Reprinted with permission from Anatomical Chart Company.

shear forces that arise from turbulent blood flow. Fibrin, platelets, and red blood cells are deposited at the site of endothelial damage and initially form a noninfected thrombus. Transient bacteremia or fungemia results when microbial pathogens adhere to the injured endocardium and thrombus. More fibrin and platelets are deposited over the by then infected vegetation, and a protective sheath develops (Fig. 21.9). This protective sheath isolates the bacteria (or fungi) from host defenses and allows the infectious agent to rapidly proliferate.

Infective endocarditis can be caused by a variety of organisms and pathologic phenomena. Four underlying phenomena include bacteremia (or fungemia), valvulitis, immunologic conditions, and emboli (Baltimore et al., 2015). The most common microorganisms leading to bacteremia associated with endocarditis in children are staphylococci and streptococci. Bacteria can enter the bloodstream through dental work (e.g., teeth cleaning, tonsillectomy, or adenoidectomy), a medical procedure (e.g., bronchoscopy), or gastrointestinal, urinary tract, or respiratory surgery.

Clinical Presentation

Children present with infective endocarditis in a variety of ways. Symptoms can develop slowly or rapidly and be subtle or quite severe. Some children do not appear ill but present with recurrent low-grade fever and nonspecific symptoms such as fatigue and weakness. Others may have flulike symptoms, such as muscle aches, joint pain, headache, tiredness, and night sweats. Patients who have fulminant endocarditis present with high, spiking fevers and appear severely ill. Some children present with a cough and shortness of breath. Gastrointestinal symptoms may be present, such as nausea, vomiting, and decreased appetite. Cardiovascular signs may include blood from small broken blood vessels in the eyes, mouth, or chest and swelling in the hands, feet, and ankles. Red, painful bumps under the skin on the fingers and toes (Osler nodes) and nontender blanching macular lesions on the palms of the hands or feet (Janeway lesions) may also be present.

Assessment and Diagnosis

Assessment includes a review of risk factors, because most children with infective endocarditis have an identifiable risk factor. Risk factors include congenital heart disease, presence of a central venous catheter, intracardiac devices such as pacemakers, implantable cardioverter-defibrillators and prosthetic devices, and rheumatic heart disease. IV drug use is also a risk factor for older adolescents, but it is not commonly seen in young children.

Diagnosis is made according to the Duke criteria (Box 21.8). Multiple blood cultures from separate venipuncture sites are obtained over several hours to 2 days to determine the bacterial pathogen. A CBC may reveal anemia and an elevated white blood cell count. CRP level and ESR may be elevated. An ECHO is performed on all patients for whom there is a reasonable suspicion of infective endocarditis. An ECHO may detect the presence of a vegetation, abscess, valvular regurgitation, and, in children with a prosthetic device, evidence of a partial dehiscence.

Box 21.8 Duke Criteria for Diagnosis of Infective Endocarditis

Major Criteria

1. Blood culture for typical microorganisms returns positive result consistent with that for infective endocarditis from two separate blood cultures *or* a single positive blood culture result for *Coxiella burnetii or* phase I immunoglobulin G antibody titer >1:8,000
2. Evidence of endocardial involvement: ECHO positive for vegetation, abscess, or partial dehiscence of prosthetic valve

Minor Criteria

1. Presence of a predisposing heart condition or IV drug use
2. Fever: temperature ≥38.0°C (100.4°F)
3. Vascular phenomena: major arterial emboli, septic pulmonary infarcts, mycotic aneurysm, intracranial hemorrhage, conjunctival hemorrhage, or Janeway lesions
4. Immunologic phenomena: glomerulonephritis, Osler nodes, Roth spots, or rheumatoid factor
5. Microbiologic evidence: positive blood culture results that do not meet major criteria *or* serologic evidence of active infection with organism consistent with infective endocarditis

Diagnosis

Diagnosis is confirmed using the Duke criteria when one of the following occurs:

- Two major criteria are present.
- One major and three minor criteria are present.
- Five minor criteria are present.

Adapted with permission from Li, J. S., Sexton, D. J., Mick, N., Nettles, R., Fowler Jr, V. G., Ryan, T., ... & Corey, G. R. (2000). Proposed modifications to the Duke criteria for the diagnosis of infective endocarditis. *Clinical Infectious Diseases, 30*(4), 633–638.

Therapeutic Interventions

Nursing care of the child with infective endocarditis focuses on assessment of the child's condition, supporting the cardiovascular system, promoting rest and providing comfort measures, administering medications, including antibiotics (The Pharmacy 21.4), monitoring for complications of the disease and from medication therapy, and teaching parents about the child's care. See the section General Therapeutic Interventions for Cardiovascular Disorders earlier for details on these interventions.

Evaluation

Expected outcomes for a child at risk for or with infective endocarditis include the following:

- Infective endocarditis is prevented in the child with identifiable risk factors, including congenital heart disease, rheumatic heart fever, and central venous catheter.

- Complications of infective endocarditis are quickly detected and treated.
- The at-risk child receives prophylactic antibiotics before dental and respiratory procedures.

Discharge Planning and Teaching

Education regarding prophylactic antibiotic therapy to prevent infective endocarditis is essential. Teach parents and children when prophylaxis is needed and the appropriate timing and dosage of any prescribed antibiotic. Prophylactic antibiotics are often prescribed for use before dental procedures (e.g., routine cleanings, tonsillectomy, adenoidectomy, and incision and drainage of infections), invasive gastrointestinal or genitourinary procedures, and procedures involving the respiratory system. Teach parents and reinforce the use of a pharmacy-supplied measuring device for administering the correct dose of prophylactic antibiotics. Teach the child and parents of young children the importance of dental hygiene and how to prevent dental caries. Inform parents of children with risk factors for endocarditis of the signs and symptoms of endocarditis and the importance of seeking early diagnosis and treatment to reduce the risk of long-term cardiovascular complications.

Cardiomyopathy

Cardiomyopathy, which means disease of the heart muscle, is a serious disorder of the heart's muscle that affects the size of the heart chambers, chamber wall thickness, and contraction and leads to ventricular systolic or diastolic dysfunction. Dilated cardiomyopathy and hypertrophic cardiomyopathy are the most common forms of cardiomyopathy in children (Lee et al., 2017).

Etiology and Pathophysiology

In dilated cardiomyopathy, the heart muscle becomes thin, the left ventricle becomes dilated, and the heart is unable to squeeze effectively, resulting in reduced cardiac output (Fig. 21.10). Dilated cardiomyopathy accounts for over 50% of pediatric cardiomyopathies (Lee et al., 2017). The most common cause of dilated cardiomyopathy is myocarditis, an inflammation of the heart muscle, which is often caused by a virus. Approximately 35% to 48% of children with dilated cardiomyopathy have evidence of myocarditis on a biopsied tissue (Lee et al., 2017). Other causes include chemotherapy exposure and metabolic diseases such as glycogen storage disease and mitochondrial storage disorders. Genetics plays a role in causing dilated cardiomyopathy. Genetic forms of dilated cardiomyopathy account for about half of all cases and can be autosomal dominant, autosomal recessive, or X-linked. Thus far, about 40 causative genes have been linked to cardiomyopathy (Mestroni, Brun, Spezzacatene, Sinagra, & Taylor, 2014). Duchenne muscular dystrophy is example of one of the rare genetic dilated cardiomyopathy diseases.

Hypertrophic cardiomyopathy accounts for approximately 42% of pediatric cardiomyopathy cases (Lee et al., 2017).

The Pharmacy 21.4	Medications Used for Prophylaxis of Infective Endocarditis			
Medication	**Classification**	**Route**	**Action**	**Nursing Considerations**
Amoxicillin	Anti-infective aminopenicillin	PO	• Binds to bacterial cell wall, causing cell death • Broader spectrum than penicillin	• Used when patient *can* take PO • Teach parents to monitor bowel function. • If diarrhea, abdominal cramping, bloody stools, or fever develop, notify physician. May be a sign of pseudomembranous colitis
Ampicillin	Anti-infective aminopenicillin	• IV • IM	• Binds to bacterial cell wall, causing cell death • Broader spectrum than penicillin	• Used when patient *cannot* take PO • Pseudomembranous colitis can occur; monitor stool output, diarrhea, abdominal cramping, and temperature for fever.
Cefazolin, ceftriaxone	Anti-infective cephalosporin	• IV • IM	Binds to bacterial cell wall, causing cell death	• Used when patient *cannot* take PO and when patient is allergic to penicillin or ampicillin • Assess patient for skin rash; notify provider immediately; Stevens–Johnson syndrome may develop.
Azithromycin, clarithromycin, clindamycin	• Bacteriostatic macrolide (azithromycin, clarithromycin) • Anti-infective lincosamide (clindamycin)	PO	Inhibits protein synthesis by binding to the 50S bacterial ribosome	• Used when patient is allergic to penicillin or ampicillin • More common side effects are abdominal pain, diarrhea, and nausea. • Administer 1 h before or 2 h after meals. • May cause elevated liver enzymes and bilirubin.

From Lexicomp. *Pediatric & Neonatal Dosage Handbook* (25th ed.), 2018.
IM, intramuscular; IV, intravenous; PO, by mouth.

In this form, enlargement (hypertrophy) of the left ventricle and ventricular septum occurs and the ventricular walls become rigid. As the hypertrophy increases, obstruction of the blood outflow tract, diastolic dysfunction of the left ventricle, and myocardial ischemia ensue. Causes of hypertrophic cardiomyopathy include inborn errors of metabolism, malformation syndromes, and other genetic mutations.

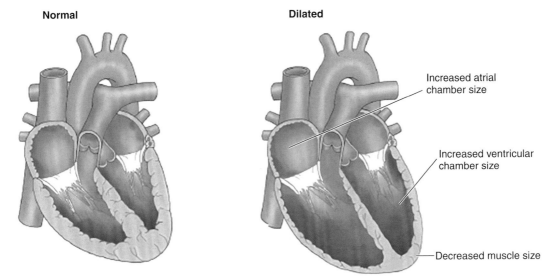

Normal   **Dilated**

Increased atrial chamber size

Increased ventricular chamber size

Decreased muscle size

Figure 21.10. Comparison of a normal heart and a heart with dilated cardiomyopathy. Reprinted with permission from Lippincott Nursing Advisor May 2016.

Assessment and Diagnosis

In dilated cardiomyopathy, 75% to 80% of children present with signs of heart failure, including tachypnea, cough, wheezing, tachycardia, weak pulses, and fatigue. Children with hypertrophic cardiomyopathy may be asymptomatic. Symptoms vary according to the degree of outflow obstruction. Symptomatic children may appear with exertional dyspnea, shortness of breath when lying supine, general fatigue, and nonspecific chest pain. In a previously healthy child, cardiac arrest or sudden death may be the presenting event for hypertrophic cardiomyopathy (Lee et al., 2017).

Diagnosis includes obtaining a family history, particularly for dilated cardiomyopathy, and a recent medical history to learn of any recent viruses the child may have had. An ECHO is done to assess the heart function, ventricle size, and pressures in the chambers of the heart. An ECG is obtained to assess for arrhythmias, including atrial fibrillation and ventricular arrhythmias. Laboratory data required include many of the same as required for the workup for heart failure.

Therapeutic Interventions

Nursing management for dilated cardiomyopathy is the same as for a child with heart failure. For children diagnosed with hypertrophic cardiomyopathy, nursing management includes monitoring the child at frequent visits for progression of disease and assessing use of medications such as beta-blockers (The Pharmacy 21.5). Patients with hypertrophic cardiomyopathy may need an implantable cardioverter-defibrillator, which has been proved effective for some children at risk for sudden death. Patients with severe or progressively worsening cardiomyopathy, despite treatment, may need a heart transplant.

Evaluation

Expected outcomes for a child with cardiomyopathy include the following:
* The child has improved heart function as evidenced by improved ejection fraction and increased ability to perform activities without worsening symptoms.

* Disease progression is slowed or prevented.
* See the section Evaluation within the section Heart Failure for expected outcomes specific to a child with heart failure.

Discharge Planning and Teaching

Use the same discharge planning and teaching points as for heart failure. In addition, refer the child and family for genetic testing and screen immediate family members for cardiomyopathy, as needed.

Kawasaki Disease

Kawasaki disease is an acute, idiopathic systemic vascular inflammatory disorder that affects infants and young children, particularly those younger than age 5 years. Kawasaki disease is the most common cause of acquired heart disease in children in developed countries, including the United States (McCrindle et al., 2017). It is an acute, self-limiting, febrile illness that can lead to coronary aneurysms in up to 25% of children affected with the disease (McCrindle et al., 2017). The disorder occurs more commonly in males than in females and more frequently in children of Asian and Pacific Islander ancestry (Singh, Vignesh, & Burgner, 2015). In fact, in children younger than age 5 years in Hawaii, Kawasaki disease occurred in 210.5 per 100,000 children of Japanese descent and in 13.7 per 100,000 white children (Holman et al., 2010). The disorder most commonly occurs in winter and in early spring.

Etiology and Pathophysiology

The exact etiology of Kawasaki disease is unknown. However, genetic influences and an infectious or viral trigger may initiate the inflammatory process. The disorder occurs in three phases: the acute phase, the subacute phase, and the convalescent phase. The acute phase is characterized by abrupt onset of fever that is not responsive to antibiotics or antipyretics and the beginning of widespread inflammation of small and medium-sized arteries. The subacute phase begins when fever has

---

The Pharmacy 21.5   Medications Used in the Treatment of Cardiomyopathy

Medication	Classification	Route	Action	Nursing Considerations
Metoprolol	Beta-blocker	PO	• Blocks stimulation of beta-1 (myocardial) adrenergic receptor sites • Decreases heart rate and blood pressure	• Abrupt withdrawal may precipitate life-threatening arrhythmias, hypertension, and myocardial ischemia. • Take apical pulse and blood pressure before administering. • Monitor intake and output, weight, and for signs of fluid overload; patient may experience worsening heart failure at onset of therapy. • Be aware of the difference between immediate-release (metoprolol) and sustained-release to metoprolol XL.

From Lexicomp. *Pediatric & Neonatal Dosage Handbook* (25th ed.), 2018.
PO, by mouth.
Also, see The Pharmacy 21.2 for additional medications used in the treatment of cardiomyopathy, including furosemide, digoxin, carvedilol, and ACEs.

subsided, and the convalescent phase is marked by complete resolution of clinical signs. The classic clinical criteria defining Kawasaki disease include fever and five principal clinical manifestations: changes of the oral cavity and lips, including a classic strawberry tongue; a polymorphous rash involving the trunk, extremities, and perineal areas; bilateral, nonpurulent conjunctivitis; erythema of the hands and feet; and cervical lymphadenopathy (often unilateral). A diagnosis is made when fever and at least four of the five clinical manifestations are present.

Clinical Presentation

A child with Kawasaki disease often presents to the pediatrician or the emergency room with prolonged fever, irritability, vomiting, diarrhea, joint pain, cough, runny nose, and weakness. The three stages of Kawasaki disease are marked by characteristic manifestations.

- The acute stage typically lasts 1 to 2 weeks and features the following manifestations: fever lasting longer than 5 days, irritability, conjunctival erythema without exudate, swollen cervical lymph nodes (unilateral), maculopapular rash on the trunk and perineal area, swollen hands and feet, diarrhea, and vomiting (Fig. 21.11). Children may not want to walk because of painful feet related to edema and joint pain. Cracked lips and a strawberry tongue may also be present. During the acute stage, myocarditis occurs in most patients and is manifested by tachycardia and diminished left ventricular function as visualized on an ECHO.
- The subacute phase begins when the fever has subsided and generally lasts several weeks. Classic signs occurring in the subacute phase include desquamation of the fingers and toes, thrombocytosis (very high platelet count), joint pain, and anorexia. This is the period when coronary aneurysms are most likely to develop and sudden death is most likely to occur.
- The convalescent phase is marked by the complete resolution of clinical signs, which typically occurs 3 months after onset. Coronary aneurysm may still be present, and myocardial infarction remains a concern.

Assessment and Diagnosis

There is no definitive test for the diagnosis of Kawasaki disease. Diagnosis is based on the presence of clinical signs. The nurse should be astute to the clinical signs and symptoms associated with each of the stages of Kawasaki disease.

Laboratory data and tests that may be useful in diagnosing Kawasaki disease in the acute phase include CRP level, ESR, alpha-1 antitrypsin level, and a white blood cell count. During the subacute phase, thrombocytosis is present and platelet levels can average 700,000.

An ECG is often obtained at diagnosis and throughout the care of a patient with Kawasaki disease. Changes in the ECG can indicate myocarditis and, later, signs of a myocardial infarction. An ECHO allows the provider to visualize any coronary involvement that may occur.

Therapeutic Interventions

Nursing care of the child with Kawasaki disease requires critical assessment and monitoring of the signs and symptoms, effects of medication therapy, and early signs of complications. It also requires monitoring the child's intake and output, administering fluids as needed to prevent dehydration, promoting comfort, providing pain relief therapies, administering and monitoring IVIG therapy and aspirin therapy as prescribed (The Pharmacy 21.6), and supporting the patient and family. See the section General Therapeutic Interventions for Cardiovascular Disorders earlier for details on these interventions.

Evaluation

Expected outcomes for a child with Kawasaki disease include the following:
- The child remains comfortable during the acute phase, when symptoms are present.
- The child has adequate periods of rest to promote recovery.
- The child is free from complications of coronary aneurysms, if present.
- The child is free from complications of aspirin therapy.

Discharge Planning and Teaching

Before the hospitalized child can be discharged, parents must demonstrate how to take the child's temperature accurately and how to properly administer aspirin therapy. Instruct parents to take the child's temperature daily via the same route (axillary, temporal, or via an ear), record it in a log, and report any fever above 38.3°C (101°F) to the provider. Because toddlers can often refuse medications, teach parents how to navigate such refusal. Inform parents that mixing the aspirin with applesauce or ice cream or hiding a chewable aspirin in yogurt or soft food are effective and acceptable methods of getting a toddler to take the medication.

Instruct parents to provide adequate rest periods for the child and to avoid allowing the child to participate in contact sports or play and other activities that can cause bleeding. Aspirin increases the risk of bleeding. Inform parents of the importance of follow-up care, particularly for cardiac complications that, if left untreated, could result in death. If coronary aneurysms are present, children should avoid strenuous activity. In addition, teach parents to postpone immunizations with live vaccines (measles, varicella) for 11 months after IVIG administration, which interferes with the child's immune response to live virus vaccines (AAP, 2017).

Hypertension

Over the past decade, it has become clear that hypertension begins in childhood and adolescence and then contributes to the early development of cardiovascular disease in adulthood. Many children and adolescents have hypertension but are asymptomatic. The odds of elevated blood pressure in children increased 27% from 1999 to 2008, after accounting for differences in age, waist circumference, ethnicity, gender, sodium intake, and body mass index (Rosner, Cook, Daniels, & Falkner, 2013).

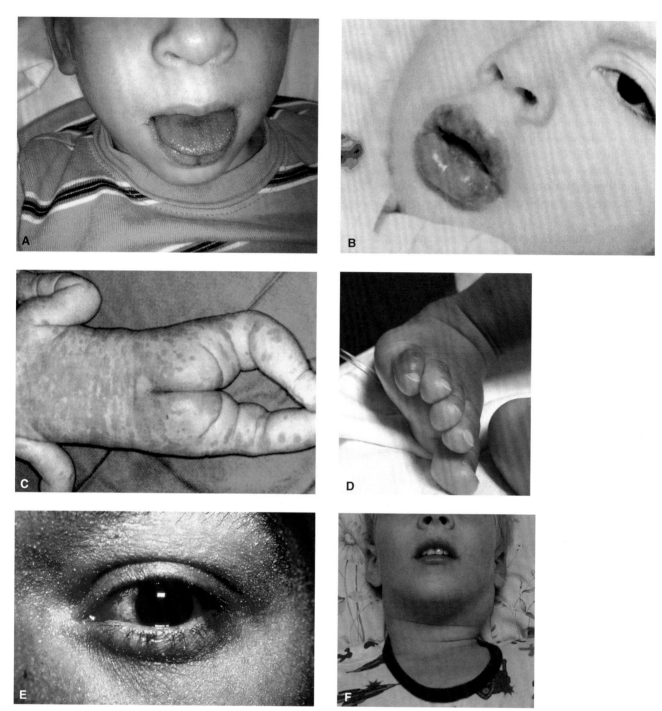

Figure 21.11. Manifestations of the acute stage of Kawasaki disease in a child. A. Strawberry tongue. **B.** Cracked lips. **C.** A maculopapular rash on the trunk. **D.** Swollen and erythematous feet. **E.** Conjunctival erythema without exudate. **F.** Swollen lymph nodes. Part A reprinted with permission from Bachur, R. G., & Shaw, K. N. (2016). *Fleisher & Ludwig's textbook of pediatric emergency medicine* (7th ed., Fig. 47.5). Philadelphia, PA: Wolters Kluwer. Parts B and C reprinted with permission from Coombs C., & Kirk, A. S. (2010). *Oski's pediatric certification and recertification board review* (1st ed.). Philadelphia, PA: Wolters Kluwer Health. Part D: Photo courtesy of Esther K. Chung, MD, MPH. From Chung, E. K., Atkinson-McEvoy, L. R., Lai, N. L., & Terry, M. (Eds.). (2014). *Visual diagnosis and treatment in pediatrics* (3rd ed., Fig. 50-6). Philadelphia, PA: Lippincott Williams & Wilkins. Part E reprinted with permission from Goodheart, H. P. (2003). *Goodheart's photoguide to common skin disorders* (2nd ed.). Philadelphia, PA: Lippincott Williams & Wilkins. Part F reprinted with permission from Gru, A. A., & Wick, M. (2018). *Pediatric dermatopathology and dermatology* (1st ed., Fig. 6.45). Philadelphia, PA: Lippincott Williams & Wilkins.

The Pharmacy 21.6   Medications Used in the Treatment of Kawasaki Disease

Medication	Classification	Route	Action	Nursing Considerations
IVIG	Immunoglobulin	IV	• A human serum fraction that contains IgG antibodies • Provides passive immunity in a variety of infections • Shown to reduce incidence of coronary complications and fever resulting from Kawasaki disease (McCrindle et al., 2017)	• Monitor HR, RR, BP, and temperature throughout and after infusion. • Monitor for signs of anaphylaxis: wheezing, chest tightness, hypotension, flushing, dizziness, nausea, vomiting, and diarrhea. • May premedicate with diphenhydramine to reduce risk of allergic response
Aspirin	• Analgesic • NSAID • Platelet aggregate inhibitor • Antipyretic	PO Rectal	• Inhibits prostaglandin production, resulting in reduced inflammation, fever, and analgesia • Decreases platelet aggregation	• Monitor for signs of bleeding. • Monitor hepatic function before and during therapy. • May cause nausea, epigastric distress, dyspepsia (indigestion)

From Lexicomp. *Pediatric & Neonatal Dosage Handbook* (25th ed.), 2018.
BP, blood pressure; HR, heart rate; IgG, immunoglobulin G; IV, intravenous; IVIG, intravenous immunoglobulin G; NSAID, nonsteroidal anti-inflammatory drug; PO, by mouth; RR, respiratory rate.

The American Academy of Pediatrics (2017) categorizes blood pressure ranges for two different age groups, children aged 1 to 12 years and children 13 years or older. Blood pressure percentiles are based on gender, age, and height. Table 21.8 defines ranges for normal blood pressure, elevated blood pressure, stage 1 hypertension, and stage 2 hypertension for each of the two age groups.

Etiology and Pathophysiology

Blood pressure is the product of cardiac output and peripheral vascular resistance. An increase in either cardiac output or peripheral vascular resistance results in an increase in blood pressure. Blood pressure may not increase if one of these two factors increases and the other decreases. Hypertension can be classified according to etiology as primary or secondary. Primary hypertension is hypertension that has no identifiable cause and is the most common type in pediatrics. It is more likely to occur in school-age children and adolescents who have a family history of hypertension and who are overweight or obese. Primary hypertension is also more common in African Americans.

Secondary hypertension is hypertension that has an identifiable cause. The most common causes of secondary hypertension in children are renal disease, endocrine disease, and renovascular disease. Renal causes include, but are not limited to, pyelonephritis, acute glomerulonephritis, nephrotic syndrome,

Table 21.8   Definition of Elevated Blood Pressure in Children

Category	Children Aged 1–12 Y	Children Aged ≥13 Y
Normal BP	Systolic and diastolic BP <90th percentile	Systolic BP <120 and diastolic BP <80 mm Hg
Elevated BP	• Systolic and diastolic BP 90th–95th percentile • OR 120/80 mm Hg to >95th percentile (whichever is lower)	Systolic BP 120–129 and diastolic BP <80 mm Hg
Stage 1 HTN	• Systolic and diastolic BP ≥95th percentile to <95th percentile + 12 mm Hg • OR 130/80–139/89 mm Hg (whichever is lower)	130/80–139/89 mm Hg
Stage 2 HTN	• Systolic and diastolic BP ≥95th percentile + 12 mm Hg • OR ≥140/90 mm Hg (whichever is lower)	≥140/90 mm Hg

BP, blood pressure; HTN, hypertension.
Reprinted with permission from Flynn, J. T., Kaelber, D. C., Baker-Smith, C. M., Blowey, D., Carroll, A. E., Daniels, S. R., ... Urbina E. M. (2017). Clinical practice guideline for screening and management of high blood pressure in children and adolescents. *Pediatrics, 140*(3).

hypoplastic kidney, polycystic kidney disease, hydronephrosis, and Wilms tumor. Endocrine causes include hyperthyroidism, Cushing syndrome, diabetes mellitus, congenital adrenal hyperplasia, and primary aldosteronism. Renovascular causes include renal artery anomalies, fibromuscular dysplasia, umbilical artery catheterization that leads to a renal artery clot, and neurofibromatosis. Hypertension due to renovascular disease results from a decrease in renal blood flow, which triggers increased plasma levels of renin, angiotensin, and aldosterone.

Children who are overweight (greater than the 85th percentile for weight) are more likely to have higher blood pressure values than do their counterparts who are not overweight. Rosner et al. (2013) found that body mass index, waist circumference, and sodium intake were independently associated with the prevalence of elevated blood pressure. Hypertension and prehypertension are more prevalent in boys than in girls. Furthermore, in the United States, Mexican American and non-Hispanic black children are more likely to have elevated blood pressure compared with non-Hispanic white children, when adjusted for age, gender, and height. Box 21.9 lists the risk factors for primary hypertension.

Clinical Presentation

Most children who have hypertension are asymptomatic. If symptomatic, children may present with headaches, visual disturbances, fatigue, epistaxis, or dizziness. The child may be overweight or obese. For children with secondary hypertension, the symptoms are most often related to the underlying cause of high blood pressure.

Assessment and Diagnosis

Children 3 years and older should have their blood pressure measured annually. Children 3 years and older who are obese, take medications known to cause hypertension, have renal disease, or have been diagnosed with aortic arch obstruction, coarctation, or diabetes should have their blood pressure checked at every health encounter (Flynn et al., 2017). Consistently measure blood pressure on the right arm with the appropriately sized cuff. The child should sit quietly for at least 5 minutes before the measurement to reduce the risk of activity falsely elevating blood pressure. For patients who have been diagnosed with or are suspected of having coarctation of the aorta, measure blood pressure on all four extremities. Assess the child's weight and height. Then compare findings with values in a blood pressure table according to gender, age, and height to determine whether hypertension is present.

Additional assessment includes taking a history to screen for possible risk factors and sources of secondary hypertension. Consider the following questions: Is there a family history of hypertension? Is the child obese? What does a typical daily nutrient intake consist of? How many servings of fruits, vegetables, dairy products, and salt-containing foods does the child typically consume? What physical activity, exercise, or sports is the child involved in? Does the child have any sleep problems, such as awakening frequently at night, loud snoring, or snoring that wakes the child up? One of the most important components in assessment and management of pediatric hypertension is distinguishing between primary and secondary hypertension. A thorough history assists the provider in making this determination.

Diagnosis of hypertension is made on the basis of blood pressure measurements taken on three separate visits that are greater than the 95th percentile for gender, age, and height (Flynn et al., 2017). Initially, all children with hypertension should have a urinalysis, chemistry panel, and a lipid profile. A renal ultrasound is recommended for children who have abnormal urinalysis or renal function test results (Flynn et al., 2017). For obese patients, additional tests are warranted. A hemoglobin A1C test (to screen for diabetes), aspartate aminotransferase and alanine aminotransferase levels (to screen for fatty liver disease), and a fasting lipid profile (to screen for dyslipidemia) are also recommended (Flynn et al., 2017).

Therapeutic Interventions

Nursing care of the child with hypertension focuses on first screening and detecting the child with high blood pressure and then assisting the family with lifestyle changes that will help control blood pressure to reduce the risk of atherosclerotic changes that can occur as a result of prolonged hypertension.

For the long term, it requires ongoing monitoring of blood pressure. Measure blood pressure in the same arm (preferably the right arm) using a manual blood pressure technique at each office visit for patients who are at risk, have borderline hypertension, or have been diagnosed with hypertension. Be sure to use the appropriate cuff size.

At initial and follow-up visits for hypertension, encourage the child and parents and teach them regarding appropriate weight goals, nutrition, exercise, and stress reduction. See the subsection Teaching, for more specific information.

Evaluation

Expected outcomes for a child with hypertension include the following:

- The child maintains an age-appropriate weight and height.
- The child and family recognize foods high in sodium.
- The child and family recognize foods to consume to maintain a low-fat diet.
- The child and family attend follow-up appointments for hypertension evaluation, treatment, and monitoring.

Box 21.9   Risk Factors for Primary Hypertension in Children

- Obesity
- Gender (boys at higher risk than are girls)
- Ethnicity: Mexican American and African American
- Family history: present in 70%–80% of all patients with primary hypertension
- Prenatal and neonatal factors: very low birth weight babies (Hovi et al., 2016)

Teaching

Teaching topics for children and adolescents include lifestyle changes (dietary modifications and weight reduction) and medication therapy, if prescribed. Teach the child and parent the importance of weight reduction and then maintaining a healthy weight. Inform parents of recommended weight ranges for various ages as the child grows. Teach and reinforce recommendations for dietary changes at each visit and when necessary. Teach families about salt substitutes and how to read food labels for sodium content. Maintaining a low-salt diet is important in managing blood pressure, particularly if the child is overweight. Encourage consumption of low-fat dairy products, fruits, and vegetables.

Help parents and children identify ways to increase activity in their daily routines. Offer examples of age-appropriate exercise and activities that include aerobic exercise (bicycling, playing outside, jumping rope, etc.). Encourage parents to limit the child's screen time (e.g., watching television or playing on the computer) and time spent on other sedentary activities. Teach older children and parents the methods for reducing and managing stress as well as the importance of avoiding smoking, alcohol, and drugs. Instruct the child and family regarding medication management and recognizing symptoms of hypertension.

Think Critically

1. The nurse is educating the parents of a young child diagnosed with Kawasaki disease. The nurse is reviewing the medications and begins to explain the rationale for aspirin. The mother looks worried and asks, "I thought young children should not ever be given aspirin. Is this safe for my child to take?" What rationale should the nurse give the family?

2. Many infants and children with congenital heart defects require increased caloric intake. Explain why increased calories are needed.

3. Describe why a child with a moderate-to-large VSD may have left-to-right shunting.

4. The nurse is caring for a 5-year-old who just underwent cardiac catheterization. List three important assessments the nurse should make in the immediate postprocedure period.

5. The nurse is caring for a newborn who has a suspected coarctation of the aorta. The physician orders four-extremity blood pressures. Why are blood pressures on all four extremities often ordered when an infant has a suspected coarctation of the aorta?

6. Elijah, a 12-year-old African American male is being seen for his annual well-care visit. Elijah's height and weight are 5 ft 2 in (157.5 cm) and 172 lb (32.6 kg). The nurse takes his blood pressure and finds it to be 148/97 mm Hg. At the end of the visit, she takes the blood pressure again and it is 145/93 mm Hg. The nurse practitioner discusses her concern for Elijah's blood pressure. What risk factors does Elijah have that raise concern for the nurse practitioner?

7. The nurse is preparing to administer prostaglandins to an infant diagnosed with tricuspid atresia. What is the purpose of a prostaglandin infusion in this situation? Why is the prostaglandin infusion necessary?

8. The nurse is assessing a newborn for possible signs of congenital heart defect. What assessment findings would the nurse encounter that would suggest a congenital heart defect?

References

American Academy of Pediatrics. (2017). *Kawasaki disease in infants and young children*. Retrieved from https://www.healthychildren.org/English/health-issues/conditions/heart/Pages/Kawasaki-Disease.aspx

Baltimore, R., Gewitz, M., Baddour, L., Beerman, L., Jackson, M., Lockhart, P., ... & Willoughby, R. (2015). Infective endocarditis in childhood: 2015 update: A scientific statement from the American Heart Association. *Circulation, 132*(15), 1487–1515.

Bjornard, K., Riehle-Colarusso, T., Gilboa, S., & Correa, A. (2013). Patterns in the prevalence of congenital heart defects, metropolitan Atlanta, 1978 to 2005. *Birth Defects Research Part A: Clinical and Molecular Teratology, 97*(2), 87–94.

Carapetis, J., Beaton, A., Cunningham, M., Guilherme, L., Karthikeyan, G., Mayosi, B., ... & Zühlke, L. (2016). Acute rheumatic fever and rheumatic heart disease. *Nature Reviews: Disease Primers, 2*, 15084.

Elumalai, G., & Thelma, U. (2016). Patent Ductus Arteriosus embryological basis and its clinical significance. *Elixir Embryology, 100*, 43433–43438.

Elias, P., Poh, C., du Plessis, K., Zannino, D., Rice, K., Radford, D., ... & d'Udekem, Y. (2018). Long-term outcomes of single-ventricle palliation for pulmonary atresia with intact ventricular septum: Fontan survivors remain at risk of late myocardial ischaemia and death. *European Journal of Cardio-Thoracic Surgery, 53*(6), 1230–1236.

Flynn, J., Kaelber, D., Baker-Smith, C., Blowey, D., Carroll, A., Daniels, S., ... & Gidding, S. (2017). Clinical practice guideline for screening and management of high blood pressure in children and adolescents. *Pediatrics, 140*(3).

Gewitz, M., Baltimore, R., Tani, L., Sable, C., Shulman, S., Carapetis, J., ... & Mayosi, B. (2015). Revision of the Jones Criteria for the diagnosis of acute rheumatic fever in the era of Doppler echocardiography: A scientific statement from the American Heart Association. *Circulation, 131*(20), 1806–1818.

Gilboa, S., Devine, O., Kucik, J., Oster, M., Riehle-Colarusso, T., Nembhard, W., ... & Marelli, A. J. (2016). Congenital heart defects in the United States clinical perspective: Estimating the magnitude of the affected population in 2010. *Circulation, 134*(2), 101–109.

Hovi, P., Vohr, B., Ment, L., Doyle, L., McGarvey, L., Morrison, K., ... & Kajantie, E. (2016). Blood pressure in young adults born at very low birth weight: Adults born preterm international collaboration. *Hypertension, 68*(4), 880–887.

Holman, R. C., Christensen, K. Y., Belay, E. D., Steiner, C. A., Effler, P. V., Miyamura, J., ... & Melish, M. (2010). Racial/ethnic differences in the incidence of Kawasaki syndrome among children in Hawai'i. *Hawaii medical journal, 69*(8), 194.

Lee, T., Hsu, D., Kantor, P., Towbin, J., Ware, S., Colan, S., ... & Addonizio, L. (2017). Pediatric cardiomyopathies. *Circulation Research, 121*(7), 855–873.

Mai, C., Riehle-Colarusso, T., O'Halloran, A., Cragan, J., Olney, R. S., Lin A., ... & Canfield, M. (2012). Selected birth defects data from population

congenital heart defects targeted for pulse oximetry screening. *Birth Defects Research Part A: Clinical and Molecular Teratology, 94,* 970–983.

Masarone, D., Valente, F., Rubino, M., Vastarella, R., Gravino, R., Rea, A., ... & Limongelli, G. (2017). Pediatric heart failure: a practical guide to diagnosis and management. *Pediatrics & Neonatology, 58*(4), 303–312.

Mestroni, L., Brun, F., Spezzacatene, A., Sinagra, G., & Taylor, M. R. (2014). Genetic causes of dilated cardiomyopathy. *Progress in pediatric cardiology, 37*(1), 13–18.

Mozaffarian, D., Benjamin, E., Go, A. S., Arnett, D., Blaha, M., Cushman, M., ... & Howard, V. J. (2016). Executive summary: Heart disease and stroke statistics-2016 update: A report from the American Heart Association. *Circulation, 133*(4), 447–454.

McCrindle, B. W., Rowley, A. H., Newburger, J. W., Burns, J. C., Bolger, A. F., Gewitz, M., ... & Kobayashi, T. (2017). Diagnosis, treatment, and long-term management of Kawasaki disease: A scientific statement for health professionals from the American Heart Association. *Circulation, 135*(17), e927–e999.

Rosner, B., Cook, N. R., Daniels, S., & Falkner, B. (2013). Childhood blood pressure trends and risk factors for high blood pressure novelty and significance: The NHANES experience 1988–2008. *Hypertension, 62*(2), 247–254.

Rossano, J., Kim, J., Decker, J., Price, J., Zafar, F., Graves, D., ... & Jefferies JL. (2012). Prevalence, morbidity and mortality of heart failure related hospitalizations in children in the United States: A population-based study. *Journal of Cardiac Failure, 18,* 459–470.

Shuler, C. O., Black, G. B., & Jerrell, J. M. (2013). Population-based treated prevalence of congenital heart disease in a pediatric cohort. *Pediatric cardiology, 34*(3), 606–611.

Singh, S., Vignesh, P., & Burgner, D. (2015). The epidemiology of Kawasaki disease: A global update. *Archives of Disease in Childhood, 100*(11), 1084–1088.

Stockmann, C., Ampofo, K., Hersh, A., Blaschke, A. J., Kendall, B. A., Korgenski, K., ... & Pavia, A. T. (2012). Evolving epidemiologic characteristics of invasive group A streptococcal disease in Utah, 2002−2010. *Clinical Infectious Diseases, 55*(4), 479–487.

Sugimoto, M., Manabe, H., Nakau, K., Furuya, A., Okushima, K., Fujiyasu, H., ... & Kajino, H. (2010). The role of N-terminal pro-B-type natriuretic peptide in the diagnosis of congestive heart failure in children. *Circulation Journal, 74*(5), 998–1005.

van der Linde, D., Konings, E., Slager, M., Witsenburg, M., Helbing, W., Takkenberg, J., & Roos-Hesselink, J. (2011). Birth prevalence of congenital heart disease worldwide: A systematic review and meta-analysis. *Journal of the American College of Cardiology, 58,* 2241–2247. doi:10.1016/j.jacc.2011.08.025

Van Velzen, C., Haak, M., Reijnders, G., Rijlaarsdam, M., Bax, C., Pajkrt, E., ... & Blom, N. (2015). Prenatal detection of transposition of the great arteries reduces mortality and morbidity. *Ultrasound in Obstetrics & Gynecology, 45*(3), 320–325.

Watson, G., Jallow, B., Le Doare, K., Pushparajah, K., & Anderson, S. T. (2015). Acute rheumatic fever and rheumatic heart disease in resource-limited settings. *Archives of Disease in Childhood, 100*(4), 370–375.

Suggested Readings

Cincinnati Children's. *Congenital heart defects.* Retrieved from https://www.cincinnatichildrens.org/patients/child/encyclopedia/defects

Newburger, J. W., Takahashi, M., & Burns, J. C. (2016). Kawasaki disease. *Journal of the American College of Cardiology, 67*(14), 1738–1749.

Rao, G. (2016). Diagnosis, epidemiology, and management of hypertension in children. *Pediatrics, 138*(2).

Toole, B. J., Toole, L. E., Kyle, U. G., Cabrera, A. G., Orellana, R. A., & Coss-Bu, J. A. (2014). Perioperative nutritional support and malnutrition in infants and children with congenital heart disease. *Congenital Heart Disease, 9*(1), 15–25.

Yim, D., Curtis, N., Cheung, M., & Burgner, D. (2013). An update on Kawasaki disease II: Clinical features, diagnosis, treatment and outcomes. *Journal of paediatrics and child health, 49*(8), 614-623.

22 Alterations in Neurological and Sensory Function

Objectives

After completing this chapter, you will be able to:

1. Compare and contrast anatomical and physiological characteristics of the neurological systems of children and adults.
2. Relate pediatric assessment findings to the child's neurological status.
3. Discuss the pathophysiology of common pediatric neurological disorders.
4. Differentiate between signs and symptoms of common pediatric neurological disorders.
5. Outline the therapeutic regimen for each of the pediatric neurological disorders.
6. Describe the pharmacological management of common pediatric neurological disorders.
7. Apply the principles of growth and development to the care of a child with a neurological disorder.
8. Create a nursing plan of care for each of the common pediatric neurological disorders.

Key Terms

Cisternogram
Conjunctivitis
Craniosynostosis
Deceleration
Deformational plagiocephaly (DP)
Encephalitis
Focal seizure
Generalized seizure
Hydrocephalus

Meningitis
Microcephaly
Paroxysmal
Periorbital cellulitis
Photophobia
Posturing
Status epilepticus
Teratogen

Brain development in the fetus and the infant is critical, because defects that occur during these stages of development contribute directly to neurological and sensory deficits that range from mild to severe and that can significantly affect the child's quality of life. Mild deficits may not manifest in any delay in motor or cognitive development, whereas severe ones can result in permanent motor and cognitive issues that require long-term care or can result in death. Knowledge of the type of defect a child has, where it is located, and what structures of the central nervous system are involved helps the nurse know what to expect in terms of the child's long-term growth and development, which the nurse can, in turn, communicate to the parents.

Careful assessment and prompt recognition of many conditions can vastly improve the outcome for many children. The nurse plays an important role in the assessment, care, and support of the child with a neurological condition. This chapter covers alterations in the neurological and sensory function that the nurse may encounter within the pediatric care setting, including structural defects, infectious disorders, seizure disorders, head trauma, headaches, eye disorders, and hearing deficits.

Variations in Anatomy and Physiology

The nervous system begins to develop sometime during the third or fourth week after conception. It begins as the ectoderm of the embryo develops into the neural plate, with the top portion differentiating into the neural tube and neural crest. These structures eventually give rise to the central nervous system (the brain and spinal cord) and the peripheral nervous system. Because these developments take place so early in pregnancy, the embryo's nervous system is highly vulnerable to genetic alterations, maternal exposure to environmental insults, and **teratogens**.

The brain and cranial structures grow and develop throughout pregnancy. Newborns enter the world with the brain and its structures intact but immature, and brain development really begins to take hold after birth. The Harvard University Center on the Developing Child (2018) indicated that in the first few years of life, more than 1 million neuronal connections are formed every second. The interaction between an infant's genetic makeup and the environment and experiences is responsible for these connections, and the infant requires a "serve and return" reciprocal relationship with adults to build the foundational brain architecture (Harvard University Center on the Developing Child, 2018). Harvard University indicated that significant adversity can impair cognitive, language, and emotional development in the first 3 years of life (2018). Poverty, child abuse, and caregiver mental illness have been found to contribute to developmental delays (Harvard, 2018), whereas structural defects, infectious disorders, exposure to toxins, and trauma can also affect a child's development.

Variations in infant and child anatomy and physiology compared with those of adults contribute to this increased vulnerability to neurological disorder or injury. The cranial and spinal anatomy of infants and children undergo frequent and significant changes over the course of several years. As the fontanelles and cranial sutures close once physical brain growth has slowed, the thickness of the skull increases as the pliability decreases, and the cervical ligaments and muscles strengthen and mature to provide more protection (Figaji, 2017).

Variations in the anatomy of other body systems in infants and young children also contribute to increased risk for neurological compromise. Because the head is relatively large, the airway is much narrower and can become compromised easily, and the chest is poorly protected, because the ribs are more horizontal to allow for lung expansion in a crowded thorax. As children grow and the abdominal cavity increases in size, the organs are allowed more space and the ribs are displaced downward while the intercostal muscles increase in strength, offering more protection to the cardiovascular system. Cerebral metabolism in infants and young children develops rapidly, because the brain requires a large portion of the body's blood to maintain growth and development, which is triggered by cortical development, synaptogenesis, and rapid myelination (Figaji, 2017). In addition, the ratio of body surface area to body weight in infants and very young children is much greater than that in adults, which contributes to their losing body heat more quickly and being at greater risk for hypothermia. The nurse must be astute in recognizing these differences and prepared to support the child's neurological, respiratory, and cardiovascular systems to promote optimal growth and development.

Assessment of the Pediatric Neurological System

Assessment of the pediatric neurological system can be a challenge, because young children and infants are not able to effectively verbalize their symptoms. A general rule is to investigate any change in behavior, because it may signify a neurological injury or disorder. Box 22.1 provides a general assessment guide to help identify any change in the neurological system of an infant or child.

Box 22.1   Assessment Guide: Identifying Neurological Changes in Children

General Assessment

1. Obtain a comprehensive birth and general health history, including whether and/or when the child has met specific developmental milestones, such as sitting up unassisted, rolling over, and walking.
2. Also obtain an accurate history of why the child is being seen—what happened? When? How? Is it getting better? Worse?
3. Obtain information regarding any medications the child is taking and whether immunizations are up to date.
4. Obtain a family history—this is important because it might provide information regarding neurological disorders that are familial.

5. Perform a general head-to-toe physical assessment, because it may elicit subtle or obvious deficiencies that signify neurological issues. Observe the child's general appearance and measure and record height, weight, HC, and vital signs. Include a complete visual inspection of the child.

Neurological Assessment

6. Observe how the child interacts with you, a parent, or others. Can the child speak clearly? What is the general mood? Does the child seem coordinated in all extremities with movement? Does the child understand and follow basic instructions? Do the child's interactions and movements seem appropriate for age?

7. Proceeding from least to most invasive, do the following:
   a. Palpate the cranium, including the anterior fontanelle, to detect any abnormality.
   b. Move a toy through the child's fields of vision while keeping the head still to assess eye movement, vision, and tracking.
   c. For an older child, test visual acuity using an age-appropriate chart.
   d. Blow on the child's face to assess for the blink reflex.
   e. Shine a penlight in each eye, separately, to assess pupillary reaction.
   f. Run a cotton swab along the surface of each extremity and the face to assess general sensation.
   g. Whisper a word and observe the child's head movement to assess hearing and vestibular function.
   h. Inspect the child's uvula, palate, and tongue for deviation, which may indicate vagal nerve insufficiency (if present, the uvula and tongue deviate toward the affected side, whereas the palate deviates away from it).
   i. Elicit the gag reflex last; infants and young children typically cry afterward because they find it invasive.

8. Assess motor development by performing the following:
   a. Observe the child playing, walking, or running to assess nerve and muscle coordination.
   b. Ask the child to squeeze your fingers and to move an extremity against resistance to assess strength.
   c. Observe the child's posture and muscle tone in one or all extremities.

9. For an older child, place a paper clip or coin in the child's hand while the eyes are closed and ask to identify it to test object discrimination.

10. Assess for the presence of primitive reflexes (e.g., Babinski's reflex should be present up to 1 year of age and absent thereafter). See Chapter 28 for gross motor developmental milestones and developmental (primitive) reflexes (Tables 28.1 and 28.2).

General Nursing Interventions for Neurological Disorders

General nursing interventions for an infant or child with a neurological disorder are aimed at maintaining function and promoting optimal growth and development. As a rule, Salehi (2018) emphasized that the nurse should always assume that a comatose or an unconscious patient can hear and therefore should talk to the patient and explain what is happening.

Maintain a Patent Airway and Effective Ventilation and Oxygenation

Maintaining the child's airway and breathing is a priority. Therefore, keep oxygen, a suction device, and the proper size of bag-valve mask at the bedside and functioning properly. Position an unconscious child to maintain the airway, such as on the side, with the chin extended, which will prevent the tongue from obstructing the airway if the child is not receiving artificial ventilation.

Maintain Adequate Hydration and Nutrition

Make sure the child maintains adequate nutrition, because injury to the neurological system may cause an increase in the metabolism and thus the need for extra calories for proper maintenance, particularly if the child has hypertonia. Feed unconscious children by gavage through a nasogastric or gastric tube while in the Fowler's or semi-Fowler's position to prevent aspiration. If the child is conscious and able to take nutrition by mouth, elicit the gag, cough, and swallow reflexes to confirm that the child can swallow. If the child is receiving intravenous (IV) fluids to rehydrate or correct electrolyte imbalances, maintain a patent IV. Children with increased intracranial pressure (ICP) may be on fluid restriction. Maintain an accurate record of intake and output to ensure that the child is receiving adequate hydration and to determine whether the child is retaining fluids, particularly if the child has a cranial injury leading to increased pressure. If a Foley catheter is present to monitor urinary output, ensure that it is patent and the site is clear and dry.

Promote Safety

Institute seizure precautions for all children with a suspected or diagnosed neurological injury or impairment. Maintain the child in the C-spine position to prevent spinal movement. Keep the side rails up at all times and padded. Ensure that trays and tables are reachable for the conscious child and that the child does not walk without assistance. If appropriate, provide the patient with a bedpan or porta-potty at the bedside to use, and bathe the patient in bed to prevent further injury from falling.

Promote Skin Integrity

Unconscious children are at risk for alteration in skin integrity because of pressure sores resulting from immobility. Frequently turn and change the position of the child to prevent sustained and unrelieved pressure on any one point. Pad bony prominences and position the limbs for protection using rolls or pillows. Use a foot board or put the child's shoes on while in bed to help prevent foot drop. Keep the skin clean and dry. Change diapers as soon as possible and cleanse the perianal area with gentle wipes or mild soap and warm water. Apply protective barriers and/or nystatin to prevent skin breakdown related to *Candida albicans*. The American Academy of Pediatrics (2009) recommended bathing the child every other day (in addition to cleaning after diaper changes) to prevent drying of the skin. In addition, apply lotion after bathing to keep the skin supple. Perform oral hygiene and apply a protective lubricant to the lips. Perform gentle massage of the skin to stimulate circulation. Finally, change the bed linen daily or when damp or wet to maintain skin integrity.

Maintain Neurological Function

The key to maintaining neurological functioning in children is to recognize changes, even subtle ones, early on and intervene as quickly as possible. Older children can verbalize symptoms, whereas younger children and infants cannot. Monitor the child closely to detect any change in behavior that might indicate that an issue is progressing or resolving. With each child, be aware of the disorder you are dealing with and anticipate potential complications so that you can prevent them. Recognizing early complications or effects of a disorder may mean the difference between optimal functioning and living with serious neurological deficits.

Although many neurological conditions allow a child to completely recover, some have long-term consequences. In the case of the latter, be aware of what resources and support the caregiver and child will need to allow for optimal functioning. Many children can still participate in daily life after suffering a serious neurological event; excellent nursing care and a comprehensive healthcare team approach are important in helping children reach their fullest possible potential.

Prevent or Manage Infection

Infants and children may have surgery related to a neurological disorder or injury. Preventing infection or managing it effectively if it does occur is a nursing priority. Keep incisions and surgical sites clean and dry and monitor the surrounding skin for signs of infection. Monitor the child's temperature for signs of fever, obtaining rectal temperatures, if possible, because they are the most accurate. Use strict aseptic technique during dressing changes. When removing tape and dressings, gently remove the tape in the direction of hair growth when possible to reduce the risk of skin trauma, disruption of wound, and infection. Apply skin protectants such as no-sting barrier films before applying tape or adherent dressings. Apply tape from the center of an incision to the outer edges to avoid tension on the skin and wound bed. As ordered, administer antibiotics or apply topical antibiotic ointments. Prevent and teach the parents to prevent the child from touching the wound or incision.

Promote Pain Relief, Comfort, and Rest

Children with neurological disorders often experience pain. Promote comfort and rest, particularly if the child has increased ICP. Children with increased ICP may be agitated and irritable; sedation with short-acting benzodiazepines (such as midazolam) is recommended, because the effects can be reversed quickly to allow for monitoring for changes in status (Sankhyan, Vykunta Raju, Sharma, & Gulati, 2010). Sedation may provide pain relief in this situation. Other pain medications that are effective include acetaminophen, ibuprofen, opioids (in uncomplicated cases), and corticosteroids to reduce inflammation that might lead to pain. Administration of osmotics such as mannitol can help reduce ICP, which also promotes comfort.

Keep the child's room at a comfortable temperature, as hyper- or hypothermia can alter the body's metabolism, subsequently leading to increased oxygen consumption. Many children with neurological conditions experience **photophobia** (hypersensitivity to light), so keeping the lights low can reduce discomfort. Soft music and soothing voices are also comforting. The irritable infant may want only the mother to touch him or her; therefore, allow parents to help whenever necessary at the bedside. Comfortable positioning, warm or cool compresses, massage, and warm baths can also help relax the child. Proper positioning can also help prevent contractures, along with using a footboard, supporting limbs with pillows and rolls, and frequent turning.

If the child is comfortable, rest can be achieved to maximize healing. Sedation medications may be instituted for the child who is highly irritable to promote rest. Stool softeners may be administered to maintain bowel movement and prevent fecal impaction.

Administer and Manage Medications

As indicated earlier and throughout the chapter, infants and children with neurological disorders receive many different medications, from anti-inflammatories to sedatives to antibiotics. Be aware of what is being administered, the proper dosage and how it is determined, and why the healthcare provider ordered it. Children frequently receive medications that have not been tested in the pediatric population, so always question why a medication is ordered if the reason is not clear. Use of a drug book or online resource provided by the facility is essential to administer medications safely. Nurses caring for children in the hospital setting must always anticipate complications for medication administration, because children may react differently than expected. Know how to prevent complications while supporting healing.

Check medications on discharge orders for accuracy and safety. Teach caregivers in a language that they understand how to administer medications at home, because this is critical for the child's safety. Teach parents how to use an oral syringe to ensure that they give the proper dosage.

Structural Defects of the Neurological System

Structural defects of the neurological system include defects in which the brain, cerebral spinal fluid tracts, spinal cord, or skull is malformed, incompletely developed, or, in some cases, absent. Structural defects covered in this chapter include cranial defects, hydrocephalus, and arteriovenous malformations. Neural tube defects, another type of structural defect, are covered in Chapter 28.

Cranial defects involve the skull bones and cranial sutures and can range from major defects that are incompatible with life to defects that are insignificant and do not require intervention. Cranial defects can be caused by premature closure of the cranial sutures, a skull that grows too quickly in relation to how fast the brain is growing, or absence of the bones that make up the skull. Craniosynostosis, deformational plagiocephaly (DP), and microcephaly are discussed in this chapter.

Craniosynostosis

Craniosynostosis is a condition of premature closure of one or more of the cranial sutures. Most commonly occurring at or before birth, craniosynostosis may occur on its own or in conjunction with other congenital anomalies.

Etiology and Pathophysiology

Simple craniosynostosis involves the premature fusion of one suture. Complex craniosynostosis involves the premature fusion of multiple sutures, which can contribute to a variety of clinical manifestations, depending on the sutures involved. Anantheswar and Venkataramana (2009) indicated that, although the exact cause of the fusion is unclear, mutations in fibroblast growth factor receptor genes may play a factor in the proliferation, differentiation, and migration of plates in the skull that lead to premature fusion.

Craniosynostosis is common in certain genetic syndromes, and its risk factors include maternal Caucasian race, advanced maternal age, male gender, maternal use of nitrosatable drugs, fertility treatments, and paternal exposure to teratogens through occupation (e.g., agriculture, automobile repair, mechanics, and forestry service).

Craniosynostosis leads to an abnormal head shape and can cause increased ICP, which, in turn, can cause brain abnormalities. The most common suture to prematurely fuse is the sagittal suture, which leads to anterior-posterior elongation with no increase in ICP or hydrocephalus. Other types of craniosynostosis, particularly those that involve fusion of more than one suture, contribute to varying head shapes, brain abnormalities ranging from mild to severe, functional and cognitive delays, facial abnormalities, eye abnormalities that can lead to blindness, and malocclusion (see Fig. 22.1 for variations of craniosynostosis).

Clinical Presentation

Clinical presentation for craniosynostosis depends on which suture or sutures are fused. The main characteristic is malformation of the head, which may be noticeable at birth. Facial structures may be affected as well, depending on the severity of the early fusion. In addition, the fontanelle may appear abnormal or may disappear completely and a raised, hard ridge may appear along the affected sutures. If untreated, symptoms may progress from cranial malformation to abnormal brain function and may manifest in developmental delays, cognitive impairment, lethargy, blindness, eye movement disorders, seizure activity, and, in rare instances, death (Mayo Clinic, 2018).

Assessment and Diagnosis

Assessment of a child with suspected craniosynostosis includes a complete developmental history to help identify any neurological deficits, a physical exam to assess for skull abnormalities, and a complete neurological exam to determine any subsequent brain abnormalities. Diagnosis is based on computed tomography (CT) scans and magnetic resonance imaging (MRI), which also help

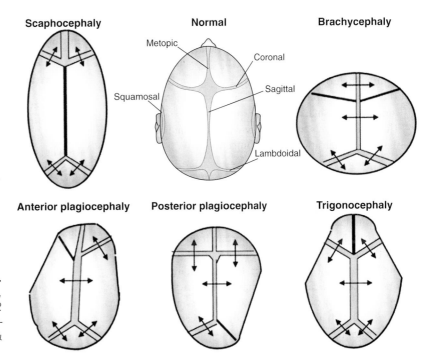

Figure 22.1. Variations of craniosynostosis. Reprinted with permission from Mongan, P., Soriano, S. G., Sloan, T. B., & Gravlee, G. P. (2013). *Practical approach to neuroanesthesia.* Philadelphia, PA: Lippincott Williams & Wilkins.

determine which sutures are fused. Genetic testing may also be offered to determine the underlying cause of the malformation, because many genetic syndromes accompany craniosynostosis.

Therapeutic Interventions

Craniosynostosis is treated by surgery to release the fused suture(s) and to achieve cosmetic improvements for facial and head deformities. Surgery is best done before the child is 6 months of age to achieve the best outcome. Endoscopic surgery is done on infants up to 6 months old and is minimally invasive, but it still requires that the child wear a helmet afterward. Open surgery is reserved for infants older than 6 months and is done to reshape moderate to severe malformations. Infants receiving open surgery are typically hospitalized for 3 or 4 days, because absorbable plates and screws are used to hold the repaired cranial sections in place.

Monitoring in the pre- and postoperative periods involves obtaining a neurological baseline and monitoring carefully to identify complications. Monitor hemoglobin and hematocrit levels for signs of blood loss because of surgery, and administer supportive transfusions of packed red blood cells or whole blood as ordered and indicated. Pain management and fluid administration are also essential during the postoperative period. Fluids may be administered intravenously initially, with the goal of beginning oral intake as soon as possible. If swollen eyelids develop, which is common, calm the child and gently cleanse the eye area. Finally, a molding helmet is indicated postoperatively for a child who has a mild deformation or has had endoscopic surgery and should be worn for 23 hours per day for 3 to 4 months (Fig. 22.2). An infant who has had open surgery does not need a helmet to form the cranium postoperatively.

Evaluation

Expected outcomes for a child with craniosynostosis include the following:

- The child is successfully treated for craniosynostosis, as evidenced by an improvement in the shape of the skull and minimal neurological complications.
- The caregiver applies the helmet as prescribed and minimal complications such as pressure spots occur.
- The child recovers from surgery with minimal pain and no signs of complications such as infection.

Discharge Planning and Teaching

Teach caregivers of children who have undergone surgery about proper wound care, basic signs and symptoms of infection, and pain relief, which is particularly important if surgery was open as opposed to endoscopic. Proper wound care aids in healing and minimizes the chance of infection. In addition, instruct caregivers on other complications that may arise as a result of surgery, depending on how extensive the cranial repair has been. Infants being treated with helmet therapy should be seen frequently, because helmets need to be changed as the infant grows. Instruct caregivers to monitor for signs of erythema, which may indicate

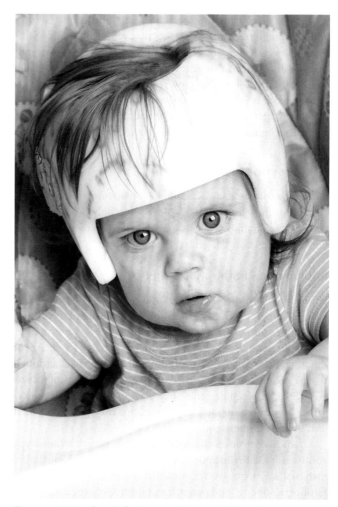

Figure 22.2. **An infant wearing a helmet to correct craniosynostosis.**

the development of pressure points as the head begins to grow, in which case the child would need a new helmet.

Deformational Plagiocephaly

Deformational plagiocephaly (DP) is a common issue and has been defined as asymmetry and flattening of the head caused by external forces on the skull (Looman & Flannery, 2012). Unwin and Dika (2017) indicted that although the 1992 "Back to Sleep" campaign was successful in reducing the number of infants dying from sudden infant death syndrome, it may have contributed to a dramatic increase in the number of infants presenting with cranial defects as a result of increased time spent in the supine position.

Etiology and Pathophysiology

Although DP may occur as a result of supine positioning for long periods of time, other conditions may contribute to its increased incidence, including premature birth, prolonged intubation, male gender, multiple-gestation pregnancies, breech position in utero, primiparous mothers, maternal age greater than 35 years, birth trauma, congenital anomalies, low activity level, developmental milestone delay, inadequate time spent in the prone position, bottle feeding, and prolonged labor (Unwin & Dika, 2017). Congenital muscular torticollis (CMT), a common musculoskeletal abnormality related to a shortening or contraction of the sternocleidomastoid muscle, is also a significant risk factor for the development of DP.

Clinical Presentation

Skull deformation is the main clinical presentation of DP, with the right occiput affected more often than the left. Depending on the severity, infants may present with varying facial abnormalities, as well, including unevenness of facial features (Unwin & Dika, 2017). Although the defects may be present at any age in infancy, DP peaks in incidence at the age of 4 months, on average, and rarely progresses thereafter, as infants by that age have typically gained adequate neck muscle control to hold their heads up, which reduces external forces on the skull. Further evaluate infants presenting with DP for the presence of central nervous system lesions, deformities of the vertebral column, craniosynostosis, and brachycephaly as differential diagnoses (Unwin & Dika, 2017). Children with DP may have developmental delays (Analyze the Evidence 22.1).

Assessment and Diagnosis

A careful history and physical assessment are both essential in determining the cause of DP. Obtain a thorough prenatal and birth history, which can help determine whether DP is related to in utero risk factors or it developed after birth. Ask parents how much time the infant spends in a supine or seated position, which may also reveal the cause. In addition, ask caregivers whether the infant demonstrates a preference for looking to one specific side coupled with a decreased range of motion in the head and neck, because these symptoms may indicate CMT-related DP. The physical assessment must focus on the skull and facial features. Palpate the fontanelles and note any bulging or ridging of the cranial sutures. Observe the infant for the presence of a head tilt, decreased range of motion, or thickening of the sternocleidomastoid muscle, which could reveal the presence of CMT.

Therapeutic Interventions

There are no specific guidelines for the treatment of DP, and management is typically conservative, including repositioning of the infant and physiotherapy, but may progress to the use of orthotics if conservative treatment fails to correct the defect. Underlying conditions that contribute to DP, such as CMT, must be treated to correct the defect. Unwin and Dika (2017) emphasized that orthotics must be worn for 20 to 23 hours a day for 2 to 6 months, depending on the severity of the defect. Age appears to be important, as research has shown that orthotics tend to be ineffective after 12 months of age, because cranial growth slows down considerably after this age (Unwin & Dika, 2017).

Evaluation

Expected outcomes for a child with DP include the following:

- The DP is recognized early and treatment begun early, minimizing long-term complications.
- The treatment for DP is successful, as evidenced by an improvement in the shape of the skull and minimal neurological complications.
- The caregiver applies the helmet as prescribed and minimal complications such as pressure spots occur.
- The child recovers from surgery with minimal pain and no signs of complications such as infection.
- The child experiences minimal cognitive and/or developmental delays as a result of DP.

Discharge Planning and Teaching

Unwin and Dika (2017) emphasized that early screening and identification of at-risk infants is important, and prevention is the key with DP. Switch infant positions frequently to prevent unnecessary force on any one part of the skull, particularly during the first 4 months of life, when infants lack the ability to position themselves. In addition, teach caregivers to place the child prone ("tummy time") for a total of 30 to 60 minutes per day to reduce skull pressure and promote motor development. Tummy time can be broken down into 10-minute increments to acclimate those infants who do not prefer this position. Placing toys on the floor or interacting with the infant while in this position can encourage mutual engagement and promote

 Analyze the Evidence 22.1

Deformational Plagiocephaly and Developmental Delays

Do children with DP have developmental delays? Research has shown a correlation between DP and developmental delays, particularly in motor skills (Laughlin, Luerssen, & Dias, 2011). However, it is not known whether there is a direct causal relationship between DP and the delay, or whether the delays are preexisting and present before the development of the defect. It may be possible that motor delays lead to decreased movement, thus rendering the infant unable to reposition the body. Unwin and Dika (2017) indicated that some literature reported that the incidence of developmental delays in children with DP was similar to that in the general population, whereas other studies have found that infants with DP are 3–4 times more likely to present with language and motor difficulties. Because research is inconclusive regarding DP and developmental delays, the nurse should perform careful screening and obtain a developmental history to detect any signs as early as possible, allowing for early intervention to take place.

development, as well. Teach parents to keep infants limited to car seats only when traveling in the car, because placement in car seats decreases infant movement and may contribute to excessive pressure on the skull. The same is true for infant swings and seats that limit movement. Prevent DP by recognizing infants at risk early and teaching caregivers the strategies to promote optimal movement.

Microcephaly

Microcephaly is an abnormally small head, which is defined as an occipitofrontal circumference greater than 2 standard deviations below the mean for age and sex (Ashwal, Michelson, Plawner, & Dobyns, 2009).

Etiology and Pathophysiology

Microcephaly is diagnosed as either primary, in which a genetic, chromosomal, or hereditary cause is implicated, or secondary, in which the defect occurs as a result of exposure to irradiation, maternal infection with toxoplasmosis, rubella, or cytomegalovirus, or maternal use of alcohol or tobacco. Feldman et al. (2012) indicated that studies have shown a correlation between maternal alcohol use and microcephaly, low birth weight, and low birth length. Trauma, metabolic disorders, and anoxia during the fetal period may also challenge brain growth and contribute to microcephaly. Presently, Zika virus (ZIKV) has received much attention as a cause of microcephaly (Analyze the Evidence 22.2).

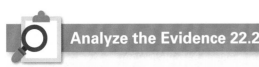

Analyze the Evidence 22.2

Zika Virus and Microcephaly

Does ZIKV cause brain malformation? Alvarado and Schwartz (2017) indicated that ZIKV has erupted as a global epidemic and has become a public health problem that has as many unanswered questions as it has answers. Beginning in 2015, several babies with microcephaly were born to mothers who reported having a rash during early pregnancy. Nearly 700 cases of the rash were diagnosed in areas of Brazil between December 2014 and April 2015, yet it was not until April 29, 2015, that the Bahia State Laboratory in Brazil reported that samples were identified as ZIKV. Confirmed by the World Health Organization (WHO) at Brazil's national reference laboratory in May 2015, ZIKV was identified as an epidemic reaching from Brazil to the Western hemisphere (Kindhauser, Allen, Frank, Santhana, & Dye, 2016). In October 2015, an unexplained increase in the number of infants born with microcephaly was reported in areas where the initial outbreak began, and in November 2015, the WHO declared a national public health emergency in Brazil after 700 cases of ZIKV-associated microcephaly were reported (Kindhauser et al., 2016).

Clinical Presentation

In addition to decreased head circumference (HC), microcephaly results in varying degrees of cognitive impairment, ranging from no or mild cognitive delay to unresponsiveness, motor impairment, and autistic behavior.

Assessment and Diagnosis

Ashwal et al. (2009) emphasized that microcephaly is indicated when a child has an HC of more than 2 standard deviations below the mean for age and gender (Fig. 22.3). To determine the presence of microcephaly, MRI is done to examine the brain in detail, because a CT scan may not provide enough information. The infant with microcephaly typically presents with global delays in cognitive and motor development that are evident from birth. Depending on the degree of the microcephaly, these delays can be mild to profound. Microcephaly can be detected by fetal ultrasound, but most pregnancies do not warrant a diagnostic ultrasound unless risk factors are present. If microcephaly runs in the family, a couple may undergo genetic testing to determine the risk of having a child with the condition to allow them to make an educated choice about having children.

Therapeutic Interventions

Because microcephaly affects brain development and has no cure, nursing care is supportive for both the infant and parents, who are facing life with a child who has special needs. Most interventions are aimed at providing support for the caregiver and minimizing complications for the infant. Monitor children with mild cases for growth and development and provide them with services, resources, and equipment to promote optimal functioning. Physical therapy and special services to help the child with learning in school are examples of the support that a child may receive.

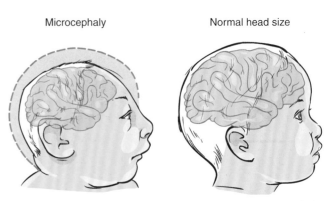

Microcephaly   Normal head size

Figure 22.3. Comparison of a child with microcephaly (left) with a child with a normal head size (right). Note how much smaller the brain is in the child with microcephaly.

Evaluation

Expected outcomes for a child with microcephaly include the following:

- The child is diagnosed early and receives the best services to promote growth and development.
- The child experiences minimal cognitive and/or developmental delays as a result of mild microcephaly.
- The caregivers receive help from support groups and services, such as respite care for those with children with severe-to-profound microcephaly.

Discharge Planning and Teaching

Educate and prepare caregivers of children with microcephaly for their role. Teach parents about their child's level of severity and the specific care their child requires. Although many cases of microcephaly are profound, infants and children in this category can experience a full lifespan. Prepare caregivers for what will ensue in terms of services and care. Inform them that respite care may be available to allow them a break to carry on their own activities of daily living. Support groups are also helpful.

Hydrocephalus

Hydrocephalus is a term derived from the Greek *hydor* (water) and *kephale* (brain) and refers to the buildup of cerebrospinal fluid (CSF) in a patient's brain. CSF is produced by the choroid plexus, a vascular lining in the ventricles of the brain. Infants produce roughly 25 mL of CSF per day, whereas older children produce between 25 and 500 mL per day. Although it is age dependent, the adult volume of CSF in the ventricles and

subarachnoid space is approximately 150 mL and is reached by the age of 5 years. Most cases of hydrocephalus involve a blockage of CSF, but the rate of formation does not change significantly or is only slightly decreased when hydrocephalus is present (Kahle, Kulkarni, Limbrick, & Warf, 2016). Once secreted, CSF circulates through the intracranial vault and spinal cord, helping buffer the brain, maintain normal chemical balance, and maintain the blood-brain barrier (Roumila, 2018). Once it has circulated through the brain and spinal column, CSF is absorbed by the arachnoid villi and lymphatic system, enters the venous system, is filtered by the kidney and liver, and then is processed and excreted in a manner similar to other fluids.

Etiology and Pathophysiology

Hydrocephalus may occur as a result of increased production of CSF, decreased ability to absorb CSF, or an obstruction of flow of CSF, all subsequently leading to an increase in ICP. *Communicating hydrocephalus* is related to increased production or decreased absorption of CSF, whereas *noncommunicating hydrocephalus* is the result of an obstruction that prevents proper flow and causes the CSF to build up in the brain. Although brain tumors, head injury, bleeding, or infection can cause hydrocephalus, Arnold-Chiari malformation types I and II are among the most common causes of noncommunicating hydrocephalus. Both types of Arnold-Chiari malformation involve a narrow foramen magnum and herniation of the cerebellar tonsils, blocking the flow of CSF through the fourth ventricle and spinal column (Fig. 22.4). Although the cause of Arnold-Chiari type I is not known and many patients with it are not symptomatic until early adulthood, Arnold-Chiari type II is most commonly associated with myelomeningocele (see earlier discussion) and

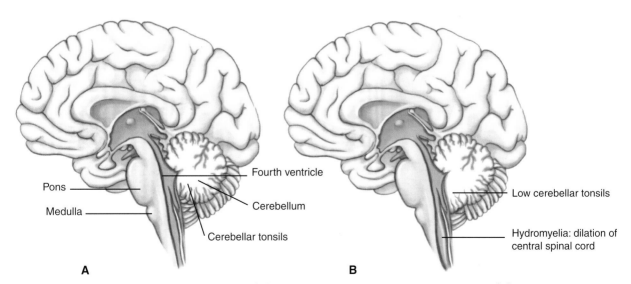

Figure 22.4. **Comparison of a normal brain (A) with a brain with a Chiari malformation (B).** Note the herniation of the cerebellum through the foramen magnum in the brain with the Chiari malformation. Reprinted with permission from Bowden, V., & Greenberg, C. S. (2013). *Children and their families* (3rd ed., Fig. 21.6). Philadelphia: Lippincott Williams & Wilkins.

is typically diagnosed at birth. Patients with type I typically present with daily headaches that encompass the entire head (Green, 2003).

Clinical Presentation

Children with hydrocephalus present differently as symptoms of hydrocephalus vary by the age, cause, and rate of development. Typical symptoms are consistent with ICP. The most prominent sign in an infant is an enlarging occipitofrontal HC. In addition, infants may exhibit the following:

- Dilated scalp veins
- Pale scalp skin and separation of cranial sutures
- Macewen's sign: tapping on the skull near the junction of the frontal, temporal, and parietal bones produces a resonant sound
- Difficulty holding the head upright
- Frontal bossing (an enlarged forehead; Fig. 22.5)
- Sunsetting eyes (Fig. 22.6)
- Bulging fontanel
- Emesis and/or poor feeding
- Irritability
- Sixth nerve palsy
- Periods of apnea

Children with hydrocephalus may present with headaches, nausea and vomiting, which may be worse in the morning upon rising, lethargy, irritability, a decline in school performance, gait disturbances, or sixth nerve palsy, in addition to other neurological sequelae.

Assessment and Diagnosis

Diagnosis of hydrocephalus can be made prenatally on the basis of an ultrasound or postnatally on the basis of a finding on physical assessment of an increase in HC inconsistent with normal growth for a child. A comprehensive physical assessment may

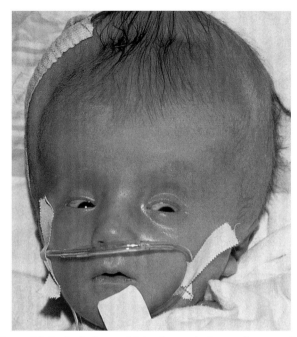

Figure 22.6. An infant with hydrocephalus and sunsetting eyes. Notice the dilated scalp veins. Reprinted with permission from Gold, D. H., & Weingeist, T. A. (2000). *Color atlas of the eye in systemic disease* (1st ed., Fig. 98.1). Baltimore: Lippincott Williams & Wilkins.

also reveal neurological deficits related to hydrocephalus. A CT scan or an MRI can indicate an enlargement of the ventricles and the presence of bleeding, and a **cisternogram** can identify any abnormality in CSF flow dynamics in the infant's or child's brain and spinal cord. Although a lumbar puncture may yield important information regarding the status of CSF, it is contraindicated in noncommunicating hydrocephalus, in which the pressure gradient in the brain is higher than that in the spinal column. This difference in the pressure gradient can cause

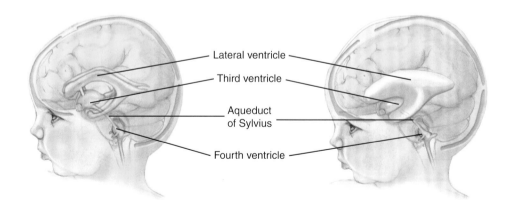

Lateral ventricle

Third ventricle

Aqueduct of Sylvius

Fourth ventricle

A   **B**

Figure 22.5. Comparison of a child with a normal brain (B) with a child with hydrocephalus (Bright). Note the enlarged ventricles and forehead in the child with hydrocephalus. Reprinted with permission from Hatfield, N. T., & Kincheloe, C. A. (2017). *Introductory maternity and pediatric nursing* (4th ed., Fig. 21.3). Philadelphia: Lippincott Williams & Wilkins.

a drop in pressure when the spinal column is accessed through a lumbar puncture, causing the brain to herniate downward. Finally, radiographs can identify a thinning or separation of the skull bones associated with increased head size.

Therapeutic Interventions

Treatment for hydrocephalus is aimed at relieving ICP by reducing ventricular size through a ventriculostomy with the surgical placement of a ventriculoperitoneal (VP) shunt. The shunt is a special catheter with a one-way valve set at a desired pressure that is placed into the lateral ventricle to drain the excess CSF. The catheter extends into the child's peritoneal cavity and is coiled to keep the shunt positioned properly in the abdomen as the child grows (Fig. 22.7). The CSF then drains into the peritoneum, where it is absorbed by the body.

Preoperatively, nursing care focuses on frequently changing the position of the child's head to prevent impaired skin integrity due to thinning of the skin of the scalp and prolonged pressure on any one area. The child also receives IV antibiotics preoperatively to prevent an infection and acetazolamide or furosemide to decrease CSF production or help remove excess fluid. In addition, it is important to obtain an HC (Priority Care Concepts 22.1) and baseline abdominal circumference before surgery, because paralytic ileus may be a complication after surgery.

Postoperatively, nursing care focuses on careful neurological assessments, daily HC measurement, and monitoring for changes in an infant's fontanelle. Irritability or a change in behavior may indicate the development of an infection such as meningitis or increased ICP. Initially, position the child flat to prevent rapid ventricular decompression. Do not elevate the head of the bed higher than 30 degrees. Also, position the child on the nonoperative side to prevent pressure on the site. Safety precautions are imperative, because the child may become disoriented with pain or fever; report fever immediately, because

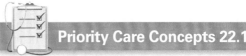

Priority Care Concepts 22.1

Measuring HC

HC is a critical variable to assess when caring for an infant or a child with the potential for increased ICP. Obtain a baseline HC when the infant or child is admitted and subsequent daily measurements to detect any change in size. To measure HC, place a nonstretchable tape measure around the most prominent part of the occiput and just above the eyebrows. Remove any braids or hair decorations to obtain the most accurate measurement. Ensure that the measuring tape is snug and read the measurement to the nearest 0.1 cm.

Normal HC measurements are as follows:

- *Birth to 3 months*: Median HC at birth is 33.9 (girls) to 40.5 (boys) cm.
- *4 to 6 months*: Median HC at 6 months is 42.2 (girls) to 43.3 (boys) cm.
- *6 months to 1 year*: Median HC at 1 year is 44.9 (girls) to 46.1 (boys) cm.

Adapted from the World Health Organization. (2019). Growth standards: Head circumference-for-age. Retrieved from https://www.who.int/childgrowth/standards/hc_for_age/en/.

IV antibiotics may need to be added or changed depending on presentation. Palpate for warmth, which may indicate an underlying infection, and monitor the incision sites for redness or drainage. Common shunt infections include *Staphylococcus aureus* and *Staphylococcus epidermidis*. Monitor for signs of peritonitis, including an elevated temperature, a rapid heart rate, and a change in the blood pressure, in addition to an increased white blood cell (WBC) count, abdominal rebound tenderness, and muscle rigidity. Nausea and vomiting may also be present.

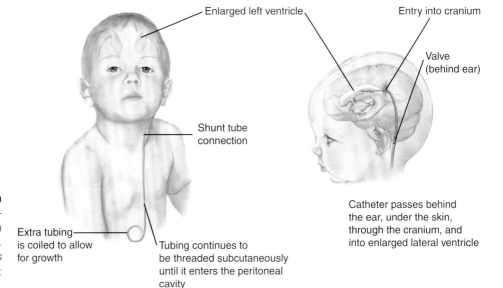

Figure 22.7. Placement of a ventriculoperitoneal shunt. Reprinted with permission from Bowden, V., & Greenberg, C. S. (2013). *Children and their families* (3rd ed., Fig. 21.5). Philadelphia: Lippincott Williams & Wilkins.

Enlarged left ventricle

Entry into cranium

Valve (behind ear)

Shunt tube connection

Extra tubing is coiled to allow for growth

Tubing continues to be threaded subcutaneously until it enters the peritoneal cavity

Catheter passes behind the ear, under the skin, through the cranium, and into enlarged lateral ventricle

Also monitor for the return of bowel sounds; a continued absence of bowel sounds coupled with an increase in abdominal circumference related to distension may indicate paralytic ileus.

Evaluation

Expected outcomes for a child with hydrocephalus include the following:

- The child experiences a reduction in CSF and subsequent reduction in head size.
- Complications from increased ICP are minimized, allowing the child to grow and develop appropriately.
- The child with a VP shunt experiences minimal complications such as infection or clotting of the shunt.
- The child and caregivers receive the resources necessary to help the child participate in activities of daily living at an optimal level.

Discharge Planning and Teaching

The placement of a VP shunt is typically for life. Although VP shunts are helpful in draining excess fluid from the ventricle of the brain and helping reduce ICP, they are not without complications. VP shunts can become infected, clogged, or kinked or develop a blood clot. VP shunts may also become displaced within the abdomen because of growth. Teach parents to watch for any change in the child's behavior, a rise in temperature, nausea and vomiting, lethargy or unresponsiveness, poor feeding, and seizure activity. In addition to infections, which are common complications, increased ICP may occur as a result of the shunt no longer draining CSF. Those in frequent contact with the child should be aware of and report any changes immediately so that treatment may be rendered. In addition, instruct parents that their child will not be able to participate in contact sports because of the risk of shunt damage.

Intracranial Arteriovenous Malformation

Intracranial arteriovenous malformations (AVMs) are congenital vascular lesions that are present at birth but not typically identified until the patient is older. El-Ghanem et al. (2016) indicated that AVMs are rare in general (between 0.06% and 0.11% of the population) and even more so in children but still count as the most frequent abnormality of intracranial circulation in childhood. AVMs are also the most common cause of spontaneous hemorrhage in children and rupture more frequently in children than in adults (El-Ghanem et al., 2016).

Etiology and Pathophysiology

Dy and Schuster (2015) indicated that AVMs are thought to arise from failure in the differentiation of vascular channels into mature arteries, capillaries, and veins. This failure occurs around the third week of embryogenesis and involves a structural defect in the formation of the arteriolar capillary network that is normally present between arteries and veins (Dy & Schuster, 2015). This defect causes an absence of communication

between capillaries and leads to an elevation in intraluminal venous pressure, eventually leading to distension and thickness of the capillaries and the forming of a vascular network that becomes a direct connection between the artery and vein (Fig. 22.8). Over time, this malformation enlarges because of pressure differentials and eventually causes hemorrhaging in some patients. The location of these malformations in children is typically in the posterior fossa, the basal ganglia, and the thalamus, leading to catastrophic outcomes when they rupture (Dy & Schuster, 2015).

Clinical Presentation

Children with AVMs may present with complaints of headaches, weakness, seizure activity, visual or swallowing difficulties, limb paralysis, bowel and/or bladder symptoms, or cognitive impairment (Dy & Schuster, 2015). A careful examination of the past medical history may lead to clues that something is wrong, yet 80% to 85% of children experience a hemorrhagic event as the initial presenting symptom (Dy & Schuster, 2015).

Assessment and Diagnosis

Because no laboratory studies can detect an AVM, neuroimaging is important in identifying the malformation. CT scans with angiography can provide details of the nature of the malformation by examining the vasculature. MRIs with or without contrast are important in detecting hemorrhaging and can provide a better view of the vascular anatomy. Conventional

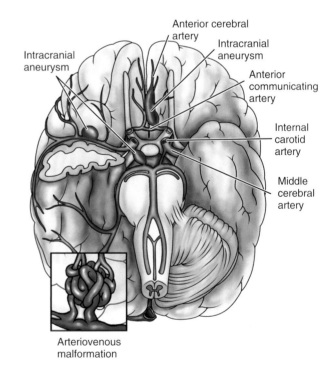

Figure 22.8. Intracranial arteriovenous malformation. Reprinted with permission from Hinkle, J. L., & Cheever, K. H. (2017). *Brunner & Suddarth's textbook of medical-surgical nursing* (14th ed., Fig. 67.5). Philadelphia: Lippincott Williams & Wilkins.

four-vessel angiography is the gold standard for diagnosis, because it can detect very small lesions, and is used in treatment planning with children (Dy & Schuster, 2015).

Therapeutic Interventions

An AVM must be obliterated to completely remove the risk of rupture and re-rupture. Microsurgical resection and radiosurgery with or without endovascular embolization may be instituted to destroy or remove the malformation, except in cases in which the risks outweigh the benefits or the therapy is determined to be ineffective (El-Ghanem et al., 2016). El-Ghanem et al. (2016) indicated that microsurgical resection is the preferred treatment, especially in cases in which urgent intervention is needed. However, technology is continually evolving and presenting other options for children with AVMs.

Evaluation

Expected outcomes for a child with an AVM include the following:

- The child is able to participate in activities of daily living at an optimal level.
- The child's AVM is identified early to allow for intervention to minimize the serious complications that arise from the malformation.
- The child recovers from surgery for the AVM with a minimum amount of pain and maximum healing.

Discharge Planning and Teaching

Numerous complications are associated with AVMs and their treatment, ranging from permanent disability to death. The inability of treatment to completely obliterate the AVM presents the continual risk of rupture. Provide coordination of care and

family education to ensure that the child has optimal supportive care and that outcome measures are focused on preventing further neurological deficits. Support groups for the child and family may be beneficial in connecting them with other families who have experienced neurological events with a child.

Infectious Disorders of the Neurological System

Infections of the neurological system can be bacterial, viral, fungal, or parasitic and can affect the brain, CSF, or spinal column. Infectious disorders of the neurological system covered in this chapter include meningitis, Reye syndrome, and encephalitis. An infectious disease that affects the neuromuscular system, botulism, is covered in Chapter 28.

Meningitis

The brain is protected by three important membranes: the dura mater, the arachnoid mater, and the pia mater (Fig. 22.9). All three layers work together to protect the brain from injury and infection by housing arterioles, venules, and CSF that bathe the brain and provide chemical functional support. Although these structures are important in preventing infection, they can become infected themselves. **Meningitis** is an infection of the meninges and is classified as septic (caused by bacterial pathogens such as *Streptococcus pneumoniae*, *Neisseria meningitidis*, *Escherichia coli*, or *Haemophilus influenzae* type B) or aseptic (caused by a known or unknown viral agent typically associated with the flu season, in the fall or winter).

Etiology and Pathophysiology

Meningitis can be acquired at any age and can be transmitted during labor and delivery or in utero. Although immunizations

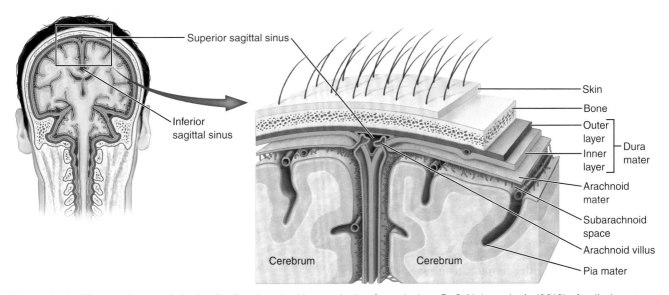

Figure 22.9. The meninges of the brain. Reprinted with permission from Archer, P., & Nelson, L. A. (2012). *Applied anatomy and physiology for manual therapists* (1st ed., Fig. 7.20). Philadelphia: Lippincott Williams & Wilkins.

for *H. influenzae* type B have been successful in almost eradicating this deadly pathogen, other organisms are still held accountable for cases of meningitis. The incidence of meningitis is the highest in infants (children younger than age 1 year) and in adolescents and young adults 16 to 23 years old, with *N. meningitidis* implicated in many cases (Centers for Disease Control and Prevention [CDC], 2017). Meningitis is passed from person to person by close contact with respiratory secretions. Septic meningitis is the result of dissemination of the pathogen from a nasopharyngeal or hematological inoculation. The pathogen travels through the CSF and embeds itself in the subarachnoid space (CDC, 2017).

Clinical Presentation

The body reacts to the invading organism with an inflammatory response and WBC proliferation, causing hyperemic meningeal tissue with exudate covering the lining, resulting in varying degrees of fever, headache, and complaints of a stiff neck, photophobia, lethargy, or irritability. Infants may not demonstrate classic symptoms, but may be inactive or slow in movement and reaction or feed poorly. *N. meningitidis* may also cause cold chills, cold hands and feet, severe muscle aches, rapid breathing, diarrhea, and a dark purple rash (Fig. 22.10; CDC, 2017).

Assessment and Diagnosis

Meningitis is diagnosed with a lumbar puncture to analyze the CSF and identify the organism. A complete blood count (CBC) is also drawn. Positive signs include an elevated WBC count and clotting deficiencies related to *N. meningitidis*. Coureuil, Join-Lambert, Lécuyer, Bourdoulous, Marullo, and Nassif (2013) indicated that the rash is associated with a high bacteria load, leading to a significant increase in vascular permeability

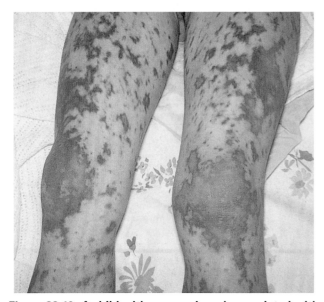

Figure 22.10. A child with a purpuric rash associated with *Neisseria meningitidis*. Reprinted with permission from Scheld, W. M., Whitley, R. J., & Marra, C. M. (2014). *Infections of the central nervous system* (4th ed., Fig. 24.23). Philadelphia: Lippincott Williams & Wilkins.

and associated with thrombosis and purpura. Manage children presenting with a purpuric rash immediately, because it indicates sepsis when it appears with other meningitis symptoms. A positive Kernig's or Brudzinski's sign indicates meningeal irritation resulting in hyperreactive reflexes.

- Kernig's sign: Lay the child supine with the hips flexed. Try to straighten a leg out—the test is positive if pain behind the knee is experienced when the leg is extended. Younger children may cry out or resist leg extension (Fig. 22.11A and B).
- Brudzinski's sign: Lay the child flat. Attempt to raise the child's head toward the chest and place the chin on the chest. Meningeal irritation is present if the child indicates pain or resistance or the child immediately flexes the hips and knees (Fig. 22.11C and D).

Therapeutic Interventions

Children with suspected meningitis are placed in an isolation room until a confirmative diagnosis regarding the pathogen can be made. Once the child is diagnosed, meningitis treatment involves diligent assessment of the child's neurological status. Closely monitor the level of consciousness and use the pediatric Glasgow Coma Scale (see Fig. 22.14 for an example). Because the child may develop seizure activity, institute seizure precautions. The child may also need to be kept NPO (nothing by mouth) if nausea and vomiting are prominent. Provide fever management and general comfort measures to help treat the malaise and headaches that may be present. Nonsteroidal anti-inflammatory medications, antipyretics such as acetaminophen, and IV antibiotics are necessary for treating bacterial meningitis. Although aseptic meningitis may present with similar symptoms, it is not as severe and is usually self-limiting, requiring only supportive care. Those in close contact with the child with septic meningitis should be placed on a course of antibiotics to present the spread of the illness.

Evaluation

Expected outcomes for a child with meningitis include the following:

- The child's neurological status returns to normal.
- The child is free of infection and other potential complications.
- Pain is adequately controlled.

Discharge Planning and Teaching

Children with meningitis may go home with medications to take once they are able to function well on their own. If IV medications are still needed, a home health nurse may follow up with the child to administer medications. Instruct the child and caregivers on any limitations that might need to be instituted during the recovery phase. Most children are able to return to school and participate in normal activities once they achieve a full recovery. Anti-seizure medications are typically not needed once the child has recovered, but some cases are more complicated and may progress into epilepsy. Instruct caregivers,

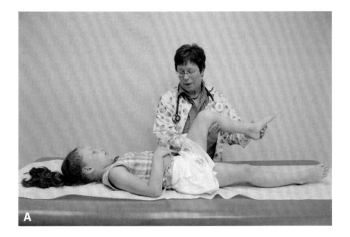
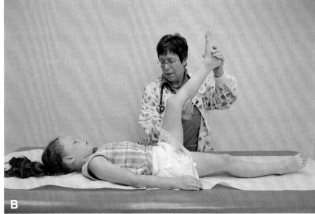
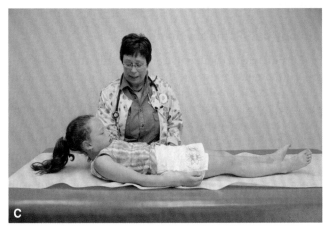
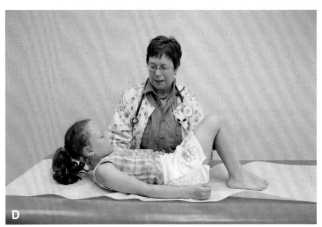

Figure 22.11. Eliciting Kernig (A and B) and Brudzinski's (C and D) signs of meningitis. Kernig sign is tested by flexing legs at the hip and knee (A), then extending the knee (B). A positive report of pain along the vertebral column and/or inability to extend knee is a positive sign and indicates irritation of meninges. Brudzinski sign is tested by the child lying supine with the neck flexed (C). A positive sign occurs if resistance or pain is met. The child may also passively flex hip and knees in reaction, indicating meningeal irritation (D). Reprinted with permission from Kyle, T., & Carman, S. (2016). *Essentials of pediatric nursing* (3rd ed., Fig. 16.14). Philadelphia, PA: Wolters Kluwer.

teachers, and the child on seizure precautions. The child should wear an identification bracelet and follow basic precautions such as not swimming unless an adult is present.

Reye Syndrome

Reye syndrome is a serious illness that is defined by rapid progression and subsequent multiorgan failure with a poor outcome. Although it is rare, early identification is necessary because it is associated with an increased chance of recovery.

In 1977, researchers followed 373 cases—of those, 42% died, whereas another 11% had residual neurological damage (Degnan, 2012). The incidence of cases has dropped over the years because caregivers have been instructed to avoid the use of acetylsalicylic acid (aspirin) in children.

Etiology and Pathophysiology

Reye syndrome occurs when aspirin is administered to a child during a viral illness. Influenza A and B and varicella are the viruses most commonly associated with Reye syndrome, although parainfluenza, measles, adenoviruses, Coxsackie viruses,

cytomegalovirus, Epstein-Barr virus, human immunodeficiency virus (HIV), hepatitis A and B, and rotavirus have been implicated as well (Degnan, 2012). Mitochondrial injury is thought to be the underlying pathophysiology. Mitochondrial damage occurs from aspirin combined with cytokines and endotoxins released during the viral illness. Oxidative phosphorylation and fatty acid beta-oxidation are inhibited, leading to a cascade of events caused by increasing levels of ammonia resulting in acute noninflammatory encephalitis and fatty degenerative liver failure.

Clinical Presentation

Children with Reye syndrome typically present in stages from 0 to 6. Children in stage 0 are relatively asymptomatic. Children in stage 1 present with vomiting that may or may not be accompanied by dehydration and are sleepy and lethargic. The syndrome progresses rapidly from there. Stage 2 is defined by restlessness, irritability, combativeness, disorientation, tachycardia, hyperventilation, dilated pupils with sluggish response, and a positive Babinski's sign. Stage 3 is defined by children who are comatose and demonstrate decorticate posturing and inappropriate response to noxious stimuli. Children who are in stage 4 are in a deep coma, demonstrate decerebrate posturing, and have fixed and dilated pupils. Stage 5 is defined by seizures, flaccid paralysis, absence of deep tendon reflexes and pupillary response, and respiratory arrest. Stage 6 is reserved for children who do not fit into the other stages because they have been given medications that alter the level of consciousness (Weiner, 2018).

Assessment and Diagnosis

Diagnosis is made with a liver biopsy, lumbar puncture, and serum tests, including liver enzyme levels, coagulation studies, blood glucose level, and ammonia levels. Diagnosis can be challenging, because Reye syndrome can mimic other metabolic diseases. The CDC has issued diagnostic criteria for Reye syndrome, which include the following: acute noninflammatory encephalopathy diagnosed with a biopsy, with altered level of consciousness, hepatic dysfunction associated with fatty liver, CSF with WBCs less than $8/mm^3$, and no other explanation for the cerebral edema and liver dysfunction (CDC, 1990). Signs and symptoms are related to increased ammonia levels, hypoglycemia, and increased serum short-chain fatty acids. The child may appear to be lethargic with vomiting and drowsiness at first and rapidly progressing to seizure activity, decreased levels of consciousness, coma, liver dysfunction, and respiratory arrest.

Therapeutic Interventions

Care is collaborative and typically takes place in a pediatric intensive care environment, where respiratory and neurological status can be monitored very closely. Owing to the risk of bleeding because of liver involvement, institute bleeding precautions in addition to seizure precautions. Administration of medications and fluids is supportive. As ordered, administer corticosteroids to decrease cerebral edema, diuretics to reduce ICP, electrolytes to correct imbalances, and insulin to increase glucose metabolism. Instruct caregivers to avoid aspirin and aspirin-containing medications in children younger than 19 years of age who present with a viral illness. Over-the-counter medications containing aspirin include sodium bicarbonate, acetaminophen/aspirin/caffeine combination medications, and bismuth subsalicylate. Instruct caregivers to always ask the healthcare provider or pharmacist about whether prescription medications contain aspirin.

Evaluation

Expected outcomes for a child with Reye syndrome include the following:

- Parents and caregivers verbalize an understanding of which over-the-counter medications contain aspirin.
- The child's neurological status returns to baseline.
- The child is free of signs and symptoms of bleeding.
- The child's liver function returns to baseline.

Discharge Planning and Teaching

Prevention of Reye syndrome is important, because by the time children exhibit symptoms, the body has already been compromised. Carefully instruct every caregiver to not administer aspirin to children unless specifically instructed to do so by the pediatrician. Acetaminophen or ibuprofen should be used to treat minor pain and fever in children. Children who do develop Reye syndrome face a long recovery and potential long-term effects that caregivers must monitor for. Educate caregivers and the child about what to watch for in terms of complications.

Encephalitis

Encephalitis is an illness similar to meningitis that is characterized by an infection surrounding the meninges with subsequent cerebral edema. It is usually viral in origin and presents as an acute febrile illness that progresses within hours to weeks, depending on the organism.

Etiology and Pathophysiology

Encephalitis is most commonly associated with arthropod-borne viruses (mosquito-bite related) and herpes simplex type I. It may also occur as a result of a fungus, bacterium, or parasite, exposure to toxins or drugs, or a complication of cancer. Systemic illnesses such as poliomyelitis, mononucleosis, and rabies also may progress to encephalitis. As with meningitis, bacterial encephalitis results in a more serious illness. Bagdure et al. (2016) conducted a study of children in the United States hospitalized with encephalitis and found that among the 7,298 children diagnosed, 40% required care in the pediatric intensive care unit and were significantly more likely to have seizure activity and an increased length of stay.

Clinical Presentation

The signs and symptoms of encephalitis are similar to those of meningitis but can progress rapidly; thus, it is important to identify the signs and make a definitive diagnosis as soon as possible. Children present with a recent history of lethargy, neck stiffness, photophobia, behavioral changes progressing rapidly to a decreased level of consciousness, flaccid paralysis, and seizure activity.

Assessment and Diagnosis

Obtain a careful history of outdoor activities and exposure to unvaccinated pets, wild animals, medications, and recent illnesses to identify a possible cause. Blood work and an MRI or CT scan are conducted to identify cerebral edema and complications related to lesions or shifts within the brain. Bykowski et al. (2015) indicated that the use of an MRI scan is more successful than a CT scan in identifying encephalitis and abnormal brain findings.

Therapeutic Interventions

Encephalitis is treated with IV antibacterials or antivirals, and antipyretics, anti-inflammatories, and antiepileptics may be ordered. Seizure precautions and close monitoring are necessary because many children with encephalitis have seizure activity.

Use neck rolls and position the child to prevent neck-vein compression, and maintain the child's body temperature in the normal range to reduce the oxygen demand caused by increased metabolism. Children with encephalitis may also demonstrate signs and symptoms related to syndrome of inappropriate antidiuretic hormone (SIADH); therefore, monitor fluid and electrolyte levels.

Evaluation

Expected outcomes for a child with encephalitis include the following:

- The child's neurological status returns to normal.
- The child is free of infection and experiences minimal or no seizure activity.
- The body temperature is adequately controlled.
- Electrolyte levels remain within age-appropriate limits, and no signs or symptoms of SIADH develop.

Discharge Planning and Teaching

Family teaching includes measures to prevent insect bites, particularly in areas where mosquitoes are common. Advise families to use insect repellents containing DEET (*N,N*-diethyl-meta-toluamide) and picaridin only in children 2 months or older and those containing oil of lemon eucalyptus only in children 3 years or older (Karwowski et al., 2016). Instruct caregivers to apply the products according to the label and to avoid applying them to the hands, eyes, mouth, or broken or irritated skin. In addition, encourage caregivers to ensure that skin treated with insect repellant is washed thoroughly with soap and water after returning indoors and before eating. Teach caregivers to avoid products containing sunscreen plus insect repellent because sunscreen requires more product and frequent reapplication to be effective, which can lead to an overexposure to the repellant in children (Karwowski et al., 2016).

Seizure Disorders

A seizure is an electrical disturbance within the brain and is classified according to the area of the brain that is affected (Fisher, Shafer, & D'Souza, 2017). Epilepsy is a condition in which one experiences seizures that are recurrent and unprovoked (El-Radhi, 2015). According to the American Epilepsy Society (AES) (2018), the incidence of epilepsy in the United States is between 5 and 8.4 cases per 1,000 persons per year, or roughly 1% of the population (2018). The AES also reports that 1 in 26 persons will develop epilepsy in their lifetime (2018). Modalsli Aaberg et al. (2017) indicated that in children, epilepsy is the most frequent neurological condition, accounting for 0.5% to 1% of the pediatric population in the United States. Seizure activity results in a variety of motor, sensory, and cognitive changes and can be a frightening event for parents and children alike.

Fisher et al. (2017) indicated that seizures are caused by large numbers of brain cells that are activated abnormally all at the same time and that their clinical manifestations depend on the person's age, sleep-wake cycle, prior brain injury, genetics, medications, and which areas of the brain are activated. Because there are as many clinical manifestations as there are areas of the brain that can be affected, classifying seizures helps to guide diagnosis and testing, treatment, and prediction of long-term prognosis (Fisher et al., 2017). The International League Against Epilepsy (ILAE) has studied seizure activity extensively over many years and has recently revised the classification system to make diagnosing types of seizures easier for clinicians (Fig. 22.12). The new classification is based on identifying where seizures begin, defining whether a patient has altered level of consciousness, and describing the type of activity that is exhibited during a seizure. The new classification system is given later.

Remember Jessica Wang in Chapter 9? She was diagnosed as having tonic-clonic seizures when she was 4 years old. What signs and symptoms did she have leading up to and during her seizures that led to this classification of seizure disorder? How are tonic-clonic seizures different from other types of seizures? What challenges did Jessica face in keeping her seizures under control?

Etiology and Pathophysiology

Many conditions place a child at risk for seizure activity. The cause of a seizure may be any of the following (Falco-Walter, Scheffer, & Fisher, 2018):

- *Structural:* a tumor, cyst, or other defect in the brain, which may be identified on neuroimaging
- *Genetic:* a specific gene or copy number variant
- *Infectious:* invasion of a microorganism (e.g., HIV, cytomegalovirus, or cerebral toxoplasmosis) that triggers a seizure in a child with epilepsy
- *Metabolic:* metabolic derangement
- *Immune:* abnormal autoimmune response
- *Unknown:* no known cause

Clinical Presentation

As mentioned previously, seizures are classified according to where they are located in the brain. **Focal seizures** are those in which the abnormal electrical activity is in only one hemisphere (side) of the brain, whereas **generalized seizures** involve both hemispheres. Children experiencing focal seizures may be aware during the seizure, may have impaired awareness, or may be unconscious. Focal seizures involving impaired awareness manifest in motor activity including (but not limited to) jerking in one extremity, lip smacking, stiffness on one side of the body, and inappropriate mannerisms. Children who have focal seizures without motor activity typically have nonmotor manifestations including (but not limited to) experiencing buzzing sounds or tingling; feeling anxious, fearful, or angry; and seeing flashing lights.

A

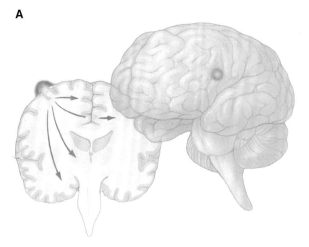

B

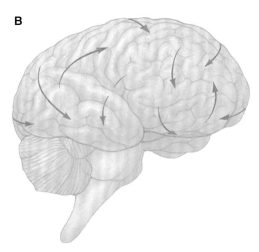

Simple
Consciousness is not impaired, can involve senses (flashing lights or a change in taste or speech) or motor function (uncontrolled stiffening or jerking in one part of the body such as the finger, mouth, hand, or foot), nausea, déjà vu feeling.

Complex
Consciousness is impaired and variable (unconscious repetitive actions), staring gaze, hallucination/delusion.

Focal evolving to generalized
Begins as focal seizure and becomes generalized.

Absence
Involve a loss of consciousness with vacant stare or unresponsiveness.

Myoclonic
Involve sudden, forceful contractions of single or multiple groups of muscles.

Clonic
Longer rhythmic jerking activity.

Tonic–clonic
Include alternate contraction (tonic phase) and relaxation (clonic phase) of muscles, a loss of consciousness, and abnormal behavior.

Atonic
Loss of muscle tone; person suddenly drops.

Figure 22.12. The updated International League Against Epilepsy seizure classification. Reprinted with permission from Ford, S. M. (2017). *Roach's introductory clinical pharmacology* (11th ed., Fig. 29.1). Philadelphia, PA: Lippincott Williams & Wilkins.

Generalized seizures, on the other hand, manifest in loss of consciousness. Generalized seizures may also present with motor or nonmotor activity. Generalized seizures with nonmotor activity may be a challenge to diagnose and are often misdiagnosed as attention-deficit/hyperactivity disorder, because the child may stop all activity and appear to be daydreaming or staring off into space. Alternatively, the child may also present with a fluttering of the eyelids, smacking the lips, or rubbing the fingers together (Kessler et al., 2017). These seizures, also known as *absence seizures*, may last just seconds and can occur many times a day, contributing to the difficulty in diagnosis. Generalized seizures with motor activity can be categorized according to the activity demonstrated by the patient. Table 22.1 provides information about the specific types of motor activity found with generalized seizures.

In addition to classification by region of the brain affected and type of clinical manifestation, seizure activity may be classified according to frequency, duration, and etiology. Thus, epilepsy, status epilepticus, and febrile seizures are discussed here.

Epilepsy

As mentioned previously, epilepsy exists when a child has seizure activity that is recurrent and unprovoked (El-Radhi, 2015). Falco-Walter et al. (2018) indicated that a child may be diagnosed with epilepsy when any one of the following conditions exists:

1. At least two unprovoked or reflex seizures occur more than 24 hours apart.
2. One unprovoked or reflex seizure occurs with a probability of having another seizure related to risk factors (e.g., abnormal activity on an encephalogram or a brain abnormality found on imaging) over the next 10 years.
3. An epileptic syndrome is present.

Epilepsy is considered resolved when the child with an age-dependent syndrome is older than the age in which the syndrome is considered active, or the child has not had seizure activity for 10 years or more and has been off all antiepileptic medications for 5 years or more (Falco-Walter et al., 2018).

Table 22.1 Generalized Seizure Motor Activity

Motor Activity	Presentation
Tonic	The body stiffens as the child loses consciousness and falls to the floor. Air is forced out of the lungs and the child may produce a grunt or groan. The child may bite the tongue or the inside of the cheek and oral secretions may be bloody or frothy.
Clonic	The arms and legs jerk rapidly and rhythmically, bending at the elbows, hips, and knees.
Tonic-clonic	A combination of both tonic and clonic activity occurs: a stereotypical seizure. The tonic phase comes first, followed by the clonic phase. As the child begins to relax, he or she may lose control over the bowel and/or bladder and, if having difficulty breathing, may be dusky or blue in color.
Myoclonic	This type of seizure is brief and may be mistaken for tics, tremors, or clumsiness. The child may have brief twitching or jerking in a muscle. Juvenile myoclonic epilepsy typically involves the neck, shoulders, and upper arms and most often begins around puberty. Lennox-Gastaut syndrome is an uncommon condition that involves myoclonic and other types of seizure activity and begins in early childhood. This condition is severe and difficult to control.
Atonic	Also known as "drop attacks," this type of seizure is associated with a complete loss of tone. The muscles become limp, and the child falls to the ground if standing. Children with these seizures are at high risk for injury; a soft helmet or other protective headgear is generally recommended. These attacks are typically brief, lasting <15 seconds.
Myoclonic-tonic-clonic	This type of seizure is a mix of myoclonic, tonic, and clonic activity. Children may experience all three together or have individual episodes of each type.
Myoclonic-atonic	A child with this type of seizure exhibits both myoclonic and atonic activity.

Status Epilepticus

Status epilepticus is a medical emergency in which a child experiences a seizure that is prolonged or a series of seizures within a short period in which the child does not recover between episodes. In the past, status epilepticus was defined as a seizure that lasted longer than 20 minutes, but now it is defined as a seizure that lasts longer than 5 minutes or a series of seizures occurring within a 5-minute period (Schacter, Shafer, & Sirven, 2013). Status epilepticus can be categorized as *convulsive* (with tonic-clonic activity) or *nonconvulsive* (in which the activity is related to prolonged absence seizures and is defined by confusion or impaired awareness in the child). Both types require immediate medical attention, but convulsive status epilepticus requires more urgent treatment to lessen the chance of serious complications. Regardless of type, children who experience status epilepticus should be transported by emergency personnel to a hospital and be given oxygen, antiepileptic medications, and IV fluids to stop the seizure activity and provide support. Some children must be placed into an induced coma to stop the seizure activity (Schacter et al., 2013).

Febrile Seizures

Febrile seizures are acute seizures triggered by a high fever. They affect 2% to 5% of the pediatric population and are the most

common form of seizures in children (Leung, Hon, & Leung, 2018). Most commonly occurring between the ages of 6 months and 3 years, febrile seizures on average peak in incidence at 18 months of age and rarely occur after 7 years of age. The ILAE defined febrile seizures as those occurring in infants older than 1 month of age in conjunction with a febrile illness in the absence of central nervous system infection or electrolyte imbalance. To be defined as a febrile seizure, body temperature must be greater than 101.2°F (38.4°C), although the increase in temperature may not occur until after the seizure Leung, Hon, & Leung (2018) stated that of the cases of febrile seizures, about 70% are simple and 30% complex. A simple febrile seizure is brief (<10 minutes) and occurs only once during a 24-hour period in an infant or a child with an otherwise unremarkable medical history (Leung, Hon, & Leung, 2018). Complex febrile seizures are prolonged (>10 minutes), have focal features, or occur more than once during the febrile illness. The prognosis for febrile seizures overall is good, although about 30% to 40% of children who have complex febrile seizures do develop epilepsy (National Institute of Neurological Disorders and Stroke, 2018). In general, simple complex febrile seizures have not been found to cause brain damage.

Assessment and Diagnosis

Seizure activity in children is diagnosed with the help of neuroimaging. A CT scan or an MRI is performed to help identify

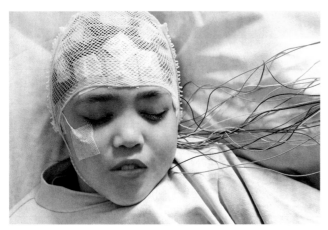

Figure 22.13. A child receiving an electroencephalogram.

the presence of abnormal electrical activity in the brain and its cause, whether central nervous system malformations, lesions, malignant neoplasms, hemorrhaging, trauma, entry of a foreign body, or edema (Fisher, Shafer, & D'Souza, 2017). An electroencephalogram (EEG) is also a standard procedure for diagnosing a seizure disorder. Children may be admitted to the hospital for this procedure, because many clinicians want to view brain activity over a 24-hour period. Electrodes are attached to the child's scalp and provide a read-out of electrical activity in the various areas of the brain during normal sleep-wake cycles and during stimulation (Fig. 22.13). Loud noises, flashing lights, and/or rapidly flashing images may be used to stimulate a child's brain. The EEG is typically combined with video monitoring of the child to correlate electrical activity of the brain with the child's behavior at any given time, which aids with diagnosis.

In addition to neuroimaging, laboratory testing is often performed to help identify the cause of the seizure activity, such as to assess for electrolyte imbalances, infection (particularly within the central nervous system), or toxicity related to medications or other potentially ingested substances. If a child has an increase in seizure activity and takes antiepileptic medications, a thorough review of the medications and their therapeutic levels is warranted.

Therapeutic Interventions

Antiepileptic drug therapy is the primary mode of treatment for children with epilepsy. Many medications are available and have varying effects on the brain. Each medication is designed to act on a specific area of the brain and thus to treat a specific type of seizure. Many children do well with monotherapy (one drug), which is optimal, but others may need polytherapy (more than one drug) to help control seizure activity. Polytherapy is typically initiated when a child is not having success with one drug, because taking multiple drugs may have a synergistic effect. Children begin on one medication at a low dose, and then the dosage is adjusted as needed according to the child's response. Any additional drugs are initiated in the same manner. Physical growth may necessitate increasing the dosage of a drug to maintain its effectiveness.

Instruct parents and children to never abruptly stop drug therapy, because doing so may trigger severe seizure activity. Clinicians choosing to discontinue any drugs must wean the child off by reducing the dosage slowly, one drug at a time. Antiepileptic drugs can be toxic, so obtain baseline measures of liver and renal function and hematological values and consistently monitor serum therapeutic drug levels every 3 to 6 months to maintain drug effectiveness and minimize adverse effects.

Children typically undergo surgery for epilepsy when a single focus area for the seizures can be identified and excised. Depending on the area excised, the child may experience minimal-to-moderate long-term effects related to cognitive, speech, language, or motor development.

Use of a vagal nerve stimulator, another treatment modality for seizures, has been found to be successful in some children 4 years and older. The device uses neuromodulation by sending regular, mild pulses of electrical energy to the brain via the vagus nerve. The device is implanted through a surgical incision, and most patients are not aware of the impulses. Vagal nerve stimulation is not a cure for epilepsy but may help reduce the severity and frequency of episodes (Shafer & Dean, 2018).

The Pharmacy 22.1 provides information regarding the most common antiepileptic medications, their uses with specific seizures, and adverse effects important for the nurse to teach the family about.

Nursing care for a child with seizures is focused on administering medications, monitoring and recording specifics about the child's behavior during seizure activity, instituting safety precautions, coordinating services for collaborative care, and supporting and educating the child and family on seizure and medication management. Obtain a detailed current and past medical history, including family history of seizures and details about the child's gestation and birth.

When a child has a seizure, document the following:

- Time of onset
- Duration
- Child's activities and behavior before onset
- Clinical manifestations, such as level of consciousness, physical activity, loss of bowel and/or bladder control, cyanosis, and sounds made by the child
- People present
- Child's state and behavior afterward (postictal period)

When a child has a seizure in the hospital setting, provide oxygen via a blow-by method, administer antiepileptic medications (in the event of status epilepticus—typically lorazepam or diazepam), monitor the airway, and monitor the heart and circulation with a pulse oximeter and a cardiac monitor. In addition, place nothing into the child's mouth during a seizure. Loosen restrictive clothing to allow for adequate circulation. When the seizure is over, place the child in the left lateral recumbent recovery position. Monitor the child's respiratory status, particularly for signs of apnea. Ensure that a suction device, oxygen, and the appropriately sized bag-valve mask are at the bedside and working. Children may be very sleepy or combative after a seizure. Allow the sleepy child to sleep while monitoring

The Pharmacy 22.1 Common Antiepileptic Drugs Used in Children

Medication	Type of Seizure	Typical Dosage	Adverse Effects
Carbamazepine (Tegretol)	• Focal: motor onset • Generalized: tonic-clonic	• Age <6 y: 10–20 mg/kg/d • Age 6–12 y: 400–800 mg/d	Drowsiness, nausea, changes in liver function, increased appetite
Valproic acid (Depakene)	• Focal: Motor onset • Generalized: Tonic-clonic	Age <10 y: • Initial dose: 10–15 mg/kg/d • Maintenance dose: 10–60 mg/kg/d	Confusion, ataxia, nystagmus, nausea, gingival hyperplasia, bleeding disorders
Phenytoin (Dilantin)	• Focal: Motor onset • Generalized: Tonic-clonic	5 mg/kg/d	Dizziness, drowsiness, uncoordinated physical movement, gingival hyperplasia
Phenobarbital (Luminal)	• Focal: Motor onset • Generalized: Tonic-clonic	• Loading dose: 15–20 mg/kg • Maintenance dose: 3–6 mg/kg/d	Hyperactivity, inattentiveness, dizziness, slurred speech, fever, rash
Fosphenytoin (Cerebyx)	Focal: Motor onset	Age 1–6 y: • Loading dose: 10–20 mg/kg • Maintenance dose: 6–8 mg/kg/d	Itchiness, dizziness, drowsiness, ataxia, nystagmus, tinnitus, bruising, nausea, vomiting, weakness
Gabapentin (Neurontin)	Focal: Motor onset	Age 3–11 y: 10–15 mg/kg/d	Dizziness, drowsiness, nausea, vomiting, viral infections, fever
Ethosuximide (Zarontin)	Generalized: Nonmotor onset	3–8 mg/kg/d	Dizziness, headache, drowsiness, anorexia, diarrhea, nausea, vomiting, aplastic anemia, sleep disturbance; avoid antacids
Topiramate (Topamax)	Focal: Nonmotor onset	1–3 mg/kg/d	Weight loss, dizziness, diarrhea, cognitive dysfunction; avoid antidepressants and antacids

status, speak in soothing tones to the child who is confused, fearful, or combative, and reorient the child on recovery.

Whenever caring for a child with a seizure disorder in the hospital, institute seizure precautions, padding the side rails and making sure they are elevated. In addition, do not allow the child to ambulate alone; assist the child with using a bedpan or bedside commode, as ordered.

Evaluation

Expected outcomes for a child with a seizure disorder include the following:

- The child is free from seizures or seizure activity is diminished.
- Medications are administered and adhered to properly by the child's parents.

- The child's parents and teachers demonstrate the correct actions to take to prevent injury when a seizure does occur.
- The child's environment is modified to remove any risk factors that may be the cause for the seizures.
- The child and family take measures to prevent infection that may lead to febrile seizure activity.
- The child experiences minimal side effects of seizure medications.
- The child and parents receive adequate support to cope with the child's condition.

Discharge Planning and Teaching

Teach the child and family about the medications the child is taking and the monitoring of specific laboratory tests and drug therapeutic levels. Teach them about safety at home and at school. Recommend that the child wear a medical alert bracelet and that the school nurse and personnel receive specific information regarding the child's daily regimen of medications. In addition, inform the parents that the school nurse should have an individualized seizure action plan for each child with epilepsy at the school (The Epilepsy Foundation, 2018). Advise them to ensure that the child's teachers are trained on what to do should a seizure happen at school. Instruct the family that the child should never swim without adult supervision. Explain the importance of the child, family, and school personnel all knowing what to do during and after a seizure, and how such collaboration and a shared focus on safety can give them a measure of control and help the child reach his or her maximum potential.

Head Trauma

Trauma to the head, whether accidental or nonaccidental (abusive), is a major cause of neurological dysfunction and death in children.

Accidental Head Trauma

Traumatic brain injury (TBI) occurs when a blow or jolt to the head causes trauma and disrupts the normal function of the brain. TBI is one of the leading preventable causes of death in the pediatric population (Geyer, Meller, Kulpan, & Mowery, 2013). The CDC reports that the incidence of TBI is distinctly elevated in two age groups: adolescents and toddlers (2018a). Motor vehicle accidents remain the number one cause of TBI in adolescents, whereas falls contribute to most of the TBI cases in toddlers (Geyer et al., 2013).

Etiology and Pathophysiology

TBI can be blunt or penetrating and is classified as primary (directly occurring from the trauma at the time of injury) or secondary (indirectly occurring from the injury sometime later). Primary TBI includes the following:

- Skull fracture (possibly with the bone penetrating into brain tissue)
- Bleeding
- Concussion (a global disruption of the brain's network)
- Contusion (a focal disruption of brain tissue—similar to a bruise)

Secondary TBI includes the following:

- Tissue ischemia and hypoxia
- Cerebral edema
- Increased ICP

Infants and toddlers are at the highest risk for direct trauma because they have an unsteady gait; a large, heavy head in proportion to the rest of the body; and a lack of reflexes, which are needed to break a fall. In addition, their skull is thinner and the brain tissue is softer.

Clinical Presentation

The effects of TBI range from mild to severe, and clinical manifestations change over time as complications develop.

Early signs of TBI include the following:

- Photophobia
- Nausea and vomiting
- Headaches
- Vertigo
- Irritability
- Lethargy
- Poor feeding (in an infant)
- Amnesia and/or confusion
- Apnea (especially in an infant)
- Altered level of consciousness (from mild to coma)
- Leakage of CSF from the ears or nose

Late signs of TBI include the following:

- Increased ICP
- Hydrocephalus
- Seizure activity
- Posturing
- Unequal or nonreactive pupils
- Ecchymosis around the eyes or the mastoid

Cardinal signs of TBI include the following:

- Diminished reflexes or return of primitive reflexes (Babinski's)
- Brainstem herniation
- Cushing's triad
- Coma

Assessment and Diagnosis

The sooner TBI is recognized, diagnosed, and treated, the better the outcome, depending on the severity of the initial injury. Use of a pediatric Glasgow Coma Scale is important to determine the child's level of consciousness (Fig. 22.14). In addition, assessment includes physical exam, CT or MRI scanning, an EEG, intracranial monitoring to determine pressure, and calculation of cerebral perfusion pressure (CPP) to determine brain function and the extent of the injury. CPP is the difference between the mean arterial pressure (MAP) and the ICP (CPP = MAP − ICP) and represents the normal pressure gradient required to deliver blood to the brain. CPP should be greater than 40 to 50 mm Hg for infants and toddlers and greater than 50 to 60 mm Hg for older children. A CPP of less than 40 mm Hg is a significant predictor of mortality in children with TBI (Kumar, Lorenc, Robinson, & Blair, 2011). The role of the nurse is paramount, because careful monitoring is necessary to detect any early changes. Nonverbal children may not be able to tell a caregiver that they are dizzy or have a headache; thus, report immediately and follow up on any change in behavior.

If bleeding is present, it is important to determine whether it is epidural, subdural, or intracerebral (Fig. 22.15). Epidural hemorrhage is between the meninges and skull and is typically arterial, exerting pressure on the brain rapidly. Subdural hemorrhage, on the other hand, is between the meninges and the

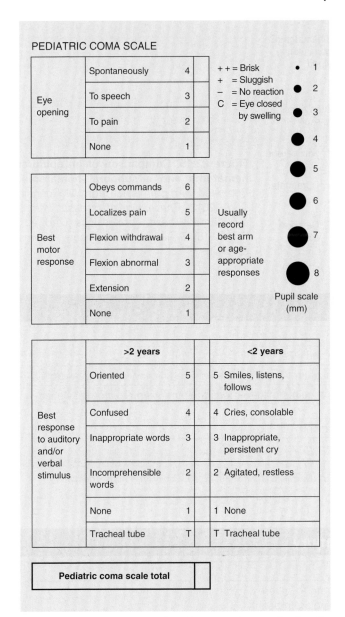

Figure 22.14. The Pediatric Glasgow Coma Scale. Reprinted with permission from Kyle, T., & Carman, S. (2016). *Essentials of pediatric nursing* (3rd ed., Fig. 16.2). Philadelphia, PA: Wolters Kluwer.

needed to arouse the child. Boxes 22.2 and 22.3 provide information about levels of consciousness and TBI classification, respectively.

Finally, assess for **posturing** and, if present, what type, because it can indicate the amount of damage present. Posturing is typically a late sign and may be accompanied by the return of primitive reflexes, such as Babinski's. Decorticate posturing, the less severe of the two types of posturing, indicates damage to one or both of the corticospinal tracts. Decerebrate posturing indicates damage to the upper portion of the brainstem and typically has a poor outcome. Figure 22.16 presents decorticate and decerebrate posturing and how they appear in patients.

Therapeutic Interventions

Management and nursing care of the child with a TBI are supportive, typically involving a "watch and wait" approach regarding long-term outcome. Priority Care Concepts 22.2 provides a list of priority nursing interventions to use when caring for a child with a TBI. Again, early intervention is associated with better outcomes and depends on careful assessment and recognizing changes early on.

Evaluation

Expected outcomes for a child with accidental head trauma include the following:

- Signs and symptoms of ICP are recognized early.
- The child receives adequate ventilation and oxygenation, and circulation is maintained.
- The child's comfort is promoted and pain is managed.
- The child's level of consciousness is closely monitored to detect any neurological changes early.
- The child's body temperature and vital signs remain within the appropriate parameter.
- The child's intake and output remain within limits that are adequate for perfusion.
- The child recovers from the injury with minimal complications.

Discharge Planning and Teaching

When the child who has a head injury is discharged from the hospital, the parents or caregivers need to receive education regarding what to observe for regarding complications. Explaining that the child may experience sleep disturbances, a change in behavior, phobias, or seizure activity will help the parents or caregivers distinguish posttraumatic symptoms from changes in the child's neurological status. Parents, caregivers, and teachers should all be trained in what to do if the child experiences seizure activity. A list of practitioners to call if there are questions is also necessary. Rehabilitation for a child who has had a head injury may be basic or complicated depending on the child's injury. Some children recover but are left with often severe long-term complications. Ensuring that the child has the proper medications, equipment, and devices needed for care

brain and is typically venous, exerting pressure slowly. Subdural hemorrhage might not be evident at first, so instruct caregivers to return to the emergency room with the child immediately if they observe any sign of change in behavior. Depending on where it is located, intracerebral hemorrhage can cause focal or diffuse disruption of the brain tissue, resulting in mild-to-severe manifestations, including death.

Children diagnosed with TBI are classified according to their Glasgow coma score and presenting criteria. Classification is important because it provides guidance regarding treatment and nursing care. In addition, assess the level of consciousness of the child, taking care to use the minimum amount of stimulation

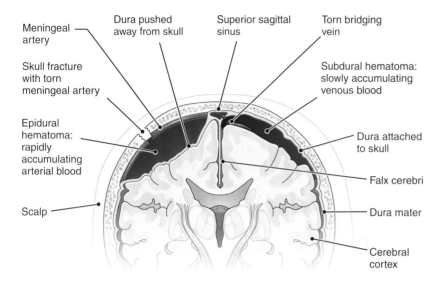

Meningeal artery

Dura pushed away from skull

Superior sagittal sinus

Torn bridging vein

Skull fracture with torn meningeal artery

Subdural hematoma: slowly accumulating venous blood

Epidural hematoma: rapidly accumulating arterial blood

Dura attached to skull

Falx cerebri

Scalp

Dura mater

Cerebral cortex

Figure 22.15. Comparison of an epidural hematoma and a subdural hematoma. Reprinted with permission from McConnell, T. H. (2013). *The nature of disease: Pathology for the health professions* (2nd ed., Fig. 19.18). Philadelphia: Lippincott Williams & Wilkins.

Box 22.2   Levels of Consciousness

Level of Consciousness	Manifestations
Clouding of consciousness	The patient appears inattentive and sleepy.
Confusion	May be disoriented to time, place, and/or person; has difficulty following commands
Obtundation	Demonstrates blunted senses; requires mild-to-moderate stimulation to arouse; sleeps more than usual
Stupor	Responds to vigorous stimulation only
Coma	Does not respond to stimuli; cannot be aroused

Adapted from Tindall, S. C. (1990). Level of consciousness. In H. K. Walker, W. D. Hall, & J. W. Hurst (Eds.), *Clinical methods: The history, physical, and laboratory examinations* (3rd ed.). Boston, MA: Butterworths.

Box 22.3   Classifications of Traumatic Brain Injury

Classification	Criteria

Symptomatic (possible TBI)	• None of the mild or moderate to severe criteria apply
	• One or more of the following are present:
	  • Blurred vision
	  • Confusion
	  • Dizziness
	  • Headache
	  • Nausea
	  • Focal neurological symptoms

Mild (probable TBI)	• Loss of consciousness (momentarily to <30 min) • Posttraumatic anterograde amnesia (momentarily to <2–4 h) • Depressed basilar or linear skull fracture with intact dura
Moderate to severe (definite TBI)	• Glasgow Coma Scale score <13 in initial 24 h • Loss of consciousness for <30 min • Hemorrhage (epidural, subdural, intracerebral, or subarachnoid) • Cerebral or hemorrhagic contusion or penetrating TBI • Brainstem injury • Death

TBI, traumatic brain injury.
Adapted from Geyer, K., Meller, K., Kulpan, C., & Mowery, B. D. (2013). Traumatic brain injury in children: Acute care management. *Pediatric Nursing, 39*(6), 283–289. Retrieved from http://0-search.ebscohost.com.catalog.llu.edu/login.aspx?direct=true&db=ccm&AN=104130316&site=ehost-live&scope=site.

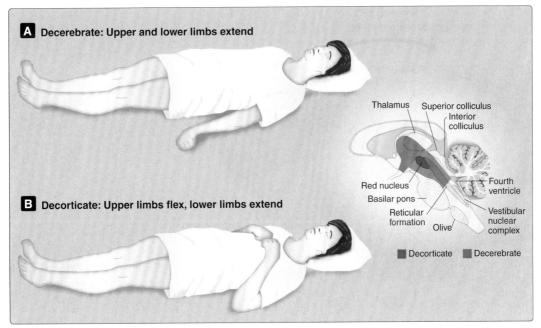

Figure 22.16. Decerebrate and decorticate posturing. Reprinted with permission from Krebs, C., Weinberg, J., Dilli, E., & Akesson, E. (2011). *Lippincott illustrated reviews: Neuroscience* (1st ed., unnumbered figure in Chapter 8). Philadelphia, PA: Wolters Kluwer.

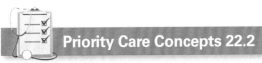

Priority Care Concepts 22.2

Traumatic Brain Injury

The following nursing interventions are priorities when caring for a child with TBI:

- Maintain adequate blood pressure, O_2 saturation level, and ventilation. Also keep body temperature within normal limits, because increased body temperature increases metabolism and oxygen consumption.
- Monitor and maintain any specific external devices used to monitor ICP, drain CSF, measure arterial blood pressure and gas levels, and manage the airway. Administer anti-seizure medications and institute seizure precautions to prevent injury.
- Monitor blood glucose level and prevent hypoglycemia, because the brain needs a constant amount of glucose for metabolism.
- Administer hyperosmolar fluids such as mannitol and hypertonic saline to draw fluid from the cellular spaces within the brain and shift it to the intervascular compartment to allow the kidneys to process and excrete it.
- Monitor for and promptly correct any electrolyte abnormalities. Children with TBI are at risk for SIADH and diabetes insipidus (DI). Monitor central venous pressure and urine output to detect changes related to SIADH or DI.
- Maintain adequate nutrition. Children with TBI have increased caloric needs. Provide them with enteral feeds if at all possible, either through a nasogastric tube or gastric feeding tube. If the child cannot be fed enterally, administer total parenteral nutrition (TPN) through a central venous line. TPN is not optimal because the presence of a central venous line can place the child at risk for a blood infection and because it requires additional glycemic control.

and medical follow-up is important. The child and family may also benefit from support groups to help them cope with potentially lifelong disability.

Nonaccidental Head Trauma

Nonaccidental head trauma occurs when an infant or a small child has been shaken or beaten by an adult. Shaken baby syndrome (SBS; also referred to as abusive head trauma) is the number one cause of brain damage in the infant population and the most common form of nonaccidental head trauma in infants in the United States.

Etiology and Pathophysiology

The National Center on Shaken Baby Syndrome (2018) indicates that 1,300 cases are reported each year, of which 25% result in death; among those who survive, 80% experience

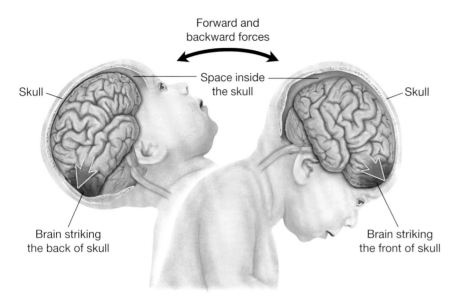

Figure 22.17. Pathophysiology of shaken baby syndrome.

permanent, and often severe, disability. The trauma to the brain occurs when the infant is shaken forcefully (Fig. 22.17). Major rotational forces and angular **deceleration** occur when the infant is shaken, leading to the shearing and tearing of tissue and vessels within the structures of the brain and leading to cerebral edema, hemorrhage, and damage. In addition to brain hemorrhage, hydrocephalus often develops. Retinal hemorrhage also occurs, because the vessels of the eyes are fragile and rupture as a result of the force. Clots begin to develop as a result of the bleeding and, coupled with the pressure from swelling, decrease the blood supply to the brain tissue, leading to tissue ischemia.

Clinical Presentation

SBS is often viewed as a silent condition, because it has very few outward clinical manifestations in the early stages. When present, its symptoms can mimic those of other illnesses and may go unchecked, such as vomiting, irritability, or increased sleeping. The most common early clinical manifestation that brings the infant to the clinician's attention is apnea.

Assessment and Diagnosis

A CT scan or an MRI is typically used to identify the damage to the brain. Most hospitals routinely include a funduscopic exam in the assessment of any infant who is brought in with reports of apnea. The funduscopic exam can reveal retinal hemorrhaging, which is often sufficient evidence to suspect SBS. Although a full workup is still necessary in such cases to rule out other potential conditions, the suspicion of SBS guides the infant's further care and prompts the launch of an investigation, as well. The nurse is essential in gathering a detailed history. As a nurse, remember that you are a mandated reporter and are responsible legally and ethically to report any suspected abuse to the proper child welfare and law enforcement agencies. In addition to reporting, objective documentation in the medical record is of utmost importance because the document may be used in court.

Therapeutic Interventions

Care of the infant with nonaccidental head trauma is generally supportive and depends on the impairment. Measures are taken to reduce ICP and prevent cardiovascular collapse, as well as to preserve as much function as possible. Family may be allowed at the bedside and are likely to need support, especially if the injuries are severe.

Evaluation

Expected outcomes for a child with nonaccidental head trauma include the following:

- The child's parents follow prevention methods for dealing with an irritable infant to help prevent injury from occurring in the first place.
- The child's ICP is normalized.
- The child experiences no injury with seizure activity.
- The child's brain receives optimal perfusion and oxygenation.
- The child experiences minimal complications related to therapy or medications.
- The child's parents receive support to cope with the situation.
- If the parent or caregiver is incarcerated as a result of the child's injury, the child is placed with family members or a foster family as soon as possible to foster a stable home environment for the child.
- The child receives the necessary medications, equipment, and resources to foster optimal functioning.

Discharge Planning and Teaching

Permanent effects of SBS include seizure activity, learning disabilities, cognitive delay, neuromotor impairment, deafness, blindness, persistent vegetative state or coma, and respirator or ventilator dependency. Some children are fairly functional, whereas others depend on total care. As previously mentioned, 80% of infants who survive SBS have permanent disability. The child's prognosis depends on the severity of the injury and the child's response to treatment. Unfortunately, some disabilities related to learning and cognition may not be apparent until later on.

Focus on prevention and take every opportunity to teach parents how to care for infants. Various programs endorsed by the CDC and the National Center on Shaken Baby Syndrome have been developed to help parents and caregivers deal with infants who cry for long periods. These programs help parents and caregivers understand why the baby is crying and how to manage the crying in positive ways, such as by giving the baby a warm bath or massage. Refer parents to these programs and to new parenting groups for support. Learn about these resources yourself and how to access them so that you can communicate this information to parents.

Headaches

Headaches are a common complaint in children and are typically related to specific illnesses or conditions. Headaches may be acute or chronic, depending on the cause, and may be accompanied by other symptoms.

Etiology and Pathophysiology

Because the pathology of headaches varies, it is important to identify specific patterns so that the cause may be determined and proper treatment rendered. Common pediatric illnesses, extracranial and intracranial diseases or conditions, vascular abnormalities, and/or psychogenic disorders can cause headaches.

Headaches may be classified as *acute, acute recurrent, chronic progressive, or chronic nonprogressive* (Blume, 2017). Acute headaches may be caused by more common illnesses, such as sinusitis, colds, and flus, or by trauma, dental disorders, or ocular conditions. Acute headaches generally dissipate when the child is recovering or the acute issue is resolved. Acute headaches may also be accompanied by other symptoms according to the underlying illness, such as fever, tenderness over the sinuses, rhinorrhea, and pharyngitis. Acute headaches may be exacerbated with chewing, localized to one area, such as with trauma, or generalized and accompanied by nuchal rigidity, such as with meningitis. Acute headaches that occur late in the day may be related to ocular abnormalities (Blume, 2017).

Acute recurrent headaches are classified as migraine headaches (Blume, 2017). The average age of onset of migraine headaches varies with the gender of the child and prevalence varies with both age and gender: the average age of onset is 7.2 years in boys compared with 10.9 years in girls. On reaching puberty (around the age of 12 years), girls are twice as likely as boys to experience migraines. Migraines are **paroxysmal** and symptoms vary by age: typical symptoms include nausea, vomiting, and abdominal pain. Pain may also be accompanied by an aura, motor weakness, vertigo, diplopia, and/or altered consciousness (Blume, 2017). Young children may not be able to verbalize pain and may demonstrate decreased activity and/or pallor with episodes. Migraine pain is of shorter duration in children than in adults: 1 hour as opposed to 4 hours, respectively. The Migraine Research Foundation (2019) indicated that although migraines may demonstrate a familial pattern in as many as 75% of children who experience migraines, there is no consistent genetic factor, with the exception of familial hemiplegic migraine. The Migraine Research Foundation also indicated that although the most common cause of migraines has been thought to be related to cerebral vessel dilation, this is no longer the case and other neuronal pathophysiology cannot be ruled out.

Chronic progressive headaches have been classified according to intracranial abnormalities and demonstrate symptoms related to increased ICP (Blume, 2017). Tumors, hematomas resulting from injury, abscesses, and hydrocephalus are all factors contributing to these types of headaches. Early morning headaches accompanied by vomiting typically occur with tumors, whereas those associated with hydrocephalus have symptoms of ICP, depending on where the CSF imbalance occurs. Infants with migraines often present with a bulging fontanel and splitting of the cranial sutures in addition to increased ICP symptoms. Seizures and focal neurological deficits may accompany headaches related to tumors and hematomas, depending on the location. Abscesses within the brain may be accompanied by chronic sinus or ear infections, although rare.

Chronic nonprogressive headaches are typically related to tension or psychiatric issues (Blume, 2017). Tension headaches are common and are typically frontal and described as tight or pressing. Anxiety in children may lead to a conversion reaction, in which the anxiety is converted to somatic symptoms in the form of headaches.

Clinical Presentation

The presentation of headaches in children can be mild to severe, depending on the cause. The location of the headache is important to determine, because this might provide information related to the cause. Headaches in children may be present in the morning and get progressively worse throughout the day, or may dissipate after the child has vomited. Nausea may accompany a headache, or the child may complain of visual disturbances, sensitivity to light, or the presence of auras. A child may present with irritability, fatigue, and changes in facial expression. In rare instances, some children with severe migraines present with paresthesias, speech or language disturbances, confusion, or amnesia. Younger children may complain of stomach upset, as well.

Assessment and Diagnosis

While assessing the nature of a headache, help the parent and child begin a headache journal to track when headaches occur, their intensity, what activity the child was involved in before the headaches occurred, and any accompanying symptoms, in addition to what treatment was taken to aid with the headaches and how effective it was. In addition, ask questions to elicit specific information regarding possible causes. While gathering information, be alert for the following red flags, which require immediate follow-up (Dao & Qubty, 2018):

- Headaches that progress in frequency and severity
- Headaches that awaken a child from sleep
- Headaches that occur early in the morning
- Headaches that become worse upon arising
- Headaches that are accompanied by nausea and/or vomiting that are unexplained (not related to flulike illnesses)
- Headaches that are persistent and located in the frontal or occipital areas
- Headaches that are accompanied by a change in gait, personality, or behavior
- Headaches that are made worse by the Valsalva maneuver

Therapeutic Interventions

Treatment for headaches is aimed at the underlying cause and may require pharmacological, surgical, and/or cognitive/behavioral therapy. Most common headaches can be treated with relaxation techniques and administration of ibuprofen or acetaminophen. Migraines can be treated in older children with serotonin agonists. In the United States, almotriptan has been approved for use in adolescents aged 12 to 17 years. For refractory migraines, tricyclic antidepressants, antiepileptic medications, or antiserotonergic medications may be ordered (Hershey & Winner, 2005). These medications are not without their adverse effects; inform the parent and the child of specific symptoms to watch for.

Evaluation

Expected outcomes for a child with headaches include the following:

- The cause of the headaches is identified and removed, allowing the child to experience relief.
- The child experiences a decrease in the number and severity of headaches.
- The child has optimal pain relief if headaches are chronic.
- The child maintains optimal functioning in school and activities of daily living.
- Behavioral interventions successfully reduce the number of headaches related to psychosomatic causes.

- Medications are successful in helping the child deal with migraines and provide relief with minimal side effects.
- All medications are taken as prescribed for maximal effect for migraines and chronic headaches.

Discharge Planning and Teaching

Discharge planning and teaching may be multidisciplinary for the child with headaches. Although most headaches resolve, those children with chronic headaches must learn how to manage them. Teach the caregiver and child about prescribed medications, because both must follow guidelines and instructions carefully for optimal relief and minimal complications. Share with the child and caregiver information about the side effects of medications and strategies to minimize them for optimal functioning. Encourage the child and family to keep a headache journal to aid in diagnosis and management of the headaches, and instruct them in what information to include. When appropriate, refer a child for behavioral therapy, which may be beneficial in treating headaches related to a psychosomatic cause.

Eye Disorders

Eye disorders in children are common and can range from mild to severe, can permanently affect vision, and can have a wide range of etiologies. Children, especially young children, may not be acutely aware of changes in vision and may not voice complaints unless there is an obvious injury. Eye disorders include structural and refractive disorders, including amblyopia, strabismus, and nystagmus, as well as nasolacrimal duct obstruction and infections of the eye.

Infections of the eye are common in childhood, with a variety of factors contributing to their development. Prompt recognition and diagnosis are necessary to initiate the proper treatment to promote comfort and prevent potential damage to vision. The most common childhood eye infections are conjunctivitis and periorbital cellulitis.

Structural and Refractive Disorders

Cotter, Cyert, Miller, and Quinn (2015) indicated that amblyopia, strabismus, and refractive errors (Table 22.2) are the most common visual disorders in preschool children 36 to 72 months old. Many children experience vision challenges as a result of a structural disorder, and the long-term outcome depends on the severity of the disorder. Refractive errors as a result of a structural disorder are the most common category and are related to problems with how light passes through the lens of the eye. Table 22.2 provides details on common structural and refractive disorders that occur in the pediatric population.

Etiology and Pathophysiology

The causes and pathophysiology of eye disorders are multifactorial and vary depending on the disorder. Some conditions are hereditary or congenital, whereas others develop later as a primary problem or a complication of another condition. The pathophysiology of an eye disorder may involve deformation of the eye itself or improper development of the internal structures. Damage to the eye from trauma may cause eye disorders. Brain disorders or damage to the optic nerve may contribute to cortical vision deficits. Blockage of the tear ducts can lead to vision or eye complications, and damage to or uneven curving of the lens or cornea can cause refractory issues. The muscles surrounding the eye may not function properly, contributing to difficulty with eye movement, or the eyelid may be affected, blocking vision. Once the cause is determined, treatment can ensue with the goal of restoring or maintaining vision as much as possible.

Amblyopia, also known as "lazy eye," is a condition that can accompany strabismus; it is blindness that occurs from disuse or decreased visual acuity in one eye and typically occurs when strabismus is not detected and corrected by 4 to 6 years of age. One eye does not receive enough stimulation, and the visual cortex responds by suppressing vision, leading to vision loss.

Clinical Presentation

Changes in behavior may indicate that a child is struggling with a vision problem and should warrant a visit to the general pediatrician for an evaluation. Depending on the cause, the child may have ptosis, strabismus, pupillary alterations, clumsiness, or poor depth perception (Martin, 2017). Younger children often cannot verbalize vision difficulty, but older children typically can describe what they are experiencing. They may squint frequently when reading or strain to view a blackboard or whiteboard in the classroom. In the case of amblyopia, the child may present with increasing vision loss in one eye.

Assessment and Diagnosis

With eye disorders, early detection is the key, because many of the disorders, particularly amblyopia, more readily respond to treatment the younger the child is. Therefore, the U.S. Preventive Services Task Force has recommended that children between 3 and 5 years of age be examined at least once to detect the presence of significant vision disorders (Cotter et al., 2015). Although early detection is important, it presents challenges, because children may not be acutely aware of changes in vision and may not report difficulties. In particular, visual acuity tests are challenging in younger children, because they do not identify letters sufficiently; so modifications must be made to successfully detect difficulty with vision (Cotter et al., 2015). Many visual acuity tests are available to screen older children, and vision screening should be part of the routine checkup.

Teachers have been instrumental in identifying vision problems in children, because many of the signs of poor vision—such as squinting to see the board, difficulty reading, or poor performance on activities requiring acute vision—are most evident in the school setting.

A comprehensive ophthalmic exam is necessary to diagnose amblyopia. The sooner it is diagnosed, the better the outcome

for the child. Any infant presenting with ptosis or strabismus should be evaluated. Acuity testing, examining the retina with a scope, evaluating binocular vision and pupillary responses, and dilated funduscopic exam are necessary to diagnose the condition.

Therapeutic Interventions

Interventions to treat structural and refractive eye disorders vary widely depending on the specific disorder. Corrective lenses may be prescribed to help improve visual acuity with any vision disorder.

Laser surgery is typically required for cataracts to remove them. As the eye in younger children is still growing, a permanent lens will not be placed until the eye has reached its maturity (Martin, 2017). Glaucoma is also treated surgically to relieve the pressure and remove obstruction.

Strabismus is typically treated with occlusion therapy, or wearing a patch over the "good" eye, to help strengthen muscles that might be weak or to enhance visual acuity by forcing the weaker eye to work independently. Surgery may be indicated for more complex cases or for those in which occlusion therapy is either not indicated or does not work successfully.

Amblyopia is preventable with early detection and treatment for the underlying cause. Once vision is lost, it cannot be regained. Treatment is typically done with occlusion therapy, but many very young children are noncompliant with it. Corrective lenses may be indicated in this situation, with one lens supporting the weaker eye. Eye muscle surgery may also be indicated to help correct alignment of the eyes to preserve vision.

Because most procedures for treating eye disorders are done on an outpatient basis, the primary role of the nurse is preparing the child and family for what to expect after surgery. Administering pain medications if needed and monitoring the status of the eye after surgery are also important responsibilities of the nurse.

Evaluation

Expected outcomes for a child with a structural or refractive eye disorder include the following:

- The condition is detected and diagnosed early and treatment initiated promptly.
- The child with a vision disorder adjusts to using corrective lenses and achieves normal vision.
- The child who has undergone surgery experiences minimal pain and complete healing, with no infection or complications.
- The child undergoing occlusion therapy complies with wearing the patch and experiences restoration or preservation of normal vision in the weak eye.

Discharge Planning and Teaching

Most children who undergo a procedure to treat a structural or refractive eye disorder are able to go home the same day, with follow-up visits scheduled to the pediatric eye specialist to

Table 22.2 Common Structural and Refractive Disorders of the Eye in Children

Disorder	Clinical Manifestations	Treatment
Astigmatism Unequal curvatures of the refractory structures of the eye (cornea or lens)	• Blurred vision at all distances that persists with corrective lenses • Headaches • Dizziness • Difficulty with reading or close work	• Corrective lenses • Routine follow-up exams to maintain vision and prevent amblyopia
Nystagmus A rapid, irregular, involuntary movement of one or both eyes; caused by a congenital (mild, persists into adulthood) or acquired neurological disorder		• Assessment for and treatment of the underlying neurological disorder • Pharmacological, optical, and/or surgical interventions

Normal Eye

Cornea
Light
Pupil
Lens
Focal points
Normal vision

Astigmatic Eye

Astigmatic cornea
Light
Pupil
Lens
Multiple focal points
Astigmatic vision

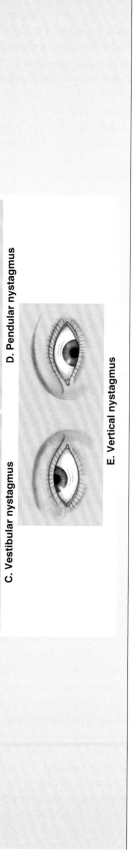

A. Jerk nystagmus

B. Downbeat nystagmus

C. Vestibular nystagmus

D. Pendular nystagmus

E. Vertical nystagmus

Strabismus (cross-eye)

The deviation of one eye from the point of fixation, usually due to muscle imbalance or paralysis; can cause blindness if not treated; refer for ophthalmological evaluation if visual fixation is not present by 3–4 mo of age

- Squinting or frowning
- Difficulty changing focus (near-far)
- Inaccurate judgment when reaching for and picking up objects
- Closing one eye
- Tilting the head from side to side
- Diplopia
- Photophobia
- Dizziness
- Headaches

- Assessment for and treatment of the underlying condition
- Occlusion therapy (patching the stronger eye)
- Surgery to stimulate the weaker eye

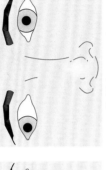
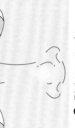

A Primary position: right esotropia   **B** Right hypertropia   **C** Right exotropia

Infantile glaucoma

A congenital increase in intraocular pressure due to defective structures related to the aqueous humor compressing the optic nerve and causing atrophy and subsequent visual impairment

- Loss of peripheral vision (infant bumps into objects not directly in front when becoming mobile)
- Buphthalmos (enlarged eye globe)
- Epiphora (excessive tearing)
- Photophobia (sensitivity to light)
- Corneal opacification (clouding)
- Blindness, if untreated

Surgery to restore the flow of aqueous humor to the canal of Schlemm

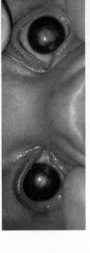

Congenital cataracts

A cloudiness or haziness of the corneal lens that may be hereditary or acquired (due to eye trauma, radiation exposure, or maternal infection with toxoplasmosis, rubella, cytomegalovirus, herpes simplex, or HIV)

- Abnormal or absent red reflex
- Epiphora
- Strabismus
- Photophobia
- Decreased visual acuity

- Corrective lenses
- Laser surgery to remove the cataract
- Surgery to remove the clouded lens (a permanent lens is not placed until the eye is fully mature)

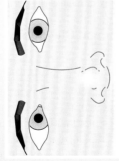

HIV, human immunodeficiency virus.

Images reprinted with permission from Nystagmus—Lippincott Nursing Advisor November 2013. Strabismus—Norris, T. L., & Lalchandani, R. (2018). *Porth's pathophysiology* (10th ed., Fig. 19.26). Philadelphia, PA: Wolters Kluwer. Infantile glaucoma—MacDonald, M. G., & Seshia, M. M. (2015). *Avery's neonatology* (7th ed., Fig. 50.4). Philadelphia, PA: Wolters Kluwer. Congenital cataracts—Wilson, M. E., Trivedi, R. H., & Pandey, S. K. (2005). *Pediatric cataract surgery* (1st ed., Fig. 2.6). Philadelphia, PA: Wolters Kluwer.

monitor progress. Teach the child's caregivers about any medications they may need to administer at home. Provide them with instructions for caring for the eye following surgery and recognizing and reporting signs and symptoms of infection and other complications.

Nasolacrimal Duct Obstruction

Congenital nasolacrimal duct obstruction (CNLDO) is a condition in which the nasolacrimal duct, or tear duct, fails to open properly, leading to obstruction and excessive tearing (epiphora).

Etiology and Pathophysiology

Tears are made in the tear gland (lacrimal gland) under the upper eyelid and are necessary to keep the eye moist. Tears drain from the eye through the upper and lower puncta and flow through the canaliculi. The canaliculi merge and empty the tears into the lacrimal sac. From there, the tears drain through the nasolacrimal duct and into the cavity of the nose. Before a baby is born, the membrane that blocks the opening between the nose and the nasolacrimal duct opens up, typically at around 6 months of intrauterine life (Perveen, Rasool Sufi, Rashid, & Khan, 2014). Failure of this canalization leads to an obstruction, causing the eye to excessively water because the tears cannot drain properly (Fig. 22.18). The tears become trapped, leading to infection (Lueder, 2015). Although the symptoms of this condition may resemble those of conjunctivitis, the pathophysiology is related to the blocked duct. Perveen et al. (2014) indicated that causes for the canalization failure are related to failure of the membrane (the valve of Hasner) to open, absent puncta, a narrow duct system, an infection, or a nasal bone that blocks the opening into the nose (Fig. 22.19).

Clinical Presentation

Perveen et al. (2014) indicated that approximately 30% of full-term infants are born with CNLDO, yet only 2% to 4% become

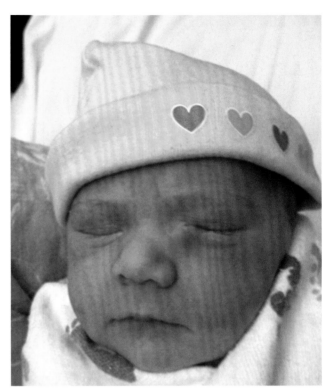

Figure 22.19. A newborn with a blocked nasolacrimal duct. Note the palpable mass in the left eye. Reprinted with permission from Nelson, L. B., & Olitsky, S. E. (2013). *Harley's pediatric ophthalmology* (6th ed., Fig. 16.1). Philadelphia, PA: Wolters Kluwer.

symptomatic. Red or chapped skin around the eyes commonly occurs, and some infants present with a palpable mass over the lacrimal sac (Lueder, 2015). In addition to epiphora, the eyelids may become red and swollen with purulent discharge and stick together as the drainage crusts.

Assessment and Diagnosis

An ophthalmologist can diagnose the condition with a careful examination. Diagnosis is typically made within a few weeks of birth when caregivers report that the newborn has notable tearing in one or both of the eyes. Infection is a common symptom, because bacteria are not properly flushed out of the eye. Perveen et al. (2014) emphasized that diagnosis can be confirmed by gently pressing over the nasolacrimal sac and observing a reflux of mucopurulent material from either punctum.

Therapeutic Interventions

Lueder (2015) emphasized that about 90% of infants with CNLDO have a spontaneous resolution of the condition within the first year of life. Treatment involves monitoring the child's eyes, performing lacrimal massage, and applying topical antibiotics to treat infections. Caregivers can perform lacrimal massage at home in conjunction with applying warm compresses to open up the membrane. Instruct caregivers to place the index finger between the inner corner of the child's eye and the side of the

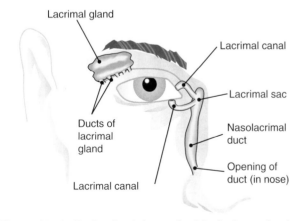

Figure 22.18. Pathophysiology of a blocked nasolacrimal duct. Reprinted with permission from Cohen, B. J. (2012). *Memmler's structure and function of the human body* (10th ed., Fig. 10.2). Philadelphia: Lippincott Williams & Wilkins.

nose and press in and down over the lacrimal sac for a few seconds (Boyd, 2015). The recommended frequency of the massage technique is 10 strokes to each eye once in the morning and once in the evening (Boyd, 2015).

If the blockage does not resolve on its own or complications such as frequent infections develop, treatment typically progresses to probing with dilation and irrigation to open the duct. Probing is considered standard and produces rapid improvement in symptoms. It involves dilating the punctal opening with an instrument and inserting a probe to open the canal. The system is then flushed with normal saline to remove any residual blockage. Perveen et al. (2014) recommended that probing be done under general anesthesia to allow the surgeon to access the delicate structures of the inner eye in a safe, controlled manner. They also suggested performing probing when the child is 6 to 18 months old for the best chance for success and by the age of 24 months at the latest.

Probing may not be indicated for or successful in some children. Stenting may then be performed to open up the drainage system. The stents are left in for 3 to 4 months and then removed. A surgical procedure known as a dacryocystorhinostomy is used when other methods have failed. It involves creating a new duct by making a fistula into the nasal cavity, either endoscopically or externally through a small incision. The endoscopic method allows the surgeon to view the intranasal bone structures and correct any abnormalities potentially contributing to the blockage without leaving an external scar. Dacryocystorhinostomy has a reported success rate of up to 93% (Jung, Kim, Cho, Paik, & Yang, 2015). Although the success rate is excellent, the procedure is invasive and is not without its complications; thus, pediatricians usually choose to treat CNLDO conventionally first.

Evaluation

Expected outcomes for a child with nasolacrimal duct obstruction include the following:

- The tear duct is opened and remains patent to allow free flow of tears.
- The child experiences treatment with minimal pain and maintains normal vision in the eye.
- The surgical site heals completely with minimal complications.
- Chronic infection and irritation of the affected eye are eliminated.

Discharge Planning and Teaching

Children who undergo only conventional treatment have no incisions to care for and should have minimal discomfort. In this case, simply instruct caregivers to administer acetaminophen as needed to relieve mild discomfort.

Most procedures used to open up the lacrimal duct are done on an outpatient basis, and the infant goes home the same day with few to no complications. Antibiotic and/or saline drops may be prescribed following surgery to prevent infection; educate caregivers about their administration. Follow-up with the pediatrician after surgery is usually on an as-needed basis.

Conjunctivitis

Conjunctivitis is an inflammation of the conjunctiva of the eye, which is the transparent membrane that covers the eyeball and lines the inner eyelid. Also known as "pink eye" because of the characteristic pink coloration of the sclera and conjunctiva of the eye that occurs in this condition, it is very common in childhood and has many causes.

Etiology and Pathophysiology

There are four main types of conjunctivitis based on etiology: bacterial, viral, allergic, and irritant. Bacterial conjunctivitis is typically caused by infection of the eye with staphylococcal or streptococcal bacteria, often as a result of touching the eyes with unclean hands. Viral conjunctivitis is usually caused by infection of the eye with a contagious virus associated with the common cold. Allergic conjunctivitis is caused by an allergic response in the eyes because of exposure to some allergen, such as pollen or pet dander. Irritant conjunctivitis is caused by exposure of the eye to chemicals that irritate it.

Clinical Presentation

In addition to the characteristic pink sclera, conjunctivitis may produce other symptoms, which vary depending on the type. Infectious (bacterial or viral) conjunctivitis typically begins in one eye and can be transferred to the other eye. Symptoms accompanying infectious conjunctivitis include the following (Fig. 22.20; Windell, 2018):

- An eye that feels itchy or gritty, as though sand were in it
- White, yellow, or green discharge that forms a crust around the eye during sleep and can make it difficult to open the eye
- A watery eye

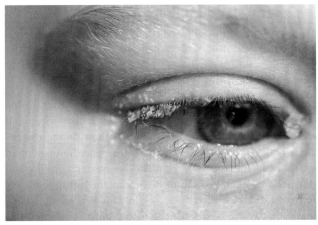

Figure 22.20. Conjunctivitis. Note the honey-colored crusts in the corner of the eye and on the eyelashes.

- A swollen eyelid
- Sensitivity to light

Conjunctivitis related to allergies or irritants is *not* contagious and affects both eyes at the same time. Allergic conjunctivitis may present as sneezing, watery eyes, and rhinitis. Irritant conjunctivitis may present as watery, itchy, or burning eyes.

Assessment and Diagnosis

Assessment of a child with suspected conjunctivitis should begin with obtaining a patient history to determine possible exposure to infectious agents, allergens, or chemical irritants. It should also include a physical and eye exam, along with vision assessment. As needed, refer children with suspected allergic conjunctivitis for an allergic workup to determine the sensitivity causing the symptoms. Cases related to irritants involve identifying what the irritant is.

Therapeutic Interventions

Children with conjunctivitis receive a variety of treatments depending on the cause. Children with the bacterial type are treated with antibiotic eye drops or ointment. Children with the viral type may be treated with home remedies to relieve discomfort.

Children with allergic conjunctivitis may be treated with antihistamines and cool compresses to soothe the symptoms, as well as desensitizing shots. In many cases, beginning desensitizing shots can help reduce the allergic response and thus reduce the amount of antihistamines required for relief.

For children with irritant conjunctivitis, gently flush the eyes with cool water to remove the irritant and reduce symptoms.

Evaluation

Expected outcomes for a child with conjunctivitis include the following:

- The cause of the condition is determined and the proper treatment initiated to prevent future cases.
- The parents and child maintain appointments for allergy shots, if ordered.
- The condition clears up and complete vision is restored once the treatment has been completed.

Discharge Planning and Teaching

Because bacterial and viral forms of conjunctivitis are highly contagious, educate children with these types of infection and their parents on avoiding contact with others during the period of infectiousness, performing frequent and thorough hand washing, avoiding contact between the eyes and hands, and undertaking other methods of preventing the spread of the infection. Inform caregivers that a child with viral conjunctivitis should *not* return to day care or school until the eye is completely clear, with no discharge. Silver (2018) emphasized that this may take up to 2 weeks as the virus works its way through the system. Children with bacterial conjunctivitis, however, can return to day care or school after 24 hours of receiving antibiotics, because the medications alter the contagious manner of the bacteria (Silver, 2018). For a child with bacterial conjunctivitis, instruct caregivers to administer the full course of antibiotic drops or ointment as prescribed by the pediatrician to completely eradicate the bacteria. Also, explain that instilling the drops or ointment is often unpleasant and that they may need to distract the child, particularly if younger, while administering the treatment. Advise them that applying warm compresses may help soothe the eye and remove discharge and crusts to help restore vision. Likewise, for a child with viral conjunctivitis, encourage the application of cold or warm compresses to the eye to relieve discomfort and to keep the eye clean (Silver, 2018).

For a child with allergic conjunctivitis, teach the family the importance of avoiding the offending allergen and keeping up with appointments for allergy shots, because the course of treatment is typically long and requires numerous visits.

For a child with irritant conjunctivitis, educate the family on how to prevent or limit the child's exposure to the irritant, such as by wearing eye goggles when swimming in a chlorinated pool. Emphasize with parents the importance of keeping the home environment free of the irritating factor.

Periorbital Cellulitis

Periorbital cellulitis, also known as "preseptal cellulitis," is a common infection of the eyelid and soft tissue surrounding the eye and is characterized by acute edema of the tissues (Pegram, 2016). Although its causative agents are not easy to identify, periorbital cellulitis must be treated promptly, because the potential for vision loss increases the longer the child goes without treatment (Harrington, 2018).

Etiology and Pathophysiology

Potential mechanisms of infection include direct inoculation due to trauma or surgery to the eye, bacteria spread from the bloodstream, or extension of an infection from the paranasal sinuses or other structures in the area. In many cases, the cause is not evident. Some cases are related to methicillin-resistant *Staphylococcus aureus* (MRSA), and can lead to blindness in the affected eye because there are no antibiotics that treat the infection successfully.

Serious complications can arise when periorbital cellulitis is untreated or when treatment is delayed. Abscesses may form, or corneal damage may lead to blindness. Secondary glaucoma, optic neuritis, or central retinal artery occlusion may also occur (Harrington, 2018). In addition, ocular motor nerves may be affected, leading to decreased movement of the eye, and intracranial complications, such as meningitis, cavernous sinus thrombosis, or abscesses within the dura or brain, may occur in severe cases (Harrington, 2018).

Clinical Presentation

In addition to the distinct swelling of the eyelid and surrounding area, children with periorbital cellulitis may also have decreased vision in the affected eye, elevated intraocular pressure, ptosis, pain on movement of the eye, a discoloration of the sclera and/or conjunctiva, and purulent nasal discharge (Fig. 22.21). Fever, headache, and increasing malaise may also be present (Harrington, 2018). Harrington (2018) emphasized that MRSA should be suspected when there are multiple orbital abscesses and/or lacrimal gland abscesses.

Assessment and Diagnosis

Children with periorbital cellulitis are treated in the hospital because of the risk and severity of complications. Assessment includes a CBC, and a WBC count greater than 15,000 (leukocytosis) is a positive finding for this condition (Harrington, 2018). In addition, blood cultures and purulent discharge should be examined to determine the potential causative agent. Imaging studies may be ordered to examine the orbit to identify abscesses, and an MRI may be completed to determine whether cavernous sinus disease is present. If the child is demonstrating neurological signs, a lumbar puncture may be performed to determine the presence of meningitis.

Therapeutic Interventions

A child with periorbital cellulitis requires IV antibiotics and is hospitalized for close monitoring. A broad-spectrum antibiotic is administered until specific coverage can be prescribed depending on culture results. Harrington (2018) suggested that IV antibiotic therapy be continued for 1 to 2 weeks and then be followed by oral antibiotics for another 2 to 3 weeks. Harrington (2018) also emphasized that systemic steroidal anti-inflammatory medications should not be administered until the child improves with antibiotic or surgical intervention. Other medications may include decongestants to decrease secretions and promote comfort for the child and glaucoma medications to reduce orbital pressure. Care is multidisciplinary, because the child may be seen by a general pediatrician; an ear, nose, and throat specialist; infectious disease specialists; radiologists, for repeat scans to determine the success of treatment; and pediatric surgeons, if surgery is indicated to drain abscesses or debride the area when fungus is the culprit of the infection. Neurologists may also care for the child if brain involvement is present.

Close monitoring is necessary to track progress of the treatment and identify any complications; thus, the nurse is important in caring for the child with periorbital cellulitis. Conduct neurological checks throughout the day and vision checks. As needed, coordinate care, administer antibiotics and other medications, and monitor the status of the child, particularly if the sinus is involved, because the airway can become compromised. Care for surgical sites, monitor drainage if a drain has been placed, and promote comfort by reducing fever and pain.

Evaluation

Expected outcomes for a child with orbital cellulitis include the following:

- Vision to the eye is retained or optimized.
- The infection is resolved through the use of antibiotics.
- The parents administer necessary medications correctly at home to eradicate the infection.
- Skin integrity around the affected eye is maintained.
- The child resumes normal activity once the infection is cleared.

Discharge Planning and Teaching

Educate the caregivers about the child's condition, medications, and other necessary treatments, which should help alleviate any anxiety they feel related to the urgency of treatment, the frequency of visits, and monitoring by the multidisciplinary team. The long-term prognosis for this condition is good if the infection is caught very early, treatment is initiated immediately, and complications are minimal.

Hearing Deficits

Hearing loss in children is caused by several factors and must be recognized early, because a child's speech, language, and social skill development may be affected. The CDC emphasized that the sooner hearing issues are identified and services are employed, the better the chance the child has to reach his or her full potential (2018b). As with vision, younger children may not be able to recognize and verbalize changes in hearing. Hearing loss in infants is particularly hard to detect. Any suspicion, however, should be followed up promptly by a practitioner trained in hearing loss diagnosis and treatment.

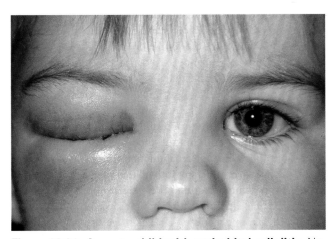

Figure 22.21. A young child with periorbital cellulitis. Notice the erythema and swelling of the right eye. Reprinted with permission from Bachur, R. G., & Shaw, K. N. (2015). *Fleisher & Ludwig's textbook of pediatric emergency medicine* (7th ed., Fig. 131.4). Philadelphia, PA: Wolters Kluwer.

Etiology and Pathophysiology

Causes of hearing loss may be genetic, acquired, or unknown. Hearing loss that is caused primarily by genetic factors is unavoidable. The CDC stated that in one out of every two cases of hearing loss in babies in the United States, genetics was a defining factor. For example, children with family members with hearing loss and infants born with certain genetic syndromes, such as trisomy 21 (Down syndrome), are at increased risk for experiencing hearing loss.

Acquired hearing loss, however, is avoidable. The WHO (2019) indicated that 60% of hearing loss in children around the world is preventable. Recognizing the causes of acquired hearing loss and instituting appropriate preventive measures are key in preserving hearing in children. According to the CDC, one in four cases of hearing loss in children is due to maternal infection during pregnancy, complications after birth, or head trauma (2018b), all of which are preventable. Infections during pregnancy associated with hearing loss in the child are primarily related to TORCH infections, which include toxoplasmosis, other (syphilis, varicella-zoster, parvovirus B19), rubella, cytomegalovirus, and herpes. Cytomegalovirus is the most common of the TORCH infections that lead to infant hearing loss. Chronic ear infections during infancy and childhood (such as otitis media) have the potential to cause hearing loss, as well. About 25% of cases of infants born with hearing loss are of unknown etiology.

Hearing loss may also be classified according to the portion of the auditory system in which the dysfunction occurs. Conductive hearing loss involves dysfunction in the ear structures responsible for transmitting sound from outside of the ear to the inner ear, including the outer ear, tympanic membrane (eardrum), and ossicles. Ear infections are the most common cause of conductive hearing loss, and such cases are typically mild, temporary, and treatable (Kids Health, 2016). Sensorineural hearing loss involves dysfunction in ear structures responsible for transducing auditory signals into nerve impulses in the inner ear (cochlear hair cells) or transmitting these nerve impulses to the brainstem (cranial nerve VIII, the vestibulocochlear nerve). Sensorineural hearing loss is typically present at birth and is usually permanent (Kids Health, 2016).

Clinical Presentation

Hearing loss in infants should be suspected if the startle reflex is absent (the infant does not startle at loud sounds), if the infant does not turn to the source of a sound after 6 months of age, or if the child does not respond when the parent calls out to him or her and lacks simple speech (such as "mama") by 1 year of age. Children with hearing loss may demonstrate a delay in speech development, have difficulty with articulating words or being understood, or not follow commands. In addition, children may frequently ask for something to be repeated or turn the volume up too high on a television. Children may also appear to be inattentive and may be misdiagnosed with attention-deficit/hyperactivity disorder before the hearing loss is recognized. If a child demonstrates such signs and symptoms or if a caregiver or teacher expresses concern, refer the child to an audiologist or other clinician trained in assessing hearing loss for follow-up.

Assessment and Diagnosis

The CDC recommends that all babies have a hearing screening no later than 1 month of age. Most hospitals evaluate hearing before a newborn has been discharged. Pediatricians also evaluate hearing when children come in for well-care visits. Hearing evaluations involve an otoscopic exam and an audiological testing. The otoscopic exam involves use of the pneumoscope to check the mobility of the tympanic membrane, followed by a more detailed tympanogram if hearing loss is detected.

When a child is old enough to cooperate and follow directions, an audiologist can perform an audiological assessment on the child to evaluate hearing. Some children may also receive a brainstem auditory evoked response (BAER) test to evaluate brainwave activity in response to certain sounds. The BAER test is typically done in a controlled clinical setting, because infants or children who cannot lie still must be sedated and require monitoring before, during, and after the exam. As with the EEG test, electrodes are attached to the scalp and the brainwaves are then recorded as sounds are introduced. Hearing loss may be diagnosed as *mild* (the child cannot hear certain sounds), *moderate* (the child cannot hear many sounds), *severe* (the child cannot hear most sounds), or *profound* (the child hears no sound).

Therapeutic Interventions

Although some types of hearing loss are mild and can be resolved by treating infections and encouraging children and adolescents to reduce the sound on their televisions and music devices, other types require care that is more involved. Those with chronic ear infections may have surgery to place myringotomy tubes in the tympanic membrane to allow for drainage and to equilibrate pressure. Some conduction disorders may be treated with a tympanoplasty or stapedectomy to restore hearing. Cochlear implants may be indicated for children with severe-to-profound hearing loss but carry the risk of meningitis (Niedermeier, Braun, Fauser, Strubinger, & Stark, 2012). Hearing aids may also be successful in amplifying sound for infants and children with mild-to-moderate loss with some amplification ability. Hearing rehabilitation consisting of auditory, listening, and speech therapy for children may be successful in helping with communication. There are also many technological devices to help children communicate and participate in school. The use of American Sign Language also helps children with hearing loss communicate with others (Fig. 22.22).

Nurses are important in identifying and recognizing speech and language patterns that might indicate a hearing issue with a child. Nurses also may detect hearing loss in young children and infants through physical assessment.

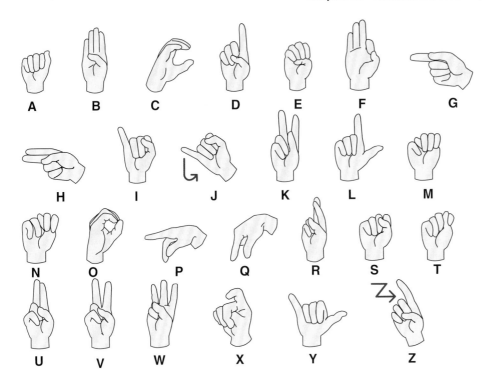

Figure 22.22. The American Sign Language alphabet. Reprinted with permission from Timby, B. K., & Smith, N. E. (2017). *Introductory medical-surgical nursing* (12th ed., Fig. 7.11). Philadelphia, PA: Wolters Kluwer.

Evaluation

Expected outcomes for a child with a hearing deficit include the following:

- The child maintains optimal hearing with the appropriate interventions and assistive devices.
- The child experiences a reduction in the frequency of ear infections.
- Speech and language development are optimal with the appropriate therapy services for support.
- The child is able to communicate with others through the use of speech, sign language, and/or assistive devices.

Discharge Planning and Teaching

Provide support for the caregivers, because learning that a child has lost his or her hearing can be difficult. Teach the family about resources that are available to help them learn to live with the hearing loss and refer the child to specialists who can help. Teach caregivers about medications that they must administer to treat infections and care that they must provide for a child who has had surgery to aid in hearing. Finally, when hearing loss is severe or profound, provide the family with a variety of strategies to enhance communication to help the child grow and develop to his or her full potential.

Think Critically

1. What can the nurse and parents or caregivers do to help promote optimal development in an infant with a cranial malformation?
2. Develop a care plan that focuses on the child who has had a VP shunt placed. How will the nurse know that the shunt is functioning properly? What types of signs and symptoms would indicate that there is a shunt malfunction?
3. What are some potential seizure triggers and how can they be eliminated to reduce the risk of seizure activity in a child with epilepsy?
4. Create a home plan of care focusing on safety for the child with epilepsy. What types of measures should the parents or caregivers incorporate into daily life to prevent serious injury?
5. What are some priorities the nurse should recognize when caring for an infant who may be a victim of SBS?
6. Develop a plan of care that focuses on helping a child cope with chronic headaches.
7. What types of interventions can the nurse initiate to improve communication for a hospitalized child who has hearing loss?

References

Alvarado, M. G., & Schwartz, D. A. (2017). Zika virus infection in pregnancy, microcephaly, and maternal and fetal health . . . what we think, what we know, and what we think we know. *Archives of Pathology & Laboratory Medicine, 141*(1), 26–32. doi:10.5858/arpa.2016-0382-RA

American Academy of Pediatrics. (2009). *Healthy children.org: Bathing & skin care.* Retrieved from https://www.healthychildren.org/English/ages-stages/baby/bathing-skin-care/Pages/default.aspx

American Epilepsy Society. (2018). *Working toward a world without epilepsy: How often does epilepsy occur in the United States?* Retrieved from https://www.aesnet.org/clinical_resources/faqs

Anantheswar, Y. N., & Venkataramana, N. K. (2009). Pediatric craniofacial surgery for craniosynostosis: Our experience and current concepts: Part-1. *Journal of Pediatric Neurosciences, 4*(2), 86–99. doi:10.4103/1817-1745.57327

Ashwal, S., Michelson, D., Plawner, L., & Dobyns, W. B. (2009). Practice parameter: Evaluation of the child with microcephaly (an evidence-based review). *Neurology, 73*(11), 887–897. doi:10.1212/WNL.0b013e3181b783f7

Bagdure, D., Custer, J. W., Rao, S., Messacar, K., Dominguez, S., Beam, B. W., & Bhutta, A. (2016). Hospitalized children with encephalitis in the United States: A pediatric health information system database study. *Pediatric Neurology, 61,* 58–62. doi:10.1016/j.pediatrneurol.2016.04.014

Blume, H. K. (2017). Childhood headache: A brief review. *Pediatric Annals, 46*(4), e155–e165. doi:10.3928/19382359-20170321-02

Boyd, K. (2015). Blocked tear duct treatment. *American Academy of Ophthalmology; Pediatric Ophthalmology Education Center.* Retrieved from https://www.aao.org/eye-health/diseases/treatment-blocked-tear-duct

Bykowski, J., Kruk, P., Gold, J. J., Glaser, C. A., Sheriff, H., & Crawford, J. R. (2015). Acute pediatric encephalitis neuroimaging: Single-institution series as part of the California encephalitis project. *Pediatric Neurology, 52*(6), 606–614.

Centers for Disease Control and Prevention. (1990). *Reye syndrome 1990 case definition: Clinical criteria.* Retrieved from https://wwwn.cdc.gov/nndss/conditions/reye-syndrome/case-definition/1990/

Centers for Disease Control and Prevention. (2017). *Meningococcal disease.* Retrieved from https://www.cdc.gov/meningococcal/surveillance/index.html

Centers for Disease Control and Prevention. (2018a). *Folic acid; Birth defects count.* Retrieved from https://www.cdc.gov/ncbddd/folicacid/global.html

Centers for Disease Control and Prevention. (2018b). *Hearing loss in children: Screening and diagnosis of hearing loss.* Retrieved from https://www.cdc.gov/ncbddd/hearingloss/screening.html

Cotter, S. A., Cyert, L. A., Miller, J. M., & Quinn, G. E. (2015). Vision screening for children 36 to <72 months: Recommended practices for the national expert panel to the national center for children's vision and eye health. *Optometry & Vision Science, 92*(1), 6–16. doi:10.1097/OPX.0000000000000429

Coureuil, M., Join-Lambert, O., Lécuyer, H., Bourdoulous, S., Marullo, S., & Nassif, X. (2013). Pathogenesis of meningococcemia. *Cold Spring Harbor Perspectives in Medicine, 3*(6). doi:10.1101%2Fcshperspect.a012393

Dao, J. M., & Qubty, W. (2018). Headache diagnosis in children and adolescents. *Current pain and headache reports, 22*(17). doi:10.1007/s11916-018-0675-7

Degnan, L. A. (2012). Reye's syndrome: A rare but serious pediatric condition. *Clinical Pediatric Pharmacist, 37*(3), HS6–HS8.

Dy, R. T., & Schuster, C. (2015). *Vascular formations of the brain and spine in children.* Retrieved from https://now.aapmr.org/vascular-malformations-of-the-brain-and-spine-in-children/

El-Ghanem, M., Kass-Hout, T., Hass, Hout, O., Alderazi, Y. J., Amuluru, K., Al-Mufti, F., . . . Gandhi, C. D. (2016). Arteriovenous malformations in the pediatric population: Review of the existing literature. *Interventional Neurology, 5,* 218–225.

El-Radhi, A. (2015). Management of seizures in children. *British Journal of Nursing, 24*(3), 152–155. Retrieved from http://0-search.ebscohost.com.catalog.llu.edu/login.aspx?direct=true&db=hch&AN=100963134&site=ehost-live&scope=site

Epilepsy Foundation. (2018). *Seizure training for school personnel.* Retrieved from https://www.epilepsy.com/living-epilepsy/our-training-and-education/seizure-training-school-personnel

Falco-Walter, J. J., Scheffer, I. E., & Fisher, R. S. (2018). The new definition and classification of seizures and epilepsy. *Epilepsy Research, 139,* 73–79. doi:10.1016/j.eplepsyres.2017.11.015

Feldman, H. S., Jones, K. L., Lindsey, S., Slyman, D., Klonoff-Cohen, H., Kao, K., . . . Chambers, C. (2012). Prenatal alcohol exposure patterns and alcohol-related birth defects and growth deficiencies: A prospective study. *Alcoholism, 36*(4), 561–744. doi:10.1111/j.1530-0277.2011.01664

Figaji, A. A. (2017). Anatomical and physiological differences between children and adults relevant to traumatic brain injury and the implications for clinical assessment and care. *Frontiers in Neurology, 8:* 685. doi:10.3389/fneur.2017.00685

Fisher, R. S., Shafer, P., & D'Souza, C. (2017). *The Epilepsy Foundation 2017 revised classification of seizures.* Retrieved from https://epilepsychicago.org/2017/01/04/2017-revised-classification-of-seizures/

Geyer, K., Meller, K., Kulpan, C., & Mowery, B. D. (2013). Traumatic brain injury in children: Acute care management. *Pediatric Nursing, 39*(6), 283–289. Retrieved from http://0-search.ebscohost.com.catalog.llu.edu/login.aspx?direct=true&db=ccm&AN=104130316&site=ehost-live&scope=site

Green, A. J. (2003). Update on Chiari malformation: Clinical manifestations, diagnosis, and treatments. *Pediatric Nursing, 29*(4), 331–335. Retrieved from http://0-search.ebscohost.com.catalog.llu.edu/login.aspx?direct=true&db=aph&AN=10596339&site=ehost-live&scope=site

Harrington, J. N. (2018). *Orbital cellulitis.* Retrieved from https://emedicine.medscape.com/article/1217858-overview

Harvard University Center on the Developing Child. (2018). *Brain Architecture.* Retrieved from https://developingchild.harvard.edu/science/key-concepts/brain-architecture/

Hershey, A. D. & Winner, P. K. (2005). Pediatric migraine: Recognition and treatment. *JAOA, Supplement 2, 105*(4).

Jung, S. K., Kim, Y. C., Cho, W. K., Paik, J. S., & Yang, S. W. (2015). Surgical outcomes of endoscopic dacryocystorhinostomy: Analysis of 1083 consecutive cases. *Canadian Journal of Ophthalmology, 50*(6), 466–470.

Kahle, K. T., Kulkarni, A. V., Limbrick, D. D., & Warf, B. C. (2016). Hydrocephalus in children. *The Lancet, 387*(10020), 788-799. doi:10.1016/S0140-6736(15)60694-8

Karwowski, M. P., Nelson, J. M., Staples, J. E., Fischer, M., Fleming-Dutra, K. E., Villanueva, J., . . . Rasmussen, S. A. (2016). Zika virus disease: A CDC update for pediatric health care providers. *Pediatrics, 137*(5). doi:10.1542/peds.2016-0621

Kessler, S. K., Shinnar, S., Cnaan, A., Dlugos, D., Conry, J., Hirtz, D. G., Hu, F., . . . Glauser, T. A. (2017). Pretreatment seizure semiology in childhood absence epilepsy. *Neurology, 89*(7). doi:10.1212/WNL.0000000000004226

Kids Health. (2016). *Hearing evaluation in children.* Retrieved from https://kidshealth.org/en/parents/hear.html

Kindhauser, M. K., Allen, T., Frank, V., Santhana, R., & Dye, C. (2016). *Zika: The origin and spread of a mosquito-borne virus.* Retrieved from https://www.who.int/bulletin/online_first/16-171082/en/

Kumar, R., Lorenc, A., Robinson, N., & Blair, M. (2011). Parents' and primary healthcare practitioners' perspectives on the safety of honey and other traditional paediatric healthcare approaches. *Child: Care, Health & Development, 37*(5), 734–743. doi:10.1111/j.1365-2214.2010.01186.x

Laughlin, J., Luerssen, T. G., & Dias, M. S. (2011). Prevention and management of positional skull deformities in infants. *Pediatrics, 128*(6), 1236–1241. doi:10.1542/peds.2011-2220

Leung, A.K.C., Hon, K. L., & Leung, T.N.H. (2018). Febrile seizures: An overview. *Published online at Drugs Context, 7:* 212536.

Looman, W. S., & Flannery, A. B. (2012). Evidence-based care of the child with deformational plagiocephaly, Part I: Assessment and diagnosis. *Journal of Pediatric Health Care, 26*(4), 242–250. doi:10.1016/j.pedhc.2011.10.003

Lueder, G. T. (2015). Nasolacrimal duct obstruction in children. *American Academy of Ophthalmology; Pediatric Ophthalmology Education Center.* Retrieved from https://www.aao.org/disease-review/nasolacrimal-duct-obstruction-4

Martin, E. F. (2017). Performing pediatric eye exams in primary care. *Nurse Practitioner, 42*(8), 41–47. doi:10.1097/01.NPR.0000520791.94940.7e

Mayo Clinic. (2018). *Craniosynostosis.* Retrieved online at: https://www.mayoclinic.org/diseases-conditions/craniosynostosis/symptoms-causes/syc-20354513

Migraine Research Foundation. (2019). *Migraine facts.* Retrieved from https://migraineresearchfoundation.org/about-migraine/migraine-facts/

Modalsli Aaberg, K., Gunnes, N., Johanne Bakken, I., Lund Søraas, C. Berntsen, A., Magnus, P., . . . Surén, P. (2017). Incidence and prevalence of childhood epilepsy: A nationwide cohort study. *Pediatrics, 139*(5), 1–10. doi:10.1542/peds.2016-3908

National Center on Shaken Baby Syndrome. (2018). *Facts.* Retrieved from https://www.dontshake.org/learn-more

Niedermeier, K., Braun, S., Fauser, C., Strubinger, R. K., & Stark, T. (2012). A safety evaluation of dexamethasone-releasing cochlear implants: Comparative study on the risk of otogenic meningitis after implantation. *Acta Oto-Laryngologica, 132*(12), 1252–1260.

Pegram, T. A. (2016). *Periorbital cellulitis (preseptal cellulitis) organism-specific therapy*. Retrieved from https://emedicine.medscape.com/article/2018322 -overview

Perveen, S., Rasool Sufi, A., S., Rashid, S., & Khan, K. (2014). Success rate of probing for congenital nasolacrimal duct obstruction at various ages. *Journal of Ophthalmic &Vision Research, 9*(1), 60–64.

Roumila, K. (2018). *Brain 101: The ventricles and CSF flow*. Retrieved from the Hydrocephalus Association, https://www.hydroassoc.org/ brain-101-the-ventricles-and-csf-flow/

Sankhyan, N., Vykunta Raju, K. N., Sharma, S., & Gulati, S. (2010). Management of raised intracranial pressure. *Indian Journal of Pediatrics, 77*(12), 1409–1416. doi:10.1007/s12098-010-0190-2

Schacter, S. C., Shafer, P. O., & Sirven, J. I. (2013). *The epilepsy foundation: Triggers of seizures*. Retrieved from www.epilepsy.com/learn/triggers-seizures

Shafer, P. O., & Dean, P. M. (2018). *Vagus nerve stimulation (VNS)*. Retrieved from https://www.epilepsy.com/learn/treating-seizures-and-epilepsy/devices /vagus-nervestimulation-vns

Tindall, S. C. (1990). Level of consciousness. In H. K. Walker, W. D. Hall, & J. W. Hurst (Eds.), *Clinical methods: The history, physical, and laboratory examinations* (3rd ed.). Boston, MA: Butterworths.

Unwin, S., & Dika, C. (2017). Deformational plagiocephaly—A focus on prevention. *The Journal for Nurse Practitioners, 13*(2), 162–169.

Weiner, D. L. (2018). *Reye syndrome clinical presentation*. Retrieved online at: https://emedicine.medscape.com/article/803683-overview

Windell, J. (2018). The eyes have it. *Community Practitioner, 91*(2), 24–26.

World Health Organization. (2019). *Deafness and hearing loss*. Retrieved from https://www.who.int/news-room/fact-sheets/detail/deafness-and-hearing-loss

Suggested Readings

Duffy, L. V., & Vessey, J. A. (2016). A randomized controlled trial testing the efficacy of the creating opportunities for parent empowerment (COPE) program for parents of children with epilepsy and other chronic neurological conditions. *Journal of Neuroscience Nursing, 48*(3), 166–174. doi:10.1097/ JNN.0000000000000199

Morrow, J., & Hunt, S. (2017). Subclinical seizures: No alternative facts here! *Canadian Journal of Critical Care Nursing, 28*(2), 45.

Newton, C. R. (2018). Global burden of pediatric neurological disorders. *Seminars in Pediatric Neurology, 27*, 10–15. doi:10.1016/j.spen.2018.03.002

Prasad, M. R., Swank, P. R., & Ewing-Cobbs, L. (2017). Long-term school outcomes of children and adolescents with traumatic brain injury. *Journal of Head Trauma Rehabilitation, 32*(1), E24–E32. doi:10.1097/ HTR.0000000000000218

Stolz, H. E., Brandon, D. J., Wallace, H. S., & Tucker, E. A. (2017). Preventing shaken baby syndrome: Evaluation of a multiple-setting program. *Journal of Family Issues, 38*(16), 2346–2367. doi:10.1177/0192513X16647985

23 Alterations in Gastrointestinal Function

After completing this chapter, you will be able to:

1. Compare and contrast anatomical and physiological characteristics of the gastrointestinal systems of children and adults.
2. Relate pediatric assessment findings to the child's gastrointestinal status.
3. Discuss the pathophysiology of common pediatric gastrointestinal disorders.
4. Differentiate between signs and symptoms of common pediatric gastrointestinal disorders.
5. Outline the therapeutic regimen for each of the pediatric gastrointestinal disorders.
6. Describe pharmacological management of common of pediatric gastrointestinal disorders.
7. Apply the principles of growth and development to the care of a child with a gastrointestinal disorder.
8. Create a nursing plan of care for each of the common pediatric gastrointestinal disorders.

Key Terms

Ascites
Atresia
Cyclic vomiting
Encopresis
Gastroschisis

Hyperbilirubinemia
Intussusception
Omphalocele
Projectile vomiting
Volvulus

The gastrointestinal tract provides a route for a child to ingest and absorb foods and fluids necessary to sustain life and promote growth and development. The gastrointestinal tract includes the mouth, esophagus, stomach, pancreas, small intestine, and large intestine. The liver plays an essential role in the metabolism of fats, proteins, and carbohydrates; the storage of vitamins A, D, E, and K; and the secretion of bile and bilirubin. The gallbladder, which is located behind the liver, stores and concentrates the bile produced by the liver. Bile is necessary to emulsify fats so that fatty acids can be absorbed.

In children, some gastrointestinal disorders produce symptoms that are short-term and interfere with nutrition and fluid

and electrolyte balance for a brief period. Examples of these alterations include appendicitis, vomiting, diarrhea, and constipation. Other alterations of the gastrointestinal system may be long-term and lead to complications that interfere with or prevent optimal nutrition and adequate growth. Gastrointestinal disorders can result from congenital defects, acquired diseases, infection, or injury. These disorders can be categorized as structural anomalies, acute gastrointestinal disorders, chronic gastrointestinal disorders, and hepatobiliary disorders, which are those that involve the liver, gallbladder, and bile ducts. This chapter describes common gastrointestinal disorders and the appropriate management and nursing care for each disorder.

Variations in Anatomy and Physiology

The gastrointestinal tract includes the mouth, esophagus, stomach, small intestine, large intestine, and pancreas. In addition, the liver, gallbladder, and spleen play important roles in the digestive processes. Figure 23.1 reviews the anatomical structures of the gastrointestinal tract. In utero, the fetus makes sucking and swallowing movements and ingests amniotic fluid. However, the gastrointestinal tract is immature at birth. The placenta provides nutrients and removes waste while the fetus grows; therefore, the processes of absorption and excretion are not necessary until after birth. Sucking is a primitive reflex that can be stimulated by stroking the lips or cheeks. Until about 6 weeks of age, the infant, although capable of sucking and swallowing, has no voluntary control over swallowing. The pediatric gastrointestinal system differs from that of the adult in several ways. Table 23.1 summarizes these differences.

Table 23.1 Summary of Pediatric and Adult Gastrointestinal Differences

Characteristic	Infant	Older Child and Adult
Swallowing	Involuntary until 6 wk of age	Voluntary
Stomach capacity	• 30–90 mL at 1 wk of age • 500 mL at 2 y of age	1,500 mL by age 16 y
Digestive enzymes	• Deficiency of amylase, lipase, trypsin at birth • Sufficient quantities present at 4–6 mo of age • Abdominal gas common	Present and functional
Liver function	• Bilirubin conjugation begins at 2–3 wk of age • Gluconeogenesis, vitamin storage, and deamination immature • Very large liver relative to body mass	• Liver function normal • Much smaller liver relative to body mass
Excretory function	Unable to control defecation	Awareness of rectum, control over defecation at 18–24 mo of age
Small intestine	200 cm at birth	6 m in an adult

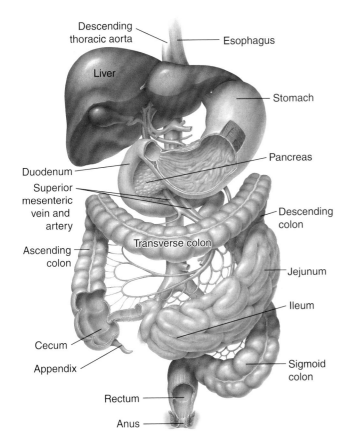

Figure 23.1. The gastrointestinal tract. Reprinted with permission from Kawamura, D., & Lunsford, B. (2012). *Abdomen and superficial structures* (3rd ed., Fig. 9.1). Philadelphia, PA: Lippincott Williams & Wilkins.

Assessment of the Pediatric Gastrointestinal System

The nursing assessment of a child with a potential or actual gastrointestinal condition involves the careful and in-depth review of many body systems and analysis of their relationship to gastrointestinal function. Table 23.2 is a guideline for performing a comprehensive assessment of the infant or child with an alteration in gastrointestinal function. Diagnostic procedures and laboratory tests are also an essential part of managing gastrointestinal disorders (Box 23.1).

Table 23.2 Assessment Guide: Pediatric Gastrointestinal System

Mouth and esophagus	• Presence of increased or decreased oral secretions • Cleft lip or cleft palate present?
Abdomen	• Inspection • Auscultation • Palpation
Nutrition	• Amount of fluid intake • Amount of food intake, including calorie count
Emesis	• Spitting up: When does it occur? Frequency? • Color of emesis? • When? Frequency? Volume?
Stool	• Color, consistency, size • Frequency: Change in stool pattern?
Heart	• Heart rate and rhythm: Tachycardia, irregular rhythm? • Heart sounds: Murmurs present? • Pulse: Weak or absent? Bounding? • Capillary refill: <2 s? >4–5 s?
Skin	• Diaphoretic? Clammy? • Warm, cool, or cold • Color: Pallor—sign of anemia; Mottled—sign of poor perfusion
Fluid status	• Edema present? Periorbital, facial, peripheral • Signs of dehydration? Poor skin turgor, dry mucous membranes. Low urine output • Weight increase or decrease? • Palpate for hepatosplenomegaly: possible fluid excess
Activity	• Sleeping more than usual? • Changes in the child's activity level?
Growth and development	• Growth patterns • Gaining adequate weight and height for age?

Box 23.1 Diagnostic Procedures and Laboratory Tests for the Gastrointestinal System

Diagnostic Procedures

• Abdominal X-rays
• Abdominal ultrasound
• Barium or contrast enema
• Barium or contrast swallow
• Computed tomography scan of the abdomen
• Endoscopy
• Intraesophageal pH probe monitoring

Laboratory Tests

• Basic metabolic panel
• Complete blood count
• Gastric pH level
• Magnesium and phosphorus levels
• Serum hepatic panel (aspartate aminotransferase, alanine aminotransferase, bilirubin, gamma-glutamyl-transferase, and alkaline phosphatase levels)
• Stool for occult blood
• Stool for ova and parasites

Maintain Effective Ventilation and Oxygenation

Some gastrointestinal disorders, such as cleft lip and palate and esophageal atresia/transesophageal fistula, place infants at higher risk for aspiration. In such cases, a priority nursing intervention is to implement aspiration precautions. Assess these infants frequently for respiratory distress and vital sign changes such as tachycardia and tachypnea, which are early signs of aspiration. Keep suction equipment and a bulb syringe immediately available at the infant's bedside to remove milk and secretions, such as mucus, that accumulate in the infant's nasopharyngeal airway. Place infants in a slightly elevated position to minimize aspiration of secretions into the trachea, particularly for feedings and for at least 30 minutes after feedings. In some cases, the infant may have to have nothing by mouth (NPO) until surgical correction takes place.

Postoperatively, continue to assess the patency of the airways and the infant's ability to maintain an effective breathing pattern. Infants are placed on a cardiorespiratory monitor to allow for early detection of abnormal respirations, heart rate, and O_2 saturations. Suction the nasopharynx as needed, avoiding any sutures present. Vigorous suctioning can irritate the mucosa, so take care to avoid mucosal damage. Often, cool mist is ordered postoperatively for the first 24 hours to moisturize secretions and the oral cavity. Reposition the infant frequently, at least every 2 hours, to allow expansion of lung fields.

During reintroduction of feedings, assess for respiratory difficulty and ensure that the infant is burped frequently, after every 15 to 30 mL of fluid, to help prevent regurgitation and aspiration.

General Nursing Interventions for Gastrointestinal Disorders

Given here is an overview of key nursing interventions that apply to gastrointestinal disorders, in general. Interventions that are specific to a given disorder are discussed within the Therapeutic Interventions section of that disorder.

Maintain Adequate Hydration and Nutrition

By their very nature, gastrointestinal disorders pose special challenges to maintaining adequate hydration and nutrition in children. Disorders that disrupt the integrity of the gastrointestinal tract, such as anorectal malformation or intussusception, require that the child be NPO until after surgical repair and return of bowel function, at which time the child may progress from clear liquids to breast milk or formula for infants and to solid foods for older children. Surgery of any type, of course, requires the child to be NPO immediately before, during, and immediately after the procedure, such as for appendicitis or Meckel diverticulum.

Conditions and surgical procedures that compromise gastrointestinal function for longer periods, such as necrotizing enterocolitis (NEC), short bowel syndrome, and biliary atresia, may require total parenteral nutrition (TPN) (Hopkins, Cermak, & Russell, 2017). TPN requires placement of a central venous access catheter and monitoring of fluid status and electrolytes upon initiation and throughout the duration of administration. Other conditions may permit the child to receive or progress to enteral tube or full gastrostomy tube feedings, with the gastrostomy tube possibly being placed during an initial surgery to correct a deformity. A gastrostomy tube provides a means of ensuring adequate nutrition while the child grows and undergoes further surgeries to correct the defect. When working with children receiving gastrostomy tube feedings, be sure to monitor weight, length, and growth and development regularly to ensure that they are receiving adequate nutrition.

Other conditions, such as vomiting, require the child to avoid solid foods for a time but allow liquids by mouth. In these cases, teach parents which liquids are appropriate to offer, such as electrolyte solutions (per provider recommendation), popsicles, sugar water (2.5 mL of sugar in 120 mL of water), gelatin water (5 mL of gelatin powder in 120 oz of water), and plain water. Also teach parents about minimum daily intake requirements. For example, a 6- to 7-lb (2.7- to 3.1-kg) infant requires a minimum of 10 oz of fluid per day, whereas a 26-lb (11.7 kg) child needs a minimum of 28 oz of fluid each day. Teach parents to monitor actual fluid intake.

Dehydration, whether primary or secondary to another condition (e.g., gastroenteritis, Meckel diverticulum, omphalocele, or NEC), is a serious challenge to a child's fluid and electrolyte balance. Oral rehydration is the first intervention for mild or moderate dehydration. Give or instruct parents to give fluids, such as Pedialyte, in 1- to 3-teaspoon increments every 10 to 15 minutes. Fluids should be given even if the child vomits, because some fluids are absorbed. The child should consume 50 mL of fluid for each kilogram of weight during the first 2 to 4 hours of oral rehydration therapy.

For cases of severe dehydration, intravenous (IV) fluids are necessary to restore fluid balance and correct volume depletion. Normal saline or lactated Ringer's solution is used to administer 10 to 20 mL/kg boluses until vital signs are stabilized. Once vital signs are stabilized, the child receives IV fluids until oral intake can begin. IV fluid intake is also based on weight, and the nurse should ensure that the child is receiving the appropriate volume of fluids per hour. Monitor the IV site for signs of infiltration during IV fluid administration. A pump is used to administer fluids to ensure more accurate delivery of volume. Electrolytes such as potassium may need to be replaced depending on the severity of dehydration and source of fluid loss.

Assess and record the urine output of children who are dehydrated or at risk of becoming dehydrated. Adequate urine output is 1 to 3 mL/kg/h for infants and 1 to 2 mL/kg for children. If a child has inadequate urine output, a fluid bolus or an increase in IV fluids may be necessary to prevent further dehydration. Obtaining the child's weight, sometimes twice a day, is necessary to assess for fluid loss and gain.

Prevention of dehydration can be attained through astute nursing care and teaching. Reduce insensible water loss by using a humidified, warm incubator instead of an infant warmer with radiant heat. If a radiant warmer must be used, monitor the infant's temperature to prevent overheating and resultant dehydration. Careful management of the child with a high or prolonged fever is also necessary to reduce insensible fluid losses and prevent dehydration. Teach parents to prevent overheating of infants by selecting appropriate clothes for the humidity and temperature. Also teach parents about car safety in hot weather, including keeping automobiles locked when not in use and never leaving a child unattended in a car for any length of time during hot or humid weather. Educate families on proper amounts of fluid for their children to take in during warm or hot days or when they are physically active during excessively hot periods.

Disruption of electrolyte balance is another common complication of gastrointestinal disorders, including omphalocele, Meckel diverticulum, NEC, and pyloric stenosis. Vomiting and gastrointestinal bleeding, as occurs with Meckel diverticulum, may result in an alteration in electrolytes, particularly sodium, potassium, and chloride, in addition to dehydration and anemia. Electrolytes can also become imbalanced when acidosis is present, such as may occur in NEC, or when they are removed due to the use of a nasogastric (NG) tube with low wall suction. Electrolyte imbalances are common in infants with pyloric stenosis. Gastric fluid is high in potassium, and frequent vomiting can lead to hypokalemia. Hyponatremia and hypochloremia are also common with this condition. Metabolic alkalosis occurs secondary to the loss of hydrochloric acid with emesis. When working with children with any of these conditions, monitor for signs of electrolyte disturbances and notify the provider of any concerning findings. IV replacement of electrolytes, including sodium, chloride, and potassium, may be necessary.

Some gastrointestinal disorders require restriction of intake of liquids or certain nutrients, which may worsen the condition, or of the amount consumed. For example, a low-sodium, low-protein diet with fluid restriction is necessary when **ascites** is present, such as may occur with cirrhosis. When fluid restriction is necessary, minimize the child's desire to drink by removing water pitches, cups, and straws from the child's sight. Educate parents and visitors on the need for fluid restriction and ask them to speak with the nurse before offering the child fluids. With peptic ulcer disease, instruct children and families to exclude any foods that exacerbate the disorder. Children with celiac disease require a diet free of gluten. Those with irritable bowel syndrome should limit fiber intake, which can worsen the condition. In the case of many gastrointestinal disorders, such as gastroesophageal reflux disease (GERD) and irritable bowel syndrome, children can only tolerate smaller, more frequent feedings.

For many children with gastrointestinal disorders, the biggest challenge is ensuring that they take in enough calories to meet their growth and development needs. When anorexia is present and the child is not consuming adequate calories, supplementation with high-calorie shakes or drinks or administration of enteral or even parenteral feedings may be necessary. For infants, higher–calorie concentration formulas are available to help increase caloric intake without increasing overall fluid intake. Powder supplements that can be mixed with regular formula to increase caloric intake are also available. Refer children who are having difficulty growing without increased calories to a dietician or nutritionist.

Many gastrointestinal disorders require that children with liver conditions, such as biliary atresia or hepatitis, be offered a high-protein, high-carbohydrate diet and may require administration of vitamins A, D, E, and K, because absorption of these vitamins is impaired when liver dysfunction is present. Children with omphalocele also require a high-protein diet, because protein losses are increased in this condition.

Positioning of the child during feeding is also important. In addition to avoiding aspiration, placing the child in a more upright position can improve feeding tolerance and avoid exacerbating certain conditions, such as GERD. In general, keep the head of the bed elevated or hold the child in an upright position during and after feedings. Avoid placing the infant in a seated position, such as an infant seat, because this increases abdominal pressure and promotes reflux. Although prone positioning decreases reflux, encourage parents to avoid positioning the infant prone because the increase in risk for sudden infant death syndrome.

Maintain Skin Integrity

Alterations caused by some gastrointestinal disorders make children's skin and other tissues more vulnerable to injury and breakdown. In omphalocele, the internal organs are eviscerated in a sac through a defect in the abdominal wall, exposing these delicate tissues to the environment. Handle this defect gently and as little as possible to prevent damage to the herniated viscera and sac. To avoid accidental injury, place the umbilical cord clamp away from the sac. Position the infant in a manner that avoids compression of the viscera. Side-lying is often the preferred position.

Cover the defect in sterile saline-soaked gauze and wrap it in plastic wrap or place it in a sterile, clear bowel bag.

In esophageal atresia, irritable bowel disease, and acute gastroenteritis (AGE), excessive moisture can result in breakdown of the skin. In esophageal atresia, before surgery, the infant may have large amounts of oral secretions, which can drain onto the neck and create a moist environment. Assess skin folds on anterior and posterior neck frequently. Keep the skin clean and dry. Also monitor the integrity of the skin on the cheeks and face where the NG or orogastric drainage tube is secured (this tube is necessary until after surgical repair to keep the esophageal pouch drained of secretions and reduce risk of aspiration).

For children with frequent diarrhea, as occurs with irritable bowel disease and AGE, breakdown of skin on the buttocks and perianal area often occurs. Keep the skin clean and dry. For younger children, change diapers or soiled underpants every 2 hours or more frequently. Assess the skin of the perineum and rectum for signs of skin breakdown with each diaper change or bowel movement. Wash the area with warm water and mild soaps or use alcohol-free, fragrance-free wipes after each soiling episode. Avoid soaps with fragrances, because these can be irritating. Apply a barrier cream or ointment to the skin after each episode of diarrhea. If the skin becomes irritated, leave the buttocks open to air for periods of time throughout the day. Air circulation helps prevent moisture accumulation. For older children, bathe in the tub daily in tepid, not hot, water. Pat the area dry. Bathing loosens stool adhering to the skin without requiring scrubbing or rubbing, which can cause additional irritation. Allow children to not wear underpants; this promotes air circulation and prevents moisture accumulation.

Any condition that causes excessive itching can also threaten skin integrity due to scratching. In biliary atresia, for example, as the disease progresses, the child may experience intense itching from accumulation of toxins (cholesterol and bile acids) in the skin. Xanthomas, yellow patches, or nodules on the skin, may appear. Tepid baths may relieve itching. Pat the skin dry, because rubbing causes further irritation. Moisturize skin with lotions. Covering the child's hands with mittens or socks is helpful to reduce the potential for irritating skin by scratching. Monitor open areas for infection and bleeding. Ursodeoxycholic acid (Actigall) is used to lower cholesterol levels but does not directly relieve pruritus.

Surgery related to a gastrointestinal disorder poses a challenge to skin integrity, as well. After surgery to repair an anorectal malformation, for instance, care centers on protection of the surgical site. As ordered, place a urinary catheter to protect the anal opening from urine. Perform dressing changes at the surgical site and keep the site clean and dry. Once the first stool is passed, the perineal and anal skin is at high risk for breakdown. Use barrier creams to protect the skin.

Prevent Infection

Some gastrointestinal disorders, such as NEC and hepatitis, are caused by infection with a microorganism. In such cases, nursing priorities include treating the infection itself (administering antibiotics as ordered) as well as preventing transmission of the infection to others and educating parents on preventing future infections. Children with NEC are placed in strict enteric precautions to prevent the spread of infection to other children on the unit. Encourage hand washing by parents and visitors. Take care to maintain aseptic technique when accessing the child's central venous access catheter. Perform dressing changes using sterile technique. In the case of hepatitis A and B, vaccines are available. Inform parents that hepatitis A vaccines are generally given at the age of 1 year. The vaccine requires two shots, 6 months apart. Hepatitis B vaccines are given in three to four shots over a 6-month period. Infants are given the first dose at birth and complete the regimen by 6 months of age. Also encourage parents to take additional preventative measures such as meticulous hand washing before handling food and after using the toilet.

Other gastrointestinal disorders, such as omphalocele, biliary atresia, and short bowel syndrome, make children more vulnerable to infections. Children with omphalocele (a condition involving internal organs eviscerating in a sac through the umbilical cord) are at increased risk of infection related to unavoidable exposure of the defect to environmental organisms. When caring for such children, use sterile gloves and sterile dressings when handling the defect and keep it contained in a sterile bag or with sterile saline-soaked gauze to reduce the risk of infection. Teach parents proper hand washing techniques, as well.

Children with biliary atresia are at increased risk for infection related to a compromised immune system. These children should avoid sick contacts, practice meticulous hand hygiene, and get adequate rest. Meticulous care of the child's central venous access catheter is essential. The child may require prolonged TPN, in which case the central line is a life-line for nutrition for the child until liver transplantation can occur. Likewise, the child with short bowel syndrome is at increased risk for infection because of altered gut flora and central line access, if present.

Children are also vulnerable to infection following surgical interventions for gastrointestinal disorders, such as repair of a cleft lip or palate and central line access for TPN. In such cases, assess the surgical site frequently for signs of infection, such as tenderness, redness, inflammation, increased secretions and drainage, or presence of pus. Clean suture lines with normal saline or sterile water to reduce the presence of bacteria. Give 5 to 10 mL of water to the child after each feeding, which helps prevent the accumulation of carbohydrates, which can encourage bacterial growth. Practice meticulous hand hygiene when caring for the child, particularly when caring for the suture line. Do not allow the child to use a pacifier after surgery, because sucking can irritate and disrupt the suture line, altering tissue integrity and leading to infection and poor healing.

Promote Pain Relief, Comfort, and Rest

Pain frequently results from gastrointestinal disorders. When caring for children experiencing pain, assess their pain level frequently with a developmentally appropriate pain scale and use both nonpharmacological and pharmacological interventions to address the pain. Nonpharmacological measures include the following:

- Providing a dark, quiet environment and minimizing interruptions
- Allowing parents to hold and comfort the child
- Allowing the child to have toys, blankets, and other comfort items within reach
- Providing massage or soft music
- Moistening the mouth with wet wash cloths or sponges regularly
- Moistening the mouth with ice chips, if allowed
- Placing the child in a position of comfort, such as side-lying on the right with knees bent or with the bed elevated

Administer medications for pain as ordered, which may range from mild analgesics such as acetaminophen to narcotics such as morphine or fentanyl, and document relief from pain. Postoperatively, children may require stronger pain medications, including narcotics and IV pain medications, to adequately relieve pain.

Promoting rest is also important in the acute phases of some gastrointestinal disorders, such as viral hepatitis. Fatigue and malaise force most children to voluntarily limit their activities during the initial phase of the illness. Offer the child age-appropriate diversional activities that require minimal effort and energy. Activities that can be done from the bed or chair, such as board games, coloring, small crafts, and reading are appropriate during the acute phase when rest is most important.

Administer and Manage Medications

A wide range of medications are used to treat gastrointestinal disorders, from antibiotics to treat appendicitis, peptic ulcer disease, and inflammatory bowel disease to analgesics to treat procedural and disease-related pain, antiemetics to treat vomiting, laxatives to treat constipation, and proton pump inhibitors to treat GERD and peptic ulcer disease. See The Pharmacy features throughout the chapter for details on specific medications.

Provide Emotional and Psychosocial Support to the Child and Parents

Whether acute or chronic, gastrointestinal disorders disrupt the lives of children and parents and pose significant emotional and psychosocial challenges. For many children, developing an acute gastrointestinal disorder, such as appendicitis, severe dehydration, intussusception, or volvulus, leads to their first hospitalization, and anxiety and fear are common. Chronic diseases such as inflammatory bowel disease can require difficult lifestyle changes such as use of colostomies and concerns over body image. Congenital anomalies such as cleft lip or palate and esophageal atresia can be overwhelming because of the emotional strain of a disfiguring condition and the multiple healthcare visits and procedures required for their repair. Receiving a diagnosis of a potentially fatal disorder, such as congenital diaphragmatic hernia (CDH), biliary atresia, or cirrhosis, can be devastating for parents.

When caring for a child with a gastrointestinal disorder, provide the child and family with emotional and psychosocial support by doing the following:

- Offer clear and concise explanations of conditions, procedures, and hospital routines.
- Give parents time to ask questions, express frustrations, and process information.
- Encourage parents to keep a journal or log of their child's care and write down questions.
- Help parents view their child as a whole person rather than focusing solely on the defect.
- Allow time for parents to touch, hold, cuddle, talk to, and bond with their child.
- Encourage parents to participate in care when possible such as feeding and bathing.
- Give parents resources on helping the child keep up with academic work.

Structural Anomalies of the Gastrointestinal Tract

Structural anomalies of the gastrointestinal tract include cleft lip and palate, Meckel diverticulum, omphalocele, gastroschisis, hernias, anorectal malformations, CDH (umbilical and inguinal), and transesophageal fistula/esophageal atresia. Although the structural anomaly can often be successfully repaired, complications from the anomaly or surgical repair can result in long-term, chronic problems.

Cleft Lip and Palate

Cleft lip and cleft palate are two separate facial defects that can occur singly or in combination. Cleft lip with or without a cleft palate is the most common craniofacial birth defect. Both defects require surgical repair to optimize nutrition and efficiency of feeding, reduce risk of infections, and promote speech development.

Etiology and Pathophysiology

During fetal development, the lip and palate normally form during the first 30 to 60 days of gestation. A cleft develops when something interferes with the normal processes of fusion of the frontonasal and maxillary processes of the face. Instead of growing together to form a normal lip and palate, the tissues remain separate, causing a cleft to form. Although the cause of cleft lip or palate is not known, genetics, folic acid deficiency, advanced maternal or paternal age, use of anticonvulsants, use of alcohol, and smoking appear to be contributing factors.

Cleft lip results when the developing tissues of the lip do not completely fuse, dividing the lip into two parts. A malalignment of the lip muscles results. A cleft lip primarily involves the upper lip (Fig. 23.2). Rarely, facial clefting can involve the lower lip. Typically, cleft lip involves the nose, resulting in distorted nostrils and nasal sill.

Cleft palate involves the hard and soft palates, or roof of the mouth. The teeth erupt in the anterior hard palate, and the posterior hard palate serves as the base of the nasal cavity. The soft palate, composed of muscles important for speech and proper function of the eustachian tubes, lies in the posterior roof of the mouth. Cleft palate may involve the soft palate only or the soft and hard palates.

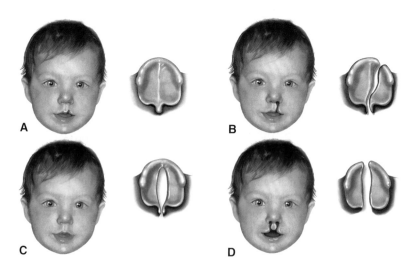

Figure 23.2. Cleft lip and palate. Cleft lip can be small and unilateral, affecting only the lip itself **(A)**, or extend all the way through the vermillion border and up into the nostril, either unilaterally **(B)** or bilaterally **(D)**, and be accompanied by cleft palate. Cleft palate can also occur independent of cleft lip **(C)**. Reprinted with permission from Kyle, T., & Carman, S. (2016). *Essentials of pediatric nursing* (3rd ed., Fig. 20.4). Philadelphia, PA: Wolters Kluwer.

The most common presentation is a left-sided unilateral cleft lip with cleft palate (Fig. 23.2B). Boys are affected more often than are girls. Most infants with cleft lip or palate are otherwise healthy and have normal intellectual development. However, 25% of infants with cleft lip or palate have additional anomalies such as neurological and cardiac anomalies and club foot. Cleft lip or palate occurs in approximately 1 in 600 to 700 live births (Rahimov, Jugessur, & Murray, 2012). American Indian, Alaskan Native, and Asian infants have a higher incidence than do Caucasian or African American infants (Lewis, Jacob, & Lehmann, 2017). The incidence is also increased in families with a prior history of cleft lip or palate.

Complications associated with cleft lip or palate include feeding difficulties, otological manifestations such as otitis media, dental and orthodontic complications, and difficulty with speech development (Lewis et al., 2017). Table 23.3 reviews these complications, the etiology of each, and appropriate nursing interventions.

Clinical Presentation

Initially, the child presents with a deformity of the lip and/or palate, which often can be seen on a fetal ultrasound. A cleft lip defect is noted at birth. Cleft palate is discovered during the newborn physical exam by palpation of the palate with the finger.

Assessment and Diagnosis

Knowing the location and extent of the defect is helpful in determining the correct method of feeding. A complete and thorough physical exam is necessary because additional defects are sometimes present when a cleft lip or palate is present.

Assessment should include not only the gastrointestinal system but also the cardiovascular, respiratory, renal, and integumentary systems, which can also be affected by a structural defect and develop complications during the postoperative phase of care. Tachycardia, delayed capillary refill, and decreased peripheral pulses can indicate inadequate fluid intake, a common problem for infants with a cleft lip or palate. Closely assess the skin for signs of breakdown. Moisture is common under the neck in babies with a cleft lip or palate because of increased secretions and frequent drooling.

Therapeutic Interventions

Cleft lip is generally repaired when the child is between the age of 2 and 6 months. A cheiloplasty is the primary cleft lip repair. A cheiloplasty involves reconstructing the muscles of the sphincter, adding length to and creating symmetry in the upper lip, and improving the symmetry and function of the nasal passages. Early repair of the lip enables the infant to form a better seal on a nipple and thus improves feeding efficiency. Advances

Table 23.3 Complications of Cleft Lip and/or Cleft Palate

Complication/Etiology	Nursing Interventions
Feeding and gastrointestinal • Inability to suck on a bottle or breast • Abdominal distension and gastrointestinal distress due to excess air taken in	• Refer to a speech pathologist, occupational therapist, or nurse specialist for assessment of sucking and recommendations for special nipples. • Refer to a lactation consultant for assistance in breastfeeding or pumping for mothers who wish to provide breast milk. • Feed the baby in an upright position and burp frequently. • Monitor weight and length to assess adequacy of nutrition and growth.
Otological • Otitis media with effusion (90% before age 1 y; Lewis et al., 2017) due to eustachian tube dysfunction • Mild-to-moderate hearing loss due to frequent otitis media	• Teach families ways to prevent ear infections. • Provide pre- and postoperative teaching on tympanoplasty, if needed. • Monitor for ear infections; teach families signs and symptoms of an ear infection and to seek treatment for infections. • Encourage families to finish antibiotic regimens when prescribed. • Recommend routine audiology screenings.
Dental and orthodontic • Abnormal pattern of tooth eruption (small, missing, or pointed teeth) due to a malformed palate • Delayed primary tooth eruption	• Refer to a dentist specializing in cleft lip and palate. • Teach caregivers to provide good oral hygiene. • Encourage tooth brushing early, upon eruption of first tooth. • Encourage a low-sugar diet. • Encourage families to ensure fluoridated water or give fluoride supplements.
Speech Impaired speech due to a malformed palate and dentition and hearing loss caused by recurrent otitis media	• Refer to a speech pathologist. • Assess language and speech development with each well-child visit.

in surgical techniques have allowed for much less scarring after the surgical repair (Fig. 23.3).

Cleft palate repair does not usually take place until the child is between the age of 9 and 18 months. A palatoplasty is performed to close the connection between the oral and nasal cavities and to reconstruct palate musculature. Because the palatoplasty is essential for normal speech development, its timing is an important consideration (Lewis et al., 2017).

Nursing care of the child with a cleft lip or palate is focused on feeding, maintaining adequate nutritional intake, preventing aspiration and infection, helping parents cope with an infant with a birth defect, preoperative and postoperative care, and assisting parents to maintain a healthy home environment.

The greatest concern for an infant with a cleft lip or palate is the ingestion of adequate calories and fluids to maintain hydration and allow for proper growth. An infant with a cleft palate does not have the ability to build up enough pressure inside the mouth to propel the liquid into the back of the mouth while sucking.

Therefore, a child with a cleft lip or palate requires a unique approach to feeding to ensure adequate calories are obtained while risk of aspiration and respiratory compromise is reduced. Instruct mothers who are breastfeeding to plug the cleft lip/palate while the baby is nursing and to elicit the letdown reflex before nursing so the baby does not have to initially suck harder to produce milk letdown. La Leche League promotes breastfeeding and can be a supportive resource for mothers who wish to breastfeed.

Instruct parents who are bottle-feeding to place the nipple of the bottle against the inside of the cheek, toward the back of the tongue. Recommend to the parents use of nipples designed for premature infants, which are slightly longer, larger, and softer than regular nipples and make it much easier for the baby to suck.

Instruct all parents to hold the infant in an upright position during feeding to facilitate swallowing and minimize the amount of formula or milk that returns from the nose and into the eustachian tubes. Box 23.2 lists strategies for feeding an infant with a cleft lip or palate. Special feeding devices that can

Box 23.2 Strategies for Feeding an Infant with a Cleft Lip or Palate

- Feed the infant with the head upright at a 45° angle.
- Use a nipple made for premature infants (larger opening) or cut an X in the tip of a regular nipple. The larger opening allows more liquid to flow out of the nipple with less suction.
- Use a squeezable bottle to facilitate getting liquid into the infant's mouth.
- Refer to a pediatric orthodontist to have an obturator made. An obturator is an appliance made to fit in the infant's mouth to cover the cleft that improves the infant's ability to suck and ingest calories without expending excess energy.
- Recommend special feeding devices, which may be beneficial for some infants (Fig. 23.4).

help the infant take in adequate fluid and calories are also available. Figure 23.4 shows examples of adaptive feeding devices for use with infants with a cleft lip or palate.

See the section Maintain Adequate Hydration and Nutrition, earlier, for guidelines on assessing fluid and calorie intake, weight, and growth and development.

As discussed, in Maintain Effective Ventilation and Oxygenation, infants with a cleft lip or palate are at increased risk for aspiration. Implement aspiration precautions with these infants, frequently assessing them for respiratory distress and vital sign changes that indicate aspiration, keeping suction equipment immediately available, holding them upright for feedings, and burping them frequently during feedings. Postoperatively, assess for patency of the airways, monitor respirations and heart rate, suction the nasopharynx gently as needed, and reposition the infant frequently, at least every 2 hours, to allow expansion of lung fields.

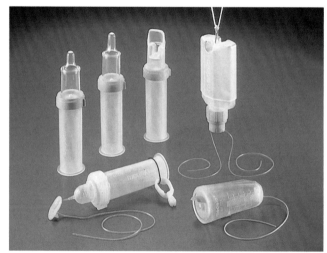

Figure 23.4. Feeding devices used for infants with cleft lip or cleft palate. Reprinted with permission from Kyle, T., & Carman, S. (2016). *Essentials of pediatric nursing* (3rd ed., Fig. 20.6a). Philadelphia, PA: Wolters Kluwer.

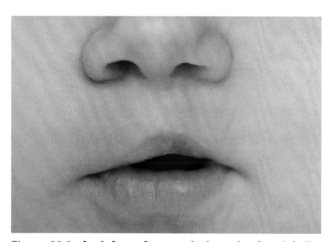

Figure 23.3. An infant after surgical repair of a cleft lip. Scarring above the lip is minimized.

The infant is also at increased risk for infection at the surgical site following repair of a cleft lip or palate. Therefore, implement measures to reduce the risk of infection when working with these infants, as described in the section Prevent Infection. These include assessing the oral cavity frequently for signs of infection, cleaning suture lines with normal saline or sterile water, giving water to the infant after each feeding to help prevent the accumulation of carbohydrates, not allowing pacifiers, and meticulous hand hygiene.

Assess the child's pain level frequently and provide nonpharmacological and pharmacological interventions to relieve pain as ordered and appropriate (see the section Promote Pain Relief, Comfort, and Rest, earlier). Adequate pain management minimizes crying, which is important because crying can cause stress on the suture line, thus altering tissue integrity.

For guidelines on addressing families' emotional and psychological needs related to gastrointestinal disorders, see the section Provide Emotional and Psychosocial Support to the Child and Parents, earlier.

Evaluation

Expected outcomes for an infant with a cleft lip or palate include the following:

- The infant maintains adequate nutritional intake and gains weight appropriately.
- The infant exhibits no signs of respiratory distress or respiratory infection.
- The infant remains free of infection in the oral cavity.
- The family demonstrates the ability to cope with and manage the infant's care.
- The infant's pain is controlled.
- The parents demonstrate proper feeding techniques.

Discharge Planning and Teaching

Begin to address the infant's home care needs well before discharge. Involve the parents in their infant's care well in advance of discharge, as well, to increase their comfort in caring for their child with unique needs at home. Early parental involvement in care also promotes bonding. Refer the parents to social services, as needed, for financial assistance, because private insurance does not always cover all costs of necessary care, such as special feeders and special formulas.

Parents may need assistance in preparing siblings for the arrival of the infant in the home. The infant will need more attention at home, and sibling rivalry is common as a result. Encourage parents to set limits with siblings, provide one-on-one times with each child, and involve siblings in the infant's care when possible. A child life specialist can be helpful in providing pictures, talking with siblings, and preparing siblings for the arrival of their new baby brother or sister.

Follow-up with a home healthcare agency may be a helpful support for parents. Encourage parents to keep follow-up appointments. Speech therapy may be necessary to help with speech development. Recommendations for plastic surgery in the future may also be warranted. Also, the infant will need regular assessment for the presence of ear infections.

Teaching topics include feeding techniques, proper positioning of the infant, how to recognize signs of infection, and how to care for the suture line. Preventing the infant from touching the suture line can be a challenge for parents. Teach parents how to bundle the infant with arms tucked in and how to use a front-sling baby carrier, which also helps immobilize the arms.

Meckel Diverticulum

Meckel diverticulum is an outpouching of the lower segment of the small intestine. Only a small percentage of people with this congenital defect become symptomatic and need surgical removal.

Etiology and Pathophysiology

Meckel diverticulum is a remnant of the embryonic yolk sac. This remnant is also referred to as the omphalomesenteric duct or vitelline duct. The omphalomesenteric duct connects the yolk sac to the gut in a developing embryo, providing nutrition until the placenta is established. Between the fifth and seventh weeks of gestation, the duct normally becomes thin and separates from the intestine. Failure to separate, be it partial or complete, results in residual structures, the most common being Meckel diverticulum. Two to three percent of all infants are born with Meckel diverticulum. In fact, Meckel diverticulum is the most common birth defect of the digestive system. Typically, a Meckel diverticulum is a 3- to 6-cm outpouching of the ileum about 50 to 75 cm from the ileocecal valve (Fig. 23.5). There is an increased incidence of Meckel diverticulum in children with other congenital anomalies, such as imperforate anus, esophageal atresia, Crohn disease, omphalocele, and various cardiovascular and neurological anomalies.

Clinical Presentation

Most children with Meckel diverticulum are asymptomatic and do not have any related problems. Many children who do develop symptoms are asymptomatic for the first year of life.

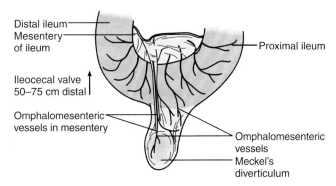

Figure 23.5. Meckel diverticulum. There is an outpouching of the ileum off of the small intestine. Modified with permission from Lawrence, P. F. (2018). *Essentials of general surgery and surgical specialties* (6th ed., Fig. 14.9). Philadelphia, PA: Wolters Kluwer.

Symptoms usually arise during the first or second year of life. The most common symptom is painless rectal bleeding. The stool is brick colored or currant jelly (red) colored. Small ulcers may form in the intestinal lining and can rupture or bleed, leading to peritonitis because of leakage into the peritoneal cavity. Meckel diverticulum can also be associated with partial or complete bowel obstruction. The diverticulum acts as the lead point of an intussusception. Younger patients usually present with obstruction. A Meckel diverticulum that becomes inflamed (diverticulitis) manifests similarly to acute appendicitis. Children with diverticulitis are often older, with a mean age of 8 years.

Assessment and Diagnosis

Assessment of the child with suspected Meckel diverticulum includes a thorough abdominal and gastrointestinal assessment. The child usually presents with bloody stool, abdominal pain and distension, and nausea and vomiting. Parents also report irritability and fatigue. Fever can also be present (Francis et al., 2016).

Diagnostic testing depends on the presentation. Laboratory tests to assess for electrolyte imbalances, dehydration, and anemia are typically performed. Imaging studies are also used to help diagnosis Meckel diverticulum. An abdominal X-ray, ultrasound, computed tomography (CT) scan, and radionuclide testing can all be used to confirm the presence of Meckel diverticulum. A Meckel scan is the imaging method of choice for a bleeding diverticulum. A radioactive substance called technetium, which is preferentially absorbed by stomach tissue, is injected intravenously. Technetium can be seen on X-rays and indicates areas where acid-secreting stomach tissue exists, including that seen in the Meckel diverticulum.

Therapeutic Interventions

Treatment for a symptomatic Meckel diverticulum is surgical resection. The mass can be removed via several different surgical techniques, including laparoscopy, double-balloon enteroscopy, and exploratory laparotomy with surgical resection.

Nursing care of Meckel diverticulum is similar to that for a child with appendicitis requiring surgical removal. Priorities of care include monitoring intake and output, monitoring for bleeding, fluid and electrolyte management, and postoperative care of the child undergoing abdominal surgery, including providing pain comfort measures.

As discussed in the section Maintain Adequate Hydration and Nutrition, earlier, vomiting and gastrointestinal bleeding may result in dehydration, anemia, and an alteration in electrolytes. Carefully measure urine output and administer IV fluids as ordered to achieve and maintain hydration. The child is NPO for surgery.

Monitoring blood loss from the rectum is a priority until the child undergoes surgical removal of the diverticulum. Stools are tested for occult blood when no obvious signs of blood are present in the stool. Occult blood is blood that is present in such small quantities that it is measurable only by laboratory testing.

A child with symptomatic Meckel diverticulum may present with signs of dehydration, anemia, and electrolyte imbalance.

As ordered, administer IV fluids to maintain hydration while the child is NPO, including fluid boluses of normal saline or lactated Ringer's to correct volume depletion. Be prepared to administer packed red blood cells, which may be ordered if the child is bleeding excessively or has a low hematocrit and hemoglobin. Replacement of electrolytes such as potassium is often necessary, as well.

Assess the child's pain level frequently and provide nonpharmacological and pharmacological interventions to relieve pain as ordered and appropriate (see the section Promote Pain Relief, Comfort, and Rest, earlier).

Evaluation

Expected outcomes for a child with Meckel diverticulum include the following:

- Electrolytes are within normal limits.
- The child achieves and maintains adequate fluid balance.
- Postoperative pain is adequately controlled.
- The abdominal wound heals without signs of infection.

Discharge Planning and Teaching

Discharge planning and teaching for Meckel diverticulum is similar to that for the child with appendicitis. See the discussion of appendicitis.

Omphalocele

Omphalocele is a congenital defect of the abdominal wall in which the internal organs eviscerate in a sac through the umbilical cord, covered by a three-layered membrane made of peritoneum, Wharton jelly, and amnion. The sac usually contains the small intestine, colon, and spleen and sometimes contains the gonads (Fig. 23.6).

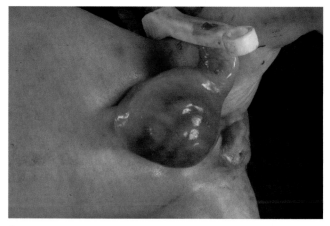

Figure 23.6. Omphalocele. Note the sac covering the abdominal contents and the umbilical cord inserting in the midline of the omphalocele. Reprinted with permission from Husain, A. N., Stocker, J. T., & Dehner, L. P. (2015). *Stocker and Dehner's pediatric pathology* (4th ed., Fig. 14.14). Philadelphia, PA: Wolters Kluwer.

Etiology and Pathophysiology

Omphalocele is a result of the failure of bowel loops to return to the abdominal cavity following physiological herniation of the umbilical cord between weeks 6 and 11 of fetal development. An omphalocele that is at least 4.5 to 5 cm and contains the liver is considered a giant omphalocele. The prevalence of omphalocele is approximately 1 per 3,000 to 4,000 live births in Western countries (Gamba & Midrio, 2014). About 775 babies in the United States are born each year with omphalocele.

Maternal risk factors for having a baby with an omphalocele include consuming alcohol, smoking more than 1 pack per day, or taking selective serotonin-reuptake inhibitors during pregnancy or being overweight or obese before or during pregnancy.

Clinical Presentation

The diagnosis of omphalocele is often made during a routine ultrasound in pregnancy. Diagnosis can also be made immediately upon delivery of the infant. There is a lack of evidence supporting cesarean section over vaginal delivery when a fetus has been diagnosed with omphalocele. Unlike those with gastroschisis, infants with omphalocele are often born full term. Immediately upon delivery, assess the infant for respiratory distress and cardiovascular stability. There is a high risk of cardiac defects associated with omphalocele. Therefore, a cardiac evaluation including auscultation, four-extremity blood pressure measurements, and peripheral pulse comparison is essential following birth. Respiratory instability (tachypnea, hypoxia, and respiratory distress) may be present as a result of unsuspected pulmonary hypoplasia, which is often found in infants with omphalocele (Gamba & Midrio, 2014). Upon delivery, dress the omphalocele with saline-soaked gauze and an impermeable dressing to minimize fluid and temperature loss and to protect the sac itself. Place an NG or orogastric tube to decompress the stomach.

Assessment and Diagnosis

Monitor urine output frequently, because increased abdominal pressure can lead to decreased perfusion to the kidneys and to kidney failure. Monitor skin and mucosal membranes for adequate moisture in cases of omphalocele and gastroschisis.

Therapeutic Interventions

Nursing care of the child with an omphalocele focuses on protecting the protruding organs and sac, preventing hypothermia, preventing infection, and providing preoperative and postoperative care, including providing comfort measures and nutritional support. Supporting the family members through the phases of care and learning to care for their child with a deformative condition is essential.

As described in the section Maintain Skin Integrity, handle the defect gently and as little as possible to prevent damage to the herniated viscera and sac, place the umbilical cord clamp away from the sac, position the child in side-lying, and cover the defect with sterile gauze or a sterile bag.

Administer antibiotics as prescribed. As noted in the section Prevent Infection, earlier, the infant is at increased risk of infection related to unavoidable exposure of the defect to environmental organisms. Use sterile gloves and sterile dressings when handling the defect, keeping it contained in a sterile bag or with sterile saline-soaked gauze, and teach parents proper hand washing techniques.

Assess the child's pain level frequently and provide nonpharmacological and pharmacological interventions to relieve pain as ordered and appropriate (see the section Promote Pain Relief, Comfort, and Rest, earlier).

As discussed in the section Maintain Adequate Hydration and Nutrition, earlier, fluid, electrolyte, and protein losses are increased in the infant with omphalocele. Fluids and electrolytes are lost through the NG tube drainage and from the intestines, with the greatest losses occurring if the sac ruptures. The infant is also NPO. Reduce insensible water loss by using a humidified, warm incubator. Establish IV access, administer IV fluids, and closely monitor urine output for adequacy (1–3 mL/kg is desired).

Monitor the infant's temperature hourly and strive to maintain a normothermic temperature. Avoid hypothermia, because it leads to vasoconstriction and decreased tissue perfusion. Heat is lost through the sac and exposed abdominal contents, particularly if the sac ruptures. Also avoid hyperthermia, because increased temperature causes increased insensible water losses. Keep the infant dry. Use a humidified incubator to maintain a normothermic environment.

Evaluation

Expected outcomes for a child with an omphalocele include the following:

- Organs and other tissues remain free of injury preceding surgery.
- Fluid balance is maintained.
- The infant's pain is effectively controlled.
- The patient's body temperature (thermoregulation) is maintained.
- The child is free of signs of infection.
- Parents demonstrate appropriate coping mechanisms.

Discharge Planning and Teaching

Infants being treated for an omphalocele are often hospitalized for an extended period of time. Because bowel motility and function are often delayed for weeks after surgery, the child remains hospitalized and receives TPN for nutritional support. Introduce feeds once bowel function returns. Give parents resources, including home care referrals, to assist them in providing care at home.

Gastroschisis

Gastroschisis is a life-threatening congenital malformation of the abdominal wall in which the intestines are outside the body via a hole beside the umbilicus (Fig. 23.7).

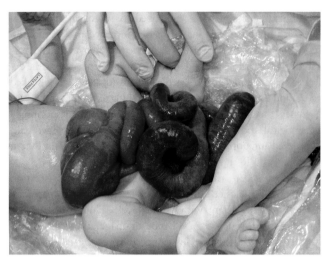

Figure 23.7. Gastroschisis. The organs exit the abdomen to the side of the umbilicus. There is no sac covering the organs, as in an omphalocele. Reprinted with permission from MacDonald, M. G., & Seshia, M. M. (2015). *Avery's neonatology* (7th ed., 41.22). Philadelphia, PA: Wolters Kluwer.

Etiology and Pathophysiology

Gastroschisis occurs early in fetal development when the abdominal muscles do not form correctly. The cause of gastroschisis is unknown. The organs exiting the body, which may include the intestines, stomach, and liver, are not covered in a protective sac and are exposed to amniotic fluid. Table 23.4 compares the characteristics of gastroschisis and omphalocele. This exposure can cause irritation, causing the intestine to twist, shorten, or become edematous.

Mothers of neonates with gastroschisis are often young. One-third of newborns with gastroschisis were born to teenage mothers (Allman et al., 2016). Women who consume alcohol or tobacco products during pregnancy are also more likely to have a child with gastroschisis. Infants with gastroschisis are more likely to be born premature and small for gestational age. Gastroschisis is associated with significant morbidity and mortality. The mortality rate is slightly below 10% (Youssef, Cheong & Emil, 2016). Common morbidities of gastroschisis include

feeding intolerance, NEC, failure to thrive, and prolonged hospitalization (Allman et al., 2016).

Clinical Presentation

Gastroschisis is diagnosed via ultrasound during pregnancy or immediately upon delivery.

Therapeutic Interventions

There is no difference in mortality or complication rates of babies with gastroschisis born vaginally vs. cesarean section. However, infants born with gastroschisis need prompt medical and nursing intervention upon delivery. The baby may be in respiratory distress upon exiting the birth canal. Placement of an endotracheal tube may be necessary to relieve respiratory distress. An NG tube is also placed to decompress the abdomen, which may reduce respiratory distress. The baby is at risk for fluid loss and requires fluid and electrolyte replacement.

Place the exposed intestines on the newborn's abdomen and cover them in a way that prevents traction on the bowel mesentery. The baby is likely to have difficulty with thermoregulation and is at risk for heat loss due to the large portion of abdominal contents outside the body. Placing the baby under a radiant warmer is necessary. A prompt surgical intervention in which the intestine is placed back in the abdominal cavity is also recommended for small defects. Larger defects require a staged surgical intervention, in which a small portion of the intestine and organs are placed in the abdominal cavity with each surgery.

Nursing care of a child with gastroschisis is similar to that for a child with omphalocele. See Therapeutic Interventions for the child with an omphalocele.

Anorectal Malformations

Anorectal malformations include imperforate anus (absence of an anal opening), cloacal malformations, and a wide spectrum of anomalies of the rectum, distal anus, urinary tract, and genital tract. Anorectal malformations are frequently associated with

Table 23.4   Comparison of Gastroschisis and Omphalocele Characteristics

Characteristic	Gastroschisis	Omphalocele
Defect diameter	2–3 cm	2–15 cm
Presence of a sac	Never	Always, but may be ruptured
Umbilical cord location	Adjacent to the defect (left side)	Attached to the sac
Malrotation	Yes	Yes
Bowel character	Inflamed, edematous	Normal
Enteral nutrition	Delayed	Normal
Additional anomalies	Uncommon	Common

anomalies of the musculoskeletal system and chromosomal abnormalities, such as trisomy 13, 18, or 21. Some infants with anorectal malformations may have vertebral, anorectal, cardiac, tracheal, esophageal, renal, radial, or limb (VACTERL) conditions.

Etiology and Pathophysiology

Several abnormalities can occur when an anorectal malformation is present. The anal passage may be stenotic or in front of where it is normally located (prolapsed). A membrane may cover the anal opening. The rectum may not connect to the anus (**atresia**). A fistula, or connection between two parts that are normally not connected, may be present. The rectum may connect to a part of the urinary tract or the reproductive system.

The exact cause of anorectal malformations is unknown. It is likely that the mutation of a variety of genes can result in anorectal malformations. Anorectal malformations have an incidence rate of 1 in 4,000 to 5,000 newborns (Iwai & Fumino, 2013). Cloacal anomalies occur exclusively in girls, at an incidence rate of 1 in 20,000 live births. Infants are rarely diagnosed prenatally. A thorough physical exam in the early newborn period can detect anomalies. The absence of an anal opening is an obvious sign of a malformation, whereas other malformations are identified after failed attempts at placing a rectal thermometer during the newborn period (Pandya, 2016).

Clinical Presentation

Newborns with an anorectal malformation are generally diagnosed in the first few days of life. Failure to pass meconium within the first 24 hours of birth may indicate an imperforate anus. When stool is present in urine, a fistula is suspected. Females may have cloacal malformations. A cloacal anomaly occurs when the rectum, vagina, and urethra form a common channel and present with one opening in the perineum.

Assessment and Diagnosis

During the newborn assessment, inspect the perineal area. Sacral anomalies and a poorly developed anal dimple are observed when anorectal malformations are present. Failure to pass meconium can indicate an anorectal malformation. Assess the infant for evidence of pain, particularly after surgery. Accurately measure and record the intake and output.

When an anorectal malformation is suspected, an abdominal–pelvic ultrasound and abdominal radiographs aid in diagnosis. A plain cross-table lateral X-ray with the infant lying prone is helpful in diagnosing some malformations. The X-ray is taken 24 hours after birth to allow time for bowel distension from swallowed air.

Therapeutic Interventions

Management of the malformation depends on its severity and the coexistence of other malformations. A simple anal stenosis may be treated nonsurgically with daily manual dilations. A surgical procedure called the posterior sagittal anorectoplasty

(PSARP) is commonly used to surgically correct anorectal malformations. This procedure is also known as a "pull-through" procedure. Timing of the surgery varies. Most infants have undergone surgical repair by 6 months of age. A temporary colostomy may be needed in the early newborn period and after surgery while the surgical site heals. Several weeks after surgery, infants need manual dilations until the anal opening is of adequate size. Colostomy takedown occurs 6 to 8 weeks after successful surgery and after the desired size of the anal opening has been achieved via dilations.

Nursing care of the infant with an anorectal malformation focuses on supporting the family and providing preoperative and postoperative care to the infant. Following a PSARP or any other surgical repair of an anorectal malformation, educate parents regarding axillary temperatures, colostomy care, and anal dilation (Priority Care Concepts 23.1).

Postoperatively, protect the surgical site by performing regular dressing changes and keeping the site clean and dry (see the section Maintain Skin Integrity, earlier). Administer antibiotics as prescribed to prevent infection.

Assess the child's pain level frequently and provide nonpharmacological and pharmacological interventions to relieve pain as ordered and appropriate (see the section Promote Pain Relief, Comfort, and Rest, earlier). Positioning the child off of the surgical site, often in a prone position, helps alleviate pain.

The infant is NPO until after surgical repair and return of bowel function. Place an NG tube and maintain to low-wall suction to decompress the stomach. Provide IV fluids or TPN until the infant is able to take breast milk or formula by mouth.

Evaluation

Expected outcomes for a child with an anorectal malformation include the following:

- The parents demonstrate effective coping with stress related to the child's condition and care.
- Fluid and electrolyte balance is maintained.
- Nutrition is adequate to achieve growth and development milestones.
- Surgical incisions heal without signs of infection.
- Adequate bowel function is achieved.
- Parents demonstrate an understanding of postoperative care, including ostomy care and dilation techniques.

Priority Care Concepts 23.1

Postoperative Care of a Child With an Anorectal Malformation

Following surgical repair for an anorectal malformation, the infant should have nothing placed in the rectum. Avoid taking the temperature or administering medications or enemas rectally.

Discharge Planning and Teaching

Caregivers need to be taught about a colostomy in cases where children have undergone a PSARP. Teaching points include emptying the colostomy bag, assessing and cleaning the site, and applying a new bag. Pediatric patients require smaller ostomy appliances than do adults. Special pediatric supplies are available for ostomy care and maintenance. Troubleshooting in the case of leakage or skin breakdown is essential. Caregivers should be able to recognize a normal-appearing stoma and an abnormal-appearing stoma and what steps to take if the stoma is abnormal.

Congenital Diaphragmatic Hernia

A CDH is a communication between the thoracic and abdominal cavities (Fig. 23.8). Abdominal contents may or may not be present in the thoracic cavity. The defect may be located at the esophageal hiatus, in the paraesophageal area, retrosternally, or in the posterolateral portion of the diaphragm.

Etiology and Pathophysiology

A CDH is caused by an incomplete fusion of the embryological elements that give rise to the diaphragm during fetal development. As a result of incomplete formation of the diaphragm, an opening or communication is present between the thoracic and abdominal cavities. The opening allows abdominal contents to enter the chest wall. The resulting communication between the thoracic and abdominal cavities leads to a compressed and often a hypoplastic lung.

The incidence rate is 1 in 2,000 to 5,000 live births. Females are twice as likely as males to be affected. Approximately 85% of CDHs are on the left side (Maheshwari & Carlo, 2017).

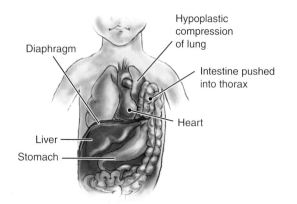

Figure 23.8. Congenital diaphragmatic hernia. The intestinal loops and part of the stomach are in the left pleural cavity. The heart and mediastinum are pushed to the right and the left lung is compressed. Reprinted with permission from Stephenson, S. R. (2012). *Obstetrics and gynecology* (3rd ed., Fig. 21.7). Philadelphia, PA: Wolters Kluwer.

Clinical Presentation

Shortly after birth, the newborn with a CDH experiences severe respiratory distress and can quickly progress to respiratory failure secondary to pulmonary hypoplasia. Tachypnea, grunting, use of accessory muscles, and cyanosis are characteristic signs of respiratory distress in the newborn with CDH. Crying worsens the respiratory distress as the abdominal organs push further into the thorax because of increased abdominal pressure, decreasing the ability of the lungs to expand. Dyspnea and cyanosis are present. Lung sounds are absent on the affected side. Heart sounds may be auscultated on the right side of the chest as a result of the heart being pushed to the right by the abdominal contents. Bowel sounds may be present in the lung fields. CDH is a life-threatening condition, and interventions to support respiratory function are implemented immediately after birth.

The infant is transferred to a neonatal intensive care unit (NICU) as soon as possible. The infant is intubated and placed on a ventilator to control respiratory function and treat respiratory failure. Conventional mechanical ventilation, high-frequency oscillation, and extracorporeal membrane oxygenation (ECMO) are the main methods used to support respiratory failure in the infant with CDH (Maheshwari & Carlo, 2017).

Once the infant has been stabilized, surgical repair can occur. Indicators of stability include use of a conventional ventilator to maintain adequate oxygenation and ventilation, low peak inspiratory pressures on the ventilator, and an oxygen requirement of less than 50% fraction of inspired oxygen (Maheshwari & Carlo, 2017). Infants should be stable for 48 hours before surgery.

Assessment and Diagnosis

Continuously monitor the infant's vital signs and frequently assess respiratory status. Remain vigilant for signs of respiratory compromise. Auscultate the lung fields for the presence of breath sounds and bowel sounds. Frequently monitor and assess heart rate and rhythm, because the infant is at risk for pulmonary hypertension and heart failure. Assess for altered mental status indicating a rising carbon dioxide level or decreasing oxygen level.

CDH can be diagnosed prenatally between 16 and 24 weeks of gestation using prenatal ultrasound in more than 50% of all cases (Maheshwari & Carlo, 2017). In the newborn, a chest X-ray is used to confirm the diagnosis.

Therapeutic Interventions

Nursing care of the child with CDH focuses on maintaining respiratory function via ventilatory support, providing preoperative and postoperative care, and supporting the parents and family through what may be a life-altering diagnosis.

Nursing care for the child with CDH involves critical care in a NICU. Parents and family members experience great stress related to admission to the NICU, emergency surgical intervention, and poor survival rates in children with CDH. Supportive care of the parents and family is essential in planning nursing care.

Continuously monitor the child via cardiorespiratory monitors and continuous pulse oximetry. Be alert to vital sign changes indicating respiratory changes. Be prepared to establish an arterial line and central venous access catheter for frequent laboratory tests and administration of fluids, vasoactive medications, and other medications to support blood pressure, treat pulmonary hypertension, and sedate the infant during the critical period. Promote decreased stimulation, which helps to keep the infant calm and abdominal pressures lower. Offer parents ongoing information and emotional support during this time.

Start IV fluids immediately to maintain hydration, as the infant is NPO for a long period of time. As the infant stabilizes, TPN is begun to provide adequate calories, fluids, and electrolytes for growth and healing.

The prognosis for CDH can be poor, particularly when a major anomaly is present and ECMO is needed to support the infant. Overall survival rate is 67% (Maheshwari & Carlo, 2017). Even when the infant survives, long-term complications and medical care can place stress on parents. For guidelines on addressing the families' emotional and psychological needs related to gastrointestinal disorders, see the section Provide Emotional and Psychosocial Support to the Child and Parents, earlier.

Evaluation

Expected outcomes for an infant with CDH include the following:

- The infant demonstrates an effective respiratory pattern following surgical correction.
- Adequate fluid and electrolyte balance is maintained.
- Nutrition is provided for adequate growth and development.
- The parents demonstrate effective coping with the stress of a child with a complex medical need.

Discharge Planning and Teaching

An infant with CDH is hospitalized for a long period, often several months. Discharge planning and teaching vary for each infant with CDH depending on the success of the surgery and complications encountered during hospitalization. Infants who survive have ongoing healthcare needs, including pulmonary, gastrointestinal, nutritional, and neurodevelopmental (Maheshwari & Carlo, 2017). Children with CDHs, even after repair, are especially prone to respiratory complications. Parents may need home healthcare referrals, wound care supplies, and early intervention services for growth and development needs.

Palliative care may be an option for parents of an infant whose condition is unresponsive to interventions or deteriorates before surgical correction. Even after surgical intervention, the postoperative course may lead to palliative care. Comfort becomes the focus of care for these infants and their families.

Esophageal Atresia/Tracheoesophageal Fistula

Esophageal atresia occurs when the upper part of the esophagus does not connect to the lower part of the esophagus, resulting in a blind pouch. Tracheoesophageal fistula is a connection between the esophagus and the trachea that allows gastric secretions to enter the airways. Most infants with esophageal atresia also have tracheoesophageal fistula.

Etiology and Pathophysiology

Esophageal atresia is a malformation resulting from the failure of the esophagus to develop as a continuous tube. Esophageal atresia occurs in approximately 1 in 4,000 neonates. Approximately 90% of infants with esophageal atresia also have a tracheoesophageal fistula (Khan & Orenstein, 2016). The exact cause is unknown, but maternal risk factors include advanced maternal age, tobacco use, low socioeconomic status, and European ethnicity.

During the fourth and fifth weeks of gestation, the foregut should lengthen, separate, and fuse into two tubes, the esophagus and the trachea. Esophageal atresia occurs when the foregut fails to lengthen, separate, and fuse normally. Instead, the esophagus ends in a blind pouch (esophageal atresia) that may be connected to the trachea by a fistula (tracheoesophageal fistula). The structural deformity can appear in several ways (Fig. 23.9).

Approximately 50% of infants with esophageal atresia also have associated anomalies such as VATER (vertebral, anorectal, tracheal, esophageal, renal, radial) syndrome or VACTERL syndrome. Cardiac (32%) and vertebral (24%) anomalies are also common in infants with esophageal atresia (Khan & Orenstein, 2016).

Clinical Presentation

Immediately following birth, the neonate has frothing and bubbling at the mouth, excessive salivation, and drooling accompanied by three classic signs: cyanosis, coughing, and choking. Frequent sneezing is noted. Feeding exacerbates these symptoms. Signs of aspiration may also be present. There is an inability to pass an NG tube or orogastric tube.

Assessment and Diagnosis

During the newborn period, assess for signs and symptoms of respiratory distress. Tachypnea, increased work of breathing, choking, and noisy breathing are indications of possible aspiration of gastric contents. Coarse lung sounds may be auscultated and indicate the presence of secretions in the lungs. Closely assess the skin for breakdown. Moisture is common under the neck in babies with esophageal fistula/atresia due to increased secretions and frequent drooling. Assess for difficulty feeding and choking with feeding.

Confirm the diagnosis by attempting to pass an NG or orogastric tube into the stomach. Resistance is met and there is failure to pass the tube when esophageal atresia is present. Radiological examination is also helpful in determining where along the esophagus the defect occurs and what type of defect is present.

Therapeutic Interventions

Initially, nursing care is focused on maintaining a patent airway, proximal pouch decompression to prevent aspiration of

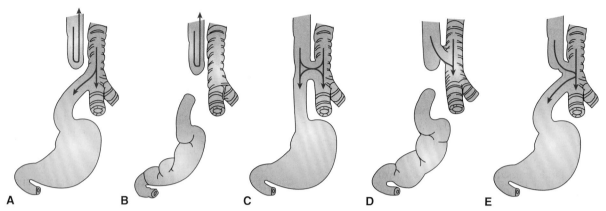

Figure 23.9. Types of esophageal fistulas. A. The proximal end of the esophagus ends in a blind pouch, whereas the distal end connects to the trachea. **B.** The esophagus is disconnected and the proximal end is a blind pouch. **C.** The proximal end connects to the trachea, as does the distal end. **D.** The proximal end of the esophagus connects to the trachea, creating a fistula, whereas the distal end is disconnected. **E.** The fistula connects to both the upper and lower ends of the esophagus. Reprinted with permission from Pillitteri, A. (2002). *Maternal and child health nursing* (4th ed., Fig. 39.5). Philadelphia, PA: Lippincott Williams & Wilkins.

secretions, administration of antibiotics to prevent pneumonia that results from aspiration of gastric contents, and providing adequate nutrition and fluids. Nursing care also includes facilitating feeding and providing postoperative care, teaching, and emotional support of the family as they prepare to care for their newborn with complex medical needs.

After diagnosis, an NG tube is inserted to suction the upper pouch and reduce pooling of secretions. Low continuous or intermittent suction removes the secretions from the pouch. As described, in Maintain Effective Ventilation and Oxygenation, take measures to prevent aspiration, such as suctioning secretions and placing the infant in a slightly elevated position. The infant is NPO until surgical correction takes place. Postoperatively, assess for respiratory difficulty during reintroduction of feedings.

As discussed in the section Maintain Skin Integrity, frequently assess skin folds on the anterior and posterior neck and the skin on the cheeks and face where the drainage tube is secured for signs of moisture or skin breakdown and keep the skin clean and dry.

As discussed in the section Maintain Adequate Hydration and Nutrition, earlier, provide IV fluids to maintain hydration before surgery and while the infant is NPO. Following surgery, TPN may be necessary until the infant is tolerating full gastrostomy tube feedings or is able to take in adequate calories via the oral route. Monitor weight, length, and growth and development regularly.

For guidelines on addressing the families' emotional and psychological needs related to gastrointestinal disorders, see the section Provide Emotional and Psychosocial Support to the Child and Parents, earlier.

Evaluation

Expected outcomes for an infant with esophageal atresia include the following:

- The child does not experience respiratory distress.
- The child achieves normal weight and growth trends.

- The parents demonstrate understanding of the care associated with esophageal atresia, surgical care, and prevention of complications.

Discharge Planning and Teaching

Once the infant is tolerating enteral feedings via a gastrostomy tube or is taking adequate fluid and calories by mouth, discharge to home is appropriate. Parents may need a referral for home care services if continuous tube feeds, supplies, or equipment is necessary in caring for the infant at home.

Teach parents the use and care of a gastrostomy tube in children who require the surgical placement of a gastrostomy tube related to difficulty swallowing, consuming oral feedings, or gaining weight (Fig. 23.10). Families need teaching and demonstration with repetitive practice regarding performing site care, administering feeds and medications, troubleshooting,

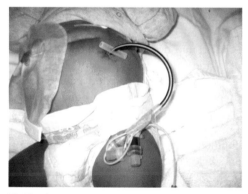

Figure 23.10. A gastrostomy tube in an infant after undergoing major abdominal surgery. Note the colostomy and upper abdominal healed incision. Reprinted with permission from Hatfield, N. T., & Kincheloe, C. (2017). *Introductory maternity and pediatric nursing* (4th ed., Fig. 30.6A). Philadelphia, PA: Wolters Kluwer.

and performing emergency procedures, such as in the case of accidental removal of the gastrostomy tube. Families also need to identify signs and symptoms of infection at the site.

Acute Gastrointestinal Disorders

Acute gastrointestinal disorders include dehydration, vomiting, diarrhea, hypertrophic pyloric stenosis, NEC, intussusception, malrotation and volvulus, and appendicitis. Acute gastrointestinal disorders have a sudden, often unexpected, onset and, although of short duration, can have complications that persist, such as with NEC.

Dehydration

Dehydration is a common complication of many pediatric illnesses. Vomiting and diarrhea are the causes of most cases of dehydration in the pediatric patient. Infants and young children are especially vulnerable to dehydration because of their inability to inform thirst and fluid needs to caregivers or access their own fluids and because of greater insensible losses due to higher body surface area–to-mass index (Powers, 2015). Early recognition and intervention are essential to reduce the risk of progression to hypovolemic shock and end-organ failure.

Etiology and Pathophysiology

Dehydration can be classified as isotonic, hypotonic, or hypertonic (Table 23.5). Regardless of the type of dehydration, the body continuously attempts to compensate for fluid and electrolyte imbalances by shifting fluid from one compartment to another. Children often have more than one type of dehydration simultaneously. Therefore, volume depletion is an important factor to consider when caring for a patient with dehydration. In this chapter, as often occurs in the literature, the terms dehydration, hypovolemia, and volume depletion are used interchangeably when referring to intravascular fluid volume deficits. However, note that the terms refer to different physiological conditions resulting from different types of fluid loss. Volume depletion is the reduction of effective circulating volume in the intravascular space. Dehydration is the loss of free water in greater proportion than the loss of sodium.

The mechanisms of dehydration can be divided into three categories: decreased intake, increased fluid output, and increased insensible losses. Dehydration in the infant and child is frequently the result of output from gastroenteritis, characterized by vomiting and diarrhea. However, vomiting and diarrhea, leading to dehydration, can also be caused by other illnesses or disease processes (Box 23.3).

Clinical Presentation

Infants and children present in various stages of dehydration. Dehydration can be classified as mild (3%–5% volume loss), moderate (6%–9% volume loss), or severe (>10% volume loss). Table 23.6 reviews the classifications and signs and symptoms of dehydration in infants and children. Mild dehydration can be difficult to detect because children appear alert and have moist mucous membranes. Moderate dehydration becomes more obvious as children appear lethargic or have periods of restlessness and irritability. Mucous membranes appear dry and skin turgor is diminished in moderate dehydration. A child with severe dehydration presents with increasing lethargy and altered level of consciousness and may be unarousable. Blood pressure is low, pulses are thready, skin turgor is poor, and urine output is minimal (oliguria) to absent (anuria). Assessment of dehydration is only an estimate. Continuous assessment and reevaluation, even after initial presentation and interventions, ensures that appropriate fluid replacement volumes are being administered.

For mild and moderate dehydration, use oral rehydration to replenish fluids and electrolytes. The goal for intake should be 50 mL of fluid for every kilogram of body weight in the first 2 to 4 hours of oral rehydration therapy. This is achieved by giving

Table 23.5 Isotonic, Hypotonic, and Hypertonic Dehydration

	Type of Dehydration		
Characteristic	**Isotonic**	**Hypotonic**	**Hypertonic**
Water vs. sodium loss	Proportional	Greater loss of sodium than water	Greater loss of water than sodium
Serum sodium level	Normal	Low	High
Fluid shift	Loss of fluid from extracellular component	Extracellular to intracellular; great extracellular dehydration	Intracellular to extracellular
Causes	Vomiting, diarrhea	• Severe, prolonged vomiting and diarrhea • Burns • Renal disease	• Diabetes insipidus • Administration of IV fluids or tube feedings with high electrolyte levels

IV, intravenous.

Box 23.3 Causes of Vomiting and Diarrhea

Causes of Vomiting

- Central nervous system causes
  - Infections such as meningitis
  - Increased intracranial pressure
- Gastrointestinal causes
  - Obstruction
  - Hepatitis
  - Liver failure
  - Appendicitis
  - Peritonitis
  - Intussusception
  - Volvulus
  - Pyloric stenosis
  - Drug toxicity
- Endocrine causes
  - Diabetic ketoacidosis
  - Congenital adrenal hypoplasia
  - Addisonian crisis
- Renal causes
  - Infection
  - Pyelonephritis
  - Renal failure

Causes of Diarrhea

- Gastrointestinal causes
  - Malabsorption
  - Intussusception
  - Irritable bowel syndrome
  - Crohn disease
  - Ulcerative colitis
  - Short gut syndrome
- Endocrine causes
  - Thyrotoxicosis
  - Congenital adrenal hypoplasia
  - Addisonian crisis

one to three teaspoons of fluid every 10 to 15 minutes. Instruct parents to continue giving fluid even if the child vomits, offering one teaspoon every 2 to 3 minutes, because small amounts of fluid may still be absorbed. If the child's condition does not improve after 4 hours of oral rehydration therapy, parents should contact the healthcare provider for further direction.

Remember Maalik Abdella in Chapter 5? Maalik was a 2-year-old with fever, vomiting, and diarrhea. What instructions did the nurse give Maalik's parents over the phone regarding oral rehydration? What did the nurse tell them to avoid giving Maalik and why?

Manage severe dehydration with IV fluids. Initially, give the child a 20-mL/kg bolus of normal saline (0.9% sodium chloride) over 30 to 60 minutes to quickly replace fluid losses.

If reassessment following the bolus reveals tachycardia, low blood pressure, or other signs of inadequate tissue perfusion, administer additional boluses of normal saline until hemodynamic stability is achieved. Generally, a child with moderate-to-severe dehydration requires 40 to 60 mL/kg of rapid fluid replacement with normal saline. Estimate the fluid volume deficit by obtaining the weight and comparing it with a very recent weight or by observing clinical signs and symptoms (Table 23.6). Replacement fluid volume is calculated on the basis of percent of dehydration and given over 24 hours. See Box 23.4 for an example of how to calculate percent of dehydration and determine replacement fluid rates. Replacement fluids are generally isotonic fluids (normal saline or lactated Ringer's). In addition to replacing lost fluids, administer maintenance IV fluids. Box 23.5 reviews how to calculate maintenance IV fluid rates in children.

Assessment and Diagnosis

See Table 23.6 for clinical assessment findings in mild, moderate, and severe dehydration. In addition, ask the parents when the last wet diaper or void was and how often the child normally voids per day to compare the child's current urine output with normal urine output. Obtain a blood pressure with the child supine and with the child standing to assess for orthostatic changes, which are present in dehydration.

Diagnosis of dehydration is made on the basis of presenting history, presenting symptoms, and laboratory values, including sodium, blood urea nitrogen, and creatinine.

Therapeutic Interventions

The priorities for nursing care are to begin rehydrating the child, determine the cause of dehydration, implement measures to stop the cause, and teach parents how to prevent future episodes of dehydration.

Following the guidelines provided in the section Maintain Adequate Hydration and Nutrition, earlier, administer oral or IV rehydration, as needed, closely monitor intake and output, and weigh the child regularly to assess for fluid loss and gain. Also, as discussed, take measures to prevent dehydration via insensible fluid losses in the hospital and teach parents how to prevent dehydration in their child at home.

Evaluation

Expected outcomes for a child with dehydration include the following:

- Urinary output is within normal limits for age.
- Adequate fluid intake for age and weight is achieved.
- Vital signs are within normal limits.
- Fluid and electrolyte balance is achieved.

Discharge Planning and Teaching

Once adequate rehydration is achieved and the child is tolerating oral intake, discharge the child to home. Before discharge, instruct the parents on which types of fluids are acceptable to

Table 23.6 Severity of Clinical Dehydration

	Severity of Dehydration		
Clinical Assessment	**Mild**	**Moderate**	**Severe**
Respirations	Normal	Normal; tachypnea	Deep, tachypnea
Pulse/heart rate	Easily palpable/regular	Normal to decreased/tachycardia	Weak to nonpalpable/ severe tachycardia
Blood pressure	Normal for age	Normal for age or decreased; older children and adolescents may have postural hypotension	Very low or undetectable
Capillary refill	Normal	Prolonged	Very prolonged
Mental status	Alert, restless, thirsty	Infants/young children: irritable, lethargic; older children/ adolescents: thirsty, restless	Difficult to arouse, unconscious; older children may be apprehensive
Eyes	Normal	Slightly sunken	Deeply sunken; dark periorbital skin tones
Fontanel	Flat, soft	Sunken	Sunken
Mucous membranes, mouth and tongue	Moist	Dry	Parched
Skin turgor	Immediate return to normal after pinching	2–3 s to return to normal after pinching; poor	3–4 s to return to normal after pinching; very poor
Tears	Present	Decreased	Absent
Urine output	Normal; slightly decreased	Decreased; dark color; increased specific gravity	Minimal or absent

Data from Bhutta, Z. (2017). Acute gastroenteritis in children. In R. Kliegman, B. Stanton, J. St. Geme, N. Schor, & R. Behrman (Eds.). *Nelson textbook of pediatrics* (20th ed., pp. 1863–1874). Philadelphia, PA: Elsevier.

use in treating dehydration at home, ways to avoid dehydration, and signs and symptoms of dehydration. Teach parents how to recognize signs such as increased lethargy, decreased urine output, and increased thirst or anorexia and that these signs indicate the need for immediate medical attention. The child should resume a normal diet once he or she has achieved adequate urine output and is alert and oriented. Instruct parents to keep oral rehydration fluids at home in case they are needed.

Box 23.4 Calculating Dehydration and Replacement Fluid Volume

Equation for calculating dehydration:

$$\%\text{dehydration} = \frac{(\text{Preillness weight} - \text{illness weight})}{\text{Preillness weight}} \times 100$$

Maalik's dehydration status:

$$\%\text{dehydration} = \frac{(11.8\,\text{kg} - 10.9\,\text{kg})}{11.8\,\text{kg}} \times 100 = 7\%\,\text{dehydration}$$

Equation for calculating replacement fluid volume:

$$1\,\text{kg} = 1\,\text{L of fluid}$$

Fluid deficit for Maalik:
11.8 kg × 7% dehydration × 10 = 826

Subtract any boluses Maalik received:
20 mL/kg (20 × 11.8 = 236 mL)

826 − 236 = 590 mL; this is the current fluid deficit

Maintenance intravenous fluids (MIVFs) for an 11.8-kg child = 1,000 + 90 = 1,090

Add the fluid deficit total and MIVF: 590 + 1,090 = 1,680 mL

1,680 mL should be given over the next 24 h as follows:

1/2 remaining deficit + 1/3 MIVF over the first 8 h = 295 + 360 = 655/8 = 81.9 mL/h

1/2 remaining deficit + 2/3 MIVF over the next 16 h = 295 + 719 = 1,014/16 = 63.4 mL/h

Box 23.5 Daily Maintenance Fluid Requirement Formula for Pediatric Patients

0–10 kg: 100 mL/kg/d (100 × kg)

11–20 kg: 1,000 mL (for the first 10 kg) + 50 mL/kg/d for each additional kilogram from 10–20 kg

>20 kg: 1,500 mL (for the first 20 kg) + 20 mL/kg/d for each additional kilogram over 20 kg

Divide the total by 24 to get the hourly intravenous fluid rate.

Vomiting

Vomiting is a very common complaint in infants and children who present to the primary care provider and to the emergency room. A large percentage of infants and children with vomiting have a self-limiting illness and a nonserious etiology. However, vomiting can become life-threatening if it is prolonged and adequate hydration and electrolytes are not provided. Furthermore, there are several life-threatening conditions in infants and children in which vomiting is the presenting symptom.

Etiology and Pathophysiology

Vomiting is a complex behavior composed of three successive activities: nausea, retching, and expulsion of stomach contents. Nausea is a sensation of impending emesis. Increased heart rate and salivation, which are autonomic changes, frequently accompany nausea. Vomiting can occur without preceding nausea, such as in **projectile vomiting** seen in children with increased intracranial pressure. Retching, also referred to as "dry heaves," is a strong, involuntary effort to vomit that does not actually expel stomach contents. Vomiting, a protective reflex, is defined as a forceful ejection of stomach contents up to and out of the mouth (Singhi, Shah, Bansal, & Jayashree, 2013).

Common causes of vomiting vary by age. The leading cause of acute vomiting in children is acute gastritis and gastroenteritis (Singhi et al., 2013). Vomiting is more frequent in young children and declines in older children. Vomiting can be categorized according to organic and nonorganic causes. Box 23.6 reviews illnesses presenting with vomiting according to age. Nonorganic causes include psychogenic vomiting, **cyclic vomiting** syndrome, abdominal migraine, and the eating disorder of bulimia.

Clinical Presentation

The child with vomiting presents in various ways and may appear well or ill, often depending on the underlying cause of vomiting. Because vomiting can be a symptom of some life-threatening diagnoses, an assessment for more serious causes is necessary (Patient Safety 23.1). If vomiting has been prolonged or frequent, dehydration may be present (see the section Clinical Presentation, under Dehydration). Assessment of the emesis contents is necessary to help determine the underlying cause.

Box 23.6 Common Causes of Vomiting According to Age

Neonate
- Reflux
- Pyloric stenosis
- Sepsis
- UTI
- Malrotation
- Esophageal atresia
- Hydrocephalus
- Milk allergy
- Inborn errors of metabolism

Infant
- Gastroenteritis
- Food poisoning
- Gastroesophageal reflux
- Coughing
- Overfeeding
- Food intolerance
- UTI
- Otitis media
- Pneumonia

Toddler/Older Child
- Gastroenteritis/gastritis
- Otitis media
- Pharyngitis
- Sinusitis
- Coughing
- Meningitis
- Toxins/poisons
- Gastroesophageal reflux

Adolescent
- Gastroenteritis/gastritis
- Appendicitis
- Ingestion
- Migraine
- Inflammatory bowel disease
- Toxins/poisons/drugs
- Obstruction

UTI, urinary tract infection.

Bloody or bilious vomiting signals a gastrointestinal bleed or an obstruction. Food particles are present in emesis when motility is slowed. Additional gastrointestinal symptoms accompanying vomiting may include diarrhea and abdominal pain. Generalized abdominal pain could indicate peritonitis or an abdominal migraine. Epigastric pain is associated with gastritis and pancreatitis. Pain in the right upper quadrant may be a symptom of cholelithiasis or pneumonia. Right lower quadrant pain can be a symptom of appendicitis, whereas generalized lower abdominal pain or suprapubic pain can be present with a urinary tract

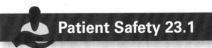

Patient Safety 23.1

Red Flags in a Child With Vomiting

Observe for the following signs in a child presenting with vomiting, which often indicate a potentially life-threatening illness. If present, address the underlying cause promptly.

- Altered mental status
- Apprehensive appearance
- Toxic appearance
- Bilious or bloody vomiting
- Inconsolable cry, excessive irritability (signs of possible meningitis, intussusception)
- Signs of severe dehydration
- Drawing up of the knees to the chest, avoidance of unnecessary movement (signs of peritonitis, intussusception)

infection (UTI). Children may also present with nonintestinal symptoms, such as sore throat, ear pain, headache, vertigo, or back pain.

Assessment and Diagnosis

Initially, assess the airway, breathing, and circulation, as well as vital signs and hydration status. Assess emesis for signs of blood. Determine how long the vomiting has been occurring. See the section Clinical Presentation, earlier, for signs and symptoms to assess for.

Therapeutic Interventions

Nursing care of the child with vomiting often focuses on first determining whether the child is dehydrated and then establishing a plan for reducing episodes of vomiting and avoiding dehydration. For a child seen in the pediatrician's office, nursing care is focused on teaching the parents how to give oral rehydration and offering reassurance of the self-limiting nature of vomiting.

The symptoms of nausea and vomiting can be treated with ondansetron in children older than 6 months. Exceeding the recommended dose of ondansetron can lead to diarrhea

(Truven Health Analytics, 2016); be aware of the age- and weight-based dosing for ondansetron (The Pharmacy 23.1).

For the first 24 hours, the child should avoid solid foods, because they are more likely to stimulate vomiting. Following the guidelines in the section Maintain Adequate Hydration and Nutrition, earlier, teach parents about minimum daily intake requirements and how to administer oral rehydration to their children at home, as well as the importance of monitoring actual fluid intake.

Evaluation

Expected outcomes for a child with vomiting include the following:

- The child is free from signs of dehydration.
- Vomiting is controlled or no longer present within 24 to 48 hours of onset.

Discharge Planning and Teaching

Children are rarely hospitalized for vomiting. Hospitalization occurs when vomiting is related to a more serious condition such as appendicitis, intestinal obstruction, or pyelonephritis. In the clinic setting, review with parents the minimum requirements for oral intake and oral rehydration techniques and encourage them to keep the child upright or side-lying to reduce the risk of aspiration during episodes of vomiting.

Gastroenteritis (Acute Diarrhea)

Gastroenteritis is an acute inflammation of any part of the stomach or intestinal tract and is often accompanied by vomiting and diarrhea. AGE, one of the most common illnesses in the United States, is most often treated in the outpatient setting. Children younger than 5 years are the most often affected, experiencing one to five episodes of gastroenteritis per year (Farthing et al., 2013).

Etiology and Pathophysiology

The specific etiology of AGE is not always identified. Viral pathogens are the most common causative agent of AGE, accounting for 75% to 90% of cases (Churgay & Aftab, 2012).

The Pharmacy 23.1 Ondansetron

Classification	Route	Action	Nursing Considerations

Antiemetic	• PO
	• IM
	• IV
		• Selective 5-HT$_3$ receptor antagonist
		• Works in the chemoreceptor trigger zone
			• Dosing depends on reason for use.
			• For gastroenteritis in children 8–15 kg:
			  ○ PO: 2 mg/dose × 1
			  ○ IV: 0.3 mg/kg/dose × 1, not to exceed 16 mg/dose
			• Monitor for agitation and anxiety with PO use.
			• Monitor for sedation and drowsiness with IV use.

IM, intramuscular; IV, intravenous; PO, by mouth.

Table 23.7 Causes of Diarrhea in Children

Etiology	Bowel Manifestations
Infection of the intestines • Viral: rotavirus, norovirus, adenovirus • Bacterial: *Escherichia coli*, *Salmonella*, *Shigella*	• Mucosa inflammation • Increased mucus secretion in the large intestine
Food sensitivity • Gluten • Cow's milk • Lactose	Decreased digestion of food
Stress, anxiety, or fatigue	Increased motility

Other causes include bacterial infection (much less common), food sensitivities, stress, and fatigue (Table 23.7). Rotavirus is the most frequent cause of AGE; however, in countries with high vaccination rates for rotavirus, norovirus is becoming the leading causative agent (Guarino et al., 2014). Risk factors for AGE include age younger than 24 months, day care attendance, exposure to sick contacts, recent travel to a foreign country, low socioeconomic status, and immunocompromised state (Guarino et al., 2014).

Clinical Presentation

Children with AGE present with mild, moderate, or severe diarrhea. In mild diarrhea, the stools are slightly increased in number and have a more liquid consistency. Children with moderate diarrhea present with multiple loose, liquid, or watery stools per day; are often irritable; feel nauseous and tend to vomit; and experience a loss of appetite. Diarrhea may be mucoid, liquid, or watery and may vary in color. Yellow, green, clear, and brown stools are common. The provider should be notified if stool with any evidence of blood or clots is present, so that the need for further workup can be determined. Tenesmus, the urge to continuously defecate, can be present. Abdominal pain and cramping are present, and the child may feel nauseous and have episodes of vomiting. Headache and myalgias are common in children with gastroenteritis.

Assessment and Diagnosis

Obtain a thorough history of the onset of diarrhea and illness, which may help determine a cause. Ask parents about recent exposure to sick contacts, travel out of the country, and day care attendance, all of which increase the risk of exposure to diarrheal illnesses, as well as recent food consumption. Assess the onset, frequency, consistency, color, and amount of stool with each episode. Assess for abdominal distension and cramping. Monitor urine output for adequacy, color, and odor. Obtain a baseline weight and assess daily thereafter while the child is hospitalized. Assess vital signs every 2 to 4 hours for changes indicating fluid volume

deficit. Assess skin integrity, particularly in the perianal area and buttocks. Diagnosis is made on the basis of the presence of diarrhea and symptoms.

Therapeutic Interventions

Nursing care of the child with AGE focuses on preventing complications such as dehydration and hypovolemic shock, maintaining fluid and electrolyte balance, and providing skin care, particularly for the diapered child, who is at high risk for loss of skin integrity.

International practice guidelines strongly recommend probiotics for the treatment of diarrhea, although the quality of evidence is low (Guarino et al., 2014). Probiotics degrade and modify dietary antigens and balance the anti-inflammatory response of cytokines. Probiotic microorganisms such as *Lactobacillus* and *Saccharomyces* are supplements, which are not regulated by the federal quality and safety standards, so their efficacy may vary. Provide families with this information before administration.

As discussed in the section Maintain Adequate Hydration and Nutrition, earlier, oral rehydration is the initial recommended treatment, with an emphasis on alleviating deficits and reducing ongoing fluid losses (Carson, Mudd, & Madati, 2016).

As covered in the section Maintain Skin Integrity, earlier, take measures to prevent skin breakdown, which frequently results from diarrhea, such as frequently changing diapers, keeping the area clean and dry, and applying barrier creams to the area.

Assess the child's pain level frequently and provide nonpharmacological and pharmacological interventions to relieve pain as ordered and appropriate (see the section Promote Pain Relief, Comfort, and Rest, earlier).

Evaluation

Expected outcomes for a child with gastroenteritis include the following:

- The child's bowel function returns to baseline.
- If an infant, urine output is 1 to 3 mL/kg/h.
- If an older child, urine output is 0.5 to 1 mL/kg/h.
- The child's electrolytes are within normal limits.
- The child's skin on the buttocks and in the perianal and rectal areas remains intact and free of breakdown.

Discharge Planning and Teaching

Teach parents about the signs and symptoms of dehydration and appropriate actions to take if dehydration is suspected. Reinforce the importance of proper hand washing and good hygiene to avoid the spread of microorganisms that cause gastroenteritis. Encourage parents to inform day care providers of their child's gastroenteritis so that the facility can take actions to prevent the spread of the infection. Teach parents that antidiarrheal agents should not be used in patients with AGE, because they delay the elimination of infectious agents from the intestines.

Hypertrophic Pyloric Stenosis

Hypertrophic pyloric stenosis is a disorder that affects young infants and is caused by elongation and thickening of the pylorus muscle, leading to hypertrophy of the pylorus (Fig. 23.11). Hypertrophy can progress to nearly complete obstruction of the gastric outlet, leading to projectile or forceful vomiting. In infancy, hypertrophic pyloric stenosis is the most common surgical cause of nonbilious vomiting.

Etiology and Pathophysiology

The circular pylorus muscle becomes hypertrophied, which results in stenosis in the passage between the stomach and duodenum. The lumen of the stomach becomes partially obstructed. Inflammation and edema narrow the pylorus even further, until complete obstruction occurs. The infant has forceful vomiting, resulting in the infant becoming dehydrated and depleted of electrolytes, which then leads to metabolic disturbances such as metabolic alkalosis secondary to loss of hydrochloric acid.

The exact etiology of hypertrophic pyloric stenosis is unclear, but it is proposedly multifactorial. Exposure to erythromycin or azithromycin during early infancy increases the risk of pyloric stenosis. The risk is highest if exposure occurs during the first 2 weeks of life but remains high if exposure occurs within the first 6 weeks of life (Eberly, Eide, Thompson, & Nylund, 2015). Environmental factors, such as maternal smoking and bottle feeding, may also increase the risk of pyloric stenosis. Maternal smoking has been shown to increase the risk by 1.2- to 2-fold (Svenningsson, Svensson, Akre, & Nordenskjöld, 2014). Bottle feeding was found to be the most significant risk factor for the onset of pyloric stenosis (Zhu, Zhu, Lin, Qu, & Mu, 2017). Other risk factors include being the first born, being born via cesarean section, and being premature (<37 weeks of gestation) (Zhu et al., 2017).

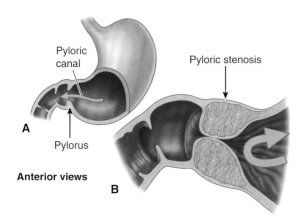

Figure 23.11. Hypertrophic pyloric stenosis. A. Normal passage through the pyloric sphincter. **B.** Flow is stopped as a result of the stenosed area. Reprinted with permission from Moore, K. L., Dalley, A. F., & Agur, A. M. R. (2017). *Clinically oriented anatomy* (8th ed., unnumbered figure in Clinical Blue Box in Chapter 5). Philadelphia, PA: Wolters Kluwer.

Hypertrophic pyloric stenosis occurs in approximately 2 to 3.5 per 1,000 live births. Prevalence varies from region to region. Males are affected 4 times more often than are females. Symptoms of hypertrophic pyloric stenosis have a sudden onset at 1 to 12 weeks of age, typically beginning around 3 to 5 weeks and rarely occurring after 12 weeks of age.

Clinical Presentation

Classically, an infant of about 3 to 6 weeks of age develops immediate postprandial, nonbilious, projectile vomiting. In addition, parents report that the infant is hungry soon after vomiting. The infant can appear emaciated and dehydrated, although recent studies demonstrate better nourishment and normal or slightly altered electrolyte balance among infants with hypertrophic pyloric stenosis, most likely as a result of advances in diagnostic imaging and increased awareness among clinicians (Taylor, Cass, & Holland, 2013).

Assessment and Diagnosis

Inspect the infant's abdomen for peristaltic waves. Upon auscultation, hyperactive bowel sounds may be present. Palpation may reveal an olive-shaped mass in the right upper quadrant. Assess vomiting episodes for amount and characteristics of emesis and presence of projectile vomiting.

Assess for signs of dehydration. Very young infants can quickly become dehydrated when vomiting episodes are large and frequent. Assess vital signs for tachycardia and tachypnea, current weight, skin turgor, fontanels, urinary output, capillary refill, and mucous membranes. The child may cry frequently due to hunger and be generally uncomfortable.

Therapeutic Interventions

Nursing care focuses on meeting the infant's fluid, electrolyte, and nutritional needs while minimizing weight loss and promoting comfort. After pyloromyotomy, nursing care is directed toward preventing infection, promoting comfort, and providing support to parents.

As noted in the section Maintain Adequate Hydration and Nutrition, earlier, monitor for signs of electrolyte disturbances and notify the provider of any concerning findings. Be prepared to administer IV replacement of sodium, chloride, and potassium, as ordered.

The infant is NPO until surgical correction takes place. Provide a pacifier to meet the infant's need to suck. Keep the infant warm and allow parents to hold and cuddle the infant for comfort.

Surgical correction is the treatment of choice for an infant with hypertrophic pyloric stenosis. A pyloromyotomy is the procedure used to correct the stenosis. During a pyloromyotomy, the pylorus muscle is split to allow passage of fluid and food into the duodenum. The procedure can be performed via a periumbilical or small, transverse upper abdominal incision (open pyloromyotomy) or laparoscopically. Both methods have been shown to be equally successful. The prognosis is good, and most infants are able to take fluids within a few hours of surgery.

Discharge home is often within 24 hours postoperatively, and the infant can typically take full-strength formula.

Nursing interventions to meet fluid and nutritional needs for a child with pyloric stenosis are similar to those used for a child with vomiting. See Maintain Adequate Hydration and Nutrition, earlier.

Evaluation

Expected outcomes for a child with hypertrophic pyloric stenosis include the following:

- The infant's electrolyte and fluid balance is restored to normal and maintained.
- Pain is controlled.
- The child is free from signs of infection at the surgical site.
- Parents demonstrate the ability to recognize postoperative complications such as infection before discharge.

Discharge Planning and Teaching

Infants are discharged home once adequate oral intake is resumed. Teach parents to monitor for signs of infection at the surgical site, including redness, swelling, and drainage, and report them or fever to the provider immediately. Teach parents to avoid placing a diaper or irritating clothing over the incision area and giving the child a tub or soaking bath until the incision is healed. Instruct them to keep the surgical site clean and dry and pat it dry after sponge baths.

Following a pyloromyotomy, infants may spit up or vomit, which does not mean the surgery was unsuccessful. Teach parents to hold the infant in an upright position when feeding and to burp the infant after every 1 to 2 oz of formula or, if breastfeeding, every 5 to 10 minutes. Parents should keep the infant in an upright position for at least 30 minutes after feeding or on the right side with the head and upper body elevated. Instruct parents to avoid playing with or rocking the infant for at least 30 minutes after feedings.

Necrotizing Enterocolitis

NEC, which is characterized by varying degrees of mucosal and transmural necrosis of the intestine, is the most lethal disorder affecting the gastrointestinal tract of newborn infants (Papillon, Castle, Gayer, & Ford, 2013).

Etiology and Pathophysiology

Although the exact pathophysiology of NEC is unknown, recent studies suggest that the epithelial barrier and prematurity combined with the inflammatory response play a role in the development of NEC (Choi, 2014). Intestinal mucosal stress and inadequate host defense and repair can result in activation of the proinflammatory cascade, which is the final common pathway of intestinal injury and NEC (Choi, 2014). Prematurity is the greatest risk factor for NEC. Other risk factors include early enteral feeding, bacterial colonization, and intestinal ischemia. However, human milk has been shown to protect against the disease.

Clinical Presentation

Infants can develop NEC anytime during the first few weeks of life, before or after enteral feedings. Feeding intolerance, vomiting, and abdominal distension may initially appear. Bloody diarrhea can be present. As the disease progresses, lethargy is noted and the infant appears quite ill. Apnea, bradycardia, and unstable vital signs are seen.

Assessment and Diagnosis

Assess for increased abdominal distension, vomiting, and characteristics of stool output indicative of NEC, such as blood in the stool. Measure abdominal circumference and assess bowel sounds every 4 hours. Small changes in abdominal circumference can indicate NEC. Report abnormal findings immediately to the provider for timely intervention.

Diagnosis is made on the basis of the presence of air in the bowel wall (pneumatosis intestinalis), as demonstrated on an X-ray of the abdomen. Blood in the stool and emesis are present. Laboratory values commonly associated with NEC include the following: decreased hemoglobin and hematocrit, leukopenia, leukocytosis, thrombocytopenia, metabolic or respiratory acidosis, and electrolyte imbalances.

Once a diagnosis is suspected, treatment includes making the infant NPO to rest the bowel, decompressing the stomach by inserting an NG tube, and antibiotic therapy. As ordered, take serial abdominal X-rays to monitor for worsening of the disease process. Measure abdominal girth often to detect changes in abdominal distension. Should perforation or necrosis occur, a bowel resection is necessary. The infant can become quite unstable during this time.

Therapeutic Interventions

Initial nursing care related to NEC focuses on prevention and early detection (Analyze the Evidence 23.1). Once the child is diagnosed with NEC, nursing care focuses on maintaining fluid and electrolyte balance, managing infection and spread of infection, and administering essential nutrition for healing and

 Analyze the Evidence 23.1

The Use of Probiotics to Prevent Necrotizing Enterocolitis

In a meta-analysis and systematic review of studies carried out to determine whether the use of probiotics decreases the incidence of necrotizing enterocolitis (NEC), Sawh, Deshpande, Jansen, Reynaert, and Jones (2016) found that the incidence of severe NEC and all-cause mortality was significantly reduced when probiotics were administered to infants <37 wk of gestation or <2,500 g. *Lactobacillus* species and *Bifidobacterium* species were the two probiotics used that decreased the incidence of NEC. *Saccharomyces boulardii* supplement used alone did not affect the incidence of NEC.

growth and development. Postoperative care and supporting the family through a time of crisis are also important aspects of managing an infant with NEC.

Fluid losses can occur quickly if necrosis leads to intestinal perforation. Monitor fluid losses closely, as well as vital signs for tachycardia, tachypnea, and hypotension. Electrolytes, too, can become imbalanced, because acidosis and loss resulting from use of an NG tube placed for low-wall suction. Therefore, monitor and replace electrolytes as ordered.

Infants with NEC are placed in strict enteric precautions to prevent the spread of infection to other infants on the unit. Educate parents and visitors on the importance of hand washing, and take care to maintain aseptic technique when accessing the infant's central venous access catheter. Perform dressing changes using sterile technique.

Because ischemia is associated with the incidence of NEC and can lead to worsening of NEC once diagnosed, adequate tissue perfusion is essential. Accurate intake and output is necessary. Assess the infant for signs of poor tissue perfusion, including tachycardia, reduced capillary refill, reduced intensity of peripheral pulses, cool skin, and decreased urine output. If sepsis occurs, the infant may need fluid resuscitation and vasopressor support to maintain perfusion.

Nutritional needs are met using TPN via a central venous access catheter until the bowel is healed and function returns, at which time oral or enteral feedings are established. The child may need a slow reintroduction to feedings for feeding tolerance to develop.

Evaluation

Expected outcomes for a child with NEC include the following:

- Fluid and electrolyte balance is maintained.
- Tissue perfusion and hemodynamic stability are maintained following surgical removal of the necrotic bowel.
- The infant is free of signs and symptoms of infection.
- Adequate nutritional intake is achieved to support growth and development.
- Tissue integrity is restored following surgical opening of the abdomen.

Discharge Planning and Teaching

Upon discharge from the hospital, the child needs frequent follow-up care to monitor weight and growth and development, as well as to monitor for signs of complications. Teaching points include feeding regimen, medications, and ostomy care (if the child leaves the hospital with an ostomy).

Intussusception

Intussusception, a potentially life-threatening condition and frequent cause of bowel obstruction, occurs when one portion of the intestine prolapses and then telescopes into another (Fig. 23.12A). It is one of the most common causes of intestinal obstruction in children 5 months to 3 years old.

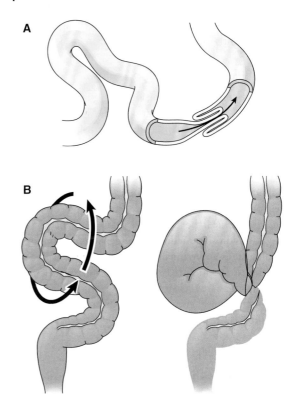

Figure 23.12. Intussusception and volvulus. A. Intussusception: the intestine pushes into itself. **B.** Volvulus: the intestine twists. Reprinted with permission from Cohen, B. J., & DePetris, A. (2016). *Medical terminology* (8th ed., Fig. 12.9). Philadelphia, PA: Wolters Kluwer.

Etiology and Pathophysiology

The most common site of intussusception is the ileocolic region of the bowel, where the ileum of the small intestine joins the colon. The upper portion of the bowel invaginates into the lower, pulling its mesentery along with it. The mesentery becomes constricted and obstructs venous return. The intussusception becomes engorged with blood and edematous. Bleeding from the mucosa leads to a bloody stool with mucus. If left untreated, intussusception can lead to intestinal infarction, perforation, peritonitis, and death.

The incidence varies from 1 to 4 per 1,000 live births. Males are affected more often than are females, with a 3:1 ratio. Approximately 90% of intussusception cases in children are idiopathic. Incidence peaks in fall and winter. Intussusception has been correlated with a prior or concurrent respiratory adenovirus infection (Kennedy & Liacouras, 2016). Eighty percent of all cases occur before the age of 24 months.

Clinical Presentation

Children present with an abrupt onset of severe, paroxysmal, colicky abdominal pain. The child may play normally and appear well between episodes of pain initially. Nausea, vomiting, and currant jelly stools or bloody stools are also common symptoms. If the intussusception is not reduced, the infant becomes weak and lethargic and appears ill. In later stages, fever and signs of peritonitis can be present.

Assessment and Diagnosis

Assess the abdomen for distension and guarding. Auscultate bowel sounds. Monitor vital signs every 4 hours or more frequently if the child presents dehydrated from vomiting and poor oral intake. Measure and record urine output. Measure and record vomitus and stool output.

Diagnosis of intussusception is made via ultrasound. Once the diagnosis is confirmed, initiate as ordered air, hydrostatic (saline), or contrast enemas under fluoroscopic or ultrasonic guidance to reduce the intussusception. The success rate of radiological hydrostatic reduction under fluoroscopic or ultrasonic guidance is approximately 80% to 95% in patients with ileocolic intussusception (Kennedy & Liacouras, 2016). When reduction enemas are unsuccessful, surgery is needed to reduce the invaginated bowel and remove any necrotic tissue that may have resulted.

Therapeutic Interventions

Nursing care of the child with intussusception focuses on decompressing the stomach, maintaining hydration and electrolytes by administering IV fluids, pain control, and monitoring the child for signs of peritonitis and shock until the reduction can be performed. Additional nursing care focuses on assisting the child to return to a normal feeding schedule once normal bowel function is achieved.

An NG tube is often placed to decompress the stomach before reduction and remains in place for a short time after the reduction. Monitor the NG tube output and patency. After reduction with an enema, monitor for signs of infection, maintain NG tube patency, and monitor for return of bowel function.

Assess the child's pain level frequently and provide nonpharmacological and pharmacological interventions to relieve pain as ordered and appropriate (see the section Promote Pain Relief, Comfort, and Rest, earlier).

The child is NPO until the intussusception is resolved. Administer IV fluids to maintain hydration and electrolyte balance. Once bowel function returns, the child may begin to breastfeed or, if bottle-fed, progress from clear liquids to full-strength formula.

Evaluation

Expected outcomes for a child with intussusception include the following:

- Adequate bowel function is achieved.
- Fluid and electrolyte balance is achieved.
- The child's pain is adequately controlled.

Discharge Planning and Teaching

Before discharge, the child should be consuming full feedings without difficulty. Teach parents to monitor for signs of infection, such as fever, fussiness, decreased oral intake, and wound drainage.

Malrotation and Volvulus

A **volvulus** is a condition in which the intestine twists upon itself as a result of gastric or intestinal malrotation. Figure 23.12B shows a volvulus.

Etiology and Pathophysiology

During the eighth week of fetal life, the stomach normally makes two rotations and ligaments form. When these rotations do not occur and ligaments do not form, the infant is at risk for gastric volvulus. Gastric volvulus is rare in children. Likewise, during the 6th to 10th weeks of fetal development, the intestinal loops grow and make several rotations along the superior mesenteric artery. When these rotations do not occur, the infant is at high risk for intestinal volvulus. Intestinal volvulus is more common than is gastric volvulus. The incidence of intestinal malrotation is 1 in 500 births (Kennedy & Liacouras, 2016). Intestinal malrotation is often associated with other abdominal wall defects, such as CDH, gastroschisis, and omphalocele.

Clinical Presentation

Vomiting is the most common symptom of volvulus. Bilious emesis is observed and signs of small bowel obstruction are present. The abdomen is firm and distended, and bloody stools may be present. Irritability related to pain is common. Abdominal pain can be colic in nature. Older children present with recurrent abdominal pain.

Assessment and Diagnosis

Perform a comprehensive abdominal exam, including inspection, auscultation, percussion, and palpation. The child may complain of recurring abdominal pain, and the abdomen is often distended and firm. Bowel sounds may be absent. Tympany is heard upon percussion. The parent often reports that the child has not had a recent bowel movement or that stools contain blood. An upper gastrointestinal series or contrast studies are used to support the diagnosis of volvulus.

Therapeutic Interventions

Emergency surgery known as a Ladd procedure is needed to untwist the bowel and restore blood flow. If necrotic bowel is present, it is removed and an ostomy may be needed while the bowel heals. Nursing care is similar to that for a child with intussusception.

Appendicitis

Acute appendicitis is the disease that most commonly requires emergency surgical treatment in children and is the abdominal diagnosis that most commonly leads to hospitalization in

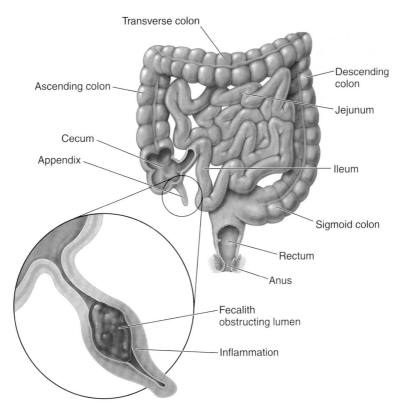

Figure 23.13. Appendicitis. Fecal matter obstructs the appendix, leading to inflammation and possible rupture. Reprinted with permission from Braun, C., & Anderson, C. (2016). *Applied pathophysiology* (3rd ed., Fig. 18.9). Philadelphia, PA: Wolters Kluwer.

children (Shah et al., 2016). Appendicitis, which is inflammation of the appendix, is often challenging to diagnose, particularly in young children. The appendix lies in the lower right quadrant of the abdomen (Fig. 23.13). The function of the appendix is unknown. However, one theory suggests that the appendix may be a storage area for "good" bacteria in the intestines. According to this theory, the bacteria are released after an episode of diarrhea, for example, and repopulate the intestinal tract with good bacteria.

Etiology and Pathophysiology

In the United States, approximately 80,000 children per year are diagnosed with appendicitis. Appendicitis is most common in older children, with peak incidence between the ages of 12 and 18 years. Boys are affected slightly more often than are girls. The peak incidence of appendicitis occurs in autumn and spring. Appendicitis accounts for more than 1 million hospital days used per year.

Acute appendicitis most likely has multiple etiologies but almost always results from an obstruction in the appendiceal lumen. Causes of obstructions include a fecalith (hard fecal mass), stenosis, parasitic infections, hyperplasia of lymphoid tissue, or a tumor. Mucus continues to be secreted and bacteria proliferate following acute obstruction, resulting in increased luminal

pressure. Elevated intraluminal pressure leads to lymphatic and venous congestion, followed by impaired perfusion to the area. Eventually, the appendix wall becomes ischemic, allowing invasion of bacteria and inflammatory infiltrates to all layers of the appendix. Necrosis occurs. Left untreated, the appendix becomes gangrenous and ruptures.

A ruptured appendix can lead to fecal and bacterial contamination of the peritoneum, leading to bacterial peritonitis. Peritonitis, if left untreated, spreads quickly and can lead to small bowel obstruction, hypovolemic shock, sepsis, and death. Early and accurate diagnosis of appendicitis is essential to minimize the risk of rupture and associated complications. Overall, the rate of rupture is 20% to 30%. However, in children younger than 3 years, the rate of rupture is 60% to 86% (Bansal, Banever, Karrer, & Partrick, 2012).

Clinical Presentation

Initially, children may present with cramping around the umbilicus, decreased appetite, nausea, and fever. Children with appendicitis often present with pain in the lower right quadrant of the abdomen. Specifically, rebound tenderness at McBurney's point is present (Fig. 23.14). As the inflammation progresses, pain becomes more intense and constant. Guarding of the abdomen, rigidity, and vomiting occur.

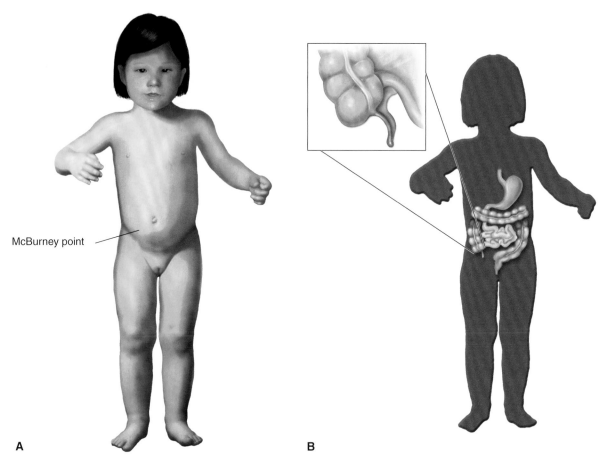

McBurney point

A   B

Figure 23.14. McBurney point. McBurney point, the area where the appendix is most commonly found, is located about one-third of the distance between the umbilicus and the anterior spine of the ilium **(A)**. Rebound tenderness over the McBurney point suggests the presence of appendicitis **(B)**. Reprinted with permission from Kyle, T., & Carman, S. (2016). *Essentials of pediatric nursing* (3rd ed., Fig. 20.14). Philadelphia, PA: Wolters Kluwer.

Rupture of the appendix can lead to sepsis and shock. Monitor vital signs for indications of septic shock and peritonitis. Specifically, monitor for increased heart and respiratory rates, fever, and decreased blood pressure, which can be signs of impending sepsis. Additional signs of a ruptured appendix include the following: guarding; abdominal distension; rapid, shallow breathing; pallor; chills; and irritability or restlessness. Notify the provider immediately if the child reports sudden, spontaneous relief of pain; this usually means the appendix has ruptured.

Assessment and Diagnosis

Assessment of pain is an essential part of determining whether appendicitis is present. Ask the child to show where the pain occurs in the abdomen. Note the intensity and location of the pain and whether rebound tenderness is present. Assess for rebound tenderness by deeply palpating the left side of the abdomen and then removing your hand quickly. If pain intensifies on the right side of the abdomen after you remove your hand, rebound tenderness is present. Recall the order of an abdominal assessment:

inspect, auscultate, and then palpate. Once appendicitis is diagnosed, avoid palpating the abdomen until after surgery to avoid increasing pain. Assess for signs of dehydration, particularly if the child has been vomiting or reports poor oral intake in the past 24 hours.

Diagnosis can be difficult in young children, who are unable to fully describe pain in the abdomen. A combination of the child's history, pain episodes, abdominal assessment, laboratory values, and an ultrasound or CT scan is used to diagnose appendicitis. Ultrasound is preferred over a CT scan because a CT scan exposes a child to radiation, whereas ultrasound does not. Ultrasound has been shown to have a greater than 90% sensitivity and specificity in the evaluation of acute appendicitis (Aiken & Oldham, 2016).

Therapeutic Interventions

Nursing care specific to appendicitis includes relieving pain and promoting comfort, maintaining hydration, administering antibiotics, monitoring and recognizing symptoms of infection, providing postoperative care of the child after removal of the appendix, and providing emotional support.

Patient Safety 23.2

Monitoring Fluid Losses From a Nasogastric Tube

Accurate measurement of output from a nasogastric (NG) tube is an essential nursing task. Loss of large amounts of stomach contents can lead to metabolic alkalosis if adequate fluid and electrolyte replacement is not administered. When large amounts of NG output are present, hydrogen and chloride ions are lost, leading to hypochloremic metabolic alkalosis and the loss of electrolytes such as potassium. Fluid replacement is often necessary to balance hydrogen, chloride, and potassium levels. Report immediately any increase in NG output so that adequate fluid replacement can be administered.

Assess the child's pain level frequently and provide nonpharmacological and pharmacological interventions as ordered and appropriate to relieve pain (see the section Promote Pain Relief, Comfort, and Rest, earlier).

The child is NPO until surgery can be performed to remove the infected or ruptured appendix. As described in the section Maintain Adequate Hydration and Nutrition, earlier, administer IV fluids as ordered to maintain hydration and electrolyte balance, continuing them postoperatively until bowel sounds return and then starting the patient on clear liquids and advancing the diet as tolerated. An NG tube is often in place to decompress the stomach following surgery. Once bowel sounds return, the NG tube is removed. Monitor and record intake and output, including NG output (Patient Safety 23.2).

Antibiotics are prescribed both preoperatively and postoperatively. Ensure timely administration of ordered antibiotics to stop the spread of infection. Monitor for side effects, including nausea and diarrhea, and allergic reactions while a child receives antibiotics. Monitor the effectiveness of therapy by assessing laboratory values, such as white blood cell count, and monitoring fever trends, pain levels, and surgical sites for signs of infection, such as redness, purulent drainage, and warmth.

For guidelines on addressing families' emotional and psychological needs related to gastrointestinal disorders, see the section Provide Emotional and Psychosocial Support to the Child and Parents, earlier.

Evaluation

Expected outcomes for a child with appendicitis include the following:

- Fluid and electrolyte balance is achieved and maintained.
- Pain is effectively managed and controlled.
- Wound healing occurs without signs of secondary infection.

Discharge Planning and Teaching

The child is discharged when adequate fluid intake is achieved and bowel function has returned. Teach parents to recognize signs and symptoms of infection at the surgical site and when to seek treatment if they suspect infection. Instruct parents on how to slowly resume a regular, nutritious diet. The child may resume activities as tolerated, except for strenuous or sports activities, which require the approval of the primary provider. Depending on the severity of the infection and surgical site healing, the child may need to rest at home for a period of time before returning to school. Encourage parents to make arrangements with the child's school so that the child does not fall behind academically.

Chronic Gastrointestinal Disorders

Chronic gastrointestinal disorders include peptic ulcer disease, gastroesophageal reflux, constipation, encopresis, Hirschsprung disease, short bowel syndrome, and inflammatory bowel disease (Crohn disease and ulcerative colitis). Chronic gastrointestinal disorders can be lifelong and can take an emotional, psychological, and financial toll on families. Nursing care often includes providing supportive resources and assisting children and families in coping with a chronic illness.

Peptic Ulcer Disease

A peptic ulcer is an erosion of the mucosal tissue in the esophagus, stomach, or duodenum. Ulcers in the stomach are often referred to as gastric ulcers, whereas ulcers in the intestine are referred to as duodenal ulcers.

Etiology and Pathophysiology

Peptic ulcers are either primary or secondary in origin. Primary peptic ulcers occur in otherwise healthy children. Secondary ulcers occur in children with preexisting illness or injury. Secondary ulcers are known as stress ulcers. Common conditions placing children at higher risk for secondary ulcers include injuries, such as burns or severe trauma, and multisystem organ failure, such as resulting from sepsis or pneumonia. Medications such as salicylates, corticosteroids, and nonsteroidal anti-inflammatory drugs also increase the risk of ulcers.

Peptic ulcer disease is highly prevalent in adults, affecting up to 10% of the population, but is less common in children. However, *Helicobacter pylori*, the main cause of peptic ulcer disease in both children and adults, is acquired early in life. *H. pylori*, a gram-negative, rod-shaped bacterium, appears to be transmitted from person to person (interpersonal route). Low socioeconomic conditions in childhood, living in a crowded home, and drinking contaminated water are risk factors for *H. pylori* (Eusebi, Zagari, & Bazzoli, 2014).

Clinical Presentation

Children with peptic ulcers present with varying symptoms according to age and location of the ulcer. Children with gastric ulcers have abdominal pain and burning, particularly on an empty stomach. The pain often awakens the child at night. Vomiting and pain after meals can also occur, particularly in the case of duodenal ulcers. Abdominal distension, anemia, and occult blood in the stool may be present.

Assessment and Diagnosis

In younger children, ask parents about feeding difficulties and crying episodes and whether blood appears in vomit, spit-up, or stool. Younger children often present with feeding difficulties, inconsolable crying, hematemesis, and melena. Assess school-age and older children for abdominal pain and distension and a feeling of abdominal fullness. Children often describe the pain as dull and aching and as lasting for minutes to hours. Establish whether eating relieves or worsens symptoms. Assess also for a family history for *H. pylori* infection.

Diagnosis is made on the basis of the history of abdominal symptoms and findings on esophagogastroduodenoscopy (EGD). An EGD is the preferred method to establish the presence of a peptic ulcer (Blanchard & Czinn, 2016). *H. pylori* can be detected in biopsy specimens obtained via the EGD.

Therapeutic Interventions

Nursing care of the child with a peptic ulcer focuses on relieving associated pain, promoting healing, teaching the parents about treatment, and assisting the child in learning stress-reduction techniques.

Stress can contribute to peptic ulcer disease. Assist the child in identifying sources of stress. Teach stress-reduction techniques. Assess coping mechanisms and give referrals for counseling and mental health services. Teach the child and family simple relaxation techniques such as rhythmic breathing and give referrals to yoga classes appropriate for children.

Medications such as proton-pump inhibitors (e.g., lansoprazole or omeprazole) and a combination of antibiotics, such as amoxicillin, clarithromycin, metronidazole, and tetracycline, are used to eradicate the infection (Garza-González, Perez-Perez, Maldonado-Garza, & Bosques-Padilla, 2014). Bismuth salts (an antidiarrheal agent) are also used in the treatment of *H. pylori*. Stress the importance of finishing antibiotic therapy as ordered with children and families.

Avoid using ibuprofen, because it irritates the gastric mucosa. If pain medication or treatment of fever is needed, administer acetaminophen. Teach parents to read over-the-counter medication labels to identify sources of ibuprofen.

Provide children and families information on nutritionally sound, age-appropriate diets, excluding foods only if they exacerbate the disorder.

Evaluation

Expected outcomes for a child with peptic ulcer disease include the following:

- The child experiences fewer episodes of pain and demonstrates evidence of pain relief.
- The child consumes adequate amounts of fluid and nutrition to meet growth and development needs.
- The child uses learned stress-reduction and relaxation techniques.

Discharge Planning and Teaching

Teach the child and parents about the importance of antibiotics and other medications in eradicating *H. pylori* and helping heal the ulcer. Stress the importance of follow-up visits. Teach adolescents and parents how to read medication labels, which medications to avoid, such as ibuprofen and aspirin-containing medications, and to seek medical advice if unsure of what a medication contains. Encourage the use of acetaminophen for pain relief. Teach parents when to seek immediate medical attention, such as if the child vomits bright red blood.

Gastroesophageal Reflux

Gastroesophageal reflux, a common physiological event, is the passage of stomach contents into the esophagus. Reflux occurs as a result of lower esophageal sphincter relaxation. Approximately 40% of infants experience gastroesophageal reflux or regurgitation (Davies, Burman-Roy, & Murphy, 2015). It is important to distinguish between gastroesophageal reflux and GERD (Patient Teaching 23.1).

Gastroesophageal reflux is common during infancy, with a peak prevalence at about 4 months of age, with two-thirds of infants regurgitating at least once a day (Baird, Harker, & Karmes, 2015). With gastroesophageal reflux, there are no signs of esophagitis or respiratory infections and caregivers do not

 Patient Teaching 23.1

Gastroesophageal Reflux and Gastroesophageal Reflux Disease

Gastroesophageal Reflux
Definition: Regurgitation or "spitting up"; no signs or symptoms of respiratory infections, excessive crying, or esophagitis
Teaching:
- Give smaller, more frequent feedings.
- Hold the infant upright after feedings for 30 min.
- Avoid placing the infant in a car seat or an infant seat after feeding, because the semi-sitting position can complicate gastroesophageal reflux.
- Thicken feedings as directed by the provider.
- Burp the infant after every 1–2 oz or after breastfeeding on each side.
- Monitor weight gain.

Gastroesophageal Reflux Disease
Definition: Regurgitation of feeds and gastric contents accompanied by poor weight gain and failure to thrive. The child may cry excessively or be persistently irritable. The infant may arch his or her neck when feeding. Respiratory symptoms include apnea, wheezing, pneumonia, cough, and cyanosis.
Teaching:
- Cover all teaching points listed in the section Gastroesophageal Reflux, earlier
- Provide medication information for histamine H_2-receptor antagonists or proton pump inhibitors.
- Teach parents about accurate dosing, frequency, side effects, and toxic effects of medications.
- Provide Nissen fundoplication preoperative and postoperative teaching.

report excessive crying. Gastroesophageal reflux is not troublesome. In other words, it does not interfere with the infant's or child's ability to gain weight and achieve growth and development milestones.

GERD is more serious than is gastroesophageal reflux. With GERD, infants fail to gain weight, may refuse to eat, are irritable, and have a history of respiratory symptoms such as wheezing, apnea, and cyanotic spells (Baird, Harker, & Karmes, 2015).

Etiology and Pathophysiology

The lower esophageal sphincter, a band of smooth muscle located at the junction of the esophagus and stomach, is the primary barrier to reflux. Reflux occurs when the esophageal sphincter relaxes too much as a result of an overdistended stomach or immature sphincter muscle and stomach contents travel up the esophagus to the pharynx (Baird, Harker, & Karmes, 2015). A smaller stomach, shorter esophagus, and an immature lower esophageal sphincter muscle in infants are contributing factors to reflux. Large-volume feedings and supine positioning predispose the infant to reflux (Baird, Harker, & Karmes, 2015). Many conditions are associated with increased risk for GERD. These include hiatal hernia, CDH, neurodevelopmental disorders, cystic fibrosis, epilepsy, congenital esophageal disorders, asthma, and prematurity (Baird, Harker, & Karmes, 2015). The incidence of gastroesophageal reflux is 3 times higher in males than in females. Although the incidence of gastroesophageal reflux is high, the incidence of GERD is much lower at 1.48 per 1,000 person-years in infants. GERD affects approximately 1.25% to 3.3% of children (Ruigómez, 2010).

Clinical Presentation

Infants present with regurgitation and vomiting, the most common signs of gastroesophageal reflux. Caregivers often report that the child is frequently hungry and irritable and at times inconsolable. Despite eating frequently, the child does not gain weight. Caregivers may also report excessive crying, arching of the neck with feeding, and respiratory symptoms such as noisy breathing (wheezing), cough, turning blue (cyanosis), and periods of apnea. The child may be seen multiple times for respiratory infections. Older children may report heartburn, epigastric pain, or regurgitation one or more times in a week.

A surgical procedure known as a Nissen fundoplication is performed for severe cases of GERD, such as those with recurrent aspiration, failure to thrive, or esophagitis. In this procedure, a valve mechanism is created by wrapping the fundus (the greater curvature of the stomach) around the distal esophagus. Stomach contents cannot enter the esophagus as long as the surgical repair is intact.

Assessment and Diagnosis

Engage parents to obtain a thorough history of feeding patterns and vomiting episodes. Observe emesis for amount, color, and consistency, noting whether blood is present. Monitor and record weight at each visit. Follow growth and development trends using a growth chart.

Diagnosis is made on the basis of the history of feeding patterns and findings from esophageal pH monitoring. The child may be admitted for pH probe and impedance probe monitoring. The pH probe measures the acidity of acid reflux, whereas the impedance probe measures both acid and nonacid reflux. A catheter is placed via the NG route and the child is monitored for 24 hours, while data are collected. The child eats and drinks normally during monitoring.

Therapeutic Interventions

Children with GERD are generally treated in the outpatient setting, such as in the clinic or provider's office. Nursing care focuses on teaching the parents about feeding, medication administration, monitoring weight gain and growth and development (if nutritional intake is in question related to excessive regurgitation and spit-up), and promoting interventions to reduce the occurrence of reflux, such as maintaining the infant in an upright position during and after feeding and burping the infant frequently. The nurse should also provide reassurance to the parents regarding normal regurgitation.

Use of medications to treat GERD varies by provider. Sometimes several medications are tried to achieve optimal outcomes and reduce gastric pH. See The Pharmacy 23.2 for a review of these mediations.

The Pharmacy 23.2 Medications Used to Treat Gastroesophageal Reflux

Medications	Classification	Route	Action	Nursing Considerations
Ranitidine (Zantac), famotidine (Pepcid), cimetidine (Tagamet)	Histamine H_2-receptor antagonists	PO	Inhibits gastric acid secretion by inhibiting the action of histamine at the H_2-receptor site; decreases symptoms of reflux	• May cause confusion, headache, dizziness, constipation, diarrhea, nausea, thrombocytopenia, bradycardia • Avoid administering within 2 h of antacids. • Administer with or without food.
Esomeprazole (Nexium), lansoprazole (Prevacid)	Proton pump inhibitors	PO	Binds to an enzyme in the presence of gastric acid, preventing the transport of hydrogen ions into the gastric lumen	• May cause dizziness, headache, diarrhea • Inform provider if diarrhea occurs. • Administer in the morning on an empty stomach.

PO, by mouth.

As noted in the section Maintain Adequate Hydration and Nutrition, earlier, interventions for the child with GERD include maintaining adequate caloric intake, providing smaller and more frequent feedings, and maintaining an upright (but not seated) position during and after feedings.

Evaluation

Expected outcomes for a child with gastroesophageal reflux include the following:

- The child is free of signs or symptoms of respiratory distress or aspiration.
- The child remains free of signs and symptoms of infection.
- The child consumes adequate amounts of nutrition to meet growth and developmental needs.
- Fluid and electrolyte levels are within normal limits.
- Parents demonstrate proper feeding, burping, and positioning techniques.

Discharge Planning and Teaching

See Patient Teaching 23.1 for teaching points to review with parents.

Constipation

Functional constipation is a common pediatric gastrointestinal disorder found in primary, secondary, and tertiary care. Approximately 3% of pediatrician visits and 25% of pediatric gastroenterology visits are for constipation (Koppen, Lammers, Benninga, & Tabbers, 2015). Symptoms of constipation can have a significant impact on the well-being and quality of life of children. Constipation is characterized by infrequent bowel movements, hard and/or large stools, painful defecation, and fecal incontinence and is often accompanied by abdominal pain (Dehghani et al., 2015).

Etiology and Pathophysiology

No organic cause is found in approximately 95% of children with constipation. Influencing factors in the pathophysiology of constipation include psychosocial factors such as major life events (parents' divorce, death of a friend or family member, moving to a new home) and behavioral disorders such as autism and attention-deficit/hyperactivity disorder. Additional influencing factors include socioeconomic status, educational level, and parental child-rearing attitudes (Koppen et al., 2015). Constipation is common in both sexes, but boys with constipation have higher rates of fecal incontinence than do girls (Hyams et al., 2016). The prevalence of constipation increases from approximately 3% in the first year of life to 10% in the second year of life (Turco et al., 2014).

The triggering event leading to constipation is most likely the universal instinct to avoid defecation because of pain or social reasons. Social reasons include fear or embarrassment of having a bowel movement at school or in public places. The longer the child holds the stool, the more water is absorbed from the colonic mucosa, causing the feces to become hard and progressively more difficult to evacuate. A vicious cycle of stool retention ensues. The rectum becomes increasingly distended, resulting in overflow fecal incontinence, loss of rectal sensation, and, finally, loss of the normal urge to defecate (Hyams et al., 2016). Furthermore, as stool accumulates in the rectum, motility in the foregut decreases, leading to anorexia, abdominal distension, and pain.

Clinical Presentation

Children present with constipation in various ways. Obvious symptoms may include difficult, painful bowel movements and, in toddlers, fecal incontinence. Significant symptoms of functional constipation are listed in the Rome IV diagnostic criteria established by the European Society for Paediatric Gastroenterology, Hepatology, and Nutrition and the North American Society for Pediatric Gastroenterology, Hepatology, and Nutrition (Box 23.7). Additional symptoms may include irritability, decreased appetite, and/or feeling full early in consumption of a meal (early satiety). These symptoms may disappear when the child has a bowel movement.

Box 23.7 Rome IV Diagnostic Criteria for Functional Constipation

For a child with a developmental age younger than 4 y, two or more of the following criteria must be present for at least a week and in the absence of organic pathology:

1. Less than two defecations per week
2. At least one episode of incontinence per week after the acquisition of toileting skills
3. History of excessive stool retention
4. History of painful or hard bowel movements
5. Presence of a large fecal mass in the rectum
6. History of large-diameter stools that may obstruct the toilet

For a child with a developmental age of older than 4 y with insufficient criteria for irritable bowel syndrome, two or more of the following criteria must be met at least once per week for at least 1 mo before diagnosis:

1. Fewer than two defecations in the toilet per week
2. At least one episode of fecal incontinence per week
3. History of retentive posturing or excessive volitional stool retention
4. History of painful or hard bowel movements
5. Presence of a large fecal mass in the rectum
6. History of large-diameter stools that may obstruct the toilet

Data from Benninga, M., Faure, C., Hyman, P. E., St James Roberts, I., Schechter, N., & Nurko, S. (2016). Childhood functional gastrointestinal disorders: neonate/toddler. *Gastroenterology, 150*(6), 1443–1455; Hyams, J., Di Lorenzo, C., Saps, M., Shulman, R., Staiano, A., & van Tilburg, M. (2016). Childhood functional gastrointestinal disorders: Child/adolescent. *Gastroenterology, 150*(6), 1456–1468.

Assessment and Diagnosis

Assess stooling patterns and characteristics of stool, including the presence of blood. Assess dietary intake for adequate intake of fluids and fiber content. Assess the abdomen for fullness, distension, and bowel sounds in all quadrants. Note the presence of any palpable mass (retained stool). Observe for hemorrhoids and anal fissures. Children may have pain and cramping in the lower abdomen.

Diagnosis is made on the basis of findings from the history, physical exam, and abdominal X-ray (conducted to assess for distended bowel or stool in the bowels).

Therapeutic Interventions

Nursing care of the child with constipation most likely takes place in the clinic or outpatient setting. The nursing care specific to constipation includes disimpaction for those who present with fecal impaction and providing maintenance therapy to prevent accumulation of stool. Educating patients and families is as important as medical therapy.

Disimpaction, if needed, is achieved by the use of enemas such as a sodium docusate enema or with high-dose oral polyethylene glycol for up to 6 days (Koppen et al., 2015). Following disimpaction, maintenance therapy is used to prevent reaccumulation of stool. Children with constipation require various medication regimens to both restore normal bowel function and maintain a regular stooling pattern. The first-line therapy for constipated children is generally polyethylene glycol. Other pharmacological interventions for preventing reaccumulation of stool include lactulose, bisacodyl, docusate sodium, and milk of magnesia (The Pharmacy 23.3).

Teach families how to recognize withholding behaviors and use behavioral and pharmacological interventions. Behavioral interventions include regular toileting; the use of diaries to track time of day, amount of stool, and difficulty defecating; and reward systems for successful evacuations of stool (Nurko & Zimmerman, 2014). Teach parents to encourage regular bowel habits by placing the child on the toilet after a meal and to provide positive reinforcement to help prevent withholding of stool. Educate families on age-specific dietary practices such as adequate fluid and fiber intake. Increasing fruit and vegetable intake and offering high-fiber snacks can increase fiber intake.

Evaluation

Expected outcomes for a child with constipation include the following:

- A routine bowel elimination pattern is established and maintained.
- The child demonstrates normal stool patterns and frequency.
- The child is free of signs of constipation.

The Pharmacy 23.3 Medications Used to Treat Constipation

Medication	Classification	Route	Action	Nursing Considerations
Polyethylene glycol (Miralax)	Osmotic laxative	PO G-tube	Draws water into the GI tract, which softens stools and increases peristalsis related to increased intestinal distension	• Effect usually occurs within 1–2 d; but in the case of impactions, it may take 3–4 d • Common side effects: fecal incontinence, flatulence, abdominal pain, nausea and bloating
Docusate sodium (Senna)	Anthraquinone stimulant laxative	PO	Metabolite of docusate sodium acts as a local irritant on the colon, stimulating peristalsis; promotes movement of water into stool, softening stool	• May cause severe diaper rash, blisters, skin sloughing in infants; avoid use in infants younger than age 1 y • Common side effects: abdominal cramping, nausea, vomiting
Magnesium hydroxide (Milk of Magnesia)	Laxative	PO Rectal	Causes an osmotic gradient, resulting in a laxative effect	• Common side effects: diarrhea, hypotension, weakness, lethargy • Contraindicated in patients with severe renal failure
Bisacodyl	Diphenylmethane stimulant laxative	PO Rectal	Alters fluid and electrolyte transport in the colon, resulting in fluid accumulation in the colon	• Common side effects: abdominal cramps, nausea

GI, gastrointestinal; G-tube, gastrostomy tube; PO, by mouth.

Encopresis

Encopresis is defined as voluntary or involuntary passage of stool into inappropriate places at least once a month for 3 consecutive months after the age of 4 years. The majority of children (65%–95%) with encopresis have a history of chronic constipation (retentive encopresis). Nonretentive encopresis is when constipation is not present. Nonretentive encopresis can be associated with emotional or psychological disturbances.

Etiology and Pathophysiology

The etiology of encopresis is multifactorial. A combination of biological, emotional, and learning factors appears to play a role in the development of encopresis. Abnormal gastrointestinal motility, hereditary predispositions, and developmental delays have been associated with the development of encopresis. Also, turmoil and conflict within the family unit have been associated with encopresis in children. Approximately 4% of children aged 5 to 6 years are diagnosed with encopresis, whereas 1.5% of children aged 11 to 12 years have the diagnosis. Risk factors for encopresis include chronic constipation after the age of 2 years, male gender, and a history of stool retention (Kammacher Guerreiro, Bettinville, & Herzog, 2014).

Clinical Presentation

Children with encopresis present with reports of underwear soiling. Parents often assume their child has diarrhea, not constipation, because of the liquid nature of the stool. For children with chronic constipation, the parent or child reports complaints of difficulty defecating, abdominal or rectal pain, impaired appetite, and urinary incontinence. Parents and children also report large bowel movements that obstruct the toilet. Increased frequency of UTIs also occurs when a child has encopresis.

Assessment and Diagnosis

See the section Assessment and Diagnosis under Constipation.

Therapeutic Interventions

Nursing care of the child with encopresis includes managing the clearance of impacted fecal material followed by short-term use of mineral oil or laxatives to prevent further constipation. Teaching parents about acceptable diets and behavioral modifications is also a priority when managing encopresis. See the section Therapeutic Interventions under Constipation.

Behavior therapy is also a part of managing encopresis. Encourage parents to reward the child for adherence to a healthy bowel regimen and to not respond to soiling with punitive measures. Punitive measures can result in the child becoming angry, ashamed, and then resistant to intervention.

Evaluation

Expected outcomes for a child with encopresis include the following:

- The child practices routine toilet sitting after morning and evening meals.

- The child and family effectively use behavior modification techniques that reward and reinforce appropriate toileting habits.
- The child is free from episodes of soiling or passage of stool at inappropriate times.

Discharge Planning and Teaching

Teaching the parents and child about regular postprandial toilet sitting and adoption of a balanced, high-fiber diet is also necessary. See the section Therapeutic Interventions under Constipation.

Hirschsprung Disease

Hirschsprung disease is a disease of the intestinal tract, usually of the rectum or sigmoid colon, in which there is absence of peristalsis and motility due to the lack of neuronal ganglion cells.

Etiology and Pathophysiology

Hirschsprung disease, also known as congenital megacolon, is a birth defect characterized by complete absence of neuronal ganglion cells (aganglionosis) in a portion of the intestinal tract. Without the neuronal ganglion cells, peristalsis cannot occur and the individual cannot pass stool. The segment of bowel affected includes the distal rectum and a variable length of contiguous proximal intestine. Approximately 80% of children diagnosed with Hirschsprung disease have short-segment disease, in which aganglionosis is restricted to the rectosigmoid colon. Long-segment disease, in which aganglionosis extends proximally to the sigmoid colon, occurs in 15% to 20% of those diagnosed (Parisi, 2015). Total colonic aganglionosis, in which aganglionic cells affect the entire large intestine, occurs in 5% of children diagnosed with Hirschsprung disease.

The prevalence of Hirschsprung disease is 1 in 5,000 births. Definitive diagnosis is made by examining tissue from a distal rectal biopsy and finding it absent of ganglion cells. In older children, anorectal manometry can be used to assist in diagnosing Hirschsprung disease. Abdominal radiographs show a dilated proximal colon with an empty rectum. A barium enema study demonstrates delayed emptying times.

Clinical Presentation

Newborns often present with symptoms such as a distended abdomen, failure to pass meconium within the first 48 hours of birth, and repeated vomiting. Older infants and children present with chronic constipation, marked abdominal distension, and palpable dilated bowel loops. A digital rectal exam reveals an empty rectal vault. A forceful passage of stool can occur after completion of the rectal exam. If left untreated, enterocolitis (inflammation of the intestines) can develop and lead to a fatal outcome if unrecognized. Symptoms of enterocolitis include fever, pain, vomiting, bloody diarrhea, and frequent, foul-smelling stools.

Treatment for Hirschsprung disease is surgical correction. The type of surgical correction is determined by the health of the child and the presence of any concurrent morbidities. A short-term colostomy may be necessary, but many children are treated successfully using a single-stage pull-through procedure (Parisi, 2015). A single pull-through procedure involves resecting the aganglionic segment and anastomosing the proximal bowel to the anus.

Assessment and Diagnosis

Assess newborns for the passage of meconium. Failure to pass meconium within 48 hours of birth requires further investigation for possible Hirschsprung disease. Abdominal distension may be present. For older infants and children, obtain a history of bowel patterns and elimination habits and assess the child's growth and development, including weight gain and loss trends. Constipation alternating with diarrhea and vomiting may also be present. Assess the consistency and color of stools, as well as for the presence of blood.

Therapeutic Interventions

Nursing care of the child with Hirschsprung disease is similar to that of any child undergoing abdominal surgery. Preoperatively, the child may be NPO or have clear fluids the day before surgery. The bowel may be evacuated before surgery using rectal irrigations. Monitor for signs of enterocolitis, infection, and increased abdominal distension. Postoperatively, maintain hydration by administering IV fluids until bowel function returns and the child has adequate oral intake. Monitor for signs of infection, and administer pain medication as prescribed. If an ostomy is present, monitor the stoma for adequate moisture, color, and output.

Evaluation

Expected outcomes for a child with Hirschsprung disease include the following:

- The child consumes adequate nutritional intake to promote growth and development.
- The child's fluid and electrolyte levels are within normal limits.
- Regular and adequate bowel function is evident.
- The child's pain is managed effectively.
- Parents demonstrate effective coping strategies while caring for their child with Hirschsprung disease.

Short Bowel Syndrome

Short bowel syndrome, also referred to as short gut syndrome, is a condition in which a large portion of the small intestine has been removed or is dysfunctional and the resulting inadequate bowel length leads to suboptimal absorption of nutrients. The actual length of small intestine required for adequate absorption of nutrients remains controversial. However, bowel length less than 100 cm in the first year of life is regarded as abnormal (Coletta, Khalil, & Morabito, 2014). Bowel length less than 40 cm requires therapy, according to most centers (Soden, 2010).

Etiology and Pathophysiology

Causes of short bowel syndrome vary according to age. In infancy, some causes include NEC, gastroschisis, volvulus of malrotation, intestinal atresia, and motility disorders. The gestational age of the child and the timing of the actual incident leading to short gut syndrome are taken into consideration when defining short bowel syndrome because significant growth of the bowel occurs in the third trimester of pregnancy and during childhood. In older children, causes of short bowel syndrome include a midgut volvulus, trauma, Crohn disease, and vascular events. Males and females are equally affected.

Short bowel syndrome can lead to intestinal failure. Intestinal failure occurs when intestinal function is insufficient to meet the body's nutrition and hydration needs (Coletta, Khalil, & Morabito, 2014). Supplementary parenteral nutrition and/or IV fluids are necessary for growth and hydration.

Clinical Presentation

Children with short bowel syndrome often have severe diarrhea related to accelerated intestinal transit, gastric acid hypersecretion, intestinal bacterial overgrowth, and malabsorption of fats and bile salts (Coletta, Khalil, & Morabito, 2014). Signs of dehydration may be present specifically when diarrhea is uncontrolled. Unintended weight loss or failure to gain weight is also seen in children with short bowel syndrome, related to the inability to absorb fats, carbohydrates, vitamins, minerals, trace elements, and fluids. Overgrowth of gut bacteria can lead to bloating and diarrhea.

Assessment and Diagnosis

Assessment of the child with short bowel syndrome includes not only examining the gastrointestinal system but also assessing the child for signs of dehydration (tachycardia, tachypnea, poor skin turgor and hypotension), signs of electrolyte imbalances and signs of infection. Assess the abdomen for bowel sounds, tenderness, distention and if pain is present. Assessment of urinary and stool losses of sodium and potassium is essential to prescribe adequate parenteral nutrition concentrations to replace sodium and potassium. Deficiencies in vitamins, iron, and trace elements are also common. Replacement via parenteral nutrition is often necessary, and assessment for consequences of vitamin and mineral deficiencies is ongoing. Table 23.8 reviews common vitamin and mineral deficiencies and the potential symptoms.

Central line infections and sepsis can also be seen in children with short bowel syndrome who are receiving parenteral nutrition. Assess for signs and symptoms of systemic infection, such as fever, tachycardia, tachypnea, irritability, and malaise.

Therapeutic Interventions

Children with short bowel syndrome often receive nutrition support via parenteral nutrition and/or enteral feeding tubes (Hopkins et al., 2017). Note that fluid and electrolyte imbalance is common in short bowel syndrome related to gastrointestinal water and salt losses, so monitor intake and output and weight carefully. Also, the child with short bowel syndrome is at increased risk for infection because of altered gut flora and central line access, if present, so follow guidelines provided in section Prevent Infection, earlier.

Table 23.8 Vitamin and Mineral Deficiencies Associated With Short Bowel Syndrome and Associated Symptoms

Vitamin or Mineral	Symptoms of Deficiency
Vitamin A	Night blindness, abnormal dryness and thickening of the conjunctiva and cornea (xerophthalmia), corneal ulcerations, dry and scaly skin, impaired immunity, infections, growth retardation
Vitamin B	Stomatitis, glossitis, cheilosis, edema, anemia, ophthalmoplegia, tachycardia or bradycardia, peripheral neuropathy, fatigue, confusion, seizures
Vitamin D	Rickets, short stature, bone fractures due to weakening or softening of the bones (osteomalacia), low calcium blood levels (which can also be associated with tetany and paresthesias)
Vitamin E	Paresthesias, tetany, ataxia, edema, depressed deep tendon reflexes, vision problems
Vitamin K	Prolonged bleeding, bruising, petechiae, ecchymosis, purpura
Iron	Pallor, glossitis, abnormally spooned nails, weakness, fatigue, difficulty concentrating, dyspnea
Zinc	Stomatitis, alopecia, poor wound healing, reddened and scaly skin rash

Evaluation

Expected outcomes for a child with short bowel syndrome include the following:

- The child remains free of central line infections.
- The child gains adequate weight and height.
- Parents demonstrate the ability to administer parenteral nutrition and tube feeds.
- Skin integrity remains intact.

Discharge Planning and Teaching

Before discharge, teach parents how to prepare and administer parenteral nutrition and how to care for the central line. Teach parents about the importance of proper hand washing and use of clean and sterile techniques while working with the child's central line. Once enteral feedings have begun, teach parents how to care for the feeding tube, manage the feeding pump, and maintain skin integrity of the face where the feeding tube is secured. Home health visits may be needed to monitor growth and development, monitor and care for the central line and feeding tube, and assist parents in troubleshooting common problems with these medical devices. Blood draws are necessary to monitor fluid and electrolyte levels.

Inflammatory Bowel Disease: Crohn Disease and Ulcerative Colitis

Crohn disease and ulcerative colitis, known as inflammatory bowel diseases, are chronic, idiopathic inflammatory disorders of the gastrointestinal tract. Approximately 15% to 20% of all cases of inflammatory bowel disease are diagnosed in childhood or adolescence (Adamiak et al., 2013).

Etiology and Pathophysiology

Inflammatory bowel disease can be separated into two disease processes: Crohn disease and ulcerative colitis. Both diseases are characterized by exacerbations and remissions.

Crohn disease primarily affects the large and small intestines but can affect the entire alimentary canal, from the mouth to the anus. In Crohn disease, some areas of the intestinal tract may be normal, whereas others are affected. In essence, the disease can skip areas of the bowel (Fig. 23.15).

Ulcerative colitis affects only the large intestine and rectal mucosa and is continuous along the colon. The disease usually begins in the rectum and can progress up the large intestine. Inflammation is limited to the mucosa. Superficial inflammation is present.

Genetic and environmental influences play a role in the development of inflammatory bowel disease. The risk of having inflammatory bowel disease ranges from 7% to 30% in a child with some family history of the disease but is 35% in a child whose parents both have the disease (Grossman & Baldassano, 2016).

Clinical Presentation

A child with Crohn disease presents with fever, fatigue, and malaise. Failure to grow is also common in Crohn disease because of suboptimal absorption of nutrients or excessive nutrient loss and inadequate caloric intake. When the stomach and duodenum are involved, the child presents with epigastric pain and vomiting. Cramping abdominal pain and abdominal distension are also seen. Perianal lesions (fissures, abscesses, and fistulas) are noted. Table 23.9 compares clinical manifestations of Crohn disease and ulcerative colitis.

A child with ulcerative colitis presents with diarrhea and with blood, mucus, and pus in the stool. Urgency, abdominal cramping, and nighttime defecation are also noted. In fulminant colitis, fever, anemia, leukocytosis, and more than five bloody stools per day are present.

Crohn disease

- Both large and small bowel involved

- Areas of normal bowel skipped

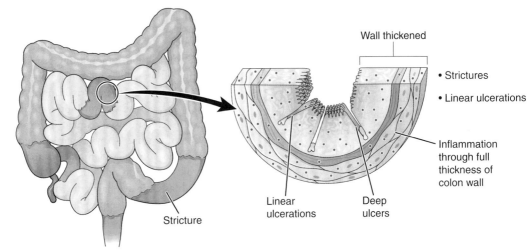

Wall thickened

- Strictures
- Linear ulcerations

Inflammation through full thickness of colon wall

Linear ulcerations

Deep ulcers

Stricture

Ulcerative colitis

- Small bowel not involved

- Continuous involvement
  –No skipped areas of normal bowel

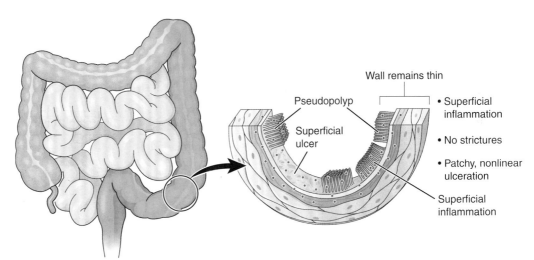

Wall remains thin

Pseudopolyp

Superficial ulcer

- Superficial inflammation

- No strictures

- Patchy, nonlinear ulceration

Superficial inflammation

Figure 23.15. Comparison of how Crohn disease and ulcerative colitis affect the intestine. Reprinted with permission from Braun, C., & Anderson, C. (2016). *Applied pathophysiology* (3rd ed., Fig. 3.30). Philadelphia, PA: Wolters Kluwer.

Table 23.9 Comparison of Clinical Manifestations for Crohn Disease and Ulcerative Colitis

Clinical Manifestation	Crohn Disease	Ulcerative Colitis
Type of lesions	Transmural (through the intestinal wall), segmental	Superficial, continuous
Anal or perianal lesions	Common	Rare
Anorexia	Can be severe	Mild to moderate
Bleeding	Absent	Present
Diarrhea	Moderate	Severe; mixed with blood and mucus
Growth suppression	Significant	Mild
Pain	Cramping abdominal pain	Pain present before and during bowel movement; relieved by passing stool and flatus
Risk of cancer	Greatly increased	Slightly increased
Weight loss	Severe	Moderate

Assessment and Diagnosis

Perform a thorough gastrointestinal assessment (Table 23.2). When flare-ups occur, assess for signs of dehydration and possible hypovolemic shock.

Diagnosis is made by clinical presentation, ruling out infectious processes, and an endoscopy and colonoscopy with biopsy. The endoscopy helps determine the extent and severity of the inflammatory process. Laboratory studies contribute to the diagnosis. Findings consistent with a diagnosis of irritable bowel disease include occult blood in the stool, anemia, elevated erythrocyte sedimentation rate, hypoalbuminemia, and an elevated white blood cell count.

Therapeutic Interventions

Nursing care of the child with inflammatory bowel disease occurs primarily in the clinic and home settings. Children may require hospitalization for flare-ups and complications from the disease and corresponding treatment.

Nursing care focuses on administering medications, monitoring nutritional status, monitoring growth status, managing diet therapy, and providing emotional support and resources to families.

Medication therapy is important in controlling inflammatory bowel disease. Antibiotics, usually metronidazole and ciprofloxacin, are used to treat infection, particularly for perianal Crohn disease. Corticosteroids and immunosuppressants are used to control inflammation and keep flare-ups under control. Assess for side effects of these medications. Side effects such as excessive hair growth, altered mood, and development of a Cushingoid appearance can be difficult for adolescents and teenagers to cope with. See The Pharmacy 23.4 for additional information regarding medications.

Although treatment with medications is usually effective in achieving remission in children, some cases of ulcerative colitis

The Pharmacy 23.4 Medications Used to Treat Inflammatory Bowel Disease

Medication	Classification	Route	Action	Nursing Considerations
Prednisone, prednisolone, hydrocortisone, budesonide	Corticosteroids	• PO • IV	Anti-inflammatory	• Administer with meals to reduce gastric irritation. • Avoid abrupt discontinuation. • Monitor for and report delayed wound healing. • Common side effects: nausea, vomiting, immunosuppression, hypertension, acne, growth suppression, altered mood, Cushingoid appearance
Azathioprine, cyclosporine, methotrexate, 6-mercaptopurine	Immuno-suppressants	• PO • IV	Immuno-suppressive effect	• Teach the child and family ways to reduce risk of infection: avoid exposure to sick people, proper hand washing technique, proper hygiene. • Common side effects: nausea, vomiting, anorexia, diarrhea, bone marrow suppression, infection, mucositis
Infliximab (Remicade), adalimumab (Humira), certolizumab (Cimzia)	• Biological therapies • Monoclonal antibodies	• IV • IM	• Neutralizes and prevents the activity of tumor necrosis factor • Anti-inflammatory and anti-proliferative effect	• Monitor for signs of infection. • Common side effects: headache, fatigue, upper respiratory infection, nausea, vomiting, abdominal pain, fever, infusion reactions
Sulfasalazine, mesalamine	Aminosalicylates	PO	Inhibits prostaglandin synthesis, resulting in a gastrointestinal anti-inflammatory effect in the colon	• Assess for rash; may cause Stevens–Johnson syndrome. • Monitor CBC and liver function tests throughout therapy. • Administer after meals. • Do not crush or chew extended-release tablets. • Common side effects: headache, nausea, vomiting, diarrhea, anorexia, rash, fever

CBC, complete blood count; IM, intramuscular; IV, intravenous; PO, by mouth.

do not respond to medication therapy. In these cases, a colectomy (surgical removal of all or part of the colon) is performed.

Offer dietary supplements such as protein shakes and high-calorie meals to ensure that caloric requirements are met. Offer several small meals a day rather than a few large meals. Increased fiber intake can increase intestinal motility, worsening diarrhea. Therefore, limit fiber intake by removing peels from fruits and avoiding serving the child nuts and large quantities of whole-grain foods.

As discussed in the section Maintain Adequate Hydration and Nutrition, earlier, TPN is ordered for children who are unable to take in sufficient calories to meet metabolic demands and maintain growth and development. TPN requires a central venous access catheter. When caring for a child on TPN, monitor fluid and electrolyte status upon initiation and throughout administration and obtain the child's weight at least weekly while on TPN.

As discussed in the section Maintain Skin Integrity, earlier, change diapers and soiled underpants frequently, wash the area with mild soap, keep the area dry and clean, and apply barrier creams to prevent skin breakdown.

For guidelines on addressing families' emotional and psychological needs related to gastrointestinal disorders, see the section Provide Emotional and Psychosocial Support to the Child and Parents, earlier.

Evaluation

Expected outcomes for a child with inflammatory bowel disease include the following:

- The child's fluid and electrolyte values are within normal limits.
- The child maintains adequate nutritional intake to meet growth and development needs.
- The child remains free of infection.
- The child adheres to the medication regimen.
- The child and parents demonstrate the ability to cope with a chronic, sometimes debilitating, disease.

Discharge Planning and Teaching

In most cases of inflammatory bowel disease, the child can be cared for at home. Provide parents with the teaching and resources they need to care for the child. If TPN is being administered at home, teach parents how to care for the central line, perform proper hand washing, and handle infusion pumps and tubing. Parents must demonstrate how to care for the central line and administer TPN before discharge and during home visits. Review with parents the signs and symptoms of infection and emergency procedures regarding the central line. Assist parents in obtaining resources such as infusion equipment and central line supplies. Make home healthcare referrals as needed.

Teach parents and the child about the importance of adhering to the medication regimen. The child should continue taking medications even when he or she feels well and is asymptomatic. Reinforce teaching about care of the child associated with altered immune systems. Instruct the child and family to avoid sick contacts while the child is taking steroids. Encourage parents to immediately report fever and exposure to infectious diseases to the provider.

Celiac Disease

Celiac disease, also known as gluten-sensitive enteropathy and nontropical sprue, is an autoimmune reaction to gluten that leads to intestinal inflammation, villous atrophy, and malabsorption (Fig. 23.16).

Etiology and Pathophysiology

Celiac disease is a chronic, irreversible disease triggered by the ingestion of gluten in genetically predisposed individuals. Gluten is a plant storage protein contained in wheat, barley, and rye. If left untreated, celiac disease can lead to inflammation of the small intestine and systemic complications. Small intestinal mucosal damage occurs in varying degrees and is typically more severe proximally than distally (Guandalini, 2017).

In the early onset of celiac disease, fat absorption is impaired, leading to the excretion of large amounts of fat in the

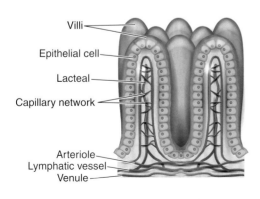

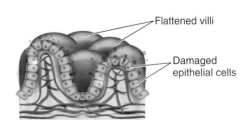

Normal villi   **Damaged villi**

Figure 23.16. Celiac disease. Intestinal villi are flattened and the epithelial walls of the intestine are damaged.

stool (steatorrhea). As a result, stools are frothy, greasy, and foul-smelling. As celiac disease progresses, changes in the villi occur, leading to malabsorption of proteins, carbohydrates, fat-soluble vitamins (A, D, E, and K), calcium, iron, and folate.

Celiac disease occurs in approximately 1% of the world's population (Fasano & Catassi, 2012). Individuals who have first-degree relatives with celiac disease are more likely to have the disease. A child with Down syndrome, Turner syndrome, Williams syndrome, or immunoglobulin A (IgA) deficiency is more likely to have Celiac disease. Individuals with type 1 diabetes mellitus, autoimmune thyroid disease, and autoimmune liver disease are also at higher risk for celiac disease.

Clinical Presentation

Infants with celiac disease often present with vomiting, diarrhea, abdominal distension, anorexia, and failure to thrive. Symptoms are most likely to appear when solid foods containing gluten are introduced to the child's diet. Children with celiac disease present with abdominal pain, constipation, and weight loss. Diarrhea and abdominal bloating are common in children. Muscle wasting and hypotonia can also be present. Skin rashes, known as dermatitis herpetiformis, may appear, particularly around the elbows, buttocks, and knees.

Assessment and Diagnosis

Assess the child for signs of abdominal discomfort and distress. Assess the frequency of vomiting and diarrhea. Assess stool for steatorrhea. Signs of poor nutritional intake may be present, such as thinning hair and nails, dry skin, weight loss, delayed cognitive development, and a failure to meet developmental milestones.

Diagnosis is made by first screening for celiac disease antibodies using a serum test called a tissue transglutaminase IgA (tTG-IgA) test. The tTG-IgA test is done while the infant or child is consuming gluten-containing foods. If the tTG-IgA test is positive, an endoscopic biopsy of the small intestine is performed to evaluate the intestinal mucosa for damage consistent with celiac disease. As part of the diagnosis, a complete blood count, ferritin levels, iron levels, and iron-binding capacity are obtained because children with celiac disease are often anemic (Snyder et al., 2016). The only treatment currently available for individuals with celiac disease is a lifelong gluten-free diet.

Therapeutic Interventions

Nursing care of the child diagnosed with celiac disease focuses on assisting parents in choosing appropriate formulas and foods, ensuring adequate fluid and nutrient intake for growth and development, and maintaining skin integrity.

Children with celiac disease require a diet free of gluten. Provide parents with food lists containing gluten-free, age-appropriate foods. Referral to a dietician experienced in gluten-free diets for nutrition consultation is often helpful. Educate parents on hidden sources of gluten as well as on how to make substitutions with potatoes, rice, buckwheat, soy, and quinoa. Instruct children, adolescents, and their parents on sources

of calcium and vitamin D, because evidence shows that this population consumes diets deficient in these nutrients (Snyder et al., 2016).

School can often be a challenge for children on a gluten-free diet. Emphasize to parents and children the need to maintain a gluten-free diet. Encourage parents to provide gluten-free alternatives for snacks at school, friends' homes, and extracurricular activities. Children are more likely to comply with a gluten-free diet if they have readily available alternatives.

Children with celiac disease should have routine anthropometric measurements and be under the care of a registered dietician. At each clinic visit, obtain and record length (height), weight, and head circumference (for children younger than age 2 years). Assess trends in growth and developmental milestones at well-visit checkups. Educate parents on age-specific milestones and encourage them to bring any concerns to the provider.

Evaluation

Expected outcomes for a child with celiac disease include the following:

- The child receives adequate nutrition to support growth and development.
- Parents demonstrate an understanding of special dietary needs required when caring for their child with celiac disease.
- The child meets growth and development milestones.
- Parents understand the importance of and adhere to follow-up appointments.

Discharge Planning and Teaching

Infants and children with celiac disease are managed in the home setting. During clinic visits, provide education on and reinforcement of dietary restrictions for celiac disease. Teach school-age children the concepts of a gluten-free diet early. Often, the entire family adopts a gluten-free diet. This can be difficult for older siblings, who may have been eating a regular diet before their sibling's diagnosis. Provide resources and support for coping with the management of a gluten-free diet.

Hepatobiliary Disorders

The liver and biliary system play vital roles in the breakdown of wastes, elimination of toxins, production of coagulation factors, and metabolism of drugs. Any disorder that affects the liver can be life-threatening. Four common pediatric liver disorders are discussed: hyperbilirubinemia, biliary atresia, hepatitis, and cirrhosis.

Hyperbilirubinemia (Jaundice)

Hyperbilirubinemia is a condition of abnormally elevated serum bilirubin level. Hyperbilirubinemia in the newborn period can be divided into two categories: physiological and pathological. Physiological jaundice is discussed here.

Etiology and Pathophysiology

Physiological jaundice (hyperbilirubinemia) is a common problem of newborns. Approximately 60% of full-term newborns and 80% of preterm newborns experience jaundice (Ambalavanan & Carol, 2017). In most cases, it is benign. Accumulation of unconjugated bilirubin causes the yellow color, or jaundice, seen in the skin and mucous membranes. Bilirubin is a product of the breakdown of red blood cells. When red blood cells are broken down or destroyed, they are separated into heme and globulin. Heme is converted to bilirubin in the liver, spleen, and bone marrow. The bilirubin is then transported to the liver, conjugated, and excreted into the bile. The bile goes through the gallbladder and into the intestines, where it is converted into a variety of pigments and excreted eventually by the kidneys. Newborns have a difficult time excreting "heme," or the colored part of the red blood cell, due to immature liver and intestinal function.

Clinical Presentation

Yellow discoloration of the skin, sclera, and mucous membranes is a sign of hyperbilirubinemia. Jaundice usually progresses in a cephalocaudal manner, starting at the face and eyes and progressing to the abdomen and feet as serum bilirubin levels rise (Ambalavanan & Carol, 2017). Jaundice is generally noticed when the newborn's serum bilirubin level reaches greater than 3 mg/dL. Infants with severe hyperbilirubinemia often present with poor feeding and lethargy. If left untreated, encephalopathy can ensue.

Assessment and Diagnosis

Assess the newborn every 8 hours for signs of jaundice, beginning with the face, eyes, and mucous membranes. Assess alertness and arousability. Assess the infant's ability to nurse or suck on a bottle. Remain alert for signs of dehydration (see the section Dehydration, earlier). Diagnosis is made by obtaining a transcutaneous bilirubin measurement or by checking a total serum bilirubin level.

Therapeutic Interventions

Nursing care of the child with physiological jaundice focuses on lowering bilirubin to acceptable levels by establishing regular feeding patterns and adequate intake and providing phototherapy when necessary, as well as educating parents regarding physiological jaundice.

Early and frequent feedings decrease bilirubin levels (Ambalavanan & Carol, 2017). Instruct parents to feed the infant every 2 to 3 hours during the newborn period. Inadequate frequency or amount of breastfeeding and dehydration can increase serum levels of bilirubin. Encourage mothers to breastfeed frequently (8–12 times a day) and, as needed, to supplement with formula to improve hydration, particularly if the mother's milk is slow to come in. Supplementing with water or sugar water is not recommended, because this can alter sodium and other electrolyte levels in the newborn.

Phototherapy reduces the amount of unconjugated bilirubin in the bloodstream by promoting excretion via the intestines

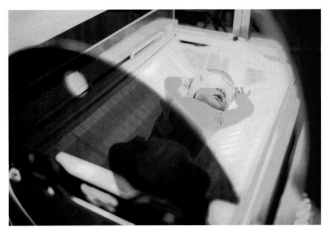

Figure 23.17. An infant receiving phototherapy.

and kidneys (Fig. 23.17). The exposure to blue light changes bilirubin into water-soluble forms that can be excreted. Phototherapy takes at least 8 to 12 hours to have an impact on bilirubin levels. Therefore, it should be initiated before levels are severely elevated. There is no consensus on what bilirubin level is needed to begin phototherapy. The American Academy of Pediatrics provides guidelines for use of phototherapy.

Regularly assess for complications of phototherapy in the child, which include loose stools, erythematous macular rash, overheating, and dehydration. Frequently monitor body temperature, and shield the infant's eyes to prevent light exposure (Patient Safety 23.3). Check total serum bilirubin levels periodically during therapy and 24 to 48 hours after discontinuation of therapy to ensure that levels have not risen.

Evaluation

Expected outcomes for an infant with physiological jaundice include the following:

- Bilirubin values are in an acceptable range.
- The infant is free of complications from phototherapy.
- The infant is free of complications associated with prolonged hyperbilirubinemia.

Discharge Planning and Teaching

Many infants with jaundice are managed at home and visit the pediatrician's office or clinic for follow-up assessment and

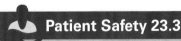

Patient Safety 23.3

Phototherapy Safety

Cover the infant's eyes during phototherapy to prevent retinal damage. When the phototherapy lights are off, such as during feeding, you may remove the eye protection. Monitor temperature frequently to prevent overheating.

bilirubin checks every 1 or 2 days for the first 10 days of life or until bilirubin levels are in an acceptable range. Teach parents the signs of dehydration and to report these immediately to the provider. Frequent feedings should continue at home. Teach parents to call the provider if the infant does not take a bottle or nurse for more than two or three scheduled feedings. Refer mothers who are breastfeeding to a lactation specialist, who can support them in breastfeeding.

Biliary Atresia

Biliary atresia is a disease characterized by progressive obstruction of the extrahepatic bile ducts (Fig. 23.18). Without treatment, biliary atresia progresses to liver failure and death.

Etiology and Pathophysiology

Anatomically, biliary atresia can occur in different forms. The most common form, accounting for approximately 85% of cases, is a complete obliteration of the entire extrahepatic biliary tree (Hassan & Balistreri, 2016). Most infants with this form of the disease are normal at birth and then develop progressive obliteration of the bile ducts several weeks into the newborn period. Approximately 1 in 10,000 to 1 in 15,000 babies are affected with biliary atresia in the United States (Hassan & Balistreri, 2016).

Clinical Presentation

Infants with biliary atresia are initially asymptomatic. At about 2 to 3 weeks after birth, jaundice may be detected. Bilirubin levels continue to rise and abdominal distension and hepatomegaly occur. Bruising, bleeding, and intense itching develop as biliary atresia progresses. Bile pigments are absent in the stool, which causes stools to appear white or clay-colored. Urine appears dark and tea-colored because of an increase in bilirubin and bile salts excreted in the urine. Failure to thrive is common.

Assessment and Diagnosis

Early diagnosis is essential to prevent or slow liver damage, which occurs rapidly in infants with biliary atresia. History, physical exam, and laboratory values are used in conjunction with a percutaneous liver biopsy and exploratory laparotomy to diagnose biliary atresia. Positive laboratory findings include elevated serum aminotransferase, alkaline phosphatase, and bilirubin levels. Prothrombin time is elevated, as are serum ammonia levels. A percutaneous liver biopsy, the most valuable procedure for diagnosing biliary atresia, reveals evidence of biliary atresia (Hassan & Balistreri, 2016). Cholangiography (an X-ray of the bile ducts to locate an obstruction) and an exploratory laparotomy are used to confirm the diagnosis.

Therapeutic Interventions

The only effective treatment for biliary atresia is a Kasai procedure. A Kasai procedure consists of removing the biliary tree and creating a Roux-en-Y hepatojejunostomy to drain bile from the portal plate directly into the jejunum (Hassan & Balistreri, 2016). Unfortunately, in the United States, the success rate, with success being defined as resolution of jaundice and a bilirubin level less than 2 mg/dL, is only 48%. Eventually, children with biliary atresia may need a liver transplant.

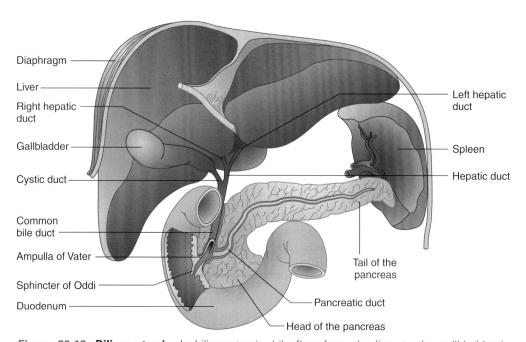

Figure 23.18. Biliary atresia. In biliary atresia, bile flow from the liver to the gallbladder is blocked, causing bile to be trapped inside the liver. Buildup of bile causes damage and scarring of the liver cells and, eventually, liver failure. Reprinted with permission from Norris, T. L., & Lalchandani, R. (2018). *Porth's pathophysiology* (10th ed., Fig. 38.1). Philadelphia, PA: Wolters Kluwer.

Nursing care for a child with biliary atresia focuses on providing supportive care, meeting nutritional needs, reducing risks of complications associated with the disease, providing postoperative care, and preparing the family for liver transplantation, if needed.

As noted earlier in the Prevent Infection section, children with biliary atresia are at increased risk for infection because of a compromised immune system and having a central line in place. Instruct parents to take the measures discussed to help prevent infection in their children.

As discussed in the section Maintain Skin Integrity, earlier, provide the child with tepid baths, pat the skin dry, and moisturize the skin with lotions to prevent itching and scratching, which can compromise skin integrity. Also, cover the hands with mittens or socks to reduce irritation of the skin from scratching.

As discussed in the section Maintain Adequate Hydration and Nutrition, earlier, offer children with liver conditions a high-protein, high-carbohydrate diet, supplement with vitamins A, D, E, and K as needed, and monitor weight and growth regularly. If caloric intake is inadequate, tube feedings or TPN may be needed.

The child is typically under the care of multiple providers, including a gastrointestinal specialist, a primary provider, a liver specialist, and, oftentimes, a nutrition team. Consistent information sharing across teams is needed to maintain the parents' trust. For guidelines on addressing families' emotional and psychological needs related to gastrointestinal disorders, see the section Provide Emotional and Psychosocial Support to the Child and Parents, earlier.

Evaluation

Expected outcomes for a child with biliary atresia include the following:

- The child consumes adequate nutrition to support growth and development.

- The child remains free of infection.
- The parents cope effectively with the child's chronic care and complex medical needs.

Discharge Planning and Teaching

Discharge planning focuses on teaching parents how to care for their child with a chronic liver condition. Teach parents about skin care, nutritional needs, monitoring for infection, and administering medications before discharge. Provide parents with resources for support groups and home care referrals if a central line, TPN, or enteral feedings are continued in the home.

Hepatitis

Hepatitis is an inflammation of the liver. Viruses are the most common cause of hepatitis, but bacterial infections, trauma, metabolic disorders, and chemical toxicity can also lead to hepatitis. Hepatitis can be self-limiting or can progress to fibrosis, cirrhosis, or liver cancer.

Etiology and Pathophysiology

Hepatitis A virus is responsible for most acute and benign forms of hepatitis. The most common causes of viral hepatitis, hepatitis A, B, C, and D viruses, are compared in Table 23.10. Cytomegalovirus, adenovirus, and Epstein–Barr virus can also cause hepatitis. Hepatitis A virus, traditionally called infectious hepatitis, is highly contagious and spread through the fecal–oral route. Approximately 50% of all cases of acute viral hepatitis are a result of hepatitis A virus. Hepatitis A virus frequently occurs in children who are in child care settings where hygiene practices are poor (Patient Teaching 23.2). Restaurants are another setting where hepatitis A virus is prevalent, because infected food handlers can spread the virus.

Table 23.10 Comparing Hepatitis Types

Hepatitis Type	Immunization Available	Prophylaxis	Primary Route of Transmission	Incubation Period (d)
A	Yes	• Hepatitis A vaccine • Immune globulin	Fecal–oral	15–19
B	Yes	• Hepatitis B vaccine • Hepatitis B immune globulin	• Needle sticks • Intravenous drug use • Birth process • Sexual activity	60–180
C	No	None	• Needle sticks • Intravenous drug use • Birth process • Sexual activity	14–160
D	No	Hepatitis B vaccine	• Needle sticks • Intravenous drug use • Birth process • Sexual activity	21–42
E	No	None	Fecal–oral	21–63

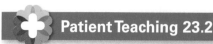

Child Care Centers and Hepatitis

Nurses can play an active role in helping staff at a child care center reduce the risk of and prevent hepatitis A virus transmission. Standards include the following:

- Hand washing after each diaper change or assisting small children to the toilet
- Disposing of diapers properly
- Dedicated areas for changing diapers, cleaning diaper-changing surfaces after each diaper change with appropriate cleaning products
- Food handlers never performing diaper changes
- Instructing parents to keep children at home for at least 2 wk after being diagnosed
- Informing parents and staff of cases of hepatitis A at the center
- Teaching parents about the symptoms of the disease
- Teaching staff to recognize signs and symptoms and report concerns to parents

Fulminant hepatitis can occur after an infection with a virus or exposure to a toxin and is characterized by massive necrosis of the liver and a decrease in liver size, which can result in death if the child does not receive a liver transplant. Ingestion of toxic levels of acetaminophen (Tylenol) is the leading cause of acute liver failure in the United States. Children with fulminant liver failure present with an acute onset of severe jaundice, elevated ammonia levels, coagulopathy, and significantly elevated liver enzyme levels. Children with fulminant liver failure become encephalopathic and comatose.

Autoimmune hepatitis is a chronic disorder, affecting mostly adolescent females. Seventy percent of those with autoimmune hepatitis are female. Children and adolescents with autoimmune hepatitis present with hepatosplenomegaly, jaundice, fever, fatigue, and chronic right upper quadrant pain. Anorexia is also common.

Clinical Presentation

Children with hepatitis present with jaundice, fever, fatigue, and abdominal pain. Nausea, vomiting, and malaise are present. Current and past medical histories typically reveal a risk factor such as recent foreign travel, sick contacts, medication use, or abdominal trauma. Other risk factors include sexual activity, IV drug use, and a recent blood transfusion. Jaundice can be observed in the skin, scleras, and mucous membranes. Laboratory values for a child with hepatitis include elevated liver enzymes, prolonged prothrombin time and partial thromboplastin time, and an elevated ammonia level.

Assessment and Diagnosis

Assess for signs of jaundice in the skin and sclera. Assess the abdomen for pain and tenderness. Note the location and intensity of pain. Obtain a short record of food intake from the parents to establish whether anorexia is present. Nausea, vomiting, malaise, and arthralgia (joint pain) can be present. Ask parents about their child's exposure to persons with hepatitis or other illnesses over the past 2 months.

Diagnosis is made on the basis of the history, physical exam, and laboratory data. A history of exposure to persons with hepatitis plays a significant role in the diagnosis. Laboratory testing includes serological testing for antigens and antibodies to hepatitis A, B, C, and D viruses. Obtain liver function studies and a complete blood count.

Therapeutic Interventions

Children with hepatitis are rarely admitted to the hospital; therefore, nursing care focuses on the home and community. Preventing the spread of infection, reducing the risk of complications, maintaining adequate nutrition, and promoting rest and comfort (see the section Promote Pain Relief, Comfort, and Rest, earlier) are part of the care plan for a child with hepatitis.

As discussed in the section Prevent Infection, earlier, inform parents of vaccination schedules for hepatitis A and B viruses and instruct them and the child to wash their hands meticulously before handling food and after using the toilet.

As discussed in the section Maintain Adequate Hydration and Nutrition, earlier, offer children with liver conditions a high-protein, high-carbohydrate diet and monitor weight and growth regularly. If caloric intake is inadequate, offer high-calorie supplemental shakes or drinks.

Evaluation

Expected outcomes for a child with hepatitis include the following:

- The child consumes adequate calories and nutrients to maintain growth and development.
- Parents cope effectively with the stress of caring for a child with a chronic condition.
- Hepatitis is not spread to the child's contacts or family.

Discharge Planning and Teaching

Teach parents how to prevent the spread of hepatitis, the importance of adequate nutrition, and ways to promote rest and comfort while the child heals during the acute phase.

Cirrhosis and Portal Hypertension

Cirrhosis is scarring of the liver caused by an underlying liver dysfunction or illness. This degenerative disease results in fibrotic changes and may lead to end-stage hepatic failure.

Etiology and Pathophysiology

Cirrhosis can have many causes. Chronic cholestasis, inborn errors of metabolism, and chronic hepatitis are the three main causes in children (Pinto, Schneider, & da Silveira, 2015). Cirrhosis can be present without definitive symptoms until the onset of liver dysfunction and portal hypertension (Pinto,

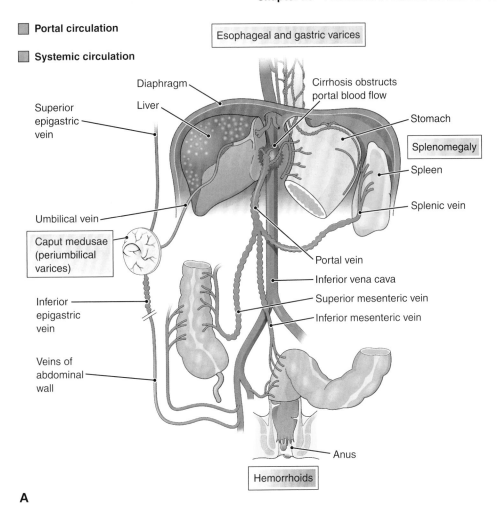

Portal circulation

Systemic circulation

Esophageal and gastric varices

Diaphragm

Cirrhosis obstructs portal blood flow

Superior epigastric vein

Liver

Stomach

Splenomegaly

Spleen

Splenic vein

Umbilical vein

Caput medusae (periumbilical varices)

Portal vein

Inferior vena cava

Inferior epigastric vein

Superior mesenteric vein

Inferior mesenteric vein

Veins of abdominal wall

Anus

Hemorrhoids

A

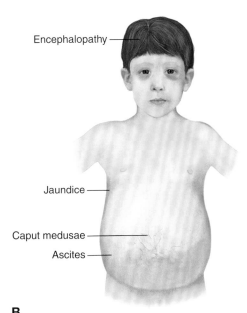

Encephalopathy

Jaundice

Caput medusae

Ascites

B

Figure 23.19. Portal hypertension. Portal hypertension can lead to multiple complications, such as esophageal varices **(A)** as well as ascites and hepatic encephalopathy **(B)**. Part A reprinted with permission from Timby, B. K., & Smith, N. E. (2017). *Introductory medical-surgical nursing* (12th ed., Fig. 47.5). Philadelphia, PA: Wolters Kluwer.

Schneider, & da Silveira, 2015). Progressive fibrosis and scarring alter blood flow in and out of the liver and can lead to portal hypertension. Portal hypertension occurs when blood pressure in the portal venous system is higher than normal physiological values. The portal venous system refers to the vessels involved in the drainage of the capillary beds of the gastrointestinal tract and spleen into the capillary bed of the liver. Portal hypertension can lead to many of the complications associated with liver failure, such as esophageal varices, gastrointestinal bleeding, ascites, splenomegaly, encephalopathy, and jaundice (Fig. 23.19).

Clinical Presentation

A child in the early stages of cirrhosis may appear normal. In up to 40% of cases, children may be asymptomatic before liver failure occurs (Beath, 2013). Early symptoms include poor weight gain, anorexia, fatigue, muscle weakness, nausea, and vomiting (Pinto, Schneider, & da Silveira, 2015). Children with advanced cirrhosis present with a cascade of progressive complications. Gastrointestinal bleeding, ascites, severe jaundice, and hepatic encephalopathy may be present. Collateral vessels, resulting from portal hypertension, may be present on the abdomen.

Assessment and Diagnosis

Assessment of the child with cirrhosis involves a multisystem approach. Assess mental status for irritability, lethargy, and fatigue. Asterixis and the Babinski reflex may be present as cirrhosis progresses. Assess the skin for jaundice, pruritus, spider nevi, xanthomas, palmar erythema, and clubbing of the nails. The child can be short of breath and tachypneic because of an enlarged abdomen compromising lung expansion. Abdominal distension is present, along with splenomegaly and a small liver diameter. Assess for nausea and vomiting, abdominal pain, diarrhea, and dyspepsia. Assess for signs of bleeding in the nose, mouth, and gums as well as for petechiae and bruising, indicating an alteration in coagulability.

Diagnosis is made on the basis of the child's history and physical exam as well as on laboratory values and a liver biopsy. Laboratory values reveal abnormal liver function test results, such as elevated aspartate aminotransferase, alanine aminotransferase, and bilirubin levels.

Therapeutic Interventions

Nursing care focuses on minimizing complications associated with cirrhosis, administering medications and monitoring for side effects, meeting nutrition needs, and providing supportive care for the child and family.

Monitor electrolytes as ordered to determine the need for electrolyte replacements. Monitor for bleeding, including bruising, petechiae, and nose bleeds. An alteration in coagulation status occurs in cirrhosis that places the child at high risk for bleeding. Minimize the risk of infection by teaching proper hand washing and educating parents to not allow visitors who are ill or have come into contact with ill persons. Pruritus is common in children with liver failure and often leads to scratching, which leads to impaired skin integrity and open wounds. Keep skin moisturized with lotion, provide warm baths (not hot baths, because they dehydrate the skin), and avoid using irritating soaps and tapes. Change the child's position frequently to avoid skin breakdown.

Take care when administering medications and monitoring for side effects because of how liver dysfunction alters metabolism. Dosage adjustments may be necessary as cirrhosis progresses and liver function declines.

As discussed in the section Maintain Adequate Hydration and Nutrition, earlier, when ascites is present, provide the child with a low-sodium, low-protein diet and restrict fluids. When anorexia is present and the child is not consuming adequate calories, enteral feedings may be necessary. Obtain daily weights to assess for fluid retention as well as proper weight gain and growth.

For guidelines on addressing families' emotional and psychological needs related to gastrointestinal disorders, see the section Provide Emotional and Psychosocial Support to the Child and Parents, earlier.

Evaluation

Expected outcomes for a child with cirrhosis include the following:

- Nutritional status is optimized.
- Electrolytes are within normal limits.
- Complications of liver failure are minimized.
  - Episodes of bleeding are minimized.
  - The child is free of signs of infection.
  - The child maintains baseline neurological status.
- Skin remains intact.
- Parents demonstrate effective coping with stress of the child's condition and chronic care needs.

Discharge Planning and Teaching

Discharge planning for a child with cirrhosis depends on which stage of liver failure the child is in. Many children are cared for at home in the early stages of cirrhosis. As liver failure progresses, the risk of complications increases. Teach parents to monitor for signs of infection, inadequate fluid intake, and bleeding. Teach them when to call the provider and when to seek medical care as complications arise. Reinforce nutrition and diet restrictions before discharge. Referral to support groups or counseling may be beneficial. Provide parents with social service contacts who can provide financial resources.

Think Critically

1. A 2-year-old child presents to the pediatrician's office with a 2-day history of fever, vomiting, and diarrhea. The nurse obtains the child's temperature, pulse, and respiratory rate. Temperature is 101.3°F (38.5°C). The child's heart rate is 156 beats/min and respiratory rate is 32 breaths/min. The child appears tired but alert and clings to the mother when the nurse is obtaining vital signs. What other assessments should the nurse make?

2. The nurse is creating a discharge plan for the parents of an 11-month-old admitted with gastroenteritis. What signs or symptoms should prompt the parents to call the pediatrician after discharge?

3. What assessment findings should the nurse most expect to find in a child who has been diagnosed with hypertrophic pyloric stenosis?

4. The nurse is caring for a child with a cleft lip and cleft palate and is reinforcing teaching and information regarding complications of these conditions. What are the complications parents should be aware of when caring for a child with a cleft lip and palate?

5. A 6-week-old boy is being seen in the pediatrician's office. The mother reports that the infant has frequent spitting-up episodes and occasional vomiting and is frequently hungry and fussy. The mother has tried giving the infant 5 oz of formula instead of 3 oz at each feeding, but the spitting up and vomiting seem worse afterward. The physician diagnoses the infant with GERD. Explain why giving a larger volume of formula with each feeding is generally not recommended for an infant with GERD.

6. A 4-year-old girl presents to the emergency room with moderate dehydration. The child weighs 42 lb (19 kg). The provider orders a fluid bolus of 20 mL/kg of 0.9 normal saline and then to start the child on maintenance IV fluids at 42 mL/h. How many milliliters should the bolus be written for? Is 42 mL/h the correct maintenance intravenous fluid (MIVF) rate for this child?

7. An 8-year-old child is being worked up for Crohn disease. At the pediatrician visit, the mother tells you that she has been reading on the Internet about inflammatory bowel disease and wonders how the pediatrician knows that her child has Crohn disease and not ulcerative colitis. Help the mother understand by comparing and contrasting the two diagnoses.

8. A mother and her newborn are being seen at the pediatrician's office for hyperbilirubinemia. The mother is tearful and states, "I thought breastfeeding was good for my baby, and the doctor just told me it can cause my baby to be jaundiced." You quickly realize the mother misunderstood the information. Explain what you would say to the mother to help clarify how breastfeeding affects bilirubin levels.

References

Adamiak, T., Walkiewicz-Jedrzejczak, D., Fish, D., Brown, C., Tung, J., Khan, K., . . . Kugathasan, S. (2013). Incidence, clinical characteristics, and natural history of pediatric IBD in Wisconsin: A population-based epidemiological study. *Inflammatory Bowel Diseases, 19*(6), 1218–1223.

Aiken, J., & Oldham, K. (2016). Acute appendicitis. In R. Kliegman, B. Stanton, J. St. Geme, N. Schor, & R. Behrman (Eds.), *Nelson textbook of pediatrics* (20th ed., pp. 1887–1894). Philadelphia, PA: Elsevier.

Allman, R., Sousa, J., Walker, M., Laughon, M., Spitzer, A., & Clark, R. (2016). The epidemiology, prevalence and hospital outcomes of infants with gastroschisis. *Journal of Perinatology, 36*(10), 901.

Ambalanvanan, N & Carlo, R. (2016). Jaundice and Hyperbilirubinemia in the Newborn. In R.Kliegman, B. Stanton, J. St. Geme, N. Schor, & R. Behrman (Eds.). *Nelson textbook of pediatrics* (20th ed., pp. 872–874). Philadelphia, PA: Elsevier.

Baird, D., Harker, D., & Karmes, A. (2015). Diagnosis and treatment of gastroesophageal reflux in infants and children. *American Family Physician, 92*(8), 705–714.

Bansal, S., Banever, G., Karrer, F., & Partrick, D. (2012). Appendicitis in children less than 5 years old: Influence of age on presentation and outcome. *American Journal of Surgery, 204*, 1031–1035.

Beath, S. (2013). End stage liver disease. *Paediatrics and Child Health, 23*(12), 535–544.

Blanchard, S., & Czinn, D. (2016). Peptic ulcer disease in children. In R. Kliegman, B. Stanton, J. St. Geme, N. Schor, & R. Behrman (Eds.). *Nelson textbook of pediatrics* (20th ed., pp. 1816–1819). Philadelphia, PA: Elsevier.

Carson, R., Mudd, S., & Madati, P. (2016). Clinical practice guideline for the treatment of pediatric acute gastroenteritis in the outpatient setting. *Journal of Pediatric Health Care, 30*(6), 610–616.

Choi, Y. (2014). Necrotizing enterocolitis in newborns: Update in pathophysiology and newly emerging therapeutic strategies. *Korean Journal of Pediatrics, 57*(12), 505–513.

Churgay, C. A., & Aftab, Z. (2012). Gastroenteritis in children: Part II. Prevention and management. *American Family Physician, 85*(11), 1066–1070.

Coletta, R., Khalil, B. A., & Morabito, A. (2014, October). Short bowel syndrome in children: surgical and medical perspectives. In *Seminars in pediatric surgery* (Vol. 23, No. 5, pp. 291–297). WB Saunders.

Davies, I., Burman-Roy, S., Murphy, M., Guideline Development Group. (2015). Gastro-oesophageal reflux disease in children: NICE guidance. *British Medical Journal, 350*, g7703.

Dehghani, S., Kulouee, N., Honar, N., Imanieh, M., Haghighat, M., & Javaherizadeh, H. (2015). Clinical manifestations among children with chronic functional constipation. *Middle East Journal of Digestive Diseases, 7*(1), 31.

Eberly, M., Eide, M., Thompson, J. L., & Nylund, C. (2015). Azithromycin in early infancy and pyloric stenosis. *Pediatrics, 135*(3), 483–488.

Eusebi, L., Zagari, R., & Bazzoli, F. (2014). Epidemiology of *Helicobacter pylori* infection. *Helicobacter, 19*(suppl 1), 1–5.

Farthing, M., Salam, M., Lindberg, G., Dite, P., Khalif, I., Salazar-Lindo, E., . . . & Krabshuis, J. (2013). Acute diarrhea in adults and children: A global perspective. *Journal of Clinical Gastroenterology, 47*(1), 12–20.

Fasano, A., & Catassi, C. (2012). Clinical practice. Celiac disease. *New England Journal of Medicine, 367*(25), 2419–2426.

Francis, A., Kantarovich, D., Khoshnam, N., Alazraki, A. L., Patel, B., & Shehata, B. M. (2016). Pediatric Meckel's diverticulum: report of 208 cases and review of the literature. *Fetal and pediatric pathology, 35*(3), 199–206.

Gamba, P., & Midrio, P. (2014). Abdominal wall defects: Prenatal diagnosis, newborn management, and long-term outcomes. *Seminars in Pediatric Surgery, 23*(5), 283–290.

Garza-González, E., Perez-Perez, G., Maldonado-Garza, H., & Bosques-Padilla, F. (2014). A review of *Helicobacter pylori* diagnosis, treatment, and methods to detect eradication. *World Journal of Gastroenterology, 20*(6), 1438.

Grossman, A. & Baldassano, R. (2016). Inflammatory bowel disease. In R. Kliegman, B. Stanton, J. St. Geme, N. Schor, & R. Behrman (Eds.). *Nelson textbook of pediatrics* (20th ed., pp. 1819–1831). Philadelphia, PA: Elsevier.

Guandalini, S. (2017). The approach to celiac disease in children. *International Journal of Pediatrics and Adolescent Medicine, 4*, 124–127.

Guarino, A., Ashkenazi, S., Gendrel, D., Vecchio, A., Shamir, R., & Szajewska, H. (2014). European Society for Pediatric Gastroenterology, Hepatology, and Nutrition/European Society for Pediatric Infectious Diseases evidence-based guidelines for the management of acute gastroenteritis in children in Europe: Update 2014. *Journal of Pediatric Gastroenterology and Nutrition, 59*(1), 132–152.

Hassan, H., & Balistreri, W. (2016). Neonatal cholestasis. In R. Kliegman, B. Stanton, J. St. Geme, N. Schor, & R. Behrman (Eds.), *Nelson textbook of pediatrics* (20th ed., pp. 1928–1936). Philadelphia, PA: Elsevier.

Hopkins, J., Cermak, S. A., & Merritt, R. J. (2018). Oral feeding difficulties in children with short bowel syndrome: A narrative review. *Nutrition in Clinical Practice, 33*(1), 99–106.

Hyams, J., Di Lorenzo, C., Saps, M., Shulman, R., Staiano, A., & van Tilburg, M. (2016). Childhood functional gastrointestinal disorders: Child/adolescent. *Gastroenterology, 150*(6), 1456–1468.

Iwai, N., & Fumino, S. (2013). Surgical treatment of anorectal malformations. *Surgery Today, 43*(9), 955–962.

Kammacher Guerreiro, M., Bettinville, A., & Herzog, D. (2014). Fecal overflow often affects children with chronic constipation that appears after the age of 2 years. *Clinical Pediatrics, 53*(9), 885–889.

Kennedy, M., & Liacouras, C. (2016). Malrotation. In R. Kliegman, B. Stanton, J. St. Geme, N. Schor, & R. Behrman (Eds.). *Nelson textbook of pediatrics* (20th ed., pp. 1803–1804). Philadelphia, PA: Elsevier.

Khan, S., & Orenstein, S. (2016). Esophageal atresia and tracheoesophageal fistula. In R. Kliegman, B. Stanton, J. St. Geme, N. Schor, & R. Behrman (Eds.). *Nelson textbook of pediatrics* (20th ed., pp. 1783–1784). Philadelphia, PA: Elsevier.

Koppen, I., Lammers, L., Benninga, M., & Tabbers, M. (2015). Management of functional constipation in children: Therapy in practice. *Pediatric Drugs, 17*(5), 349–360.

Lewis, C., Jacob, L., & Lehmann, C. (2017). The primary care pediatrician and the care of children with cleft lip and/or cleft palate. *Pediatrics, 139*(5), e20170628.

Maheshwari, A., & Carlo, W. (2017). Diaphragmatic hernia. In R. Kliegman, B. Stanton, J. St. Geme, N. Schor, & R. Behrman (Eds.). *Nelson textbook of pediatrics* (20th ed., pp. 862–864). Philadelphia, PA: Elsevier.

Nurko, S., & Zimmerman, L. (2014). Evaluation and treatment of constipation in children and adolescents. *American Family Physician, 90*(2), 82–90.

Pandya, S. (2016). Anorectal malformations. *NeoReviews, 17*(5), e251–e262.

Papillon, S., Castle, S. L., Gayer, C. P., & Ford, H. R. (2013). Necrotizing enterocolitis: Contemporary management and outcomes. *Advances in Pediatrics, 60*(1), 263–279.

Parisi, M. A. (2015). Hirschsprung disease overview. In M. Adam, H. Ardinger, R. Pagon, et al., (Eds.), *GeneReview*. Seattle, WA: University of Washington.

Pinto, R., Schneider, A., & da Silveira, T. (2015). Cirrhosis in children and adolescents: An overview. *World Journal of Hepatology, 7*(3), 392.

Powers, K. (2015). Dehydration: Isonatremic, hyponatremic, and hypernatremic recognition and management. *Pediatrics in Review, 36*(7), 274–285.

Rahimov, F. Jugessur, A., & Murray, J. (2012). Genetics of nonsyndromic orofacial clefts. The *Cleft Palate-Craniofacial Journal, 49*(1), 73–91.

Ruigómez, A., Wallander, M. A., Lundborg, P., Johansson, S., & Rodriguez, L. A. (2010). Gastroesophageal reflux disease in children and adolescents in primary care. *Scandinavian Journal of Gastroenterology, 45*(2), 139–146.

Sawh, S., Deshpande, S., Jansen, S., Reynaert, C., & Jones, P. (2016). Prevention of necrotizing enterocolitis with probiotics: A systematic review and meta-analysis. *PeerJ, 4*, e2429.

Shah, S., Sinclair, K., Theut, S, Johnson, K., Holcomb III, G., & Peter, S. (2016). Computed tomography utilization for the diagnosis of acute appendicitis in children decreases with a diagnostic algorithm. *Annals of Surgery, 264*(3), 474–481.

Singhi, S. C., Shah, R., Bansal, A., & Jayashree, M. (2013). Management of a child with vomiting. *The Indian Journal of Pediatrics, 80*(4), 318–325.

Snyder, J., Butzner, J., DeFelice, A., Fasano, A., Guandalini, S., Liu, E., & Newton, K. (2016). Evidence-informed expert recommendations for the management of celiac disease in children. *Pediatrics, 138*(3), e20153147.

Soden, J. (2010). Clinical assessment of the child with intestinal failure. *Seminars in Pediatric Surgery, 19*(1), 10–19.

Svenningsson, A., Svensson, T., Akre, O., & Nordenskjöld, A. (2014). Maternal and pregnancy characteristics and risk of infantile hypertrophic pyloric stenosis. *Journal of Pediatric Surgery, 49*(8), 1226–1231.

Taylor, N., Cass, D., & Holland, A. (2013). Infantile hypertrophic pyloric stenosis: Has anything changed? *Journal of Paediatrics and Child Health, 49*(1), 33–37.

Truven Health Analytics. (2016). *Micromedex 2.0.* Retrieved from http://www.micromedexsolutions.com

Turco, R., Miele, E., Russo, M., Mastroianni, R., Lavorgna, A., Paludetto, R., . . . & Romano, C. (2014). Early-life factors associated with pediatric functional constipation. *Journal of Pediatric Gastroenterology and Nutrition, 58*(3), 307–312.

Youssef, F., Cheong, L., & Emil, S. (2016). Gastroschisis outcomes in North America: A comparison of Canada and the United States. *Journal of Pediatric Surgery, 51*(6), 891–895.

Zhu, J., Zhu, T., Lin, Z., Qu, Y., & Mu, D. (2017). Perinatal risk factors for infantile hypertrophic pyloric stenosis: A meta-analysis. *Journal of Pediatric Surgery, 52*(9), 1389–1397.

Suggested Readings

Carson, R., Mudd, S., & Madati, P. (2016). Clinical practice guideline for the treatment of pediatric acute gastroenteritis in the outpatient setting. *Journal of Pediatric Health Care, 30*(6), 610–616.

KidsHealth. *Orofacial clefts.* Retrieved from https://kidshealth.org/en/parents/cleft-lip-palate.html

Koppen, I., Lammers, L., Benninga, M., & Tabbers, M. (2015). Management of functional constipation in children: Therapy in practice. *Pediatric Drugs, 17*(5), 349–360.

24 Alterations in Genitourinary Function

The genitourinary system consists of the kidneys and urinary structures (Fig. 24.1), as well as the reproductive organs. The kidneys and urinary system are responsible for vital functions such as removing waste products and maintaining fluid and electrolyte balance. Infections, structural disorders, and disease processes can alter genitourinary function. Disruption of the kidneys and urinary organs can pose a significant threat to the health and well-being of children.

Variations in Anatomy and Physiology

All urinary tract and reproductive organs are present at birth. However, a child's genitourinary organs mature over time. Differences between the pediatric and adult genitourinary systems can be categorized as differences in renal and urethral structure, renal and urinary function, and reproductive organ structure and function.

465

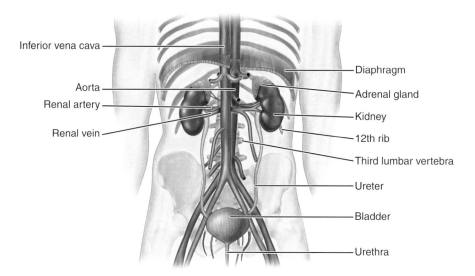

Figure 24.1. The kidneys and urinary structures. Reprinted with permission from Cohen, B. J., & Hull, K. (2014). *Memmler's the human body in health and disease* (13th ed., Fig. 22.1). Philadelphia, PA: Wolters Kluwer.

Structurally, the kidney is large in relation to the size of the abdomen until the child reaches adolescence. Consequently, the kidneys of the child are less well protected from injury by the fat padding and ribs until late adolescence or adulthood. The urethra is shorter in females than in males throughout the lifespan, and, in the female infant and young child, the urethral opening is very close to the rectum. These factors lead to an increased risk of bacteria entering the urethra and subsequent urinary tract infections (UTIs) in female infants and young girls. Male infants and young boys are at increased risk of UTI compared with adult men because of a much shorter urethra.

The renal system does not reach functional maturity until around 2 years of age. However, all the nephrons (Fig. 24.2) that make up the kidney are present at birth. In the infant and young toddler, the glomerular filtration rate (blood flow through the kidneys) is much slower than that in the adult. In a newborn, it is as low as one-third to one-fourth that of an adult (Otukesh, Hoseini, Rahimzadeh, & Hosseini, 2012). The immature kidney is less able to concentrate urine and reabsorb amino acids, which puts the infant and young toddler at increased risk for dehydration during episodes of fluid loss or decreased fluid intake, such as during an episode of gastroenteritis. The normal ranges for blood urea nitrogen (BUN) and serum creatinine levels of the healthy infant or toddler are generally less than those of the older child or adult. Bladder capacity also increases with age and reaches the usual adult capacity of about 270 mL by 1 year of age. Urine output in an infant or child is much less per day than that of an adult, although an infant or toddler may void as often as 9 or 10 times a day. By the age of 3 years, the average number of voids per day is the same as that of an adult, about three to eight voids per day.

Reproductive organs are immature at birth and only fully mature, in most children, in adolescence. Female adolescents undergo many hormonal changes during puberty, which account for some of the reproductive concerns encountered in the pediatric population.

Assessment of the Pediatric Genitourinary System

Assessment of the pediatric genitourinary system includes an examination of the genitalia, assessment of urine characteristics, and assessment for pain or discomfort in the abdomen, flank, or back during urination or in the genitalia. When renal dysfunction is suspected, assessing for the presence of edema is also necessary. Table 24.1 provides guidelines for the assessment of the genitourinary system. Box 24.1 reviews expected urinary output according to age. Diagnostic procedures and laboratory values to consider when assessing the genitourinary system are listed in Box 24.2.

General Nursing Interventions for Genitourinary Disorders

Given here is an overview of key nursing interventions that apply to genitourinary disorders, in general. Interventions that are specific to a given disorder are discussed within the section Therapeutic Interventions Within Genitourinary Disorders.

Maintain Adequate Hydration

Maintaining adequate hydration in a child with renal dysfunction can be challenging because of factors such as disinterest in drinking and changes in tastes of fluids and foods. Intravenous (IV) access is often necessary for the child hospitalized with

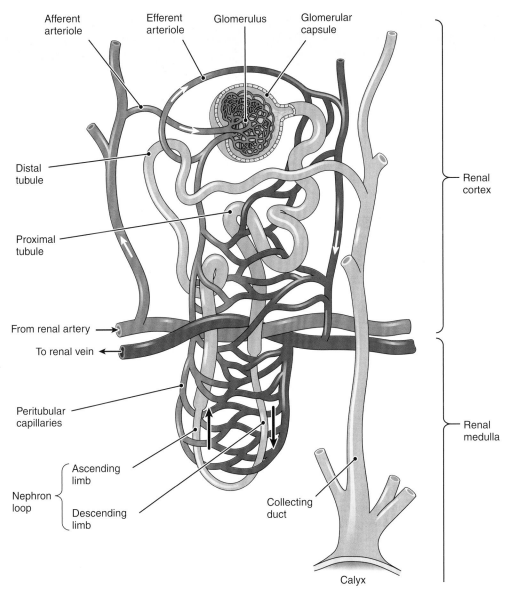

Afferent arteriole
Efferent arteriole
Glomerulus
Glomerular capsule
Renal cortex
Distal tubule
Proximal tubule
From renal artery
To renal vein
Peritubular capillaries
Renal medulla
Nephron loop
Ascending limb
Descending limb
Collecting duct
Calyx

Figure 24.2. Nephron. Nephrons, the functional unit of the kidney, are responsible for filtering water and wastes across the glomerular capillaries to maintain fluid and electrolyte balance and pH balance. There are approximately 1 million nephrons in each kidney. Reprinted with permission from Cohen, B. J. (2012). *Memmler's the human body in health and disease* (12th ed., Fig. 22.3). Philadelphia, PA: Wolters Kluwer.

renal disorders. Administer IV fluids as prescribed, and be vigilant in ensuring the rate is accurate for age, weight, and current volume status. Children in renal failure are often prescribed IV fluids at low rates, such as one-quarter maintenance rate. Assess for volume overload in the child receiving IV fluids, particularly when the child is also eating and drinking.

Maintain Normal Fluid and Electrolyte Balance

Children with renal disorders may present with an array of fluid volume disturbances, from varying degrees of dehydration to massive fluid overload. Maintain strict records of intake and output.

For the child who is dehydrated and needs an increase in fluid intake, provide IV fluids as ordered. Normal saline or lactated Ringer's solution is used for fluid boluses, such as the case in a child with hemolytic uremic syndrome (HUS) who presents with dehydration. For children who need increased oral intake, provide fluids the child prefers and offer them in special cups. Provide smaller volumes at more frequent intervals to make fluid consumption less overwhelming.

For the child on fluid restriction, such as in chronic renal failure, plan the child's intake for the entire 24 hours to ensure the child has fluids with meals, with medications, and when feeling thirsty. Be sure to count foods that have high fluid content, such as gelatin and fruit-flavored ice pops, in the daily

Table 24.1 Assessment Guide: Pediatric Genitourinary System

Urine and voiding characteristics	• Color, clarity, strong odor? • Amount of urine per day? • Number of times a day the child has wet diapers or urinates?
Pain or discomfort	• Pain when urinating? • Pain in the abdomen, back, or flank area? • Pain in the genital area?
Genitalia	• Location of the urethra on the glans penis? • Testes present or palpable in the scrotum? • Discharge or drainage from the penis? • Discharge or drainage from the urethra or vagina? • Lesions on the genitalia?
Edema	• Edema of the genital area? • Edema of the face, trunk, hands, or legs? Severity of the edema?

Box 24.2 Diagnostic Procedures and Laboratory Tests for the Genitourinary System

Diagnostic Procedures

• Computed tomography
• Cystoscopy
• Intravenous pyelogram
• Magnetic resonance imaging
• Radionuclide cystography
• Renal biopsy
• Ultrasound (renal or bladder)
• Voiding cystourethrogram

Laboratory Tests

• Blood urea nitrogen
• Creatinine
• Urinalysis
• Urine culture
• Urine electrolytes

fluid intake. Use containers with volume measurements on them, such as medicine cups, to accurately measure fluids. Provide fluids in smaller cups for the appearance of a full cup vs. a half-empty cup. Encourage parents and visitors to avoid drinking in front of the child who is on fluid restriction. Ensure that parents and visitors understand the daily fluid restrictions and the importance of maintaining them.

Electrolyte levels may be imbalanced, varying from very low to potentially fatally high, such as hyperkalemia in renal failure. Electrolyte supplements may be prescribed for states of low electrolyte levels, such as hypokalemia. When administering supplements, monitor laboratory values for response to supplementation and to ensure that the values remain within normal limits. Teach the child and parents which foods contain necessary electrolytes. For example, in the case

Box 24.1 Expected Urine Output According to Age

As a child grows, the kidney becomes more efficient at concentrating urine. Therefore, urine output per kilogram of body weight decreases as the child ages.

Infant: 1–3 mL/kg/h
Child: 0.5–1 mL/kg/h (a 1-y-old voids about 400–500 mL/d)
Adolescent: 40–80 mL/h (800–1,400 mL/d)

of a child who requires an increase in potassium, teach parents about foods high in potassium, such as dairy products, citrus fruits, potatoes, and tomatoes. When electrolyte restrictions, such as a sodium restriction, are ordered, the child and parents may benefit from a list or printed guideline of foods to avoid. Parents may be unaware of common foods that contain sodium, potassium, calcium, or phosphorus, all electrolytes that may be imbalanced in a child with renal dysfunction.

Meet Nutritional Requirements

Children with renal dysfunction often have loss of appetite or may become disinterested in eating. Allow children to choose appropriate foods for meals and snacks. Offer choices when possible. Present small portions. Allow adequate time for consumption of meals and snacks so the child does not feel pressured or rushed to consume food. Socialization or eating with family or friends may improve the child's appetite. Offer highest calorie meals at the time of day when the child is most hungry or has the greatest appetite. Provide high-calorie shakes or puddings for children who need increased caloric intake. These foods require less energy to consume. For children on restricted diets, such as a low-sodium or low-phosphorus diet, teach them what foods they are allowed to have and do not offer foods they cannot consume. Weigh the child weekly to monitor for increased growth.

Prevent Infection

Impaired renal function places the child at risk for infection. Children who undergo surgical procedures are at risk for infection related to open wounds and incisions. Monitor the child for signs of infection, including fever, malaise, and an elevated white blood cell count. Strict aseptic technique is essential during invasive procedures. Meticulous hand washing is necessary. Instruct family members and visitors in good hand hygiene techniques. Encourage visitor limitations and restrictions when the risk of infection is high to reduce potential exposure to germs and bacteria.

Promote Bladder Emptying

Assess the child for the ability to adequately empty the bladder. Consider the child's history and characteristics of lower urinary symptoms to establish a baseline. Assess for a history of encopresis, constipation, or fecal impactions that could have a negative impact on bladder emptying. Assess for bladder distension by palpation. Measure postvoid residual urine volume via catheterization to get a baseline of urine volume retained. A bladder scan can assist in determining an approximate volume of retained urine.

Encourage the parents and the child to maintain adequate hydration. Use a clock and chart to schedule regular voiding times, such as every 2 hours in preschool and school-age children. Use positive reinforcement or a reward system when the child achieves goals for emptying the bladder. For children who are unable to completely empty their bladder, because of anatomical, physiological, or developmental reasons, teach the parent and/or the child the technique of clean intermittent catheterization to allow for regular complete emptying of the bladder.

Promote Pain Relief, Comfort, and Rest

For children with genitourinary conditions that cause pain, such as a UTI, testicular torsion, paraphimosis, and conditions requiring surgical correction with an incision, administer prescribed medications for pain relief. Use a developmentally appropriate pain scale to assess pain before medication administration and for follow-up assessments. Bladder spasms are common in conditions such as UTI and following surgical correction of bladder exstrophy. Administer antispasmodics as ordered. Nonpharmacological interventions for pain may include positioning; heat or cold therapy (when acceptable for the clinical condition); and providing diversional activities, such as play, movies, arts and crafts and, for older children, peer visits, when appropriate.

Adequate rest is essential for healing. Rest reduces the production of metabolic wastes, which put extra stress on the kidneys to excrete them. Bed rest may be ordered for children with certain conditions, such as glomerulonephritis, nephrotic syndrome, and bladder exstrophy before surgery. Explain to older children and parents of infants and young children the importance of bed rest. Provide quiet activities to minimize energy expenditure and stress on the kidneys. Encourage quiet activities such as listening to relaxing music, watching a movie, and coloring.

Promote Healing of Incisions and Prevent Skin Breakdown

Children on bed rest have an increased risk for skin breakdown. Pad bony prominences and apply skin protectant to the heels, elbows, and sacral areas. Use a sacral border to protect the sacrum. Elevate the legs and feet on pillows while the child is lying in bed. Ensure that beds and chairs are free of food crumbs, small toys, and other objects that can cause pressure injury. Ensure that IV tubing is positioned off of the patient. Keep linens clean and dry. For children on prolonged bed rest, use low-flow air mattresses or special mattresses to help reduce the potential for pressure injury.

Monitor incisions and other surgical sites for signs of infection, and keep the skin surrounding them clean and dry. Use strict aseptic technique during dressing changes. To the extent possible, when removing tape and dressings, gently remove the tape in the direction of hair growth, to reduce the risk of skin trauma and disruption of the wound. Apply skin protectants, such as no-sting barrier films, before applying tape or adherent dressings. Apply tape to the outer edges of an incision to avoid tension on the skin and wound bed. Partner with the parents to ensure that the child does not touch the wound or incision.

Provide Emotional and Psychosocial Support to the Child and Family

When body image is distorted as a result of edema, children may refuse to look in the mirror, refuse to participate in care, or begin to not care about grooming and appearance. Assist children to maintain a normal appearance by setting routines for grooming, encouraging the use of scarves or hats to lessen the appearance of edema, and allowing them to wear their own pajamas in the hospital, rather than hospital gowns. Encourage teenagers to journal to express their feelings and assist with coping. Body image may also be a concern for children who have urinary diversion devices and openings, such as a vesicostomy. Partner with the child and parents to promote a positive body image by helping them choose clothes that cover or hide the device or appliance.

Administer and Manage Medications

A variety of medications are administered when a child has a renal disorder. Be aware of medications, such as antibiotics used in the treatment of infections associated with the kidneys or urinary tract, that may need dosage adjustment when renal function is decreased. Examples of these medications include gentamicin, vancomycin, ciprofloxacin, and trimethoprim/sulfamethoxazole. When administering diuretics, strictly monitor and record intake and output. Assess the child for signs of dehydration resulting from liberal use of diuretics. Note the presence of any tachycardia, hypotension, decreased skin turgor, or decreased urine output and report it to the provider.

Genitourinary Disorders

Genitourinary disorders in infants, children, and adolescents occur as a result of abnormalities in fetal development, genetic influences, neurological deficits, infectious processes, or trauma. A large proportion of genitourinary disorders in infants are congenital defects, whereas older children are most often affected by enuresis and UTIs. Although some disorders only affect the urinary tract, many others may have a long-term effect on the kidneys and renal function if treated inadequately or left untreated. Disorders affecting the reproductive system require early diagnosis and treatment to preserve future reproductive capabilities.

Urinary Tract Infection

UTIs are a common problem in children. UTI is most often the result of bacteria entering the urethra and ascending to the bladder. **Cystitis** is a UTI that involves the urethra or bladder. Pyelonephritis is a UTI that involves the ureters, renal pelvis, or renal parenchyma.

Etiology and Pathophysiology

UTIs affect approximately 2.6% to 7.5% of febrile children annually (Sood et al., 2015). The most common causative agent for UTIs is *Escherichia coli* (Flores-Mireles, Walker, Caparon, & Hultgren, 2015). Other common causative agents include *Klebsiella pneumoniae*, *Staphylococcus*, *Enterococcus faecalis*, group B *Streptococcus*, *Pseudomonas aeruginosa*, and *Candida*.

  Risk factors for UTI in children include congenital genitourinary conditions, female gender, lack of circumcision in boys, immature host defenses, and a prior history of UTI (Sood et al., 2015). Other risk factors associated with increased risk of UTI include poor hygiene, inadequate cleaning after having a bowel movement, and urinary stasis. Urinary stasis can be caused by an anatomical or functional abnormality, such as a **neurogenic bladder**. Children with constipation also have an increased risk of recurrent UTI (Shaikh et al., 2016).

Clinical Presentation

UTI may present with nonspecific symptoms, making diagnosis difficult. However, timely detection is important, because a delay in recognition and treatment can lead to life-threatening complications. Symptoms depend on the location of the infection and the age of the child. Children younger than age 2 years who present with fever of unknown origin should be tested for a UTI because symptoms in the infant and young child tend to be nonspecific. Many UTIs are asymptomatic and are discovered on routine examinations. Table 24.2 reviews presenting signs and symptoms of a UTI by age group.

Remember Ellie Raymore, the 3-year-old in Chapter 4 with vesicoureteral reflux (VUR) and a UTI? What symptoms of a UTI did Ellie exhibit? What type of UTI did Ellie develop? Why was it so important that Ellie's mom seek treatment early for Ellie? What were some challenges in diagnosing and treating Ellie for a UTI?

Assessment and Diagnosis

Assessment of the child with a possible UTI includes a review of systems, particularly focusing on voiding patterns, urine characteristics, and recent history of incontinence or enuresis. Assess for history of recurrent UTIs. Assess for quality, quantity, and frequency of voiding. Assess infants and young children for fever, poor feeding, irritability, and ill appearance, because urinary symptoms are difficult to determine in a child who cannot communicate. Vital sign findings, particularly low blood pressure, can indicate a more severe UTI. Assess the child's hydration status by evaluating oral intake, skin turgor, and mucous membranes.

  Perform an abdominal assessment, particularly assessing for masses, tenderness, and distension. Flank pain, costovertebral pain, and suprapubic pain may be present. Assess for urinary frequency, urgency, and dysuria. Assess for risk factors such as frequent bubble baths, wiping in the wrong direction (girls), sexual activity (adolescent girls), and a history of constipation.

  Adolescents may deny symptoms of a UTI if they are sexually active for fear of disclosing this information to parents.

Table 24.2	Clinical Manifestations of Urinary Tract Infections by Age
Age Group	**Signs and Symptoms**
Neonates (birth to 1 mo)	Jaundice, fever, failure to thrive, poor feeding, vomiting, irritability
Infants and toddlers (1 mo–3 y)	Poor feeding, fever, vomiting, strong-smelling urine, abdominal pain, irritability
Preschoolers (3–6 y)	Vomiting, abdominal pain, fever, loss of appetite, strong-smelling urine, enuresis, urinary symptoms such as dysuria, frequency, urgency
School-age children (6–12 y)	Fever, vomiting, abdominal pain, flank or back pain, foul-smelling urine, enuresis, urinary symptoms such as dysuria, frequency, urgency, incontinence
Adolescents (10–21 y)	Same as for school-age children. Girls may have concurrent vaginitis or a sexually transmitted infection.

Assessing and questioning the adolescent without the parents present may be necessary to gather accurate information and elicit concerns for a UTI.

Diagnostic tests include examination of a urine specimen for the presence of bacteria. Screening for a UTI can be done with a dipstick. A dipstick that is positive for nitrites or leukocyte esterase signals the presence of gram-negative bacteria or white blood cells, respectively. Obtaining a clean-catch urine specimen is appropriate if the child is old enough to properly do this. If not, obtaining urine by catheterization is preferred. Diagnosis of a UTI cannot be established reliably through a culture collected in a bag (Roberts et al., 2016). However, urine collected in a bag can be used to perform a urinalysis. If the urine obtained in a bag is positive for leukocytes or nitrites, then a specimen obtained via catheterization is necessary for a urine culture (Roberts et al., 2016).

A renal and bladder ultrasound may be performed in children with recurrent UTIs to assess for renal scarring or structural defects that increase the risk of UTIs. A voiding cystourethrogram (VCUG) may also be performed after the UTI is cleared to assess for VUR. However, the American Academy of Pediatrics no longer recommends a VCUG after the first UTI during infancy (Roberts et al., 2016). A VCUG is indicated if the renal and bladder ultrasound reveals hydronephrosis, renal scarring, or other concerns for VUR.

Therapeutic Interventions

Begin antibiotic therapy, as ordered, after collecting a urine sample. Current treatment recommendations are for a 7- to 14-day course of antibiotics (Roberts et al., 2016). Antibiotic therapy is based on the child's signs and symptoms, severity of illness, age, and sensitivity of the cultured organism. Common antibiotics used in the treatment of UTIs include trimethoprim sulfamethoxazole, ciprofloxacin, amoxicillin, and ceftriaxone. Hospitalization for IV antibiotic therapy may be necessary for children who appear ill and cannot tolerate oral antibiotic therapy.

Restoring and maintaining adequate hydration is essential in treating a child with a UTI. Fever and inadequate intake related to decreased appetite can lead to dehydration. Adequate fluid intake is also essential to flush the kidneys and bladder of organisms. For children who present with dehydration, hospital admission and IV fluid therapy may be necessary.

Pain, burning, and spasticity during urination can be relieved with phenazopyridine. However, this drug should only be used on a short-term basis (no more than 2 days) while on antibiotic therapy (Fisher, 2017).

Evaluation

Expected outcomes for a child with a UTI include the following:

- The child is free from infection.
- Pain is adequately controlled.
- The child remains hydrated.
- Urine is of normal color, clarity, and volume.
- Parents verbalize and demonstrate ways to reduce the risk of UTI.

Discharge Planning and Teaching

Most children with UTIs are treated at home. Teaching about UTI includes ensuring parents understand the importance of completing the entire antibiotic regimen even though symptoms may be resolved soon after starting the antibiotic. Failure to complete the entire course of antibiotics may result in recurrence of the UTI and may lead to antibiotic resistance. Teach parents the amount (volume) of fluid needed each day for the age and weight of the child. An adequate amount of fluid intake for 24 hours is equivalent to the maintenance fluid rate for the age plus additional fluids when fever or additional fluid losses are present (refer to Chapter 23). Encourage parents to avoid giving children carbonated or caffeinated beverages, because these may irritate the bladder mucosa. Teach prevention strategies (Box 24.3).

Enuresis

Enuresis is continued incontinence of urine past the age of toilet training. Some children may have **diurnal enuresis** (daytime loss of urinary control), **nocturnal enuresis** (nighttime bedwetting), or both. Enuresis is a distressing condition and can impact a child's emotional well-being and behavior.

Etiology and Pathophysiology

Enuresis can be categorized as primary or secondary. Primary enuresis occurs when the child has never had a dry night. An estimated 80% of children have primary enuresis (Elder, 2016). Possible causes of primary enuresis include small bladder capacity, nocturnal polyuria, disorder of sleep arousal, and idiopathic causes. Secondary enuresis occurs in children who have been reliably dry for at least 6 months but begin bedwetting. The exact cause of secondary enuresis is unknown. Likely factors include unusually stressful events (parents' divorce, new sibling, etc.), constipation, and suboptimal daytime voiding habits.

The prevalence of enuresis gradually declines during childhood. In the United States, approximately 25% of children wet the bed at the age of 4 years. By the age of 7 years, 5% to 10%

Box 24.3 Preventing Urinary Tract Infections in the Pediatric Population

- Encourage children to drink enough fluid.
- Have children wear loose-fitting cotton underwear, which reduces the incidence of perineal irritation.
- Avoid having children wear tight-fitting jeans or pants.
- Teach girls to wipe from front to back after voiding.
- Encourage children to avoid long periods of holding urine.
- Remind young children to use the toilet frequently. Watch for cues such as the "pee dance," crossing legs, and holding the genital area.
- Discourage frequent bubble baths and use of hot water in tub baths. Chemicals in bubble bath solution and hot water can irritate the urethra.

wet the bed, and by the age of 10 years, fewer than 5% wet the bed. Enuresis is more common in boys than girls.

Clinical Presentation

Children with diurnal enuresis may present with clinical manifestations of urgency, frequency, constant dribbling, and involuntary loss of control even after voiding. Nocturnal enuresis is manifested by reports of bedwetting.

Assessment and Diagnosis

A thorough history, including family history of enuresis, recent stressors or changes in lifestyle, and toilet training history, can assist in the diagnosis of enuresis. Assess whether the child has met growth and development milestones in the development of bladder control (Growth and Development Check 24.1).

Diagnostic tests include a urinalysis and urine culture to assess for a possible UTI. The urinalysis reveals the urine specific gravity, which provides information about the child's ability to concentrate urine. A urine culture may reveal an asymptomatic UTI. Other possible diagnoses, such as diabetes insipidus, diabetes mellitus, and renal insufficiency, should be ruled out in children who present with enuresis and polyuria or **oliguria**, or less than the normal amount of urine. An ultrasound of the urinary tract and postvoiding residual measurements may also be obtained to rule out structural abnormalities leading to enuresis.

Therapeutic Interventions

A multifaceted approach is most effective in the treatment of enuresis. Treatment approaches for enuresis include fluid restriction, bladder exercises, timed voiding, enuresis alarms, and

Growth and Development Check 24.1

Milestones in the Development of Bladder Control

Age (y)	Milestone
1½	Passes urine at regular intervals
2	Verbalizes when he or she is urinating
2½	Can hold urine; knows when he or she needs to void
2½–3½	Achieves nighttime control of urine
3	Holds urge to void when preoccupied with play or activities; uses bathroom by himself or herself
5	Prefers privacy; is able to initiate urination regardless of fullness of bladder; voids approximately 7 times a day

medications. Enuresis alarms have been shown to be effective in the treatment of enuresis. Studies demonstrate the effectiveness of bell and pad conditioning alarms. A large study using bell and pad conditioning alarms in 2017 by Apos et al. demonstrated an overall 76% success rate in achieving dryness for 14 consecutive days. Medications used in the treatment of enuresis include desmopressin, tricyclic antidepressants, and antispasmodics. Medications are reviewed in The Pharmacy 24.1.

The Pharmacy 24.1 Medications for Enuresis

Medication	Classification	Route	Action	Nursing Considerations
Desmopressin	Antidiuretic hormone	PO	Antidiuretic effect; enhances reabsorption of water in the kidneys	Monitor sodium levels for hyponatremia.
Imipramine	Tricyclic antidepressant	PO	Anticholinergic and antispasmodic effects	• Treatment should not exceed 3 mo. • Obtain baseline EKG before starting therapy. • Monitor child for cardiotoxicity, seizures, hepatic dysfunction, and neutropenia. • Side effects include dry mouth, nausea, constipation, tachycardia, postural hypotension, insomnia, lethargy.
Oxybutynin	Anticholinergic	PO	Antispasmodic effect	• Monitor for dizziness, drowsiness, constipation, dry mouth, and nausea. • Monitor voiding pattern. • Monitor intake and output.

From Lexicomp. *Pediatric & Neonatal Dosage Handbook* (25th ed.), 2018.
EKG, electrocardiogram; PO, by mouth.

Evaluation

Expected outcomes for a child with enuresis include the following:

- The child and family use one or more interventions to control nighttime wetting.
- The child has an increased number of dry nights.

Discharge Planning and Teaching

Children with enuresis are treated in the outpatient setting. Before beginning treatment, assess the parent's and the child's motivation and readiness for interventions. The child must be an active participant in the treatment plan to achieve successful resolution of enuresis.

Suggest using a reward system. Set realistic goals for the child and reinforce dry days or nights with stickers on a chart. Plan rewards when the child reaches milestones, such as a week of dry days or nights.

Structural Defects of the Genitourinary System

Structural defects of the urinary and reproductive system may interfere with urinary flow and possibly affect reproductive function. Structural defects discussed in this section include the following: phimosis, cryptorchidism, inguinal hernia and hydrocele, testicular torsion, hypospadias and epispadias, and congenital hydronephrosis.

Phimosis

In **phimosis**, the foreskin of the penis cannot be retracted (Fig. 24.3). Phimosis is normal in the newborn period. Over time, the prepuce (foreskin) naturally becomes retractable because of keratinization of the inner foreskin and intermittent erections. However, phimosis can be pathological after the newborn and toddler periods.

Etiology and Pathophysiology

At birth, phimosis is physiological. During neonatal development, adhesions form leading to the inner epithelial lining of the foreskin fusing to the glans. Over time, there is lysis of the adhesions between the prepuce and glans and the phimotic ring loosens. By the age of 3 years, 90% of uncircumcised boys have a fully retractable prepuce (Drake, Rustom, & Davies, 2013).

Paraphimosis occurs when the foreskin is retracted and the prepuce cannot be pulled back over the glands. Venous stasis occurs in the retracted foreskin, leading to edema and severe pain. The foreskin cannot be pulled back over the glands.

Clinical Presentation

Children with phimosis present with irritation or bleeding from the opening of the prepuce, erythema or edema of the penis, discharge, and/or dysuria. Pain and a swollen penis are characteristic of paraphimosis.

Assessment and Diagnosis

Assessment includes obtaining a brief history, including the onset of symptoms such as erythema, edema, irritation, or discharge from the penis. Assess for signs of bleeding. Ask the parents whether they have noted blood in the diaper or underwear. Inspect the penis for abnormal scarring or a white ring around the penis. Erythema and edema of the foreskin and glans (balanoposthitis) or only the glans (**balanitis**) may be present.

Therapeutic Interventions

Topical steroid creams may be prescribed for phimosis. Typically, the topical steroid cream, such as betamethasone, is applied twice daily for 2 to 8 weeks. Application of steroid cream can hasten the natural retraction of the foreskin without systemic side effects (Drake et al., 2013).

Paraphimosis is a medical emergency. A reduction of the prepuce or a small dorsal incision to release the foreskin is necessary to restore blood flow to the prepuce area. Circumcision is also used to treat both phimosis and paraphimosis.

Evaluation

Expected outcomes for a child with phimosis include the following:

- The child is free of infection around the penis.
- Skin integrity is restored to normal and maintained.
- Parents understand proper care and hygiene for the uncircumcised boy.
- Preschool-age and older boys are able to appropriately retract the foreskin and clean the penis during each bath or shower.

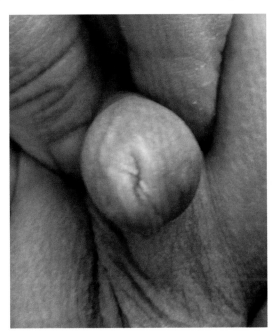

Figure 24.3. Phimosis. Note that the foreskin is unable to be retracted. Reprinted with permission from Graham, S. D., & Keane, T. E. (2015). *Glenn's urologic surgery* (8th ed., Fig. 16.2). Philadelphia, PA: Wolters Kluwer.

Discharge Planning and Teaching

Phimosis is treated in the outpatient setting. Educating parents regarding normal physiological changes in the uncircumcised male is necessary. Inform parents of proper hygiene (Box 24.4). Educate parents about signs and symptoms of paraphimosis and the need to seek immediate medical treatment if it occurs. Review the signs of balanitis and infection.

Cryptorchidism

Cryptorchidism (undescended testes) occurs when one or both of the testes fail to descend through the inguinal canal into the scrotum.

Etiology and Pathophysiology

During fetal development, the testes develop in the abdomen and descend into the scrotal sac during the seventh to ninth months of gestation. The cause of undescended testicles may be mechanical, hormonal, enzymatic, or chromosomal. Approximately 4.5% of boys have undescended testicles at birth, with a higher incidence in premature boys because the testicles normally descend during the later weeks of gestation. The majority of cases of undescended testicles resolve spontaneously by 2 months of life, when there is a temporary testosterone surge that results in significant penile growth (Elder, 2016). If the testicles do not descend by 4 months of age, they will remain undescended and interventions are needed to correct the problem (Elder, 2016).

Undescended testicles should be corrected. If the testicles remain undescended, possible complications include poor testicular growth, associated hernia, torsion of the testis, infertility, testicular malignancy, and the potential for psychological consequences of an empty scrotal sac (Elder, 2016).

Clinical Presentation

A child with undescended testes has no clinical manifestations other than the absence of testicles in the scrotal sac.

Box 24.4 Proper Hygiene in the Uncircumcised Male

- In newborns and infants, change the diaper frequently.
- Wash the penis daily with mild soap and water.
- In newborns, the foreskin does not normally retract; do not force it to do so.
- In the older infant, when the foreskin easily retracts, retract the foreskin and clean around the glans with mild soap and water once a week. Dry the area before replacing the foreskin.
- Always replace the foreskin after retraction.
- Preschool-age boys are able to learn to retract the foreskin and clean the penis during each bath or shower.
- Avoid bubble baths, which can cause irritation.

Undescended testes can present in one of four ways: abdominal (nonpalpable), peeping, inguinal gliding, or ectopic. Peeping refers to testes that are abdominal but can be pushed partially into the inguinal canal. Inguinal gliding refers to testes that can be pushed into the scrotum but retract immediately. Ectopic testes are located in a superficial inguinal pouch or in the perineum.

Assessment and Diagnosis

A physical exam can establish the diagnosis of cryptorchidism. The child should be completely undressed and calm. Palpate the child's scrotum and inguinal canal using your dominant hand while your nondominant hand is positioned over the pubic tubercle and pushes inferiorly toward the scrotum.

Therapeutic Interventions

An orchiopexy is performed to correct cryptorchidism. During an orchiopexy, an inguinal incision is made and mobilization of the testis and spermatic cord and correction of an indirect inguinal hernia are performed. Typically, orchiopexies are performed on an outpatient basis, and approximately 98% of procedures are successful in correcting undescended testicles (Elder, 2016).

Evaluation

Expected outcomes for a child with cryptorchidism include the following:

- The incision heals without signs of infection.
- Postoperative pain is effectively managed.
- Parents verbalize understanding of incision and postoperative care.
- The child (if an adolescent) and parents verbalize an understanding of the need for regular testicular exams once the child reaches puberty.

Discharge Planning and Teaching

Following an orchiopexy, teach parents to monitor for signs of infection and bleeding at the surgical site. Instruct parents to keep the incision clean and dry.

Inguinal Hernia and Hydrocele

An inguinal hernia occurs when an intra-abdominal structure, such as the intestine, protrudes through a defect in the abdominal wall. Hydrocele is a condition in which there is fluid in the scrotal sac.

Etiology and Pathophysiology

An inguinal hernia is one of the most common conditions seen in the pediatric population. Surgical correction of an inguinal hernia is the most common surgical procedure performed in the pediatric population.

Hydrocele is present in about 1% to 2% of neonates. In most cases of hydrocele, the hydrocele is noncommunicating and resolves spontaneously by reabsorption by the age of 1 year (Elder, 2016).

Priority Care Concepts 24.1

An Incarcerated Inguinal Hernia

A child with an incarcerated inguinal hernia requires immediate medical attention and intervention to prevent ischemia to the incarcerated bowel. Be alert for signs of an incarcerated hernia; in infants, these include acute onset of colicky pain, irritability, feeding intolerance, abdominal distention, and vomiting (Aiken & Oldham, 2016). Older children present with abdominal pain and a nonfluctuant mass in the inguinal region that is firm and cannot be reduced.

Clinical Presentation

A child with an inguinal hernia or hydrocele presents with a palpable, round, smooth, nontender mass in the scrotum or inguinal area. Parents may also report noticing an intermittent bulge or protrusion in the groin or swelling in the scrotum. Parents may report noticing the bulge more when the infant is crying or straining, when increased intra-abdominal pressure forces the hernia downward and outward.

Assessment and Diagnosis

Assessment and diagnosis of the infant or child with an inguinal hernia or hydrocele involves a physical exam of the abdomen, inguinal area, and scrotum (Priority Care Concepts 24.1). Transillumination of the scrotum confirms that the fluid-filled mass is a hydrocele. Hydroceles that persist beyond 12 to 18 months are likely communicating and should be surgically repaired (Elder, 2016).

Therapeutic Interventions

An inguinal hernia generally requires surgical correction. The surgery is an elective, outpatient procedure at an early age (after 3 months of age to reduce anesthesia risks). If **incarceration** (a condition in which the hernia is unable to be reduced and blood flow is compromised) occurs, the hernia is repaired emergently to avoid ischemic injury to the affected bowel and abdominal contents. A hydrocele is surgically corrected in a manner similar to that of an inguinal hernia.

Postoperatively, administer pain medication as ordered. If a spinal or regional block was used during the surgery, pain may be minimal. Routine incision care is necessary to prevent infection. Typically, the incision is covered with a protective sealant rather than with a dressing. In cases of emergency surgery for an incarcerated hernia, the child may need IV antibiotics and a nasogastric tube for a short time after surgical correction.

Evaluation

Expected outcomes for a child with an inguinal hernia and/or a hydrocele include the following:

- The child's pain is controlled postoperatively.
- The surgical incision heals without signs of infection.
- Skin integrity is restored to normal.
- The child is free of complications from an incarcerated inguinal hernia.

Discharge Planning and Teaching

Before discharge, instruct parents on incision care and ways to prevent surgical site infection. Reinforce the importance of hand washing before and after diaper changes and toileting. Frequent diaper changes and meticulous cleaning of the diaper area help reduce the risk of infection. Review with parents the signs and symptoms of infection, which include redness, increased pain at the surgical site, swelling, drainage, and fever. Reassure parents that edema and bruising are common and normal after surgery.

Testicular Torsion

Testicular torsion is an emergency condition in which the testicle rotates, twisting the spermatic cord and cutting off blood supply to the scrotum. Torsion is caused by inadequate fixation of the testes within the scrotum, allowing excessive mobility of the testes.

Etiology and Pathophysiology

Testicular torsion is uncommon before the age of 10 years. Torsion is the most common cause of testicular pain in boys 12 years and older (Elder, 2016). Torsion occurs in approximately 1 in 4,000 males under the age of 18 years annually (Lemini et al., 2016).

Minor genital trauma, sporting injuries, exercise, and sexual activity can lead to testicular torsion. A congenital deformity, known as bell clapper deformity, increases the risk of testicular torsion. Bell clapper deformity is when the tunica vaginalis attaches high on the spermatic cord, leaving the testes free to rotate and twist.

Clinical Presentation

Sudden onset of severe pain followed by scrotal and inguinal swelling are classic presenting symptoms in testicular torsion (Lemini et al., 2016). Radiating pain, nausea and vomiting, and scrotal wall erythema are also found. Symptoms can occur at any time but generally occur when the child is sleeping or inactive.

Assessment and Diagnosis

A detailed history regarding the cause, onset, and activities surrounding pain and swelling of the scrotum is helpful in diagnosing testicular torsion. The testes are tender and often difficult to examine. The testes are often found to be positioned transversely in the scrotum, instead of laterally. Normal cremasteric reflex is usually absent in testicular torsion and is one of the most consistent findings in boys with torsion (Lemini et al., 2016). Cremasteric reflex, elicited by stroking the inner thigh, normally results in an immediate contraction of the cremaster muscle that pulls up the ipsilateral testes. Diagnosis is made on the basis of symptoms and physical exam.

Therapeutic Interventions

Treatment of testicular torsion requires prompt surgical exploration and detorsion of the affected area. Once the testicles are untwisted (detorsion), an orchiopexy is performed to prevent future episodes of torsion. An orchiopexy involves moving the affected testicle to the correct location in the scrotum and suturing it in place. The most important indicator of testicular salvage is time; males who underwent surgical correction of testicular torsion within 6 hours of the onset of symptoms were most likely to have successful restoration of blood flow and return of spermatogenesis (Ramachandra, Palazzi, Holmes, & Marietti, 2015). When surgical exploration and correction occur within 6 hours of onset of symptoms, salvage rates are over 90%, compared with only 50% if symptoms have been present over 12 hours before surgical exploration (Ramachandra et al., 2015). If blood flow cannot be restored to the testicle or necrosis has occurred, an orchiectomy is performed.

Evaluation

Expected outcomes for a child with testicular torsion include the following:

- Blood flow is restored to the scrotum and testicles.
- The incision is free of signs of infection.
- The child is free of pain following surgical correction.
- Anxiety and fear are reduced following surgical correction of testicular torsion.

Discharge Planning and Teaching

Incision care and pain management are priorities during discharge preparation and teaching. The child often goes home the same day following surgical correction. Reinforce with the child and family that the child should avoid heavy lifting for 4 weeks postoperatively and strenuous activity for at least 2 weeks following surgery. Educate the adolescent regarding the importance of testicular self-exams.

Parents and adolescents often wonder about the effect on fertility following testicular torsion. Provide psychological support for the child and family and reassure parents that when torsion involves only one testicle and prompt surgical correction is performed, fertility should not be affected.

Hypospadias and Epispadias

Hypospadias is a urethral defect in which the opening of the urethra is on the ventral side of the penis rather than at the end of the penis. **Epispadias** occurs when the urethral opening is on the dorsal side of the penis. Figure 24.4 compares a normal urethral opening with epispadias and hypospadias.

Etiology and Pathophysiology

Hypospadias is a congenital anomaly of the penis in which the urethral opening occurs on the ventral side of the penis because of an abnormal closure of the urethral folds during weeks 8 to 14 of gestation (Canon, Mosley, Chipollini, Purifoy, & Hobbs,

2012). Specifically, the prepuce, termed the dorsal hood, develops incompletely, such that the foreskin is on the sides and dorsal aspect of the penis but deficient or absent ventrally. Hypospadias affects 1 in 250 newborns.

The exact causes of hypospadias and epispadias are unknown. However, evidence shows that low birth weight, maternal hypertension, and multiple pregnancies are associated with a higher incidence of the defect (Van Rooij et al., 2013). Incidence is also increased in children with anorectal malformations and congenital heart disease. Hypospadias also occurs in conjunction with congenital chordee. A family history of hypospadias increased the risk by 7- to 10-fold, suggesting a genetic component (Van Rooij et al., 2013). The incidence also appears to increase due to in utero exposure to estrogenic or antiandrogenic hormones (Elder, 2016).

Clinical Presentation

Hypospadias and epispadias are typically observed soon after birth, either on physical exam or when the neonate begins voiding. Urine is seen coming from the dorsal (epispadias) or ventral (hypospadias) side of the penis. In hypospadias, the urethral meatus can be found anywhere along the course of the ventral surface of the penile shaft, from the tip of the glans to the

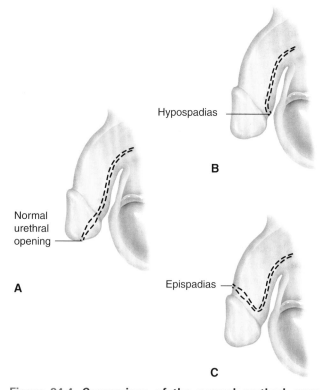

Figure 24.4. Comparison of the normal urethral opening with those in hypospadias and epispadias. A. Normal urethral opening. **B.** Urethral opening on the ventral side of the penis (hypospadias). **C.** Urethral opening on the dorsal side of the penis (epispadias). Reprinted with permission from Stewart, J. (2017). *Anatomical Chart Company atlas of pathophysiology* (4th ed., unnumbered figure in Chapter 14). Philadelphia, PA: Wolters Kluwer.

perineum. In epispadias, the urethral meatus is found anywhere along the course of the dorsal surface of the penile shaft.

Assessment and Diagnosis

Assessment for hypospadias or epispadias should include a thorough exam of the genitalia, because there may also be other anomalies or defects present. Parents may report an unusual urine stream. Assess the penis for placement of the urethral meatus. Inspect for **chordee**, a fibrous band causing the penis to curve downward. Assess for the presence of testicles in the scrotal sac. Cryptorchidism and inguinal hernias often occur with hypospadias.

Diagnosis can be made by prenatal ultrasound or on physical exam at birth.

Therapeutic Interventions

Circumcision should be avoided because the foreskin is often used in the repair of the defect. The treatment for hypospadias and epispadias is surgical correction. The defects are usually corrected during infancy, preferably between 6 and 12 months of age, when the risk of general anesthesia is similar to that of older children (Elder, 2016). If left uncorrected, the child may have a deformity of the urine stream, infertility (if the urethral meatus is proximal), and self-esteem and body image issues related to the abnormal appearance of the genitalia. The goal of surgical correction is to provide an appropriately placed meatus that allows for normal voiding and ejaculation.

Surgical correction involves moving the meatus to the glans penis and reconstructing the urethra as needed, depending on the location of the defect. Most repairs are accomplished in one surgery. Severe or complicated defects may require two or more surgeries to fully correct.

Evaluation

Expected outcomes for an infant with hypospadias or epispadias include the following:

- Pain is controlled effectively.
- The incision heals without signs of infection.
- The stent or catheter remains in place and free of complications until healing occurs.
- Parents cope effectively with the need for their child to undergo surgery.

Discharge Planning and Teaching

The child is often discharged the day of or the day after surgery. Parents need instructions regarding care of the surgical site, double diapering, medication administration, and signs of infection. Patient Teaching 24.1 reviews discharge teaching points for parents.

Teach parents how to double diaper, a method used to protect the urethra and stent or catheter after surgery. Double diapering helps keep the surgical site clean and free from infection. The inner diaper contains stool and the outer diaper collects urine, keeping stool away from the incision site. Place a smaller diaper inside a larger diaper. Cut a hole or cross-shaped slit in the front of the smaller diaper. Place both diapers under the

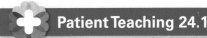

Patient Teaching 24.1

Care of the Child After Hypospadias or Epispadias Repair

- Do not bathe the child in a tub until the stent or catheter is removed.
- Use the double-diapering technique to protect the stent and reduce the risk of stool contamination at the surgical site.

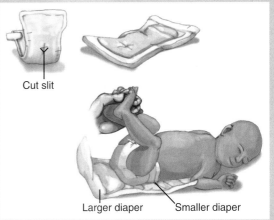

Cut slit

Larger diaper   Smaller diaper

Figure reprinted with permission from Kyle, T., & Carman, S. (2016). *Pediatric nursing clinical guide* (2nd ed., Fig. 3.6). Philadelphia, PA: Wolters Kluwer.

- Avoid holding the child in a straddle position such as on the hip.
- Limit the child's activity for 2 wk after surgery, restricting activities that put pressure on the surgical site. For example, do not allow the child to play on riding toys.
- Encourage adequate fluid intake. Use special cups and provide fluids the child prefers.
- Observe for signs of infection such as fever, swelling at the site, redness, drainage, strong or foul-smelling urine, or a change in the flow or stream of urine.
- Call the provider if urine is seen leaking from any area other than the penis.
- Complete the entire course of prescribed antibiotics.

child. Carefully bring the penis and catheter or stent through the hole in the smaller diaper. Fasten the smaller diaper. Then fasten the larger diaper, making sure the tip of the catheter or stent is inside the larger diaper.

Bladder Exstrophy

Bladder exstrophy occurs when the bladder extrudes through the lower abdominal wall.

Etiology and Pathophysiology

The incidence of bladder exstrophy is approximately 1 in 35,000 to 40,000 live births. Females are affected more often than are males, by a ratio of 2:1. During fetal development, failure of the abdominal wall to close leads to protuberance of the bladder and a wide separation of the rectus muscles and symphysis pubis.

Clinical Presentation

Bladder exstrophy is noted immediately following delivery. The posterior bladder protrudes through the lower abdominal wall (Fig. 24.5). A red, moist bladder lies on the lower abdomen, displacing the umbilicus downward and separating the rectus muscles.

Assessment and Diagnosis

Assessment of the child with bladder exstrophy includes a physical exam of the bladder on the abdominal wall. Draining urine is visible. Skin surrounding the bladder may be excoriated from frequent or continuous contact with urine. Assessment of the genitalia may reveal a malformed urethra in females and an unformed or malformed penis with epispadias in males.

Diagnosis may be made prenatally with ultrasound. Diagnosis is also made at delivery depending on the physical appearance of the abdomen.

Therapeutic Interventions

Cover the exposed bladder with plastic wrap or a sterile plastic bag to keep the bladder mucosa moist (Elder, 2016). Keep the infant in the supine position. Change soiled diapers immediately to prevent contamination of the bladder with stool. Give the infant a sponge bath rather than submerging him or her in water to prevent pathogens from the bath water from entering the exposed bladder. Use protective barrier creams on the surrounding skin to prevent breakdown from contact with urine.

Surgical intervention is necessary to repair bladder exstrophy. The goal of surgery is to achieve urinary continence and preserve renal function. Untreated bladder exstrophy results in total urinary incontinence and puts the child at higher risk of

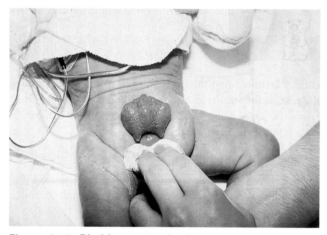

Figure 24.5. Bladder exstrophy in a newborn. Note that the bladder is bright red. Reprinted with permission from Kyle, T., & Carman, S. (2016). *Essentials of pediatric nursing* (3rd ed., Fig. 21.1). Philadelphia, PA: Wolters Kluwer.

bladder cancer, specifically adenocarcinoma (Elder, 2016). Primary closure of the bladder and abdominal wall usually occurs within 48 to 72 hours of birth. Some children with complex bladder exstrophy require multiple surgeries to establish urinary continence.

Postoperative nursing care for the child with a bladder exstrophy repair centers on maintaining immobilization and proper alignment, avoiding abduction of the infant's legs, pain management, monitoring peripheral circulation, providing pain relief, and meticulous skin care. The pelvis is immobilized to facilitate healing. Internal and external fixation devices are used to maintain immobilization. Effective pain management is a priority to help maintain immobilization. Bladder spasms are common and are treated with antispasmodics such as oxybutynin or belladonna and opioid suppositories. Maintain aseptic technique during wound care and dressing changes.

Routinely monitor and record urine output from ureteral drains every 2 to 4 hours. Assess for changes in urine output that could indicate obstruction of the drains, such as decreased or absent urine output. Urine or blood draining from the urethral meatus and increased intensity of bladder spasms may also indicate obstruction. Small amounts of blood or blood clots are common for the first few days after surgery but should dissipate.

Evaluation

Expected outcomes for an infant with bladder exstrophy include the following:

- The incision heals without signs of infection.
- Skin integrity is restored.
- Pain is effectively managed.

Discharge Planning and Teaching

Discharge planning and teaching for a child with bladder exstrophy focuses on establishing urinary continence, preventing infection, and maintaining skin integrity. Parents may need assistance in learning how to hold the baby. Review dressing and wound care with the parents, along with the signs and symptoms of infection. Emphasize the need to immediately notify the provider if there are signs of infection or a change in urinary output. Long-term care includes addressing social and sexual issues. Parents may also need assistance in coping with the child's incontinence.

Establishing urinary continence is often more difficult in children with bladder exstrophy. Multiple procedures may be necessary to achieve urinary continence. Some children may require urinary diversion devices when surgery is not successful. Encourage parents to toilet train the child for bowel movements at the age-appropriate time when urinary continence is not successful.

Vesicoureteral Reflux Disease

VUR occurs when there is retrograde flow of urine from the bladder into the ureters and, in severe cases, into the renal pelvis and calyces. Reflux of urine occurs during bladder contraction when voiding.

Etiology and Pathophysiology

VUR affects 1% to 3% of all infants and children. VUR occurs in about 30% of female children presenting with a febrile UTI (Elder, 2106). VUR appears to be an autosomal dominant trait. Approximately 35% of siblings of children with VUR have VUR as well. In addition, about 50% of children born to women with a history of VUR also have VUR of varying grades.

Backflow of urine (reflux) may occur in one or both ureters. If reflux occurs when the urine is infected, the kidney is exposed to bacteria and pyelonephritis may result. VUR is graded using the International Classification of Vesicoureteral Reflux grades of I to V (Fig. 24.6). Grade I is characterized by mild reflux into the distal ureter, and grade V is characterized by severe dilation of the ureter and pelvis of the kidney (Elder, 2016). VUR may be primary or secondary. Primary VUR results from a congenital malformation or abnormality at the vesicoureteral junction. The abnormality results in an incompetent valve that allows urine to backflow into the ureter. Secondary VUR results from other structural or functional problems, such as a neuropathic bladder or bladder outlet obstruction.

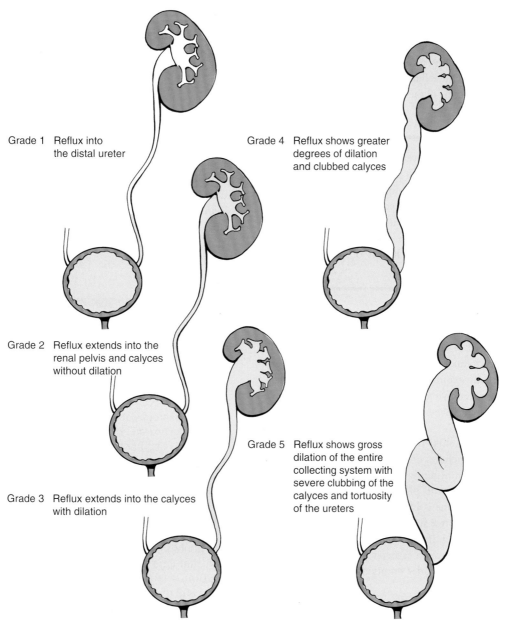

Grade 1 Reflux into the distal ureter

Grade 2 Reflux extends into the renal pelvis and calyces without dilation

Grade 3 Reflux extends into the calyces with dilation

Grade 4 Reflux shows greater degrees of dilation and clubbed calyces

Grade 5 Reflux shows gross dilation of the entire collecting system with severe clubbing of the calyces and tortuosity of the ureters

Figure 24.6. International Classification of Vesicoureteral Reflux grades I to V. Notice in grade I that there is no dilation of the ureter and that the urine does not reach the kidney during backflow. In grade V, there is severe dilation of the ureter and backflow of urine into the kidney. Modified with permission from Brown, L. J., Coller, R. J., & Miller, L. T. (2018). *BRS pediatrics* (2nd ed., Fig. 11.4). Philadelphia, PA: Wolters Kluwer.

Clinical Presentation

Children with VUR may be asymptomatic (when no UTI is present). Symptoms associated with VUR are the same as in a UTI. VUR is usually discovered during evaluation for a UTI. The average age of diagnosis is 2 to 3 years, and 80% of those diagnosed are female (Elder, 2016).

Assessment and Diagnosis

Assessment of the child with VUR includes obtaining a history of urinary symptoms such as dysuria, frequency, urgency, nocturia, and hematuria. Fever and back, flank, or abdominal pain may also be present. Medical history of the child with VUR may include recurrent UTIs, congenital defects, and a family history of VUR. Palpate the abdomen for the presence of a mass if hydronephrosis is suspected.

A VCUG and renal ultrasound are used to diagnose VUR and grade the severity of the reflux. A renal ultrasound provides information on the structure of the kidney and whether scarring is present.

Remember Ellie Raymore, the 3-year-old with VUR in Chapter 4? Why was Ellie prescribed trimethoprim-sulfamethoxazole before her diagnosis with a UTI was confirmed? Discuss two teaching points to review with Ellie's mother regarding the administration of prophylactic antibiotics for a 3-year-old. Why did Ellie's history of VUR place her at higher risk for a UTI?

Therapeutic Interventions

Children with grade I or II VUR often have spontaneous resolution of urinary reflux (Elder, 2016). Children with grade III, IV, or V usually require surgical intervention. Surgical correction involves removing the ureters from the bladder and reimplanting them elsewhere in the bladder wall to regain functionality.

Nursing care of the child who has undergone surgery to reimplant the ureters includes urinary catheter care, monitoring urinary output, administering medications, and managing pain. A urinary catheter is in place for several days postoperatively. Initially, the urine is bloody, but it returns to clear within 2 to 3 days. Monitor urine output for blood clots or signs or increased bleeding. If urine output decreases or stops, notify the provider, because the catheter may need to be irrigated to ensure adequate bladder emptying and reduce pressure on the implanted ureters.

Medications include antibiotics, antispasmodics, and pain medication (Analyze the Evidence 24.1). Bladder spasms are common following surgical correction of VUR. Oxybutynin is often prescribed to control bladder spasms. Antispasmodics can cause constipation. Ensure adequate fluid intake once IV fluids are discontinued and promote intake of fiber.

Evaluation

Expected outcomes for a child with VUR include the following:

- The child remains free of a UTI.
- Renal scarring is minimized in severe cases of reflux.
- The child remains free of postoperative complications following surgical correction of VUR.

Discharge Planning and Teaching

Children with low-grade VUR are managed in the outpatient setting. Reinforce the importance of prophylactic antibiotic administration, if prescribed, to help prevent UTIs. Instruct parents to give prophylactic antibiotics at bedtime because of urinary stasis overnight. Parents of toddlers or children who refuse to take medications may need assistance to develop strategies for successful administration.

For children with VUR, preventing UTIs and pyelonephritis is the goal. Teach parents and children appropriate perineal hygiene. Reinforce the importance of hand washing after toileting. Teach the child to empty the bladder completely. Encourage parents to use a time-voiding technique during the day (the child uses the bathroom at timed intervals throughout the day). Promote regular bowel movements to avoid constipation, which can hinder complete bladder emptying, and ensure adequate fluid intake.

Reinforce with parents and older children the importance of seeking prompt medical assessment and treatment at the first

---

 Analyze the Evidence 24.1

Do Prophylactic Antibiotics Reduce Urinary Tract Infections in Children With Vesicoureteral Reflux?

Historically, prophylactic antibiotics have been prescribed for children with vesicoureteral reflux (VUR) to reduce the risk of or prevent recurrent urinary tract infections (UTIs) and thus lessen the risk of renal scarring, which can occur as a result of a UTI. In recent years, the use of prophylactic antibiotics has been challenged on the basis that it does not reduce the risk of recurrent UTIs or renal scarring.

A randomized, double-blind, placebo-controlled trial with trimethoprim-sulfamethoxazole was carried out in an attempt to answer the question (Hoberman et al., 2014). A total of 607 children were enrolled in the study; 302 received prophylaxis, and 305 received the trimethoprim-sulfamethoxazole. The study concluded that, among children aged 2 to 71 mo who had grade I to IV VUR, antimicrobial prophylaxis was associated with reduced risk of UTI recurrence but was not associated with a reduced risk of renal scarring.

signs of a UTI or fever. Recurrent, untreated infections place the child at high risk for renal scarring and renal damage.

Discharge instructions for children who had ureteral reimplantation to correct VUR include educating the parents on the importance of taking prophylactic antibiotics as prescribed and the use of antispasmodics for bladder spasm and pain relief. The child should avoid active play for 3 weeks postoperatively. Reinforce the need for follow-up appointments and reporting any signs of infection, such as fever, back pain, and swelling or redness at the surgical site.

Renal Disorders

Alteration in renal function can be caused by a number of acquired disorders. Bacterial infections and autoimmune dysfunction can lead to renal insufficiency. Obstructive disorders such as VUR can lead to renal dysfunction. Untreated disorders can ultimately lead to renal failure. Sometimes, even when treated appropriately, children develop acute or chronic renal failure.

Hydronephrosis

Hydronephrosis occurs when the pelvis and calyces of the kidney become dilated because urine cannot drain from the kidney (Fig. 24.7). Hydronephrosis can occur as a congenital defect, as a result of obstructive uropathy, or secondary to VUR.

Etiology and Pathophysiology

Anatomical abnormalities such as urethral strictures and stenosis at the ureterovesical or ureteropelvic junction account for the majority of cases of hydronephrosis in children. Risk factors for congenital hydronephrosis include maternal

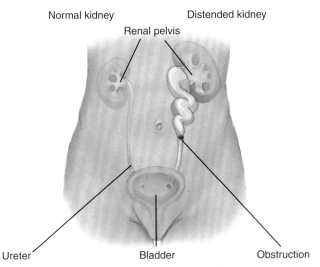

Figure 24.7. Hydronephrosis. Note that the ureter and kidney are dilated. Reprinted with permission from Kyle, T., & Carman, S. (2016). *Essentials of pediatric nursing* (3rd ed., Fig. 21.4). Philadelphia, PA: Wolters Kluwer.

oligohydramnios or polyhydramnios and elevated levels of serum alpha-fetoprotein.

Clinical Presentation

Children with hydronephrosis may be asymptomatic in the early stages. In infants and young children, a mass may be palpated on the affected side. Abdominal pain, flank pain, and hematuria can also be present. Recurrent UTI and pyelonephritis may be present in children with hydronephrosis. Children who develop renal insufficiency as a result of hydronephrosis may present with failure to thrive, vomiting, diarrhea, and other nonspecific signs and symptoms (Elder, 2016).

Assessment and Diagnosis

Assessment of a child with suspected hydronephrosis includes obtaining information regarding the present illness, chief complaints, and ultrasound findings in utero. Assess for signs of failure to thrive, including parent reports of difficulty feeding, failure to gain weight, irritability, not meeting growth and development milestones, and sleepiness. Assess for hematuria and signs of a UTI. Palpate the abdomen for enlarged kidneys or a distended bladder. Assess and monitor blood pressure.

Congenital hydronephrosis may be diagnosed during a prenatal ultrasound. Other imaging studies, such as a renal ultrasound, contrast VCUG, or an IV pyelogram, may be used to diagnose hydronephrosis.

Therapeutic Interventions

Treatment of the underlying cause of hydronephrosis is essential to prevent long-term complications such as renal insufficiency, hypertension, and renal failure. When hydronephrosis is caused by an acute obstruction, a urinary catheter is placed to promote drainage and relieve pressure in the kidneys. Surgical interventions vary depending on the location and type of obstruction. A **pyeloplasty** (removal of an obstructed segment of the ureter with reimplantation in the renal pelvis) and valve repair or reconstruction of the tract are common surgical interventions.

Evaluation

Expected outcomes for a child with hydronephrosis include the following:

- The child remains free of signs of UTI.
- The child remains free of complications such as renal insufficiency or renal failure.

Discharge Planning and Teaching

Children with hydronephrosis are at risk for complications such as UTI and sepsis. Teach parents the signs and symptoms of UTI and infections. Parents should observe for adequate urine output and adequate daily intake of fluids. Reinforce the importance of meticulous care of the perineal area. Encourage parents to keep appointments with the pediatric urologist or nephrologist, because long-term care may be necessary.

Nephrotic Syndrome

Nephrotic syndrome is a group of symptoms that indicate kidney damage and results in too much protein from the body in the urine. Causes of nephrotic syndrome can be congenital, primary (the most common type), or secondary. Congenital nephrotic syndrome is rare and affects infants in the first 3 months of life. Primary nephrotic syndrome begins in the kidneys and affects only the kidneys. Secondary nephrotic syndrome is caused by other diseases.

Etiology and Pathophysiology

Nephrotic syndrome occurs as a result of increased glomerular basement membrane permeability. Increased glomerular permeability results in larger plasma proteins passing through the glomerular basement membrane, resulting in an excess loss of protein (albumin) in the urine and decreased albumin in the bloodstream. Proteins lost in nephrotic syndrome and found in the urine tend to be exclusively albumin in nephrotic syndrome. Hypoalbuminemia (decreased albumin in the bloodstream) results in a change in osmotic pressure that allows fluid to shift from the bloodstream into the interstitial tissues. Edema results from this fluid shift. As fluid shifts to the interstitial tissues, there is a decrease in blood volume in the vascular space. Decreased blood volume triggers the kidneys to conserve sodium and water, resulting in an even further increase in edema. The loss of proteins in the bloodstream triggers the liver to increase production of lipoproteins, leading to hyperlipidemia. Hyperlipidemia results because the kidneys are unable to excrete excess lipids via urine. Immunoglobulins are lost in the urine, leaving the child potentially immunosuppressed and less able to fight infections. Figure 24.8 depicts the pathophysiology of nephrotic syndrome.

Congenital nephrotic syndrome, also referred to as infantile nephrotic syndrome, is caused by an inherited genetic defect. Secondary nephrotic syndrome results from a disease, medications, or toxins that alter kidney function. Common diseases that can cause secondary nephrotic syndrome include diabetes, systemic lupus erythematosus, hepatitis, malaria, and human immunodeficiency virus. Henoch–Schönlein purpura, a disease in which small blood vessels become inflamed and leak, can also cause nephrotic syndrome. Medications such as ibuprofen, aspirin, and other nonsteroidal anti-inflammatory drugs can cause nephrotic syndrome.

Primary nephrotic syndrome, referred to as idiopathic, manifests in three ways: minimal change disease, focal segmental glomerulosclerosis, and membranoproliferative glomerulonephritis. Minimal change disease, the most common type of idiopathic nephrotic syndrome, involves damage to the glomeruli that can only be seen with an electron microscope. Minimal change disease accounts for approximately 85% of cases of nephrotic syndrome (Niaudet & Boyer, 2016). Focal segmental glomerulosclerosis is scarring of the parts of individual glomeruli. Membranoproliferative glomerulonephritis occurs when antibodies build up in the glomeruli, causing thickening and damage. Minimal change disease is the focus of this discussion.

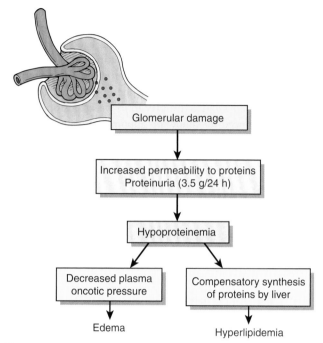

Figure 24.8. Pathophysiology of nephrotic syndrome. Loss of proteins results in decreased osmotic pressure, leading to edema and an increase in synthesis of proteins by the liver, leading to hyperlipidemia. Reprinted with permission from Grossman, S., & Porth, C. M. (2013). *Porth's pathophysiology* (9th ed., Fig. 41.14). Philadelphia, PA: Wolters Kluwer.

Clinical Presentation

A child with nephrotic syndrome typically presents with generalized edema. Parents often do not seek medical treatment until the edema is noticeable. Classically, edema develops over a period of several weeks. Parents report swollen eyes and face when the child awakens that resolves during the day as the fluid shifts to the abdomen and lower extremities (Fig. 24.9). Parents report that the child's clothing has been fitting snugly and shoes tightly, particularly in the afternoon and evening, as edema shifts. Parents note pallor, irritability, malaise, and anorexia. Urine output may be decreased and may appear frothy or foamy. In cases of severe fluid overload, respiratory distress may be present related to the development of a pleural effusion.

Assessment and Diagnosis

Assessment of the child with suspected nephrotic syndrome includes inspecting for the presence of edema, assessing the skin, obtaining measurements of height, weight, and vital signs, and noting respiratory changes. Edema can be periorbital, generalized, or abdominal (ascites). Progression of this disease results in **anasarca** or massive edema. Inspect the skin for pallor, shiny or tight appearance, and breakdown due to severe edema. Document the child's height and weight and compare them with recent values. Blood pressure may be normal, decreased, or, if renal failure is present, increased. Assessment of the respiratory system may reveal tachypnea, increased work of breathing,

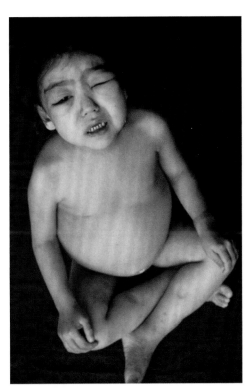

Figure 24.9. Edema resulting from nephrotic syndrome.
In children with nephrotic syndrome, periorbital and facial edema is present, particularly on rising in the morning. Note, too, the distended abdomen and pitting edema in the legs of this child. Reprinted with permission from Salimpour, R. R., Salimpour, P., & Salimpour, P. (2013). *Photographic atlas of pediatric disorders and diagnosis* (1st ed., unnumbered figure). Philadelphia, PA: Wolters Kluwer.

and decreased breath sounds in the lower lobes, suggesting a pleural effusion is present.

Diagnosis is made on the basis of history, symptoms, and laboratory findings. A urinalysis reveals marked proteinuria (3+ to 4+ proteins) and, in some cases, mild hematuria. Serum albumin levels reveal hypoalbuminemia (albumin < 2.5 g/dL) and low serum protein levels. Serum cholesterol and triglyceride levels are elevated. As nephrotic syndrome progresses, BUN and creatinine levels become elevated. A renal ultrasound is performed to check for structural abnormalities that could cause nephrotic syndrome. A renal biopsy may be performed to assess for renal failure and other causes of nephrotic syndrome.

Therapeutic Interventions

Treatment of nephrotic syndrome may be outpatient, or, if severe edema or an infection is present, inpatient. Therapeutic interventions focus on reducing edema, decreasing proteinuria, managing symptoms, improving nutrition, and preventing complications such as infection.

Medications used in the treatment of nephrotic syndrome include corticosteroids, immunosuppressants, diuretics, and antihypertensives (The Pharmacy 24.2). Corticosteroids are the primary treatment for nephrotic syndrome. Approximately

85% to 90% of children with nephrotic syndrome go into remission with an 8-week course of treatment with corticosteroids (Larkins, Kim, Craig, & Hodson, 2015). Corticosteroids have reduced the mortality rate of nephrotic syndrome to about 3% (Hahn, Hodson, Willis, & Craig, 2015). If corticosteroids are not effective, cytotoxic agents such as cyclophosphamide may be used to stimulate remission. Diuretics, furosemide, for example, are prescribed to promote diuresis. IV albumin may be prescribed for children with severe hypoalbuminemia. Immunosuppressants such as cyclosporine and tacrolimus are used in cases of nephrotic syndrome that do not respond to corticosteroids. In children with hypertension related to nephrotic syndrome, angiotensin-converting enzyme inhibitors such as enalapril may be prescribed to treat hypertension and reduce further kidney damage.

Nursing care for the child with nephrotic syndrome focuses on medication administration, supportive care, and prevention of complications. Goals for nursing management include promoting adequate nutrition, preventing infection, and promoting diuresis. Administering prescribed medications at the scheduled time is essential to maintaining adequate drug levels in the body, particularly for patients receiving immunosuppressant therapy. Closely monitor for side effects of corticosteroids, such as increased appetite, moon face, increased hair growth, abdominal distention, and mood swings. Corticosteroids can also cause adverse effects such as hypertension and hyperglycemia. Routine monitoring of blood pressure and fasting blood glucose levels are often necessary during corticosteroid therapy. When diuretics have been prescribed, monitor urine output, heart rate, and blood pressure to assess for hypovolemia from excessive fluid shifts. Monitor for signs of hypokalemia, an adverse effect of loop diuretics, and administer potassium supplements as ordered. Weigh the patient daily. Assess for resolution of edema. Oral fluid restriction may be necessary during the acute phase of nephrotic syndrome.

Supportive care includes promoting rest, providing emotional support, and helping the child to meet nutritional and fluid needs. Adequate rest is essential for healing. Encourage quiet play, such as coloring, reading, watching movies, and playing board games. Adjust the child's daily schedule depending on the amount of fatigue the child has. Signs of fatigue include irritability and withdrawal. Limit visitors when necessary and promote a quiet environment. Provide emotional support for children and parents. Parents may be overwhelmed in coping with a child who has a chronic disease and requires hospitalization, particularly if frequent relapses occur. Promote the child's independence by offering choices when possible, such as allowing the child to select food and drinks for meals and activities for the day. Fluids are not usually restricted for children with nephrotic syndrome unless severe edema or renal failure is present. Body image disturbance may be present because of weight gain and edema. See nursing care for the child with renal disorders.

Preventing complications such as infection and skin breakdown are priorities in the nursing care of the child with nephrotic syndrome. Loss of immunoglobulins in the urine and

The Pharmacy 24.2 Medications Used to Treat Nephrotic Syndrome

Medication	Classification	Route	Action	Nursing Considerations
Prednisone, methylprednisolone	Corticosteroids	• PO • IV	Suppresses inflammation and normal immune response	Monitor: • Blood pressure for increases • Weight with long-term use • Electrolytes • Serum glucose • Growth with long-term use • Signs and symptoms of infection with long-term use
Cyclophosphamide	Alkylating agent	• PO • IV	• Prevents cell division by cross-linking DNA strands and decreasing DNA synthesis • Immunosuppressant activity	Monitor: • For nausea and vomiting • For hemorrhagic cystitis • CBC • Platelet count • BUN
Cyclosporine, tacrolimus, mycophenolate	Immunosuppressants	• PO • IV	Decreases immunological response, decreasing the glomerular filtration rate and affecting the permeability of the glomerular basement membrane to albumin	Monitor: • For hypertension, nausea, vomiting, and abdominal discomfort • Renal function • Hepatic function • For gingival hyperplasia; encourage regular dental exams • Serum drug levels to avoid toxic effects of elevated drug levels • Patient instructions: take at the same time each day • Avoid grapefruit juice
Furosemide	Loop diuretic	• PO • IV	Inhibits reabsorption of sodium and chloride from the proximal and distal tubules and ascending loop of Henle, resulting in sodium-rich diuresis	Monitor: • Urine output following administration • Potassium levels (patient may require potassium replacement) • Weight, daily • For orthostatic hypotension
Enalapril	Angiotensin-converting enzyme inhibitor	PO	Blocks the conversion of angiotensin I to angiotensin II, which decreases blood pressure, decreases aldosterone secretion, slightly increases potassium, and causes sodium and fluid loss	• Monitor blood pressure for hypotension. • Medication may interact with OTC medications; have the patient check with provider before taking any OTC medications. • Adverse effects include cough, nausea, diarrhea, headache, and dizziness.

From Lexicomp. *Pediatric & Neonatal Dosage Handbook* (25th ed.), 2018.
BUN, blood urea nitrogen; CBC, complete blood count; IV, intravenous; OTC, over-the-counter; PO, by mouth.

the administration of corticosteroids place the child at increased risk of infection. Signs of infection may be masked by corticosteroid therapy. Monitor vital signs for early detection of infection. Encourage the family to limit the child's social contacts, including visitors at the hospital and at home, to avoid exposure to individuals with respiratory illnesses and communicable diseases. Monitor the child's white blood cell count as ordered when cytotoxic medications are prescribed. Cytotoxic medications such as cyclophosphamide may cause bone marrow suppression. Skin breakdown can occur as a result of massive edema and decreased skin integrity related to corticosteroid administration. Skin breakdown increases the risk of infection. Ensure that the child is turned or repositioned frequently and keep the skin clean and dry. Use therapeutic mattresses such as low–air loss mattresses or alternating pressure air mattresses to reduce the risk of skin breakdown.

Evaluation

Expected outcomes for a child with nephrotic syndrome include the following:
- Fluid and electrolyte balance is restored and maintained.
- Dietary guidelines are followed and nutritional requirements are met.
- Skin remains intact.

Discharge Planning and Teaching

A child may not be able to return to school immediately following discharge from the hospital. Assist parents in locating resources for tutoring and establishing a plan for the child to return to school. Teach parents the importance of avoiding exposing their child to sick contacts and taking precautions to protect the child with decreased immunity. Educate parents on the importance of avoiding taking their child to malls, sporting arenas, grocery stores, and other public areas where the risk of infection is increased. Reinforce the need for a no-salt-added diet while the child is symptomatic or is on corticosteroid therapy. Review the side effects of corticosteroids, including the potential for increased appetite and weight gain. Stress the need to control the child's caloric intake to prevent excessive weight gain.

Explain to parents the potential for relapses. Many children who initially achieve remission with corticosteroid therapy relapse and require repeated courses of corticosteroids. Children who receive repeated treatment for multiple relapses should have periodic bone density tests, because corticosteroids can weaken bones and lead to osteoporosis.

Acute Poststreptococcal Glomerulonephritis

Acute **glomerulonephritis** describes the pathological process characterized by inflammation and cellular proliferation of the glomeruli not caused by a direct infection of the kidneys (VanDeVoorde, 2015). There are numerous causes of glomerulonephritis. For the purposes of this discussion, acute poststreptococcal glomerulonephritis, the most common glomerulonephritis in children worldwide, is the focus.

Etiology and Pathophysiology

Poststreptococcal glomerulonephritis occurs following exposure to group A beta-hemolytic Streptococcus (GAS). The exact GAS antigens that form the immune complexes that are known to induce the pathological changes of poststreptococcal glomerulonephritis are not known. Also unclear is the mechanism of immune complex injury to the glomeruli. However, there is a common pathway of inflammatory response in the glomerulus that results in the clinical manifestations of acute poststreptococcal glomerulonephritis (Fig. 24.10). The presence of immune complexes leads to complement deposition, infiltration of leukocytes, and proliferation of the structural mesangial cells of the glomerulus (VanDeVoorde, 2015). Capillary perfusion becomes impaired as a result, reducing glomerular filtration. This causes water and sodium retention, leading to an increase in extracellular fluid volume and fluid overload. In addition, there is accumulation of potassium, urea, and organic acids, all byproducts of metabolism and normally filtered in the urine.

Poststreptococcal glomerulonephritis typically affects children 4 to 12 years old. The latency period after a group A streptococcal infection varies from 1 to 2 weeks after pharyngitis to

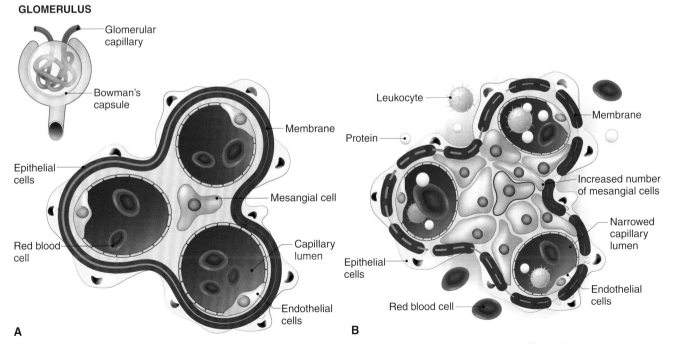

GLOMERULUS

A

B

Figure 24.10. Pathophysiology of glomerulonephritis. A. A normal glomerulus. **B.** A glomerulus affected by poststreptococcal glomerulonephritis.

3 to 6 weeks after a skin infection (VanDeVoorde, 2015). More than 450,000 cases of glomerulonephritis occur annually, with most in children in developing countries where skin infections such as impetigo are common (VanDeVoorde, 2015). However, poststreptococcal glomerulonephritis is the most common glomerulonephritis in children in the United States.

Clinical Presentation

Commonly, children present with the classic triad of glomerulonephritis: gross hematuria, edema, and hypertension (VanDeVoorde, 2015). Children may present with increased work of breathing or a cough related to cardiopulmonary congestion. Blood pressure is elevated for age. In a child presenting with acute hypertension, headache, irritability, lethargy, and seizures indicate acute encephalopathy related to high blood pressure. Generalized edema is present. Urine appears bloody and dark. Other common signs and symptoms of acute poststreptococcal glomerulonephritis include fever, lethargy, headache, decreased urine output, and abdominal symptoms such as abdominal pain, vomiting, and anorexia.

Assessment and Diagnosis

Assessment of the child with suspected glomerulonephritis includes a review of recent illnesses, particularly for pharyngitis (sore throat) or strep throat. Assess the child's respiratory status, noting tachypnea, increased work of breathing, and crackles on auscultation, indicating fluid overload. Assess for edema, which may be mild. The cause of the edema is from excessive fluid and sodium retention, not massive protein losses. Therefore, ascites is not usually present. Obtain a blood pressure reading and note elevation for age and sex. Hypertension also results from excessive fluid and salt retention. A gallop may be heard when assessing heart sounds, indicating possible fluid overload. Assessment of urine reveals hematuria, and urine may appear tea-colored, cola-colored, or a dirty green color.

Laboratory tests conducted in the diagnostic workup for glomerulonephritis include urinalysis, serum BUN and creatinine levels, a complete blood count, serum protein levels, serum complement levels, and erythrocyte sedimentation rate. Positive results include evidence of proteinuria and hematuria on urinalysis, normal or elevated BUN and creatinine levels, elevated white blood cell count, and elevated erythrocyte sedimentation rate, indicating inflammation or infection. Hemoglobin and hematocrit levels may reveal anemia in the acute phase of glomerulonephritis because extracellular fluid is diluting the serum. Serum complement levels, particularly C3, may be decreased, indicating a recent infection. An antistreptolysin (ASO) titer and DNAse B antigen titer are also obtained. If *Streptococcus* is the causative agent leading to glomerulonephritis, laboratory values will reveal elevated ASO and DNAse B antigen titers.

Therapeutic Interventions

There is no specific treatment for glomerulonephritis. Therapeutic interventions are aimed at managing hypertension and maintaining fluid volume. If a current streptococcal infection is present, antibiotic therapy is initiated.

Nursing care includes monitoring fluid status, promoting rest, preventing skin breakdown, preventing infection, meeting nutritional requirements, and providing emotional support to the child and family. Bed rest is required during the acute phase of glomerulonephritis. Because of edema and prolonged bed rest, there is increased potential for skin breakdown in dependent areas and other pressure areas. Medications specific to symptoms such as hypertension are administered.

Evaluation

Expected outcomes for a child with glomerulonephritis include the following:

- Fluid and electrolyte balance is restored and maintained.
- Skin remains intact throughout illness.
- The child maintains preillness body weight and consumes enough calories to maintain nutritional status.
- The child's kidney function returns to baseline.

Discharge Planning and Teaching

Children with glomerulonephritis are hospitalized for several days to a week, depending on the severity of symptoms. Children are often discharged before complete resolution of the disorder. It may take up to 3 weeks for hematuria and hypertension to resolve and even longer for the complete resolution of glomerulonephritis. Discharge planning includes teaching parents about medication administration (including side effects), signs and symptoms of complications, and dietary restrictions and requirements. Teach parents the proper way to take the child's blood pressure and when to report elevations in blood pressure to the provider. Teach parents how to assess urine for blood and protein if ordered. Instruct the parents and child to avoid sick contacts, including those with mild respiratory symptoms. Rest is essential for healing. Assist parents in developing a plan for adequate rest and return to daily activities, including school and extracurricular activities.

Hemolytic Uremic Syndrome

HUS is a thrombotic microangiopathy that is characterized by thrombocytopenia, hemolytic anemia, and acute renal failure. HUS is one of the main causes of acute kidney injury (AKI) in children. HUS is broadly classified as typical (after diarrhea or diarrhea positive) and atypical. Typical HUS is usually preceded by an episode of diarrhea and mainly caused by Shiga toxins or verotoxins. Atypical HUS is familial or sporadic and is caused by a dysregulation of the alternative complement pathway. Typical HUS is discussed in this text.

Etiology and Pathophysiology

The majority of cases of HUS, approximately 60%, are caused by a verotoxin-producing strain of *E. coli*, O157:H7 (Picard et al., 2015). *Streptococcus pneumoniae, Shigella dysenteriae,* and other types of bacteria may also cause HUS. Shiga-like toxin producing bacteria are transmitted by contaminated food and water. *E. coli* O157:H7 is commonly found in undercooked meat (usually beef) and unpasteurized milk and apple cider (Van Why & Avner, 2016). Other modes of transmission include cross-contamination of foods from unwashed cutting boards, petting zoos, swimming in contaminated pools, lakes, or ponds, and contaminated vegetables such as lettuce, bean sprouts, and raw spinach (Van Why & Avner, 2016).

Following ingestion of contaminated food, the bacteria colonize in the colon and adhere to the enterocyte brush border. The bacteria release toxins called Shiga toxins or verotoxins that damage the intestinal wall, already harmed by *E. coli* colonization. Both Shiga toxin and verotoxin damage the endothelial cell walls. In the kidney, capillary and arteriolar endothelial damage leads to localized thrombosis in the glomeruli, causing a significant decrease in the glomerular filtration rate. Damage to the glomeruli also causes increased glomerular permeability. Shiga toxin also directly activates platelet to promote their aggregation, particularly in areas of microvascular injury, leading to thrombocytopenia (Van Why & Avner, 2016).

HUS occurs most often in preschool- and school-age children, primarily affecting children younger than age 5 years, but can occur at any age. In the United States, the annual incidence of HUS resulting from Shiga toxin–producing *E. coli* is approximately two to three cases per 100,000 children.

Clinical Presentation

A child with typical HUS presents with sudden onset of pallor, irritability, weakness, and lethargy following a case of gastroenteritis, respiratory tract infection, or a UTI. The preemptive gastroenteritis is described by parents as the child having abdominal pain, fever, vomiting, and diarrhea that may have been bloody. Parents report the diarrhea lasting up to 7 days. The child also presents with vomiting, abdominal pain, anorexia, mild jaundice, and edema or ascites (Van Why & Avner, 2016).

Assessment and Diagnosis

Assessment of the child with HUS begins with a thorough history for recent exposure to possible contaminated food or water. Determine whether risk factors such as ingestion of ground beef or a recent visit to a pool, water park, or petting zoo are present. Assessment of the urine and urine output may reveal oliguria or anuria and the presence of blood. Overall general appearance of the child may reveal pallor, edema, or a toxic appearance. Assess the abdomen for pain, discomfort, and possible ascites. Obtain a full set of vital signs. If dehydration is present as a result of recent diarrhea, vomiting, decreased intake, or fluid shifts, tachycardia and hypotension may be present.

Diagnosis of HUS is based on the presence of the classic triad of microangiopathic hemolytic anemia, thrombocytopenia, and AKI. Laboratory tests are needed to confirm these symptoms. Laboratory results indicate microangiopathic anemia (hemoglobin < 10 g/dL) and a low platelet count. Platelets are rapidly consumed in thrombi that are formed during HUS.

High serum levels of lactate dehydrogenase (LDH) are noted. Elevated LDH levels reflect diffuse tissue ischemia and damage. Elevated serum creatinine levels, low glomerular filtration rates, microscopic hematuria, and proteinuria are present in HUS, indicating kidney involvement.

Therapeutic Interventions

There is no specific treatment for HUS. Symptomatic treatment and care are provided to prevent complications from renal failure. Care of the child with HUS is the same as care for the child in acute renal failure. See the section Renal Failure for care.

Evaluation

Expected outcomes for a child with HUS include the following:

- Hydration is restored and fluid balance is maintained.
- Electrolyte balance is restored and maintained.
- The child's kidney function returns to baseline.

Discharge Planning and Teaching

Discharge teaching focuses on teaching parents about medications, diet, and fluid restrictions and how to reduce the risk of HUS. Medications, diet, and fluid restrictions are the same as in acute renal failure. Ways to reduce the risk of HUS include avoiding contaminated beef, washing hands thoroughly after handling raw or undercooked beef, and ensuring that raw meat does not come into contact with cooked beef. Teach parents to use separate utensils when preparing raw beef and serving cooked beef to avoid contamination. Encourage them to use separate cutting boards or to thoroughly wash and dry a single cutting board when preparing raw vegetables and beef at the same time. Encourage the use of meat thermometers to ensure that beef has reached the appropriate temperature to kill bacteria before serving.

Renal Failure

Renal failure occurs when the kidneys are unable to concentrate urine and adequately excrete waste products. Renal failure can be acute or chronic and has multiple etiologies. Acute renal failure develops over days to weeks and may be reversible. Chronic renal failure develops gradually over months to years and is permanent, resulting in lifelong dialysis or the need for a kidney transplant.

Etiology and Pathophysiology

Both acute and chronic renal failure are characterized by **azotemia**, accumulation of nitrogenous wastes in the blood, and, often, oliguria. In renal failure, the kidney is unable to excrete metabolic waste products, which consequently build up to toxic levels and can lead to death if untreated.

Acute kidney injury (AKI) is the current term used to describe acute renal failure. AKI is a clinical syndrome characterized by sudden onset in which rapid deterioration of kidney function results in the inability of the kidneys to rid the body of waste products and maintain fluid and electrolyte balance (Sreedharan & Avener, 2016). AKI can be caused by prerenal, intrinsic (actual kidney damage), or postrenal factors. Prerenal AKI, the most common type of AKI in infants and young children, is the result of decreased circulating arterial volume, which leads to decreased perfusion to the kidney and an inadequate glomerular filtration rate. Hypovolemia secondary to dehydration, hemorrhage, or sepsis is a common cause of prerenal failure in children. Intrinsic AKI results from primary damage to the kidney structures from inflammation, toxins, drugs, infection, or decreased blood supply. Glomerulonephritis, HUS, and acute tubular necrosis are common causes of intrinsic AKI. Postrenal AKI results from obstruction of the urinary tract. Conditions that can lead to postrenal AKI include neurogenic bladder, urolithiasis, and tumors that obstruct the outflow of urine. In infants, congenital conditions such as posterior urethral valves account for the majority of cases of AKI (Sreedharan & Avener, 2016).

Chronic kidney disease (CKD; chronic renal failure) is present if at least one of the following criteria is met (Levey et al., 2002):

1. Kidney damage for greater than 3 months as defined by structural or functional abnormalities of the kidney with or without a decrease in glomerular filtration rate, manifested by one or more of the following features:
   a. Abnormalities in the composition of the blood or urine.
   b. Abnormalities in imaging test findings.
   c. Abnormalities in kidney biopsy findings.
2. Glomerular filtration rate less than 60 mL/min/1.73 m^2 for greater than or equal to 3 months, with or without the other signs of kidney damage described earlier.

CKD is staged I through V on the basis of the glomerular filtration rate. Stages II through V have progressively lower glomerular filtration rates. Children with stage I CKD have a normal or increased glomerular filtration rate (>90 mL/min/1.73 m^2), whereas children with stage V CKD have a glomerular filtration rate less than 15 mL/min/1.73 m^2 or are on dialysis. CKD may result from congenital, acquired, inherited, or metabolic kidney disease. In children younger than age 5 years, CKD is most commonly the result of renal hypoplasia, dysplasia, or obstructive uropathy (Sreedharan & Avener, 2016). In children older than 5 years, acquired diseases such as glomerulonephritis and inherited disorders are the predominant causes of CKD.

AKI is seen in 2% to 3% of children admitted to pediatric tertiary care centers and up to 8% of infants admitted to neonatal intensive care units (Sreedharan & Avener, 2016). CKD affects approximately 18 in 1 million children (Sreedharan & Avener, 2016).

Clinical Presentation

Children with AKI present with a sudden onset of symptoms, whereas children with CKD present with a gradual onset of symptoms (Box 24.5). The symptoms are a result of electrolyte imbalances, uremia, and imbalanced fluid status. Hyponatremia affects the central nervous system and can cause symptoms such as headache, fatigue, and lethargy. Fluid overload can

---

Box 24.5 Clinical Presentation: Acute vs. Chronic Renal Failure

Acute Renal Failure
- Urine: dark or gross hematuria, oliguria
- Neurological: headache, fatigue, lethargy, confusion
- Respiratory: crackles, increased work of breathing
- Cardiovascular: pallor, gallop heart sounds, hypertension or hypotension (depending on cause of renal failure)
- Gastrointestinal: nausea, vomiting

Chronic Renal Failure
- Urine: oliguria or anuria
- Neurological: fatigue, malaise, headache, decreased mental alertness or inability to concentrate
- Cardiovascular: hypertension, edema, chronic anemia
- Gastrointestinal: poor appetite, nausea, vomiting
- Musculoskeletal: short stature, fractures with minimal trauma, rickets
- Growth and development: failure to thrive

---

cause respiratory compromise, resulting in the child presenting with increased work of breathing and crackles on auscultation of the lungs. The child appears pale and may be nauseated and vomit. Urine output is decreased, and urine may be dark in color.

Children with CKD appear with symptoms similar to those of children with AKI but may also have musculoskeletal symptoms such as short stature and a history of bone fractures. Urine output may be absent (**anuria**).

Assessment and Diagnosis

Assessment of the child with renal failure includes obtaining a thorough history to assess for risk factors such as a history of vomiting or diarrhea, recent pharyngitis, recent exposure to nephrotoxic drugs, shock, trauma, and urological abnormalities such as congenital hydronephrosis. Assess for signs indicating altered volume status, whether hypovolemia or hypervolemia. Signs of hypovolemia include tachycardia, hypotension, poor skin turgor, dry mucous membranes, and poor peripheral circulation. Signs of hypervolemia include hypertension, gallop or murmur, peripheral edema, and crackles when auscultating the lungs. Assess the child's abdomen and flank for signs of masses. Clinical manifestations of imbalanced electrolytes may be present during the assessment (Table 24.3).

Diagnosis of renal failure is based on blood chemistry results and a urinalysis. Positive chemistry results include hyperkalemia, hyperphosphatemia, increased BUN and creatinine levels, and hypocalcemia. A urinalysis may reveal hematuria, proteinuria, infection, altered specific gravity and osmolarity, and acidic urine. Imaging studies such as ultrasound and computed tomography are used to assess the kidney structure, renal blood flow, renal perfusion, and overall function. A kidney biopsy may be performed to examine the glomeruli, identify the specific

Table 24.3 Electrolyte Imbalances in Acute and Chronic Renal Failure

Electrolyte Imbalance	Cause	Clinical Manifestations	Therapeutic Interventions
Hyperkalemia	• Inability to adequately excrete potassium • In metabolic acidosis, potassium moves from intracellular to extracellular fluid (increasing serum levels)	• Muscle weakness • Peaked T waves • Widening of QRS • Dysrhythmias	• Eliminate potassium intake • Administer polystyrene sulfonate (PO or rectally) • Administer chloride or calcium gluconate IV • Administer dextrose and insulin IV • Administer sodium bicarbonate • Dialysis, if other methods are not effective
Hyponatremia	Accumulation of fluid (kidneys cannot excrete adequate amounts of fluid in the oliguric or anuric phase)	• Muscle cramps • Nausea and vomiting • Headache • Confusion • Fatigue, drowsiness • Loss of consciousness • Seizures	• Restrict fluids • Replace sodium • Hypertonic saline (sodium < 120 mEq/L or seizures are present) • Dialysis
Hypocalcemia	• Phosphate binds calcium, and hyperphosphatemia depresses serum calcium concentrations. • Calcium is deposited in the bone and extraskeletal tissue.	• Tetany • Muscle cramping • Muscle tingling • Muscle twitching or stiffness • Positive Chvostek sign	• Oral phosphate binders • Low-phosphorus diet • Calcium gluconate or calcium chloride IV if tetany is present • Dialysis
Hyperphosphatemia	Normally kidneys remove phosphate from the blood and it is excreted in the urine. Renal failure results in the inability to remove phosphorus from the body.	Manifestations result from the effects of hypocalcemia. See hypocalcemia CNS symptoms: altered mental status, delirium, obtundation, coma, seizures, paresthesias	Same as for hypocalcemia

CNS, central nervous system; IV, intravenous; PO, by mouth.

disease process, and determine the amount of damage that has occurred and whether it is reversible.

Therapeutic Interventions

Treatment of AKI depends on the underlying cause. Therapeutic interventions are geared toward minimizing or preventing further renal damage while maintaining homeostasis and fluid and electrolyte balance. Monitor blood pressure and administer antihypertensives as prescribed. Maintain strict intake and output and monitor urine specific gravity as ordered. Monitor for hypotension when administering diuretics and when urine output is restored, because diuresis and fluid loss may be significant. Monitor serum electrolyte levels as ordered and assess for clinical manifestations of imbalances such as hyperkalemia and hypocalcemia.

Treatment of CKD focuses on slowing the progression of kidney disease, replacing absent or diminished kidney function, preventing complications, and promoting growth and development. CKD is irreversible and may result in the need for permanent dialysis. The method of dialysis (peritoneal dialysis, hemodialysis, or continuous renal replacement therapy, CRRT) is selected on the basis of the child's age and hemodynamic stability. Eighty-eight percent of children younger than age 5 years are treated with peritoneal dialysis, whereas 54% of children older than 12 years are treated with hemodialysis (Sreedharan & Avner, 2016). CRRT is reserved for children who are hemodynamically unstable and in the intensive care unit.

Nursing care of the child with AKI is focused on preventing complications, achieving and maintaining fluid and electrolyte balance, preventing infection, and administering medications. Provide emotional support for the child and family during treatment for AKI. Help minimize or prevent complications such as further kidney damage, altered electrolyte levels, and fluid overload by encouraging the parents and child to comply with the treatment regimen. Educate the parents and child regarding the importance of following fluid requirements and dietary restrictions, such as sodium, potassium, and phosphorus restrictions, to prevent electrolyte disturbances. Nephrotoxic drugs are avoided to prevent further kidney damage (Priority Care Concepts 24.2).

During AKI, the kidney's ability to excrete drugs is impaired. Be aware of medications that may need dosing adjustments for renal impairment. Monitor drug levels as ordered to prevent toxicity, particularly if kidney function is rapidly deteriorating. Familiarize yourself with the signs of toxicity for drugs that the child is prescribed that are normally cleared by the kidneys. Report signs of toxicity to the provider immediately.

During AKI, the child has high metabolic demands and may be at risk for malnutrition. Recommended caloric intake should be specific to each child based on metabolic demand, age, height, and weight. Collaborate with a dietician to assist the child and family with making menu choices that meet carbohydrate, fat, protein, and caloric needs. The child may need parenteral nutrition or enteral feedings for a short time while recovering from AKI.

Both children with AKI and those with CKD are at high risk for infection. Compromised immunity, altered nutritional status, and numerous invasive procedures such as central line placement put the child at increased risk for hospital-acquired infections. See the section Prevent Infection, within the larger section General Nursing Interventions for Genitourinary Disorders, earlier, for ways to prevent infection.

Nursing care of the child with CKD is focused on promoting fluid and electrolyte balance, assisting the child to achieve adequate and optimal nutrition, and preventing complications associated with renal dysfunction and dialysis. The child with CKD is typically on multiple medications, including vitamin replacements, vitamin D supplements, antihypertensives, and diuretics (The Pharmacy 24.3).

Children with renal disease often must have dietary restrictions and requirements. A diet low in sodium, potassium, and phosphorus is recommended. Increased calcium intake and adequate protein intake are necessary. Educate the parents and child regarding foods to avoid or eat in restricted amounts. Box 24.6 reviews foods to avoid or limit to achieve a diet low in sodium, potassium,

and phosphorus. Encourage consumption of complex carbohydrates and fruits and vegetables low in potassium. For children with CKD, oil, hard candy, sugar, honey, and jelly may be recommended to add calories to achieve adequate caloric intake.

Complications associated with CKD include adverse effects of hemodialysis, such as hypotension, a rapid shift in fluid and electrolyte levels, and disequilibrium syndrome. Assess for potential complications while the child is undergoing hemodialysis (Priority Care Concepts 24.3).

Complications of peritoneal dialysis include peritonitis, hyperglycemia, pain, leakage at the catheter site, and respiratory symptoms. Clinical manifestations of peritonitis include cloudy dialysate, abdominal pain or tenderness, fever, foul-smelling drainage, and constipation. Lessen the child's pain during inflow or outflow by slowing the rate of inflow and ensuring the volume is appropriate for the child's size. Warm the dialysate before instilling to minimize cramping caused by cold dialysate. Repositioning the patient during outflow to reduce the risk of the omentum entering the catheter can lessen pain. Respiratory symptoms such as shortness of breath and decreased breath sounds often result from abdominal fullness during the dwell time, which is the time during which the solution is in the child's abdomen during peritoneal dialysis. Assist the child to a position of comfort to reduce respiratory symptoms. Monitor the child for potential complications of peritoneal dialysis before, during, and after treatments.

Children with CKD often experience depression, anxiety, and embarrassment because they are perceived as being different from their peers. Differences include poor growth and short stature related to metabolic abnormalities, delayed pubertal onset, and delayed scholastic achievement. Children with CKD may also feel isolated from their peers as a result of missing school for appointments, illness, and dialysis. Encourage the parents to seek counseling for their child. Encourage older children to become involved in age-appropriate activities or organizations such as scouts, youth groups, or clubs.

Evaluation

Expected outcomes for a child with AKI include the following:

- The child's kidney function returns to baseline.
- The child's fluid and electrolyte balance is restored and maintained.
- The child's fluid balance is restored and maintained.
- The parents and child implement effective coping strategies throughout the illness.
- The child remains free of complications, such as infection, of AKI.

Expected outcomes for a child with CKD include the following:

- The child maintains an adequate fluid volume.
- The child's electrolyte levels are stable for the degree of CKD.
- Nutritional requirements are met while adhering to dietary restrictions.
- The child achieves growth and development milestones.
- The child maintains a positive body image.

The Pharmacy 24.3   Medications Used to Treat Chronic Renal Failure

Medication	Classification	Route	Action	Nursing Considerations
Calcitriol	Vitamin analog (vitamin D^3)	PO	Replaces calcitriol, which kidneys do not produce	• Ensure calcium supplement is provided. • Monitor calcium levels as ordered. • Do not administer with other vitamin D supplements because of increased risk of hypercalcemia.
Epoetin alfa	Antianemic	• SQ • IV	Stimulates erythropoiesis (production of red blood cells in the bone marrow)	Monitor: • Blood pressure for hypertension • Hemoglobin and hematocrit during therapy
Nephrocaps	Vitamin	PO	Replaces vitamin C, thiamine, riboflavin, niacin, vitamin B_6, folic acid, vitamin B_{12}, biotin, pantothenic acid	OTC vitamins may contain harmful elements; educate parents to only use prescribed supplements.
Calcium carbonate, calcium acetate, sevelamer hydrochloride	Phosphate binders	PO	Reduces the bioavailability of phosphate in the intestinal tract	• Take with food. • Avoid aluminum-containing phosphate binders.
Enalapril, lisinopril	Angiotensin-converting inhibitors	PO	Blocks the conversion of angiotensin I to angiotensin II, which decreases blood pressure, decreases aldosterone secretion, slightly increases potassium, and causes sodium and fluid loss	• Monitor blood pressure for hypotension. • May interact with OTC medications; have the patient check with provider before taking any OTC medications. • Adverse effects include cough, nausea, diarrhea, headache, and dizziness.
Losartan	Angiotensin II blocker	PO	Blocks the vasoconstricting and aldosterone-secreting effects of angiotensin II, thus lowering blood pressure by allowing relaxation of blood vessels	Monitor: • Blood pressure immediately before administering • For signs of hypotension: dizziness, fainting
Furosemide (Lasix)	Loop diuretic	• PO • IV	Inhibits reabsorption of sodium and chloride from the proximal and distal tubules and ascending loop of Henle, resulting in sodium-rich diuresis	Monitor: • Urine output following administration • Potassium levels (patient may require potassium replacement) • Weight, daily • For orthostatic hypotension

From Lexicomp. *Pediatric & Neonatal Dosage Handbook* (25th ed.), 2018.
IV, intravenous; OTC, over-the-counter; PO, by mouth; SQ, subcutaneous.

Box 24.6 Nutritional Information for the Child With Renal Disease

High-Sodium Foods
• Soups (especially canned soups)
• Processed lunch meat (salami, ham, bologna)
• Hot dogs
• Sauces (tomato sauce, spaghetti sauce, barbeque sauce, gravy)
• Pickles
• Smoked meats (bacon, ham, corned beef)
• Potato chips
• Seasonings

High-Potassium Foods
• Dairy products (milk, ice cream, pudding, yogurt)
• Peanuts
• Vegetables (celery, dried beans, spinach, tomatoes, potatoes, leafy greens, lima beans)
• Fruits (citrus fruits, bananas, pears, nectarines, melons, raisins, avocados, prunes, dates, figs)
• Salt substitutes (avoid those containing potassium)

High-Phosphorus Foods
• Sausage
• Hot dogs
• Chocolate
• Nuts
• Peanut butter
• Dried beans
• Peas
• Dairy products (milk, cheese, yogurt, pudding, ice cream)

Priority Care Concepts 24.3

Recognizing Sudden Complications of Hemodialysis

Children who are receiving hemodialysis are at risk for hypotension, sudden and rapid fluid and electrolyte exchange, and disequilibrium syndrome. Monitor for the signs of these complications:

- Hypotension: tachycardia, dizziness, sudden nausea and vomiting, and abdominal cramping
- Rapid change in fluid and electrolyte state: dizziness, muscle cramps or twitching, and nausea and vomiting
- Disequilibrium syndrome: blurred vision, headache, restlessness, altered level of consciousness, muscle twitching, and nausea and vomiting

Discharge Planning and Teaching

In preparation for discharge to home, parents need education regarding medication administration, proper technique for measuring blood pressure, and signs and symptoms of progressive renal failure. Reinforce the need for follow-up appointments. Ensure that parents understand how to properly administer medications, including proper dosage and timing.

Dietary counseling is often necessary before the child goes home. A dietician, in collaboration with the provider, can provide instruction on dietary needs and restrictions.

For patients with CKD, the parents and child (if older) must understand the necessity for long-term treatment and keeping follow-up appointments. Make referrals to appropriate home care nursing agencies as needed for things such as dialysis catheter care and occupational and physical therapy. Provide the family with resources for contacting school personnel who can guide the family in making arrangements for the child to return to school and attend classes around dialysis appointments or, perhaps, be homeschooled and/or tutored. Provide families with resources related to financial support and support groups within the community.

Parents of a child who will be receiving peritoneal dialysis at home need education on how to use a peritoneal dialysis automated cycler or how to perform manual peritoneal dialysis. Allow adequate time for teaching and return demonstration so that parents are comfortable with the procedure before discharge. Parents must understand the potential complications and when to report findings such as symptoms of peritonitis to the provider.

Think Critically

1. A child with a diagnosed inguinal hernia is being seen for increased irritability, vomiting, not tolerating feedings, and being inconsolable, according to the mother. What should the nurse be immediately concerned about? What interventions should the nurse anticipate?

2. A 4-year-old who recently visited a petting zoo is diagnosed with HUS. Explain to the parents how visiting a petting zoo puts the child at increased risk of HUS.

3. A teenage girl comes to the pediatrician's office complaining of difficulty urinating, urinating very frequently, and abdominal pain. The physician orders a urine dipstick test, and the findings reveal positive nitrites and positive leukocytes. Are these results of concern? Why? What would you anticipate the next orders to be?

4. Differentiate between enuresis and encopresis.

5. The parents of an infant with cryptorchidism are receiving preoperative teaching. The dad asks you what an orchiopexy is. How would you explain what happens in an orchiopexy?

6. A 10-year-old child has been diagnosed with acute poststreptococcal glomerulonephritis. The child is very edematous but does not have ascites. Explain what the underlying cause of edema in glomerulonephritis is and why ascites is not present.

7. A 20-month-old girl has had three UTIs in the past 4 month. The physician orders a VCUG and a renal ultrasound to assess for VUR. Why is it important to diagnose VUR early?

8. An 8-year-old who has been diagnosed with renal failure is being treated in the hospital for an unrelated infection. The child complains of a headache. The mother asks whether her child can have a dose of ibuprofen for his headache. What concerns do you have about administering ibuprofen to a child in renal failure?

References

Aiken, J., & Oldham, K. (2016). Inguinal hernias. In R. Kliegman, B. Stanton, J. St. Geme, N. Schor, & R. Behrman (Eds.), *Nelson textbook of pediatrics* (20th ed., pp. 1903–1909). Philadelphia, PA: Elsevier.

Apos, E., Schuster, S., Reece, J., Whitaker, S., Murphy, K., Golder, J., . . . & Gibb, S. (2017). Enuresis management in children: Retrospective clinical audit of 2861 cases treated with practitioner-assisted bell-and-pad alarm. *The Journal of Pediatrics, 193*, 211–216.

Canon, S., Mosley, B., Chipollini, J., Purifoy, J. A., & Hobbs, C. (2012). Epidemiological assessment of hypospadias by degree of severity. *The Journal of Urology, 188*(6), 2362–2366.

Drake, T., Rustom, J., & Davies, M. (2013). Phimosis in childhood. *British Medical Journal, 346*, f3678.

de Camargo, M., Henriques, C., Vieira, S., Komi, S., Leão, E., & Nogueira, P. (2014). Growth of children with end-stage renal disease undergoing daily hemodialysis. *Pediatric Nephrology, 29*(3), 439–444.

Elder, J. (2016). Bladder exstrophy. In R. Kliegman, B. Stanton, J. St. Geme, N. Schor, & R. Behrman (Eds.), *Nelson textbook of pediatrics* (20th ed., pp. 2575–2577). Philadelphia, PA: Elsevier.

Elder, J. (2016). Cryptorchidism. In R. Kliegman, B. Stanton, J. St. Geme, N. Schor, R. Behrman (Eds.), *Nelson textbook of pediatrics* (20th ed., pp. 2592–2593). Philadelphia, PA: Elsevier.

Elder, J. (2016). Hypospadias. In R. Kliegman, B. Stanton, J. St. Geme, N. Schor, & R. Behrman (Eds.), *Nelson textbook of pediatrics* (20th ed., p. 2586). Philadelphia, PA: Elsevier.

Elder, J. (2016). Obstruction of the urinary tract. In R. Kliegman, B. Stanton, J. St. Geme, N. Schor, & R. Behrman (Eds.), *Nelson textbook of pediatrics* (20th ed., pp. 2567–2575). Philadelphia, PA: Elsevier.

Elder, J. (2016). Testicular (spermatic cord) torsion. In R. Kliegman, B. Stanton, J. St. Geme, N. Schor, & Behrman, R (Eds.), *Nelson textbook of pediatrics* (20th ed., p. 2595). Philadelphia, PA: Elsevier.

Fisher, D. (2017). *Pediatric urinary tract infection: Clinical presentation.* Retrieved from: https://emedicine.medscape.com/article/969643-clinical

Flores-Mireles, A. L., Walker, J. N., Caparon, M., & Hultgren, S. J. (2015). Urinary tract infections: Epidemiology, mechanisms of infection and treatment options. *Nature Reviews Microbiology, 13*(5), 269.

Hahn, D., Hodson, E. M., Willis, N. S., & Craig, J. C. (2015). Corticosteroid therapy for nephrotic syndrome in children. *Cochrane Database Syst Rev, 3,* CD001533.

Hoberman, A., Greenfield S. P., Mattoo, T. K., Keren, R., Mathews, R., Pohl, H. G., . . . Carpenter, M. A; RIVUR Trial Investigators. (2014). Antimicrobial prophylaxis for children with vesicoureteral reflux. *New England Journal of Medicine, 370*(25), 2367–2376.

Larkins, N., Kim, S., Craig, J., & Hodson, E. (2015). Steroid-sensitive nephrotic syndrome: An evidence-based update of immunosuppressive treatment in children. *Archives of Disease in Childhood, 101*(4), 404–408.

Lemini, R., Guanà, R., Tommasoni, N., Mussa, A., Di Rosa, G., & Schleef, J. (2016). Predictivity of clinical findings and Doppler ultrasound in pediatric acute scrotum. *Urology Journal, 13*(4), 2779–2783.

Levey, A., Coresh, J., Bolton, K., Culleton, B., Harvey, K., Ikizler, T., . . . & Levin, A. (2002). K/DOQI clinical practice guidelines for chronic kidney disease: Evaluation, classification, and stratification. *American Journal of Kidney Diseases, 39*(2 suppl 1):i-ii+S1-S266.

Niaudet, P., & Boyer, O. (2016). Idiopathic nephrotic syndrome in children: Clinical aspects. *Pediatric Nephrology,* 1–52. doi:10.1007/978-3-642-27843-3_24-1

Otukesh, H., Hoseini, R., Rahimzadeh, N., & Hosseini, S. (2012). Glomerular function in neonates. *Iranian Journal of Kidney Diseases, 6*(3), 166.

Picard, C., Burtey, S., Bornet, C., Curti, C., Montana, M., & Vanelle, P. (2015). Pathophysiology and treatment of typical and atypical hemolytic uremic syndrome. *Pathologie Biologie, 63*(3), 136–143.

Ramachandra, P., Palazzi, K., Holmes, N., & Marietti, S. (2015). Factors influencing rate of testicular salvage in acute testicular torsion at a tertiary pediatric center. *Western Journal of Emergency Medicine, 16*(1), 190.

Roberts, K., Downs, S., Finnell, S., Hellerstein, S., Shortliffe, L., Wald, E., . . . & Okechukwu, K. (2016). Reaffirmation of AAP clinical practice guideline: The diagnosis and management of the initial urinary tract infection in febrile infants and young children 2–24 months of age. *Pediatrics, 138*(6). doi:10.1542/peds.2016-3026

Shaikh, N., Hoberman, A., Keren, R., Gotman, N., Docimo, S. G., Mathews, R., . . . & Carpenter, M. A. (2016). Recurrent urinary tract infections in children with bladder and bowel dysfunction. *Pediatrics, 137*(1), e20152982.

Sood, A., Penna, F., Eleswarapu, S., Pucheril, D., Weaver, J., Wagner, J., . . . & Elder, J. (2015). Incidence, admission rates, and economic burden of pediatric emergency department visits for urinary tract infection: Data from the nationwide emergency department sample, 2006 to 2011. *Journal of Pediatric Urology, 11*(5), 246.e1–246.e8.

Sreedharan, R., & Avener, E. (2016). *Renal failure.* In R. Kliegman, B. Stanton, J. St. Geme, N. Schor, & R. Behrman (Eds.), *Nelson textbook of pediatrics* (20th ed., pp. 2539–2546). Philadelphia, PA: Elsevier.

VanDeVoorde, R. G., III. (2015). Acute poststreptococcal glomerulonephritis: The most common acute glomerulonephritis. *Pediatrics in Review, 36*(1), 3.

Van Rooij, I., van der Zanden, L., Brouwers, M., Knoers, N., Feitz, W., & Roeleveld, N. (2013). Risk factors for different phenotypes of hypospadias: Results from a Dutch case-control study. *BJU International, 112,* 121–128.

Van Why, S., & Avner, E. (2016). Hemolytic uremic syndrome. In R. Kliegman, B. Stanton, J. St. Geme, N. Schor, & R. Behrman (Eds.), Nelson textbook of pediatrics (20th ed., pp. 2507–2510). Philadelphia, PA: Elsevier.

25 Alterations in Hematological Function

Variations in Anatomy and Physiology

Caring for children with hematological disorders requires an understanding of the hematological system and its function. The hematological system incorporates all of the components of blood: erythrocytes (red blood cells, RBCs), leukocytes (white blood cells, WBCs), and thrombocytes (platelets), as well as the plasma, or liquid portion, that carries the cellular components. Understanding the jobs of the components is critical.

Erythrocytes transport oxygen and carbon dioxide through the hemoglobin (Hgb) molecules within these cells. Hgb is composed of two sets of polypeptides (the alpha and beta chains, which form the protein), globulin, and heme, which is composed of four atoms of iron per molecule. A key variation in children is the presence of fetal Hgb until 4 to 6 months of life. At this time, it is replaced by adult Hgb or one of the variants.

WBCs are responsible for infection control and immunological regulation. The WBCs are granulocytes and agranulocytes. Granulocytes include neutrophils, the most abundant of the granulocytes. Neutrophils are primarily the first line of defense that battle or phagocytize bacterial invaders. The other two types of granulocytes are eosinophils, which function in allergic reactions, and basophils, which have function in parasitic infections and a protective function in creating pathways for the phagocytes to move to sites of inflammation. The agranulocytes are lymphocytes and monocytes. Lymphocytes are small, less powerful phagocytes and are the first responders in viral infections. During a bacterial or immune-regulated process, lymphocytes become T cells and B cells. Monocytes, which are the most powerful phagocytizers and which become macrophages, phagocytize viral and bacterial infections. In addition, monocytes have a longer life than do neutrophils and lymphocytes.

Thrombocytes and other clotting factors in the plasma, such as fibrinogen, factors I, II to V, VII, VIII, IX, and X, are the key to clotting. These platelets and coagulation factors aggregate to seal tissues from injury and to protect from hemorrhage by sealing blood vessels (see Table 26.2 for age-specific complete blood count [CBC] values).

Assessment of the Pediatric Hematological System

When the nurse is assessing the hematological system, analyzing the CBC is a critical starting point. High or low blood cell counts can indicate certain blood disorders. Moreover, if erythrocytes, which carry oxygen via their Hgb molecules to the tissues, are small (microcytic) and pale (microchromic), they cannot carry as much oxygen because of a lower iron capacity. This low iron carrying capacity results in a child who tires easily and has tachypnea and tachycardia to compensate for the lower oxygen delivery. As hypoxia lingers, the child will not grow, develop, or increase in cognitive abilities as well as a child who has adequate oxygen saturation levels (93%–98%, supplemented, or up to 100% without supplementation).

A component of the CBC known as the differential is the breakdown of the leukocytes or WBCs by type. These cells are the key to the immune response and the first line in the anti-inflammatory process. In bacterial infections, neutrophils proliferate first to start battling the infective bacterial agent. Therefore, an increased neutrophil count is a key indicator that a bacterial infection is present and the immune response is beginning. If the number of lymphocytes is elevated, it usually indicates a viral infection. These smaller infectious agents are phagocytized by lymphocytes. As the infection continues, monocytes begin to proliferate and transform into macrophages to continue the battle as the neutrophils and lymphocytes wane. With certain bacterial infections, the number of lymphocytes is low, overall, and atypical lymphocytes may appear on the report. These are the helper and killer T cells. The B cells are responsible for cellular immunity and make the immunoglobulins. When the leukocyte count is low, it indicates that the child has limited defenses and is susceptible to infection, as in a child undergoing treament for leukemia or a child with aplastic anemia.

Thrombocytes (platelets) are essential in clot formation. Thus, a low laboratory thrombocyte count, as well as increased clotting times, can indicate petechiae, ecchymoses, purpura, or spontaneous to prolonged bleeding.

General Nursing Interventions for Hematological Disorders

When a child has a hematological disorder that limits the erythrocyte function, less oxygen is delivered to the tissues and the body fatigues easily. Given here are general interventions for addressing hematological disorders in children.

Maintain Adequate Oxygenation

When erythrocyte function is compromised because of a lack of RBCs or Hgb, RBCs cannot bind and transport enough oxygen to the organs and tissues. The body attempts to compensate with tachycardia and tachypnea. So it is important to assess the child for fatigue, rapid heart rate and breathing, and poor tissue perfusion, as evidenced by cool extremities, mottling, and sluggish capillary refill. When these signs are present, encourage the child to conserve energy and rest to maintain oxygenation to the tissues. If oxygen saturation levels get below 93%, administer additional oxygen (maintain oxygen saturation levels from 93% to 98% when the child is on supplemental oxygen) or, when the Hgb level is less than 9 to 10 g/dL, prepare to transfuse packed RBCs. Teaching about iron-rich foods (red meats, green leafy vegetables, raisins, and dried beans), which promote iron absorption, and encouraging consumption of such foods may help the child increase intake and build reticulocytes and erythrocytes. If iron supplements are required, instruct the child to take them between meals, take fruits and juices containing vitamin C or ascorbic acid, use a straw or dropper to prevent teeth staining, and avoid tea for 1 hour before and after the dose to decrease the tannins from binding the iron. An indication that the iron is being absorbed is the appearance of tarry, black stools and improved Hgb levels within a month.

Polycythemia, a state of increased RBCs, can also occur. This increase in cells occurs from prolonged hypoxia. The body produces more cells to make up for the poor circulating oxygen levels. Having too many RBCs slows the circulation and increases venous congestion, which makes the heart work harder than normal. Assess for increased cardiac workload, elevated blood pressure, headaches, stroke, and pulmonary hypertension with congestion and dyspnea for this issue.

Maintain Adequate Hydration

Adequate circulatory fluid volume is needed to carry and transport the blood cells within the plasma. Inadequate hydration impairs the circulatory flow of oxygen to the tissues and makes the heart work harder than desired. In children, the Holliday-Segars formula is used to calculate daily fluid requirements:

- For infants 3.5 to 10 kg, the daily fluid requirement is 100 mL/kg.
- For children 11 to 20 kg, the daily fluid requirement is 1,000 mL plus 50 mL/kg for every kilogram over 10.

- For children weighing more than 20 kg, the daily fluid requirement is 1,500 mL plus 20 mL/kg for every kilogram over 20, up to a maximum of 2,400 mL daily.
- Note that this calculation does not apply to newborn infants (i.e., from 0 to 28 days after full-term delivery).

Maintain Adequate Tissue Perfusion

In addition to adequate oxygenation and hydration, adequate tissue perfusion is required to deliver the oxygen and nutrients needed to the tissues and organs of the body and to remove waste products from them. To ensure sufficient tissue perfusion, maintain a urine output of 1 to 3 mL/kg/h, a warm skin temperature, a skin color that is without cyanosis, and a capillary refill that is brisk (3 seconds or greater).

Prevent Infection or Control Promptly

When alterations in WBCs occur, the child may not be able to mount a normal inflammatory response to fight off illness or infection. The nurse must protect the child from exposure to infectious agents with the following:

- Performing strict hand washing
- Restricting visitors with known upper respiratory infections
- Using chlorhexidine preparation with a vigorous friction when applying the antiseptic to the skin and intravenous ports when giving injections
- Removing raw meats, vegetables, and fruits from the child's diet
- Assessing for wounds that are open and not healing
- Having a child with an absolute neutrophil count of 500 or less wear a mask in public and avoid crowds

Monitoring the child's temperature is also very important because, in some cases, febrile reactions occur when the WBC count is low. An elevated WBC count is associated with infection and cancer.

Prevent or Control Bleeding

If a child has insufficient platelets or absent or deficient coagulation factors, the child is at high risk for hemorrhage. Internally, hemorrhaging can result in a hemorrhagic stroke, bleeding into the joint spaces, or gastrointestinal bleeding. External hemorrhage is visible blood loss. To stop the bleeding, encourage rest of the injured area, apply ice and direct pressure (compression) to it, and elevate it, as indicated by the acronym RICE (rest, ice, compression, elevation).

The nurse may need to administer platelets or other coagulation factors. If the bleeding occurs in a joint, the blood in the joint space can cause tissue damage. So once the bleeding stops, restoring normal range of motion and function is very important. In some cases, the body goes into a process of generating coagulation factors spontaneously and an anticoagulant may be used to keep clots from occurring.

Maintain Thermoregulation and Prevent Cold Stress

In infants, exposure to cold increases the metabolic demand and tissue oxygenation needs. Therefore, keep the infant warm to maintain tissue perfusion and keep the oxygen delivery optimal.

Prevent or Control Pain

Pain is an issue in sickle cell disease, because the infarcts from vasoocclusion produce **ischemia**, which is a lack of oxygen in the tissues. Pain alters the quality of life of individuals when it is constant. For a child with a hematological condition, transfusions of healthy blood cells into the circulation can be a key to pain control. Maximizing positioning, using warm compresses to vasodilate, and using biofeedback can also reduce pain. Medications may also be needed.

Educate the Patient and Family on Therapies and Care

The nurse must prepare the family for home care and educate them on medications, treatments, and home care needs. Depending on the condition, home care can range from administering oral medications, such as hydroxyurea and iron supplements, to administering chelating agents or replacement coagulation factors intravenously or subcutaneously.

The families need to be aware of when to seek medical attention and when to handle care at home, by making minor adjustments. Patients with sickle cell anemia must seek medical attention when infections occur because they can trigger a vasoocclusive crisis. Children with hemophilia must receive coagulation factors if bleeding, but the family may need to implement RICE therapy at home before administering the factor or going to the hospital.

Teach the parents of a child with severe anemia to recognize increased fatigue and loss of energy as indications for the need for a transfusion. Early detection of such signs can help prevent the anemia from getting severe before an intervention is initiated.

Provide Appropriate Developmental Care and Promote Optimal Health

When a child has any kind of illness, promoting normal development and growth is important. Help children continue to achieve their developmental milestones as they confront their illness, particularly those related to language, cognition, and motor function. A child with a bleeding disorder still needs to walk. Children with low RBC counts need to have oxygenation and perfusion maintained through exchange transfusions or periodic transfusions to keep their Hgb levels up to prevent cognitive impairment. Adequate oxygenation is essential for normal physical growth and cognitive functioning.

Provide Psychosocial Support and Engage a Support System

Having a child with a chronic illness puts a large stress burden on the family unit. The family may be divided by hospital stays and the demands of care. Siblings who are not ill may experience jealousy over the attention parents give the child who is affected by a chronic condition. Therefore, teach the family to cope by having parents take time together as a couple and set aside special time for each child.

Encourage the family to seek out family members and friends who can help care for the child with the chronic illness and allow the family some down time. Refer the family to associations or organizations associated with their child's condition, such as the Cooley's Anemia Foundation, Sickle Cell Anemia Foundation, and Hemophilia Society, for support and information about research trends. By networking, they can find others dealing with their same issues and have outlets to vent frustrations and joys.

Anemias

Anemias are conditions in which mature erythrocytes are decreased in number or volume or impaired in function. In some conditions, this decrease in RBCs may be accompanied by an increase in immature RBCs, known as reticulocytes, in the circulation. Yet these cells are not as good at carrying oxygen as the mature ones. Sickle cell disease is a type of hemoglobinopathy, or disease of the Hgb, that shortens the RBC lifespan and causes the cell to become sickle shaped, which results in occlusions in the microcirculation. Beta-thalassemia, also known as Cooley's anemia, occurs as a result of a failure of the beta chains to form, which leads to rapid cell lysis. Aplastic anemia results from a congenital or acquired bone marrow failure in which no erythrocytes are produced in the bone marrow. The following discussion elaborates on each condition in more detail.

Sickle Cell Disease

Sickle cell disease is a group of diseases associated with the presence of an abnormal Hgb gene known as the Hgb sickle (*Hgb S*) gene, which results in sickle-shaped RBCs that tend to clump together, leading to occluded blood vessels, impaired oxygen delivery, pain crises, premature RBC death, and anemia.

Etiology and Pathophysiology

Sickle cell disease occurs when a person inherits two abnormal Hgb genes instead of two normal adult Hgb *(Hgb A)* genes, with at least one of the two abnormal genes being the Hgb sickle *(Hgb S)* variant. There are several abnormal variants of the Hgb gene in addition to *Hgb S*, and the type of sickle cell disease present depends on the combination of these variants in the gene pair. The most common type of sickle cell disease is sickle cell anemia, in which both members of the Hgb gene pair are *Hgb S* genes *(Hgb^{SS})*; sickle cell anemia accounts for 60% to 65% of infants diagnosed with a sickle cell disease

(Noronha, Sadreameli, & Strouse, 2016). Known as the homozygous form of sickle cell disease, *Hgb^{SS}* is considered the most severe type, with a median lifespan in the 40s. The heterozygous forms include *Hgb^{SC}* and variations containing *Hgb S* and beta-thalassemia (Noronha et al., 2016).

The *Hgb S* gene variant is an autosomal recessive trait, which means that the child with sickle cell anemia has received the gene from each parent. Individuals who have one normal adult Hgb gene *(Hgb A)* and one *Hgb S* gene, giving them the heterozygous *Hgb^{AS}* genotype, are said to be carriers of the sickle cell trait and do not have the disease itself. The carriers of the trait are usually asymptomatic because of having a lower percentage of hemoglobin S, meaning that they do not have a sickling response to physiological stress. Yet, they can pass the sickle cell trait on to their children.

When both the mother and the father are carriers of the trait, each child that they have has a 25% chance of having a normal genotype *(Hgb^{AA})*, a 25% chance of having a genotype homozygous for *Hgb S (Hgb^{SS})* and thus of having sickle cell anemia *(Hgb^{SS}* is estimated to occur in one out of every 400 to 600 African American births), and a 50% chance of being a carrier of the sickle cell trait *(Hgb^{AS}*; Noronha et al., 2016; Porth, 2015). See Figure 25.1 for a depiction of this genetic transmission.

Recall that Natasha Austin in Chapter 12 was diagnosed with sickle cell anemia. Did Natasha's parents have sickle cell disease or the sickle cell trait? What type of genetic transmission did Natasha have?

Sickle cell disease occurs most frequently in people of African descent and less frequently in people of Hispanic, Middle Eastern, Mediterranean, and Asian descent. It is very important that families receive genetic counseling so they understand how the disease is transmitted and the risks of having a child with sickle cell disease.

When an infant is born with sickle cell disease, the fetal Hgb protects the child for the first 4 to 6 months from the sickling. Once the fetal Hgb disappears, the aberrant *Hgb S* gene results in RBCs becoming crescent or sickle shaped (Fig. 25.2) because of endothelial changes during periods of physiological stress triggered by hypoxia, acidosis, dehydration, fever, and hypothermia (Manwani & Frenetti, 2013; Porth, 2015).

The sickling is due to Hgb within the cells crystalizing, and the RBC can revert to its usual discoid shape once the triggering condition has passed. Sickling can occur multiple times in the same RBC, until it breaks down or no longer returns to the discoid shape. Sickled RBCs have a propensity to adhere to each other and surrounding structures, and once there is enough of them, they begin to clog the vascular circulation, a process known as vasoocclusion (Porth, 2015).

According to Noronha et al. (2016), when the RBCs that are sickling are greater than 30% of the total volume of RBCs

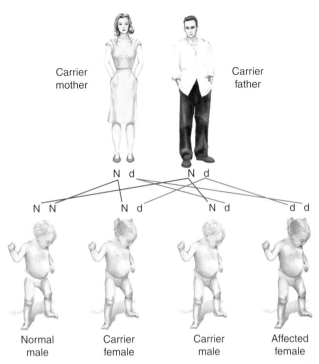

Figure 25.1 Genetic transmission of sickle cell anemia: Autosomal recessive inheritance. Reprinted with permission from Kyle, T., & Carman, S. (2016). *Essentials of pediatric nursing* (3rd ed., Fig. 27.2). Philadelphia, PA: Lippincott Williams & Wilkins.

and the total Hgb volume is 10g/dL or less, there is an increase in vasoocclusion and thickening of the circulating blood. The rigid crescent cells stick together, obstruct the tiny microvessels, and block the blood flow, preventing the delivery of oxygen and nutrients to the tissues in that area (Fig. 25.3). When this infarction occurs, it produces severe pain and damage or death to the tissues deprived of the oxygen (Porth, 2015). Once the cell is permanently sickled, it dies prematurely, with a lifespan much less than the normal 120 days. This shortened lifespan results in a lower-than-normal RBC count, producing hemolytic

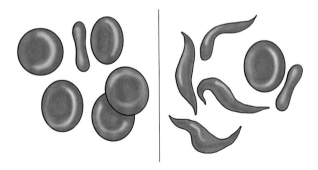

Figure 25.2 Red blood cell shape. Sickled cells and discoid cells. Reprinted with permission from Wilkins, E. M. (2016). *Clinical practice of the dental hygienist* (12th ed., Fig. 68.2). Philadelphia, PA: Lippincott Williams & Wilkins.

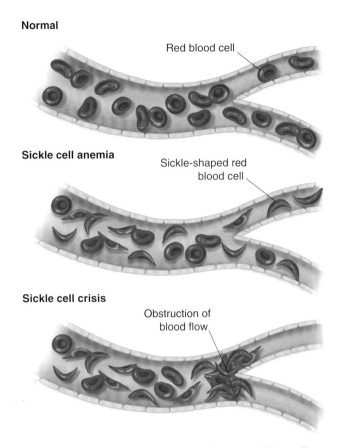

Figure 25.3 Obstruction of blood flow in sickle cell anemia. Sickled red blood cells do not circulate through the capillaries as easily as normal red blood cells, which are discoid. The obstruction of blood flow results in pain. Reprinted with permission from Cohen, B. J. (2007). *Medical terminology* (5th ed.). Philadelphia, PA: Wolters Kluwer.

anemia. These lysed RBCs become either circulatory debris that is absorbed by the spleen and liver or an occlusive mass in the circulatory bed. They also release free iron into the circulation, which can deposit in organs and tissues, causing damage. Thus, sickle cell disease results in tissue death and injury by two pathways—occlusion and hemolysis—with all tissues and organs susceptible to the damage.

Clinical Presentation

The first manifestation of sickle cell disease is often a vasoocclusive crisis. Vasoocclusion produces a painful crisis, which is the most frequent cause of hospitalization in children and adolescents with sickle cell disease.

The vasoocclusion robs the tissues of oxygen and results in ischemic infarcts at the site of the occlusion, ensuing in cellular death, which is extremely painful and can occur anywhere the blood flows. Figure 25.4 shows the areas of involvement in a child with sickle cell disease.

In children younger than 5 years of age, the vasoocclusive crisis frequently affects the bones in the hands and feet, resulting

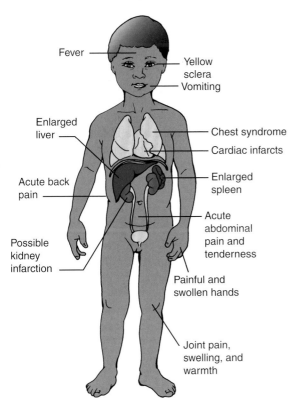

Fever

Yellow
sclera

Vomiting

Enlarged
liver

Chest syndrome

Cardiac infarcts

Acute back
pain

Enlarged
spleen

Acute
abdominal
pain and
tenderness

Possible
kidney
infarction

Painful and
swollen hands

Joint pain,
swelling, and
warmth

Figure 25.4 Systemic effects of sickle cell disease. Sickle cell disease affects many different areas of the child's body. Reprinted with permission from Pillitteri, A. (1999). *Maternal and child health nursing: Care of the childbearing and childrearing family* (3rd ed.). Philadelphia, PA: Lippincott-Raven.

in dactylitis (Fig. 25.5; hand-foot syndrome). The infarct of the bone marrow spaces produces edematous, erythematous extremities. The dactylitis is very painful and can lead to ulcerations of the tissues similar to venous and arterial insufficiency ulcers.

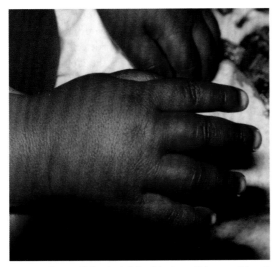

Figure 25.5 Dactylitis. A child with dactylitis resulting from a vasoocclusive crisis. Reprinted with permission from Kyle, T., & Carman, S. (2016). *Essentials of pediatric nursing* (3rd ed., Fig. 24.11). Philadelphia, PA: Lippincott Williams & Wilkins.

Another common area for vasoocclusive crisis in toddlers and preschoolers is the brain, where a cerebral vascular infarct can occur, producing neurological tissue injury. The child may have a stroke or silent cerebral ischemia (SCI) that may be unrecognized or produce debilitating paralysis, aphasia, seizure, headache, facial droop, and even death. The nurse must pay careful attention to neurological assessment of these children and seek emergency assistance for them when any suspected alterations are noted. Children with sickle cell disease are at risk for SCI and chronic anemia for impaired cognition. Transfusions and exchange transfusions are part of the emergency intervention for SCI (Noronha et al., 2016). Similar to dactylitis, the peak age of SCI occurs between birth and 5 years.

Acute chest syndrome is a complication of sickle cell disease that occurs as a result of sickling occlusion in the pulmonary vessels, emboli from infarcted bone marrow, or an infectious change that damages the lung tissue. This condition results in chest pain, hypoxemia, dyspnea, tachypnea, cough, fever, wheezing, radiographic infiltrates, and respiratory distress. The onset can be subtle or sudden respiratory compromise. It is very serious and should be treated as a medical emergency. Acute chest syndrome mimics pneumonia, but the chest radiograph shows infarcted infiltrates rather than empyema or purulent areas.

The coronary vessels are susceptible to infarcts just as the brain and lungs are. Children may have infarcts that kill tissue in the cardiac muscle. The infarct is caused by sickle cell obstruction, not plaques, as in atherosclerosis.

The gastrointestinal organs also may be affected by vasoocclusion and hemolysis. The spleen absorbs the damaged and lysed cells and slowly become fibrotic and nonfunctional, a condition known as asplenia. This damage produces a splenic sequestration that is chronic and leads to increased infection risk because the spleen stops filtering infectious agents and trapping debris. The acute form of splenic sequestration is a medical emergency in which the spleen suddenly absorbs a vast volume of blood and depletes the circulatory volume, resulting in shock and abdominal distension. Treatment of asplenia requires a splenectomy.

In the liver and hepatic system, hemolysis and sludge in the bile ducts and gallbladder lead to gallstones. The repeated infarcts of vasoocclusion and excessive absorption of cells lead to hepatomegaly; a fibrotic, damaged liver (sickle hepatopathy); and, in some cases, cirrhosis or liver failure. Children experiencing these complications have jaundice, amber urine, and hyperbilirubinemia (bilirubin levels ranging from 13 to 76 mg/dL).

The genitourinary tract is also impacted by vasoocclusion. Males may have painful erections, a condition called priapism. The infarct occurs in the penile circulation, and blood is unable to flow in or out of penis.

The priapism is not related to sexual stimulation. Repeated priapisms can result in erectile dysfunction. The testicles and ovaries are also susceptible to the poor circulatory flow and can sustain damage, causing infertility.

Hemolysis and infarcts in the kidneys can produce inefficient glomerular filtration and renal tubular dysfunction, resulting in the inability to concentrate the urine. Enuresis develops because the urine output is greater than bladder capacity. Unlike other cases of enuresis, restricting oral fluids before bedtime is not advisable. Hydration is essential to maintain the blood flow. Teach parents to get the child up to go to the bathroom periodically to prevent bedwetting.

The altered filtration results in hematuria. The RBCs are not reabsorbed and are excreted in the urine. The urine color is amber to red tinged.

Another complication is retinal detachment due to repeated infarcts from vasoocclusion. Retinal ischemia leads to serious retinal disease and visual acuity changes, ending in retinal detachment.

In Chapter 12, Natasha experienced many episodes of vasoocclusive crisis during her childhood. What serious vasoocclusive complication did she experience when she was 14 years old? What signs and symptoms did she develop? What other vasoocclusive complications did Natasha experience, earlier in her life?

Assessment and Diagnosis

Diagnosis of sickle cell disease is based on both clinical presentation (described earlier) and diagnostic testing (Box 25.1). Often, children with sickle cell disease are diagnosed at birth with the newborn screen.

Box 25.1 Diagnostic Tests for Sickle Cell Disease

- Hgb electrophoresis:
  - Is the most diagnostic test for sickle cell disease
  - Determines the types of Hgb present and the percentage of each in the circulating blood (i.e., Hgb A, Hgb F, and Hgb S)
  - Guides treatment by determining the percentage of the variant Hgb
- Sickledex:
  - Is used for routine screening before surgery to prevent a sickle cell crisis in an undiagnosed patient when under anesthesia
  - Cannot differentiate between the disease state and the trait
- Complete blood count:
  - Is used as a diagnostic tool to visually detect the presence of sickled RBCs
  - Is not optimal for detecting the condition, because the cells may not be visualized, although present
  - Allows identification of RBC morphology

In the United States, the prevalence of multiracial descent makes identifying those at risk for having sickle cell disease challenging. For that reason, all patients should have a sickle cell screen before surgery and the results documented to alert the healthcare team to potential surgical complications associated with this condition. For example, hypoxia, which occurs commonly in the surgical setting, can trigger a sudden and severe crisis in an individual with sickle cell disease. Knowing ahead that a patient has this risk factor allows the nurse and other members of the healthcare team to take extra measures to prevent this complication.

Therapeutic Interventions

The key to treatment of sickle cell disease is addressing the triggers of sickling—the conditions that cause the erythrocytes to change shape from discoid to crescent or sickle. Therefore, take measures to prevent hypoxia, infections that produce fever and acidosis, and dehydration. Other interventions for sickle cell disease include pain management, medications to increase fetal Hgb (hydroxyurea) or bind iron (deferoxamine), bone marrow transplantation, and providing psychosocial support to the child and family. These are discussed in detail later.

To help prevent hypoxia, maintain the child's oxygen saturation levels at 93% or above. Also, prepare patients for surgical procedures that can result in hypoxia. Before surgical procedures that may lower the oxygen tension, administer a transfusion of packed RBCs. The aim of this transfusion is to have a higher concentration of non-sickle than sickling cells. Keep the percentage of sickle cells in the circulatory flow below 30% and the Hgb volume greater than 10 g/dL to lower the risk of the child having a vasoocclusive crisis. Patients may need transfusions at other times, as well. In some situations, the patient receives a transfusion simply to correct the blood Hgb concentration and volume. Other times, the patient may need an exchange transfusion to remove the sickled cells and replace them with normal Hgb[AA] cells. Transfusions are also used in treating strokes, priapisms, and, in some cases, acute chest syndrome, splenic sequestration, and other complications of sickle cell disease.

To prevent infections, make sure the child with sickle cell disease receives prophylactic antibiotics and regular vaccines to protect from illness, particularly when asplenic and exposed to infections. Early treatment is necessary for any signs of infection. Viral illnesses, many of which may be prevented with immunizations, can trigger an aplastic crisis, which is an autoimmune response following a viral infection that stops bone marrow production. Hyperhemolytic crisis is also associated with an infectious process that causes the RBCs to break down excessively.

Hydration is very important because it helps prevent vasoocclusion by moving the RBCs through the vessels and vascular bed, which prevents sickled cells from aggregating and clogging the microcirculation. During a vasoocclusive crisis, providing intravenous hydration with an isotonic solution increases the hydrostatic pressure and volume and improves blood flow. Prevent dehydration by maintaining the child's fluid intake at

1,600 mL/m² or at 1.5 times the normal fluid needs for age and weight. If using the Holliday-Segar formula for fluid requirements, calculate the child's fluid needs and then multiply it by 1.5. For example, to calculate the recommended fluid intake for a child with sickle cell disease whose normal needed fluid intake for age and weight is 800 mL, complete the following:

800 mL × 1.5 = 1,200 mL × 0.033814 (to convert to ounces) = 40.58 oz

Therefore, in this case, the nurse should instruct parents to provide the child with about 5 to 6 (8-ounce) cups of fluid daily. The fluids can come in a variety of forms: 3 (90-mL) water popsicles (1 cup), 1 bowl of soup, juice, water, and ice cream.

Pain management for sickle cell disease should focus on general comfort measures and medication (How Much Does It Hurt? 25.1). Apply warm compresses using devices such as a heat therapy pump to help vasodilate the painful areas for 15 to 20 minutes. A systematic review revealed that cognitive behavioral therapy, acupuncture, biofeedback, massage, and aquatic therapy have been studied as nonpharmacological therapies for pain management in patients with sickle cell disease. The most significant intervention was cognitive behavioral therapy (Williams & Tanabe, 2016), which is a form of psychotherapy that changes how individuals view and cope with pain. Nonsteroidal anti-inflammatory drugs are also used as an adjunct to potentiate the effects of opioids in pain control. However, they have side effects that may increase the risk for heart complications and stroke, as well as gastrointestinal bleeding.

In 2017, hydroxyurea, also known as hydroxycarbamide, was approved by the U.S. Food and Drug Administration (FDA) as a medication for treating children with sickle cell disease (The Pharmacy 25.1). The recommended initial daily dose for children 2 years of age and older is 20 mg/kg (FDA, 2017). The benefits of hydroxyurea for treating sickle cell disease are that it increases the level of fetal Hgb and reduces the incidence of vasoocclusive crisis, promotes splenic function, and reduces the incidence of stroke and acute chest syndrome (Hankins et al., 2014; Nottage et al., 2014). The Baby Hug study tested, over a 2-year period, the effects of hydroxycarbamide/hydroxyurea on infants with sickle cell disease who were 9 to 18 months of age. The statistically significant findings revealed decreased pain and dactylitis in the study participants. The fetal Hgb level was increased (Wang et al., 2011). The

How Much Does It Hurt? 25.1

Pain Management During Vasoocclusive Crisis

Frequent assessment of pain in children with sickle cell disease in vasoocclusive crisis is important. These children have extremely severe pain and need to feel confident that their pain will be controlled. The delivery of pain medication may be patient-controlled analgesia, oral, or intermittent intravenous dosing with opioids (e.g., codeine, oxycodone, and morphine). Meperidine is contraindicated in pain treatment for sickle cell anemia because of the risk of a chemical reaction that may lead to a seizure. In the climate of opioid addiction and crisis, the nurse must practice diligent pain management, balancing the needs of pain relief and prevention of drug overuse and misuse (Smith, 2014).

adverse effect of hydroxyurea is neutropenia, but it reverses if the medication is stopped for a week (Noronha et al., 2016; Nottage et al., 2014; Wang et al., 2011). Monitoring the absolute neutrophil count and WBC levels is a key nursing intervention for this therapy, in addition to the earlier measures for the prevention of infection.

Deferoxamine therapy may be used if hemolysis results in high levels of free iron (The Pharmacy 25.2). This chelating agent given by subcutaneous infusion binds the iron and makes it excretable in the urine. Instruct the child and parents to report any side effects, such as urinary changes (especially urinary tract infections), oliguria, dark color of the urine as a sudden change, blurred vision or halos around lights, swelling of the throat or difficulty breathing, signs of infection (especially bladder and urinary tract infections) or infection at the insertion site, and diarrhea or watery stools. Also inform the patient and family that the child should take vitamin C when taking deferoxamine to maximize the iron-binding capacity of this medication.

The only curative therapy for sickle cell disease is a bone marrow transplantation, specifically autologous stem cell therapy with a human leukocyte antigen (HLA)-matched sibling donor (Meier, Dioguardi, & Kamani, 2015; Thompson, Ceja,

The Pharmacy 25.1 Hydroxyurea

Classification	Route	Action	Nursing Considerations
Antineoplastic agent	PO	• Increases RBC Hgb F levels • Increases RBC water content • Alters adhesion of RBCs to endothelium	• Monitor Hgb F levels. • Monitor CBC, reticulocyte count, and platelet count. • Monitor for neutropenia and thrombocytopenia (signs of toxicity). • Do not open capsules.

CBC, complete blood count; Hgb F, fetal hemoglobin; PO, oral; RBC, red blood cell.
Adapted from Taketomo, C. K., Hodding, J. H., & Kraus, D. M. (2018). *Pediatric & neonatal dosage handbook* (25th ed.). Hudson, OH: Lexicomp.

& Yang, 2012). Researchers in one study reported on more than 1,200 transplantations in patients with sickle cell disease and found that the highest survival rates occurred in patients who received a transplant from an HLA-matched unaffected sibling donor (Meier et al., 2015). Despite its potential for being curative, transplantation is the least-used modality for treatment of sickle cell disease and its risks versus benefits have not been adequately studied (Oringanje, Nemecek, & Oniyangi, 2016).

The use of umbilical cord stem cells is another potential area of cure that needs to be explored more because of the increased availability of cord blood stem cells. Engraftment is slower with cord blood than with peripheral or bone marrow stem cells. Yet, the rate of graft-versus-host disease (GVHD) is lower in cord blood stem cell transplants. HLA-matched sibling cord blood stem cells and unmatched cord blood stem cells have been used (Thompson et al., 2012).

Finally, help the patient and family cope with this chronic and life-threatening condition. Encourage the family to seek emotional support and involvement from one another and from their extended support system. Chronic illness is very stressful on the family, and many divorces occur under these challenges. The Sickle Cell Foundation is a supportive association that helps keep families aware of treatment innovations and funding for research activities to improve care.

Natasha (in Chapter 12) required many hospitalizations and interventions to treat her sickle cell anemia. What medications did Natasha take regularly for her condition? What major surgery did she undergo at the age of 4 years related to her sickle cell anemia? What interventions were performed during her most recent hospitalization, at the age of 14 years, and why?

Evaluation

Expected outcomes for a child with sickle cell disease include the following:

- The child's oxygen saturation level is maintained at 93% or greater.
- The child maintains adequate hydration.
- Infection is prevented or treated effectively.
- The child's pain is controlled.
- Tissue damage is prevented or minimized.
- If needed, the child is prepared effectively for a transfusion or exchange transfusion.
- The transition to home care is seamless, with the family meeting the child's needs.
- The child is emotionally sound and obtaining growth and developmental milestones.

Discharge Planning and Teaching

When planning the discharge of a child with sickle cell disease, teaching the family to maintain hydration levels is very important. The child needs to be given the required amount of fluid per day in milliliters and cups. To help ensure that the child takes in the full required amount, the daily total can be divided by the number of hours the child is awake to provide an hourly intake goal. For example, if a child is to have 1,674 mL in a day and is awake about 12 hours per day, divide the total by 12 hours, which results in an hourly intake goal of about 140 mL. The family also needs to have an idea of the variety of forms the fluid can take and their approximate volume. A single popsicle is 90 mL, and a double or twin popsicle is 180 to 200 mL. An 8-oz cup is 240 mL, and a 4-oz cup is 120 mL; thus, a small bowl of soup is about 120 mL. In particular, the family needs to know how many 4-oz cups (14 cups) and 8-oz cups (7 cups) should be consumed daily.

The Pharmacy 25.2   Deferoxamine

Classification	Route	Action	Nursing Considerations
Chelating agent	• SQ • IV	• Binds to iron in the tissues and is removed by the kidneys • Slows accumulation of hepatic iron	Monitor: • Growth • Serum iron and ferritin levels and total iron-binding capacity Monitor for: • Tachycardia and shock • Acute respiratory distress • Visual and hearing disturbances • Local injection site infection • Urinary tract infections or insults

IV, intravenous; SQ, subcutaneous.
Adapted from Taketomo, C. K., Hodding, J. H., & Kraus, D. M. (2018). *Pediatric & neonatal dosage handbook* (25th ed.). Hudson, OH: Lexicomp.

Review with the family their plan for getting medications filled and proper administration of the medications. Discuss the use of analgesics at home, including the importance of safely storing narcotics out of the child's reach, of only parents administering them, and of protecting them from unprescribed use. Teach the family the purpose of each medication, side effects to watch for, and when to notify the prescriber about issues.

Teach patients and families to avoid potential triggers for hypoxia, such as high altitudes and planes that are not pressurized. Teach the family to get the child immunized, including annual influenza vaccines and a pneumovax every 5 years, and to avoid exposing the child to crowds when cold and influenza viruses are rampant. Teach the child to use a hand sanitizer and wash hands frequently. Stress that the child should avoid touching the mouth, nose, and eyes unless the hands have just been washed. Educate the family to seek medical attention promptly when the child has a fever of 100.5°F to 101°F (38.1°C–38.3°C) or greater or demonstrates signs of an infection, such as diarrhea, vomiting, sore throat, cough, or congested nose or chest.

Inform the family of the signs of a stroke or splenic sequestration and when to go to the emergency room versus the primary care provider. Urgent signs and symptoms include severe pain not relieved by home medications, chest pain and congestion that is getting rapidly more severe, inability to speak, drooling, inability to move one side of the body, seizure activity, and altered level of consciousness or orientation.

Beta-Thalassemia (Cooley Anemia)

Beta-thalassemia is another chronic hemoglobinopathy. This condition is caused by abnormal beta chains in the Hgb, which destabilize the RBCs and lead to their rapid destruction. It is characterized by severe anemia and cellular or tissue damage from free iron buildup.

Etiology and Pathophysiology

Beta-thalassemia is an autosomal recessive trait in which the beta chains are defective in the Hgb molecule. Beta-thalassemia affects people of Mediterranean (Greek and Italian), Middle Eastern, and Asian descent. This alteration in the Hgb molecule results in a very unstable cell membrane, which causes the Hgb molecule to easily disintegrate in the circulation and the erythroblast to be destroyed in bone marrow or erythrocytes to be destroyed in the circulation.

Clinical Presentation

The rapid destruction of RBCs results in a severe hemolytic anemia, and the futile **erythropoiesis**, or production of RBCs by the bone marrow, results in hyperplasia of bone marrow in the extramedullary sites (Fig. 25.6). The cortical bone is thin and new bony growth forms over it, which changes the maxilla and frontal lobe bones of the face (Fig. 25.7).

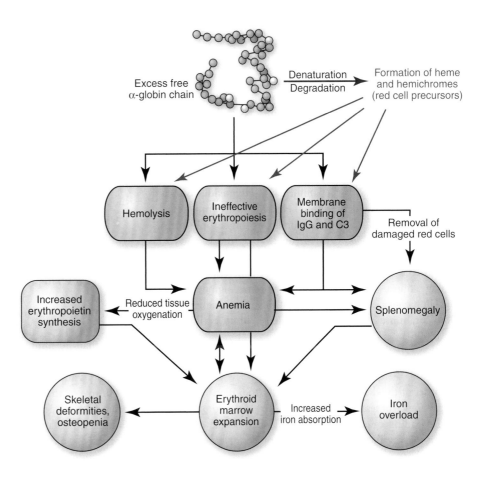

Figure 25.6 Pathophysiology of beta-thalassemia. The effects of the defective chains of the hemoglobin molecule in beta-thalassemia. C3, complement 3; IgG, immunoglobulin G. Reprinted with permission from Vigorita, V. J. (2015). *Orthopaedic pathology* (3rd ed., Fig. 12.6A). Philadelphia, PA: Lippincott Williams & Wilkins.

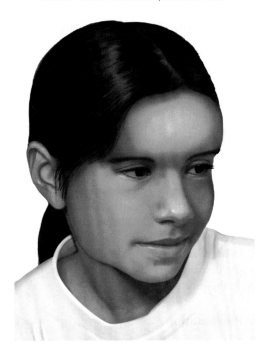

Figure 25.7 Clinical manifestations of beta-thalassemia.
The characteristic pattern of maxillary prominence ("chipmunk face") and frontal lobe prominence in a child with beta-thalassemia. Reprinted with permission from Kyle, T., & Carman, S. (2016). *Essentials of pediatric nursing* (3rd ed., Fig. 24.12). Philadelphia, PA: Lippincott Williams & Wilkins.

The iron overload is also due to increased gastrointestinal absorption and frequent transfusions. Other marrow-producing bones, such as the ribs, pelvis, long bones, and vertebrae, develop osteopenia and osteoporosis from overworking to make RBCs that do not last (Porth, 2015).

As discussed with sickle cell disease, hemolysis releases free iron (**hemosiderin**) into the circulation, along with cellular debris, which is absorbed into the spleen (causing splenomegaly) and liver (causing hepatomegaly). **Hemosiderosis** and **hemochromatosis** emerge as the hemosiderin accumulates and continues to amass. The hemochromatosis and chronic anemia cause cardiac damage (cardiomyopathy), cirrhosis and liver failure, and endocrine dysfunction due to deposits in the pituitary, thyroid, and adrenal glands and the pancreas that worsen with age. Short stature and yellow or bronze pigmentation of the skin are also common manifestations (Cunningham et al., 2004; Ibrahim et al., 2016; Porth, 2015; Rund & Rachmilewitz, 2005).

Assessment and Diagnosis

The onset of the disease occurs around 4 to 6 months with the disappearance of fetal Hgb. Cardiac failure and cardiomyopathy are the leading cause of death in beta-thalassemia, and better detection is available with tissue Doppler imaging (Ibrahim et al., 2016).

Therapeutic Interventions

The key to therapeutic management in a child or adult with beta-thalassemia is transfusion, chelation, or bone marrow transplantation. With the instability of the RBCs, children need frequent replacement of RBCs. The lysis and hemosiderin levels make it essential to chelate and remove the free iron from the body to prevent hemochromatosis. When treated with both transfusion therapy and chelation therapy with deferoxamine to control excessive iron, children experience more normal growth patterns and fewer complications such as liver disease, cardiac damage, along with the other complications caused by iron overload and chronic anemia (Cunningham et al., 2004; Ibrahim et al., 2016; Rund & Rachmilewitz, 2005). The best hope to resolve the problems of beta-thalassemia is an HLA-matched sibling bone marrow transplantation. Each of the therapies is discussed in more detail here.

Transfusion Therapy

From an early age, transfusion therapy is required for normal RBC function and to counteract the damage of the iron overload. Newer transfusion techniques include leukodepletion, testing for infectious agents, and minimizing the optimal level of Hgb to 9 to 10 g/dL (Rund & Rachmilewitz, 2005).

Preparing the child and family for multiple and repeated blood transfusions requires detailed education. Explain to the family that the RBCs produced are not effective and need to be replaced. The child may need a transfusion every other week, monthly, or quarterly to maintain an Hgb level of 9 to 10 g/dL. Many children receive central venous access devices (CVADs) to prevent frequent intravenous catheterizations for these transfusions. Infection prevention is a critical goal with a CVAD. The child will receive packed RBC transfusions, which require that the child have a type and crossmatch test.

The unit of packed RBCs is kept in a special laboratory blood refrigerator until 30 minutes before beginning the transfusion. Unit refrigerators are for food storage and should not be used for blood storage. The blood is checked out of the blood bank by hospital personnel. To prevent a transfusion reaction, the blood type must be verified (Patient Safety 25.1). Next, the unit is connected to an infusion set and primed. The tubing infusion set may have saline to prime it before running the packed cells through the line. The transfusion should be administered on an infusion pump to maintain the infusion rate, and precautions must be taken to prevent fluid overload (Patient Safety 25.1).

Once the tubing has been primed and packed RBCs are at the tip of the catheter, the infusion is ready to begin (Priority Care Concepts 25.1). Note that the infusion should begin no more than 30 minutes after the blood was checked out of the blood bank. Before starting the blood, obtain a baseline set of vital signs and thoroughly assess the child.

If any of the signs or symptoms of a transfusion reaction occur (Box 25.2), stop the transfusion, start infusing saline, and call for help. Stay with the child and assess the child frequently. Contact the physician along with the blood bank. Collect urine at the child's next voiding and blood to assess for a transfusion

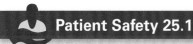

Patient Safety 25.1

Blood Transfusions

Keep in mind two key safety measures when assisting with a blood transfusion. First, verify that the units of blood to be administered match the patient to avoid a transfusion reaction, to make sure it is the correct unit for the patient. Two registered nurses should assess the blood bags and the patient's identification at the bedside to verify that they match.

Second, ensure that the proper transfusion rate is set to prevent fluid overload. The usual transfusion rate is 5 mL/kg/h. A typical transfusion volume is 10 mL/kg. One unit of blood is estimated to contain 240 to 350 mL of packed RBCs.

Box 25.2 Signs of a Transfusion Reaction

- Fever or chills (a temperature change of more than 2°F or 1.11°C)
- Flushing, itching, or rash
- Low back pain
- Tachycardia, hypotension, tachypnea, shock, or death
- Wheezing
- Dyspnea, cough, chest tightness, or cyanosis
- Nausea, vomiting, or abdominal pain
- Headache
- Jugular vein distension or peripheral edema

reaction. The patient may receive diphenhydramine and acetaminophen. For febrile nonhemolytic transfusion reactions, some 50% to 80% of patients have orders to pretreat with diphenhydramine and acetaminophen. However, the results show no significance in masking reactions when used to pretreat before administering a transfusion (Geiger & Howard, 2007).

Chelation Therapy

To reduce the iron overload, chelation (pronounced key-lay-shun) therapy is used, with administration of deferoxamine parenterally or the newer agents deferiprone and deferasirox orally.

Deferoxamine has been used to treat iron overload for decades (The Pharmacy 25.2). Its side effects include lack of compliance,

Priority Care Concepts 25.1

Blood Transfusions

1. Begin the infusion and stay with the child for the first 15 to 20 minutes of the infusion.
2. Recheck the vital signs at the end of 15 minutes.
3. Know and watch for the signs of a transfusion reaction (Box 25.2).
4. Encourage the parents and the child to call for the nurse if any signs of itching, pain, or shortness of breath occur.
5. Return in 15 minutes to reassess the child.
6. After 30 minutes of infusion, check on the child at the next 30-minute interval and then hourly until the unit is infused.
7. The transfusion should be completed within 4 hours of the blood having left the blood bank.
8. Reassess the child at the end of the infusion and again 1 hour following the transfusion.

delayed growth, urinary tract problems, reddish color to urine, oliguria, diarrhea, nausea, visual disturbances and halos around lights, local injection site infection or pain, and common signs of allergic reaction, such as rash and difficulty breathing. Taking vitamin C with the deferoxamine helps with iron binding, but excessive intake of vitamin C can increase the risk for heart failure.

Deferiprone has severe side effects, most notably damage to the myelocytes leading to severe agranulocytosis and neutropenia, which can result in a life-threatening infection. Other side effects include liver failure, petechiae, swelling around the eyes, nausea, vomiting, diarrhea, abdominal pain, changes in appetite (anorexia), weight gain, reddish-brown urine, joint and back pain, headache, increased intracranial pressure, lightheadedness, anaphylactic shock, seizures, tachycardia, urticaria, and elevated liver enzyme levels (Physician's Digital Reference [PDR], 2018).

Deferasirox (The Pharmacy 25.3) causes transient acute renal insufficiency (elevated creatinine level, proteinuria, and hematuria), nausea, vomiting, diarrhea, abdominal pain, headache, fever, upper respiratory infection (sore throat, cough, nasopharyngitis, bronchitis, influenza, and pharyngolaryngeal pain), and an elevated alanine transaminase (ALT) level (Al-Kuriashy & Al-Gareeb, 2017; PDR, 2018). Moreover, according to the online Prescriber's Digital Reference (PDR), the side effects of deferasirox are serious enough to have warranted this drug receiving a black box warning from the Federal Drug Agency for renal and hepatic failure for pediatric patients (2018).

Deferasirox is excreted in the stool, whereas deferoxamine and deferiprone are excreted in the urine (Al-Kuriashy & Al-Gareeb, 2017). The key difference, however, is that deferasirox has been shown to be significantly better than deferoxamine at reducing iron overload. The levels of cardiac- and hepatic-stored iron were also lower in patients who took deferasirox than in those who took deferoxamine because of the longer half-life of the drug (Al-Kuriashy & Al-Gareeb, 2017).

When administering deferasirox, monitor the patient's Child-Pugh score for liver impairment level and estimated glomerular filtration rate, creatinine level, and creatinine clearance for kidney function. Be alert for signs of dehydration, which is associated with renal function decline. Monitor the results of liver function tests, including ALT, aspartate transaminase, and bilirubin levels. Observe for signs of severe gastrointestinal

The Pharmacy 25.3 Deferasirox

Classification	Route	Action	Nursing Considerations
Chelating agent	PO	Binds iron, creating a complex excreted in the feces	• Monitor for acute renal failure. • Monitor for acute hepatic failure. • Take on an empty stomach when taking tablets for dispersion and liquid preparations. • Maintain adequate hydration.

PO, oral.
Adapted from Taketomo, C. K., Hodding, J. H., & Kraus, D. M. (2018). *Pediatric & neonatal dosage handbook* (25th ed.). Hudson, OH: Lexicomp.

problems, including ulceration, hemorrhage, irritation, and perforation. Be sure to administer the tablets with a light meal and at the same time each day. If the child requires the tablet to be crushed and sprinkled in food to take, put it in applesauce, yogurt, or soft food and administer immediately. Avoid using serrated blade crushers with these medications. Make sure the child is not taking any aluminum-containing antacids with the dose. Administer tablets for dispersion or liquid preparations on an empty stomach, and suspend them in a set volume of fluid on the basis of dose (PDR, 2018).

Deferiprone is available as an oral tablet or a solution and may be given with or without food. For the liquid preparation, measure the dose and add 10 to 15 mL of water to it for administration. Do not administer iron, aluminum, zinc, or other mineral supplements within 4 hours of administering this chelating drug. Instruct parents to protect this medication from light and extreme temperatures and to discard it if not all used in 5 weeks. Monitor for the adverse effects of this medication listed earlier, especially for agranulocytosis and neutropenia.

Educate the child and family on whichever drug therapy is used and its side effects. Greater patient compliance and a longer half-life are making the new drug deferasirox look more favorable as a therapy option. However, care management is essential to successful reduction of iron overload, no matter the specific medication used. Bahnasawy, El Wakeel, El Beblawy, and El-Hamamsy (2017) found that supervised care improved compliance and serum iron ferritin levels when using chelation therapy.

Other Therapies

Most children with beta-thalassemia have splenectomies. Care of the child during the recovery from abdominal surgery includes early ambulation, deep breathing, positioning to relieve pain, pain control with diversional methods, and analgesics. Prophylactic antibiotic therapy is an ongoing part of care either continuously until 5 years of age or sporadically for invasive procedures and outbreaks.

Growth hormone replacement therapy may be required to address short stature and to help children maximize their growth potential. The growth hormone is given subcutaneously daily or weekly until the child reaches adult height. The major concern is the increased risk of colon cancer and Hodgkin lymphoma.

Transplantation of the bone marrow, peripheral blood, or cord blood stem cells offers the only cure for beta-thalassemia. The decision families and children with beta-thalassemia face on whether to continue with chelation therapy and transfusions or to have a stem cell or bone marrow transplantation with risks of GVHD is a huge one. Patient and family satisfaction with transplantation has shown to be significantly higher as time goes by without a graft-versus-host reaction (Orrù et al., 2012). For further details, see the discussion of this therapy for sickle cell disease in the section Therapeutic Interventions, earlier.

To address nutritional needs, zinc and folic acid supplements may be administered to enhance erythropoiesis. However, evidence in the literature is limited as to the effectiveness of such supplements in children with sickle cell disease and beta-thalassemia. Hydroxyurea is recommended because of its potentiation of fetal Hgb.

Chronic anemia makes the heart work harder. Therefore, cardiomyopathy frequently develops in patients with beta-thalassemia. It leads to congestive heart failure and, with hemochromatosis of the heart and lungs, makes cardiac failure the leading cause of death. Encourage the family to seek support through the Cooley's Anemia Foundation.

Evaluation

Expected outcomes for a child with beta-thalassemia include the following:

- The child's Hgb level remains in the range of 9 to 10 g/dL.
- Adequate tissue oxygenation and perfusion are maintained.
- Tissue damage is prevented with adequate chelation therapy.
- No transfusion complications occur.
- Infection is prevented.
- Tissue function is maintained.
- The child and family report coping well and being engaged in psychosocially supportive activities.

Discharge Planning and Teaching

Providing teaching on the home care needs of a child on deferoxamine is very important. Instruct the parents on how to work the infusion device and prime the infusion set. Teach them how to prepare and load the medication into a syringe and administer it subcutaneously. Remind them to give the child a dose of vitamin C before starting the chelation infusion. Educate the child and parents on adverse reactions associated with the medication, such as the red-orange urine. Teach them to assess the injection site on the abdomen for signs of infection, including redness, swelling, drainage, and heat. Instruct them to be alert for altered urinary function or signs and symptoms of a urinary tract infection, which could impact the excretion of the medication.

If the patient is taking the oral chelation therapy, teach the parents and child to use proper dosing, to have the child drink plenty of fluids with the medication, and to monitor for side effects. The gastrointestinal complications, which can range from ulceration to perforation, may produce bleeding. Encourage the child and family to be aware of tarry stools, which indicate old or upper gastrointestinal tract bleeding, and bright red blood in the stool, which indicate fresh or lower gastrointestinal tract bleeding. Have them observe, as well, for color changes associated with liver injury, including yellow sclera and amber-gold urine.

Also teach the family to monitor for signs of anemia and the need for a transfusion. Signs of altered cardiac output they should monitor for include: poor urinary output, cold extremities, mottled to cyanotic peripheral coloring, and decreased pulses and capillary refill. With splenic dysfunction or removal, they should observe for generalized signs and symptoms of infection.

Aplastic Anemia (Fanconi Anemia)

Aplastic anemia is a condition of complete bone marrow suppression or failure that produces **pancytopenia**, a condition in which all three blood cellular component (RBCs, WBCs, and platelets) are low or absent (Barone et al., 2015). The red marrow is replaced by a fatty yellow substance. This condition can be congenital or acquired.

Etiology and Pathophysiology

Congenital aplastic anemia, also known as Fanconi anemia, has an autosomal recessive gene transmission. Acquired aplastic anemia is believed to occur following an insult to the body that destroys the bone marrow, such as by one of the following mechanisms (Barone et al., 2015):

- An autoimmune response
- An infection
- Exposure to chemicals: paints, plastics, petroleum products, shellacs, dyes, or benzenes
- Pharmacological agents: chloramphenicol, antibiotics that suppress bone marrow, antineoplastic agents, sulfonamides, cimetidine, or anticonvulsants
- Radiation

The autoimmune process suspected in acquired aplastic anemia has been attributed to self-reactive T cells that obliterate the bone marrow blood-forming cells (erythropoietin, leukopoietin, and thrombopoietin). As a result, the rich, red bone marrow is replaced by a fatty yellow substance (Risitano & Perna, 2011).

Clinical Presentation

Fanconi anemia is an autosomal recessive disorder that causes aplastic anemia and other congenital birth defects (Fig. 25.8). It is associated with skeletal defects of the arms, hips, legs, toes, fingers, and spine such as missing bones, distorted bones, polydactyly, and scoliosis. Genitourinary problems associated with Fanconi anemia include kidney deformities, missing kidney, hypospadias, epispadias, cryptorchidism, exstrophy of the bladder and other bladder issues, and sexual dysfunction. Associated sensory dysfunctions include deafness and malformation of the eyelid or ear. Other issues include café au lait spots (brown patchy skin; Fig. 25.9), cardiac defects (ventricular septal

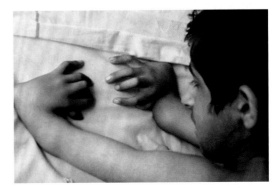

Figure 25.8 Congenital skeletal deformity in Fanconi anemia. Reprinted with permission from Salimpour, R. R., Salimpour, P., & Salimpour, P. (2013). *Photographic atlas of pediatric disorders and diagnosis* (1st ed., unnumbered figure). Philadelphia, PA: Wolters Kluwer.

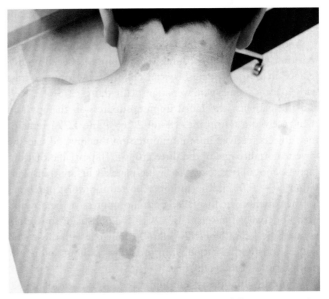

Figure 25.9 Café au lait spots. Café au lait spots on the back of a child with neurofibromatosis type 1. Reprinted with permission from Biller, J. (2017). *Practical neurology* (5th ed., color plate 37.1). Philadelphia, PA: Wolters Kluwer.

defect), short stature, delayed growth and maturation, microcephaly, and intellectual disability.

Acquired aplastic anemia presents in a manner similar to that of leukemia. It is associated with symptoms of pancytopenia, including excessive fatigue and weakness, lack of energy, and a change in behavior due to anemia; recurrent upper respiratory infections that never completely go away, febrile episodes, and lesions that remain erythemic, open, and unhealing because of leukopenia; and excessive bruising, petechiae, or epistaxis or gum bleeding as a result of thrombocytopenia.

Assessment and Diagnosis

In addition to observation of the signs described earlier, diagnosis of aplastic anemia is typically based on a CBC, with pancytopenia being a positive finding.

Therapeutic Interventions

As with the other anemia disorders, HLA-matched bone marrow or stem cell transplantation is the best option for a cure clinically (Barone et al., 2015; Bhella et al., 2018). The adverse effects of transplantation are rejection (GVHD) and failure to implant. A matched donor is the best source for transplantation, as found in a study by Yagasaki et al. (2010). In this study, 1 out of 30 matched sibling donor grafts were rejected, compared with 3 out of 31 unmatched donor grafts. None of the matched sibling donees had acute grade II to IV GVHD, compared with 37% of the unmatched donees ($P < 0.001$). Yet, chronic GVHD developed in one of the matched siblings and eight of the unmatched recipients, giving a clinically significant difference. As noted in the discussion of this study, these results were comparable to those of prior studies, showing that a long-term survival rate of 5 to 10 years was considered good for either bone marrow donor source, even though not statistically significant between matched and unmatched donors and recipients (Yagasaki et al., 2010).

Another study, by Gupta et al. (2017), in which more current transplantation procedures were involved, revealed no difference in mortality rate between children and young adults with aplastic anemia who were transplanted first (215 of 2,169) and the patients who failed immunosuppression therapy and then received a transplant (180 of 2,169). The 1,774 remaining subjects received immunosuppression therapy and had the lowest mortality rate of the three groups. The variable that did increase mortality rate was receiving platelets before transplantation ($P = 0.002$). The authors reported the worst outcomes for the patients who first failed immunosuppressive therapy and then underwent transplantation with the transplant source being umbilical cord blood ($P \leq 0.05$) compared with those who underwent transplantation with cord blood without failing immunosuppression therapy first.

Clinically, immune system suppression is the treatment goal to reduce the attack on the **hematopoiesis**, or the production of blood components by the bone marrow, and is done using antithymocyte globulin (ATG) most often or antilymphocyte globulin (ALG) and cyclosporin (Bhella et al., 2018; Risitano

& Perna, 2011; Yagasaki et al., 2010). Other treatments may include androgens and corticosteroids (Risitano & Perna, 2011). In severe aplastic anemia, Barone et al. (2015) suggested starting treatment with either a bone marrow transplantation from a matched family donor if available or immunosuppressive therapy with ATG and cyclosporin. If the child's bone marrow responds to treatment with ATG and cyclosporin, the cyclosporin is administered over 12 months, with gradual tapering to maintain the therapeutic response. If relapse occurs following treatment with ATG and cyclosporin, the child may get another ATG and cyclosporin treatment if no donor is available for bone marrow transplantation.

The administration of ATG or ALG is similar to that of a blood component. Monitor the patient for adverse reactions during the infusion, checking vital signs every 15 minutes for an hour. Then, check every 30 minutes for an hour and hourly thereafter during and after the infusion. Monitor and treat the patient with corticosteroids following the infusion to prevent a serious complication, serum sickness. Serum sickness occurs about a week after the child was infused and exhibits symptoms similar to a transfusion reaction.

Although not a common treatment, androgen therapy may be used. When androgens are administered to a prepubertal male child, puberty is induced. Therefore, the growth plates seal, the child stops growing, the voice changes, the gonadal organs grow and change, and facial, pubertal, and underarm hair appear. A 6-year-old, for example, might suddenly experience physical puberty and sexual development while having the mentality of a preschooler. This is the age of best buddies, collections, Boy Scouts, beginning to compete, and understanding rules. Children this age usually do not like members of the opposite sex and see them as weird. Therefore, when administering androgen therapy to prepubertal male child, provide teaching and emotional support to the child and family to help the child adapt to the body changes at this age and into puberty.

The child's hematological needs are treated the same for Fanconi anemia and acquired aplastic anemia as for leukemia. Promote normal growth and development in children with congenital anomalies associated with Fanconi anemia. Engage them in exercises to build fine and gross motor skills, such as the following: working puzzles, pasting, scissor cutting, finger painting, stacking blocks, picking up small items such as raisins and pieces of cereal, feeding themselves, performing gait exercises, rolling over, holding oneself up on the forearms and lifting the chest off of the floor, practicing sitting balance, standing, and weight-bearing on the legs as appropriate. Work with children with sensory problems to help them maximize visual and auditory abilities with glasses, hearing aids, or cochlear implants as needed. Provide education and care regarding any renal issues. If a baby has epispadias or hypospadias, teach the parents to delay circumcision until it is repaired.

Monitor the child's absolute neutrophil and WBC counts for signs of neutropenia. Place the child on neutropenic precautions. With anemia, encourage the child to conserve energy and monitor oxygenation and tissue perfusion. Note any signs of tachypnea or tachycardia, which could indicate compensation for the poor RBC count. Provide thrombocytopenic care for petechiae, bruising, or bleeding, and avoid intramuscular injections and rectal assessment of temperature, which could cause deep tissue injury and hemorrhage.

Evaluation

Expected outcomes for a child with aplastic anemia include the following:

- The child experiences no sepsis, hemorrhage, or life-threatening anemic event.
- Treatment is successful, and red bone marrow is produced.
- For a child with Fanconi anemia, developmental milestones are optimized or mastered.

Discharge Planning and Teaching

The discharge instructions for a child receiving immunosuppressive therapy with ALG or ATG should focus on preventing serum sickness with corticosteroids. Because corticosteroids are foul tasting, instruct parents to try different methods for making them more palatable to the child, such as adding a flavored syrup to them, giving a strongly flavored chaser after administering them, and placing them as far back in the buccal space as possible for liquid preparations and on the tongue for tablets.

If a prepubertal male child is receiving androgen therapy, prepare the family for the pubertal changes and short stature that occurs from epiphyseal growth plates sealing as a result of the treatment; refer them to an endocrinologist for guidance, if needed. Help them learn about using safety razors for shaving the facial hair that develops with puberty.

Pancytopenia indicates a need to assess tissue perfusion and conserve energy. Teach the child and family leukopenia precautions to protect the child from infections. In addition to the infection prevention measures covered earlier for sickle cell disease and beta-thalassemia, neutropenic precautions are initiated when the absolute neutrophil count drops below 1,000 and become very strict when it drops below 500. Have the child wear a face mask when in public; avoid raw fruits, vegetables, and meats; remove live plants from the household because of mold spores; avoid contact with ill people; and observe closely for wounds that remain open and unhealed. Provide thrombocytopenia home care instructions on managing epistaxis, observing for signs of gastrointestinal bleeding, using a very soft toothbrush or cloth to clean the teeth and prevent gingival bleeding, avoiding rough housing or horse play, and avoiding monkey bars or other areas that would place the child at risk for a fall that could lead to internal hemorrhage.

If congenital birth defects are present with Fanconi anemia, a multidisciplinary plan of care is needed, including speech therapy, audiology, physical therapy, and occupational therapy. Provide care for sensory disorders, and provide resources to help the family learn to use sign language to communicate with a deaf child. Teach the family about hearing aid care and

replacing batteries. Instruct parents to keep batteries out of reach of a toddler because ingesting them would result in a medical emergency. If the child is visually impaired, provide instructions to the family on assisting with corrective lenses or functional training for blindness. Encourage the child and family to use facilities that specialize in educating students who have sensory deficits, such as state schools for the deaf and blind. Provide teaching on maximizing orthopedic function, preventing contractures, and using assistive devices to potentiate activities of daily living. Teach the family how to work on strengthening the child's core and assisting with gross motor, fine motor, and language development. Provide exercises and activities that they can incorporate in their home care activities.

Bleeding Disorders

Bleeding disorders can result in visible hemorrhage or internal bleeding. External hemorrhage is very frightening to parents and the public. Since the emergence of the human immunodeficiency virus (HIV) and acquired immune deficiency syndrome, people are fearful of blood. Learn appropriate contact precautions to prevent disease spread, and be prepared to intervene when a bleeding episode occurs. Know how to assess for and treat internal bleeding; initial signs and symptoms may be sudden pain and tissue swelling.

Hemophilia

Hemophilia is a bleeding disorder that is usually inherited and involves a deficit in a coagulation factor, specifically, factor VIII (FVIII) or factor IX (FIX). In some cases, the patient may have a family history of the condition, such as a member who bled to death following a seemingly minor surgery or injury. In other cases, there is no family history of the disease—it just develops unexpectedly in an individual. Either way, the diagnosis is a matter of concern for the family.

Etiology and Pathophysiology

Hemophilia is a coagulopathy in which the child is born without an essential coagulation factor. Figure 25.10 illustrates the coagulation pathway or cascade that leads to the formation of a clot.

Hemophilia A, known as classic hemophilia, is caused by a deficiency in FVIII in the coagulation pathway. It is the most common form of hemophilia and is an X-linked recessive disorder. Hemophilia B, or Christmas disease, is a FIX deficiency in the coagulation pathway. Both forms of hemophilia are typically inherited by sons from mothers who are carriers of the trait (Fig. 25.11). In a couple where the father is unaffected and the mother is a carrier of the trait, any male offspring has a 50% chance of having the disease and any female offspring has a 50% chance of being a carrier of the trait. Overall, with any given birth, this couple would have a 25% chance of having a boy who has hemophilia, a 25% chance of having a girl who is a carrier, a 25% chance of having a boy who is unaffected,

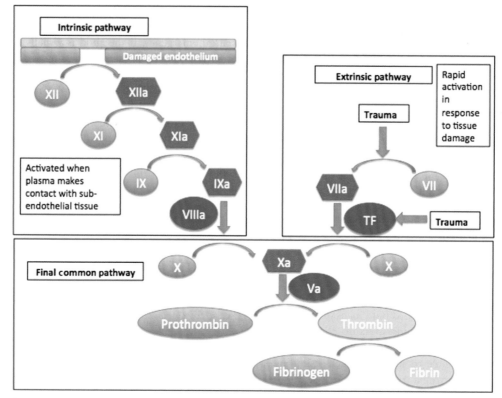

Figure 25.10 Coagulation cascade. The coagulation pathway that leads to blood clot formation. Reprinted with permission from Bucklin, B. A., Baysinger, C. L., & Gambling, D. (2016). *A practical approach to obstetric anesthesia* (2nd ed., Fig. 24.6). Philadelphia, PA: Lippincott Williams & Wilkins.

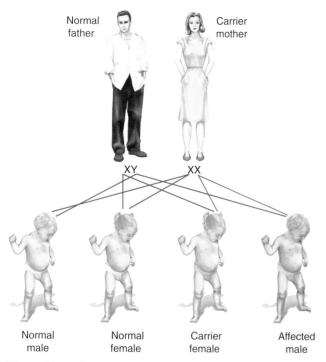

Figure 25.11 Genetic transmission of hemophilia: X-linked recessive inheritance. Reprinted with permission from Kyle, T., & Carman, S. (2016). *Essentials of pediatric nursing* (3rd ed., Fig. 27.3). Philadelphia, PA: Lippincott Williams & Wilkins.

and a 25% chance of having a girl who is unaffected. Genetic odds are just that: a statistical probability. Therefore, despite these odds, a couple with an unaffected father and a carrier mother may have four children and all of them have the hemophilia genotype.

Clinical Presentation

When a child is born with an abnormally low or absent level of a coagulation factor, the ability to clot is impaired. The deficiency factor results in spontaneous or traumatic bleeding. These children can have hemophilia that ranges in severity from mild (>5% to ≤40% FVIII or FIX activity) to moderate (1% to 5% FVIII or FIX activity) to severe (<1% FVIII or FIX activity), based on the amount of factor produced and used (Zappa, Mc-Daniel, Marandola, & Allen, 2012, p. e141). Hemorrhages in a child with hemophilia are typically contained within the tissues and commonly occur in a joint when the synovial capsule sustains friction that damages capillaries, resulting in an acute joint bleed. In a child with severe hemophilia, activities as mild as throwing a ball, walking across a grassy lawn briskly, and lifting and tugging on the shoulder joint may cause bleeding. In a child mildly affected with hemophilia, more intense trauma, such as a fall or bumping into a wall while walking at school, is required to trigger a bleed. Obviously, cuts, falls, and injuries that open the flesh result in a prolonged and excessive bleeding episode.

The acute bleed is associated with swelling, pain, redness, and, eventually, ecchymotic or purpuric coloration. After the bleeding is controlled, the joint is swollen and painful, with limited movement, a condition called hemarthrosis.

Assessment and Diagnosis

In addition to observing for signs and symptoms of hemophilia-associated bleeding, monitoring laboratory values for prothrombin time (PT), partial thromboplastin time (PTT), and hemophilia factor levels is critical both in initial assessment and to determine whether coagulation factor replacement therapy is working. PT and PTT are both tests that measure the time required to form a clot (coagulate) and thus the presence and function of various clotting factors. Specifically, PT measures the time required for extrinsic clotting factors to perform their part in coagulation, which is normally 11 to 13.5 seconds in children. PTT measures the time required for intrinsic clotting factors, which include FVIII and FIX, to perform their part in coagulation, which is normally 25 to 35 seconds. Hemophilia factor assays measure the blood levels of specific coagulation factors that are deficient in hemophilia (FVIII and FIX). Increased PT and PTT and decreased levels of coagulation factors may indicate hemophilia.

Therapeutic Interventions

The mainstay of treatment is factor replacement (The Pharmacy 25.4). For patients with severe hemophilia A, the recommendation for prophylactic treatment with FVIII is about 3 times weekly of 20 to 50 U/kg. Children with mild or moderate hemophilia A may get prophylactic treatment but are more likely to get factor on demand with injury. FVIII on-demand treatment varies in dose depending on the type of bleed: for joint hemorrhages, 40 to 50 U/kg every 12 to 24 hours; for large muscle hemorrhages, intracranial bleeds, or other severe hemorrhages, 50 U/kg continuously to intermittent infusions every 8,

12, or 24 hours (Zappa et al., 2012). Another source calculated that the dosage of FVIII of 1 U/kg would increase the plasma factor concentration 2%, that a child with severe bleeding needs an increase in plasma factor concentration of 80% to 100%, and that a child with moderate bleeding needs an increase in plasma factor concentration of 40% (Marcdante & Kliegman, 2015).

Similarly, children with severe hemophilia B (Christmas disease) are treated with FIX, but the dose range is broader and less consistent, around 40 to 100 U/kg. The on-demand doses of pediatric FIX are also less consistent, ranging from 30 to 100 U/kg every day. A child with an intracranial or serious bleed may be given a continuous infusion or intermittent doses up to every other day (Zappa et al., 2012). A dose of 1.5 U/kg of FIX raises the plasma concentration 1%, with an increase of 80% to 100% needed for a severe bleed and an increase of 30% to 40% needed for a mild-to-moderate event (Marcdante & Kliegman, 2015).

Preparing the factor for administration depends on how it is supplied. Because the factor is very expensive, if the ordered dose is slightly less than a vial when reconstituted, contact the prescriber and request authorization to give the entire vial to avoid waste.

At one time, the factor was obtained from large pools of human plasma. Many donors would sell their blood for use in producing the factor. During this time, those with hemophilia were greatly affected by infectious outbreaks of HIV and hepatitis B, C, and D. New procedures in producing the recombinant factor for replacement have reduced the viral transmission.

Unfortunately, the factor has inhibitors that develop as part of an immune reaction in deficient individuals. These inhibitors prohibit the factor from adequately producing coagulation. New procedures to counteract the inhibitors are being developed and are used to form clots in the presence of these inhibitors. If the prothrombin level is high and not responding to the

The Pharmacy 25.4 Factor VIII

Classification	Route	Action	Nursing Considerations
Antihemophilic agent	IV	• Provides the protein factor VIII, needed for clotting • Activates factor X, which converts prothrombin to thrombin, which in turn converts fibrinogen to fibrin, forming a clot	• Administer within 3 hours of reconstitution. • Administer in a separate line. • Do not mix with other medications or IV fluids. • Ensure that the child is vaccinated against hepatitis B virus. • Monitor for anaphylaxis.

IV, intravenous.
Adapted from Taketomo, C. K., Hodding, J. H., & Kraus, D. M. (2018). *Pediatric & neonatal dosage handbook* (25th ed.). Hudson, OH: Lexicomp.

factor replacement, the patient is likely continuing to hemorrhage as a result of the inhibitors, which are immunoglobulin G antibodies. The coagulation is achieved by administering agents that produce clotting in spite of the factor deficit, such as factor VIIa, activated prothrombin complex concentrate (Gringeri et al., 2011; Marcdante & Kliegman, 2019).

Although factor replacement is the priority to stop bleeding, treating hemorrhages also includes local measures. Teach the family and child the mnemonic RICE. "R" is for rest. The child should stop using the joint that is bleeding. "I" refers to the need to ice the area, which causes vasoconstriction and slows the blood loss. "C" indicates compression. Applying pressure to the site of the bleeding helps to slow and stop the bleeding to the area. "E" stands for elevate the injured area, which also helps to slow the blood loss. Teach the family to have ice packs, gallon bags of frozen alcohol and water in a 50/50 concentration, or frozen vegetables in the freezer ready to use at all times. Ace bandages may be used to apply compression, as well as direct hand compression. School nurses must also be prepared to care for the child at school and have the needed supplies to treat bleeding episodes. Gloving is important with any body fluid exposures.

Another key treatment is desmopressin acetate (DDAVP), which increases the FVIII level to three to four times the circulating level in those with mild or moderate hemophilia A (The Pharmacy 25.5). Teach patients how to administer this medication intranasally. The child must clear the nasal passages before dosing. DDAVP is a synthetic antidiuretic hormone. It causes the body to retain water and may cause hyponatremia, hypertension, and congestive heart failure. Teach patients using this medication to report inadequate urine output or if there is a urinary or respiratory tract infection while using it. Some patients may be placed on a fluid restriction, especially when at risk for water intoxication.

For dental procedures, administration of aminocaproic acid helps with clot formation by blocking fibrinolysis. The child's dentist should plan and supervise the shedding of deciduous teeth and administer aminocaproic acid to the child ahead of time. The child may also be given factor replacement and be scheduled for deciduous teeth pulling to control bleeding with this common preschool or school-age occurrence.

Evaluation

Expected outcomes for a child with hemophilia include the following:

- The child maintains normal PT, PTT, and coagulation factor levels.
- The child maintains full range of motion in all joints.
- The child engages in developmentally appropriate activities that offer a low risk of injury that could lead to bleeding.
- The child and family demonstrate an understanding of appropriate risk prevention measures, medication administration, and identification of signs of various types of bleeding.
- The child and family have a strong social support system in place.

Discharge Planning and Teaching

At discharge, teach the family how to identify signs of bleeding and proper actions to take in response. Review with them the current plan of care for exercise and regaining motion in any joint that has had bleeding. Stress the importance of active range of motion over passive because it decreases the risk of bleeding due to overextending the joint. Suggest that they use exercises such as taping a reward at a challenging height and having the child walk the arm up the wall to reach it for an involved upper extremity joint. Educate the family on and evaluate their knowledge of prophylactic and treatment factor replacement and RICE intervention for active bleeding at home (Patient Teaching 25.1). Discuss growth and developmental milestones and provide anticipatory guidance as appropriate for the child's age level. If the child has mild or moderate hemophilia, include information on DDAVP. The National Hemophilia Foundation is a good source of information to help the family learn about the condition and resources. A detailed discussion of these topics is included later.

Teach the family how to diligently assess for and identify the signs of intracranial, gastrointestinal, and renal bleeding. Intracranial bleeding may be indicated by a sudden severe headache, nausea and vomiting, dizziness, visual disturbances, changes in

The Pharmacy 25.5 Desmopressin

Classification	Route	Action	Nursing Considerations
• Antihemophilic agent • Hemostatic agent	• IN • IV • PO	• Increases plasma levels of von Willebrand factor • Increases plasma levels of Factor VIII	• Monitor for hyponatremia-induced seizures. • Monitor fluid intake in young children to prevent water intoxication. • Monitor electrolytes. • Monitor for nasal scarring with intranasal use.

IN, intranasal; IV, intravenous; PO, oral.
Adapted from Taketomo, C. K., Hodding, J. H., & Kraus, D. M. (2018). *Pediatric & neonatal dosage handbook* (25th ed.). Hudson, OH: Lexicomp.

Patient Teaching 25.1

Administering Factor VIII

Inform parents that if their child is injured, they may need to give clotting factor at home. It is important for them to know the steps to administer the clotting factor to their child, which are listed here. Explain that once their child is old enough, he or she can learn to self-administer the clotting factor.

1. Use the child's central line or port for venous access.
2. If no CVAD is available, use a butterfly needle.
3. Add diluent to the factor powder.
4. Roll the vial in your hands or gently tip it to invert it back and forth until the powder is dissolved.
5. Draw the reconstituted factor into the syringe and administer it intravenously via infusion or intravenous push.

---

motor function or gait, or seizures. Any head injury needs to be evaluated. Vomit that has the appearance of coffee grounds or contains bright red blood denotes upper abdominal or stomach bleeding. Unexplained abdominal pain or swelling and stool changes that are black and tarry or bright red may indicate gastrointestinal hemorrhage. Urine with a red, bloody to an amber-orange character may be a sign of bleeding.

One of the most frequent sites for bleeding in children with hemophilia is in the joints. A joint injury can lead to a severe deformity and a frozen joint. Movement is essential to maintain function and mobility. Therefore, once the bleeding is controlled, encourage parents to perform active range of motion exercises involving the affected joint. Active range of motion is better than passive because using passive could stretch the joint too far and cause synovial injury to recur. The injured joint is likely to be very painful, but stress to the parents the importance of the child engaging in activities that require the full range of motion in the joint. Having the child reach for a toy or stretch the hand high on the wall to retrieve a sticker, washable tattoo, or other appropriate reward can motivate the child to perform active range of motion in the shoulder or elbow joint. Playing with a ball and rolling it forward and back with the foot can assist the child in using full range of motion in the knee joint. Interdisciplinary collaboration with physical and occupational therapists can also help the child maintain joint motion.

Provide the child and parents with anticipatory guidance related to helping the child meet upcoming developmental milestones. Discuss immunizations that the child will need to receive, and explain that they will need to be administered subcutaneously instead of intramuscularly to prevent muscle bleeding. For parents of children who are ready to begin standing, walking, and toddling, provide directions on preventing injuries. Encourage parents to allow walking only on intact carpeted areas, to pad or cover fireplaces, and to remove furniture with sharp corners to make any falls and bumps as benign as possible. Sewing padding in the pants to protect knees and hips may be needed to prevent hemorrhage while allowing the child to gain these skills.

Once the child is old enough to participate in team sports, inform the parents of the risks of the child engaging in activities that involve contact or have a high likelihood of injury, such as baseball, soccer, and football. Suggest that they encourage the child to swim, golf, and participate in such activities as the scholar's bowl, chess team, and journalism club. When the child reaches puberty and needs to begin shaving, encourage the use of an electric razor. Teach the family that the child should take acetaminophen for pain and avoid nonsteroidal anti-inflammatory drugs, such as aspirin, naproxen, and ibuprofen, which inhibit platelet function.

Von Willebrand Disease

Von Willebrand disease is genetic bleeding disorder that occurs when the individual is deficient in the von Willebrand factor (vWF). Once believed to be a carrier state of hemophilia A, it is now known as a completely separate disease state. The vWF works directly with FVIII in the coagulation pathway.

Etiology and Pathophysiology

Von Willebrand disease is autosomal dominant (Fig. 25.12). The vWF helps with coagulation in two key ways. First, it acts as a link between the subendothelial collagen and platelets. Second, it binds to FVIII in the circulation and safeguards it from clearing the circulation too fast. There are three levels of von Willebrand disease. Type 1 involves insufficient amounts of vWF. Type 2 involves the quality of vWF being poor and is known as a dysproteinemia. Type 3 involves the total absence of vWF. Most people with von Willebrand disease have type 1, with a mild-to-moderate deficit of vWF (Marcdante & Kliegman, 2015).

Clinical Presentation

This condition is characterized by mucosal bleeding, epistaxis, gingival bleeding, excessively large bruising, with the width of the bruise averaging the size of the palm of the child's hand, and telangiectasias (Fig. 25.13). In young pubertal females, this condition can manifest as serious hemorrhage during the menstrual cycle, a condition known as menorrhagia. Occasionally, in severe cases, in which FVIII levels are very low, the patient may experience hemarthrosis, like a person with hemophilia.

Assessment and Diagnosis

Assessment and diagnosis are similar as for hemophilia. In addition to the PT and PTT tests and coagulation factor assays (described in the Assessment and Diagnosis section of hemophilia, above), assessment includes assays of vWF level and activity. Low vWF levels and activity indicate von Willebrand disease; by contrast, these same measures are normal in hemophilia (Marcdante & Kliegman, 2019).

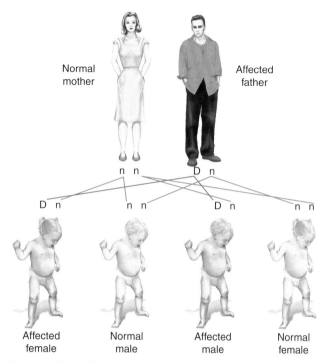

Figure 25.12 Genetic transmission of von Willebrand disease: Autosomal dominant inheritance. If a child has one von Willebrand gene, clinical symptoms are present. Reprinted with permission from Kyle, T., & Carman, S. (2016). *Essentials of pediatric nursing* (3rd ed., Fig. 27.1). Philadelphia, PA: Lippincott Williams & Wilkins.

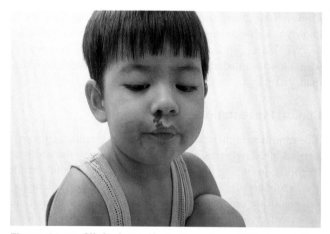

Figure 25.13 Clinical manifestation of von Willebrand disease: Nose bleed in a child.

Therapeutic Interventions

Treating von Willebrand disease is accomplished by prophylactic and scheduled doses of DDAVP and human antihemophilic factor (FVIII)/vWF complex (Franchini, Targher, & Lippi, 2007). Antihemophilic factor/vWF may also be administered on demand, following an injury that causes significant bleeding. In such cases, when ordered, administer this treatment as soon as possible following the injury.

Control nose bleeds by applying pressure to the nose. If the physician or primary care provider approves, pack the nares with nasal spray containing epinephrine to help vasoconstrict the area. Applying sterile lubricating gel helps prevent crusting in the nares after bleeding has stopped. If bleeding occurs in the eyes, clean the blood from the eyes with saline drops. As with hemophilia, avoid giving intramuscular injections and assessing temperature rectally, which can injure the tissues and result in bleeding.

Evaluation

Expected outcomes for a child with von Willebrand disease include the following:

- Bleeding episodes are managed promptly and effectively, with minimal blood loss.
- Menorrhagia in females is significantly decreased.
- The child maintains normal PT, PTT, and coagulation factor levels.
- The child maintains full range of motion in all joints.
- The child and family demonstrate an understanding of appropriate risk prevention measures, medication administration, and identification of signs of various types of bleeding.

Discharge Planning and Teaching

Discharge teaching includes many of the same measures discussed in caring for an individual with hemophilia or aplastic anemia, above. Teach parents and children how to treat epistaxis and other types of bleeding. For epistaxis, instruct them to apply direct pressure to the nose, keep the child's head upright, and apply an ice pack over the nose and on the neck. Direct them to administer DDAVP and FVIII/vWF as indicated. Educate pubertal females on how to manage menorrhagia. In some cases, birth control may be used to lighten menstrual periods or avoid them altogether. Some may use prophylactic factor replacement or DDAVP to control bleeding.

Disseminated Intravascular Coagulation

Disseminated intravascular coagulation (DIC) is a condition characterized by systemic coagulation throughout the bloodstream (due to thrombosis from stimulated thrombin) and consequent hemorrhage (due to fibrinolysis stimulated by plasmin), which uses up all the available coagulation factors. DIC is a secondary consequence in children that occurs because of some severe disease process or injury that is associated with hypoxia, acidosis, shock, burns, or sepsis and that is heralded by simultaneous bleeding and clotting. It is an emergency for an already ill child.

Etiology and Pathophysiology

DIC has many causes and may develop as a complication of any of the following: sepsis, shock, cancer, obstetrical conditions (placenta abruption, fetal demise syndrome, preeclampsia/eclampsia, or amniotic fluid embolism), burns, massive trauma, snake bites, heat stroke, or transfusion reactions (Marcdante & Kliegman, 2019; Porth, 2015; Schub & Balderrama, 2018). Regardless of the specific etiology, DIC involves the widespread formation of clots throughout the circulation, with many small blood vessels becoming occluded. The intrinsic and extrinsic coagulation pathways are activated and exhausted. Once the coagulation factors and platelets are consumed, bleeding results.

Clinical Presentation

Clinically, the patient may experience peripheral thrombosis (positive Homan's sign), excessive bleeding from a venipuncture, oozing from old entry sites, petechiae, ecchymoses, purpura, epistaxis, gingival bleeding, gastrointestinal or pulmonary hemorrhage, tachycardia, hypotension, and muscle, back, or chest pain (Marcdante & Kliegman, 2019; Porth, 2015; Schub & Balderrama, 2018). Signs that may indicate an intracranial bleed or clot include a sudden headache, slurred speech, and asymmetrical movements (Marcdante & Kliegman, 2019; Porth, 2011; Schub & Balderrama, 2018).

Assessment and Diagnosis

Assessment includes observation of the clinical signs discussed earlier, as well as laboratory tests related to clotting time and blood cell counts, such as PT, PTT, and CBC (including platelet count). The diagnosis is confirmed when laboratory test results reveal thrombocytopenia, low fibrinogen levels, and elevated PT, PTT, and D-dimer levels.

Therapeutic Interventions

Treatment of a child with DIC is focused on maintaining oxygenation and tissue perfusion, correcting acidosis, and replacing depleted coagulation factors. As ordered, administer intravenous platelets, fresh frozen plasma, and cryoprecipitate. Administer heparin or low-molecular-weight heparin to keep the coagulation factors that are being replaced from activating and continuing the hemorrhage (Marcdante & Kliegman, 2019; Porth, 2011; Schub & Balderrama, 2018).

Nursing care should include ongoing assessment of patients for signs and symptoms of microvascular clot formation and possible emboli; altered mental state; sudden hypoxia; shortness of breath; hemoptysis, hematemesis, or other types of hemorrhage; tachycardia related to volume depletion; and hypotension. Monitor the results of laboratory studies such as platelet count, PT, and PTT. Assist with therapy and treatment of the underlying disease that triggered the process of DIC (Schub & Balderrama, 2018).

Evaluation

Expected outcomes for a child with DIC include the following:

- Intravascular coagulation is stopped, and the child returns to homeostasis.
- The child has no embolism that causes permanent impairment.
- If bleeding occurs, it is rapidly controlled and the child survives this life-threatening event.

Discharge Planning and Teaching

A child who is being discharged following DIC will likely continue taking heparin, low-molecular-weight heparin, or another anticoagulant at home for a period of time. Teach the child and parents how to take the medication, the side effects to monitor for, and what laboratory tests are required to monitor levels weekly or monthly, depending on therapy length. Instruct the child to slowly resume activities when the bleeding risk has subsided.

Think Critically

1. What nursing interventions should be implemented for a 3-year-old who has been admitted in vasoocclusive crisis with wheezing and shortness of breath?
2. What are some pain control measures to implement for a child with vasoocclusive crisis?
3. When preparing a child for chelation therapy with deferoxamine, what interventions need to be initiated?
4. When administering a transfusion of packed RBCs to a child with beta-thalassemia, what signs and symptoms would indicate a transfusion reaction? What would be the nurse's priority action?
5. A child is preparing to be discharged following ATG therapy for acquired aplastic anemia. Develop a plan of care for the child's discharge.
6. You are counseling a couple on the genetic transmission of hemophilia. The male has mild hemophilia; the female is without the trait. What are the odds that any given son born to them will have the disease? What are the odds that any given daughter born to them will be a carrier? How would these odds change if the female were a carrier of the trait, in addition to the male having the disease?
7. What measures should a nurse implement for a 4-month-old with a bleeding disorder who is coming in for immunizations?
8. What nursing interventions should be used for epistaxis?
9. A teenaged girl with von Willebrand disease is having menorrhagia. What assessment findings would indicate that she needs a blood transfusion?
10. A child with DIC is experiencing chest pain, shortness of breath, tachypnea, tachycardia, sweating and lightheadedness, and declining oxygen saturation levels. What should the nurse do first?

References

Al-Kuriashy, H. M., & Al-Gareeb, A. I. (2017). Comparison of deferasirox and deferoxamine effects on iron overload and immunological changes in patients with blood transfusion-dependent β-thalassaemia. *Asian Journal of Transfusion Science, 11*, 13–17.

Bahnasawy, S. M., El Wakeel, L. M., El Beblawy, N., & El-Hamamsy, M. (2017). Clinical pharmacist-provided services in iron-overloaded beta-thalassaemia major children: A new insight into patient care. *Basic & Clinical Pharmacology & Toxicology, 120*, 354–359.

Barone, A., Lucarelli, A., Onofrillo, D., Verzegnassi, F., Bonanomi, S., Cesaro, S., . . . Saracco, P. (2015). Diagnosis and management of acquired aplastic anemia in childhood. Guidelines from the Marrow Failure Study Group of the Pediatric Heamato-Oncology Italian Association. *Blood Cells, Molecules, and Diseases, 55*, 40–47.

Bhella, S., Majhail, N. S., Betcher, J., Costa, L. J., Daly, A., Dandoy, C. E., . . . Seftel, M. D. (2018). Choosing wisely BMT: American Society for Blood and Marrow Transplantation and Canadian Blood and Marrow Transplant Group's List of 5 Tests and Treatments to Question in Blood and Bone Marrow Transplantation. *Biology of Blood and Marrow Transplantation, 24*, 909–913.

Cunningham, M. J., Macklin, E. A., Neufeld, E. J., Cohen, A. R., & Thalassemia Clinical Research Network. (2004). Complications of β-thalassemia major in North America. *Blood, 104*(1), 34–39.

Food and Drug Administration (2017). FDA approves hydroxyurea for the treatment of pediatric patients with sickle cell. Retrieved from: https://www.fda.gov/drugs/resources-information-approved-drugs/fda-approves-hydroxyurea-treatment-pediatric-patients-sickle-cell-anemia

Franchini, M., Targher, G., & Lippi, G. (2007). Prophylaxis in von Willebrand disease. *Annals of Hematology, 86*, 699–704.

Geiger, T.L. & Howard, S.C. (2007). Acetaminophen and diphenhydramine premedication for allergic and febrile nonhemolytic transfusion reactions: Good prophylaxis or bad practice? *Transfusion Medicine Reviews, 21*, 1–12.

Gringeri, A., Lundin, B., von Mackensen, S., Mantovani, L., Mannucci,P., & The ESPRIT Study Group. (2011). A randomized clinical trial of prophylaxis in children with hemophilia A (the ESPRIT Study). *Journal of Thromosis and Haemostasis, 9,* 700–710.

Gupta, A., Fu, P., Hashem, H., Vatsayan, A., Shein, S., & Dalal, J. (2017). Outcomes and health care utilization in children and young adults with aplastic anemia: A multiinstitutional analysis. *Pediatric Blood and Cancer, 64*, 1–7. doi:10.1002/pbc.26704

Hankins, J. S., Aygun, B., Nottage, K., Thornburg, C., Smeltzer, M. P., Ware, R. E., & Wang, W. C. (2014). From infancy to adolescence: Fifteen years of continuous treatment with hydroxyurea in sickle cell anemia. *Medicine, 93*(28), 1–5.

Ibrahim, M. H., Azab, A. A., Kamal, N. M., Salama, M. A., Ebrahim, S. A., Shahin, A. M., . . . Abdalla, E. A. A. (2016). Early detection of myocardial dysfunction in poorly treated pediatric thalassemia children and adolescents: Two Saudi centers experience. *Annals of Medicine and Surgery, 9*, 6–11.

Manwani, D., & Frenetti, P. S. (2013). Vaso-occlusion in sickle cell disease: Pathophysiology and novel targeted therapies. *Blood, 122*, 3892–3898.

Marcdante, K. J., & Kliegman, R. M. (2019). *Nelson's essentials of pediatrics* (8th ed.). Philadelphia, PA: Elsevier.

Meier, E. R., Dioguardi, J. V., & Kamani, N. (2015). Current attitudes of parents and patients toward hematopoietic stem cell transplantation for sickle cell anemia. *Pediatric Blood and Cancer, 62*(7), 1277–1284.

Noronha, S., Sadreameli, S. C., & Strouse, J. J. (2016). Management of sickle cell disease in children. *Southern Medical Journal, 109*(9), 494–502.

Nottage, K. A., Ware, R. E., Winter, B., Smeltzer, M., Wang, W. C., Hankins, J. S., . . . Aygun, B. (2014). Predictors of splenic function preservation in children with sickle cell anemia treated with hydroxyurea. *European Journal of Haematology, 93*, 377–383. doi:10.1111/ejh.12361

Oringanje, C., Nemecek, E., & Oniyanga, O. (2016). Hematopoietic stem cell transplantation for people with sickle cell disease (Review). *Cochrane Library: Cochrane Database of Systematic Reviews, 5*, 1–11.

Orrù, S., Orrù, N., Manolakos, E., Littera, R., Caocci, G., Giorgiani, G., . . . La Nasa, G. (2012). Recipient CTLA-4*CT60-AA genotype is a prognostic factor for acute graft-versus-host disease in hematopoietic stem cell transplantation for thalassemia. *Human Immunology, 73*(3), 282–286.

Physician's Digital Reference. (2018). Retrieved from http://www.pdr.net

Porth, C. M. (2015). *Essentials of pathophysiology* (4th ed.). Philadelphia, PA: Wolters Kluwer Lippincott Williams & Wilkins.

Risitano, A. M., & Perna, F. (2011). Aplastic anemia: Immunosuppressive therapy in 2010. *Pediatric Reports, 3*(s2:e7), 14–17.

Rund, D., & Rachmilewitz, E. (2005). Beta-thalassemia. *The New England Journal of Medicine, 353*(11), 1135–1146.

Schub, E., & Balderrama, D. (2018). *Quick lessons . . . Disseminated intravascular coagulation*. Glendale, CA: Cinahl Information Systems|Ebsco, Inc.

Taketomo, C. K., Hodding, J. H., & Kraus, D. M. (2018). *Pediatric & neonatal dosage handbook* (25th ed.). Hudson, OH: Lexicomp.

Thompson, L. M., Ceja, M. E., & Yang, S. P. (2012). Stem cell transplantation for treatment of sickle cell disease: Bone marrow versus cord blood transplants. *American Journal of Health- System Pharmacists, 69*, 1295–1303.

Wang, W. C., Ware, R. E., Miller, S. T., Iyer, R. V., Casella, J. F., Minniti, C. P., . . . Thompson, B. W. (2011). Hydroxycarbamide in very young children with sickle-cell anaemia: A multicentre, randomised, controlled trial (BABY HUG). *Lancet, 377*, 1663–1672.

Williams, H., & Tanabe, P. (2016). Sickle cell disease: A review of nonpharmacological approaches for pain. *Journal of Pain and Symptom Management, 51*(2), 163–177.

Yagasaki, H., Takahashi, Y., Hama, A., Kudo, K., Nishio, N., Muramatsu, H., . . . Kojima, S. (2010). Comparison of matched sibling-donor BMT and unrelated donor BMT in children and adolescents with severe aplastic anemia. *Bone Marrow Transplant, 45*, 1508–1513.

Zappa, S., McDaniel, M., Marandola, J., & Allen, G. (2012). Treatment trends for haemophilia A and B in the United States: Results from the 2010 practice patterns survey. *Haemophilia, 18*, e140–e153.

Suggested Readings

Marcdante, K. J., & Kliegman, R. M. (2019). *Nelson's essentials of pediatrics* (8th ed.). Philadelphia, PA: Elsevier.

Muscari, M. E. (2015). *Lippincott's review series: Pediatric nursing* (5th ed.). Philadelphia, PA: Wolters-Kluwer Health|Lippincott Williams & Wilkins.

Oliver, M. M. (2015). *Pediatric nursing made incredibly easy!* Philadelphia, PA: Wolters-Kluwer Health|Lippincott Williams & Wilkins.

26 Oncological Disorders

Objectives

After completing this chapter, you will be able to:

1. Explain the differences between pediatric and adult cancers.
2. Identify and differentiate between signs and symptoms of various types of pediatric cancer.
3. Discuss the adverse effects of treatment for cancer.
4. Identify signs and symptoms of oncologic emergencies.
5. Describe the psychological impact of a pediatric cancer diagnosis on the family.
6. Prepare a developmentally appropriate teaching plan for children diagnosed with cancer and their families.
7. Plan nursing interventions for the child undergoing chemotherapy treatment.

Key Terms

Aniridia
Apoptosis
Chloroma
Diaphysis
Intrathecal
Leukocoria

Metaphysis
Neoplasm
Oncogenesis
Proto-oncogene
Tumor suppressor gene

Although cancer is the leading cause of disease-related mortality in children older than 1 year, the incidence of cancer is rare. Pediatric cancers represent only 1% of all cancer cases in the United States (Asselin, 2016). In children and adolescents younger than age 20 years, it is estimated that 15,590 will be diagnosed in the next year and that 1,780 of those diagnosed will not survive (National Cancer Institute, 2018). Over the years, the survival rate for pediatric cancer has increased by as much as 20%. In the past 10 years, brain tumors have replaced leukemia as the leading cause of death from cancer in children and adolescents 1 to 19 years old (Curtin, Minino, & Anderson, 2016). The current 5-year average survival rate for all pediatric cancers is 83% in children 14 years and younger and 84.2% in adolescents aged 15 to 19 years old. Certain types of pediatric cancer have higher survival rates, such as acute lymphocytic leukemia at 90% for children 14 years and younger and Non-Hodgkin lymphoma (NHL) at 90.6% for children 14 years and younger (Siegel, Miller, & Jemal, 2018). Because the survival rate has increased, healthcare providers are focusing on the health and quality of life of childhood cancer survivors.

Having a child diagnosed with any type of cancer is devastating for a family. Treatment is complex, requiring multiple hospital stays. Most children diagnosed with cancer are treated at a pediatric hospital that is a member of the Children's Oncology Group (American Cancer Society [ACS], 2016c). Often, the locations of these hospitals require families to travel long distances for their children's treatment. Nurses should be keenly aware of the emotional distress of the child and family that occurs with a life-threatening illness. Nurses can ensure that not only the medical needs of the child and family are met but the psychological needs, as well.

Variations in Anatomy and Physiology

The genes involved in **oncogenesis** are the same in both children and adults. **Proto-oncogenes** regulate cell growth, division, and differentiation. Under certain conditions, proto-oncogenes mutate to form oncogenes, which allow for unchecked cellular growth and lack of differentiation, resulting in malignancy. A second type of gene, the **tumor suppressor gene** is also involved in oncogenesis. Tumor suppressor genes are involved in cell growth and normal cell death, or **apoptosis**. Uncontrolled regulation of tumor suppressor cells results in a **neoplasm**, which may be malignant or benign (Worth, 2016).

The process of oncogenesis is the same in children and in adults. However, the etiology of cancer varies greatly between children and adults. The reason for the formation of oncogenes in children is largely unknown. Only 5% of cases of pediatric cancer are associated with inherited genetic mutations or certain genetic syndromes (National Cancer Institute, 2018). Genetic mutations can also occur during fetal development, resulting in certain types of cancers.

Childhood Versus Adult Cancers

The types of cancer common in childhood differ greatly from those that typically occur in adults. Cancers that occur in childhood typically arise from embryonic cells, the lymphohematopoietic system, or the central nervous system (CNS). Adult cancers typically arise from the epithelial layer of organs, which is associated with breast, colon, lung, and prostate cancers (Asselin, 2016). The etiology of childhood cancers is not well understood and is thought to be multifactorial, whereas the majority of adult cancers are due to environmental exposure, making these types of cancer preventable.

Because so little is known about the causes of childhood cancers, they are difficult to prevent. However, nurses can educate parents and children on living a healthy lifestyle as a means of cancer prevention. Children and adolescents should receive all recommended immunizations, eat a nutritious diet, stay active, and prevent exposure to radiation by avoiding unnecessary X-rays and computed tomography (CT) scans. Table 26.1 shows a comparison of childhood and adult cancers.

Syndromes Associated With Pediatric Cancer

Certain genetic conditions are associated with increased risk of cancer in childhood. These conditions account for fewer than 5% of all pediatric cancers (Asselin, 2016). Children with neurofibromatosis type 1 or 2 have an increased risk of optic gliomas and peripheral nerve tumors. Those with von Hippel–Lindau disease are at increased risk of kidney and pancreatic cancer. The risk of leukemia is increased in children with Down syndrome.

Other Factors Associated With Pediatric Cancer

There are many theories as to the causes of some pediatric cancers. Diet and exposure to electromagnetic fields, pesticides, or chemicals from parental occupations have been studied as possible causes for childhood cancer, but these studies have not produced any statistically significant evidence. Viruses have been shown to be associated with certain types of cancer. The human papillomavirus is associated with cervical cancer. The Epstein–Barr virus is associated with NHL, although this association is less clear (Asselin, 2016).

Assessment of the Child for Oncological Disorders

Symptoms of cancer in children and adolescents are often nonspecific. Most children with cancer present with fatigue and weight loss. Other signs and symptoms include petechiae, bruising, pain, pallor, and recurrent infections. Signs and symptoms of cancer often mimic those of other childhood illnesses, resulting in a delay in diagnosis. Because of this delay, many

Table 26.1	Comparison of Childhood and Adult Cancers	
	Childhood Cancer	**Adult Cancer**
Origin	Embryonic cells, blood cells, central nervous system	Epithelial cells
Part of the body affected	Tissues, bone marrow components	Solid organs
Cause	Not well understood	Mainly due to environmental toxins
Prevention	Human papillomavirus vaccine; most not preventable	Most are preventable through screening and limiting exposure to toxins
Response to treatment	Highly responsive	Less responsive

Data from American Cancer Society, 2016c.

types of childhood cancer have metastasized by the time the child receives the proper diagnosis.

Take a careful health history of the child's presenting illness. Enquire about the location and intensity of any pain, using the appropriate pain scale. Ask whether the child or adolescent has had any recent and/or recurrent infections. Determine whether fever is present. Note any unusual bruising or petechiae. Assess the conjunctiva and mucous membranes for pallor, indicating anemia. Palpate for hepatosplenomegaly. Assess for swelling around the joints or other areas of the extremities.

General Nursing Interventions for the Child Undergoing Treatment for Cancer

Care of the child with cancer requires a multidisciplinary team that includes nurses, physicians, oncologists, radiation oncologists, surgeons, nutritionists, social workers, physical therapists, child life specialists, psychologists, and others. Working as a team is imperative to achieve desired outcomes for the child and family. Treatments include surgery, chemotherapy, radiation, and, possibly, hematopoietic stem cell transplantation (HSCT).

Children diagnosed with cancer need long-term follow-up. Survival rates for pediatric cancer have increased, and many of the long-term side effects of treatment are unknown. Morbidity in childhood cancer survivors includes problems such as secondary neoplasms, growth retardation, infertility, and cardiomyopathy related to chemotherapy (Seth, Singh, Setj, & Sapra, 2017). In addition to measuring growth and development and physical effects of treatment, healthcare providers must evaluate long-term psychosocial effects of cancer on the child. Childhood cancer survivors are at risk for anxiety disorder and post-traumatic stress disorder (McDonnell et al., 2017). Regular follow-up is needed to monitor growth and development and quality of life and to monitor for complications.

Treatment for children with cancer often includes participation in clinical trials. Clinical trials evaluate the effectiveness of a new treatment on childhood cancers. Children with newly diagnosed cancer, cancers that are difficult to treat, or recurrent cancer may be eligible for clinical trials. Refer families interested in information about clinical trials to the National Institutes of Health's National Cancer Institute (n.d.) (https://ccr.cancer.gov/pediatric-oncology-branch).

Caring for the Child on Chemotherapy

Children with malignant tumors or cancer of the blood or lymph nodes are treated with chemotherapy. Chemotherapy is given intravenously, orally, and, if required for treatment, via the **intrathecal** route. Most children requiring chemotherapy have a central line placed (see Fig. 6.5). Having a central line decreases the number of needlesticks a child experiences and lowers the chances of infiltration.

Patient Safety 26.1

Chemotherapy Administration Standards

To prevent errors in the preparation and administration of chemotherapy, including that for pediatric patients, the safety standards from the American Society of Clinical Oncology and the Oncology Nursing Society include, but are not limited to, the following:

- Chemotherapy must be prepared by a trained pharmacist.
- Parenteral chemotherapy orders must be electronic or preprinted.
- No verbal orders may be accepted for chemotherapy, other than to stop an infusion.
- Before the administration of chemotherapy, the child and family are provided with education regarding treatment plan and potential side effects of chemotherapy.
- Chemotherapy may only be administered by nurses specially trained in chemotherapy administration.
- Before administration, a second nurse trained in chemotherapy administration must identify the patient, medication, dose, route, amount of fluid to be administered, and drug expiration date.
- The nurse should double glove and wear a gown when administering chemotherapy.
- All equipment used in the administration of chemotherapy should be disposed of in specially marked puncture-resistant containers.

Data from Neuss, M. N., Gilmore, T. R., Belderson, K. M., Billett, A. L., Conti-Kalchik, T., Harvey, B. E., . . . Polovich., M. (2017). 2016 updated American Society of Clinical Oncology/Oncology Nursing Society chemotherapy administration safety standards, including standards for pediatric oncology. *Oncology Nursing Forum, 44*(1), 31–43.

Chemotherapy can be toxic to the child as well as to the healthcare provider who prepares and administers it. Healthcare settings have protocols to ensure safe handling and administration of chemotherapy. Nurses administering chemotherapy should educate themselves on chemotherapy administration safety standards (Patient Safety 26.1).

Chemotherapy works in relation to the cell cycle (Fig. 26.1). Some chemotherapeutic agents are not cell cycle–specific, meaning that they work no matter which phase of division the cell is in. Other agents work only during a specific phase of the cell cycle. Most treatment regimens use a combination of cell cycle–specific and cell cycle–nonspecific agents.

Chemotherapy dosing is based on body surface area. Accurate measurements of weight and height are required to ensure

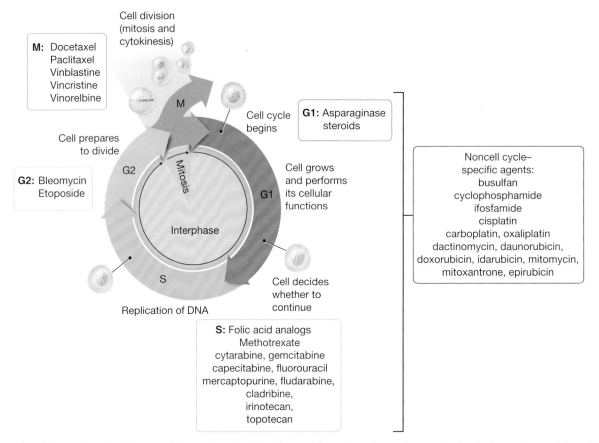

Figure 26.1. The cell cycle. Phases of the cell cycle. G1: ribonucleic acid and protein synthesis; S: deoxyribonucleic acid synthesis; G2: resting phase, in which the cell differentiates or dies; M: mitotic cell division. Shown in boxes are the chemotherapeutic agents grouped according to the phase of the cell cycle in which each is active. Modified with permission from Wingerd, B. (2013). *Human body* (3rd ed., Fig. 3.16). Philadelphia, PA: Wolters Kluwer. Data from Sweet, B. (2015). *Handbook of applied therapeutics* (9th ed., Fig. 89.1). Philadelphia, PA: Wolters Kluwer.

that the dose is correct. Body surface area can be calculated using a nomogram (Fig. 26.2). On the nomogram, locate the child's height in centimeters on the left and the child's weight in kilograms on the right. The surface area is in the middle. Draw a straight line between the weight and height points. Where the line crosses the middle column is the child's body surface area in meters squared (m²).

An additional way to calculate surface area is to use a formula. To calculate the child's body surface area, take the square root of the height in centimeters multiplied by the weight in kilograms and divided by 3,600. For example, a child who is 165 cm tall and weighs 52.27 kg has a body surface area of 1.55 m².

Understanding and monitoring for the side effects of chemotherapy are an important part of the nurse's role when caring for the child receiving chemotherapy. Myelosuppression is one of the most significant side effects of chemotherapy. To effectively monitor for myelosuppression, you must first understand the normal blood count values (Table 26.2). Closely monitoring for the effects of myelosuppression as well as other side effects of chemotherapy can prevent detrimental outcomes.

Monitor for Infection

When the white blood cell (WBC) count is decreased, the child is at risk for infection. Note subtle changes in the child, such as a flushed face, warm extremities, tachycardia, and tachypnea. Monitor the child's temperature, and report any temperature of 100.5°F (38.05°C) or greater to the healthcare provider. Do not take rectal temperatures in children undergoing treatment for cancer. Inserting a thermometer into the rectum may cause small tears, introducing a portal for infection. Ensure that the child has no fresh flowers in the room and does not consume fresh fruits or vegetables. Do not allow anyone with an illness to visit the child. Administer granulocyte colony–stimulating factor as ordered.

Another potential source of infection in the child receiving chemotherapy is the central venous catheter (CVC), through which the chemotherapy is administered. Bloodstream infections are a serious complication of chemotherapy. These infections often start in the CVC (Yacobovich et al., 2015). When changing the CVC dressing, assess for redness, swelling, and drainage. Notify the healthcare provider immediately if any of these is present.

If the child is suspected of having an infection, the healthcare provider will most likely order cultures of the blood, urine,

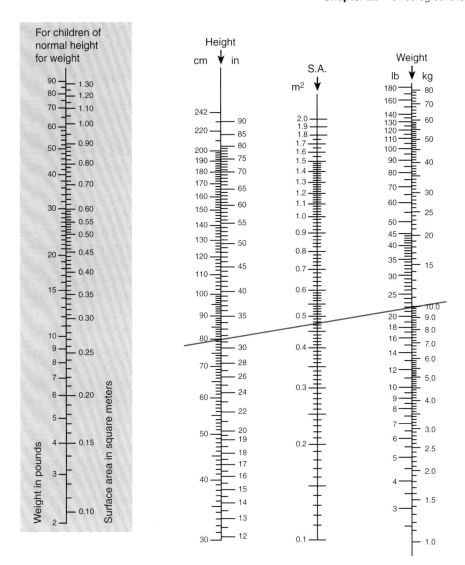

Figure 26.2. Nomogram. Draw a straight line between the child's height and weight. Determine where the line between the height and weight intersects the surface area line. This intersection is the child's body surface area. Reprinted with permission from Bowden, V. R., & Greenberg, C. S. (2015). *Pediatric nursing procedures* (4th ed., Fig. 6.1). Philadelphia, PA: Wolters Kluwer. S.A. stands for surface area.

Table 26.2 Normal Complete Blood Count Values by Age

Age	Hemoglobin (g/dL)	Hematocrit (%)	White Blood Cells (×10³/mL)	Platelets (×10³/μL)
1–6 mo	13.9–12.6	44–36	10.8–11.9	150–350
6 mo–2 y	12.0	36	6.0–17.0	150–350
2–6 y	12.5	37	5.0–15.5	150–350
6–12 y	13.5	40	4.5–13.5	150–350
12–18 y	14.0–14.5	41–43	4.5–13.5	150–350

Data from Hughes, H. K., & Kahl, L. K. (Eds.). (2018). *The Harriet Lane handbook* (21st ed.). Philadelphia, PA: Elsevier.

and sputum. Obtain the specimens as ordered. Administer antibiotics as ordered. Monitor the child closely to prevent sepsis and septic shock (refer to Chapter 6).

 In Chapter 6, Abigail Hanson was showing signs and symptoms of an infection after her first round of chemotherapy. Her absolute neutrophil count (ANC) was 288. How does the ANC affect the child's risk for infection? What were the nursing interventions implemented for Abigail? Tom, Abigail's nurse, was vigilant in monitoring her and her status improved. What if Abigail had become bradycardic and bradypneic? What should Tom have done?

In addition to monitoring for infection in the hospital, parents should know how to avoid infection after discharge (Patient Teaching 26.1). Education also includes when it is necessary to call the healthcare provider.

Manage Anemia

Myelosuppression from chemotherapy affects the production of red blood cells (RBCs). Monitor the hemoglobin and hematocrit levels. Assess for signs and symptoms of anemia, such as pallor and fatigue. Encourage the child to eat foods rich in iron.

Patient Teaching 26.1

Preventing Infection at Home in the Child Receiving Chemotherapy

General Guidelines
- Avoid taking the child to crowded areas.
- Have the child wear a mask if in public.
- Avoid having the child around people with known illnesses.
- Avoid the child receiving live virus vaccines or being exposed to those who have received a live virus vaccine in the past month.
- Do not take the child's temperature rectally.
- Avoid the child eating fresh fruit or vegetables.
- Have the child perform oral hygiene as directed.

When to Call the Healthcare Provider
Parents of children receiving chemotherapy should call the physician in the following circumstances:

- The child has a temperature of 100.5°F (38.05°C) or greater.
- There is any redness, swelling, or drainage around the CVC insertion site.
- The child becomes pale, listless, or lethargic.
- The child has episodes of vomiting that are not well controlled with medication.
- Any time there is a concern.

Administer blood transfusions and epoetin alfa as ordered (The Pharmacy 26.1).

Prevent Hemorrhage

Platelets are also affected by myelosuppression. Assess for petechiae, purpura, and bruising. Monitor for signs and symptoms of internal bleeding, such as fatigue, weakness, tachycardia, dyspnea, and diaphoresis. Notify the healthcare provider immediately if any of these symptoms are present.

Interventions to decrease bleeding include having the child participate in low-impact activities, such as coloring or board games, to prevent accidental trauma. Avoid administering rectal medications and taking the child's temperature rectally. Limit the number of procedures that require needlesticks, such as lumbar punctures and bone marrow aspirations. If these procedures are necessary, apply pressure to the site for at least 15 minutes after the procedure. Administer platelets as ordered.

Manage Nausea and Vomiting

Chemotherapy-induced nausea and vomiting is one of the most common complaints in children undergoing treatment for cancer (McCulloch, Hemsley, & Kelly, 2018). Severe nausea and vomiting affect the nutritional status of the child on chemotherapy. To help manage nausea and vomiting, administer antiemetics 15 to 30 minutes before a chemotherapy infusion and every 4 to 6 hours after the infusion as ordered. Antiemetics are most effective when given around the clock for 24 to 48 hours after the infusion.

Nonpharmacological therapies that may help alleviate nausea and vomiting include ginger root, peppermint oil, acupuncture, and craniosacral therapy. Also, cluster nursing care to decrease interruptions to the child, dim the lights, and reduce the amount of noise in the child's room.

Promote Pain Relief

The child undergoing treatment for cancer is subjected to different diagnostic procedures, such as a bone marrow biopsy, tissue biopsy, and lumbar puncture. These procedures are uncomfortable at the least. Promote pain relief during and after these procedures by administering medications as ordered and providing nonpharmacological interventions such as distraction (How Much Does It Hurt? 26.1). If the ordered pain management regimen is not adequate, contact the healthcare provider.

 In Chapter 6, a child life specialist worked with Abigail Hanson before her lumbar puncture to explain the procedure. If Abigail had been 8 years old instead of 4 years old, how would the child life specialist have explained the procedure differently? How can the child life specialist help with pain management after procedures? What interventions can nurses provide for pain management if a child life specialist is not available?

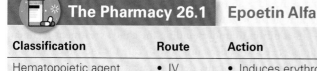

The Pharmacy 26.1 Epoetin Alfa

Classification	Route	Action	Nursing Considerations
Hematopoietic agent	• IV • SQ	• Induces erythropoiesis by stimulating erythroid progenitor cells • Induces the release of reticulocytes from the bone marrow	• Monitor hemoglobin levels. • Dosing schedules are individualized.

IV, intravenous; SQ, subcutaneous.

Adapted from Taketomo, C. K., Hodding, J. H., & Kraus, D. M. (2018). *Pediatric & neonatal dosage handbook* (25th ed.). Hudson, OH: Lexicomp.

How Much Does It Hurt? 26.1

Pain Management for Bone Marrow Aspiration and Lumbar Puncture

Nurses should help with pain control during procedures such as a bone marrow aspiration or lumbar puncture. Giving any pain medications as ordered and applying an anesthetic cream, such as lidocaine and prilocaine, to the site helps the child to better cope with having multiple procedures. Use the developmentally appropriate pain tool to assess pain both before and after the procedure.

In addition to procedural pain, the child on chemotherapy may experience pain from the cancer itself. Children with acute lymphoblastic leukemia (ALL) may experience bone pain, whereas children with solid tumors may experience pain related to compression of structures near the tumor. The side effects of chemotherapy can also be painful. Stomatitis is painful and, if severe, may require systemic pain medication.

Maintain Adequate Nutrition

The causes of nutritional deficit are multifactorial in the child on chemotherapy. Weight loss occurs in over 60% of children treated for cancer (McCulloch et al., 2018). Nausea, vomiting,

and pain due to mucositis are the most common causes of poor intake. Altered smell, altered taste, and loss of appetite are other causes of poor nutrition during treatment. Psychological changes such as anticipated nausea and negative impact of the hospital environment can also affect the child's appetite (Klanjsek & Pajnkihar, 2016).

Interventions to promote adequate nutritional intake focus on treating the underlying cause. Monitor the child's weight and intake and output daily to determine nutritional status. Maintain good oral hygiene. Inspect the oral mucosa, noting any breakdown. Provide pain relief for mucositis with analgesic mouth rinses and medications as ordered (Analyze the Evidence 26.1). Administer antiemetics as ordered to manage nausea and vomiting. Identify any smells that bother the child and try to avoid them. Provide foods that the child wants. Encourage the family to maintain regular meal times. Dieticians are part of the multidisciplinary team that cares for children with cancer. Often, a full nutritional assessment is needed, with recommended interventions from the dietician.

Promote Growth and Development

Children undergoing treatment for cancer spend a great deal of time in the hospital. Part of the nurse's role is promoting growth and development while the child is receiving treatment. Providing developmentally appropriate activities while the child is hospitalized is important to keep the child engaged. Provide nutritious meals and snacks to promote growth. Encourage families to maintain routines as much as possible while in the

Analyze the Evidence 26.1 Honey to Prevent and Treat Mucositis

Bulut and Tufecki (2016) conducted a study to determine the effectiveness of honey to treat and prevent mucositis. The study was quasi-experimental, with both experimental and control groups. The study population consisted of 83 children aged 6 to 17 y diagnosed with leukemia or lymphoma.

The control group received routine mouth care, whereas the experimental group used honey for mouth care. The honey was swabbed on the oral mucosa and

swallowed. The researchers compared compliance with mouth care and routine brushing between the two groups, which were similar. The researchers found that there was no initial difference in the recovery of mucositis up to day 4 of treatment. After day 4, the experimental group using the honey had a much quicker recovery than did the control group. The average recovery of the group using honey was 14 d, whereas the average recovery of the control group was 19 d.

hospital. Promote healthy sleep by minimizing interruptions at night. Provide opportunities for social interaction to prevent feelings of isolation, which is especially important for school-age children and adolescents.

When not in the hospital and as long as their WBC count is adequate, children should participate in normal daily activities. Encourage parents to inform teachers about the child's treatment. Some types of cancer and their treatments may affect the child's cognitive abilities. Explain to parents and teachers how the child's treatment may affect his or her school performance.

Provide Education

Providing education to families is an important part of caring for children with cancer (Patient Teaching 26.2). Teach children, if developmentally appropriate, parents, and other family members about the child's diagnosis, treatment plan, side effects of treatment, and which symptoms warrant a call to the healthcare provider. Because this information can be overwhelming and difficult to absorb, convey it to families multiple times, especially at the beginning of treatment.

In addition to understanding the child's treatment regimen, parents need to understand how to care for the child's CVC at home. Have the parents demonstrate a dressing change before discharge from the hospital after initial diagnosis. Teach the parents signs and symptoms of a CVC infection and when to call the healthcare provider.

Provide Emotional and Psychosocial Support to the Child and Family

Social and emotional support help children and families cope with the diagnosis of cancer and the side effects of treatment. Side effects that affect the child's body image, such as hair loss or amputation, are difficult to accept, especially for school-age children and adolescents (Fig. 26.3). Provide opportunities for children to be with others their age who are undergoing the same types of treatment. Allow children to express feelings

---

 Patient Teaching 26.2

Education for Families Caring for Children With Cancer

When providing patient education to families caring for children with cancer, the nurse should do the following:

- Provide written information regarding the child's diagnosis.
- Ensure the family has a written treatment plan discussing medications, procedures, and other necessary information.
- Help the family to create a calendar of healthcare provider appointments, blood draws, and infusions.
- Discuss the common side effects of chemotherapy, including the following:
  - Nausea and vomiting
  - Alopecia
  - Stomatitis
  - Fatigue
  - Loss of appetite
  - Immunosuppression
  - Diarrhea
  - Easy bruising
- Inform the parents to contact the healthcare provider when any of the following occur:
  - The child has a temperature of 100.5°F (38.05°C) or greater.
  - The child has difficulty breathing.
  - The child has excessive vomiting.
  - There is any redness, swelling, or drainage around the CVC insertion site.
  - The child becomes pale, listless, or lethargic.
  - The child has episodes of vomiting that are not well controlled with medication.
  - There is skin breakdown in the perianal area.
  - Any time there is a concern.

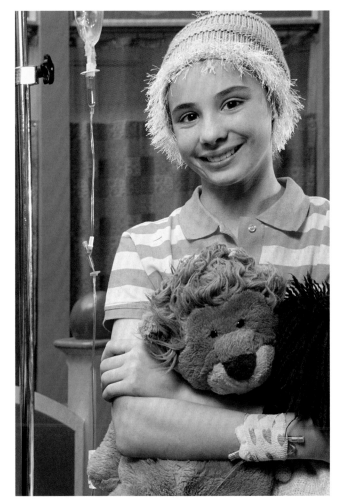

Figure 26.3. Body image. One of the side effects of chemotherapy is hair loss, which can have an effect on body image, especially in adolescents.

about their diagnosis and treatment. Give families information about support groups for both children and families. Connect families with social workers and counselors as needed.

Oncological Emergencies

Oncological emergencies can occur as a result of either the cancer itself or treatment. The most common oncological emergencies result from treatment of the cancer, hormonal imbalances, metabolic disturbances, or invasive tumor compression (Pi et al., 2016). Learn to recognize signs and symptoms of oncological emergencies early to decrease morbidity and mortality.

Tumor Lysis Syndrome

Tumor lysis syndrome occurs after treatment for cancer begins and has the potential to be life-threatening. In this condition, metabolic abnormalities occur as a result of the breakdown of malignant cells. Tumor lysis syndrome occurs more frequently in cancers of the blood and lymph, as well as in bulky tumors (Pi et al., 2016). When the malignant cell is destroyed, intracellular contents are released into the bloodstream. Release of potassium, phosphorus, and nucleic acids results in severe metabolic disturbances, such as hyperkalemia, hyperphosphatemia, hypocalcemia, and hyperuricemia.

Monitor vital signs and electrolyte levels to detect metabolic disturbances early. Hydrate the child with intravenous fluids at double the normal maintenance rate for 24 hours before chemotherapy infusions. Notify the physician if the child is exhibiting signs and symptoms such as dysrhythmias, seizures, nausea, vomiting, tetany, muscle cramps, or increased blood urea nitrogen (BUN) and creatinine levels. Early intervention is necessary to reduce morbidity and mortality (Pi et al., 2016). Treat with allopurinol as ordered (The Pharmacy 26.2).

Sepsis

Infection can progress quickly to sepsis in the immunocompromised child. Children with an ANC of less than 500 are at increased risk for sepsis. Monitor the child with infection for subtle changes indicating a worsening condition. Monitor the child for changes in skin color from flushed to pale. Children with an infection may be tachycardic and tachypneic. Changes such as bradycardia and bradypnea are ominous signs. The child with sepsis typically has cool and possibly mottled extremities. Diagnosis is confirmed with positive blood cultures. Metabolic acidosis is often present.

The goal is to prevent sepsis. Administer antibiotics as ordered for the child with an infection. If the child shows any signs and symptoms of progressing to sepsis, notify the healthcare provider immediately. Administer fluids and maintain ventilation to prevent shock.

Superior Vena Cava Syndrome

Superior vena cava syndrome is a group of symptoms resulting from compression of the superior vena cava by a mediastinal mass. Symptoms include dyspnea, cough, headache, and edema in the neck and upper extremities (Richardson, Rupasov, & Sharma, 2018). Diagnosis is confirmed with a chest radiograph and CT. Pleural effusion is often present. Superior vena cava syndrome can present as an emergency requiring intubation. Treatment is based on the underlying type of cancer and can involve surgery, chemotherapy, and radiation.

Increased Intracranial Pressure

Increased intracranial pressure can result from a primary tumor, metastases, or surgical procedures. Signs and symptoms of increased intracranial pressure include vomiting with position changes, vision changes, headaches, behavior changes, and seizures. Monitor children at risk for increased intracranial pressure and notify the healthcare provider immediately if the child exhibits any symptoms. Lack of prompt intervention can result in herniation of the brainstem. More detail on increased intracranial pressure is provided in the discussion on brain tumors.

Caring for the Child Undergoing Radiation

Radiation kills not only the malignant cells but also some of the normal cells surrounding the radiation site, specifically the squamous cells. Daily skin assessments are an important

---

The Pharmacy 26.2 **Allopurinol**

Classification	Route	Action	Nursing Considerations
Uric acid–lowering agent	• PO • SQ	• Acts on purine catabolism • Reduces production of uric acid	• Maintain adequate hydration. • Begin 1–2 d before initiation of chemotherapy. • Doses based on body surface area • Monitor for skin rash. • Monitor liver enzymes.

PO, by mouth; SQ, subcutaneous.

Adapted from Taketomo, C. K., Hodding, J. H., & Kraus, D. M. (2018). *Pediatric & neonatal dosage handbook* (25th ed.). Hudson, OH: Lexicomp.

part of the care for children receiving radiation therapy. Assess for redness, scaliness, and breakdown at the site of radiation. Ensure that the skin is clean and dry. Do not use fragranced soap or moisturizers on the child. Skin is more photosensitive during radiation therapy. Educate families that children should wear long sleeves and pants or clothing with sunscreen protection. In addition, teach families to apply sunscreen with a sun protection factor of at least 50 to the child when outside.

Radiation therapy can also cause nausea, vomiting, fatigue, and appetite changes. Interventions for these side effects of radiation are the same as for the child receiving chemotherapy.

Caring for the Child Undergoing a Hematopoietic Stem Cell Transplantation

HCST, sometimes called bone marrow transplantation, is used as either a rescue strategy or treatment for cancer. During this procedure, stem cells are infused into the child after a period of intense chemotherapy and radiation. The stem cells migrate to the child's bone marrow to establish normal hematopoiesis. Autologous transplantations use the child's own stem cells and are used to treat relapse of lymph and blood cancers, as well as some solid tumors. Allogeneic transplantations involve stem cells from a donor and are used to treat hematological cancers, as well as other genetic disorders (Velardi & Locatelli, 2016c). Care of the child undergoing HSCT is involved and complex. The information provided here is a brief overview.

Before Transplantation

Before an HSCT, the child receives high-dose chemotherapy and radiation. The goal is to eradicate the child's hematopoietic system as well as suppress the immune system. This therapy targets the T cells to decrease the potential for transplantation rejections (Velardi & Locatelli, 2016b). During the preparation phase of transplantation, the child is at risk for severe infection and other complications. Protective isolation in a positive-pressure room is required. The child should not have

any visitors during this time. Prophylactic antibiotics, antifungals, and immunoglobulins may be ordered. Once the preparation is complete, the child receives an infusion of hematopoietic cells.

After Transplantation

The child is at risk for severe complications during the posttransplantation phase. The child is at risk for infection immediately after transplantation due to severe myelosuppression. Morbidity and mortality are most often caused by graft-versus-host disease (GVHD) (Velardi & Locatelli, 2016a). Acute GVHD occurs within the first 3 months of transplantation. Symptoms include an erythematous maculopapular rash, anorexia, nausea, vomiting, diarrhea, and liver dysfunction (Velardi & Locatelli, 2016a). Acute GVHD is treated with immunosuppressive drugs, such as cyclosporine or tacrolimus (The Pharmacy 26.3). Chronic GVHD occurs later than 3 months after transplantation or is acute GVHD that persists. Treatment and prognosis depend on the organs involved. Other late effects of HSCT include growth retardation due to total body irradiation, hypothyroidism, and secondary cancers (Velardi & Locatelli, 2016a).

Care of the Dying Child

Despite advances in treatment, an estimated 1,200 children die each year from pediatric cancers (Siegel et al., 2018). Children with advanced-stage or recurrent cancer undergo extensive therapy, often involving experimental therapies. These cancers and their treatments are painful and have devastating effects on the child's and family's quality of life. The child suffers both physiologically and psychologically. Palliative care implemented early in the child's diagnosis can mitigate suffering and ensure that the child receives optimum symptom management (Kaye et al., 2018; Ranallo, 2017). When treatment is failing and death is eminent, the child is placed in hospice care. Hospice care is focused on quality at the end of life and requires that parents understand that their child will most likely not survive the next 6 months (Ranallo, 2017).

The Pharmacy 26.3 Cyclosporine and Tacrolimus

Classification	Route	Action	Nursing Considerations
Immunosuppressive agent	• PO • IV	Inhibits production and release of interleukin-2	• Monitor serum drug levels. • Monitor renal and hepatic function. • Monitor complete blood count. • Do not give with grapefruit juice.

IV, intravenous; PO, by mouth.

Adapted from Taketomo, C. K., Hodding, J. H., & Kraus, D. M. (2018). *Pediatric & neonatal dosage handbook* (25th ed.). Hudson, OH: Lexicomp.

Care of the Child

Pain management is the most important intervention for the child at the end of life. Nurses serve as advocates for the child to ensure optimal symptom management during end-of-life care. Make the child as comfortable as possible. During end-of-life care, doses of analgesics are not limited, to ensure adequate pain control (Jassal, 2015). Every child requires different interventions, because death is unpredictable. Allow the child to have comfort items. Answer the child's questions on a developmentally appropriate level. Set goals for care in collaboration with both children and their families. Assess the child at regular intervals and evaluate the outcomes of interventions.

Care of the Family

Making sure the child receives optimal pain management is the biggest stressor for families, especially for mothers, of a dying child (Mariyana, Allenidekania, & Nurhaeni, 2018). Help alleviate this stress by explaining to families the plan for pain control. Explain terms such as *palliative care* and *hospice*. Help families to understand that their child is at the end of life. Provide support during discussions about do-not-resuscitate orders. Allow the family to have a religious figure present if desired. Ensure that any siblings are involved in the explanations and care of the child if developmentally appropriate. Siblings often feel ignored during this time. Help parents to focus on their other children, as well. Families coping with the death of a child from cancer may need counseling. Refer the family to services and support groups.

Leukemia

Leukemia is the most frequently diagnosed type of cancer in children, affecting over 3,800 children per year in the United States (Whitehead, Metayer, Wiemels, Singer, & Miller, 2016). ALL and acute myelogenous leukemia (AML) are the two most common types of leukemia in childhood, with ALL being the more common of the two, accounting for 77% of the cases (Tubergen, Bleyer, Ritchey, & Friehling, 2016).

Over the past 35 years, the incidence of childhood leukemias in the United States has increased by 55% (Whitehead et al., 2016). Research efforts are being directed toward identifying causes of childhood leukemia. The causes are thought to be multifactorial, beginning with prenatal exposure and continuing with postnatal cellular mutations.

Although no definitive causes have been found, researchers have discovered that children who are breastfed, have siblings, have been in day care, and have been fully immunized are at decreased risk of developing leukemia (Schuz & Erdmann, 2016). Stimulating the immune system through immunizations, maternal antibodies, and exposure to other children prevents the immune system from overreacting and thus may prevent the mutations that cause leukemia, which are hypothesized to result from this overreaction. Conversely, prenatal exposure to environmental toxins and postnatal exposure to pesticides, tobacco smoke, and traffic-related pollution increase the risk for the development of leukemia (Whitehead et al., 2016).

Acute Lymphoblastic Leukemia

ALL is the most common form of cancer in the United States in children and adolescents, accounting for 20% of all pediatric cancers. The highest incidence of ALL is in males 1 to 4 years old and children of Hispanic ethnicity (Siegel et al., 2017). The overall survival rate of children with ALL is 80%, with children with certain subsets of ALL reaching a 98% survival rate (Cooper & Brown, 2015).

Prognosis depends on factors present at the time of diagnosis. Children diagnosed from ages 1 to 10 years with a WBC count of less than 50,000 have a better prognosis than do children and adolescents outside of these parameters. CNS or testicular involvement suggests a more aggressive form of ALL, placing the child or adolescent at high risk and indicating the need for more aggressive treatment (Cooper & Brown, 2015).

Etiology and Pathophysiology

ALL is a cancer of the WBCs in which immature, nonfunctioning WBCs dominate bone marrow production. Lymphoblasts are the immature WBCs that proliferate in ALL. Lymphoblasts are unable to function correctly, compromising the immune system. Because of the high production of lymphocytes in ALL, the bone marrow is unable to produce adequate numbers of RBCs and platelets, leading to anemia and the presence of petechiae. Lymphoblasts infiltrate the bones and the lymph nodes, causing bone pain and diffuse lymphadenopathy. If the lymphoblasts infiltrate the CNS, vomiting, headaches, or seizures may occur.

Clinical Presentation

The symptoms associated with ALL are of acute onset. Common presenting symptoms of ALL include fatigue, pallor, fever, anorexia, and low-grade fevers. Additional findings include bone pain, bruising, petechiae, and hepatosplenomegaly.

 In Chapter 6, Abigail Hanson had common presenting signs of ALL. What signs and symptoms did she have? How are Abigail's symptoms related to the pathophysiology of ALL?

Assessment and Diagnosis

A child who presents with symptoms consistent with ALL should have a diagnostic workup (Box 26.1). A complete blood cell count with differential is most likely the first test to be done. The WBC count helps determine the child's risk category (see Table 26.2 for normal WBC count ranges by age). A

bone marrow biopsy is needed to definitively diagnose ALL. A proportion of lymphoblasts to total WBCs of greater than 25% is diagnostic for ALL (Friehling, Ritchey, Tubergen, & Bleyer, 2016). The child diagnosed with ALL should have a lumbar puncture to determine whether there is CNS involvement.

Therapeutic Interventions

Treatment begins once ALL is diagnosed. Treatment for ALL consists of three phases occurring over 2 to 3 years. The first phase of treatment is called induction and lasts for 4 weeks. In this phase of treatment, the goal is to induce remission (The Pharmacy 26.4). Remission is indicated by a reduction of the number of lymphoblasts in the bone marrow to less than 5% of the total number of WBCs and a return to normal blood counts (Friehling et al., 2016).

During this phase, monitor for side effects of treatment. Give antiemetics as ordered. Monitor for blood in emesis, urine, and stool. Administer blood products as ordered.

The second phase of treatment is termed the consolidation phase. During this phase, the child receives systemic chemotherapy as well as CNS prophylaxis to either eradicate leukemic cells in the CNS or prevent CNS relapse. Multiple rounds of

---

Box 26.1   Laboratory and Diagnostic Tests for ALL

- Complete blood cell count with differential
  - Positive findings: elevated WBC count, decreased hemoglobin and hematocrit levels, and possibly decreased platelet count
- Peripheral blood smear
  - Positive finding: lymphoblasts
- Bone marrow biopsy
  - Positive finding: >25% lymphoblasts
- Lumbar puncture
  - Positive finding: infiltration of leukemic cells into the CNS

The Pharmacy 26.4   Medications for ALL Remission Induction

Medication	Classification	Route	Action	Nursing Considerations
Prednisone	Glucocorticoid	• PO • IV	• Suppresses the immune system by reducing activity of the lymphatic system • Antitumor effects through induction of cell death in immature lymphocytes	• Used in combination regimens to treat cancer • Dosed by body surface area Monitor: • Blood pressure • Weight • Serum glucose
L-asparaginase	Antineoplastic	• IM • IV	Cytotoxic to leukemia cells through reduction of the exogenous asparagine source	• Have emergency equipment available Monitor: • CBC • For anaphylaxis • For nausea, vomiting
Vincristine	• Antineoplastic • Mitotic inhibitor	IV	• Arrests cell growth at metaphase • Works on the M and S phases of cell division	Monitor: • Serum electrolytes • Hepatic function • For neurological effects such as peripheral neuropathy • For constipation
Daunorubicin	• Antitumor • Antibiotic	IV	• Causes disruption in DNA and RNA synthesis • Not cell cycle–specific	• May turn urine red Monitor for: • Cardiac arrhythmias • Congestive heart failure

CBC, complete blood count; DNA, deoxyribonucleic acid; IM, intramuscular; IV, intravenous; PO, by mouth; RNA, ribonucleic acid.
Adapted from Taketomo, C. K., Hodding, J. H., & Kraus, D. M. (2018). *Pediatric & neonatal dosage handbook* (25th ed.). Hudson, OH: Lexicomp.

intrathecal chemotherapy are given during this stage, requiring multiple lumbar punctures. Pain control is important during this phase.

The final phase of treatment for ALL is the maintenance phase, which lasts 2 to 3 years. This phase consists of rounds of intensive chemotherapy followed by rounds of less toxic treatment. The goal of this phase is to eliminate any residual disease.

Nursing management of ALL focuses on administering chemotherapy as well as on monitoring for side effects of treatment and complications of disease. Teaching children and families about the treatment regimen and anticipated side effects is an important part of the nurse's role when caring for a child with ALL. The child with ALL undergoes procedures such as a bone marrow biopsy and a lumbar puncture. Understand your role in these procedures in addition to preparing the child and family for what to expect. Refer to the section General Nursing Interventions for the Child Undergoing Treatment for Cancer, earlier, for further information.

Evaluation

Throughout the course of treatment for ALL, evaluate the outcomes of treatment and nursing interventions. Evaluation of treatment depends on the child's phase of treatment and whether any complications occurred. General expected outcomes for a child undergoing treatment for ALL include the following:

- The child achieves and maintains adequate nutritional intake.
- Fever is absent.
- Nausea and vomiting are controlled with medications.
- No signs and symptoms of bleeding are present.
- Complete blood count is normal.

Discharge Planning and Teaching

Discharge planning and teaching differ depending on the events that happened while the child with ALL was in the hospital. The most important information for the nurse to teach is when the parents should call the healthcare provider. If the child is being discharged after a round of chemotherapy, instruct parents to call the healthcare provider if the child has a temperature of 100.5°F or greater, continued nausea and vomiting, or any blood in the emesis, urine, or stool.

Acute Myelogenous Leukemia

AML differs from ALL in the type of cell that is affected. This type of leukemia affects the myelocytes rather than the lymphocytes. AML accounts for 11% of all childhood leukemias, with the greatest incidence occurring in children 15 to 19 years old. The survival rate is 60% to 70% (Tubergen, Bleyer, Friehling, & Ritchey, 2016).

AML does not respond to treatment as well as ALL does, and children or adolescents with AML generally have prolonged hospital stays. Chemotherapy regimens for AML are intense and often result in hemorrhage or sepsis due to prolonged bone marrow suppression (Tubergen et al., 2016). Many children with AML require a bone marrow or stem cell transplantation for survival.

Etiology and Pathophysiology

In AML, the bone marrow produces an excessive number of myeloblasts. These myeloblasts are immature, nonfunctioning myeloid cells. The cells in the bone marrow are replaced by the malignant myeloblasts, resulting in depletion of functional WBCs, RBCs, and platelets.

Clinical Presentation

Children with AML present with symptoms similar to those of ALL due to bone marrow failure. Those with AML also present with subcutaneous nodules. Some may present with signs and symptoms of disseminated intravascular coagulation. Children with certain types of AML present with **chloromas**, which are tumors made up of leukemic cells that are outside of the bone marrow.

Assessment and Diagnosis

Bone marrow biopsy and bone marrow aspiration are procedures used to distinguish ALL from AML. In these procedures, special staining of the cells helps identify abnormal and myelogenous cells which indicate AML.

Therapeutic Interventions

Treatment for AML is similar to that for ALL. Nursing interventions focus on monitoring and treating the side effects of treatment.

Evaluation

Expected outcomes for a child with AML are similar to those for a child with ALL. Refer to the section Evaluation for ALL, earlier.

Discharge Planning and Teaching

Discharge planning and teaching for a child with AML is similar to those for a child with ALL. Refer to the section Discharge Planning and Teaching for ALL, earlier.

Lymphoma

Lymphoma is a type of cancer involving the lymphocytes. There are two broad categories of lymphoma, Hodgkin lymphoma and NHL. Lymphoma is the third most common cancer in children and the most common cancer in adolescents aged 15 to 19 years (Hochberg, Giulino-Roth, & Cairo, 2016). Hodgkin lymphoma and NHL are not similar other than they both involve the lymphocytes. The clinical presentation and treatment are different for each classification.

Hodgkin Lymphoma

Hodgkin lymphoma accounts for approximately 15% of all cancers in adolescents aged 15 to 19 years. In younger children, Hodgkin lymphoma accounts for only 4% of all cancers (Hochberg et al., 2016). No matter the age, the presenting symptoms of Hodgkin lymphoma are the same (Englund et al., 2018). Males have a higher incidence among younger children, but this discrepancy disappears as children get older.

Children with early-stage disease have a 5-year survival rate of 95%. Those with advanced disease have a survival rate of 90%. Relapse may occur, and when it does, it tends to occur within 3 years of diagnosis but has been known to occur up to 10 years after diagnosis (Hochberg et al., 2016).

Etiology and Pathophysiology

Although there is no known cause of Hodgkin lymphoma, antigens for Epstein–Barr virus have been found in Hodgkin lymphoma cells, indicating the virus may play a role in the cancer's development. Hodgkin lymphoma involves the B lymphocytes and is characterized by the presence of Reed–Sternberg (RS) cells. RS cells are B lymphocytes that have lost most of their immune function, resulting in immune system abnormalities. Typically, RS cells are surrounded by different proportions of lymphocytes, eosinophils, and plasma cells, creating a palpable infiltrate (Hochberg et al., 2016). The disease can start anywhere in the body but most commonly starts in the lymph nodes, specifically the lymph nodes in the chest, neck, or under the arms, and spreads through the lymph system (ACS, 2017). Hodgkin lymphoma rarely occurs below the diaphragm.

Clinical Presentation

Children and adolescents with Hodgkin lymphoma typically present with swollen, painless, and rubbery-feeling lymph nodes in the cervical or supraclavicular region (Fig. 26.4). Depending on the extent of the disease at diagnosis, other symptoms may be present. If the lymph nodes of the chest are involved, the child or adolescent may experience dyspnea and cough. Chest pain may result from the pressure exerted by the enlarged nodes. General symptoms can also include fever, drenching night sweats, and weight loss.

Assessment and Diagnosis

Determine which general symptoms the child is experiencing. Cough and dyspnea indicate a mediastinal mass. On assessment, clusters of rubbery lymph nodes are palpable in the child with Hodgkin lymphoma. Palpate the abdomen. The presence of hepatosplenomegaly indicates advanced disease (Hochberg et al., 2016). Laboratory and diagnostic tests confirm the diagnosis of Hodgkin lymphoma (Box 26.2). Once the diagnosis is confirmed, staging occurs (Table 26.3). The stage of lymphoma determines the treatment.

Box 26.2   Laboratory and Diagnostic Tests for Hodgkin Lymphoma

- Chest X-ray
  - Positive finding: mediastinal mass
- Lymph node biopsy
  - Positive finding: RS cells and abnormal lymphocytes
- CT scans of the neck, chest, and pelvis
  - Determines extent of disease
- Bone marrow biopsy
  - Positive finding: bone marrow involvement, indicating advanced disease
- Complete blood count
  - Indicates bone marrow and immune function
- Erythrocyte sedimentation rate
  - Indicates the amount of inflammation

Table 26.3   Stages of Hodgkin Lymphoma

Stage	Clinical Manifestations
I	Involvement of a single node or a single extralymphatic site
II	Involvement of two or more lymph nodes on the same side of the diaphragm or one lymph node and one extralymphatic site on the same side of the diaphragm
III	Involvement of lymph nodes on both sides of the diaphragm; possible involvement of the spleen
IV	Diffuse involvement of extralymphatic organs and/or tissues

Data from Hochberg, J., Giulino-Roth, L., & Cairo, M. (2016). Lymphoma. In R. M. Kliegman, B. F. Stanton, J. W. St. Geme III, N. F. Schor, & R. E. Behrman (Eds.), *Nelson's textbook of pediatrics* (20th ed.). Philadelphia, PA: Elsevier, Saunders.

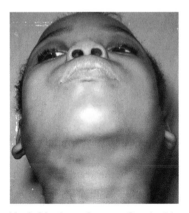

Figure 26.4. Hodgkin lymphoma. Cervical lymphadenopathy associated with Hodgkin lymphoma. Reprinted with permission from Werner, R. (2012). *Massage therapist's guide to pathology* (5th ed., Fig. 6.4). Philadelphia, PA: Wolters Kluwer.

Therapeutic Interventions

Combination chemotherapy in conjunction with low-dose radiation is the treatment for Hodgkin lymphoma (The Pharmacy 26.5). Explain to the child and parents the side effects of treatment and interventions used to manage the side effects.

Evaluation

Evaluation of a child with Hodgkin lymphoma depends on the site of the tumor or tumors. General expected outcomes include the following:

- Dyspnea is absent.
- The child achieves and maintains adequate nutritional intake.
- Fever is absent.
- Nausea and vomiting are controlled with medications.
- No signs and symptoms of bleeding are present.

Discharge Planning and Teaching

Initial discharge teaching focuses on educating the family on the disease and its treatment. Ensure that the family has a written treatment plan. Discuss with the family members infection prevention at home and when to call the healthcare provider.

Non–Hodgkin Lymphoma

NHL refers to a group of lymphomas in which there is uncontrolled proliferation of abnormal lymphocytes (Uzunova & Burke, 2015). NHL is the second most common type of cancer in adolescents aged 15 to 19 years. More than 70% of adolescents diagnosed with NHL have advanced disease at diagnosis, indicating the aggressive nature of childhood NHL (Hochberg et al., 2016). The current survival rate for NHL overall is more than 80%, but this rate varies depending on the subtype of NHL (Uzunova & Burke, 2015).

Etiology and Pathophysiology

The cause of NHL is unknown. However, there is an association between NHL and other factors that weaken the immune system. Inherited immunodeficiency disorders, acquired immunodeficiency disorders, and previous bone marrow transplantation are associated with an increased risk of NHL (Uzunova & Burke, 2015). In addition, autoimmune disorders such as rheumatoid arthritis, systemic lupus erythematosus, and celiac disease are associated with a moderately increased risk of NHL (Uzunova & Burke, 2015).

There are four major subtypes of NHL. NHL can arise from either immature B or T lymphocytes or mature B or T lymphocytes. The four major subtypes are further divided on the basis of the cell of origin and antigens present on the cellular surface

---

The Pharmacy 26.5 — Common Chemotherapeutic Agents Used in Hodgkin Lymphoma

Medication	Classification	Route	Action	Nursing Considerations
Cyclophosphamide	Alkylating agent	IV	• Prevents cell division by decreasing DNA synthesis	• Provide adequate hydration. • Monitor for hemorrhagic cystitis and hematuria. • Avoid extravasation because of vesicant properties.
Doxorubicin	• Antitumor • Antibiotic	IV	• Causes disruption in DNA and RNA synthesis • Not cell cycle–specific	• May turn urine red Monitor for: • Cardiac arrhythmias • Congestive heart failure
Bleomycin	• Antitumor • Antibiotic	IV	• Causes disruption in DNA and RNA synthesis • Not cell cycle–specific	Monitor: • Pulmonary function tests • Renal function • Hepatic function • For fever and chills within the first 24 h of infusion
Methotrexate	Antimetabolite	• PO • IV	• Folate antimetabolite inhibits DNA synthesis • Cell cycle–specific for the S phase	Monitor: • CBC • Hepatic function • For photosensitivity

CBC, complete blood count; DNA, deoxyribonucleic acid; IV, intravenous; PO, by mouth; RNA, ribonucleic acid.
Adapted from Taketomo, C. K., Hodding, J. H., & Kraus, D. M. (2018). *Pediatric & neonatal dosage handbook* (25th ed.). Hudson, OH: Lexicomp.

(Hochberg et al., 2016). B-cell lymphomas are more common in the United States than are T-cell lymphomas (ACS, 2016d).

Clinical Presentation

The signs and symptoms associated with NHL depend on the subtype. Tumors are generally present outside of the lymph system, most commonly in the liver, spleen, bone marrow, skin, and thymus (Uzunova & Burke, 2015). NHL has an acute onset, with typically only a few days to weeks from onset of symptoms to diagnosis (Hochberg et al., 2016). Symptoms relate to the site of involvement. Other symptoms that may be seen are indicative of B-cell involvement, such as fever, weight loss, and night sweats.

NHL can present as an oncological emergency. If a mediastinal mass is present, the blood flow or airways may be blocked. A spinal cord tumor could cause spinal cord compression, resulting in paralysis. Tumor lysis syndrome may also occur, resulting in severe electrolyte disturbances (refer to the section Oncological Emergencies).

Assessment and Diagnosis

Conducting a thorough history and physical assessment is important to the diagnosis of NHL. Determine whether the child has a history of congenital or acquired immunodeficiency or autoimmune disorders. Observe for cough and dyspnea. Inspect for ascites. Palpate for diffuse lymphadenopathy, hepatosplenomegaly, and abdominal masses.

There are no abnormal peripheral blood tests that indicate NHL. Diagnostic tests confirm the diagnosis of NHL. Cross-sectional imaging with either a CT scan or a magnetic resonance imaging (MRI) can confirm diagnosis and help with staging (Table 26.4). A lymph node biopsy determines the pathology and helps guide treatment decisions.

Therapeutic Interventions

Treatment of NHL depends on the pathology and subtype. Each subtype requires different combinations of chemotherapy. Administer chemotherapy as ordered and monitor for side effects of treatment. Specifically, monitor for signs and symptoms of tumor lysis syndrome.

Evaluation

Expected outcomes for a child with NHL are similar to those for a child with Hodgkin lymphoma. Refer to the Evaluation section for Hodgkin lymphoma, earlier.

Discharge Planning and Teaching

Discharge planning and teaching for a child with NHL are similar to those for a child with Hodgkin lymphoma. Refer to the section Discharge Planning and Teaching for Hodgkin lymphoma.

Solid Tumors

A solid tumor is an abnormal mass of cells and may be malignant or benign.

Table 26.4 Stages of Non–Hodgkin Lymphoma

Stage	Clinical Manifestations
I	• A single tumor; no involvement of the mediastinum or abdomen
II	• A single tumor with regional node involvement • Multiple node involvement on the same side of the diaphragm • A primary gastrointestinal tract tumor
III	• Two single tumors on either side of the diaphragm • Two or more lymph nodes involved on either side of the diaphragm • A primary intrathoracic tumor
IV	• Any of these in addition to central nervous system or bone marrow involvement

Data from Hochberg, J., Giulino-Roth, L., & Cairo, M. (2016). Lymphoma. In R. M. Kliegman, B. F. Stanton, J. W. St. Geme III, N. F. Schor, & R. E. Behrman (Eds.), *Nelson's textbook of pediatrics* (20th ed.). Philadelphia, PA: Elsevier, Saunders.

Brain Tumors

Brain tumors are the second most common type of cancer in children and adolescents. The incidence is highest in children younger than age 5 years. Mortality for children with a brain tumor is around 30% (Ater & Kuttesch, 2016). Prognosis depends on the location, malignancy, and type of tumor. Tumors that are at the surface of the brain are easier to remove than those deep within the brain structure. Tumors that are aggressive and invasive are harder to treat. Morbidity is high in survivors of childhood brain tumors and is primarily due to the neurological side effects of the tumor, as well as the surgery to remove the tumor.

Brain tumors can be benign or malignant. Benign tumors are slow growing and have well-defined borders. Malignant brain tumors can be aggressive and have no borders, invading the surrounding brain tissue (Chan, Pole, Mann, & Colantonio, 2015). Children with either type of brain tumor can have lifelong neurological effects, depending on the location of the tumor, the ability to fully remove the tumor, and any additional treatment that may be needed.

Etiology and Pathophysiology

The pathophysiology of brain tumors is not well understood. Some genetic syndromes, such as neurofibromatosis, Li–Fraumeni syndrome, and tuberous sclerosis, increase the risk for childhood brain tumors (ACS, 2016e). However, the cause of most brain tumors is not known.

Brain tumors can occur anywhere within the brain (Fig. 26.5). The most common types of tumors in children younger than 14 years old are pilocytic astrocytomas and medulloblastoma/

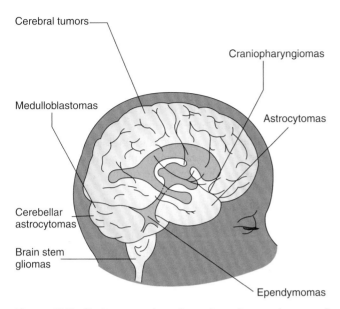

Cerebral tumors

Craniopharyngiomas

Medulloblastomas

Astrocytomas

Cerebellar
astrocytomas

Brain stem
gliomas

Ependymomas

Figure 26.5. Brain tumor locations. Locations and types of the most common brain tumors in children. Reprinted with permission from Pillitteri, A. (2002). *Maternal and child health nursing* (4th ed., Fig. 53.5). Philadelphia, PA: Lippincott Williams & Wilkins.

primitive neuroectodermal tumors. In children older than 14 years, the most common types of tumors are pilocytic astrocytomas and pituitary tumors (Ater & Kuttesch, 2016).

Clinical Presentation

Clinical manifestations of brain tumors vary with the tumor location. The tumor occupies space and exerts pressure on the brain, resulting in signs and symptoms of increased intracranial pressure. See Table 26.5 for the most common types of brain tumors in children, along with features and clinical manifestations of each.

Assessment and Diagnosis

Take a careful health history for a child suspected of having a brain tumor. Enquire about the onset and duration of symptoms. Determine whether the child has had any of the symptoms common to brain tumors, such as the following:

- Headaches
- Vomiting, particularly with position changes, such as getting out of bed
- Behavior changes

Table 26.5   Selected Types of Childhood Brain Tumors

Type of Tumor	Features	Clinical Manifestations
Medulloblastoma, PNET	• Most common type of tumor • Arises from embryonal cells • Fast growing • Located in the cerebellum • More common in children younger than 10 y old	• Headaches • Nausea/vomiting • Ataxia • Behavioral changes • Changes in appetite
Pilocytic astrocytoma	• Arise from astrocytes that make up the supportive tissue of the brain • Located in cerebral hemispheres • Low-grade astrocytoma • Do not spread • Slow growing • Enclosed within a cyst	• Headaches • New-onset seizures • Memory loss
Pituitary tumor (craniopharyngioma)	• Located near the pituitary gland • May involve the optic nerve • Benign • Large at the time of diagnosis	• Headaches • Delayed development • Vision changes • Obesity
Ependymoma	• Arise from the ependymal cells lining the ventricles of the brain • Located within or next to the ventricles • 30% in children younger than 3 y old • Various rates of growth	• Increased head circumference in infants • Irritability • Ataxia • Double vision • Facial asymmetry

PNET, primitive neuroectodermal tumor.
Data from American Brain Tumor Association. (2014). *Brain tumors in children.* Retrieved from http://www.abta.org/adolescent-pediatric/brain-tumors-in-children.html; Ater, J. L., & Kuttesch J. F., Jr. (2016). Brain tumors in childhood. In R. M. Kliegman, B. F. Stanton, J. W. St. Geme III, N. F. Schor, & R. E. Behrman (Eds.), *Nelson's textbook of pediatrics* (20th ed.). Philadelphia, PA: Elsevier, Saunders.

- Ataxia
- Diplopia
- New-onset seizures
- Weakness

Complete a thorough neurological exam appropriate to the child's developmental age. Determine whether the child is awake and alert. Observe gait for steadiness. Observe for head tilt, often present in young children with brain tumors. Note any facial asymmetry. Observe for nystagmus when conducting the cardinal fields of gaze test. Assess that the pupils are equal, round, and reactive to light and accommodation. In infants, palpate the anterior fontanelle, noting any fullness. Assess reflexes for hyperreflexia, which can indicate increased intracranial pressure.

Children suspected of having a brain tumor typically need to have an MRI done. Tumors are better delineated with an MRI rather than with a CT. Some children have a positron emission tomography scan to determine whether abnormal areas on the MRI are likely to be tumors (Ater & Kuttesch, 2016). A thorough ophthalmological exam should be done, especially if the tumor is near the optic nerve. A lumbar puncture is indicated to determine the extent of the disease. Measurement of beta-human chorionic gonadotropin and alpha-fetoprotein in the cerebrospinal fluid (CSF) can assist in the diagnosis of certain types of brain tumors.

Therapeutic Interventions

Treatment of a child with a brain tumor depends on the type, size, and location of the tumor. Most tumors require surgery to remove part or all of the tumor. Some types of tumors require chemotherapy and radiation to shrink the tumor before surgery is an option. Only certain chemotherapeutic agents cross the blood–brain barrier to treat CNS tumors (The Pharmacy 26.6). Therefore, radiation is often used in conjunction with chemotherapy to treat brain tumors. Radiation is targeted specifically to the site of the tumor to avoid negative neurological effects.

Additional therapies being tested for children with brain tumors include targeted therapy and immunotherapy. Targeted therapy includes treatment with monoclonal antibodies in which the medication distinguishes between cancer cells and healthy cells, causing fewer side effects. Immunotherapy, using vaccines to treat tumor cells, is currently in clinical trials to determine the effectiveness of the treatment (ACS, 2016e).

Nursing management of children with brain tumors includes both preoperative and postoperative care, in addition to administering chemotherapy and managing the side effects of chemotherapy and radiation.

The Pharmacy 26.6 — Common Chemotherapeutic Agents Used in Children With Brain Tumors

Medication	Classification	Route	Action	Nursing Considerations
Cisplatin	Alkylating agent	IV	• Inhibits DNA synthesis • Cell cycle–nonspecific	• Provide adequate hydration. Monitor: • For hemorrhagic cystitis and hematuria • Hearing, at baseline and after treatment
Etoposide	Mitotic inhibitor	IV	• Arrests cell growth in the S phase and early G1 phase	• Have emergency equipment available. Monitor: • For anaphylaxis • Bilirubin, albumin levels
Lomustine (CCNU)	Alkylating agent (nitrosourea)	PO	• Inhibits DNA and RNA synthesis • Able to cross the blood–brain barrier	Monitor: • CBC • Hepatic function • Pulmonary function
Irinotecan	Topoisomerase inhibitor	• PO • IV	• Binds to DNA, preventing religation of a cleaved DNA strand • Cell cycle–specific for the S phase	Monitor for: • Hypotension during infusion • Chills, fever, headache • Diarrhea, dehydration

CBC, complete blood count; DNA, deoxyribonucleic acid; IV, intravenous; PO, by mouth; RNA, ribonucleic acid.

Adapted from Taketomo, C. K., Hodding, J. H., & Kraus, D. M. (2018). *Pediatric & neonatal dosage handbook* (25th ed.). Hudson, OH: Lexicomp.

Preoperative Care

Preoperatively, nurses should assess the child routinely and monitor for any changes in status. Implement interventions to minimize events that could cause increased intracranial pressure (Box 26.3).

Before the surgery, reinforce information provided by the surgeon. Explain that the child will be in the intensive care unit and possibly on a ventilator after surgery. The child may be in a coma or in a semialert state for a few days after surgery. If any hydrocephalus is present, the neurosurgeon may place a ventriculoperitoneal shunt (refer to Chapter 22).

Make sure the parents and child have a tour of the hospital. Explain to parents the visiting policy in the intensive care unit. Answer any questions that the parent or child may have. Explain that the child will have his or her head shaved over the surgical site and determine whether the child would rather have the entire head shaved instead.

Postoperative Care

Postoperative care consists of keeping the child comfortable and monitoring for signs and symptoms of complications. Position the child so that he or she is lying on the nonaffected side of the head. Maintain the height of the bed as ordered by the physician; usually the child is positioned in the low- or semi-Fowler's position. Monitor the surgical site for blood or leakage of CSF. If the child has an external ventriculoperitoneal shunt, maintain the shunt at the level ordered by the surgeon (refer to Chapter 22).

Maintain fluid balance. Continue to monitor for signs of increased intracranial pressure in the postoperative period (Priority Care Concepts 26.1). Administer mannitol as ordered to decrease cerebral edema. Assess for pain with the appropriate pain tool and administer analgesics as ordered. Monitor neurological status. Assess orientation, speech, and cranial nerves. Assess that pupils are equal, round, and reactive to light and accommodation bilaterally. Report any abnormal signs to the healthcare provider.

Evaluation

Continually evaluate the child postoperatively. Expected outcomes before discharge for a child with a brain tumor include the following:

- The child is oriented as appropriate for age.
- Pain is controlled with oral analgesics.

Priority Care Concepts 26.1

Increased Intracranial Pressure

Goals for the postoperative child include the following:

- Maintain fluid balance.
- No signs of worsening increased intracranial pressure are present.
- The child is oriented as appropriate for age.
- Pain rating is at an acceptable level.
- No signs or symptoms of infection at the surgical site are present.

  Surgery to remove a brain tumor may result in cerebral edema. It is critical that nurses monitor for signs and symptoms of worsening cerebral edema and intervene quickly. Without intervention, the cerebral edema can cause the brainstem to herniate. Critical signs include the following:

- Unequal pupils
- Bradycardia
- Irregular respirations
- Widening pulse pressure

  Nurses should implement interventions to minimize changes in intracranial pressure (Box 26.3) and immediately notify the healthcare provider of any changes in the child's status.

- The child achieves and maintains adequate nutritional intake.
- Neurological status is intact.
- Nausea and vomiting are absent.
- The child is able to ambulate independently.

Discharge Planning and Teaching

Before discharge, explain to the family when to call the healthcare provider. If the child experiences a fever over 100.4°F, continued vomiting, headaches, weakness, or vision changes, parents should call the healthcare provider. Parents should take the child to the emergency room if the child experiences a sudden change in the level of consciousness, has uncontrollable seizures, or shows signs of irregular breathing.

Educate parents and children that recovery from surgery to remove a brain tumor is often a long process. Although the long-term survival rate for children with brain tumors is as high as 70%, up to 50% have long-term neurological sequelae (Ater & Kuttesch, 2016). Long-term sequelae may include seizures, cognitive delay, altered mobility, and sensory deficits. If the tumor was located near the pituitary gland, the child may experience delayed or absent onset of puberty and other endocrine disorders.

Children who are survivors of brain tumors will most likely need lifelong care with a team of specialists. Multidisciplinary

---

Box 26.3 Nursing Interventions to Prevent Increased Intracranial Pressure

- Minimize stimuli in the child's hospital room.
- Keep the lights low.
- Cluster nursing care to minimize disturbance.
- Administer stool softeners as ordered to decrease straining with bowel movement.
- Assess pain levels with appropriate pain tool and administer analgesics as needed.
- Minimize the amount of crying in an infant.

teams with specialist physicians, nurses, physical therapists, speech therapists, and others provide the greatest opportunity for optimal outcomes for the child and family.

Neuroblastoma

Neuroblastoma arises from the embryonal cells of the peripheral nervous system, often beginning in utero (Zage & Ater, 2016). Neuroblastoma is the most common solid tumor in children outside of brain tumors, and the most frequent in children younger than 5 years old (Mullassery & Lotsy, 2015; Lukscha et al., 2016). The median age of diagnosis is 22 months. Although only 8% of all pediatric cancers are neuroblastomas, this type of cancer is responsible for 15% of all pediatric deaths from cancer (Newman & Nuchtern, 2016).

Etiology and Pathophysiology

Neuroblastoma is part of a family of tumors called peripheral neuroblastic tumors. The tumors arise from the neuroectodermal embryonic cells (Lukscha et al., 2016). These tumors are heterogeneous and can exhibit spontaneous regression or aggressive metastatic disease. There is no known etiology. Families report a family history of neuroblastoma in 1% to 2% of children with neuroblastomas. Neuroblastoma is associated with other disorders, such as Hirschsprung disease, neurofibromatosis type 1, and central hypoventilation syndrome (Zage & Ater, 2016). Neuroblastoma can occur anywhere in the sympathetic nervous system but most commonly occurs in the medulla and the adrenal gland (Fig. 26.6). Tumors can infiltrate to surrounding structures, and metastasis occurs to the lymph and bone marrow (Mullassery & Lotsy, 2015).

Clinical Presentation

Clinical presentation depends on the site of the tumor and extent of disease. Tumors presenting in the perinatal period or in children younger than 18 months old have a higher rate of spontaneous regression. Older children are more likely to have metastatic disease at the time of diagnosis (Newman & Nuchtern, 2016).

Some children with neuroblastoma are asymptomatic, and their tumors are found incidentally. Neuroblastoma in the adrenal gland presents with asymmetric abdominal swelling. Bowel and bladder function may be affected because of compression from the tumor. General symptoms include fever, malaise, pain, and anorexia. Children with metastatic disease may exhibit periorbital ecchymosis, often called "raccoon eyes" (Mullassery & Lotsy, 2015). Other signs of metastatic disease include orbital proptosis, bluish subcutaneous nodules, and bone pain.

Assessment and Diagnosis

Assessment includes a thorough history and physical exam. During the history, determine whether there is a family history of neuroblastoma. Ask what symptoms the child is experiencing and when they started. Elicit information about bowel and bladder function and ease of respirations to determine whether the tumor is compressing other organs.

Inspect for bruising and swelling around the eyes. Note any signs of bone marrow involvement, such as anemia or petechiae. Palpate the abdomen, noting the presence, size, and location of any mass. Auscultate the lungs, noting any respiratory distress. Palpate for lymphadenopathy, noting the location, size, and consistency of palpable lymph nodes.

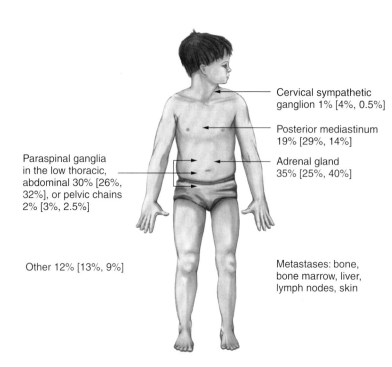

Cervical sympathetic ganglion 1% [4%, 0.5%]

Posterior mediastinum 19% [29%, 14%]

Paraspinal ganglia in the low thoracic, abdominal 30% [26%, 32%], or pelvic chains 2% [3%, 2.5%]

Adrenal gland 35% [25%, 40%]

Other 12% [13%, 9%]

Metastases: bone, bone marrow, liver, lymph nodes, skin

Figure 26.6. Neuroblastoma. The most common sites of neuroblastoma in children. Reprinted with permission from Constine, L. S., Tarbell, N. J., & Halperin, E. C. (2016). *Pediatric radiation oncology* (6th ed., Fig. 6.2). Philadelphia, PA: Wolters Kluwer. Data from Vo, K. T., Matthay, K. K., Neuhaus, J., et al. (2014). Clinical, biologic, and prognostic differences on the basis of primary tumor site in neuroblastoma: A report from the International Neuroblastoma Risk Group project. *Journal of Clinical Oncology, 32,* 3169–3176.

An ultrasound is performed initially with a follow-up CT scan or MRI to determine the extent of the disease. A 24-hour urine test shows elevated tumor markers such as the catecholamine metabolites homovanillic acid and vanillylmandelic acid, confirming the diagnosis of neuroblastoma. A tumor biopsy is necessary to determine the stage of the tumor (Table 26.6). The biopsy is done with the initial resection of the tumor. A CT of the chest and abdomen determines the presence of metastatic disease. A bone marrow biopsy is performed to rule out bone marrow involvement.

Therapeutic Interventions

Treatment for neuroblastoma depends on the stage of the disease and the presence of cytogenetic markers. Stages 1 and 2 generally require surgery only. The treatment for stage 4S is observation because this type of neuroblastoma may undergo spontaneous regression. Stages 3 and 4 require chemotherapy and radiation, in addition to chemotherapy. Biological therapy and targeted immunotherapy are used with recurring neuroblastoma to enhance outcomes for children in this population (Newman & Nuchtern, 2016).

Nursing interventions relate to preoperative and postoperative care of the child undergoing surgical resection of neuroblastoma.

Table 26.6 International Neuroblastoma Staging System

Stage	Characteristics
1	• The tumor is local with good margins. • All visible tumor is removed by surgery. • Lymph nodes outside the tumor are not involved.
2A	• The neuroblastoma is unilateral, but not all of the tumor can be resected. • Lymph nodes outside the tumor are not involved.
2B	• The neuroblastoma is unilateral and may or may not have been completely resected. • Regional lymph nodes are involved.
3	The neuroblastoma is not widespread but has one of the following characteristics: • The tumor has crossed the midline, and lymph nodes nearby may be involved. • The tumor is unilateral but has spread to contralateral lymph nodes. • The tumor is midline and spreading bilaterally across.
4	There is widespread metastasis.
4S	• The child is younger than 1 y. • The primary tumor is localized with metastasis limited to the skin, liver, and bone marrow.

Data from American Cancer Society. (2018). *Neuroblastoma stages and prognostic markers.* Retrieved from https://www.cancer.org/cancer/neuroblastoma/detection-diagnosis-staging/staging.html.

Postoperative care is specific to the site of the surgery. Abdominal surgery is the most common. Implement interventions such as incentive spirometry, splinting of the incision, and ambulation. If the child needs further treatment, such as chemotherapy and radiation, monitor and manage the side effects of treatment.

Evaluation

Initial outcomes focus on the postoperative child. Expected outcomes before discharge for a child with neuroblastoma include the following:

- Fever is absent.
- No signs or symptoms of infection at surgical site are present.
- Lungs are clear to auscultation bilaterally.
- If developmentally appropriate, the child can ambulate independently.
- The child achieves and maintains adequate nutritional intake.
- Positive bowel sounds are present in all four quadrants.

Discharge Planning and Teaching

Educate parents on signs and symptoms of infection and when to call the healthcare provider. For children with stage 3 or 4 neuroblastoma, discuss oncology follow-up appointments. Educate the parents and child, if appropriate, on the side effects of chemotherapy and radiation. Provide phone numbers and websites of support groups, especially for children with a poor prognosis.

Wilms Tumor

Nephroblastoma, otherwise known as Wilms tumor, is the most common malignant renal tumor and the second most common abdominal tumor in childhood. More than 75% of the cases occur in children younger than 5 years old, with the mean age at diagnosis being 3 years. The survival rate is greater than 90% (Daw, Huff, & Anderson, 2016). However, prognosis depends on the stage of the tumor and extent of metastasis. Morbidity from treatment of Wilms tumor can occur up to 25 years after diagnosis (Romao & Lorenzo, 2015). Long-term complications include sterility in females, bowel obstruction, and liver or renal damage.

Etiology and Pathophysiology

Wilms tumor is thought to arise from the renal mesenchyme as undifferentiated cells (Daw et al., 2016). In about 2% of cases there is a family history, but there is generally no known cause of Wilms tumor. Genetic mutations are commonly found. Wilms tumor is typically unilateral and may be associated with other congenital abnormalities, such as **aniridia** and genitourinary disorders (Fig. 26.7). Metastasis occurs in the lungs, brain, bones, and lymph nodes.

Clinical Presentation

Most Wilms tumors are found incidentally by a parent or a healthcare provider during a routine exam. Children are often

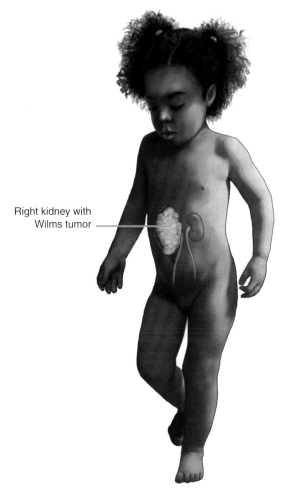

Right kidney with
Wilms tumor

Figure 26.7. Wilms tumor. Wilms tumor is typically unilateral. Reprinted with permission from Kyle, T., & Carman, S. (2016). *Essentials of pediatric nursing* (3rd ed., Fig. 24.18). Philadelphia, PA: Wolters Kluwer.

asymptomatic at the time of diagnosis. Up to 20% of children present with flank pain, hematuria, fever, and/or hypertension (Irtan, Erlich, & Pritchard-Jones, 2016).

Assessment and Diagnosis

Obtain a thorough history of the presenting illness. Determine whether the parents discovered the abdominal mass and, if so, how and when it was first noticed. Ask about a history of disorders associated with Wilms tumor, such as aniridia, genitourinary disorders, or Beckwith–Wiedemann syndrome. Enquire whether there is hematuria, fever, irritability, or pain. Determine whether the mass is causing other symptoms related to compression of organs, such as difficulty breathing, constipation, or urinary retention.

Take the child's vital signs, noting any hypertension or fever. Inspect the abdomen for asymmetry. Auscultate the lungs for adventitious lung sounds. Auscultate for bowel sounds in all four quadrants, noting hypoactive or absent bowel sounds. Palpate the abdomen, noting the size and location of any abdominal mass (Patient Safety 26.2).

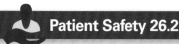

Patient Safety 26.2

Assessment of Children With Wilms Tumor

Do not palpate the child's abdomen after the initial assessment. Wilms tumors can rupture easily, resulting in seeding of the tumor and metastasis. Handle the child carefully when bathing or changing diapers. To ensure limited abdominal palpation, place a sign over the child's bed stating, "DO NOT PALPATE ABDOMEN." Make a note in the electronic medical record, as well.

Abdominal ultrasound and CT of the abdomen are used to distinguish a Wilms tumor from other abdominal masses. The CT is also used to show the extent of disease. Doppler imaging is used to determine renal vein or inferior vena cava involvement. Screening for lung metastasis is done with a chest CT. Diagnosis and staging of Wilms tumor begin with imaging before surgery and are confirmed with a nephrectomy (Table 26.7).

Table 26.7 Staging of Wilms Tumor

Stage	Characteristics
I	• The tumor is contained within one kidney. • The tumor is fully resected without breaking the renal capsule. • There is no lymph node involvement.
II	• The tumor extends beyond the kidney to the fatty tissue or blood vessels. • The tumor is completely resected. • There is no lymph node involvement.
III	The tumor is not fully resected. One or more of the following is present: • Spread to the lymph nodes of the abdomen or pelvis • Microscopic tumor deposits found along the inner lining of the abdomen • Tumor spillage either preoperatively or intraoperatively • Biopsy before nephrectomy • Extension of the tumor into the inferior vena cava • Regional lymph node involvement
IV	Metastasis occurs through the blood to the liver, lungs, brain, bones, and distant lymph nodes.
V	There is bilateral kidney involvement.

Data from American Cancer Society, 2016b; Daw, N. C., Huff, V., & Anderson, P. M. (2016). Neoplasms of the kidney. In R. M. Kliegman, B. F. Stanton, J. W. St. Geme III, N. F. Schor, & R. E. Behrman (Eds.), *Nelson's textbook of pediatrics* (20th ed.). Philadelphia, PA: Elsevier, Saunders.

Therapeutic Interventions

Treatment for Wilms tumor involves a nephrectomy. The stage of the tumor determines whether the child needs additional chemotherapy and radiation. Chemotherapy and radiation may be given before surgery to shrink the tumor. However, the more common practice is to administer chemotherapy and radiation after surgery.

Nursing interventions focus on care of the child after a nephrectomy. Postoperative interventions are related to abdominal surgery. The nurse should monitor for signs and symptoms of infection at the incision site, encourage deep breathing and the use of an incentive spirometer, and prompt the patient to ambulate as ordered. Monitor kidney function of the remaining kidney through BUN and creatinine levels, glomerular filtration rate, and electrolyte levels. Monitor blood pressure and urine output and assess for edema.

Implement general interventions related to the side effects of chemotherapy and radiation for children who require additional treatment after surgery.

Evaluation

Initial outcomes focus on the postoperative child. See the Evaluation section for neuroblastoma.

Discharge Planning and Teaching

Educate parents on warning signs to look for at home. Discuss signs and symptoms of infection at the surgical site. Inform parents of signs of problems with the remaining kidney, such as oliguria and edema. Write down follow-up appointments with the nephrologist and oncologist. Educate the parents and child, if appropriate, on the side effects of chemotherapy and radiation. Provide phone numbers and websites of support groups, especially for children with a poor prognosis.

Retinoblastoma

Retinoblastoma is a malignant tumor involving the retina. It is the most common intraocular tumor in children. The incidence of retinoblastoma is approximately 1 in 18,000 live births around the world (Khaqan, 2017). Retinoblastoma is most commonly diagnosed in children younger than 5 years of age, with 2 years being the median age at diagnosis (Tarek & Herzog, 2016). The 5-year survival rate for retinoblastoma in the United States is 95% (Siegel et al., 2018).

Etiology and Pathophysiology

Retinoblastoma can be either inherited or sporadic. Sporadic retinoblastoma is the result of a genetic mutation and is always unilateral. Inherited retinoblastoma results from a loss or mutation of the retinoblastoma gene and can be either unilateral or bilateral (Tarek & Herzog, 2016). Seventy-five percent of retinoblastoma cases are unilateral (Ortiz & Dunkel, 2016).

Tumors grow from the inner layer of the retina and extend into the vitreous cavity of the eye. Tumors can spread to the optic nerve and the CNS. Sites of distant metastasis include lungs, bone, and bone marrow.

Clinical Presentation

Leukocoria (Fig. 26.8), often called the "cat's eye" reflex, is the most common presenting sign of retinoblastoma. In this condition, the pupil has a white reflex rather than red and is often noticed by parents in a photograph taken with the use of flash photography. Strabismus commonly accompanies leukocoria. Signs that indicate more advanced disease include vision loss, orbital inflammation, and proptosis.

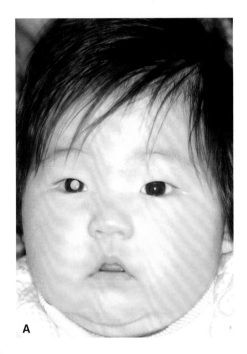

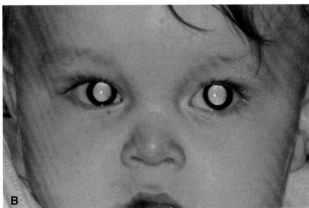

Figure 26.8. Retinoblastoma. A. Unilateral leukocoria is the most common presenting symptom. **B.** Bilateral leukocoria typically indicates an inherited retinoblastoma. Reprinted with permission from Shields, J. A., & Shields, C. L. (2015). *Intraocular tumors: An atlas and textbook* (3rd ed., Figs. 18.103 [A] and 15.5 [B]). Philadelphia, PA: Wolters Kluwer.

Assessment and Diagnosis

Conduct a thorough health history to determine whether there is a family history of retinoblastoma. Ask what signs the parent noticed and when they began. Assess that the pupils are equal, round, and reactive to light. Note the presence of leukocoria. Inspect for swelling or proptosis. Assess for strabismus.

Diagnosis is confirmed by a thorough ophthalmological exam conducted under anesthesia (Tarek & Herzog, 2016). A CT or MRI is done to determine the extent of the tumor and assist with staging of the disease (Table 26.8). A lumbar puncture or bone scan to determine metastasis is conducted only if warranted by assessment findings.

Therapeutic Interventions

The goal of treatment for retinoblastoma is to preserve the eye and vision. Treatment depends on the size and location of the tumor. Newer treatments, such as intra-arterial and intravitreal chemotherapy, have positive results without the side effects of systemic chemotherapy (Khaqan, 2017). Plaque radiation, in which a small radiation disc is placed near the tumor, also shows positive results when used in combination with chemotherapy and can be used in both unilateral and bilateral disease (Ortiz & Dunkel, 2016). Enucleation, removal of the eye, may be necessary for unresponsive or recurrent tumors.

Intra-arterial and intravitreal chemotherapy may have minimal side effects, such as fatigue and leukopenia. Teach parents about good hand washing to prevent infection. Children with metastatic disease require systemic chemotherapy. Implement general nursing interventions related to the care of a child on chemotherapy.

Table 26.8 Staging of Retinoblastoma

Stage	Characteristics
A	Tumors are 3 mm or less and not near important optic structures.
B	Tumors are >3 mm but are still only in the retina.
C	Tumors are well defined but spread under the retina or into the vitreous cavity.
D	• Tumors are large or are poorly defined with widespread seeding in the vitreous cavity. • Retinal detachment may occur.
E	• Tumor is large and extends near the front of the eye. • Bleeding may be present. • There is little to no chance of saving the eye.

Data from American Cancer Society. (2015). *How is retinoblastoma staged?* Retrieved from https://www.cancer.org/cancer/retinoblastoma/detection-diagnosis-staging/staging.html

If the child requires enucleation, postoperative care includes observing the pressure dressing over the orbital socket for bleeding. Perform dressing changes with saline rinses as ordered. Conduct a pain assessment using a developmentally applicable tool and administer pain medication as appropriate.

Evaluation

Evaluation depends on the treatment the child receives. Expected outcomes after surgery for a child with retinoblastoma include the following:

• Fever is absent.
• No signs or symptoms of infection at surgical site are present.
• Pain is at a level that is tolerable for the child.
• The child achieves and maintains adequate nutritional intake.
• The parents verbalize an understanding of care at home.
• The parents demonstrate a dressing change.

For a child not requiring surgery, expected outcomes center on managing the side effects of chemotherapy. See the section Caring for the Child on Chemotherapy, earlier.

Discharge Planning and Teaching

Discuss with parents the need for follow-up appointments with the oncologist and the ophthalmologist. Children requiring surgery have more frequent follow-up appointments in the first year. After 6 months, the child can be fitted with a prosthetic eye, if desired. Children requiring only chemotherapy should have routine ophthalmological exams to assess for tumor recurrence. Discuss protection of the remaining eye, such as using sports goggles and ensuring routine eye exams. Educate parents that when the child is older, genetic counseling is warranted.

Bone Tumors

Osteosarcoma and Ewing sarcoma are the most commonly diagnosed bone tumors in children (Fig. 26.9). Both are typically diagnosed in children 10 to 20 years old. See Table 26.9 for an overview of the differences between osteosarcoma and Ewing sarcoma.

Osteosarcoma

Osteosarcoma is the most commonly diagnosed bone tumor in children and adolescents. At the time of diagnosis, 15% to 20% of patients present with metastasis to the lungs (Taran, Taran, & Malipatil, 2017). The peak incidence of osteosarcoma occurs during the adolescent growth spurt. Adolescents diagnosed with osteosarcoma tend to be taller than their peers (Arndt, 2016a).

Etiology and Pathophysiology

The etiology of osteosarcoma is not well understood. Children with hereditary disorders such as retinoblastoma, Li–Fraumeni syndrome, and Rothmund–Thomson syndrome are predisposed to the development of osteosarcoma (Taran et al., 2017).

The increase in incidence of osteosarcoma during the adolescent growth spurt suggests a correlation with rapid bone proliferation (Taran et al., 2017). Tumors grow at the **metaphysis**, with the most common sites being the distal femur, proximal tibia, and proximal humerus (Lee, 2018).

Clinical Presentation

Pain is the most common presenting symptom. Soft-tissue swelling, a limp, and pathological fracture may also be present. Pain may wake the child up at night. Osteosarcoma typically occurs in active adolescents. The pain and swelling are often intermittent and attributed to sports or to other injuries. Because of the nature of the pain, the adolescent often delays seeking treatment for up to 6 months. Any injury that appears to be a joint sprain or strain that does not respond to conservative therapy should be evaluated.

Assessment and Diagnosis

Determine whether the child has any hereditary conditions that place him or her at increased risk for osteosarcoma. Ask when the symptoms started, the nature of the pain, and what relieves the pain. Enquire whether the pain has interfered with mobility and activity. Inspect the affected area for swelling. Palpate for tenderness and warmth. Assess the range of motion of the affected joint.

An initial X-ray may be performed to determine the cause of the pain and swelling. An MRI of the primary lesion indicates the lesion's size and proximity to blood vessels and nerves and assists with staging. A CT scan of the chest determines whether there is metastasis to the lungs. A bone scan shows whether there is metastasis to the bones. A tissue biopsy, performed after imaging, confirms the diagnosis (Lee, 2018).

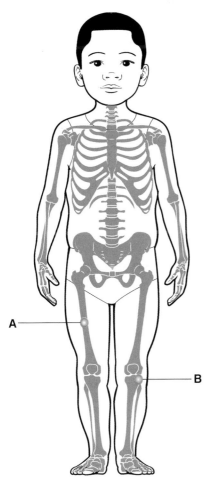

Figure 26.9. Bone tumors. A. Ewing sarcoma most commonly occurs in the shaft, or diaphysis, of a long bone. **B.** Osteosarcoma most commonly occurs near the growth plate at the end, or epiphysis, of a long bone. Modified with permission from Lee, E. (2017). *Pediatric radiology: Practical imaging evaluation of infants and children* (1st ed., unnumbered figure in Chapter 23). Philadelphia, PA: Wolters Kluwer.

Table 26.9 Comparison of Osteosarcoma and Ewing Sarcoma

Clinical Feature	Osteosarcoma	Ewing Sarcoma
Typical age at diagnosis	• Age 10–20 y • More common during growth spurts	Age 10–20 y
Races affected	• All races • Higher incidence in African-Caribbean children	Primarily Caucasian
Gender affected	Higher incidence in males	Higher incidence in males
Location of tumor	Metaphyses of long bones	Diaphyses of long bones
Treatment	• Lungs • Bones	• Lungs • Bones
Survival rates	• 65% 5-y survival rate without metastasis • <20% 5-y survival rate with metastasis at diagnosis	• 61% 5-y survival rate without metastasis • 20%–30% 5-y survival rate with metastasis at diagnosis

Data from Arndt, 2016a ; Lee, V. (2018). Bone tumours in childhood and adolescence. *Paediatrics and Child Health, 28*(4), 164–168; Siegel, R. L., Miller, K. D., Jemal, A. (2018). Cancer statistics, 2018. *CA: A Cancer Journal for Clinicians, 68*(1), 7–30.

Therapeutic Interventions

Chemotherapy is given before surgical resection of the tumor to increase the chances of limb salvage rather than amputation. Combination chemotherapy includes doxorubicin, cisplatin, and high-dose methotrexate (Arndt, 2016a; Lee, 2018). Postoperative treatment consists of chemotherapy for up to 6 months. Prognosis depends on the sites of metastases, initial response to chemotherapy, and whether the tumor was fully resected.

Provide routine postoperative care. Acknowledge the presence of phantom limb pain and give pain medications as ordered. If the adolescent had an amputation, nursing interventions need to focus on body image (Growth and Development Check 26.1). Allow the adolescent to mourn the loss of the limb. Encourage the adolescent to have a prosthetic fitted as soon as possible. Refer the family to support groups, counselors, social workers, and physical therapists.

Evaluation

Expected outcomes for an adolescent receiving treatment for osteosarcoma include the following:

- No signs or symptom of infection at the surgical site are present.
- The adolescent can ambulate independently or with crutches, as ordered.
- The adolescent achieves and maintains adequate nutritional intake.
- The adolescent's output is appropriate for age.
- Pain is at a level acceptable for the adolescent.

For an adolescent requiring amputation, expected outcomes include the following:

- The adolescent begins to accept the loss of the limb.
- The adolescent verbalizes his or her feelings.
- The adolescent demonstrates proper care of the stump.
- The adolescent performs appropriate self-care.
- If a leg is amputated, the adolescent demonstrates proper crutch walking.

 Growth and Development Check 26.1

Identity Versus Role Confusion

The adolescent is in Erikson's stage of identity versus role confusion. An amputation can cause significant identity concerns for the adolescent. Most adolescents diagnosed with osteosarcoma are active, often in sports. The loss of a limb changes the abilities of the adolescent and may cause an identity crisis. Nurses should ensure that the adolescent talks with other adolescents who have lost limbs and have prosthetics. Although it will take time to incorporate this change into a new identity, talking with others will help adolescents see that, although different, they can still participate in some sports and other activities, as well as socialize with their friends.

Discharge Planning and Teaching

If applicable, teach the parents and adolescent how to care for the stump at home. Ensure that the adolescent is able to demonstrate proper crutch walking. Discuss follow-up appointments for chemotherapy. Refer adolescents requiring amputation for a prosthetic fitting. Amputees require follow-up with the orthopedic surgeon, as well.

Ewing Sarcoma

Ewing sarcoma is rarer than osteosarcoma and most commonly found in the bone. However, some extraskeletal tumors share the same immunological traits and are known as members of the Ewing sarcoma family of tumors (Lee, 2018). The most common age of diagnosis for Ewing sarcoma is 15 years. However, the age range is wider for Ewing sarcoma than for osteosarcoma, with Ewing sarcoma occasionally seen in children younger than 10 years of age.

Etiology and Pathophysiology

The etiology of Ewing sarcoma is not known. Ewing sarcoma consists of small, round, blue cells and is differentiated from other cancers with the same types of cells, such as lymphomas, through histological stains and microscopic examination (Arndt, 2016a). The most common sites of Ewing sarcoma are the pelvis, spine, chest wall, and **diaphysis** of the long bones.

Clinical Presentation

The clinical presentation of Ewing sarcoma is similar to that of osteosarcoma. However, children with Ewing sarcoma may also present with fever, weight loss, and fatigue (Lee, 2018). As with osteosarcoma, pain may be associated with a sports injury, resulting in delayed diagnosis. Common sites of metastasis at diagnosis include the lungs, bones, and bone marrow.

Assessment and Diagnosis

Determine the history of the present illness, including when and where the pain began. Enquire whether other symptoms are present. Ask whether the child has a history of other forms of cancer. Inspect and palpate the area of pain for swelling.

Diagnosis begins with an initial X-ray, which is followed by an MRI. A CT scan of the chest, a bone scan, and a bone marrow biopsy are performed to identify any areas of metastasis. Biopsy of the tumor confirms the diagnosis of Ewing sarcoma.

Therapeutic Interventions

Combination chemotherapy is given for 14 days before resection of the tumor. Medications used include doxorubicin, cyclophosphamide, and vincristine. Chemotherapy resumes after surgery. If complete resection of the tumor is not possible, radiation is added to the treatment regimen. Long bone tumors in the extremities may require amputation.

Nursing interventions are similar to those for osteosarcoma. In addition, the child should avoid weight bearing until the treatment is complete. Teach crutch walking while the child is in the hospital. The treatment for Ewing sarcoma is more intense and may require longer hospital stays than is the case for those with osteosarcoma. Ensure that the child has developmentally appropriate activities while in the hospital.

Evaluation

See the Evaluation section for osteosarcoma.

Discharge Planning and Teaching

In addition to providing the same discharge planning and teaching as for osteosarcoma, inform the child and parents that the child will require close, long-term follow-up because of the potential late effects of treatment, such as a second malignancy or late relapses up to 10 years after treatment (Arndt, 2016a).

Soft-Tissue Tumors

Soft-tissue tumors are sarcomas that arise from the connective tissues, such as the muscles, nerves, and blood vessels (Dangoor et al., 2016). The most common soft-tissue tumor in children is rhabdomyosarcoma.

Rhabdomyosarcoma

Rhabdomyosarcoma arises from muscle tissue. About 3% of all childhood cancers are rhabdomyosarcomas (Arndt, 2016b). These tumors can occur anywhere in the body, but the most common sites are the head and neck, genitourinary tract, extremities, and orbit (Figs. 26.10 and 26.11). Most cases are diagnosed in children younger than age 10 years, with the peak incidence occurring in those younger than 6 years old (Wasti, Mandeville, Gatz, & Chisolm, 2018). Prognosis depends on the age of the child and the stage of the tumor at diagnosis. The 5-year survival rate for children younger than 15 years old is about 70%. For children older than 15 years, the 5-year survival rate is 45% (Siegel et al., 2018).

Etiology and Pathophysiology

The etiology of rhabdomyosarcoma is largely unknown. Hereditary syndromes with an increased risk of cancers, such as neurofibromatosis type I and Li–Fraumeni syndrome, also have an increased risk of rhabdomyosarcoma. Rhabdomyosarcoma tumors arise from the same embryonic cells as skeletal muscle but fail to differentiate. The cells resemble other round cell tumors, such as Ewing sarcoma, neuroblastoma, and NHL (Arndt, 2016b). Histological studies are needed for a definitive diagnosis.

Clinical Presentation

Clinical presentation of rhabdomyosarcoma depends on the site of the tumor (Table 26.10). Generally, symptoms are caused by obstruction or organ displacement by the tumor.

Assessment and Diagnosis

Obtain a thorough health history from the caregivers, including the symptoms the child is experiencing. Ask when the symptoms started and whether they have gotten worse over time. Determine

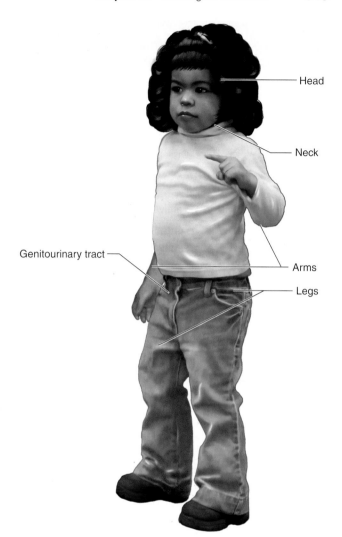

Figure 26.10. Rhabdomyosarcoma. Common sites of rhabdomyosarcoma in children. Reprinted with permission from Kyle, T., & Carman, S. (2016). *Essentials of pediatric nursing* (3rd ed., Fig. 24.17). Philadelphia, PA: Wolters Kluwer.

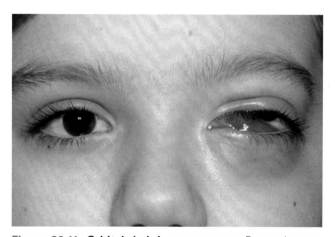

Figure 26.11. Orbital rhabdomyosarcoma. Proptosis seen with orbital tumors in rhabdomyosarcoma. Reprinted with permission from Nelson, L. B., & Olitsky, S. E. (2013). *Harley's pediatric ophthalmology* (6th ed., Fig. 19.27A). Philadelphia, PA: Wolters Kluwer.

Table 26.10 Clinical Presentation of Rhabdomyosarcoma

Origin of Tumor	Clinical Presentation
Nasopharynx	• Nasal congestion • Mouth breathing • Epistaxis • Difficulty swallowing
Face	• Swelling • Pain • Paralysis of cranial nerves
Neck	• Difficulty swallowing • Difficulty breathing
Orbital (Fig. 26.11)	• Proptosis • Periorbital edema • Pain • Visual acuity change
Middle ear	• Pain • Hearing loss • Chronic otorrhea • Cranial nerve paralysis
Larynx	• Difficulty swallowing • Croup-like cough • Stridor
Thorax	Painless mass
Genitourinary tract	• Hematuria • Recurrent urinary tract infections • Urinary obstruction
Testicles	• Mass in the scrotum • Painless
Vaginal canal	• Grape-like mass bulging through the vaginal opening • Vaginal bleeding

Data from Arndt, 2016b.

Priority Care Concepts 26.2

Maintain a Patent Airway

Children with tumors of the larynx, head, neck, or thorax are at risk for airway compression, which can result in respiratory distress. Be sure to monitor for signs and symptoms of respiratory distress, including the following:

• Stridor
• Increased work of breathing
• Adventitious lung sounds
• Tachypnea
• Bradycardia
• Pale or cyanotic skin

Intervention is necessary to prevent respiratory failure. Nurses should monitor the child's respiratory status closely for minor status changes.

Therapeutic Interventions

Treatment is based on the stage of the tumor, tumor histology, and the amount of tumor able to be resected (Arndt, 2016b). Children with rhabdomyosarcoma require surgery as well as chemotherapy and radiation. The type of chemotherapy used varies depending on the stage and size of the tumor.

Nursing interventions include routine postoperative care for the site of surgery. Assess for side effects of radiation and chemotherapy. Implement general interventions for a child on chemotherapy.

Evaluation

Evaluation of a child with rhabdomyosarcoma depends on the site of the tumor. Expected outcomes for a child with a tumor of the head, neck, or larynx include the following:

• The child maintains a patent airway.
• Adequate air movement is present in all lung fields.
• Adventitious lung sounds are absent.
• O_2 saturation level remains at 95% or above.

Expected outcomes for a child with a tumor of the bladder include the following:

• No hematuria is present.
• No signs or symptoms of a urinary tract infection are present.
• The child maintains a rate of urine output of 1 to 2 mg/kg/h.

Routine postoperative evaluation is appropriate for all children with rhabdomyosarcoma. Monitor for the side effects of chemotherapy and radiation. Evaluate the effectiveness of nursing interventions related to the side effects of chemotherapy and radiation.

Discharge Planning and Teaching

Discuss the treatment plan with the parents. Owing to the intense nature of the chemotherapy and radiation, ensure that the parents understand when to call the healthcare provider. Plan follow-up appointments for the child with the surgeon, oncologist, and radiation oncologist.

whether there is a family history of hereditary syndromes that increase the child's risk of cancer. Inspect the child for visible masses. For children with tumors of the head, neck, throat, or chest, assess for respiratory distress (Priority Care Concepts 26.2). Auscultate the lungs, noting any adventitious lung sounds. Palpate for masses, lymphadenopathy, and hepatosplenomegaly. For suspected facial, ear, orbital, and neck tumors, assess the cranial nerves. Note abnormal findings. Other abnormal findings on physical assessment relate to the location of the tumor.

Definitive diagnosis is determined by biopsy, microscopic appearance, and immunohistochemical stains (Wasti et al., 2018). Other diagnostic tests, such as CT, MRI, bone scan, and bone marrow aspiration, determine metastasis and help with staging (Table 26.11). Lymph node biopsy is also done to determine the extent of the disease.

Table 26.11 Staging of Rhabdomyosarcoma

Stage	Characteristics

1	• The tumor originated in a favorable site, such as the following:
	  ○ Orbit
	  ○ Head and neck
	  ○ Genitourinary tract (except the bladder)
	• The tumor may have spread to nearby lymph nodes.
	• No distant metastasis has occurred.

2	• The tumor originated in an unfavorable site, such as the following:
	  ○ Bladder
	  ○ Parameningeal site
	  ○ Extremity
	  ○ Other sites not mentioned in stage 1
	• The tumor is <5 cm.
	• There is no evidence of any metastasis.

3	• The tumor originated in an unfavorable site. • Tumor is <5 cm and has spread to nearby lymph nodes. *or* • The tumor is 5 cm or larger with no evidence of metastasis.
4	• The tumor originated from any site. • The tumor is any size. • Widespread metastasis has occurred.

Data from: Wasti, A. T., Mandeville, H., Gatz, S., & Chisolm, J. C. (2018). Rhabdomyosarcoma. *Paediatrics and Child Health, 28*(4), 157–163; Arndt, 2016, American Cancer Society, 2014.

Think Critically

1. Explain some of the key differences between pediatric and adult cancers.
2. List and prioritize nursing interventions for children experiencing the side effects of chemotherapy.
3. What are the biggest risks for children experiencing stomatitis, nausea, and vomiting as side effects of chemotherapy?
4. Discuss the progression from infection to sepsis.
5. What are ways to help children and adolescents cope with the emotional and social side effects of cancer?
6. What are the common presenting signs and symptoms of leukemia?
7. Why have bone tumors typically metastasized by the time they are diagnosed?

References

American Cancer Society. (2016a). *Do we know what causes brain and spinal cord tumors in children?* Retrieved from https://www.cancer.org/cancer/brain-spinal-cord-tumors-children/causes-risks-prevention/what-causes.html

American Cancer Society. (2016b). *How is Wilms tumor staged?* Retrieved from https://www.cancer.org/cancer/wilms-tumor/detection-diagnosis-staging/staging.html

American Cancer Society. (2016c). *What are the differences between cancers in adults and children?* Retrieved from https://www.cancer.org/cancer/cancer-in-children/differences-adults-children.html

American Cancer Society. (2016d). *What is non-Hodgkin lymphoma?* Retrieved from https://www.cancer.org/cancer/non-hodgkin-lymphoma/about/what-is-non-hodgkin-lymphoma.html

American Cancer Society. (2016e). *What's new in research and treatment for brain and spinal cord tumors in children?* Retrieved from https://www.cancer.org/cancer/brain-spinal-cord-tumors-children/about/new-research.html

American Cancer Society. (2017). *What is Hodgkin lymphoma?* Retrieved from https://www.cancer.org/cancer/hodgkin-lymphoma/about/what-is-hodgkin-disease.html

Arndt, C. A. S. (2016a). Malignant tumors of the bone. In R. M. Kliegman, B. F. Stanton, J. W. St. Geme III, N. F. Schor, & R. E. Behrman (Eds.), *Nelson's textbook of pediatrics* (20th ed.). Philadelphia, PA: Elsevier, Saunders.

Arndt, C. A. S. (2016b). Soft tissue tumors. In R. M. Kliegman, B. F. Stanton, J. W. St. Geme III, N. F. Schor, & R. E. Behrman (Eds.), *Nelson's textbook of pediatrics* (20th ed.). Philadelphia, PA: Elsevier, Saunders.

Asselin, B. L. (2016). Epidemiology of childhood and adolescent cancers. In R. M. Kliegman, B. F. Stanton, J. W. St. Geme III, N. F. Schor, & R. E. Behrman (Eds.), *Nelson's textbook of pediatrics* (20th ed.). Philadelphia, PA: Elsevier, Saunders.

Ater, J. L., & Kuttesch J. F., Jr. (2016). Brain tumors in childhood. In R. M. Kliegman, B. F. Stanton, J. W. St. Geme III, N. F. Schor, & R. E. Behrman (Eds.), *Nelson's textbook of pediatrics* (20th ed.). Philadelphia, PA: Elsevier, Saunders.

Bulut, H. C., & Tufecki, F. G. (2016). Honey prevents oral mucositis in children undergoing chemotherapy: A quasi-experimental study with a control group. *Complementary Therapies in Medicine, 29*, 132–140.

Chan, V., Pole, J. D., Mann, R. E., & Colantonio, A. (2015). A population based perspective on children and youth with brain tumors. *BMC Cancer, 15*(1007), 1–9.

Cooper, S. L., & Brown, P. A. (2015). Treatment of pediatric acute lymphoblastic leukemia. *Pediatric Clinics of North America, 62*, 61–73.

Curtin, S. C., Minino, A. M., & Anderson, R. N. (2016). Declines in cancer death rates among children and adolescents in the United States, 1999–2014. *NCHS Data Brief, 257*, 1–7.

Daw, N. C., Huff, V., & Anderson, P. M. (2016). Neoplasms of the kidney. In R. M. Kliegman, B. F. Stanton, J. W. St. Geme III, N. F. Schor, & R. E. Behrman (Eds.), *Nelson's textbook of pediatrics* (20th ed.). Philadelphia, PA: Elsevier, Saunders.

Dangoor, A., Seddon, B., Gerrand, C., Grimer, R., Whelan, J., & Judson, I. (2016). UK guidelines for the management of soft tissue sarcomas. *Clinical Sarcoma Research, 6*(20), 1–26.

Englund, A., Glimeliusb, I., Rostgaardd, K., Smedbyb, K. E., Elorantab, S., Molinc, D., . . . Lyngsie Hjalgrim, L. (2018). Hodgkin lymphoma in children, adolescents and young adults—A comparative study of clinical presentation and treatment outcome. *Acta Oncologica, 57*(2), 276–282.

Friehling, E., Ritchey, A. K., Tubergen, D. G., & Bleyer, A. (2016). Acute lymphoblastic leukemia. In R. M. Kliegman, B. F. Stanton, J. W. St. Geme III, N. F. Schor, & R. E. Behrman (Eds.), *Nelson's textbook of pediatrics* (20th ed.). Philadelphia, PA: Elsevier, Saunders.

Hochberg, J., Giulino-Roth, L., & Cairo, M. (2016). Lymphoma. In R. M. Kliegman, B. F. Stanton, J. W. St. Geme III, N. F. Schor, & R. E. Behrman (Eds.), *Nelson's textbook of pediatrics* (20th ed.). Philadelphia, PA: Elsevier, Saunders.

Irtan, S., Erlich, P. F., & Pritchard-Jones, K. (2016). Wilms tumor: "State-of-the-art" update, 2016. *Seminars in Pediatric Surgery, 25*, 250–256.

Jassal, S. S. (2015). Symptom control in paediatric palliative care. *Paediatrics and Child Health, 26*(2), 87–88.

Kaye, E. C., Gushue, C. A., DeMarsh, S., Jerkins, J., Sykes, A., Lu, Z., . . . Baker, J. N. (2018). Illness and end-of-life experiences of children with cancer who receive palliative care. *Pediatric and Blood Cancer, 65*, e26895.

Khaqan, H. A. (2017). Recent advances in the treatment of retinoblastoma. *Opthomology Update, 15*(3), 254–257.

Klanjsek, P., & Pajnkihar, M. (2016). Causes of inadequate intake of nutrients during the treatment of children with chemotherapy. *European Journal of Oncology Nursing, 23*, 24–33.

Lee, V. (2018). Bone tumours in childhood and adolescence. *Paediatrics and Child Health, 28*(4), 164–168.

Lukscha, R., Castellani, M. R., Collini, P., De Bernardi, B., Conte, M., Gambini, C., . . . Tonini, G. P. (2016). Neuroblastoma (peripheral neuroblastic tumors). *Critical Reviews in Oncology/Hematology, 107*, 163–181.

Mariyana, R., Allenidekania, A., & Nurhaeni, N. (2018). Parents' voice in managing the pain of children with cancer during palliative care. *Indian Journal of Palliative Care, 24*, 156–161.

McCulloch, R., Hemsley, J., & Kelly, P. (2018). Symptom management during chemotherapy. *Paediatrics and Child Health, 28*(4), 190–195.

McDonnell, G. A., Salley, C. G., Barnett, M., DeRosa, A. P., Werk, R. S., Hourani, A., . . . Ford, J. S. (2017). Anxiety among adolescent survivors of pediatric cancer. *Journal of Adolescent Health, 61*, 409–423.

Mullassery, D., & Lotsy, P. D. (2015). Neuroblastoma. *Paediatrics and Child Health, 26*(2), 68–72.

National Cancer Institute. (2017). *Cancer in children and adults*. Retrieved from https://www.cancer.gov/types/childhood-cancers/child-adolescent-cancers-fact-sheet

National Cancer Institute: Center for Cancer Research. (n.d.). *Pediatric oncology branch*. Retrieved from https://ccr.cancer.gov/pediatric-oncology-branch

Newman, E. A., & Nuchtern, J. G. (2016). Recent biologic and genetic advances in neuroblastoma: Implications for diagnostic, risk stratification, and treatment strategies. *Seminars in Pediatric Surgery, 25*, 257–264.

Ortiz, M. V., & Dunkel, I. J. (2016). Retinoblastoma. *Journal of Child Neurology, 31*(2), 227–236.

Pi, J., Kang, Y., Smith, M., Earl, M., Norigian, Z., & McBride, A. (2016). A review in the treatment of oncologic emergencies. *Journal of Oncology Pharmacy Practice, 22*(4), 625–638.

Ranallo, L. (2017). Improving the quality of end-of-life care in pediatric oncology patients through the early implementation of palliative care. *Journal of Pediatric Oncology Nursing, 34*(6), 374–380.

Richardson, B., Rupasov, A., & Sharma, A. (2018). Superior vena cava syndrome. *Journal of Radiology Nursing, 37*, 36–40.

Romao, R. L. P., & Lorenzo, A. J. (2015). Renal function in patients with Wilms' tumor. *Urologic Oncology: Seminars and Original Investigations, 34*, 33–41.

Tubergen, D. G., Bleyer, A., Friehling, E., & Ritchey, A. K. (2016). Acute myelogenous leukemia. In R. M. Kliegman, B. F. Stanton, J. W. St. Geme III, N. F. Schor, & R. E. Behrman (Eds.), *Nelson's textbook of pediatrics* (20th ed.). Philadelphia, PA: Elsevier, Saunders.

Tubergen, D. G., Bleyer, A., Ritchey, A. K., & Friehling, E. (2016). The leukemias. In R. M. Kliegman, B. F. Stanton, J. W. St. Geme III, N. F. Schor, & R. E. Behrman (Eds.), *Nelson's textbook of pediatrics* (20th ed.). Philadelphia, PA: Elsevier, Saunders.

Schuz, J., & Erdmann, F. (2016). Environmental exposure and risk of childhood leukemia: An overview. *Archives of Medical Research, 47*, 607–614.

Seth, R., Singh, A., Setj, S., & Sapra, S. (2017). Late effects of treatment in survivors of childhood cancers: A single-centre experience. *Indian Journal of Medical Research, 146*, 216–223.

Siegel, R. L., Miller, K. D., Jemal, A. (2017). Cancer statistics, 2017. *CA: A Cancer Journal for Clinicians, 67*(1), 7–30.

Siegel, R. L., Miller, K. D., Jemal, A. (2018). Cancer statistics, 2018. *CA: A Cancer Journal for Clinicians, 68*(1), 7–30.

Tarek, N., & Herzog, C. E. (2016). Retinoblastoma. In R. M. Kliegman, B. F. Stanton, J. W. St. Geme III, N. F. Schor, & R. E. Behrman (Eds.), *Nelson's textbook of pediatrics* (20th ed.). Philadelphia, PA: Elsevier, Saunders.

Taran, S. J., Taran, R., & Malipatil, N. B. (2017). Pediatric osteosarcoma: An updated review. *Indian Journal of Medical and Paediatric Oncology, 38*, 33–43.

Uzunova, L., & Burke, A. (2015). Update on non-Hodgkin lymphoma in children. *Paediatrics and Child Health, 26*(2), 57–62.

Velardi, A., & Locatelli, F., (2016a). Graft-versus-host disease, rejection, and venooclusive disease. In R. M. Kliegman, B. F. Stanton, J. W. St. Geme III, N. F. Schor, & R. E. Behrman (Eds.), *Nelson's textbook of pediatrics* (20th ed.). Philadelphia, PA: Elsevier, Saunders.

Velardi, A., & Locatelli, F. (2016b). Late effects of hematopoietic stem cell transplantation. In R. M. Kliegman, B. F. Stanton, J. W. St. Geme III, N. F. Schor, & R. E. Behrman (Eds.), *Nelson's textbook of pediatrics* (20th ed.). Philadelphia, PA: Elsevier, Saunders.

Velardi, A., & Locatelli, F (2016c). Principles and clinical indications of hematopoietic stem cell transplantation. In R. M. Kliegman, B. F. Stanton, J. W. St. Geme III, N. F. Schor, & R. E. Behrman (Eds.), *Nelson's textbook of pediatrics* (20th ed.). Philadelphia, PA: Elsevier, Saunders.

Wasti, A. T., Mandeville, H., Gatz, S., & Chisolm, J. C. (2018). Rhabdomyosarcoma. *Paediatrics and Child Health, 28*(4), 157–163.

Whitehead, T. P., Metayer, C., Wiemels, J. L., Singer, A. W., & Miller, M. D. (2016). Childhood leukemia and primary prevention. *Current Problems in Pediatric and Adolescent Health Care, 46*, 317–352.

Worth, L. L. (2016). Molecular and cellular biology of cancer. In R. M. Kliegman, B. F. Stanton, J. W. St. Geme III, N. F. Schor, & R. E. Behrman (Eds.), *Nelson's textbook of pediatrics* (20th ed.). Philadelphia, PA: Elsevier, Saunders.

Yacobovich, J., Ben-Ami, T., Abdalla, T., Tamary, H., Goldstein, G., Weintraub, M., . . . Revel-Vilk, S. (2015). Patient and central venous catheter related risk factors for blood stream infections in children receiving chemotherapy. *Pediatric Blood Cancer, 62*, 471–476.

Zage, P. E., & Ater, J. L. (2016). Neuroblastoma. In R. M. Kliegman, B. F. Stanton, J. W. St. Geme III, N. F. Schor, & R. E. Behrman (Eds.), *Nelson's textbook of pediatrics* (20th ed.). Philadelphia, PA: Elsevier, Saunders.

Suggested Readings

McCulloch, R., Hemsley, J., & Kelly, P. (2018). Symptom management during chemotherapy. *Paediatrics and Child Health, 28*(4), 190–195.

National Cancer Institute. *Childhood cancer*. Retrieved from https://www.cancer.gov/types/childhood-cancers

National Pediatric Cancer Foundation. *Facts about childhood cancer*. Retrieved from https://nationalpcf.org/facts-about-childhood-cancer/

27

Alterations in Musculoskeletal Function

Objectives

After completing this chapter, you will be able to:

1. Compare and contrast anatomical and physiological characteristics of the musculoskeletal systems of children and adults.
2. Relate pediatric assessment findings to the child's musculoskeletal status.
3. Discuss the pathophysiology of common pediatric musculoskeletal disorders.
4. Differentiate between signs and symptoms of common pediatric musculoskeletal disorders.
5. Outline the therapeutic regimen for each of the pediatric musculoskeletal disorders.
6. Describe pharmacological management of common pediatric musculoskeletal disorders.
7. Apply the principles of growth and development to the care of a child with a musculoskeletal disorder.
8. Discuss the priority care concepts for each of the common pediatric musculoskeletal disorders.

Key Terms

Abduction
Dysplasia
Epiphysis
Genu
Idiopathic
Ligament

Osteoblasts
Periosteum
Tendon
Valgus
Varus

Variations in Anatomy and Physiology

The musculoskeletal system of children differs from that of adults in three main areas: the growth of bone, the nature or characteristics of bone, and the alignment of bones. At birth, the newborn body consists of 300 bones. Most of these bones begin as temporary cartilage and then fuse and ossify, starting at 2 to 3 years of age, to form the 206 bones in the adult body. The sutures of the skull initially remain open to allow for growth of the brain and skull. The posterior fontanel usually closes by 2 months of age. The average age of anterior fontanel closure is 13 months, and most are closed by 24 months

(Kiesler & Ricer, 2013). The ossification center at the greater trochanter appears at 3 years of age in girls and 6 years of age in boys, whereas the secondary pubic ossification center appears during puberty (9–11 years of age in girls and 13–16 years of age in boys). These ossification centers are important for determining bone age and skeletal maturity.

The presence of the growth plate is the most notable musculoskeletal difference between children and adults (Fig. 27.1). Rapid growth occurs in the long bones at the growth plate. During periods of growth, cartilage cells in the **epiphysis** are ossified by **osteoblasts** (immature bone cells); this process continues until the age of the early 20s, when the growth plate

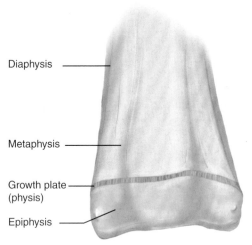

Figure 27.1. Anatomic areas of growing bone. Reprinted with permission from Kyle, T., & Carman, S. (2016). *Essentials of pediatric nursing* (3rd ed., Fig. 22.1). Philadelphia, PA: Wolters Kluwer.

completely ossifies (National Cancer Institute, n.d.). Although the growth plates allow for rapid growth, which accelerates the healing process, injuries involving the growth plate or long bones are of concern because they may affect growth and remodeling of the bone.

Bones in children are more porous and less dense than bones in adults. They are more elastic, allowing for greater deformation to occur before breaking. Commonly, rather than break, the elastic pediatric bone buckles (compresses or bulges in on itself), as did David Torres's in Chapter 3. The periosteal sleeve surrounding a child's bone is thicker than an adult's, which allows the bone to restrain a displacement. This also allows the bone to heal itself from the inside (Poduval, 2015; University of British Columbia, 2012). Ligaments and tendons of children are stronger than bones until they reach puberty.

Lower limb alignment alters as children grow. Foot arches are not developed in younger children, resulting in flat feet, which can be a normal finding until the age of 6 years. Walking with the feet turned inward (intoeing or being "pigeon-toed") can be a normal gait pattern for children up to 8 years old. Toddlers have a **varus** alignment of the knee, resulting in a "bow-leg" appearance and waddling gait until about 2 years of age. This alignment begins to straighten as the child grows but can become a **valgus** alignment, causing "knock-knees" until approximately 7 years of age (American Academy of Orthopaedic Surgeons [AAOS], n.d.a; Poduval, 2015).

Assessment of the Pediatric Musculoskeletal System

Musculoskeletal disorders can present at birth or be acquired later in childhood. Some musculoskeletal disorders have genetic components, some result from trauma, and some are **idiopathic**. Other disorders may result in musculoskeletal abnormalities; likewise, musculoskeletal disorders may affect other body systems. Table 27.1 provides a guide for assessing the pediatric musculoskeletal system. Management of musculoskeletal disorders may be short term or long term and may require hospitalization or be completely outpatient based. Depending on the nature of the disorder, treatment may consist of observation, bracing, casting, traction, surgery, and/or medication.

General Nursing Interventions for Musculoskeletal Disorders

Given here is an overview of key nursing interventions that apply to musculoskeletal disorders, in general. Interventions that are specific to a given disorder are discussed within the Therapeutic Interventions section of that disorder.

Promote Pain Relief, Comfort, and Rest

Children with musculoskeletal disorders may experience discomfort that can interfere with activities, function, and/or sleep. Encourage the child to rest when indicated, especially in the immediate postoperative period. Assist the child to achieve positions of comfort. Use pillows or towels to support the extremities, lower back, neck, or shoulders. Administer pain medications as ordered and supplement with developmentally appropriate nonpharmacological pain control techniques such as deep breathing, distraction, and imagery.

Prevent Infection

Children with open wounds secondary to injury or with surgical incisions are susceptible to infection. Assess the wound or incision for redness, edema, drainage, and approximation of the edges. Assess the child for fever. Maintain strict asepsis and meticulous hand washing. Teach the child and family to adhere to strict hand washing practices.

Maintain Body Alignment and Function

Some musculoskeletal disorders alter body alignment and function. For some disorders, surgical intervention may restore body alignment and function. Assist children to maintain body alignment and function through proper positioning, ambulation, and posture. Reinforce proper use of assistive devices. Postoperatively, reposition at least every 2 hours and support positioning with pillows or towels.

Promote Physical Ability

Children with musculoskeletal disorders may also experience alterations in physical abilities. Encourage children to be active in developmentally and physically appropriate ways. Assess the child's range of motion and physical abilities. Encourage early ambulation in the postoperative period. Assist the family with identifying appropriate activities and resources to promote the child's physical ability (e.g., therapeutic recreation, YMCA, physical therapy, and community centers).

Table 27.1 Assessment Guide: Pediatric Musculoskeletal System

Assessment Area	Assessment
General questions	• Does the child have pain or stiffness in any muscles or joints? • Does the child have difficulty getting dressed without help (for school-age children and older)? • Does the child have difficulty going up or down stairs (for preschool children and older)? • Describe the child's daily activities. • Is the child meeting developmental milestones? • What sports does the child play? • Does the child wear protective equipment during sports or recreational play? • Have there been any recent events or traumas? • Is there a family history of disorders of the musculoskeletal system?
Body alignment	• Observe the child's posture. • Observe symmetry of limbs, shoulders, hips, and body movements. • Observe limb alignment, noticing whether limbs are the same length and whether there are abnormal alignments (curvatures such as bow legs or knock-knees). • Observe the alignment of the spine for curvature (have the child bend at the waist, and note spine curvature or rib hump).
Gait	• Observe the child walking to note any abnormalities (e.g., feet turning inward, walking on the outer edges of the feet, walking on toes, ataxia). • Inquire about changes in mobility (increases or decreases). • Observe for limping. • Inquire about pain with walking.

Range of motion	• Observe flexion and extension of joints:
	   ◦ Neck
	   ◦ Shoulders
	   ◦ Elbows
	   ◦ Wrists
	   ◦ Fingers
	   ◦ Hips
	   ◦ Knees
	   ◦ Ankles
	   ◦ Toes
	• Observe for symmetry and smoothness of movements (note any spasticity or laxness).
	• Feel for masses.
	• Observe for inflammation, redness, and crepitus (can grinding or clicking noises be heard?).

Promote Growth and Development

Children being treated for musculoskeletal disorders may be immobile, inactive, or hospitalized for long periods; therefore, promoting growth and development during this time is a necessity. Provide developmentally appropriate activities that actively engage the child. Provide anticipatory guidance to the family members and encourage them to provide activities that will promote growth and development for the next stages. Encourage students to continue with school work if appropriate. Encourage friends and family to visit and/or communicate with children who are hospitalized or immobilized when appropriate.

Educate Families on Therapeutic Interventions

Most musculoskeletal disorders require some degree of therapeutic intervention. Educate the child and family about nonsurgical and surgical treatment options, as well as pharmacological interventions. Prepare the child and family for pre- and postintervention care and activity.

Congenital and Developmental Musculoskeletal Disorders

Some musculoskeletal disorders, such as pectus excavatum, polydactyly, syndactyly, and clubfoot, are congenital, meaning that they manifest at birth. Others, such as osteogenesis imperfecta (OI), Blount disease, and developmental dysplasia of the hip (DDH), only manifest as the child develops.

Pectus Excavatum

Pectus excavatum is a congenital deformity that causes the ribs and sternum to grow abnormally such that the breastbone (sternum) goes inward, producing a depression or concave

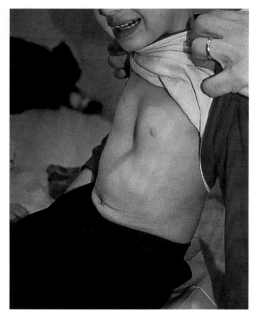

Figure 27.2. Pectus excavatum. Note the depression in the chest wall at the xiphoid process. Reprinted with permission from Kyle, T., & Carman, S. (2016). *Essentials of pediatric nursing* (3rd ed., Fig. 22.15). Philadelphia, PA: Wolters Kluwer.

appearance (Fig. 27.2). This deformity is also known as sunken or funnel chest.

Etiology and Pathophysiology

The cause of the deformity is unknown, although some familial tendencies have been noted (~35% of children with pectus excavatum have family members with the same deformity). Pectus excavatum is also associated with other conditions, such as Marfan syndrome, Poland syndrome, rickets, and scoliosis. Boys are affected with this condition 3 times more often than girls.

Clinical Presentation

Pectus excavatum is usually noticed at birth, but its degree of severity typically increases during growth spurts. Many children with this condition are physiologically asymptomatic. Children who experience more severe deformities may have cardiopulmonary difficulties resulting from pressure of the chest on the heart and lungs.

Assessment and Diagnosis

In addition to chest deformities, assess for symptoms of cardiopulmonary difficulties in children with this condition. Children may experience fatigue, exercise intolerance, chest pain, coughing, wheezing, frequent respiratory infections, and palpitations. Chest X-rays and computed tomography (CT) scans are helpful in providing information about the chest asymmetry. The physical appearance of this deformity often leads to alterations in body image and low self-esteem (Hebra, 2017). Assess affect and social support systems. An echocardiogram and pulmonary function test can provide information about cardiopulmonary

function in children experiencing complications. A consult with a cardiologist and pulmonologist might also be indicated.

Therapeutic Interventions

No treatment is indicated for children who are asymptomatic. Surgery is the indicated treatment when symptoms of cardiopulmonary compromise arise. The goal of surgery is to reshape the sternum and relieve pressure on the chest. During surgery a bar is inserted into the chest to maintain the structure. The nurse plays a key role in preparing the child and family for surgery and the postoperative period.

Postoperative care priorities are pain management, breathing exercises, and mobility. Deep breathing may be difficult in the immediate postoperative period. Teaching the child how to splint the chest with a pillow or stuffed animal while coughing and taking deep breaths will help minimize pain. Physical therapy is indicated to strengthen the weak chest wall muscles. A high-fiber diet and laxatives may be necessary postoperatively, because constipation is reported as a common complication following pectus excavatum repair (Hebra, 2017).

Evaluation

Expected outcomes for a child with pectus excavatum include the following:

- The child has no cardiopulmonary compromise.
- The child undergoes fusion of the chest postoperatively (if surgery is required).
- The child has successful removal of the stabilizing bar after fusion, if applicable.
- The child has a positive body image.

Discharge Planning and Teaching

Children should maintain a straight posture and avoid lifting for the first month postoperatively. They can resume normal activities after 3 months but should not participate in contact sports for 6 months. The bar that was inserted during surgery is usually removed after 2 years, once the bones in the chest have had time to fully fuse. Prepare the child and family for a future surgery to remove the bar. Recovery following the bar removal surgery is usually shorter and less traumatic for most children than that following the original surgery to repair the deformity.

Polydactyly and Syndactyly

Polydactyly and syndactyly are the most common congenital anomalies of the hand and foot (Malik, 2012; Lennox, 2016).

Etiology and Pathophysiology

Polydactyly is a genetic condition resulting in extra digits on the hands and/or feet. Syndactyly is a genetic condition in which the digits fail to separate and thus have a fused or webbed appearance. Both conditions can occur alone or in combination with other disorders. In both conditions, the digits can be composed of skin, soft tissue, bone, joints, or any combination of these. Syndactyly often involves nerves and muscles.

Clinical Presentation

As noted, polydactyly presents as extra digits on the hands and/or feet, whereas syndactyly presents as webbed digits.

Assessment and Diagnosis

Radiological studies are necessary to determine the nature of the defect. Ultrasound can be used for prenatal imaging.

Therapeutic Interventions

Treatment involves surgical correction consisting of removal of extra digits with polydactyly or separation of fused digits with syndactyly. Depending on the degree of structures involved, surgery can be complex and varies from child to child and from digit to digit. Postoperatively, casting may be necessary to immobilize the area and promote healing. Occupational and physical therapy may be indicated to assist the child with movement, strength, and adaptations (Whose Job Is It, Anyway? 27.1).

Evaluation

Expected outcomes for a child with polydactyly or syndactyly include the following:
- The child has proper pain control and an absence of infection following surgery.
- The child has optimal function of the hand or foot and digits.
- The child has a positive body image and self-esteem.

Discharge Planning and Teaching

Following surgery, the child's extremity may be placed in a cast or splint. Teach the family to keep the cast dry and to avoid putting anything inside the cast to prevent skin breakdown and infection.

Osteogenesis Imperfecta

OI is a disorder affecting collagen that results in fragile bones that break easily.

Etiology and Pathophysiology

OI is a genetic disorder of too little or poor quality of type I collagen. It can be carried on either a dominant or recessive gene or be the result of a spontaneous gene mutation. Collagen is the

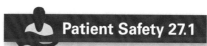

Patient Safety 27.1

Blood Pressure Cuffs

Compression of a blood pressure cuff can be enough to cause a fracture in many children with OI. Collaborate with the healthcare provider before assessing blood pressure on children with OI.

protein of the body's connective tissue that bones are formed around. There are eight types of OI, varying in symptoms and severity. Type I is the most common and the mildest form. It is the type discussed in this chapter (National Organization of Rare Disorders [NORD], 2007).

Clinical Presentation

Children with OI often begin to experience bone fractures, even with minor injuries, once they begin walking. This continues until puberty, when the frequency of fractures may decline.

Assessment and Diagnosis

Assess children suspected of having OI for signs of fractures, including inability to move the affected area, swelling, bruising, and pain (Patient Safety 27.1). Note any muscle weakness. Assess for bone deformities, which can result from repeated fractures. Assess height and note whether the child is of short stature. Assess the face for a triangular shape. Assess the sclera for blue tinting, another manifestation of OI. Assess hearing, because hearing loss is a common manifestation of OI. Diagnosis is made through clinical evaluation and history, skin biopsy to detect collagen, and genetic testing. Radiological studies are used to detect bone fractures and stages of healing. Multiple fractures, in various stages of healing, can be common (Patient Safety 27.2).

Therapeutic Interventions

Treatment is often palliative, involving managing the presenting symptoms or fractures. Physical therapy exercises, especially hydrotherapy, are beneficial to strengthen muscles supporting the weak bones. Children may need mobility aids.

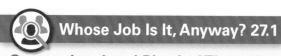

Whose Job Is It, Anyway? 27.1

Occupational and Physical Therapists

Occupational therapists work with children needing assistance with upper extremity exercises and adaptations and activities of daily living. Physical therapists work with children needing assistance with lower extremity exercises and adaptations.

Patient Safety 27.2

Distinguishing OI from Child Abuse

Children with OI often present with multiple fractures in various stages of healing. This may raise a red flag for the nurse to suspect child abuse. Conduct a thorough history and physical assessment to obtain accurate information.

Surgery to insert rods into the long bones may be indicated to strengthen long bones. Bisphosphonate drugs may be used to promote bone formation and decrease the need for surgery. Clinical trials are currently being conducted examining the effectiveness of growth hormone and bone marrow transplantations in the treatment of children with OI. Growth hormone is proving to be effective in increasing collagen in this population (NORD, 2007). There are not yet results on the effectiveness of bone marrow transplantation. If surgery is performed, provide routine postoperative care.

Evaluation

Expected outcomes for a child with OI include the following:
- The child has minimal fractures and optimal healing of injuries.
- The child has minimal complications or deformities from fractures.
- The child's caregivers promote growth and development.

Discharge Planning and Teaching

Children with OI need to participate in physical activities and exercise to encourage bone growth and strength. Educate the child and parents about the importance of engaging in non–weight-bearing or low-impact activities. Teach the family to avoid contact sports.

Fractures can occur easily in children with OI, even with normal daily activities. Teach parents about proper handling of an infant with OI. When changing diapers, parents should lift the infant from under the hips rather than pull the infant up by the legs. When picking the child up, parents should not lift under the arms but by the trunk. Teach parents about possible clinical therapy options, including medications and surgery (The Pharmacy 27.1).

Blount Disease

Blount disease (tibia vara), sometimes referred to as bowed legs, is a growth disorder involving an inward turning of the lower leg that worsens over time.

Etiology and Pathophysiology

Blount disease results from a disorder of the tibial growth plate. Bowed legs are a normal occurrence in toddlers and typically straighten naturally by 2 years of age; if the alignment has not straightened by the age of 3 years, Blount disease is suspected. Blount disease is often associated with excess body weight (obesity), early walking, vitamin D deficiency, and a genetic component. Children with Blount disease are at risk for joint degeneration and recurrence of the deformity (AAOS, n.d.a).

Clinical Presentation

The child with Blount disease has an inward turning of the lower leg. Leg length discrepancy and knee pain may also be present.

The Pharmacy 27.1   Bisphosphonates

Medication	Route	Action	Nursing Considerations

Pamidronate (Aredia)	IV	• Shortens the life of the osteoclasts and prolongs the life of the osteoblasts
		• Slows down bone resorption and promotes bone production
			• Give IV every 3–4 mo (over 1–3 d)
			• Monitor IV site during infusion
			• Excreted (50%) by the kidney
			• May cause flulike symptoms: fever and myalgia
			
			Monitor:
			• Urinary output to assess kidney function
			• Serum laboratory levels periodically:
			  ○ Electrolytes
			  ○ Phosphates
			  ○ Calcium
			  ○ Magnesium

Alendronate (Fosamax)	PO	• Shortens the life of the osteoclasts and prolongs the life of the osteoblasts
		• Slows down bone resorption and promotes bone production
			• Give PO once a week in the morning on an empty stomach, 30 min before meals or lying down (to minimize GI discomfort)
			• Excreted (50%) by the kidney
			• May cause flulike symptoms: fever and myalgia
			
			Monitor:
			• Urinary output to assess kidney function
			• Serum laboratory levels periodically:
			  ○ Electrolytes
			  ○ Phosphates
			  ○ Calcium
			  ○ Magnesium

GI, gastrointestinal; IV, intravenous; PO, by mouth.

Data from Osteogenesis Imperfecta Foundation. (2015). *Questions and answers about bisphosphonates.* Retrieved from http://www.oif.org/site/PageServer?pagename=BisphosQandA

Assessment and Diagnosis

With the child standing and walking, assess the curvature of the lower leg. Note any abnormalities in gait. Assess for discrepancies in length between the two legs. Assess for knee pain in the affected limb. Radiological studies are used to examine the nature and degree of the deformity.

Therapeutic Interventions

For children younger than 4 years, treatment consists of bracing, which may be effective if initiated early. Children who continue to have bowing despite bracing and adolescents with Blount disease require surgical treatment. Surgical treatments either arrest growth at the growth plate or reshape the tibia. Depending on the type of surgery performed, the child may have a cast or an external frame applied following surgery.

Postoperatively, frequently assess the neurovascular status of the child with a cast or an external frame (skin color, peripheral pulses, edema, skin temperature, capillary refill, ability to move the foot and toes). In particular, note the following:

- The tibia is particularly susceptible to compartment syndrome; therefore, if a cast is applied postoperatively, assessing neurovascular status (Priority Care Concepts 27.1 and 27.2) is the highest priority.
- Adolescents with Blount disease are at high risk for developing deep vein thrombosis (DVT) following surgery and secondary to obesity; assessing for symptoms of DVT is a high priority (leg pain, swelling, redness, and warmth).

 Priority Care Concepts 27.1 Cast Care

- After a plaster cast is first applied, it remains wet for 12–24 h. Handle a wet cast with an open palm to prevent indentations that can cause pressure on the skin.
- Elevate the casted area above the level of the heart to reduce swelling.
- Applying ice to the outside of the cast can help reduce swelling.
- Assess for drainage (bleeding), which may occur in postoperative patients from the incision site. Circle the area of drainage and monitor for increases in drainage.
- Assess the five P's of tissue ischemia. Alterations could indicate that the cast is too tight, which could result in compartment syndrome (Campagne, 2017).
  1. **Pain:** Assess the location, duration, and quality of the child's pain.
  2. **Pulses:** Assess the quality of peripheral pulses distal to the casted extremity.
  3. **Pallor:** Assess for pallor or cyanosis to areas distal to the casted extremity, as well as capillary refill.
  4. **Paresthesia:** Assess whether the child is experiencing numbness or tingling, and assess the child's ability to experience tactile stimuli distal to the casted extremity.
  5. **Paralysis:** Assess the child's ability to move areas distal to the casted extremity.
- Assess for signs of infection, including foul odors and drainage from the cast, fever, and warmth over the cast (hot spots).
- Assess the tightness of the cast; there should be enough space to fit one or two fingers between the edge of the cast and the child's extremity at both ends of the cast.
- Assess the edges of the cast. These edges are usually rough and can cut or dig into the child's skin, causing irritation or breakdown. Rough edges should be covered with the stockinette, padded tape, or moleskin by securing one edge of the tape inside the cast and wrapping it over the rough edge to secure the other side to the outside of the cast (petaling).
- Keep the cast clean and dry. Wet casts lead to skin breakdown, which leads to infection.
  - Sponge baths are recommended.
  - If showers are allowed, cover the cast with a plastic covering.
  - Never immerse the cast in water.
  - Avoid vigorous exercise and long periods outside in hot weather, which result in sweating.
- Teach the child and the parents not to put anything inside the cast.
  - Caution parents that small children should not be given small toys that can be put inside the cast without direct supervision.
  - As the healing process progresses, skin inside the cast begins to itch. Teach the child and the parents not to insert anything inside the cast to scratch the itch or to use lotions or powders in an attempt to relieve itching.
  - A hair dryer on the cool setting can be used to relieve itching.
- When it is time to remove the cast, prepare the child and the parents.
  - Teach the child that the cast remover is very loud, but does not hurt and will not cut the child.
  - Refer to the cast removal device as a "cast remover" instead of a cast "saw." Even school-age children and adolescents conjure images of a saw that will cut their extremity off during cast removal. The loud vibrating machine is frightening and elicits fear in children of all ages. To facilitate cooperation and alleviate anxiety, using the term "cast remover" is more developmentally appropriate.
  - When the cast is removed, the skin underneath may be dry and scaly, and the extremity may be smaller than before because it has not been used for a while.
  - Lotion can be used to rehydrate the area if the skin is intact.

Data from Nursing File. (2010). *Nursing interventions: Post cast application and cast removal*. Retrieved from http://nursingfile.com/nursing-care-plan/nursing-interventions/nursing-interventions-post-cast-application-and-cast-removal.html

Priority Care Concepts 27.2   Compartment Syndrome

The muscle groups in the body are divided into sections; each section is kept in place by tight bands called fascia, which do not stretch. Compartment syndrome occurs when trauma or other conditions cause swelling and pressure inside one of those muscle group sections (compartments). Without the ability to expand, circulation to the tissue inside that section (compartment) is impaired and can become necrotic (or die). Compartment syndrome can occur following casting of an injured extremity because (a) the cast itself becomes tight as it dries, and (b) the healing process causes edema as fluid and white blood cells flood the area to facilitate healing. Compartment syndrome is most likely to occur in the areas of long bones; forearm injuries are the second most common. Signs of compartment syndrome include the following:

- Pain out of proportion to the injury and unrelieved by opioids (the earliest and cardinal sign)
- Pain with passive movement (early sign)
- Persistent deep aching pain (early sign)
- Paresthesia (tingling), usually within 30 min of the onset

- Tense or hard area around the compartment
- Pallor
- Decreased sensation (later sign)
- Muscle weakness (2–4 h after onset)
- Paralysis (late sign)

Assessing the five P's of tissue ischemia is an effective method for providing early indicators for risks of compartment syndrome. Although the symptoms may not be specific to compartment syndrome, they alert the nurse to changes in the child's condition. The most sensitive indicator is pain. Document and report these signs, in addition to alterations in neurovascular status, to the healthcare provider immediately. Compartment syndrome is considered a medical emergency and must be evaluated for immediate intervention to avoid permanent damage.

The definitive diagnosis is made by measuring the pressure in the compartment with a manometer. Management of compartment syndrome includes removing the cast and surgically relieving the pressure with a fasciotomy (cutting the fascia to allow for expansion of the compartment).

Data from Stracciolini, A., & Hammerberg, E. M. (2018). *Acute compartment syndrome of the extremities.* Retrieved from https://www.uptodate.com/contents/acute-compartment-syndrome-of-the-extremities

- If an external frame is applied, assess the pin sites for redness, swelling, edema, and drainage. Note the color and odor of any drainage. Cleaning pin sites is often required to prevent infection; follow the prescribed procedure (various protocols exist for pin site maintenance regarding the type of medium to clean with and the frequency of cleaning).

Evaluation

Expected outcomes for a child with Blount disease include the following:
- The child has a straightened leg with full range of motion and equal leg length.
- The child is able to ambulate without difficulty or discomfort.
- The child and family strive for healthy weight management.
- The child has a positive body image and self-esteem.

Discharge Planning and Teaching

Children with Blount disease require some form of clinical therapy, so prepare the child and family for clinical therapy options. Many of these children struggle with excess body weight, which, in addition to being a risk factor for the disease, can also complicate treatment options. Educate the child and family about healthy eating choices, physical activity, and weight management. Children may have altered body images due to

the disease process, body weight issues, and the presence of an external frame applied during surgery, if applicable. Provide support to the child and the family. Support groups or interaction with other children can help the child with compliance and socialization.

Congenital Clubfoot

Clubfoot (talipes equinovarus) is a congenital disorder in which the foot is twisted (Fig. 27.3). This condition occurs in approximately 1 in 1,000 births and is more common in boys than in girls. About half of all children with this disorder are affected bilaterally.

Etiology and Pathophysiology

Clubfoot is believed to have a genetic factor due to familial tendencies, but the exact cause is still unknown (Texas Scottish Rite Hospital for Children, n.d.).

Clinical Presentation

In clubfoot, the heel of the affected foot tilts in and down, and the forefoot turns in so that the bottom of the foot faces inward or upward. The foot and calf on the affected side are often smaller than those on the unaffected side, and the affected Achilles tendon is shorter. Without treatment, children may have difficulty wearing shoes or walking and may experience pain when walking.

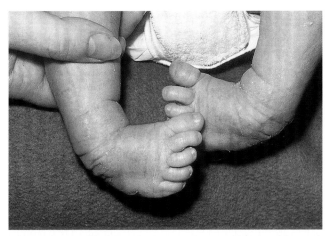

Figure 27.3. Clubfoot. Note the inverted heel, ankle equinus, and forefoot adduction in this infant with bilateral clubfoot. Reprinted with permission from Kyle, T., & Carman, S. (2016). *Essentials of pediatric nursing* (3rd ed., Fig. 22.18). Philadelphia, PA: Wolters Kluwer.

Assessment and Diagnosis

Assessment of clubfoot is noting the appearance of the foot at birth. The heel tilts in and down and the forefoot turns in. Diagnosis is usually made at birth, but the condition can be diagnosed in utero with ultrasound. Radiologic studies are used to determine the extent of the deformity.

Therapeutic Interventions

The birth of a child with physical abnormalities can be devastating to parents. Provide emotional support to the family, who may be grieving the loss of their idea of a perfect child. Nonsurgical treatment should begin early (within the first few weeks of birth) for the best outcomes.

Serial casting using the Ponseti method is the preferred nonsurgical treatment and has a 95% success rate. This method involves weekly stretching of the foot followed by the application of a long leg cast (extending from the thigh to the toes) to hold the foot in place. Weekly casting continues until the foot gradually reaches the desired corrected position; this can take from 4 to 8 weeks. Once the correction of the foot is achieved, the tightened tendon is lengthened. This procedure is completed percutaneously using a local anesthetic and making a small incision at the heel. A final cast is worn for 3 weeks to allow the tendon to heal. The child then wears a brace for 2 to 4 years to maintain the foot correction (Global Clubfoot Initiative, 2018).

The French functional physical therapy method is another popular nonsurgical treatment with a high success rate. This method involves daily stretching, massaging of the foot by a trained physical therapist to gradually place the foot into the desired position, and then taping the foot to a molded plastic splint. This daily routine continues until the child is 2 years old (Texas Scottish Rite Hospital for Children, n.d.). Compliance with these nonsurgical methods is paramount. Recurrence

of the clubfoot is a complication. If nonsurgical methods do not work, or recurrence of the deformity occurs, then surgery is indicated.

Surgical correction of clubfoot involves realigning the bones, releasing tendons and soft tissues, and inserting a pin to maintain the new bone position. A long leg cast is applied to protect the limb and allow healing. Prepare the family for surgery, if necessary. When surgery is necessary, provide routine postoperative care with an emphasis on pain management. The surgical procedure is extensive, causing severe pain in the immediate postoperative period. Assess for pain frequently and medicate routinely for the first 24 hours postoperatively. Provide cast care and assessment of neurovascular status (Priority Care Concepts 27.1).

Evaluation

Expected outcomes for a child with clubfoot include the following:
- The child's foot maintains proper foot alignment with full range of motion.
- The child attains full mobility and progresses to ambulation without difficulty.
- The child has no recurrence of clubfoot.

Discharge Planning and Teaching

Clinical therapy is extensive and time consuming. Parental involvement and compliance are critical for successful results. Provide family teaching about the condition and treatment options. Emphasize the importance of keeping appointments for nonsurgical treatments. Teach the family about cast and brace care as applicable.

Developmental Dysplasia of the Hip

DDH is the inadequate coverage of the ball of the socket of the hip joint or a dislocation of the ball from the socket (Fig. 27.4). In some cases, the ball can slip in and out of the socket, which is a condition known as a dislocatable or unstable hip.

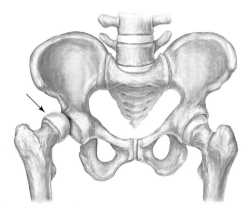

Figure 27.4. Developmental dysplasia of the hip. Reprinted with permission from Kyle, T., & Carman, S. (2016). *Essentials of pediatric nursing* (3rd ed., Fig. 22.19). Philadelphia, PA: Wolters Kluwer.

Etiology and Pathophysiology

DDH can occur during or after birth, but it is most often diagnosed in the first year of life during the newborn exam. In some cases, it is not noticed until the child begins walking. DDH is not painful for young children and does not limit physical development. The exact cause is unknown, but DDH is more common in the following: babies who are born breech, babies with a family history, babies who are swaddled with their legs straight, girls rather than boys, and firstborn babies (Wheeless, 2017).

Clinical Presentation

DDH is often first suspected in the newborn nursery when preliminary diagnostic assessments are performed. Infants with DDH exhibit limited hip movement (especially **abduction**), a difference in leg lengths (Galeazzi sign), and uneven skin folds on the thigh of the affected limb (Fig. 27.5). A palpable and audible click or clunk can be noted as the femoral head moves out of the acetabulum (Ortolani and Barlow signs; Fig. 27.5). Older children (who are walking) have an abnormal, limping gait (Trendelenburg gait).

Assessment and Diagnosis

Assessment is considered the most important means of detecting DDH. If DDH is not detected on assessment of the newborn, periodic screenings are recommended until the child reaches 2 years of age. The Ortolani test (Box 27.1) is considered the most important test to detect **dysplasia** (Kotlarsky, Haber, Bialik, & Eidelman, 2015). The Barlow test is used to detect an unstable hip that can be dislocated out of the acetabulum. Both of these tests should be negative by 3 months of age.

Ultrasound and radiological exams provide definitive diagnoses. Ultrasound is the preferred technique for confirming diagnosis and for assessing high-risk infants, but it is not recommended for universal diagnostic screening. Standard pelvic X-rays are the preferred diagnostic tool for infants 4 to 6 months of age (AAOS, 2014; Kotlarsky et al., 2015).

Therapeutic Interventions

Early treatment is essential for successful correction of DDH. The goal is to initiate treatment as soon as possible, before the child reaches 4 years of age. Prepare the family by presenting

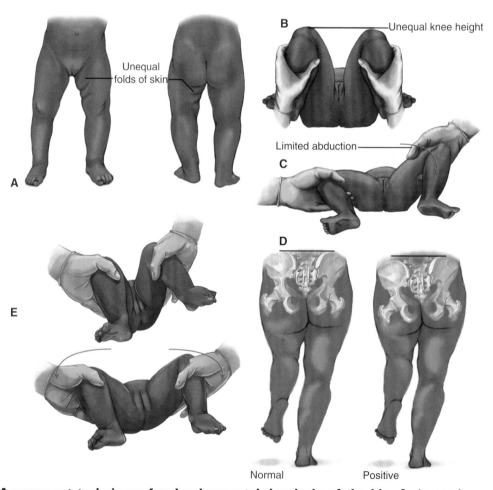

Figure 27.5. Assessment techniques for developmental dysplasia of the hip. A. Assess for asymmetry of the thigh and gluteal folds. **B.** Assess for unequal knee height related to femur shortening. **C.** Note any limitation in hip abduction. **D.** Note whether the pelvis or hip drops when the leg is raised (positive Trendelenburg sign). **E.** Feel for a "clunk" when adduction and depression of the femur dislocate the hip (Barlow test). Assess for a clunk when the dislocated hip is abducted and relocated (Ortolani sign). Reprinted with permission from Kyle, T., & Carman, S. (2016). *Essentials of pediatric nursing* (3rd ed., Fig. 22.20). Philadelphia, PA: Wolters Kluwer.

Box 27.1 How to Perform the Ortolani and Barlow Tests

Ortolani Test

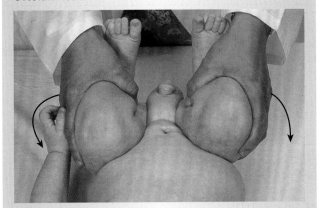

Reprinted with permission from Bickley, L. S. (2016). *Bates' guide to physical examination and history taking* (12th ed., Fig. 18.32). Philadelphia, PA: Wolters Kluwer.

1. With the infant in a supine position, flex the infant's knees and hips 90°.
2. Place your hands on the infant's knees with your thumbs on the medial thigh.
3. With your fingers, gently push upward on the lateral thigh and greater trochanter with abduction.
4. If the hip is dislocated, there will be a palpable clunk.

Barlow Test

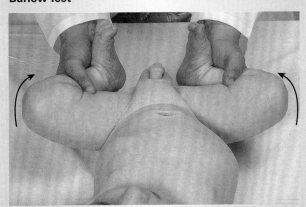

Reprinted with permission from Bickley, L. S. (2016). *Bates' guide to physical examination and history taking* (12th ed., Fig. 18.33). Philadelphia, PA: Wolters Kluwer. Wheeless, C. R. (2017). *Wheeless' textbook of orthopaedics*. Retrieved from wheelessonline.com

1. With the infant in a supine position, flex the infant's knees and hips 90°.
2. Grasp the hip and gently adduct the leg while gently applying downward lateral pressure.
3. If the hip is unstable, you will feel the femoral head slip over the rim of the acetabulum.

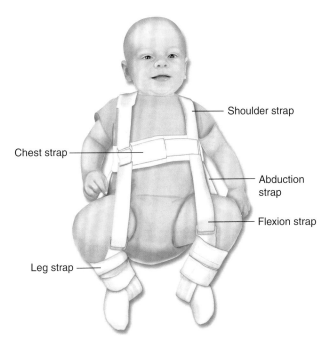

Figure 27.6. Pavlik harness.

months. Several braces are currently used, with the Pavlik harness being the most widely used (Fig. 27.6). The purpose of the Pavlik harness is to position the hips in alignment with the joint in an abducted position. The harness is worn full time (24 h/d) for 3 to 4 months. If the results are positive, the infant may continue to wear the harness at night for another 4 to 6 weeks (International Hip Dysplasia Institute, n.d.).

For children aged 6 to 24 months, a closed-reduction surgery is indicated. This procedure is performed under general anesthesia so that the surgeon can direct the head of the femur into the acetabulum without making a surgical incision. The child is placed in a spica cast to maintain alignment of the hip in the joint while the tissues repair. Before a closed reduction, the child may be placed in overhead (Bryant) traction (International Hip Dysplasia Institute, n.d). The purpose of traction is to stretch the ligaments and bring the head of the femur to the acetabulum to make the closed reduction more successful and to reduce the risk of avascular necrosis (AVN; Priority Care Concepts 27.3; Sabinski, Murnaghan, & Snyder, 2006). The use of traction before a closed reduction is controversial (Analyze the Evidence 27.1) and has been declining because its effectiveness has been challenged over the years (Kotlarsky et al., 2015).

In older children (>2 years) or children for whom a closed reduction has been unsuccessful, an open reduction may be necessary. This surgical procedure typically involves an incision allowing the surgeon to open the hip joint so that excess tissue can be removed and the head of the femur can be replaced into the acetabulum. Children older than 12 to 15 months often require bone repair or reshaping or adjustment of the hip socket or femur. This is an additional surgical procedure, which requires a cut in the bone (osteotomy) at the same time as the open reduction. Pins or plates and screws are placed to hold the bones in place until they heal. Following an open reduction and osteotomy, the child is placed in a spica cast for 6 to 8 weeks to maintain alignment until the bone heals (Kotlarsky et al., 2015).

relevant clinical therapy options, which depend on the age of the child and the response to treatment.

Nonsurgical treatments such as bracing are approximately 90% successful for correcting DDH in children younger than 6

Priority Care Concepts 27.3   Types of Traction and Traction Care

Types of Traction

- **Skin Traction:** A pull is applied to the skin that indirectly puts traction on the bone and muscle.
  - **Bryant (overhead):** used with DDH and femur fractures with children younger than age 2 y old. The hips are flexed to 90°, and the buttocks are elevated slightly off the bed.
  - **Buck:** used for knee immobilization, hip fractures, and LCP disease. The leg is extended in a straight line.
  - **Russel:** used for femur fractures. The hip and knee are flexed, and the knee is suspended with a sling.
- **Skeletal traction:** A pull is applied directly to the bone with surgically placed pins through the bone.
  - **Skeletal cervical:** used for cervical spine injury
  - **Halo:** used for head and neck traction after cervical injury or preoperatively for children with kyphosis
  - **90-90:** used for femur or tibia fractures. A pin is placed in the femur, and the lower leg is placed in a boot. Both the hip and the leg are flexed at 90°.

Note: Provide developmentally appropriate toys and activities for children in traction (hang mobiles or activity centers from the traction frame used in Bryant traction; give activity books to older children, etc.).

Principles of Traction Care

- Positioning
  - Maintain supine position.
  - Straight alignment
- Countertraction
  - Keep the bed flat.
  - No more than 20° elevation; no sitting up
- Friction
  - The footplate of the child's apparatus (or the piece of the traction attached to the child) must not be touching the end of the bed.
  - Gravity and weight of the traction often pulls the child down in the bed; therefore, frequent repositioning is required.
  - Weights must be "free hanging" and kept away from the floor, bed, and child.
  - The child's heels should not be digging into the mattress.
- Continuous use: Never remove traction without physician orders.
- Neurovascular status
  - Have the child periodically move the ankles and feet (flexion, extension, and rotation).
  - Change positions frequently (keep the child supine, but tilt from side to side).
  - Assess neurovascular status (e.g., skin color, peripheral pulses, edema, skin temperature, capillary refill, ability to move extremity, ability to feel tactile sensations, tingling, and numbness).
  - Protect pressure points (sheepskin inside splints or boots).

Data from Byrne, T. (2006). *Zimmer traction handbook.* Retrieved from dl.icdst.org/pdfs/files/0257acaa982f0f0b2e7294a80a41d032.pdf

Evaluation

Expected outcomes for a child with DDH include the following:
- The child has successful reduction of the hip.
- The child achieves full range of motion of the hip.
- The child ambulates without difficulty or pain.

Discharge Planning and Teaching

Teach parents how to care for their child while the child is in the Pavlik harness. A T-shirt should be worn underneath the harness at all times to prevent skin irritation and breakdown from the straps rubbing against the skin. Show parents how to

Analyze the Evidence 27.1   Traction in the Management of DDH

A review of the literature reveals relatively equal numbers of supporters for overhead traction, with results showing more successful closed reduction of DDH and decreased risk of AVN, and those who find that traction makes no difference in patient outcomes (Sabinski et al., 2006). Of the 17 studies reviewed, all were published between 1978 and 2000.

One more recent study investigating the effectiveness of presurgical overhead (Bryant) traction on the management of DDH was conducted in 2006. The study compared two groups of children: those receiving traction (*n* = 107) and those not receiving traction (*n* = 48). Researchers followed up the children until they were 14 y old.

Results of the study showed that traction significantly reduced the risk of growth disturbance, and the

researchers recommend traction for all children before closed reduction of DDH (Sabinski et al., 2006).

The most recent study was a retrospective comparison of patients treated with closed reduction with and without traction from 1980 to 2009. Researchers followed up 342 patients younger than 3 y old for an average of 10.4 y. Patients in both the traction and nontraction groups were further evaluated according to age groups (<1 y, 1.5 y, and <2 y). Traction was used in 276 hips.

The researchers found that there was no difference in achieving successful closed reduction between the two groups at any age. Results showed no difference in AVN between the two groups across all ages (Sucato, De La Rocha, Lau, & Ramo, 2017).

check the skin (especially in the folds and creases) every day for redness, irritation, and breakdown. Emphasize that the child should stay in the harness the prescribed amount of time (most children remain in the harness 23–24 h/d). If the doctor allows the child to come out of the harness, teach parents how to correctly reapply the harness. Teach parents how to sponge bathe the infant who is in the harness full time. Diapers should be fastened underneath the straps.

Children who require surgical correction of the hip are placed in a spica cast (a cast covering one or both legs and extending to the mid torso, wrapping around the body, with an opening in the groin for toileting). See Priority Care Concepts 27.1 for general cast care guidelines. Cast care specific to the spica cast is unique regarding toileting and movement. When moving a patient in a spica cast, if the cast has an abductor bar (a bar placed between the legs to keep the legs apart and the hips in the abduction position), do not use the bar to turn, lift, or transfer the child. Teach parents how to assist a child in a spica cast with toileting, as follows:
- If the child wears diapers:
  - Tuck the diaper inside the cast on all sides.
  - Use a smaller diaper inside a larger one for more absorption.
- If the child is toilet-trained:
  - Cover the groin area opening of the cast with waterproof tape.
  - Cover the groin area opening with a plastic lining during elimination.

Acquired Musculoskeletal Disorders

In addition to the congenital and developmental disorders already discussed, children may develop acquired musculoskeletal disorders as a result of nutritional deficiency, infection, or unknown cause. These include rickets, slipped capital femoral epiphysis (SCFE), Legg–Calvé–Perthes (LCP) disease, osteomyelitis, and scoliosis.

Rickets

Rickets is a disease of growing bone in children and adolescents in which young bone fails to calcify.

Etiology and Pathophysiology

The classic type of rickets is caused by a dietary deficiency of vitamin D, often compounded by lack of exposure to sunlight. The incidence of rickets in the United States is very low because infant formulas and milks are fortified with vitamin D. Almost all cases of rickets are seen in children who are exclusively breastfed, have dark skin, have limited exposure to sunlight, and do not receive vitamin D supplementation. Rickets can also be associated with other malabsorption disorders and end-stage renal disease (Schwarz, 2017).

Clinical Presentation

Most children with rickets are diagnosed by 1 year of age. Children may have weakness or an inability to walk.

Assessment and Diagnosis

Assessment of rickets often consists of identifying symptoms. Assess for weakness and difficulty with walking. Note deformities of the skeleton, such as **genu** varum, kyphosis, or protruding chest. Radiological studies confirm the nature and degree of bone deformities. In addition to the vitamin D deficiency, serum calcium and phosphorus levels are also typically low in rickets.

Therapeutic Interventions

Children with rickets are treated with supplemental vitamin D (The Pharmacy 27.2). If skeletal deformities are present, corrective procedures may be necessary.

Evaluation

Expected outcomes for a child with rickets include the following:
- The child maintains healthy vitamin D levels.
- The child has increased exposure to sunlight.
- The child demonstrates no muscle weakness.
- The child has minimal bone deformities.

Discharge Planning and Teaching

Teach parents about diet options for their child that contain vitamin D (e.g., fortified dairy products, eggs, fatty fishes,

---

The Pharmacy 27.2 **Vitamin D3 (Calciferol and Cholecalciferol)**

Classification	Route	Action	Nursing Consideration
Fat-soluble vitamin	PO	• Absorbs calcium and phosphorus • Assists with building bone and keeping bone strong	• May contain peanut and soy products. • Avoid other products containing magnesium (supplements, antacids). • Calciferol closely resembles calcitriol; be careful not to take other products containing calcitriol. • If a dose is missed, do not take a double dose. • Vitamin D is fat-soluble; therefore, it can build up in the body. Take as directed and avoid other supplements containing vitamin D.

PO, by mouth.

Data from Drugs.com. (2018). *Vitamin D3*. Retrieved from https://www.drugs.com/mtm/vitamin-d3.html

sardines, chicken livers) and calcium (e.g., fortified formulas and cereals for infants) but provide anticipatory guidance as the growing child's diet advances. Provide education about vitamin D supplementation to parents who will be administering the medication at home. Teach parents that sunlight increases vitamin D absorption, and encourage them to provide the child with daily outdoor activity time.

Slipped Capital Femoral Epiphysis

SCFE is the most common hip disorder in adolescents. It is a condition in which the ball at the head of the femur slips off the neck of the bone at the growth plate (Fig. 27.7).

Etiology and Pathophysiology

SCFE most commonly develops during adolescent growth spurts (10–14 years of age in girls and 12–16 years of age in boys). It can occur gradually over time or acutely following an injury. SCFE is more common in boys than in girls. Conditions that place children at higher risk for developing SCFE include overweight or obesity, renal disease, thyroid disease, pituitary disorders, and family history. A child who has a slip to one hip has a 25% chance of developing SCFE in the other hip (AAOS, n.d.d; Peck, 2010; Pediatric Orthopaedic Society of North America, n.d).

Clinical Presentation

Children with SCFE complain of intermittent pain to the hip, groin, or knee of the affected side. The child may limp. SCFE can be classified as stable, meaning the child can walk, or as unstable, meaning the child is unable to walk.

Assessment and Diagnosis

Any school-age child who is limping and complaining of pain to the groin, hip, or knee area should be considered for further evaluation of SCFE (Peck, Voss, & Voss, 2017). Assess for pain to the groin, hip, or knee. Observe the child for limping during ambulation. Limping and pain often increase after activity. Observe for an outward turning of the affected leg. Assess for limited range of motion in the affected leg, particularly with internal rotation. Diagnosis is confirmed with radiological studies.

Therapeutic Interventions

SCFE is considered a medical emergency; therefore, when a child presents with symptoms, encourage the child to immediately take weight off of the affected leg. Inform the child and family that, following confirmation of the diagnosis, the child should not be allowed to bear weight to prevent further damage to the hip (Peck, 2010). Educate the child and family about the importance of not walking or bearing weight on the hip (Patient Safety 27.3). Provide the child with developmentally appropriate activities to keep the child stimulated during times of bed rest or inactivity. Prepare the child and family for surgery. Following surgery, provide routine postoperative care.

SCFE is considered a medical emergency because the slipping of the femoral head limits blood supply to the area, which can lead to AVN. Early diagnosis and treatment is necessary to stabilize the hip and prevent complications. Surgical treatment is necessary to secure the head of the femur back into place (in situ pinning). Surgery is scheduled as soon as possible once diagnosis is confirmed (usually the day of diagnosis or the following day). The surgeon places a screw percutaneously across the growth plate to maintain positioning of the femoral head.

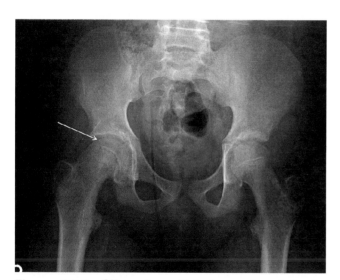

Figure 27.7. Slipped capital femoral epiphysis. A radiograph of the pelvis shows a slipped capital femoral epiphysis on the patient's right side, as indicated by the arrow. Reprinted with permission from White, A. J. (2016). *The Washington manual of pediatrics* (2nd ed., Fig. 25.18). Philadelphia, PA: Wolters Kluwer.

Patient Safety 27.3

Management of SCFE

Preventing further damage to the hip is a priority of care. The degree of activity restriction varies by physician preference; the literature is inconsistent regarding best practice. The ultimate goal is to maintain patient safety by preserving hip function, avoiding falls, and minimizing future injury (Healio, 2012).

- Some physicians suggest strict bed rest because even just flexing the hip 90° by siting can result in further damage to the hip.
- Some physicians allow the patient bathroom privileges with crutches, reasoning that this minimal non–weight-bearing activity provides comfort and decreased anxiety to the patient.
- Some physicians report that patients who are not experienced with crutches are more likely to fall and cause further damage because of their inability to properly use crutches; therefore, they allow bathroom privileges without crutches.

In more severe cases, the bone may need to be cut and repositioned before being secured into place (AAOS, n.d.d).

Evaluation

Expected outcomes for a child with SCFE include the following:
- The child has no further damage from AVN to the affected hip.
- The child has no injury following surgery.
- The child has full range of motion and mobility following healing of the hip after surgery.

Discharge Planning and Teaching

Postoperatively, the child uses crutches for 6 weeks and is only allowed toe-touch weight bearing on the affected side. A physical therapist teaches the patient proper use of crutches and exercises to strengthen the affected hip. Reinforce proper use of crutches following physical therapy teaching. Inform the child and the parent that the child is restricted from sports and vigorous activities for at least 6 weeks.

Legg–Calvé–Perthes Disease

LCP disease (or Perthes) is a self-limiting condition in which the blood supply to the head of the femur is temporarily disrupted, causing AVN or death of the bone cells (Fig. 27.8).

Etiology and Pathophysiology

As shown in Table 27.2, LCP disease occurs in four stages lasting several years (International Perthes Study Group, 2016).

LCP occurs in children aged 6 to 10 years, affecting boys 4 to 5 times more than girls. The disorder is most common in Caucasian children. The exact cause of LCP is unknown. Suspected risk factors include environmental and genetic causes. Conditions that place children at risk for developing LCP include low birth weight, trauma, low socioeconomic conditions, exposure to tobacco smoke, positive family history, and coagulation disorders (NORD, 2016).

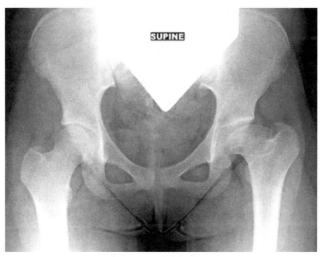

Figure 27.8. Legg–Calvé–Perthes disease. A radiograph of the pelvis showing Legg–Calvé–Perthes disease in the right hip. Reprinted with permission from Kline-Tilford, A. M., & Haut, C. (2015). *Lippincott certification review: Pediatric acute care nurse practitioner* (1st ed., Fig. 19.1). Philadelphia, PA: Wolters Kluwer.

Clinical Presentation

Children typically first present complaining of a limp with or without pain. Pain may be present in the hip, thigh, or knee.

Assessment and Diagnosis

Observe the child's gait, noting any limping. Assess for pain in the hip, thigh, or knee. Question the child about experiencing intermittent, sudden, squeezing, or tight pain in the leg that would indicate muscle spasms. Observe for loss of muscle mass to the front thigh of the affected leg, as well as shortening of the affected limb. Assess for limited hip mobility when moving the leg away from the body and turning the leg inward. Definitive diagnosis is made with X-rays (AAOS, n.d.c; NORD, 2016).

Table 27.2   Stages of Legg–Calvé–Perthes Disease

Stage	Process	Duration	Events
1	Avascular necrosis	Several months	• Blood supply is cut off from the femoral head, damaging osteoblasts and osteoclasts. • The femoral head becomes flattened or deformed.
2	Fragmentation/ resorption	1–2 y	• Dead bone is removed by the body and replaced with new, softer bone. • The new bone is weak and susceptible to fracture.
3	Reossification	Several years	Stronger bone develops and forms into the proper shape of the round head of the femur.
4	Healing	N/A	• Bone regrowth is complete, and the femoral head is reshaped. • The femoral head may not be fully round depending on the extent of the damage that occurred during stage 2 and the age of the child at the onset of the disease.

Therapeutic Interventions

Prepare the child and family for clinical therapy options depending on the child's age. Educate the child and the family that the recovery time for LCP is very long; it takes several years before the bone regrowth is totally complete.

Bisphosphonate medications are being tested in the management of LCP to slow or stop the natural process of bone loss and the preservation of bone density. Studies are investigating whether these medications can slow down femoral head collapse in LCP. At this time, there are no conclusive results from these clinical trials (NORD, 2016).

The ultimate goals of treatment are to relieve pain, protect the shape of the femoral head, and restore hip movement. Treatment strategies are based on the child's age at diagnosis, because healing and bone regrowth change as children mature (Table 27.3). Thus, compared with older children, younger children are able to heal faster, have more time to regrow bone, and require less aggressive treatment modalities.

Evaluation

Expected outcomes for a child with LCP include the following:
- The child has optimal pain control.
- The child's femoral head shape is protected.
- The child's hip movement is restored.
- The child's bone density is preserved.

Discharge Planning and Teaching

Following surgery, the child is placed in a cast for 6 weeks to allow the hip to rest and repair (International Perthes Study Group, 2016). Provide routine postoperative care. See Priority Care Concepts 27.1 for general cast care guidelines. Upon cast removal, physical therapy is initiated to strengthen the hip muscles.

Osteomyelitis

Osteomyelitis is an inflammation of the bone secondary to bacterial infection.

Etiology and Pathophysiology

Staphylococcus aureus is the most common organism responsible for infections that lead to osteomyelitis. Although the infection can originate in the blood, half of osteomyelitis infections result from a trauma, surgery, or insertion of a foreign body. Motor vehicle accidents and sports injuries have contributed to a rise in osteomyelitis in recent years. Osteomyelitis is the second most common infection in children with sickle cell disease (Kishner, 2016).

Clinical Presentation

Osteomyelitis often presents with general and vague symptoms of fever, chills, malaise, and fatigue. Children may complain of bone pain and difficulty bearing weight on the affected limb or lifting, if an upper extremity is involved.

Assessment and Diagnosis

The child with osteomyelitis displays typical signs of infection to the affected site. Assess the area for swelling, redness, and warmth. Assess the child's muscle strength in the affected limb, and compare strength bilaterally. Assess the range of motion in all extremities. The affected limb may have limited mobility. Assess for signs of decreased sensation (tingling or numbness) distal to the infection site. Assess for perfusion (e.g., skin color, peripheral pulses, edema, skin temperature, capillary refill).

Laboratory testing is used to confirm inflammatory processes. A complete blood count typically reveals an increased white blood cell count in children with this condition. C-reactive protein levels and erythrocyte sedimentation rates are also likely to be elevated. Obtain blood culture specimens as ordered to identify the causative infecting organism; however, causative organisms are only identified in 50% of cases. Bone biopsy provides a definitive diagnosis of the causative organism (Kishner, 2016).

Therapeutic Interventions

The treatment for osteomyelitis is antibiotics (The Pharmacy 27.3). Obtain blood culture specimens before the

Table 27.3   Treatment Options for Legg–Calvé–Perthes Disease by Age

Age (y)	Interventions
<6	• Observation and encouraging rest • Anti-inflammatory medications for pain • Restrictions on running and jumping • Walking aids (crutches, walker, wheelchair)
6–8	• Treatment of symptoms • Brace or traction to further limit movement of the affected limb • Possibly surgery, to immobilize the affected limb (controversial; efficacy compared with nonsurgical treatment is being studied)
8–11	Surgery (reshaping either the head of the femur or the shape of the acetabulum) necessary because of most of the femoral head being affected
>11	Surgery (reshaping either the head of the femur or the shape of the acetabulum) necessary because of most of the femoral head being affected (new types of surgeries are being investigated to compare outcomes with those of traditional methods)

The Pharmacy 27.3 — Antibiotics Used to Treat Osteomyelitis

Medication	Classification	Route	Action	Nursing Considerations
Cefazolin	Cephalosporin	IV	Active against many gram + cocci	• Administer IV intermittent infusion over 30–60 min • Monitor for rash
Nafcillin	Penicillinase-resistant penicillin	IV	Active against many gram + cocci	• Administer IV intermittent infusion over 30–60 min • Monitor for rash
Clindamycin	Anti-infective	• IV • PO	Active against most aerobic and anaerobic gram + cocci	• Administer IV intermittent infusion over 30 min • Monitor for gastrointestinal upset (diarrhea, cramps)
Vancomycin	Anti-infective	• IV • PO	Active against gram + organisms	• Administer IV over at least 60 min Monitor: • IV site closely (irritating to tissue) • For signs of anaphylaxis • Kidney function (intake and output) • Hearing (can be ototoxic)

IV, intravenous; PO, by mouth.

Data from Vallerand, A. H., & Sanorki, C. A. (2017). *Davis's drug guide for nurses* (15th ed.). Philadelphia, PA: F. A. Davis.

child begins antibiotic therapy because it can interfere with bacterial growth (Centers for Disease Control and Prevention, 2015). Initially, intravenous (IV) administration of a broad-spectrum antibiotic is initiated. If the blood culture results identify a specific organism, the antibiotic is changed as needed to one that is effective against the specific causative agent. There are some variations regarding the type and length of antibiotic therapy. Traditionally, the child received IV antibiotics for 4 to 8 weeks. Recent studies have shown that shorter courses of IV antibiotics (several days) followed by 3 weeks of oral antibiotics are effective (Castellazzi, Montero, & Esposito, 2016; Dodwell, 2013; Kalyoussef, 2016).

Assess the child frequently for changes in status (e.g., temperature, perfusion, or sensation). Assess the IV site frequently because IV antibiotics can be irritating to the vein. Administer IV antibiotics using the five rights of medication administration. Monitor the child carefully for responses to antibiotic therapy. Provide comfort measures to children with fevers (e.g., applying cool cloths to and removing extra bedding and blankets from the child who is febrile).

Evaluation

Expected outcomes for a child with osteomyelitis include the following:
• The child is free from fever and infection.
• The child's laboratory values return to normal.
• The child does not have deformities secondary to the infection.

Discharge Planning and Teaching

Provide home care instructions regarding antibiotic medications. Teach the parents how to monitor for signs of infection such as fever or redness and pain to the area.

Scoliosis

Scoliosis is a progressive condition of lateral curvature of the spine greater than 10° with rotation of the vertebrae, resulting in the spine having an S-shaped appearance.

Etiology and Pathophysiology

Scoliosis may be classified by the location of the curvature (thoracic or lumbar) and by the cause: congenital, neuromuscular, or idiopathic. Each of these causes is discussed here.

Congenital scoliosis is caused by an embryological malformation in which the vertebrae fail to develop or separate, causing curvature as one area of the spine lengthens at a slower rate than the rest. Congenital scoliosis is detected at an earlier age than the other types and is often associated with other congenital anomalies.

Neuromuscular scoliosis is a curvature of the spine secondary to neurological disease of the central nervous system or muscles. This type of scoliosis can occur at any age but tends to progress more rapidly than the other types. Compression of internal organs due to the severity of the curve is more likely with neuromuscular scoliosis.

Idiopathic scoliosis is the diagnosis given when all other causes have been ruled out and thus indicates a lateral curvature resulting from no known cause. This is the most common type of scoliosis, composing 80% of all cases. Although the exact cause is unknown, there are familial tendencies associated with this type of scoliosis, and gene markers have been identified (Richards, Sucato, & Johnston, 2014). Idiopathic scoliosis may be further categorized by age of onset:

• Infantile: occurring in children younger than 3 years
• Juvenile: occurring in children 3 to 10 years old
• Adolescent: occurring in children older than 10 years

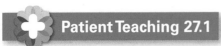

Patient Teaching 27.1

Things That Do *Not* Cause Scoliosis

- Bad posture or slouching
- Sleeping position
- Lack of calcium
- Carrying heavy items:
  - Backpacks
  - Books
  - Purses

Adapted from Texas Scottish Rite Hospital for Children. (n.d.). *What is scoliosis?* Retrieved from https://scottishritehospital.org/care-and-treatment/scoliosis-and-spine

Adolescent idiopathic scoliosis (AIS) is the most common type of childhood scoliosis and most often manifests around the time of puberty during adolescent growth spurts. AIS occurs equally in boys and in girls, but curves in girls are 8 times more likely to progress (American Association of Neurological Surgeons [AANS], 2007).

Parents may have mistaken beliefs about what can cause scoliosis. Be prepared to address these in your education (Patient Teaching 27.1).

Clinical Presentation

Scoliosis typically manifests with truncal asymmetry, uneven shoulders, raised hips, and a rib hump (Fig. 27.9). Most children do not complain of back pain, although studies show that about 23% of children report back pain. Half of the children who do complain of back pain have underlying conditions (AANS, 2007).

Assessment and Diagnosis

Screening for scoliosis can detect curves and facilitate early intervention. Scoliosis screening involves assessing for visual signs of misalignment and asymmetry. Scoliosis screening may be done by school nurses for children in fifth and seventh grades. This screening is mandated in some states but is controversial (Analyze the Evidence 27.2), because the U.S. Preventive Services Task Force has recommended against routine screenings (USPSTF, 2004). When screening, address the following questions while the child is in a standing position:

- Do the child's clothes hang evenly?
- Is the child's head in midline?
- Are the shoulders even?
- Are the shoulder blades even?
- Are the hips the same height?

In addition, perform the Adam's forward-bending test:

1. Have the child bend forward until the spine is horizontal.
2. Examine the child from the rear.
3. Note whether one side of the back appears higher than the other.
4. Note whether the spine is curved or straight.

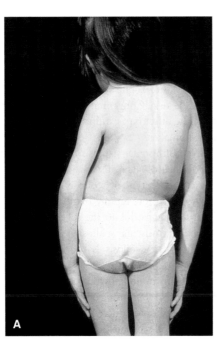

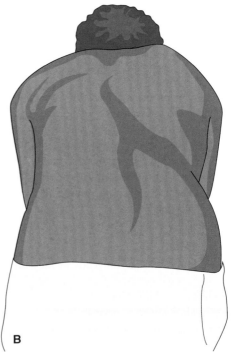

Figure 27.9. Scoliosis. A. Note right shoulder, scapula, and hip elevation, as well as discrepancy in waist curvature. **B.** Note right upper back hump. Reprinted with permission from Kyle, T., & Carman, S. (2016). *Essentials of pediatric nursing* (3rd ed., Fig. 22.30). Philadelphia, PA: Wolters Kluwer.

Analyze the Evidence 27.2 Routine Screening for AIS

Against Routine Screening	For Routine Screening
In 2004, the U.S. Preventive Service Task Force (UTPSTF) recommended against routine screening for AIS. The rationale against routine screening stated that there was lack of evidence to support that screening was accurate to detect AIS, and that mandatory screenings led to unnecessary interventions. The task force additionally found that early screenings did not result in improved outcomes. The evidence used by the task force to make the recommendations consisted of a small number of studies from 1994 through 2002, and the strength of the evidence was not evaluated (UTPSTF, 2004).	In 2008, the Scoliosis Research Society, American Association of Orthopaedic Surgeons, Pediatric Orthopaedic Society of North America, and American Academy of Pediatrics endorsed a statement supporting screening for AIS twice for girls, in grades 5 and 7, and once for boys, in either grade 8 or 9. The review of literature by this group found that there was not conclusive evidence for or against routine scoliosis screening. The support for screening by this group is based primarily on expert opinion and experience. The experts of this group maintain that screening is an accurate and reliable way to detect spinal curves. Most importantly, early detection results in improved outcomes, because brace therapy is effective in altering the natural history of the deformity (Richards & Vitale, 2008). More recent research has found that screened students were accurately identified significantly more often than unscreened students, and that bracing is effective if scoliosis is identified, suggesting that routine screening is effective (Labelle et al., 2013; Nakaishi & Nield, 2015).

A scoliometer, a simple tool that measures the degree of truncal rotation, can also be used to increase the accuracy of screenings.

Diagnosis is confirmed through radiologic studies, including X-rays, CT scans, and magnetic resonance imaging. Radiological studies allow for the curve to be measured and evaluated in terms of degrees, severity, location, skeletal maturity, and potential for progression. This information is used to determine treatment options.

Therapeutic Interventions

Refer adolescents who have abnormal or questionable screening results for further evaluation. Prepare the adolescent and the family for clinical therapy options, including bracing and surgery. For children requiring bracing, teach about the importance of compliance with brace therapy for effective outcomes.

For adolescents requiring surgical correction, postoperative care priorities focus on neurovascular status, positioning, and pain management. Children are maintained on bed rest the night after surgery and are encouraged to be sitting up on postoperative day 1. Many physicians prefer to have patients walking on postoperative day 1. The typical length of stay following a spinal fusion is 3 to 5 days. Many studies have examined the effectiveness of multimodal pain management and early ambulation, and the results show that this technique can decrease the length of stay from 5 days to 3.7 days without an increased risk of complication or readmission (Muhly et al., 2016).

Assess the child's neurovascular status frequently because during surgery the child may lose a significant amount of blood and the correction of the spinal curvature can result in sensory changes. Neurovascular assessment includes evaluation of skin color, peripheral pulses, edema, skin temperature, and capillary refill. In addition, assess the child's ability to move the lower extremities (e.g., wiggle toes, bend the knees, raise the leg) and feel stimuli (does the child complain of numbness or tingling?).

Turn the child every 2 hours using a logrolling technique (Fig. 27.10). Take special care to keep the back straight.

Assess pain frequently. Patient-controlled analgesia and epidural analgesia are common methods of pain management following spinal fusion surgeries. If the child is receiving IV medications postoperatively, provide medication on a routine basis. Use nonpharmacological pain management techniques, as well.

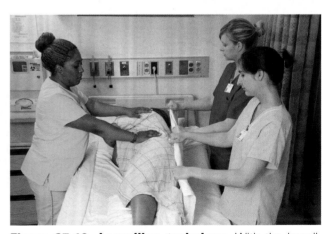

Figure 27.10. Logrolling technique. With the logrolling technique, the patient's arms are crossed and the spine aligned. The entire body is turned at the same time to avoid any twisting or bending. Reprinted with permission from Hinkle, J. L., & Cheever, K. H. (2017). *Brunner & Suddarth's textbook of medical-surgical nursing* (14th ed., Fig. 70-8). Philadelphia, PA: Lippincott Williams & Wilkins.

Treatment of scoliosis with bracing or spinal fusion is necessary for those whose curves are at risk of worsening and for those with severe curves at the time of diagnosis. Treatment options take into consideration remaining growth potential, the severity of the curve at diagnosis, and the pattern and location of the curve. Curves less than 25° do not require treatment. Curves 30° to 45° in an actively growing child are treated with bracing. This treatment is only effective if the child has not reached skeletal maturity. Growing adolescents with curves 45° to 50° are treated with surgical correction (Richards et al., 2014).

Several types of braces are available to correct scoliosis or prevent further progression of spinal curvature. The literature is not conclusive about which brace is most effective. Studies do indicate, however, that bracing itself, regardless of what specific device is used, is 80% effective when used in full compliance (AANS, 2007). Achieving successful outcomes depends on achieving a proper fit and the child wearing the brace 16 to 23 h/d until growth stops. Treatment regimens vary regarding the length of time children should wear the brace. Some braces are made only for nighttime wear. Research shows that wearing a brace full time is more effective than wearing it part time (AANS, 2007; Richards et al., 2014).

Surgical correction for AIS is called spinal fusion. This correction involves straightening the spine, supporting it with rods, and fusing the spine with a bone graft at the curved area for support (Fig. 27.11). The rods stabilize the spine while the bone graft fuses the vertebrae together (AANS, 2007).

Evaluation

Expected outcomes for a child with scoliosis include the following:
- The child has improved spinal alignment.
- The child has no signs of cardiopulmonary compromise.
- The child resumes full activities.
- The child has a positive body image and self-esteem.

Discharge Planning and Teaching

Following surgical correction of scoliosis, the child's movement and activities are restricted. Teach the child and the parents about activity restrictions, which include no bending or twisting of the torso, returning to school in 2 to 4 weeks, and resuming normal activities gradually over 3 months to 1 year. Teach about how to manage pain at home. Educate the parents on how to gradually reduce the child's pain medication dosage and frequency as the child's pain decreases over 1 to 2 weeks. Also provide adolescent patients, in particular, with support on handling body image concerns (Growth and Development Check 27.1).

Musculoskeletal Injuries

Musculoskeletal injuries are common among children and adolescents. They include strains and sprains, fractures, and overuse syndromes.

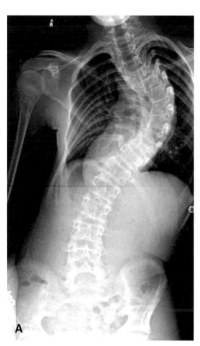
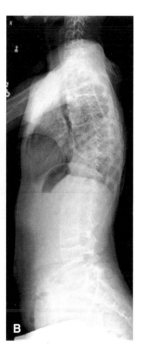
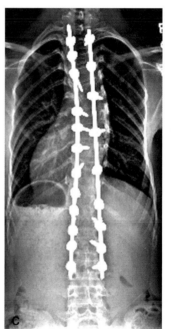
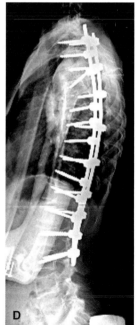

Figure 27.11. Spinal fusion to correct scoliosis. A and B. Radiographs showing thoracic and lumbar scoliosis before spinal fusion. **C and D.** Radiographs showing the same patient 1 year after surgery in which rods were inserted and fused to the vertebrae. Reprinted with permission from Bridwell, K. H., & DeWald, R. L. (2011). *Textbook of spinal surgery* (3rd ed., Fig. 105.4). Philadelphia, PA: Lippincott Williams & Wilkins.

Growth and Development Check 27.1

Addressing Body Image Concerns in Adolescents

Adolescents with scoliosis are in Erikson's stage of identity versus role confusion. The priority concern is body image and fitting in with peers. Provide adolescents with support and education about the condition and treatment. Adolescents who require bracing will be reluctant to be compliant because they will fear looking different from their peers. Provide resources with suggestions on ways to decorate the brace or clothes that disguise braces. The first question adolescents ask about spinal fusion surgery is "How big will my scar be?" Educate the child on physical aspects of the surgery including scar size, lack of curve following surgery, and increase in height following surgery.

Strains and Sprains

A strain is a stretched or torn muscle or **tendon**. Rest is recommended to allow a strain to heal. A sprain is an injury to a **ligament** caused by force exceeding the ligament's strength or ability not to break under pressure.

Etiology and Pathophysiology

Children's ligaments are stronger than their bones (unlike adults) as a protective measure to prevent bones from breaking. Common areas for sprains are ankles, knees, and shoulders. Children most at risk for sprains are those who engage in activities with jumping and "cutting" motions and those who have had previous sprains (Canares & Lockhart, 2013).

Clinical Presentation

Children with sprains often present with pain and swelling to the affected site. They may complain of difficulty bearing weight or moving the area.

Assessment and Diagnosis

When a child presents with a possible sprain, assess the area for pain and swelling. Assess for limitations in range of motion and ability to bear weight, if applicable. Radiological studies may be indicated if a fracture is suspected.

Therapeutic Interventions

Management of sprains for the first few days involves using the RICE technique:
- **R**est: Do not bear weight on the affected area for 48 to 72 hours.
- **I**ce: Apply ice packs for 10 to 20 minutes at least 3 times a day.

- **C**ompression: Wrap the area with elastic bandage to reduce swelling.
- **E**levation: Elevate the area above the level of the heart while resting and applying ice to reduce swelling.

Nonsteroidal anti-inflammatory drugs (NSAIDs) can be used to provide analgesia and reduce swelling. If the sprain is severe enough to prohibit ambulation, the child may need to see a healthcare professional, who may immobilize the area for 10 to 14 days. A brace, splint, or walking shoe may be used. Physical therapy may be consulted to facilitate recovery.

Evaluation

Expected outcomes for a child with a strain or sprain include the following:
- The child does not have further injury or deformity.
- The child has adequate pain control.
- The child has full range of motion and recovery from the injury.

Discharge Planning and Teaching

Teach the child with a strain or sprain to rest the area as much as possible. Teach the child to not put weight on the affected extremity. Teach the child and the family how to apply the RICE technique. Teach the child and the family that compliance with treatment is the most successful way to promote healing and prevent further injury.

Fractures

A fracture is a broken bone.

Etiology and Pathophysiology

In children, fractures most commonly occur from falls. Children's bones are more porous and more likely to buckle or bow under compression than to break completely. Because the **periosteum** is thicker and stronger, pediatric fractures are more stable and more likely to heal on their own. However, the presence of the open growth plate places children at higher risk for complications with healing and deformity (Dinolfo, 2004).

Remember 12-year-old David Torres from Chapter 3, who experienced a fractured bone? Which bone did David fracture? How did he fracture it? What symptoms caused his mother to take him to the emergency room? What interventions did his nurse, Gabriella, perform to address these symptoms? What medication was ordered for David's pain?

Fractures to the upper extremities are the most common in children. Because of increased activity and decreased coordination, children younger than 4 years are at high risk for fractures. One of the most common fractures in children younger than

4 years is the "toddler fracture," which is a nondisplaced spiral fracture of the tibia. This is a twisting injury that occurs in walking toddlers during normal activities (Patient Safety 27.4). Types of fractures are described in Box 27.2.

Clinical Presentation

Fractures may present with pain, swelling, and inability to move the extremity. Symptoms vary depending on the severity and location of the fracture. Visible deformity may be present.

Assessment and Diagnosis

Assess for signs of fracture, including swelling, pain, obvious deformities or abnormal positioning, and inability to move the injured area. Obtain a history of how the injury occurred.

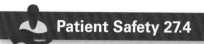

Patient Safety 27.4

A Fracture That May Indicate Abuse

The toddler fracture is an accidental twisting injury, typically to the lower extremities in ambulating toddlers during normal activities (e.g., sliding down a slide and getting the leg caught). Twisting injuries in nonambulating children should raise a red flag indicating potential child abuse (Souder, 2018).

Assess for neurovascular status below the area of injury (e.g., skin color, peripheral pulses, edema, skin temperature, capillary refill, ability to move, sensation to touch, tingling, and

Box 27.2 Types of Fractures

- **Nondisplaced (hairline):** A fracture in which the bone cracks rather than breaking into two separate pieces
- **Displaced:** A complete fracture in which the bone breaks into two or more pieces and changes position such that the ends of the bone are not in alignment
- **Complete (transverse):** A break across the entire section of bone at a 90° angle
- **Oblique:** A break across the entire section of bone at a diagonal angle
- **Comminuted:** A fracture involving the bone breaking into several fragments

- **Closed:** A fracture in which the bone does not break through the skin
- **Open:** A fracture in which the bone breaks through the skin
- **Greenstick:** An incomplete fracture in which the bone bends and only breaks on the convex side
- **Buckle (torus):** An incomplete fracture in which one side of the bone is compressed because of an impact, causing the other side of the bone to bend away from the growth plate
- **Spiral:** A twisting break across a bone

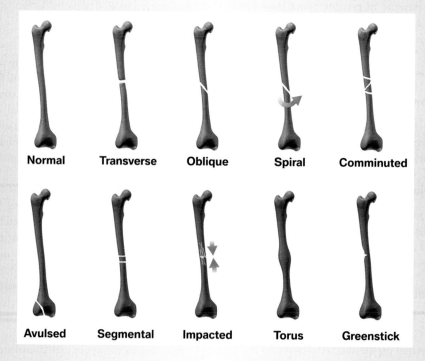

| Normal | Transverse | Oblique | Spiral | Comminuted |

| Avulsed | Segmental | Impacted | Torus | Greenstick |

Data from American Society for Surgery of the Hand. (2012). *Fractures in children.* Retrieved from www.assh.org/handcare/hand-arm-injuries/Fractures-in-Children; Singh (n.d.). *Different types of fractures—A simple classification of fractures.* Retrieved from http://boneandspine.com/types-fracturesa-simple-classification-fractures-long-bones/

numbness). Radiological studies are necessary to determine the location and degree of the fracture.

For the child placed in a cast, assess neurovascular status. Be alert to changes that can indicate compartment syndrome. Assess for signs of infection, including fever, warmth over the cast, pain, foul odor, and drainage.

Therapeutic Interventions

Fractures most commonly follow an accidental injury. If possible, immobilize the area above and below the injured area before moving the child after an injury. Treatment should focus on reduction of the fracture (putting the bone back in place) and immobilization. Reduction may be done closed (without surgery) or open (surgically), depending on the severity of the injury. Prepare the child and the family for reduction. The child may need to be sedated or receive pain medication before a reduction. Immobilization may be accomplished with a splint, a cast, or traction (Figs. 27.12 and 27.13).

Infection prevention is important in the care of children with fractures to prevent osteomyelitis, especially in children with open fractures. Keep the wound covered and maintain aseptic technique and proper hand washing.

Evaluation

Expected outcomes for a child with a fracture include the following:
- The child has successful reduction of the fracture.
- The child has minimal deformity from the healed fracture.
- The child has full range of motion and function to the healed area.
- The child has no infection and optimal pain control.

Discharge Planning and Teaching

If the child is placed in traction or a cast, provide proper care and patient and family teaching (Priority Care Concepts 27.1–27.3). Teach the child's parents how to manage pain at home. Educate the parents on how to gradually reduce the child's pain medication dosage and frequency as the child's pain decreases over 1 to 2 weeks.

Overuse Syndromes

Overuse injury is microtrauma damage to bone, muscle, or tendon subjected to repetitive stress without sufficient time to heal.

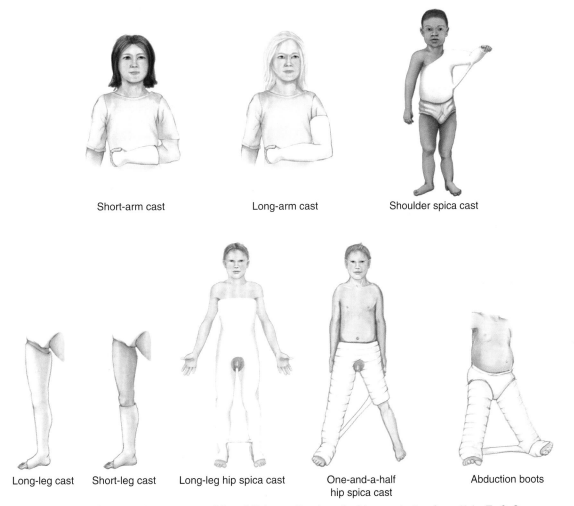

Short-arm cast   Long-arm cast   Shoulder spica cast

Long-leg cast   Short-leg cast   Long-leg hip spica cast   One-and-a-half hip spica cast   Abduction boots

Figure 27.12. Selected casts used in children. Reprinted with permission from Kyle, T., & Carman, S. (2016). *Essentials of pediatric nursing* (3rd ed., Fig. 22.4). Philadelphia, PA: Wolters Kluwer.

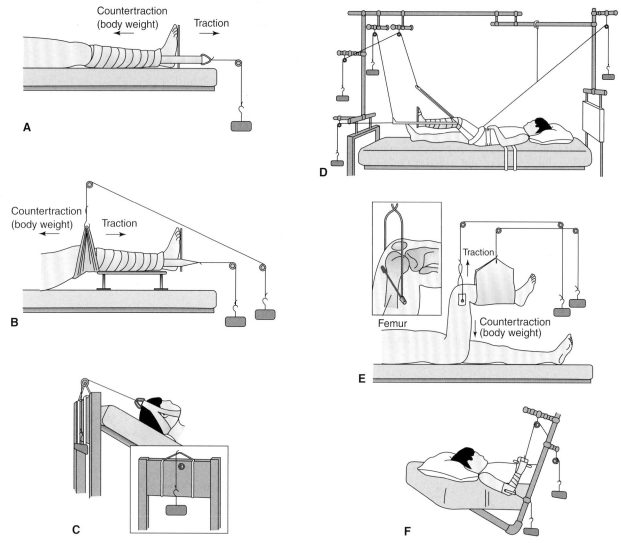

Figure 27.13. Types of traction. Types of skin traction: **A.** Buck extension, **B.** Russell, and **C.** cervical skin traction. Types of skeletal traction: **D.** balanced suspension, **E.** 90°, and **F.** Dunlop traction with pin insertion. Reprinted with permission from Silbert-Flagg, J., & Pillitteri, A. (2017). *Maternal and child health nursing* (8th ed., Fig. 51.5). Philadelphia, PA: Wolters Kluwer.

Etiology and Pathophysiology

The damage in overuse syndromes occurs in four stages:

1. Pain after physical activity
2. Pain during physical activity without restricting performance
3. Pain during activity that restricts performance
4. Chronic, unremitting pain, even at rest

Most overuse injuries are sports related and 50% of sports medicine injuries are overuse injuries (AAOS, n.d.b). Children are at higher risk for these injuries than are adults because they are still growing. Participation in childhood sports and recreational activities has increased in the past decade. Latest studies estimate that between 21 and 29 million children between the ages of 6 and 17 years participate in regular organized sports. With this increased participation in activity, sports and recreation injuries have also increased. From 2001 to 2009, 2.7 million children were treated for sports-related injuries, head injuries increased 62%, and football concussions more than doubled (Kelley & Carchia, 2013).

Clinical Presentation

The most common childhood overuse injuries include (AAOS, n.d.b) Sever disease, Osgood–Schlatter disease, patellar tendonitis, throwing injuries in the elbow, and stress fractures. Each of these is discussed here.

Sever disease, also known as osteochondrosis or apophysitis, is an inflammatory condition of the growth plate in the calcaneus (heel bone) resulting in heel pain. This is the most common cause of heel pain in children and is most often noted during the adolescent growth spurt. The most common cause is repetitive running and jumping activities that stress the foot on impact with the ground. Treatment includes rest, stretching, NSAIDs, and good shoes for support; heel pads for extra cushion are also helpful. A walking boot may be necessary if walking is affected. Recurrence is common, especially if the sports activity continues, but once the growth plate closes, the condition does not return.

Osgood–Schlatter disease involves pain at the front of the knee due to inflammation of the growth plate at the upper end of the tibia. This results from repetitive running and jumping activities. Treatment involves limiting activity, stretching, and immobilization (with a cast or brace) if walking is affected. This condition disappears after the adolescent growth spurt (about 14 years of age in girls and 16 years of age in boys). Compliance with treatment is essential because continued overuse can result in a fracture without proper healing.

Patellar tendonitis, also known as jumper's knee, involves pain in the patella (lower portion of the knee cap) caused by repetitive contraction of the quadriceps muscle. Repetitive stress to the patellar tendon can irritate and injure the growth plate. This results from activities involving repetitive jumping. Treatment involves rest, applying ice to the knee intermittently for 2 to 3 hours for the first 48 to 72 hours after the injury, and NSAIDs. This injury can result in a fracture if not allowed to heal.

Throwing injuries in the elbow, such as medial apophysitis and osteochondritis dissecans, occur from repeated stress to the growth areas of the elbow and are treated with rest.

Stress fractures occur when muscles become fatigued and transfer the overload of stress to the bone. If too much stress is on the bone, it cannot build up new bone fast enough and a crack forms. Stress fractures usually occur in the weight-bearing bones of the lower legs and feet. These fractures require 6 to 8 weeks to heal. Rest and casting or bracing are required to rest the injured bone. Stress fractures can become reinjured if they do not heal properly, leading to fractures that are larger and harder to heal.

Assessment and Diagnosis

Obtain a history of use and injury to the affected area. Assess the affected area for pain, swelling, and movement.

Therapeutic Interventions

These injuries are initially treated using the RICE technique. NSAIDs are useful for reducing inflammation. Stretching exercises and support devices may be prescribed. Physical therapy may be consulted to provide additional exercises to strengthen the area.

Evaluation

Expected outcomes for a child with an overuse injury include the following:
- The child has optimal pain control.
- The child does not experience deformity of the affected area.
- The child does not experience recurrence of the injury.
- The child does not experience long-term damage to the area.

Discharge Planning and Teaching

Teach the parent and the child that resting the area and compliance with the therapeutic interventions is necessary for optimal recovery and prevention of deformity and long-term damage (Patient Safety 27.5). Teach the parents about administering NSAIDs. Teach the child and the parents how to implement the RICE technique and how to properly use any support devices.

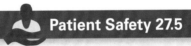

Patient Safety 27.5

Preventing Childhood Overuse Injuries

The increased participation of America's youth in organized and recreational sports has led to an increase in overuse injuries. Several factors contribute to this phenomenon, including the increased tendency for children to participate in year-round sports, become members of multiple sports teams simultaneously, and specialize early in one sport. These factors can lead to overtraining and burnout, which cause fatigue and overuse to the body, leading to injury. Recommendations from the American Academy of Pediatrics Council of Sports Medicine and Fitness to prevent overtraining, burnout, fatigue, and injury include the following (Brenner & The Council on Sports Medicine and Fitness, 2007):
- Limit activities to one sporting activity at a time.
- Limit activities to 5 d/wk, with at least 1 d off.
- Take at least 2–3 mo off per year between activities to allow injuries to heal, refresh the mind, and work on conditioning and strength.
- Prepare multisport athletes:
  - Young athletes who participate in a variety of sports have fewer injuries and play sports longer than those who specialize in one sport before puberty.
  - Multisport athletes who participate in two or more sports emphasizing the same body part (e.g., swimming and baseball) are at increased risk for overuse injuries compared with those who participate in sports that emphasize different body parts (e.g., swimming and soccer).

Think Critically

1. If a healthcare provider fails to recognize and treat a child's infection as osteomyelitis, what complications might result?

2. A 12-year-old boy who learns that he has developed osteomyelitis after having a cast for a fractured ulna states, "This is all my fault. They told me not to put anything inside my cast and I didn't listen." How should the nurse best respond to this patient?

3. When caring for a child with acute compartment syndrome, the limb should be maintained at a level no higher than the heart (as opposed to elevating the limb above the heart, as is typically done immediately postoperatively or after casting). What is the rationale for the positioning of the extremity in both of these cases?

4. A 14-year-old select team baseball pitcher has been diagnosed with medial apophysitis (pitcher's elbow). Considering the child's age and developmental stage and the recommended treatment for this injury, what are the

major obstacles and concerns the nurse should take into account when educating the child and family?

5. A 2-year-old child presents to the emergency department with a fractured tibia. There are no bruises or external injuries noted. The mother is holding the child and providing comfort; the child is consoled in her arms. X-rays reveal multiple fractures in various stages of healing. The current tibial X-ray shows a spiral (twisting) fracture. What questions should you ask the mom? What things should you consider in this situation?

6. Maintaining spinal alignment is a high priority following a spinal fusion for children with AIS. What is the significance of this positioning?

7. Following spinal fusion surgery to correct AIS, early movement is essential. Why is mobility important specifically for these patients?

References

American Academy of Orthopaedic Surgeons. (n.d.a). *Bowed legs (Blount's disease).* Retrieved from https://www.orthoinfo.org/en/diseases--conditions/bowed-legs-blounts-disease/

American Academy of Orthopaedic Surgeons. (n.d.b). *Overuse injuries in children.* Retrieved from https://orthoinfo.aaos.org/en/diseases--conditions/overuse-injuries-in-children/

American Academy of Orthopaedic Surgeons. (n.d.c). *Perthes disease.* Retrieved from https://www.orthoinfo.org/en/diseases--conditions/perthes-disease/

American Academy of Orthopaedic Surgeons. (n.d.d). *Slipped capital femoral epiphysis.* Retrieved from https://www.orthoinfo.org/en/diseases--conditions/slipped-capital-femoral-epiphysis-scfe/

American Academy of Orthopaedic Surgeons. (2014). *Detection and management of pediatric developmental dysplasia of the hip in infants up to six months of age: Evidence-based clinical practice guidelines.* Retrieved from http://www.aaos.org/research/guidelines/DDH/GuidelineFINAL.pdf

American Association of Neurological Surgeons. (2007). *Scoliosis.* Retrieved from www.aans.org/Patients/Neurosurgical-Conditions-and-Treatments/Scoliosis

Brenner, J. S., & The Council on Sports Medicine and Fitness. (2007). Overuse injuries, overtraining, and burnout in child and adolescent athletes. *Pediatrics, 119*(6), 1242–1249.

Campagne, D. (2017). *Compartment syndrome.* Retrieved from http://www.merckmanuals.com/professional/injuries-poisoning/fractures/compartment-syndrome

Canares, T. L., & Lockhart, G. (2013). Sprains. *Pediatrics in Review, 34*(1), 47–49.

Castellazzi, L., Montero, M., & Esposito, S. (2016). Update on the management of pediatric acute osteomyelitis and septic arthritis. *International Journal of Molecular Sciences, 17*(6), 855. doi:10.3390/ijms17060855

Centers for Disease Control and Prevention. (2015). *Clinician guide for collecting cultures.* Retrieved from https://www.cdc.gov/antibiotic-use/healthcare/implementation/clinicianguide.html

Dinolfo, E. A. (2004). Fractures. *Pediatrics in Review, 25*(6), 218–219. doi:10.1542/pir25-6-218

Dodwell, E. R. (2013). Osteomyelitis and septic arthritis in children: Current concepts. *Current Opinion in Pediatrics, 25*(1), 58–63. doi:10.1097/MOP.0b013e32835c2b42

Global Clubfoot Initiative. (2018). *The Ponseti method.* Retrieved from http://globalclubfoot.com/ponseti/

Healio. (2012). *Slipped capital femoral epiphysis: Controversies and current treatment options.* Retrieved from https://www.healio.com/orthopedics/pediatrics/news/print/orthopedics-today/%7B760790f6-1b9e-4e72-a309-f1f5c954a841%7D/slipped-capital-femoral-epiphysis-controversies-and-current-treatment-options

Hebra, A. (2017). *Pectus excavatum.* Retrieved from https://emedicine.medscape.com/article/1004953-overview

International Hip Dysplasia Institute. (n.d.). *Child treatment methods.* Retrieved from https://hipdysplasia.org/developmental-dysplasia-of-the-hip/child-treatment-methods/

International Perthes Study Group. (2016). *Perthes disease.* Retrieved from www.perthesdisease.org/perthes-disease-about

Kalyoussef, S. (2016). *Pediatric osteomyelitis.* Retrieved from https://emedicine.medscape.com/article/967095-overview#a4

Kelley, B., & Carchia, C. (2013, July 11). Hey, data data—Swing! *ESPN The Mag.* Retrieved from http://www.espn.com/espn/story/_/id/9469252/hidden-demographics-youth-sports-espn-magazine

Kiesler, J., & Ricer R. (2013). The abnormal fontanel. *American Family Physician, 15*(67), 2547–2552.

Kishner, S. (2016). *Osteomyelitis.* Retrieved from https://emedicine.medscape.com/article/1348767-overview

Kotlarsky, P., Haber, R., Bialik, V., & Eidelman, M. (2015). Developmental dysplasia of the hip: What has changed in the last 20 years? *World Journal of Orthopedics, 6*(11), 886–901.

Labelle, H., Richards, S. B., DeKleuver M., Grivas, T. B., Luk, K. D. K., Wong, H. K., . . . Fong, D. Y. T. (2013). Screening for adolescent idiopathic scoliosis: An information statement by the scoliosis research society international task force. *Scoliosis, 8*(17). doi:10.1186/1748-7161-8-17

Lennox, L. (2016). *Supernumerary digit.* Retrieved from https://emedicine.medscape.com/article/1113584-overview

Malik, S. (2012). Syndactyly: Phenotypes, genetics and current trends. *European Journal of Human Genetics, 20*(8), 817–824.

Muhly, W. T., Sankar, W. N., Ryan, K. Norton, A., Maxwell, L. G., DiMaggio, T., . . . Flynn, J. M. (2016). Rapid recovery pathway after spinal fusion for idiopathic scoliosis. *Pediatrics, 137*(4), e1–e9. doi:10.1542/peds.2015.1568

Nakaishi, L., & Nield, L. S. (2015). Are school scoliosis screening examinations necessary and effective? *Consult Pediatricians, 14*(12), 560–562.

National Cancer Institute. (n.d.). *Bone development and growth.* Retrieved from https://training.seer.cancer.gov/anatomy/skeletal/growth.html

National Organization of Rare Disorders. (2007). *Osteogenesis imperfecta.* Retrieved from https://rarediseases.org/rare-diseases/osteogenesis-imperfecta/

National Organization of Rare Disorders. (2016). *Legg calve perthes disease.* Retrieved from https://rarediseases.org/rare-diseases/legg-calve-perthes-disease/

Pediatric Orthopaedic Society of North America. (n.d.). *Slipped capital femoral epiphysis (SCFE).* Retrieved from http://orthokids.org/Condition/Slipped-Capital-Femoral-Epiphysis-(SCFE)

Peck, D. (2010). Slipped capital femoral epiphysis: Diagnosis and management. *American Family Physician, 82*(3), 258–262.

Peck, D. M., Voss, L. M., & Voss, T. T. (2017). Slipped capital femoral epiphysis: Diagnosis and management. *American Family Physician, 95*(12), 779–784.

Poduval, M. (2015). *Skeletal system anatomy in children and toddlers.* Retrieved from https://emedicine.medscape.com/article/1899256-overview?pa=Egkgz22x2ncmEkGz5J54llaYJlANWcMW2h0b09ncLFm731KBGnDVtXmyop%2FIRHZDX8MwC0EECwzp432Skuf9qw%3D%3D

Richards, B. S., & Vitale, M. G. (2008). Screening for idiopathic scoliosis in adolescents: An informative statement. *Journal of Bone and Joint Surgery, 90*(1), 195–198. doi:10.2106/JBJS.G.01276

Richards, B. S., Sucato, D. J., & Johnston, C. E. (2014). Scoliosis. In J. A. Herring (Ed.), *Tachdjian's pediatric orthopaedics* (5th ed., pp. 206–291). Philadelphia, PA: Elsevier Saunders.

Sabinski, M., Murnaghan, C., & Snyder, M. (2006). The value of preliminary overhead traction in the closed management of DDH. *International Orthopedics, 30*(4), 268–271.

Schwarz, S. M. (2017). *Rickets.* Retrieved from https://emedicine.medscape.com/article/985510-overview

Souder, C. (2018). *Tibia shaft fracture—Pediatric.* Retrieved from https://www.orthobullets.com/pediatrics/4026/tibia-shaft-fracture--pediatric

Sucato, D. J., De La Rocha, A., Lau, K., & Ramo, B. A. (2017). Overhead Bryant's traction does not improve the success of closed reduction or limit AVN in developmental dysplasia of the hip. *Journal of Pediatric Orthopedics, 37*(2), e108–e113. doi:10.1097/BPO.0000000000000747

Texas Scottish Rite Hospital for Children. (n.d.). *What is clubfoot?* Retrieved from https://scottishritehospital.org/care-and-treatment/clubfoot-and-foot-disorders?utm_source=google&utm_medium=cpc&utm_campaign=FY18&utm_term=%7Bkeyword%7D&utm_content=TRG&c

University of British Columbia. (2012). *The basic types of pediatric fractures, differences from adults and care as a primary care physician.* Retrieved from http://learnpediatrics.sites.olt.ubc.ca/files/2012/04/fractures.pdf

U.S. Preventive Services Task Force. (2004). *Idiopathic scoliosis in adolescents: Screening.* Retrieved from https://www.uspreventiveservicestaskforce.org/Page/Document/RecommendationStatementFinal/idiopathic-scoliosis-in-adolescents-screening

Wheeless, C. R. (2017). *Wheeless' textbook of orthopaedics.* Retrieved from wheelessonline.com

Suggested Readings

Ebraheim, N. A. (2014, March 25). *Barlow and Ortolani test, congenital hip dislocation—Everything you need to know.* [Video file]. Retrieved from https://www.youtube.com/watch?v=imhI6PLtGLc

Grivas, T. B., Hresko, M. T., Labelle, H., Price, N., Kotwicki, T., & Maruyama, T. (2013). The pendulum swings back to scoliosis screening: Screening policies for early detection and treatment of idiopathic scoliosis—current concepts and recommendations. *Scoliosis, 8,* 16. doi:10.1186/1748-7161-8-16.

Launay, F. (2015). Sports-related overuse injuries in children. *Orthopaedics & Traumatology: Surgery & Research, 101*(1), S139–S147. doi:10.1016/j.otsr.2014.06.030

Lazoritz, S. (2010, July). What every nurse needs to know about the clinical aspects of child abuse. *American Nurse Today, 5*(7). Retrieved from https://www.americannursetoday.com/what-every-nurse-needs-to-know-about-the-clinical-aspects-of-child-abuse/

Lyden, S. (2011). Uncovering child abuse. *Nursing Management, 41,* 1–5. doi:10.1097/01.NURSE.0000396601.75497.26

Morey, S. S. (2001). AAP develops guidelines for early detection of dislocated hips. *American Family Physician, 63*(3), 565–568.

Torlincasi, A. M., & Waseem, M. (2018). Compartment syndrome, extremity. *StatPearls* [Internet]. Retrieved from https://www.ncbi.nlm.nih.gov/books/NBK448124/

28 Alterations in Neuromuscular Function

After completing this chapter, you will be able to:

1. Compare and contrast anatomical and physiological characteristics of the neuromuscular systems of children and adults.
2. Relate pediatric assessment findings to the child's neuromuscular status.
3. Discuss the pathophysiology of common pediatric neuromuscular disorders.
4. Differentiate between signs and symptoms of common pediatric neuromuscular disorders.
5. Outline the therapeutic regimen for each of the pediatric neuromuscular disorders.
6. Describe the pharmacological management of common of pediatric neuromuscular disorders.
7. Apply the principles of growth and development to the care of a child with a neuromuscular disorder.
8. Create a nursing plan of care for each of the common pediatric neuromuscular disorders.

Key Terms

Anencephaly
Developmental milestone
Developmental reflexes
Encephalocele
Fine motor
Gross motor

Hypertonia
Hypotonia
Muscular atrophy
Neural tube defect (NTD)
Palsy
Spina bifida

Variations in Anatomy and Physiology

The peripheral nervous system (PNS) and the muscular system together make up the neuromuscular system. The PNS consists of 12 pairs of cranial nerves, which emerge from the brain, and 31 pairs of spinal nerves, which emerge from the spinal cord and branch into smaller nerves that travel to various parts of the body. The PNS has both sensory and motor functions. It delivers impulses from sensory receptors in the skin and special sense organs via sensory (afferent) neurons to the spinal cord and brain to process sensations and delivers impulses from the spinal cord and brain via motor (efferent) neurons out to muscles to initiate movement. The muscular system comprises the muscles of the body, which contract and relax to produce movement in bones, organs, blood vessels, the respiratory tract, and the heart, as well as to help maintain posture and generate body heat. Together, these two systems help a person move and perform functions necessary for daily life.

Although the structures of the pediatric neuromuscular system are fully formed by birth, they are immature and do not fully develop until close to adulthood, with the majority of the development of both **gross motor** and **fine motor** skills taking place in the first 2 years of life (Aubert, 2015). Maturation of the neuromuscular system takes place gradually. This process starts at conception, continues after birth, and is complete at some point during older childhood or adolescence. Unlike adults, children have varying motor and neurological capabilities depending on their age. Knowledge of these age-related differences is crucial when assessing a pediatric patient for neuromuscular disorders.

When assessing a pediatric patient for neuromuscular disorders, it is helpful to have an understanding of age-specific **developmental milestones**, which can indicate whether a child is developing normally. Developmental milestones are a progression of expected accomplishments that occur along a predicted pathway, such as sitting, walking, and talking. These milestones are attained in a fairly linear manner, with attainment of each developmental milestone helping to prepare the child for attaining the next milestone. For example, a child typically progresses from sitting independently to pulling to stand, taking steps while holding on, and then walking independently.

Although this pathway is predictable, meaning that most children must sit independently before they can pull to stand, there is also a wide degree of variability. For example, a child can begin walking as early as 8 to 9 months of age or as late as 18 months of age. When a child is later than usual in attaining a developmental milestone, parents are often concerned. However, if all other areas of development are on target, there is usually no reason to be concerned.

Developmental milestones occur in several domains: gross motor, fine motor, social/behavioral, and cognitive. A thorough assessment covers all domains, because the domains overlap and influence each other. For example, a cognitive delay can influence gross and/or fine motor skill attainment. If a child is not curious about his or her surroundings, the child will not be stimulated to explore and move, which may affect gross and fine motor skills. See Table 28.1 for examples of some gross motor milestones and the expected age of attainment for each.

Table 28.1 Gross Motor Developmental Milestones and Expected Age of Attainment

Gross Motor Developmental Milestone	Expected Age of Attainment
Lifts head 45° when prone	Birth to 3 mo
Rolls over	5–6 mo
Sits independently	5–8 mo
Pulls to stand	9 mo
Walks independently	9–16 mo
Climbs stairs without assistance	2–2½ y
Pedals a tricycle	3 y
Hops on one foot	4 y
Climbs stairs using alternating feet	4 y

Data from Graber, E. G. (n.d.). *Childhood development.* Retrieved from https://www.merckmanuals.com/professional/pediatrics/growth-and-development/childhood development#v1084884.

Many intrinsic and extrinsic factors can interrupt the development of or even damage the maturing nervous system, resulting in long-term consequences. One example of an intrinsic factor affecting development would be a genetic defect. Extrinsic factors include toxins found in the environment, such as lead. Ideal development takes place in a safe and nurturing environment in which a child is given the opportunity to explore, learn, practice, and repeat learned behaviors. Exposure to environmental toxins, such as lead, parental mental illness, such as depression, and parental substance abuse can negatively affect a child's development.

Similar to developmental milestones, developmental reflexes can serve as indicators of a child's developmental status. An infant is born with **developmental reflexes**, sometimes referred to as primitive reflexes, which often disappear soon after birth. Developmental reflexes are present as early as 34 weeks after conception and, other than the parachute reflex, disappear in the first few months of life (Table 28.2). If a reflex can be elicited in a child who is beyond the age at which the reflex should have resolved, this can be a cause for concern and further evaluation.

Assessment of the Pediatric Neuromuscular System

Although an assessment of the neuromuscular system varies depending on the patient's age, it should start with a thorough history. Included in it should be the prenatal, perinatal, neonatal, and family and relevant developmental history of the child. The birth history is important because any factor that could potentially affect the developing brain or cardiopulmonary system of the neonate could adversely affect the oxygen status, causing injury to the brain and resulting in neuromuscular deficits. A prenatal history should cover any maternal infections that could affect the developing brain of the fetus (such as Zika or cytomegalovirus), prescription or illicit drug or alcohol exposure, results of any abnormal prenatal ultrasound studies, maternal history of previous pregnancies and complications, and presence of typical fetal movements. The perinatal history addresses the time right before delivery and immediately afterward. It is important to know the gestational age of the child; complications with birth (such as footling or breech presentation, prolonged labor, fetal distress, or high-risk delivery method); measurements of the neonate's weight, length, and head circumference at birth; Apgar scores; whether any resuscitation was needed after delivery; and results of the newborn metabolic screening. The newborn metabolic screening, which is done shortly after birth, can identify several disorders that can be life-threatening or cause long-term developmental sequelae.

For older infants and children, inquire about feeding and/or swallowing difficulties, delayed milestones, frequent falls that are not age appropriate, activity intolerance, a history of frequent respiratory infections such as aspiration pneumonia, frequent muscle cramps, and muscle wasting.

When assessing the neuromuscular system of the pediatric patient, it is imperative to have a solid understanding of the developmental milestones and when those milestones should be attained. If a child was born prematurely, his or her

Table 28.2 Developmental Reflexes

Reflex	Description	Expected Age at Appearance	Expected Age at Resolution
Moro (startle)	With the infant supine, gently lift the infant off the bed by the arms. When the shoulders are off the bed but the majority of the head is still on the bed, let go of the arms. The infant should "startle," with the arms flaring outward and abducting.	34–36 wk PCA	5–6 mo
Asymmetric tonic neck	With the infant supine and calm, turn the infant's head to one side. The infant should extend the arm and leg on the side the head has been turned toward and flex the arm on the other side (fencing stance).	38–40 wk PCA	2–3 mo
Trunk incurvation	With the infant prone, stroke along the spine on one side. The infant should turn the hips toward the side that is stroked.	38–40 wk PCA	1–2 mo
Palmar grasp	Place a finger in the palm of the infant's hand. The infant should close the fingers around your finger. If you attempt to pull away, the infant should tighten the grip.	38–40 wk PCA	5–6 mo
Plantar grasp	Place a finger below the infant's toes on the plantar surface. The infant's toes should curl around your finger.	38–40 wk PCA	9–10 mo
Rooting	Stroke the infant's cheek. The infant should turn to that side and make sucking movements.	38–40 wk PCA	2–3 mo
Parachute	With the infant held in an upright position with the infant's back to you, quickly move the infant forward, as if falling suddenly. The infant's arms should extend in front as if to break the fall.	8–9 mo PCA	Persists throughout life

PCA, postconceptional age.
Kotagal, S. (2018). Detailed neurological assessments of infants and children. In D. R. Nordli (Ed.), *UpToDate*. Retrieved June 20, 2019 from https://www.uptodate.com/contents/detailed-neurologic-assessment-of-infants-and-children?search=Detailed%20neurological%20 assessments%20of%20infants%20and%20children.&source=search_result&selectedTitle=1~150&usage_type=default&display_rank=1

chronological age should be corrected according to gestational age. What is normal at one age can be a delay at another age. Any delay in achieving a milestone, or regression after achieving a previous milestone, is cause for further investigation. The American Academy of Pediatrics has identified several evidence-based developmental screening tools that can be used to assess for developmental delays in pediatric patients. More

information regarding appropriate developmental screening tools can be found in Table 28.3 and at www.screeningtime .org/star-center/#/screening-tools.

Because evaluation of the child's neuromuscular system often involves observing gross motor, fine motor, and cognitive functions, your approach to assessment depends on the age of the child. Infants are often comfortable with a new face as

Table 28.3 Developmental Screening Tools

Tool	Child's Age at Screening	How the Tool Is Administered
Ages and Stages Questionnaire (ASQ-3)	1 mo to 5½ y	The parent completes a 30-item questionnaire covering the child's communication, gross motor, fine motor, problem-solving, and personal-social development.
Parents' Evaluation of Developmental Status (PEDS)	Birth to 8 y	The parent completes a 10-item questionnaire covering the child's development, behavior, and social-emotional areas.
Child Development Inventory (CDI)	18 mo to 6 y	The parent completes questionnaire covering the child's self-help, social, motor, language, and overall development.

Data from Screening Time. (n.d.). *Screening tools*. Retrieved from https://screeningtime.org/star-center/#/screening-tools.

long as their parent is close by. Toddlers, and occasionally some preschool children, are better observed from a distance and without their awareness. As you are talking with the parent and obtaining the child's history, observe the toddler or preschool child walking, playing with toys, drawing on paper, and interacting with the parent. This approach should give you valuable information regarding the child's gross motor, fine motor, problem-solving, and cognitive abilities. Older children are usually comfortable with the exam, especially if you can relate the exam to a game or familiar activity. A thorough physical assessment of the pediatric patient includes assessment of the cranial nerves, motor function, sensory function, reflexes, gait (if age appropriate), and head and spine.

Assessment of the cranial nerves is essential when assessing the neuromuscular function of your patient; however, how you assess the pediatric patient differs from how you would an adult patient (Table 28.4). The cranial nerves have both motor and sensory functions. Adult patients can cooperate with

Table 28.4 Cranial Nerve Assessment in Adults and Infants

Cranial Nerve		How to Assess	
No.	Name	Adult	Infant
I	Olfactory	Have the patient close the eyes and attempt to identify by smell common substances with distinctive scents, such as coffee and soap.	Expose the patient to a noxious odor and observe the reaction.
II	Optic	Perform visual acuity and funduscopic exams.	Observe the infant's ability to regard a person's face, make eye contact, reach for an object, and see objects as they are introduced into the peripheral field of vision. Also observe whether the pupils are equal and reactive.
III	Oculomotor	Move an object through the patient's visual fields and observe the patient's pupil reaction and extraocular movements as the patient tracks it.	• Move a brightly colored toy through the infant's visual fields and observe the patient's ability to track it. • Observe whether the pupils are equal and reactive and the opening of the eyelids symmetric (i.e., absence of ptosis). • Observe for the corneal light reflex.
IV	Trochlear	Observe the extraocular movements as the patient looks down and inward.	• Observe for symmetric eye movements (note that in patients younger than 2 mo, it is not unusual to have "wandering eyes"). • Move a brightly colored toy through the infant's visual fields and observe the patient's ability to track it. • Observe for the corneal light reflex.
V	Trigeminal	• Motor function: Ask the patient to clench the jaw. • Sensory function: Touch areas of the face (along sensory tracts) to assess feeling.	For infants and younger children, you are only able to assess the sensory function, by observing the infant's response to light touch on the face.
VI	Abducens	Observe the patient's ability to move the eyes laterally.	• Observe for symmetric eye movements (note that in patients younger than 2 mo, it is not unusual to have "wandering eyes"). • Move a brightly colored toy through the infant's visual fields and observe the patient's ability to track it. • Observe for the corneal light reflex.
VII	Facial	• Motor function: Ask the patient to make various facial expressions, close the eyes tightly, and smile and/or frown. • Sensory function: Assess the patient's ability to identify different foods by taste alone.	• Motor function: Observe for symmetry and fullness in facial expression during crying. • Sensory function: For older children, assess the response to a salt solution put on the lateral sides of the tongue.

(continued)

Table 28.4 Cranial Nerve Assessment in Adults and Infants (*continued*)

Cranial Nerve		How to Assess	
No.	**Name**	**Adult**	**Infant**
VIII	Vestibulocochlear	• Check hearing by rubbing your fingers together near each of the patient's ears. • Check the patient's balance with the eyes closed.	Observe for the infant's ability to startle to loud noises, show interest in an unfamiliar noise, and turn to a familiar voice.
IX	Glossopharyngeal	• Motor function: Observe the patient's ability to swallow. • Sensory function: Assess the patient's ability to feel touch on the tympanic membrane, in the ear canal, and on the posterior tongue and to taste on the back of the tongue.	Observe the infant for strength and quality of cry, ability to perform sucking and swallowing in a coordinated manner, and the presence of the gag reflex.
X	Vagus	• Motor function: Observe the patient's ability to move and use the palate, pharynx, and larynx. • Sensory function: Observe the patient's ability to feel touch in the pharynx and larynx.	Observe the infant for strength and quality of cry, ability to perform sucking and swallowing in a coordinated manner, and the presence of the gag reflex.
XI	Accessory	Have the patient shrug the shoulders and turn the head left and right against resistance to assess the function of the sternocleidomastoid and upper trapezius muscles, respectively.	Observe the infant for the ability to perform coordinated movement of shoulders and turning the neck against resistance.
XII	Hypoglossal	Ask the patient to stick his or her tongue out.	Observe the infant for symmetrical movement of tongue.

Data from Bickley, L. S., & Szilagyi, P. G. (2003). *The nervous system in Bates' guide to physical examination and history taking.* Philadelphia, PA: Lippincott Williams & Wilkins.

instructions during assessment of motor function and verbalize their responses to sensory stimuli. Depending on the developmental level of your pediatric patient, you may need to alter your examination to elicit a response and may rely more on observation. Infants and toddlers, for example, are unable to respond to commands, but you may obtain much information about them through observation and altering your exam to fit the developmental level of the patient.

If you have the opportunity, start your assessment while the child is playing and interacting with others. Some children relish in the opportunity to show off their gross and fine motor skills, but others shy away. Younger children are often more comfortable on their caregiver's lap, and your exam will be much easier and more accurate if the child is calm.

The posture of the pediatric patient can reveal much about how well the neuromuscular system is functioning. Notice how the infant holds the body. Is it symmetrical? Are the muscles similar in size? Asymmetry of the upper and/or lower body can indicate that the infant is not using one side of the body, as is often seen in hemiparesis or cerebral **palsy** (CP). Does the infant have persistent arching of the back? Some intermittent arching can be normal, but arching that is persistent can indicate a brain

injury. Are there any abnormal, involuntary movements, such as tics or tremors? Does the infant keep a clenched fist during wakefulness? Although a closed fist is normal during sleep, it is an abnormal finding during wakefulness. Several neurological disorders that originate along the corticospinal tract are associated with abnormal involuntary movements.

Assess muscle tone by putting a joint through its full range of motion passively. The amount of resistance felt is the muscle tone. An infant with low muscle tone, **hypotonia**, is likely to lie supine with the legs abducted in a frog-leg position and produce little to no resistance during passive range of motion. Owing to the lack of muscle tone, often the joint is hyperextensible. On the other end of the spectrum, an infant with increased muscle tone, known as **hypertonia**, is likely to have increased resistance to passive movement of the joint that is either spastic or quick to recoil. If the child is old enough, you can actively assess muscle strength by asking the child to move a body part against resistance. For example, with the child sitting on the exam table with legs relaxed and hanging over the side of the table, put your hands on the child's lower legs and ask the child to extend, or straighten, the legs while you resist the movement. The amount of movement the child is able to accomplish is an estimate of muscle strength. Muscle strength is assessed on a 5-point scale (Kotagal, 2018):

- Grade 0/5: No muscle movement
- Grade 1/5: A small flicker of movement
- Grade 2/5: Movement with gravity eliminated
- Grade 3/5: Movement against gravity
- Grade 4/5: Movement against gravity and with some external force applied
- Grade 5/5: Movement against gravity and with good external force applied

Coordinated movements of the muscular system require full integration of the motor system, the cerebellar system, the vestibular system, and the sensory system. A deficit in any of these systems can result in a lack of coordinated movements. Most tests used with adults to assess coordination cannot be used with young children because they lack the cognitive ability to understand the commands. A thorough assessment of coordination involves assessing for accuracy in rapid, alternating movements, point-to-point touching, and gait. A common test for rapid, alternating movements involves the patient hitting the thighs with the hands, alternating between the palmar surface and the dorsal surface, as quickly as possible. For point-to-point touching, ask the patient to spread the arms out to the sides and hold them at shoulder level. With the patient's eyes closed, ask the patient to touch the tip of the nose with the index finger, alternating between the left and right arms. Most children are not able to complete these tests until they are of school age. Growth and Development Check 28.1 describes how to assess coordination in pediatric patients at each level of development.

The PNS has both motor and sensory functions, and so a full neurological exam includes an assessment of both motor and sensory function. However, assessment of a child's sensory function can be limited by the child's level of development. Exam of the sensory system of an older child or adult involves assessment of the patient's ability to feel pain, temperature, vibration, light touch, and proprioception and to distinguish between sharp and dull sensations. Exam of the sensory system in a younger child may be limited to assessment of pain, because the child often lacks the cognitive ability and language skills to follow directions.

Another area to evaluate when assessing the neuromuscular system is tendon reflexes. To best elicit a tendon reflex, tap the tendon of the relaxed and partially flexed muscle. A normal response is indicated by an involuntary flexion and extension of the muscle. The reflex can be evaluated as intact (normal response), absent or diminished, exaggerated, or asymmetric. An intact reaction is an indication of an intact neurological system. Any other response is considered abnormal and warrants further evaluation.

The tendons commonly assessed in the pediatric patient include the following:

- Biceps: With the forearm flexed at a 90° angle, the biceps tendon is found anterior to the elbow.
- Triceps: Again, with the forearm flexed at a 90° angle, the triceps tendon is found posterior to the elbow.

- Brachioradialis: This tendon is found on the distal forearm, just before the wrist.
- Patellar: This tendon is found just below the knee.
- Achilles: This tendon is found on the posterior ankle.

 Growth and Development Check 28.1

Assessing Coordination at Each Level of Development

Infants

When assessing a young child, look for smooth, purposeful, age-appropriate movements. The younger the child, the more uncoordinated the movements may appear. For example, when a caregiver is holding a 2-mo-old infant, the infant may reach and attempt to touch the caregiver's face. It may take several attempts to touch the face, and the infant may "overshoot" several times. Although these movements may appear uncoordinated, they are age appropriate for a 2-mo-old.

Toddlers

Once a child has begun to walk, observing gait is a good way to assess coordination. For toddlers, it is helpful to know how long the child has been walking. For the first couple of months of independent walking, the child's gait is uncoordinated and unsteady. After that, however, the gait should appear smooth and steady.

Preschoolers

Beginning around the age of 3 or 4 y, a child is able to participate in a more in-depth assessment of coordination. Assess the child's gait while the child is walking and running. Some children are able to participate with the heel-to-toe assessment. For this test, ask the child to walk a straight line, placing the heel of the forward foot immediately in front of the toes of the rear foot. Most preschool children are also able to stand on one foot and hop, although some may only do it when they are sure that the examiner is not watching. Often, enlisting the help of an older sibling, who is often eager to perform, entices the younger child to participate. A good understanding of developmental milestones is helpful when assessing a child's coordination.

School-Age and Older Children

The older child is often able to participate in assessment in the same manner as an adult. When assessing an older child for coordination, observe the gait for smooth, fluid, alternating movements of both the upper and lower extremities. The posture should be upright. In addition to the heel-to-toe walk, ask the child to walk only on the toes and then only on the heels. The older child is also able to perform rapid, alternating movements and point-to-point touching as in the adult examination.

Assessment of reflexes in the pediatric patient requires practice and skill. Patients often anticipate the involuntary response and can find it difficult to relax. An adult patient can often cooperate with instructions to relax or can be distracted. For the younger pediatric patients, this can be difficult. Infants, although not necessarily afraid of the examiner, often do like being held still. They are often in constant motion, and their muscles are not relaxed. Toddlers do not want a stranger touching them and pull away, tensing their muscles in their struggle to break free. You must know the exact spot to locate a tendon and strike at just the right moment to get a response. A preschool or an older child often participate if you make the exam a game and effectively distract the child. For example, lead the child to believe you are going to tap the right patellar tendon but tap the left patellar tendon, instead. If the child is focused on the right leg, the left leg is often relaxed.

When examining infants, assess for the presence of developmental reflexes. As mentioned previously, most of the developmental reflexes disappear within a few months of birth. Consider it abnormal if a reflex cannot be elicited at a time it should be present, is present at a time it should be absent, or is asymmetrical (Kotagal, 2018).

Next, examine the head and spine. Begin with observation. Assess for symmetry of the head and face, shape of the head, and any abnormal facial characteristics. For children younger than age 2 years, measure the head circumference and plot on an appropriate growth chart. An infant's head can often look too large for the body, causing concern; plotting the head circumference on an appropriate growth chart, such as the growth charts available at www.cdc.gov/growthcharts/, can alleviate such concerns. Record the measurement as a percentile based on gender and chronological age. Ideally, you should follow the child's growth over time, rather than just taking a one-time measurement. Some children have rather large or small heads in relation to their height, but this is not always a cause for concern. If a child is consistently in the same percentile, this is usually indicative of normal growth. However, it can be concerning if a child's growth crosses over two or more percentiles, whether it is increasing or decreasing in size. It is also helpful to measure the parent's head circumference, because head size can be genetically influenced.

For children younger than age 2 years, exam of the head includes evaluation of the suture lines and fontanels. The infant skull consists of eight bones. The joints where these bones come together are called suture lines. In the infant, these sutures are filled with a flexible membranous tissue that allows for compression of the skull during vaginal delivery and helps accommodate the rapid brain growth that occurs in the first year of life. The sutures are often very easily felt during the first month of life but then become more difficult to feel. The sutures ultimately close and the bones of the skull fuse together by the age of 2 years.

A fontanel is created when two major suture lines intersect, causing a larger, round area of membranous tissue. An infant has an anterior and a posterior fontanel. The posterior fontanel is formed where the occipital and parietal bones come together

and closes within the first 2 months of life. The anterior fontanel is formed where the parietal and frontal bones come together. This fontanel stays open longer than the posterior fontanel, often closing sometime between 6 and 18 months of age. Delay in closure of the fontanels can indicate a metabolic disorder such as hypothyroidism or increased intracranial pressure, which can be caused by a number of conditions. Premature closure of the sutures, which can be detected by a decreasing head circumference percentile and a closed anterior fontanel, is called craniosynostosis and must be corrected surgically to avoid causing increased intracranial pressure, which can ultimately cause brain damage.

Examine the spine from the base of the skull to the coccyx. The spine should be relatively straight, with some mild curvature from anterior to posterior, forming the normal curvature of the spine. A lateral curvature, or an exaggerated anterior-posterior curvature, may be indicative of scoliosis. The skin covering the spine should be intact and without dimples or tufts of hair, which can suggest a tethered cord, occult spina bifida, or a dermoid cyst. Palpate along the spine and note any areas of tenderness.

General Nursing Interventions for Neuromuscular Disorders

Given here is an overview of key nursing interventions that apply to neuromuscular disorders, in general. Interventions that are specific to a given disorder are discussed within the Therapeutic Interventions section of that disorder.

Promote Skin Integrity

Alterations caused by some neuromuscular disorders make children's skin and other tissues more vulnerable to injury and breakdown. Children with CP, muscular dystrophy, and severe spinal cord injury who require the use of a wheelchair for mobility are at high risk for skin breakdown from ill-fitting chairs and devices. Reposition the child frequently while the child is in the chair and assess pressure points such as the coccyx, sacrum, and elbows. Ill-fitting braces can cause pressure injury or altered skin integrity. Assess the skin under braces frequently and teach parents to do so at home. As the child grows or gains weight, new braces may be needed. Encourage parents to assess fit as the child grows.

Maintain Effective Ventilation

Children with neuromuscular disorders often have respiratory dysfunction due to either the inability to clear secretions or, as in the case of botulism or in spinal cord injury, the inability to maintain a patent airway or an adequate respiratory rate. Nursing interventions to promote effective ventilation include clearing the airway, positioning the child to provide an open airway, and using noninvasive ventilation devices such as bilevel positive airway pressure (BIPAP) or even intubation and mechanical ventilation.

Methods to aid airway clearance vary depending on the cause, acuity, and severity of obstruction. In severe, acute cases, airway obstruction can be caused by excessive production of mucus and other secretions, such as in a patient with spinal muscular atrophy (SMA) who has a respiratory infection. Children may require frequent nasotracheal or oropharyngeal suctioning. More general interventions include chest percussion (chest physiotherapy) and postural drainage. Cough assist machines and intrapulmonary percussive ventilation may be used to assist with achieving adequate cough and removal of mucus and secretions. Place patients with muscular dystrophy or CP in an upright, seated position and assist them with frequent position changes to help move secretions and clear the airway.

When muscle weakness is severe enough that the child cannot maintain adequate chest expansion for optimal oxygenation and ventilation, noninvasive ventilation strategies such as continuous positive airway pressure or BIPAP may be used. Children with severe spinal cord injuries, particularly at the level of vertebra C6 or above, and those with severe botulism may require intubation and mechanical ventilation. Assess patients receiving ventilation, whether noninvasive or invasive, for adequate chest rise, respiratory rate, and aeration. Perform frequent mouth care for the child to reduce the risks of ventilator-associated pneumonia and mucosal breakdown. Reposition the child frequently to avoid pressure injury. Secure tubing and airway devices to avoid accidental removal or disconnection by the child.

Prevent Falls

Many children with neuromuscular disorders are able to ambulate, either independently or with assistive devices. However, depending on the level of muscle weakness or impairment, the child may be at high risk for falls. Children who are mobile should wear appropriate braces when ambulating. Ensure an environment free of fall risks by removing objects that could be tripped over, providing adequate space between furniture and walls, and encouraging the child to use (or assisting the child with using) handrails when available.

Maintain Adequate Nutrition

Children with neuromuscular disorders may have difficulty consuming enough calories because of a lack of appetite, difficulty swallowing related to muscle weakness, or both. Allow children who are able to feed by mouth to choose appropriate foods for meals and snacks. Offer choices when possible. Present small portions. Allow adequate time for consumption of meals and snacks so that the child does not feel pressured or rushed to consume food. Socialization or eating with family or friends may improve the child's appetite. Offer the highest calorie meals at the time of day when the child is most hungry or has the greatest appetite. Provide high-calorie shakes or puddings for children who need increased caloric intake. These foods require less energy to consume.

Place children who consume food by mouth and are at risk for aspiration or difficulty swallowing, such as those with CP, in an upright position for each feeding and snack. Place food far back in the mouth to overcome tongue thrust or movement that can push food forward. Offer soft or blended foods and allow extra time for chewing and swallowing. Use adaptive handles or feeding utensils as needed and encourage the development of self-feeding skills.

Some infants and children may require nutrition via a gastrostomy or jejunostomy tube. The caloric needs of these children vary depending on growth and energy expenditure. Formula type is based on the child's age and tolerance. Supplements such as vitamin D may be necessary in some children who require chronic tube feedings.

No matter which route of nutrition the child needs, monitor the child's height and weight. Weigh the child weekly during times of illness and at every pediatrician visit.

Promote Pain Relief, Comfort, and Rest

Children with neuromuscular disorders can have a wide range of pain and discomfort, depending on the etiology and comorbidities of the disease. For example, spasticity is common in children with CP. Spasticity can cause pain. Antispasmodics such as baclofen are given to reduce spasticity. Braces can also be used to promote extremity alignment, which can help reduce spasticity and pain. Physical therapy and stretching, several times a day, are often performed to reduce spasticity. Properly fitted assistive devices, such as wheelchairs, are necessary, not only for safety but also to promote comfort and reduce the risk of pressure injury, which can cause pain.

When caring for children experiencing pain, assess their pain level frequently with a developmentally appropriate pain scale and use both nonpharmacological and pharmacological interventions to address it. Nonpharmacological measures include the following:

- Providing a dark, quiet environment and minimizing interruptions
- Allowing parents to hold and comfort the child
- Allowing the child to have toys, blankets, and other comfort items within reach
- Providing massage or soft music
- Placing the child in a position of comfort, such as side-lying on the right with knees bent or lying supine with the head of the bed elevated

Administer medications for pain as ordered, which may range from mild analgesics such as acetaminophen to narcotics such as morphine or fentanyl, and document relief from pain.

Provide Emotional and Psychosocial Support to the Child and Parents

Whether congenital or acquired, neuromuscular disorders disrupt the lives of children and parents and pose significant emotional and psychosocial challenges. For many children, developing an acquired neuromuscular disorder, such as botulism or spinal cord injury, leads to their first hospitalization, and anxiety and fear are common. Congenital diseases such as CP, spina bifida, muscular dystrophy, and SMA can require difficult lifestyle changes in the family, such as the use of a wheelchair, modifications to the home for the disabled child, and adjustment to changes in body image, which is particularly a concern in adolescents. Receiving diagnosis of a potentially fatal disorder, such as muscular dystrophy or SMA, can be devastating for parents.

When caring for a child with a neuromuscular disorder, provide the child and family with emotional and psychosocial support by doing the following:

- Offer clear and concise explanations of conditions, procedures, and hospital routines.
- Give parents time to ask questions, express frustrations, and process the information they receive.
- Encourage parents to keep a journal or log of their child's care and to write down questions.
- Help parents view their child as a whole person rather than focus solely on the disease.
- Allow time for parents to touch, hold, cuddle, talk to, and bond with their infant when the infant's condition allows.
- Encourage parents to participate in care when possible, such as feeding and bathing the infant.
- Give parents resources for working with the child's school to keep up with academic work.
- Provide resources on support groups, counseling, and grief groups specific to the child's condition and diagnosis.

Cerebral Palsy

CP is the most common physical disability in childhood (Centers for Disease Control and Prevention [CDC], n.d.-e; Moreno-De-Luca, Ledbetter, & Martin, 2012; Reddihough, 2011). CP is an umbrella term for a complex, multifactorial, nonprogressive but permanent disorder of the brain that affects a person's ability to move. There are varying degrees of disability, from mild gait disturbances to an inability to walk or talk, but all will have some deficit in their ability to move and maintain proper posture.

Etiology and Pathophysiology

CP results from the developing brain either failing to form correctly or receiving some type of insult, such as a prenatal stroke or maternal infection, that causes permanent damage to the brain and results in an inability to control one's muscles and movement. This damage can also impair a person's sensory functions, perception, cognitive ability, and communication (Reddihough, 2011). CP can be classified as congenital or acquired. Congenital CP is thought to be caused by damage to the developing brain before or during birth and accounts for 85% to 90% of all cases (CDC, n.d.-e). Although often the exact cause of congenital CP is unknown, there are several known risk factors, including the following (CDC, n.d.-e):

- Low birth weight
- Premature birth
- Multiple births
- Use of infertility procedures
- Maternal infections
- Jaundice or kernicterus

- Maternal thyroid disorder, seizure disorder, or intellectual disability
- Birth complications

Acquired CP, which is much less common, occurs within the first 28 days of life and is often caused by an infection such as meningitis, head trauma, or any condition that can cause cerebrovascular bleeding, such as sickle cell disease, stroke, an arteriovenous malformation, or a bleeding disorder. Infants who do not receive an injection of vitamin K after birth are at risk for developing vitamin K deficiency bleeding. If this bleeding occurs in the brain, there is a high risk for developing CP.

CP has also been classified into four main types depending on the distinctive symptoms produced by each: spastic, dyskinetic, ataxic, and mixed. Spastic CP is the most common type, affecting approximately 80% of children with CP (CDC, n.d.-e). In spastic CP, the muscles are stiff, rigid, and difficult to move. The increased muscle tone makes performing smooth, coordinated movements very difficult. Dyskinetic CP involves muscles that alternate between increased tone and decreased tone, making any voluntary movement very difficult. Individuals with dyskinetic CP vary between very slow, difficult movement to very rapid, jerky movements. Ataxic CP involves difficulty with coordination and steady gait. A combination of more than one type of CP is mixed CP.

Clinical Presentation

Because CP is a disorder of movement caused by some type of brain defect or injury, children with CP often present with a developmental delay, usually a gross and/or fine motor delay. Having either increased or decreased muscle tone makes it difficult to perform movements that are necessary for development (Fig. 28.1). Depending on the degree of spasticity or dyskinetic movements, the infant may present with feeding difficulties in the first few days to weeks of life. In addition, the brain defect or injury may also make the child predisposed to seizures or cognitive delay.

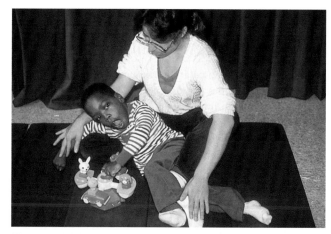

Figure 28.1. A child with cerebral palsy. A physical therapist works with a child who has cerebral palsy. Note the scissoring of the legs. Reprinted with permission from Hatfield, N. T., & Kincheloe, C. (2017). *Introductory maternity and pediatric nursing* (4th ed., Fig. 35-9). Philadelphia, PA: Lippincott Williams & Wilkins.

Assessment and Diagnosis

Assessment for CP includes exam for developmental delays and periodic formal screenings with a valid and reliable developmental screening tool (Table 28.3) during routine well-care visits at the primary care provider's office in the first 2 years of life. At such visits, subtle delays can be identified and evaluated early.

On physical exam, the child may have increased or decreased muscle tone with spastic, uncoordinated movements. In addition to gross and fine motor delays, the child may have cognitive delays, as well. Often, children with CP also fail to thrive because of difficulties with chewing and swallowing. As mentioned before, CP is multifactorial and often an exact cause cannot be identified. Depending on the child's symptoms, a diagnosis may be made on the basis of physical exam and developmental screening. At times, it may be beneficial for the child to undergo an X-ray (Fig. 28.2), computed tomography (CT) scan, or magnetic resonance imaging (MRI); electroencephalogram; metabolic studies; or genetic testing (CDC, n.d.-e).

Therapeutic Interventions

As soon as a child is identified as having a developmental delay, the child should be referred for further evaluation by a developmental physician, occupational therapist, physical therapist, and/or speech therapist. Treatment for the delays can be started before a diagnosis of CP is made.

Evaluation

Expected outcomes for a child with CP include the following:

- The child attains maximum physical abilities.
- The child engages in activities that promote and maximize growth and development.
- The child receives adequate nutrients and calories to achieve and maintain normal growth and development.
- The child and family use communication techniques necessary for successful communication.
- The child engages in social, academic, and recreational activities appropriate for development.

Discharge Planning and Teaching

Parents or caregivers of a child with CP often require much support and many resources related to physically and emotionally caring for their child. Children with CP also require support in the community. A case manager is often involved to help secure both financial and physical resources for the child and family. Braces, customized wheelchairs, and adaptive devices are often needed and can be costly (Fig. 28.3).

Early intervention programs can be helpful to both the child and the family. Families can learn how to meet the child's special needs, including occupational, speech, and educational needs. Once the child enters school, he or she may need an individualized education plan to maximize learning and mobility in the school setting.

Teach parents about the disease and about the child's current and potential special needs. Children with CP often take several different medications, including those to prevent seizures and manage spasticity. Teach parents how to administer these medications and about the side effects of each medication. Encourage parents to seek regular dental care for their child, because enamel defects and malocclusion are common dental problems in children with CP. Gingival hyperplasia can also occur when anticonvulsants are prescribed.

Children with CP are often physically but not intellectually disabled. They may need adaptive and assistive technology to foster communication and promote mobility. Assist parents in finding resources to obtain these devices and learning how to use them.

Teach parents the importance of safety devices and how to use them while caring for their child. Gait belts, safety belts, adaptive car seats that allow safe travel, and special strollers and wheelchairs are all devices that a child with CP might need.

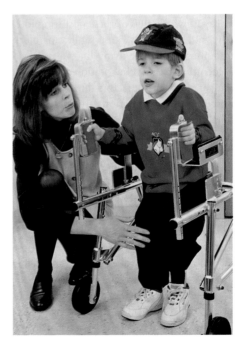

Figure 28.3. A child with cerebral palsy using a gait trainer. Reprinted with permission from Weber, J. R., & Kelley, J. H. (2017). *Health assessment in nursing* (6th ed., Fig. 31-30). Philadelphia, PA: Lippincott Williams & Wilkins.

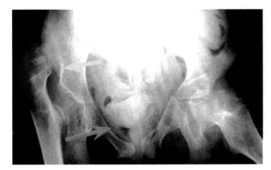

Figure 28.2. Hip deformity in cerebral palsy. A boy with cerebral palsy developed an adduction deformity (*red arrow*) and a secondary dislocation (*yellow arrow*) of the right hip. Reprinted with permission from Staheli, L. T. (2015). *Fundamentals of pediatric orthopedics* (5th ed., Fig. 1-57B). Philadelphia, PA: Lippincott Williams & Wilkins.

Congenital Neuromuscular Disorders

Congenital neuromuscular disorders affect the nerves, particularly the peripheral nerves, as well as the skeletal muscles, such as those in the trunk, arms, and legs. Congenital neuromuscular disorders covered in this chapter include **neural tube defects (NTDs)** such as spina bifida, muscular dystrophy, and SMA.

Neural Tube Defects

NTDs are congenital defects of the brain and spinal cord. Spina bifida, encephalocele, and anencephaly are NTDs discussed in this chapter.

Etiology and Pathophysiology

The neural tube refers to the brain and spinal cord. During embryogenesis, the neuroepithelium, which eventually becomes nerve tissue and differentiates into the brain and spinal cord, folds around from the anterior midline and fuses posteriorly in what will become the dorsal side of the embryo. When fusion does not occur, it can leave an open area along the neural tube (i.e., the brain and/or the spinal cord), where this central nervous tissue is not encased and protected. Often, this results in the nervous tissue being contained in a sac outside the body, known as an open NTD. Alternatively, the defect may be occult and not easily observed because the skin covers it, in which case it is called a closed NTD. This lack of closure of the neural tube affects further growth and development of the nervous tissue. NTDs typically occur around 17 to 27 days after conception, before the woman is aware of the pregnancy (Stone & Fieggen, 2006). The most common NTDs are spina bifida, encephalocele, and anencephaly.

The incidence of NTDs worldwide is approximately 300,000 per year, with 3,000 of these occurring in the United States (CDC, n.d.-d). NTDs cause significant morbidity and mortality. Although there are many known risk factors, often there is no identifiable cause. In addition to genetic influences, the following are known risk factors for NTDs: in utero exposure to valproic acid, trimethoprim, carbamazepine, phenytoin, phenobarbital, methotrexate, or aminopterin; folate deficiency; maternal diabetes; maternal obesity; and hyperthermia early in conception (Best, 2016; Brand, 2006; Bonhotal, 2015; Cameron & Moran, 2009). In addition, these factors are believed to be additive, meaning that each additional risk factor increases the likelihood of development of an NTD.

Although the causes of NTDs are multifactorial, folate deficiency was identified as a major risk factor for NTDs and, in 1992, the U.S. Public Health Service recommended that all women of childbearing years take a 400-μg supplement of folic acid daily (Williams et al., 2015). By 1998, U.S. food manufacturers were mandated to fortify any grain, such as cereal, bread, or rice, with folic acid if the food label identified the food as "enriched." Folic acid fortification has led to a significant reduction in the occurrence of NTDs overall; however, they are still prevalent in Hispanic women, who experience a higher occurrence rate of NTDs compared with non-Hispanic white and black women.

Spina Bifida

Spina bifida is the most common NTD, affecting more than 1,600 children per year in the United States (Williams et al., 2015). Failure of the neural tube to fuse in the lower spinal area results in open vertebral arches, which can result in a sac protruding from the spinal area or a lesion that is covered with skin, resulting in a "hidden" lesion (Adzick, 2013; Barker, Saulino, & Caristo, 2002). There are three types of spina bifida (Fig. 28.4):

- Spina bifida occulta (Fig. 28.4B): In this type, there is no obvious protrusion and the skin is intact. It involves only a bony abnormality. Often, there is a hair tuft in the area of the defect.
- Spina bifida with meningocele (Fig. 28.4C): In this type, there is an obvious protrusion that involves only the meninges.
- Spina bifida with myelomeningocele (Fig. 28.4D): In this type, there is an obvious protrusion and the sac contains both meninges and spinal cord.

Because the delicate nervous tissue is not enclosed within the spine or covered by skin in spina bifida, it is exposed to amniotic fluid and vulnerable to trauma throughout gestation and during the birth process, further increasing risk of damage and infection. Although children with spina bifida have varying degrees of neurological impairment, there is typically some form of permanent paralysis (complete or incomplete) below the level of the defect, which also affects bowel and bladder control, contributes to orthopedic difficulties, and potentially predisposes the child to cognitive disabilities. These infants are typically taken to surgery within 24 to 36 hours of birth to close the open area of their spine to prevent trauma and infection (Stone & Feiggen, 2006). Fetal surgery is becoming more common, and infants who undergo fetal surgery for spina bifida often have better neurological outcomes (Moldenhauer & Adzick, 2017).

It is also common for children with spina bifida to have another central nervous system defect called a Chiari II malformation. In a Chiari II malformation, previously called an Arnold-Chiari malformation, the cerebellum pushes through the foramen magnum and presses into the spinal canal, resulting in increased pressure on the cerebellum and brainstem (Brand, 2006).

Hydrocephalus is another condition that is associated with spina bifida, occurring in approximately 80% of infants born with spina bifida. Hydrocephalus occurs when the cerebrospinal fluid does not drain properly, resulting in enlarged ventricles. Clinically, the child may have a progressively enlarging head circumference, widely spaced sutures, a bulging fontanel, vomiting, irritability, and lethargy. This leads to increased intracranial pressure if the fluid is not drained. A shunt is often inserted into a ventricle and the fluid is then drained into the neck or abdomen. This shunt is permanent and may need several revisions over the course of the child's life (Barker et al., 2002; Stone & Fieggen, 2006).

Encephalocele

Encephalocele is a form of NTD in which the skull fails to properly fuse during the third or fourth week of gestation, resulting in a protrusion of the brain and cranial membranes anywhere along the midline of the skull, from the nose to the back of the neck (Fig. 28.5). The most common location is at

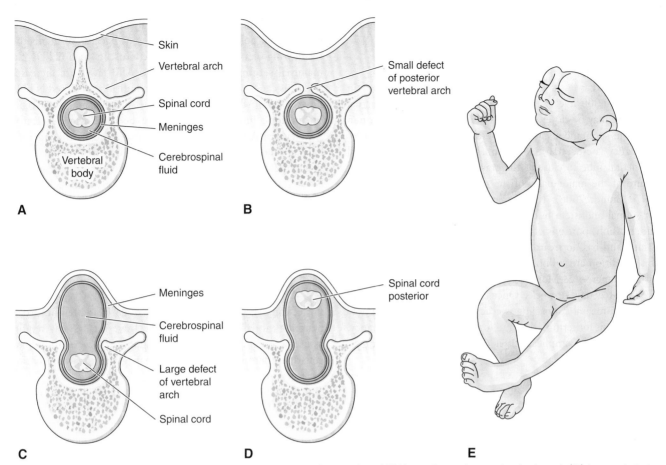

Figure 28.4. Neural tube defects. Cross-section studies of the spine. **(A)** Normal vertebra and spinal cord. **(B)** In occult (minimal) spina bifida (spina bifida occulta), the posterior vertebral arch fails to form. It is usually asymptomatic. **(C)** In spina bifida with meningocele, the meninges protrude through the defect. **(D)** In spina bifida with myelomeningocele, the meninges and spinal cord protrude through the defect. **(E)** In anencephaly, almost all of the brain and spinal cord fail to form. Reprinted with permission from Stephenson, S. R., & Dmitrieva, J. (2017). *Obstetrics and gynecology* (4th ed., Fig. 22.10). Philadelphia, PA: Wolters Kluwer.

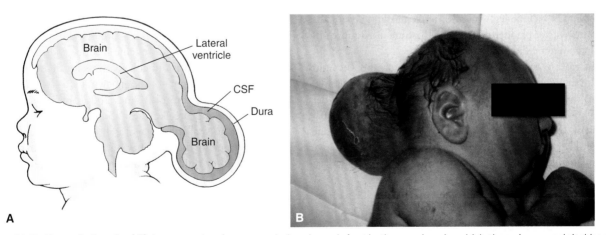

Figure 28.5. Encephalocele. (A) An example of an encephalocele, a defect in the cranium in which there is an occipital herniation, causing a protrusion; in this case, of the meninges alone. CSF, cerebrospinal fluid. **(B)** A newborn with a large occipital encephalocele. Part A reprinted with permission from Siegel, A., & Sapru, H. N. (2018). *Essential neuroscience* (4th ed., Fig. 2.6C). Philadelphia, PA: Lippincott Williams & Wilkins. Part B reprinted with permission from Kline-Fath, B., Bahado-Singh, R., & Bulas, D. (2015). *Fundamental and advanced fetal imaging* (1st ed., Fig. 15-7). Philadelphia, PA: Wolters Kluwer.

the base of the skull. The incidence of encephalocele is approximately 1 in 12,200 babies per year (CDC, n.d.-c).

Anencephaly

Anencephaly is less common than is spina bifida, occurring in 1.2 per 10,000 live births (Best, 2016). However, the actual incidence may be closer to 1 in 1,000, because this defect often results in spontaneous abortion, fetal death, or termination of pregnancy (Best, 2016). Anencephaly is caused by a failure of the neural tube to close at the cranial end, which results in a failure of the major parts of the brain to develop (Bonhotal, 2015; Brand, 2006). Most infants with anencephaly have a functional brainstem but lack the major portion of their brain and, possibly, portions of their skull (Fig. 28.4E). Anencephaly is fatal and has no treatment, and the majority of babies with this condition are stillborn or die within the first few hours of birth (Cameron & Moran, 2009). A very small number may live for a few days or weeks. Once the diagnosis of anencephaly is made, prenatal counseling is crucial. Families need to know their options for termination and for continuing the pregnancy, about potential complications if the pregnancy is continued, and about palliative care.

Clinical Presentation

An open NTD presents with the nervous tissue encased in a sac on the outside of the body, somewhere along the spinal column or midline of the skull. Although open NTDs are much more serious, closed NTDs are more difficult to diagnose. In closed NTDs, the defect is covered by skin and the disability from the defect is much more subtle, so they are usually not diagnosed until much later. They can also be discovered as an incidental finding and is not associated with any defects or physical limitations. On physical exam, an infant with a closed NTD may have a dimple or pit, patch of hair, or a pigmented lesion anywhere along the spine, but most commonly in the lower spine (Bickley & Szilagyi, 2003). Signs and symptoms suggestive of a closed NTD include leg weakness, **muscular atrophy** of the legs, and bowel or bladder difficulties. These are often more obvious in an older child.

Most cases of anencephaly are diagnosed prenatally. The fetus or infant presents with a significant portion of the skull missing, whereas the remainder of the body may be well developed. Because an infant with anencephaly most likely has a functional brainstem, the primitive reflexes of suck, swallow, and breathe are typically present. Infants with less function require palliative care and are likely to die soon after birth.

Assessment and Diagnosis

NTDs are typically diagnosed through prenatal screening. Routine prenatal care includes a screening maternal blood test for alpha-fetoprotein (AFP) or a 2D ultrasound (Brand, 2006; Cameron & Moran, 2009). Use of either of these screening tests varies depending on gestational age and number of fetuses. A 2D ultrasound can identify the loss of the normal curvature of the skull in anencephaly after 12 weeks of gestation. Often, polyhydramnios is present because of ineffective swallowing of amniotic fluid by the fetus. In open NTDs, the maternal serum and amniotic fluid AFP levels are increased and thus can be used to detect this condition. In closed NTDs, however, the AFP level does not rise in either maternal serum or amniotic fluid and thus cannot be used as an indicator. An elevated APF level can also be associated with congenital defects other than NTDs, such as gastroschisis, omphalocele, congenital kidney disease, or fetal distress or demise (Cameron & Moran, 2009). With higher quality ultrasound technology, the need for obtaining maternal serum or amniotic fluid AFP level has all but been eliminated. If any abnormality is found on screening AFP or 2D ultrasound, diagnosis is often made with a 3D ultrasound.

Therapeutic Interventions

Protection of exposed neural tissue is essential to prevent further neurological damage and infection. These infants may require resuscitation at birth and ongoing support for ventilation, oxygenation, thermoregulation, fluid management, and prevention of infection.

Infants with spina bifida diagnosed prenatally require a cesarean birth to protect the extruded sac from further damage. If the lesion is in the thoracic region, the infant may have respiratory compromise and require ventilatory support. Keep the infant on his or her side while suctioning, drying, and assessing for respiratory insufficiency. If the infant requires intubation, make the accommodations needed to prevent pressure on the lesion while the infant is supine.

The infant with an NTD faces challenges with thermoregulation, fluid management, and infection. Large open lesions allow for increased heat and fluid loss. Cover the lesion with a sterile, nonpermeable gauze soaked in warm normal saline to help prevent heat and fluid loss and protect the delicate membrane encasing the nervous tissue until the lesion can be surgically corrected.

Because the infant likely has neurological impairment below the level of the lesion, neurogenic bladder and/or bowel is of concern. Although it is difficult to assess for neurogenic bowel in a newborn, assessment of the anal wink is a good predictor of functional bladder control (Brand, 2006). Elicit the anal wink by gently stroking the skin near the anus; observe for a contraction of the anal sphincter muscle. Pay careful attention to urinary output in the early newborn period. Address urinary retention and/or fluid imbalances promptly to prevent further problems.

Protecting the lesion from infection is critical both before and after surgery. If the lesion is in the lower spine region, keeping stool away from it can be difficult. If possible, place a nonpermeable drape with an adhesive edge in between the lesion and the buttock area to prevent stool from getting in the lesion.

To monitor for development of hydrocephalus, take serial head circumference measurements, which involve measuring the circumference from the forehead to the widest part of the occipital region, and plot the results on a validated growth chart by gestational age and gender. This can help distinguish normal growth from the accelerated head circumference growth that occurs with hydrocephalus. Infants with hydrocephalus also have signs of increased intracranial pressure: a bulging fontanel, widening sutures, lethargy, emesis, and sunset eyes.

Evaluation

Expected outcomes for a child with an NTD include the following:

- The child maintains mobility using an adaptive device such as a walker, crutches, or a wheelchair.
- Skin integrity is maintained and the child remains free of pressure injury.
- Urinary continence is maintained and the risk of kidney damage is minimized.
- The child engages in social, academic, and recreational activities that promote development and positive self-esteem.

Discharge Planning and Teaching

Parents of children with an NTD are provided with teaching topics on how to use any adaptive devices ordered, as well as how to maintain skin integrity and prevent pressure injury.

Muscular Dystrophy

Muscular dystrophy is a group of related inherited diseases that may begin early in life or later and are characterized by progressive muscle weakness due to muscle fiber degeneration and muscle wasting. Onset can be sudden at birth or gradual, but all cases are terminal. Progression varies from a few to many years.

Etiology and Pathophysiology

There are eight identified disorders of muscular dystrophy, but only the two most common forms—Duchenne muscular dystrophy (DMD) and Becker muscular dystrophy (BMD)—are discussed here. Each form of muscular dystrophy has a unique muscular involvement, age at diagnosis, gender affected, and severity of impairment. All are related to a defect in specific genes. Most other forms of muscular dystrophy affect both males and females equally, whereas DMD and BMD are X-linked, affect only males, and are often discussed together because of their similarities. The genetic defect of DMD and BMD affects dystrophin, a protein that provides muscles their ability to be strong and stable over time and allows the myofibers to function appropriately. Without this protein, the muscle fibers break down and lose their function. DMD and BMD together affect approximately 15 out of every 100,000 males (Birnkrant et al., 2018; CDC, n.d.-a). DMD is often diagnosed before the age of 5 years, whereas BMD is typically diagnosed from 7 to 12 years of age.

Clinical Presentation

Children with DMD or BMD present with generalized muscle weakness, usually noticed first in the proximal muscles of the arms and legs (CDC, n.d.-a). They may be overly clumsy, have difficulty climbing stairs, demonstrate calf muscle hypertrophy, and/or toe walk (Fig. 28.6). They may not be able to keep up with peers in age-appropriate activities. It is important to have a good understanding of the developmental milestones when assessing a child for these complaints to rule out age-related normal behavior. Children with DMD often present with Gower sign, which can be diagnostic for DMD (Fig. 28.7). Because children with DMD have weakness in their thighs, they often have difficulty getting from the floor to a standing position. They use their arms to help get on all fours and then use their arms to "walk" up their thighs until they can get in an upright position. As the disease progresses, the child experiences a loss of ambulation and impairment in respiratory and cardiac function because the associated muscles lose strength and function. Muscular dystrophy is a progressive loss of muscular function that often results in death by respiratory and/or cardiac failure.

Assessment and Diagnosis

Any child with a gross motor delay, muscle weakness, impaired ability or inability to navigate stairs at the appropriate age, clumsiness, and a positive Gower sign needs further diagnostic workup. Diagnosis is often made with an evaluation by both a pediatric neuromuscular specialist and a genetic specialist.

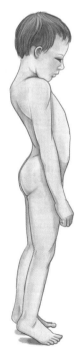

Figure 28.6. Characteristic posture of a child with Duchenne muscular dystrophy (DMD). Along with the typical toe gait, the child develops a lordotic posture as DMD causes further deterioration. Reprinted with permission from Hatfield, N. T., & Kincheloe, C. (2017). *Introductory maternity and pediatric nursing* (4th ed., Fig. 40.10). Philadelphia, PA: Wolters Kluwer.

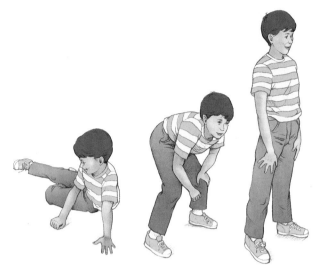

Figure 28.7. Gower sign. To check for Gower sign, place the patient in the supine position and ask him or her to rise. A positive Gower sign—an inability to lift the trunk without using the hands and arms to brace and push—indicates pelvic muscle weakness, as occurs in muscular dystrophy and spinal muscular atrophy. Reprinted with permission from Lippincott Williams & Wilkins (2011). *Lippincott's visual nursing: A guide to diseases, skills, and treatments* (2nd ed.). Philadelphia, PA: Wolters Kluwer.

In light of these physical findings, an elevated creatinine kinase (CK) level further raises the suspicion for DMD and should prompt a referral to a genetic specialist. A normal CK level all but eliminates the possibility for DMD, and alternative diagnoses should be investigated.

A definitive diagnosis for DMD or BMD is made through molecular genetic testing, which identifies deletions or mutations in the DMD gene. Before the availability of genetic testing, diagnosis was made through muscle biopsy. Although most patients are now diagnosed through genetic testing, muscle biopsy is still used in specific situations when genetic testing is not conclusive (Darras, 2018a).

Therapeutic Interventions

Early diagnosis and initiation of therapy are essential. The progressive loss of muscle function can be slowed with the use of glucocorticoids. These medications are started early on in the disease process and have been shown to delay loss of ambulation, prevent scoliosis, and preserve lung function (Birnkrant et al., 2018).

Physical therapy, including both passive and active exercises, helps maintain muscle strength and prevent contractures. Chest wall exercises improve lung function.

Children with DMD or BMD can have significant morbidity from respiratory complications. As the chest wall muscles deteriorate, pulmonary function is compromised, resulting in atelectasis, mucous plugs, pneumonia, respiratory inefficiency, and respiratory failure. Monitor respiratory function periodically with pulmonary function tests (PFTs),

which allow monitoring of forced vital capacity (FVC) over time. PFTs can usually be performed validly by around the age of 5 or 6 years. PFTs can identify decreases in FVC even before clinical symptoms of dyspnea are evident. If a child is unable to complete an adequate PFT, a sleep study can be performed as an alternative. Other therapies to help maintain lung function and minimize complications include exercises to increase lung volume, assisted coughing, and daytime and/or nighttime ventilatory support, which can be noninvasive or invasive (as with a tracheostomy).

As the disease progresses, home pulse oximetry can serve as an adjunct measurement to assess lung function. O_2 saturation levels lower than 95% should prompt the use of more aggressive interventions, such as assisted cough, to decrease the incidents of mucous plugging, atelectasis, and, ultimately, pneumonia (Birnkrant, Bushby, Bann, Apkon et al., 2018). Patients in the late stages of disease require ventilatory support to prolong survival and ease symptoms of respiratory insufficiency. Changes in the FVC noted in serial PFTs or an abnormal sleep study can indicate the need for additional ventilatory support.

Respiratory infections can be especially devastating to a child with DMD or BMD, particularly after losing ambulation. Encourage parents to make sure their child receives all recommended vaccines in accordance with the CDC guidelines (CDC, 2016; Ward & Birnkrant, 2018), with special emphasis on yearly influenza vaccination, as well as pneumococcal vaccination.

Dystrophin deficiency in the heart results in a weak myocardium that is unable to keep up with the physiological demands of the heart, leading to cardiomyopathy, arrhythmias, and cardiac failure (Birnkrant, Bushby, Bann, Apkon et al., 2018). An annual cardiac exam, electrocardiogram, and cardiovascular MRI are recommended to monitor cardiac function. It is also important for the child to have these tests done before undergoing any procedure that requires anesthesia, to minimize complications. Changes in cardiac function are more difficult to observe if the patient is not ambulatory, which makes the cardiac testing essential.

A cardiologist should be involved early on in the care of a child with DMD or BMD to monitor for cardiac changes and intervene early. Medications can be used to slow the decline in cardiac function (The Pharmacy 28.1).

The use of glucocorticoids has been shown to improve neuromuscular outcomes but is also associated with adverse effects on bone health. Long-term use of glucocorticoids predisposes a child to osteoporosis. Coupled with the fact that children with DMD or BMD have progressively weakening muscles, the risk of osteoporosis is compounded. Both vertebral fractures and fractures of the long bones are common even in low-level trauma. Annual spine radiographs are recommended to monitor for vertebral fractures, because some vertebral fractures can be asymptomatic but also predictive of future fractures. If a vertebral fracture is identified, intravenous bisphosphonate therapy has been shown to be beneficial to bone mineral density and prevention of future fractures (Birnkrant, Bushby, Bann, Apkon et al., 2018).

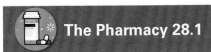

The Pharmacy 28.1 — Medications Used to Treat Cardiac Dysfunction in Muscular Dystrophy

Medication	Classification	Route	Action	Nursing Considerations
Furosemide	Loop diuretic	• PO • IV	Inhibits reabsorption of sodium and chloride from the proximal and distal tubules and ascending loop of Henle, resulting in sodium-rich diuresis	• Typically ordered at onset of cardiac dysfunction • Monitor urine output following administration. • Monitor potassium; may require potassium replacement. • Perform daily weights. • Monitor for orthostatic hypotension.
Losartan	• Angiotensin receptor blocker • Antihypertensive	• PO	Blocks angiotensin II from binding to its receptors on muscles surrounding blood vessels, which causes vasodilation, decreasing blood pressure and improving heart failure	• If symptomatic: typically ordered to begin immediately • If asymptomatic: typically ordered to begin by the age of 10 y • Monitor blood pressure for hypotension. • Adverse effects include chest pain, diarrhea, fatigue, and dizziness.
Enalapril, captopril	• ACE inhibitors • Antihypertensive	• PO • IV	• Blocks the conversion of angiotensin I to angiotensin II, which decreases blood pressure, decreases aldosterone secretion, slightly increases potassium, and causes sodium and fluid loss • In heart failure, also decreases peripheral resistance, afterload, preload, and heart size	• If symptomatic: begin immediately • If asymptomatic: begin by the age of 10 y • Monitor blood pressure for hypotension. • May interact with OTC medications; have patient check with provider before taking any OTC medications. • Adverse effects include cough, nausea, diarrhea, headache, and dizziness.
Carvedilol	Beta-1-selective adrenergic blocker	• PO • IV	• Blocks beta-adrenergic receptors in the heart and juxtaglomerular apparatus, which decreases the influence of the sympathetic nervous system on these tissues • Decreases the excitability of the heart, which decreases cardiac output and release of renin, which in turn lowers blood pressure	• Typically ordered at onset of cardiac dysfunction • Check apical pulse prior to administration. If less than 90 beats/min, do not administer medication; consult the provider. • Monitor blood pressure before administration.

ACE, angiotensin-converting enzyme; IV, intravenous; OTC, over-the-counter; PO, by mouth.

Children with DMD or BMD are prone to many nutritional complications. The progressive muscle weakness limits mobility, which, in turn, decreases energy expenditure, making the child prone to obesity. This can be compounded for those on long-term glucocorticoids, because these medications are known to increase hunger and caloric intake. Swallowing and nutrient absorption can be affected by muscular weakness along the gastrointestinal tract, leading to decreased caloric intake, weight loss, and malnutrition. Regular assessment of growth parameters and nutrition can identify problems with weight gain or loss, malnutrition, and feeding difficulties. Some children with DMD or BMD require a feeding tube to maintain their caloric requirements (Ward & Birnkrant, 2018).

Evaluation

Expected outcomes for a child with muscular dystrophy include the following:

- The child maintains optimal mobility for the stage of disease process.
- The child engages in activities that promote and maintain a positive self-image and self-esteem.
- The child receives adequate calories and nutrients to maintain appropriate height and weight.
- The child participates in activities of daily living, including bathing, feeding, oral care, and dressing as much as possible.
- Exposure to disease and illness is minimized.
- The child remains injury free.
- The child and family develop and use effective coping skills in managing the child's diagnosis and terminal illness.

Discharge Planning and Teaching

Parents of children with muscular dystrophy are provided with teaching topics on passive and active range of motion exercises, glucocorticoid administration and adverse effects (such as osteoporosis and bone fractures), signs of respiratory failure and cardiac compromise to monitor for, and nutritional guidelines.

Spinal Muscular Atrophy

SMA, an inherited disorder, causes loss of motor function throughout all muscles of the body. There are different types of SMA, but all have a mutation in the survival motor neuron. Children with SMA often die of related complications, such as pneumonia or respiratory failure.

Etiology and Pathophysiology

SMA is a genetically inherited disorder that causes progressive loss of motor function through degeneration of the motor neurons in the anterior horn cells of the spinal cord. Specifically, there is a mutation in the survival motor neuron (*SMN*) 1 gene. All humans have two forms of the *SMN* gene: *SMN1* and *SMN2*. The *SMN1* gene produces a fully functional SMN protein, which is essential for the functioning of the motor neurons in the anterior horn cells. When this genetic defect alters the *SMN1* gene, it is unable to produce the SMN protein. The *SMN2* gene is left to produce the SMN protein, but it produces a much less functional form of the SMN protein. The result is progressive, symmetrical muscle weakness and atrophy of the proximal muscles (shoulders, hips, and back) leading to premature death. The degree of severity varies significantly, which can delay diagnosis in the milder cases. It is an autosomal recessive mutation with an incidence rate of 1 in 6,000 to 1 in 11,000 infants and is the leading cause of infant death due to genetic causes (Kolb et al., 2017; Kolb & Kissel, 2011; Lin, Kalb, & Yeh, 2015).

SMA type 1, also referred to as infantile onset, is the most severe type and has the earliest onset. Approximately 50% of patients with SMA have type 1. The onset of disease is in infancy, usually before the age of 6 months (National Organization of Rare Disorders [NORD], 2012). Without intervention, these children do not live past the age of 2 years. These infants are not able to sit unassisted and have progressive difficulty swallowing, feeding, and breathing. The etiology of respiratory insufficiency and failure in these children is two-fold: a weakness of the intercostal muscles affecting the ability of the child to inhale and exhale appropriately and general immobility.

SMA type 2 is typically diagnosed a little later than is type 1, from ages 6 to 12 months. These children can usually sit unassisted and possibly stand but will likely never walk. Similar to children with type 1, these children often have swallowing and chewing difficulties and respiratory insufficiency. In addition, they may present with scoliosis or other symptoms of generalized bone weakness.

SMA type 3 is diagnosed later in childhood and is associated with much less severe symptoms. Although these children are able to walk, they fall frequently and may have difficulty navigating stairs at 2 to 3 years of age (NORD, 2012). Children with SMA type 3 often lose their ability to walk as the disease progresses and need the aid of a wheelchair at some point. Because they have impaired mobility, they are prone to scoliosis and obesity.

Type 4 is similar in severity to type 3 but is diagnosed after the age of 18 years.

Clinical Presentation

Infants with SMA type 1 or 2 present with varying degrees of motor delays, hypotonia, and absent reflexes (Fig. 28.8). Infants with type 1 show delays in rolling over or sitting independently, whereas infants with type 2 may be able to sit unassisted and possibly stand but will not be able to walk. Because type 3 is often diagnosed in later childhood, children who develop it typically achieves higher motor function than do those with type 1 or 2; however, they may report a regression of previously learned milestones, which is always a cause for concern.

Children with SMA may also present with or develop signs of impending respiratory failure. Infants with SMA may present with inadequate weight gain, which is likely due to reduced caloric intake resulting from difficulties with chewing and swallowing, which commonly occur in infants with SMA. Children with SMA may also present with scoliosis, contractures, and lax joints due to muscle weakness and gross motor delays, resulting in immobility.

Assessment and Diagnosis

Assessment and diagnosis of SMA usually begin with observation of the clinical symptoms of motor delay, such as in rolling over, sitting unsupported, standing, or walking. Obtain a thorough family and developmental history and physical exam. If there is a family history of SMA, asymptomatic children can

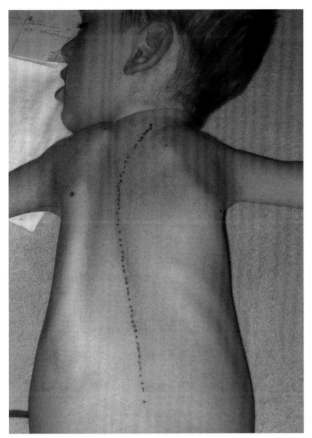

Figure 28.8. A child with spinal muscular atrophy (SMA). SMA type 1 (acute Werdnig-Hoffmann disease). This young boy has SMA type 1. The muscle wasting is evident and he is developing scoliosis. Reprinted with permission from Baum, V. C., & O'Flaherty, J. E. (2015). *Anesthesia for genetic, metabolic, and dysmorphic syndromes of childhood* (3rd ed., unnumbered figure in Chapter 18). Philadelphia, PA: Wolters Kluwer.

also undergo genetic molecular testing to identify the *SMN1* deletion. Before the availability of genetic testing, diagnosis was made by muscle biopsy and electromyography. These are no longer necessary in most cases because genetic testing is now the gold standard.

Owing to their increased risk of developing respiratory insufficiency and failure, children with SMA should have regular assessment of their O_2 saturation level through pulse oximetry and end-tidal carbon dioxide level through capnography. They may also benefit from periodic sleep studies to assess for hypoventilation.

Therapeutic Interventions

Early initiation of physical therapy, regardless of the severity of the disease, has been shown to improve outcomes in children with SMA. Physical therapy has been shown to improve function and delay deterioration through a combination of exercises, stretching, braces, and orthotics. Even for children with SMA so severe that they have difficulty sitting, such therapy can

be beneficial, such as use of assistive devices to help the child maintain an upright position.

Respiratory failure is usually the cause of death in children with SMA type 1 or 2 (Kolb & Kissel, 2015). Pulmonary interventions should be started early and proactively to improve long-term survival in children with SMA. Chest physiotherapy, which includes percussion, vibration, and positioning, and mechanical insufflation-exsufflation are essential for prophylaxis and as interventions during times of respiratory illness (Mercuri et al., 2018). These measures facilitate drainage and airway clearance, which are impaired in children with SMA because of immobility and muscle weakness. For those who demonstrate an ineffective cough, perform oral suction in conjunction with chest physiotherapy. Hypoventilation, as evidenced by low oxygen saturation level, elevated carbon dioxide level, or abnormal results from a sleep study, often responds well to noninvasive ventilation (Mercuri et al., 2018). In certain situations, a tracheostomy may be considered for long-term pulmonary support.

Scoliosis is very common in children with SMA type 1 or 2, with an incidence rate of 60% to 90% before the age of 4 years (Mercuri et al., 2018). Depending on the degree of spinal curvature, this condition can also impair respiratory function. A rigid trunk brace can be used to support a sitting position but cannot stop the progression of the curvature in the spine. Surgery to straighten the spine with hardware is often indicated to improve trunk balance for sitting and to improve respiratory function.

Children with SMA often have difficulties with swallowing, dysphagia, reflux, and constipation. Infants may have difficulty coordinating an efficient suck-swallow and tire easily during feedings, resulting in inadequate weight gain. These infants may also be predisposed to frequent aspiration due to reflux and dysphagia, causing aspiration pneumonia. A video swallowing study should be done even if no symptoms are prevalent. Infants with significant reflux may require a Nissen fundoplication. Enteral feedings through a nasogastric or gastrostomy tube are common and have been shown to improve survival age (Mercuri et al., 2018). Enteral feedings allow the infant to receive necessary calories without expending excessive calories and reduce the risk of aspiration.

Currently, randomized placebo-controlled studies are being conducted to evaluate medications to alter the progression of the disease. Although most of these medications are still in clinical trial, some are just beginning to receive approval of the U.S. Food and Drug Administration (Finkel et al., 2018). Until these medications become more widely available, pharmacological interventions used in children with SMA will remain limited to countering the effects of the disease rather than slowing its progression (The Pharmacy 28.2).

Evaluation

Expected outcomes for a child with SMA include the following:

- The child engages in age- and developmentally appropriate activities to promote brain and cognitive development.
- The child maintains an effective breathing pattern and gas exchange.

The Pharmacy 28.2   Medications Used to Treat Spinal Muscular Atrophy

Medication	Classification	Route	Action	Nursing Considerations
Albuterol	Beta-2 adrenergic agonist	PO, inhale	Facilitates breathing by the following: • Decreasing airway resistance • Dilating the lower airways • Increasing expiratory flow in the smaller airways	• Monitor heart rate for tachycardia. • May make the patient shaky after use • Monitor for signs of toxicity.
Azithromycin	Antibiotic	PO, inhale	Treats bacterial respiratory infections, such as pneumonia by killing or inhibiting the growth of bacteria	• Diarrhea and abdominal cramping should be reported to provider. • Monitor liver and renal labs.
Ranitidine, famotidine, cimetidine	H_2 receptor antagonists	PO	Treats gastroesophageal reflux by inhibiting gastric acid secretion via inhibiting the action of histamine at the H_2-receptor site	• May cause confusion, headache, dizziness, constipation, diarrhea, nausea, thrombocytopenia, bradycardia • Avoid administering within 2 h of antacids. • Administer with or without food.
Omeprazole, lansoprazole	Proton pump inhibitors	PO	Treats gastroesophageal reflux by binding to an enzyme in the presence of gastric acid, preventing the transport of hydrogen ions into the gastric lumen	• May cause dizziness, headache, diarrhea • Inform provider if diarrhea occurs. • Administer in the morning on an empty stomach.

H_2, histamine 2; PO, by mouth.

• The child remains free from pressure injuries.
• The child and family adapt to the child's declining health status.
• The child receives adequate caloric and nutrient intake to achieve and maintain appropriate weight and height.

Discharge Planning and Teaching

A patient with SMA is generally admitted to the hospital for respiratory complications. Discharge planning for these hospitalizations often includes assisting the family to secure necessary equipment such as portable suction machines, suction catheters, cough assist machines, and even a BIPAP machine and associated equipment. Oxygen may also be needed in the home. Other discharge planning needed may include securing an appropriate hospital bed, if needed, and home nursing visits.

Teaching topics for a child with SMA and his or her family include how to care for skin to prevent pressure injury (particularly important as the child gets older and less mobile), respiratory therapy treatments such as administering oxygen, and use of the cough assist machine, intrapulmonary percussive ventilator, and nasopharyngeal and oropharyngeal suctioning. It is important to direct parents to support groups for families who have children diagnosed with SMA.

Parents may need assistance seeking financial and insurance resources for the care and equipment needed to properly care for their child.

Acquired Neuromuscular Disorders

Acquired neuromuscular disorders are not inherited but occur as a result of an exposure, infection, or injury. Acquired neuromuscular disorders can cause weakness, fatigue, or even loss of the use of the muscles and motor function. Acquired disorders included in this chapter are spinal cord injury, Guillain-Barré syndrome, and botulism.

Spinal Cord Injury

Spinal cord injury is damage to the spinal cord that results in loss of physical and/or sensory function. Children younger than age 15 years account for approximately 3% to 5% of all spinal cord injuries in the United States (Powell & Davidson, 2015). Adolescents account for the majority of spinal cord injuries (Piatt, 2015). Motor vehicle accidents (both vehicle and pedestrian) are the cause of greater than 50% of spinal cord injuries (Piatt, 2015). Firearms, sports-related injuries, falls, and abuse are other potential causes of spinal cord injury.

Etiology and Pathophysiology

Two factors determine the type of lesion that results: the mechanism of injury and the direction of the forces. Children have very mobile, elastic spines. Although fractures are rare because of the elasticity, transfer of energy or force leading to spinal distortion allows the spine to maintain its structural integrity but leads to significant damage to the spinal cord. SCIWORA (spinal cord injury without radiographic bone abnormality) is more common in children than in adults.

Children are prone to specific kinds of spinal cord injuries as a result of the flexibility and extreme mobility of their spinal column. In children younger than age 8 years, the most mobile section of the spine is the cervical spine (C1 to C3). Vertebrae are not completely ossified in children younger than age 9 years and the facet joints of the vertebrae slide over each other more easily. Neck muscles are often not strong enough to adequately support the relatively large head in young children. Ligaments supporting the neck and spinal column are extremely elastic and allow for much stretching between the vertebrae. However, the spinal cord does not stretch accordingly. Injuries to vertebrae C1 to C3 are more likely to occur in children younger than 8 years of age, whereas injuries to vertebrae C4 to C6 occur more often in children 9 to 15 years old.

Types of injuries include hyperflexion, rotation, hyperextension, and compression injuries. Hyperflexion injuries occur when there is extreme bending forward of the neck, such as in whiplash. Hyperflexion can cause tears or avulsions and fractures of the vertebral body, as well as dislocation and subluxation. Rotational injuries can cause unstable spinal fractures and unilateral facet dislocation. Hyperextension (e.g., resulting from a forceful punch under the chin) may result in ligament tears and avulsion fractures of vertebral bodies. Compression injuries can result in fractures and often occur when a child falls from a height.

The extent of neurological damage may be complete or incomplete. A complete lesion means there is an absence of motor and sensory function below the injury (Figs. 28.9 and 28.10). Recovery of normal function of muscles below the level of injury is unlikely. In cases of complete spinal cord disruption, neurogenic shock and spinal shock occur simultaneously. An incomplete lesion implies some residual motor or sensory function below the level of injury. Patients may have an array of symptoms depending on the individual nerve pathways involved. Some degree of recovery is likely, depending on the degree of spinal cord injury.

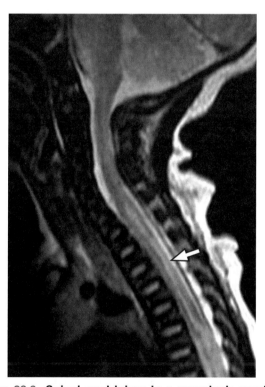

Figure 28.9. Spinal cord injury in a paraplegic newborn girl after a difficult delivery. Note the bright streaks (*arrow*) in the lower cervical and upper thoracic spinal cord, which represent lesions caused by cord ischemia and/or infarction. Reprinted with permission from Lee, E. (2017). *Pediatric radiology: Practical imaging evaluation of infants and children* (1st ed., Fig. 4-50A). Philadelphia, PA: Wolters Kluwer.

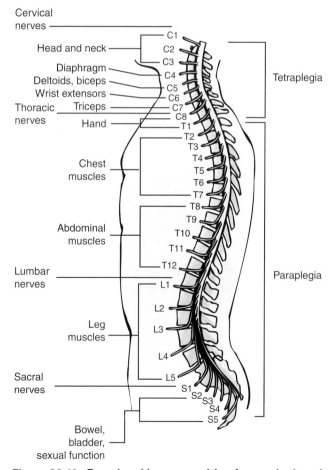

Figure 28.10. Functional losses resulting from spinal cord injury at various vertebral levels. Adapted with permission from Hickey, J. V. (2009). *Clinical practice of neurological and neurosurgical nursing* (6th ed., p. 411). Philadelphia, PA: Lippincott Williams & Wilkins.

Clinical Presentation

Children present with varying symptoms depending on the level of the injury and whether the injury is complete or incomplete. Children who present with a complete lesion have loss of sensory, motor, and autonomic function below the level of the injury. A child with an incomplete lesion presents with varying degrees of sensory, motor, and autonomic function below the level of the injury. Injuries to vertebrae T6 and above can result in autonomic dysfunction (dysautonomia), causing loss of bladder and bowel control, hypotension, and loss of thermoregulatory control (Priority Care Concepts 28.1).

Spinal shock, or spinal cord concussion, can occur at the time of injury. A transient suppression of nerve function below the level of injury occurs. The child may become flaccid and lose reflexes below the level of the injury. A full assessment of function cannot be made until spinal shock resolves, usually after 72 hours but can last much longer.

Neurogenic shock, a life-threatening event, can also occur when there is loss of vasomotor tone and sympathetic innervation of the heart. Hypotension, bradycardia, and peripheral vasodilation are present in neurogenic shock. Paralysis of the diaphragm may result in respiratory compromise.

Children with spinal cord injury often have other concurrent injuries, such as head trauma, bleeding, abdominal trauma, or internal injuries that may lead to hypovolemic shock. A thorough assessment is necessary to determine whether multiple injuries are present.

Assessment and Diagnosis

A detailed neurological exam of motor function, reflexes, and sensory function is necessary to establish the initial level of injury. Radiographic imaging of the cervical spine, thoracic and lumbar spine, and sacral spine are obtained to determine whether fractures of the vertebral column are present. CT scans and MRI are also used to determine the level and extent of

Priority Care Concepts 28.1

Autonomic Dysreflexia

Autonomic dysreflexia can occur in injuries at T6 or above. A full bladder, constipation, pain, skin issues such pressure ulcers, tight clothing, cuts and bruises, menstrual cramps and abdominal conditions such as gastric ulcers and peritonitis can all trigger an autonomic dysreflexia episode. Symptoms include headache, hypertension, dysrhythmias, facial flushing, flushing above the level of the injury, and sweating.

Priorities of care include sitting the patient upright, removing the trigger or stimulus, emptying the bladder, and monitoring the blood pressure every 2–5 min. If hypertension continues, administer antihypertensives as ordered.

injury. Figure 28.9 shows an MRI of a newborn girl with a spinal cord injury.

Therapeutic Interventions

Initially, the child is placed in a cervical collar and the body is immobilized on a backboard to protect the child from further injury of the spinal column from movement. The child remains immobilized until sufficient radiographic evidence either confirms injury or shows that there is no injury. Treatment of neurogenic shock includes intravenous fluid resuscitation, atropine for bradycardia, and inotropes such as norepinephrine for hypotension. Children with cervical spine injuries may require respiratory support such as intubation and mechanical ventilation.

A child may be placed in an external fixation device to stabilize a cervical spine injury or may require surgery to repair or internally fixate fractures or deformities of the spinal column. If compression (caused by a clot, hematoma, herniated disk, or other lesion) is present in an incomplete lesion, surgical decompression of the spinal cord and nerve roots may be performed.

Therapeutic interventions for children with spinal cord injury should be developmentally based, using appropriate strategies to maximize independence across the spectrum of physical and emotional maturity levels (Powell & Davidson, 2015). Partnering with the family is emphasized given the central role of parents and family in the child's life, particularly when the child may no longer be able to achieve independence in activities as a result of the spinal cord injury.

Interventions include astute monitoring of vital signs, respiratory status, and vital capacity to determine whether neurogenic shock or autonomic dysreflexia are occurring. Intake and output as well as bladder and bowel function are closely monitored if the risk of autonomic dysreflexia is present. The provider is notified immediately if signs of shock or autonomic dysreflexia are present.

Common interventions for children with spinal cord injury are often focused on preventing complications and reducing sequelae resulting from the injury. Spasticity, neurogenic bowel and bladder, dysautonomia, pressure injury, and nutritional deficits are often present in children with spinal cord injury. Spasticity is managed with physical therapy, stretching, splinting, and/or medications such as baclofen, diazepam, tizanidine, and clonidine (Powell & Davidson, 2015). Dysautonomia (autonomic dysreflexia and temperature regulation) is managed with early assessment of symptoms, timely intervention to reduce the trigger, and education in prevention (Powell & Davidson, 2015). Children with impaired temperature regulation are susceptible to poikilothermia. Poikilothermia occurs when the child assumes the temperature of the outside environment as a result of a disruption of afferent input to thermoregulatory centers and impaired control of the distal sympathetic nervous system (Powell & Davidson, 2015). Children at risk for poikilothermia must be protected from extreme temperatures.

Neurogenic bladder management includes promoting continence, preserving renal function, and preventing life-threatening complications such as urosepsis resulting from a urinary tract infection. Clean, intermittent catheterization is the standard of care for children with a neurogenic bladder (Powell & Davidson, 2015). Neurogenic bowel is managed by establishing a bowel regimen and may include the use of stool softeners, laxatives, enemas, and suppositories. See General Nursing Interventions for Neuromuscular Disorders.

Evaluation

Expected outcomes for a child with spinal cord injury include the following:

- Adequate ventilation and oxygenation is achieved.
- Hemodynamic stability is achieved during the acute phase of spinal cord injury.
- Skin integrity is maintained.
- The child remains free from complications such as pressure injury and contractures.
- The child receives adequate caloric and nutrient intake to maintain growth.
- Bowel and bladder control is established and maintained.
- The child and family effectively cope with and adapt to the child's disability.

Discharge Planning and Teaching

Many children with spinal cord injury are discharged to an inpatient rehabilitation facility once they are medically stable and able to begin rehabilitation. Partner with parents to determine which facility best meets their needs. Once the child is ready to be discharged home, home care needs such as enteral feeding supplies, gastrostomy tube supplies, respiratory supplies (oxygen, tracheostomy supplies, and ventilator), adaptive devices, and home modifications are assessed for and obtained. Social services, family counseling, and support groups are often helpful for the child and family as they reintegrate into school and social activities. Safety issues are identified both in the home and vehicle before discharge.

Guillain-Barré Syndrome

Guillain-Barré syndrome, also known as acute inflammatory demyelinating polyradiculoneuropathy, is a disorder in which an autoimmune response in the body results in an attack on the PNS, resulting in inflammation and demyelinization of the peripheral nerves. Guillain-Barré syndrome causes progressive weakness and areflexia and can lead to acute neuromuscular paralysis and respiratory failure. The brain and spinal cord remain unaffected during the autoimmune response.

Etiology and Pathophysiology

The cause of Guillain-Barré syndrome is not fully understood, but it is believed to be triggered by a recent viral or bacterial infection such as an upper respiratory infection or acute gastroenteritis with fever. Approximately 70% of cases occur 1 to 3 weeks after an acute infection (Kumbhar, Kumbhar, Sale, & Kawade, 2016). The most common antecedent infections include *Campylobacter jejuni, Helicobacter pylori, Haemophilus influenzae,* and *Mycoplasma pneumoniae.*

Clinical Presentation

Children with Guillain-Barré syndrome present with ascending hypotonia, numbness, pain, paresthesia, and decreased or absent deep tendon reflexes. Infants and young children may present with respiratory distress, irritability, and feeding difficulties, whereas older children initially have pain, numbness, and weakness. Weakness progresses bilaterally from the feet to the chest and neck. Weakness may progress over days up to 4 weeks. Some children develop acute ataxia and are unable to walk. In some cases, the muscles of the respiratory system and the ability to swallow may become impaired enough that the child requires respiratory support such as intubation and mechanical ventilation.

Assessment and Diagnosis

Guillain-Barré syndrome is diagnosed by assessment of motor function and degree of areflexia as well as a cerebral spinal fluid analysis. Children may have minimal weakness to the legs only or may be totally paralyzed in all extremities. A lumbar puncture is performed to obtain cerebrospinal fluid. Cerebrospinal fluid analysis reveals an elevated protein level of more than twice the normal value (Sarnat, 2018). Bacterial cultures and viral cultures usually return negative results. Electromyography tests show acute muscle denervation. MRI findings of the spinal cord are abnormal and may reveal thickening of the cauda equina and intrathecal nerve roots with gadolinium enhancement (Sarnat, 2018).

Assess the child for signs of respiratory distress such as dyspnea, inability to adequately manage and clear secretions, weak cough, signs of inadequate respiratory effort such as tachypnea, minimal chest rise, and changes in color. Autonomic nervous system dysfunction can occur in children with Guillain-Barré syndrome. Monitor the child for episodes of tachycardia, bradycardia, sweating, bowel and bladder dysfunction, and changes in blood pressure.

Therapeutic Interventions

Therapeutic interventions for Guillain-Barré syndrome include treatment with immune globulin, plasmapheresis, pain management, and physical therapy. Treatment with intravenous immune globulin (IVIG) is the preferred clinical therapy for Guillain-Barré syndrome. A common protocol is IVIG 0.4 mg/kg/d for 5 consecutive days (Sarnat, 2018). If IVIG is ineffective or the child cannot receive IVIG, plasmapheresis is an alternative treatment.

Nursing care of the child with Guillain-Barré syndrome includes monitoring the respiratory status for acute decompensation, providing nutritional support, preventing complications such as pressure injury, and providing emotional support to the child and parents. Use of a continuous cardiorespiratory monitor is necessary to assess the child's cardiorespiratory status, particularly in the early stages of Guillain-Barré syndrome. An incentive spirometer is often used to monitor the child's respiratory effort and ability to achieve adequate inspiratory volumes. Enteral feeding via a nasogastric tube may be necessary during the acute stages, when swallowing may be difficult or a gag reflex is absent, to provide adequate caloric intake.

Proper positioning including good alignment and frequent turning (every 2 hours) helps prevent complications of immobility. Keep the skin warm and dry, particularly if the child is frequently diaphoretic. Change linen and use wicking underpads to draw moisture away from the child's skin. Float the heels and position the child off of pressure points.

Evaluation

Expected outcomes for a child with Guillain-Barré syndrome include the following:

- The child's oxygenation and ventilation remain within normal limits.
- The child's nutritional needs are met.
- The child remains free of pressure-related injury and complications of immobility.
- The child's neuromuscular function returns to baseline.
- The child and parents are provided emotional support and coping strategies.

Discharge Planning and Teaching

Teaching points while the child is hospitalized include assisting the parents to understand the progression of the disease and ways they can support their child during the illness. The child may not be able to communicate for a period of time or reposition himself or herself. Teach parents proper ways to communicate and reposition the child who is unable to do so. Parents also need to learn how to assist the child in performing exercises learned in physical therapy. Encourage parents to allow children to perform activities of daily living such as brushing their teeth, combing their hair, and dressing themselves. Discharge planning includes preparing the child and parents for possible outpatient physical rehabilitation sessions several times a week during the early recovery period. The child may need frequent follow-up visits with the primary care provider to monitor recovery and ensure that the child is progressing in strength and that peripheral nerve function is returning as expected. Homeschooling may be necessary until the child has regained the strength to walk and participate in daily activities in the school setting.

Botulism

Botulism is a rare but serious neuroparalytic illness resulting from toxins produced by *Clostridium botulinum* bacteria. Infant botulism, the most common clinical form in the United States, affects approximately 70 to 100 infants annually (Rosow & Strober, 2015).

Etiology and Pathophysiology

Botulism is caused by a potent neurotoxin produced by *C. botulinum* and strains of *C. butyricum* and *C. baratii,* which are anaerobic, spore-forming bacteria. Botulism is classified according to the type of transmission: foodborne, infant, wound, adult intestinal colonization, or iatrogenic. Infant botulism is discussed in this chapter. Infant botulism affects children ranging in age from less than 1 week to 1 year, with up to 95% of cases occurring in children younger than 6 months of age (Rosow & Strober, 2015).

Botulism is characterized by symmetric descending flaccid paralysis of the muscles under both autonomic and voluntary control. Beginning in the muscles supplied by the cranial nerves, progressive muscle weakness and then paralysis develop. In many cases of botulism, the source is never confirmed. However, potential sources of the spores, which lead to the disorder, include honey, rural and farm areas where contaminated dust and soil are more prevalent, and, possibly, construction sites (Rosow & Strober, 2015). Infants are more susceptible to intestinal colonization by the botulism spores because of the immaturity of their gut flora (Rosow & Strober, 2015).

Clinical Presentation

An infant with botulism may present with signs and symptoms such as poor feeding, diminished suckling, drooling, a weak cry, and a floppy appearance as a result of neck and peripheral weakness (Fig. 28.11). The infant may be constipated because of decreased motility. Respiratory symptoms such as decreased chest rise, tachypnea, and hypoxia may be present, depending on the severity of toxicity. If untreated, the illness might progress to descending paralysis of the respiratory muscles, arms, and legs.

Assessment and Diagnosis

Assessment of the child with botulism focuses on the child's neuromuscular function and respiratory function. Often, the first sign of botulism is constipation, although this sign is often overlooked. Parents often report poor feeding. Breastfeeding mothers may report having engorged breasts because the

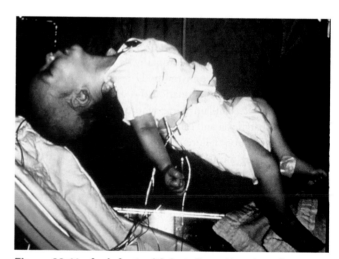

Figure 28.11. An infant with botulism. Note how floppy the infant is when picked up. Image provided courtesy of the Centers for Disease Control and Prevention.

infants' suck is too weak to empty the breasts of milk. Children with botulism typically appear weak, hypotonic, and lethargic. Assess the child for drooling, which parents may overlook as a symptom, as well, attributing it to teething. Assess the child's respiratory effort, which could indicate potential problems with oxygenation and ventilation. When the chest muscles become too weak, the child may need respiratory support such as intubation and mechanical ventilation.

Diagnosis is made on the basis of findings from the child's history, which may reveal a potential source of ingestion of spores, such as a farm or rural setting; clinical observation; and a stool sample, specifically a positive finding for botulinum toxin.

Therapeutic Interventions

Treatment and therapeutic interventions are specific to the severity of symptoms from botulism toxicity. Supportive care is the standard treatment for a child with botulism. Respiratory support with an artificial airway and mechanical ventilation may be necessary. Frequent turning and repositioning may be necessary to avoid pressure injury in an infant who is too weak to move. Depending on the severity of symptoms, a child may be given the botulism immune globulin, an anti-botulism toxin antibody (The Pharmacy 28.3).

Evaluation

Expected outcomes for a child with botulism include the following:

- The child's airway remains patent.
- The child regains maximum mobility.
- Parents verbalize foods to avoid, such as honey.

Discharge Planning and Teaching

Teaching topics for the parents of a child diagnosed with botulism include how the disease occurs and how to prevent recurrence of the disease. For children who receive botulism immune globulin, immunizations may need to be delayed until the child has fully recovered muscle strength and tone. Live vaccines are usually delayed 6 months because the immune globulin may interfere with the effectiveness of the vaccine.

The Pharmacy 28.3 — Antispasmodic Medications

Medication	Classification	Route	Action	Nursing Considerations
Botulism immune globulin	Immunoglobulin G; antitoxin	IV	Consists of human-derived anti-botulism toxin antibodies	• Used in children younger than 1 y old • Observe for development of a rash, the most common adverse effect. • Immunizations may need to be delayed or rescheduled following administration.

Think Critically

1. Explain how the neuromuscular system of an infant differs from the neuromuscular system of an adult.
2. You are teaching the parents of a newborn what to expect as the child grows in the first year of life. You want to provide anticipatory guidance for safety. When should the parents expect the baby to roll over?
3. Name some risk factors that are associated with an increased risk of CP.
4. The nurse in the neonatal intensive care unit has just received an admission. The baby was just born with an NTD known as a meningomyelocele that has not been surgically corrected. What are some of the most important interventions this nurse must do?
5. The nurse is taking care of a 10-year-old boy with DMD. He was diagnosed at the age of 4 years. For the past 2 years, he has been in a wheelchair. During the initial assessment, the nurse notes that his O_2 saturation level is consistently between 95% and 96%. What additional piece of information would the nurse want to know to determine whether he needs to have additional ventilatory support during sleep?
6. The nurse is caring for a child with a C6 spinal cord injury. Suddenly the child becomes flushed, bradycardic, and hypertensive and complains of a severe headache. What are the priority interventions for this child?

References

Adzick, N. S. (2013). Fetal surgery for spina bifida: Past, present, future. *Seminars in Pediatric Surgery, 22*, 10–17.

Aubert, E. J. (2015). Motor development in the normal child. In J. S. Tecklin (Ed.), *Pediatric physical therapy* (5th ed., pp. 15–67). Baltimore, MD: Lippincott Williams & Wilkins.

Barker, E., Saulino, M., & Caristo, A. M. (2002). A new age for childhood diseases: Spina bifida. *RN, 65*(12), 33–39.

Best, R. G. (2016). Anencephaly. *Medscape.* Retrieved from https://emedicine.medscape.com/article/1181570-overview#a1

Bickley, L. S., & Szilagyi, P. G. (2003). *The nervous system in Bates' guide to physical examination and history taking.* Philadelphia, PA: Lippincott Williams & Wilkins.

Birnkrant, D. J., Bushby, K., Bann, C. M., Alman, B. A., Apkon, S. D., & Blackwell, A. (2018). Diagnosis and management of Duchenne muscular dystrophy, part 2: Respiratory, cardiac, bone health, and orthopedic management. *Lancet Neurology, 17*(4), 347–361. doi:10.1016/S1474-4422(18)30025-5

Birnkrant, D. J., Bushby, K., Bann, C. M., Apkon, S. D., Blackwell, A., Brumbaugh, D., . . . Weber, D. R. (2018). Diagnosis and management of Duchenne muscular dystrophy, part 1: Diagnosis, and neuromuscular, rehabilitation, endocrine, and gastrointestinal and nutrition management. *Lancet Neurology, 17*(3), 251–267. doi:10.1016/S1474-4422(18)30024-3

Birnkrant, D. J., Bushby, K., Bann, C. M., Apkon, S. D., Blackwell, A., Colvin, M. K., . . . Ward, L. M. (2018). Diagnosis and management of Duchenne muscular dystrophy, part 3: Primary care, emergency management, psychosocial care, and transitions of care across the lifespan. *Lancet Neurology, 17*(5), 445–455. doi:10.1016/S1474-4422(18)30026-7

Bonhotal, S. (2015). Screening and risk factors for anencephaly. *The Journal for Nurse Practitioners, 11*(3), 371–372.

Brand, M. C. (2006). Part 2: Examining the newborn with an open spinal dysraphism. *Advances in Neonatal Care, 6*(4), 181–196.

Cameron, M., & Moran, P. (2009). Prenatal screening and diagnosis of neural tube defects. *Prenatal Diagnosis 29*, 402–411.

Centers for Disease Control and Prevention. (2016). *Recommended vaccines by disease.* Retrieved from https://www.cdc.gov/vaccines/vpd/vaccines-diseases.html

Centers for Disease Control and Prevention. (n.d.-a). *Basics about muscular dystrophy.* Retrieved from https://www.cdc.gov/ncbddd/musculardystrophy/facts.html

Centers for Disease Control and Prevention. (n.d.-c). *Facts about encephalocele.* Retrieved from https://www.cdc.gov/ncbddd/birthdefects/encephalocele.html

Centers for Disease Control and Prevention. (n.d.-d). *Folic acid & neural tube defects: Data & statistics.* Retrieved from https://www.cdc.gov/ncbddd/birthdefectscount/data.html

Centers for Disease Control and Prevention. (n.d.-e). *What is cerebral palsy.* Retrieved October 13, 2018, from https://www.cdc.gov/ncbddd/cp/facts.html

Darras, B. T. (2018a). Duchenne and Becker muscular dystrophy: Clinical features and diagnosis. In M. C. Patterson, H. V. Firth & J. F. Dashe (Eds.), *UpToDate.* Retrieved December 22, 2018, from https://www.uptodate.com/contents/duchenne-and-becker-muscular-dystrophy-clinical-features-and-diagnosis?search=muscular%20dystrophy&source=search_result&selectedTitle=1–150&usage_type=default&display_rank=1#H2598900557

Finkel, R. S., Mercuri, E., Meyer, O. H., Simonds, A. K., Schroth, M. K., Graham, R. J., . . . Sejersen, T. (2018). Diagnosis and management of spinal muscular atrophy: Part 2: Pulmonary and acute care; medications, supplements and immunizations; other organ systems; and ethics. *Neuromuscular Disorders, 28*, 197–207.

Kolb, S. J., & Kissel, J. T. (2011). Spinal muscle atrophy: A timely review. *Archives of Neurology, 68*(8), 1–11. doi:10.1001/archneurol.2011.74

Kolb, S. J., & Kissel, J. T. (2015). Spinal muscle atrophy. *Neurologic Clinics, 33*(4), 831–846. doi:10.1016/j.ncl.2015.07.004

Kolb, S. J., Coffey, C. S., Yankey, J.W., Krosschell, K., Arnold, W. D., Rutkove, S. B., . . . Kissel, J. T. (2017). Natural history of infantile-onset spinal muscular atrophy. *Annals of Neurology, 82*(6), 883–891. doi:10.1002/ana.25101

Kotagal, S. (2018). Detailed neurological assessments of infants and children. In D. R. Nordli (Ed.), *UpToDate.* Retrieved June 20, 2019 from https://www.uptodate.com/contents/detailed-neurologic-assessment-of-infants-and-children?search=Detailed%20neurological%20assessments%20of%20infants%20and%20children.&source=search_result&selectedTitle=1–150&usage_type=default&display_rank=1

Kumbhar, S. G., Kumbhar, S. K., Sale, M. S., & Kawade, R. (2016). Clinical profile of childhood Guillian-Barre syndrome: A retrospective study. *International Journal of Healthcare & Biomedical Research, 4*(3), 19–25.

Lin, C., Kalb, S. J., & Yeh, W. (2015). Delay in diagnosis of spinal muscular atrophy: A systematic literature review. *Pediatric Neurology, 53*, 293–300.

Mercuri, E., Finkel, R. S., Muntoni, F., Wirth, B., Montes, J., Main, M., . . . Sejersen, T. (2018). Diagnosis and management of spinal muscular atrophy: Part 1: Recommendations for diagnosis, rehabilitation, orthopedic and nutritional care. *Neuromuscular Disorders, 28*, 103–115.

Moldenhauer, J. S., & Adzick, N. S. (2017). Fetal surgery for myelomeningocele: After the Management of Myelomeningocele Study (MOMS). *Seminars in Fetal & Neonatal, 22*(6), 360–366.

Moreno-De-Luca, A., Ledbetter, H., & Martin, C. L. (2012). Genetic insights into the causes and classification of the cerebral palsies. *The Lancet, 11*, 283–287.

National Organization of Rare Disorders. (2012). *Spinal muscle atrophy.* Retrieved from www.rarediseases.org/rare-diseases/spinal-muscular-atrophy

Piatt, J. H. (2015). Pediatric spinal injury in the US: epidemiology and disparities. *Journal of Neurosurgery: Pediatrics, 16*(4), 463–471.

Powell, A., Davidson, L. (2015). Pediatric spinal cord injury: A review by organ system. *Physical Medicine and Rehabilitation Clinics of North America, 26*(1), 109–132.

Reddihough, D. (2011). Cerebral palsy in childhood. *Australian Family Physician, 40*(4), 192–196.

Rosow, L. K., & Strober, J. B. (2015). Infant botulism: Review and clinical update. *Pediatric Neurology, 52*(5), 487–492.

Sarnat, H. (2018). Guillain-Barré syndrome. In R. Kliegman, B. Stanton, J. St. Geme, N. Schor, & R. Behrman (Eds.), *Nelson textbook of pediatrics* (20th ed.). Philadelphia, PA: Elsevier.

Screening Time. (n.d.). *Screening tool.* Retrieved from https://screeningtime.org/star-center/#/screening-tools

Stone, P., & Fieggen, G. (2006). Spina bifida: An ongoing challenge. *Professional Nursing Today, 10*(1), 42–46.

Ward, L. M., & Birnkrant, D. J. (2018). An introduction to the Duchenne muscular dystrophy care considerations. *Pediatrics, 142*(s2), S1–S4.

Williams, J., Mai, C. T., Mulinare, J., Isenburg, J., Flood, T. J., Ethen, M., . . . Kirby, R. S. (2015). Updated estimates of neural tube defects prevented by Mandatory Folic Acid Fortification-United States, 1995-2011. *MMWR: Morbidity and Mortality Weekly Report, 64*, 1–5.

Suggested Readings

Centers for Disease Control and Prevention. (n.d.). *Botulism: Information for health professionals.* Retrieved from https://www.cdc.gov/botulism/health-professional.html

Centers for Disease Control and Prevention. (n.d.). *Cerebral palsy: What is cerebral palsy.* Retrieved from https://www.cdc.gov/ncbddd/cp/facts.html

Centers for Disease Control and Prevention. (n.d.). *Muscular dystrophy: Duchenne muscular dystrophy care considerations.* Retrieved from https://www.cdc.gov/ncbddd/musculardystrophy/care-considerations.html

29 Alterations in Integumentary Function

Variations in Anatomy and Physiology

The skin is the barrier between the external environment and the internal structures of the body. The infant's skin is thinner than that of an older child or adult, placing the infant at greater risk for injury and infection. In addition, this thinner skin more rapidly absorbs topical medications. The infant has a greater relative body surface area (BSA) than does an adult and thus is more prone to insensible fluid loss and heat loss through the skin. Owing to the infant's thin dermis and lack of subcutaneous tissue, the infant's blood vessels are closer to the surface of the skin, which decreases thermoregulation, placing the infant at risk of overheating or becoming hypothermic more quickly. The dermis and the epidermis are more loosely connected in the infant, allowing for easier skin breakdown. The skin becomes more like that of an adult by the late school-age to adolescent years.

Hair follicles are present at birth and are distributed over the body with the exception of the palms, soles, and lips. **Vellus hair**, which is fine and unpigmented, is present at birth over most of the body. **Terminal hair**—mature hair, typically thick, coarse, and pigmented—is found on the scalp, eyelashes, and eyebrows in the young child. The onset of puberty stimulates the conversion of vellus hair to terminal hair in the axillae, beard, and pubic area.

Sebaceous glands are present at birth. These glands produce sebum, which serves to lubricate the scalp and the skin. During adolescence, the sebaceous glands increase the production of sebum in response to hormones. This increased sebum is the cause of acne in some adolescents.

The **eccrine glands**, which are sweat glands that release water to the surface of the skin and help regulate body temperature, are present over the whole body but are more prominent on the palms of the hands and on the soles of the feet. These glands are underdeveloped in infants, preventing them from sweating to increase heat loss. The immature eccrine glands place infants at increased risk of hyperthermia. The **apocrine glands** are a type of sweat gland located in the axillae and pubic region. These glands remain inactive until puberty, at which time they become responsible for body odor.

Assessment of the Pediatric Integumentary System

Taking a thorough health history helps determine the type of rash, lesion, or injury present. Enquire about the onset of any rash. Determine whether the child has other signs and symptoms of illness, such as rhinitis, pain, or fever. Is pruritus associated with the rash? Has the child been exposed to anyone with the same type of rash? Does the child have any known allergies? If so, has the child come into contact with any allergens? For lesions such as petechiae or purpura, enquire whether the child has a history of thrombocytopenia or immune suppression. If the child presents with a bite or a wound, enquire about the mechanism of injury.

Assessment of the skin consists mostly of inspection and palpation. Make sure the assessment is conducted with proper lighting to adequately see lesions and wounds. Assess the skin for color, noting hyper- or hypopigmentation, which is often associated with healing wounds, especially in children with dark skin. Palpate the skin for temperature, moisture, and texture. Assess skin turgor. If lesions are present, note the size, type, location, and distribution. Inspect and palpate rashes, describing them by color, size, type, distribution, and whether they are flat or raised. Inspect injuries for depth, debris, and drainage. Inspect the skin borders of the wound.

General Nursing Interventions for Integumentary Disorders

Most children with integumentary disorders are cared for as outpatients. Exceptions to this include children with severe bites, partial- or full-thickness burns, or complications of infections. Nursing care focuses on preventing infection, promoting skin integrity and comfort, and providing education to the parents about treatment and prevention.

Prevent Infection

Primary skin lesions can become infected without proper care and education. Assess for signs and symptoms of infection such as erythema, drainage, and odor. Assess skin temperature for increased warmth around the lesion or wound. Assess for signs and symptoms of systemic infection such as fever, increased heart rate, malaise, and decreased alertness.

Apply antibiotic ointment and perform dressing changes as ordered. If necessary, administer systemic antibiotic as ordered. Teach parents the signs and symptoms of infection. Educate parents and children on how to prevent infection, such as by performing appropriate hand hygiene, keeping lesions covered if appropriate, and not scratching the affected area.

Promote Skin Integrity

Infants and children are at risk for problems with skin integrity because of the anatomy of their skin. Skin breakdown can occur as a result of moist environments, pressure, or mechanical damage, such as due to scratching. Assess the skin at regular intervals, noting areas of redness, which may indicate pressure areas. If the child has decreased mobility, reposition him or her every 2 hours. Perform frequent diaper changes as appropriate. Ensure that linens are clean and dry. Implement measures to prevent scratching, including covering lesions, applying soothing creams, and keeping nails trimmed short.

Promote Comfort

Many integumentary disorders create some discomfort in the form of localized pain or itching. Teach parents how to provide comfort measures at home. For skin disorders that cause itching, the parent may place the child in a lukewarm bath, using a commercial oatmeal bath product, if desired. Instruct the parent to pat the skin dry, not rub it. Apply antibiotic ointment, hydrocortisone cream, or moisturizers while the skin is still damp. Avoid soaps and moisturizers with fragrances, dyes, or alcohol. Administer oral antihistamines as directed by the healthcare provider. Treat rashes or minor injuries that cause pain with acetaminophen or ibuprofen, as directed by the healthcare provider. Have the child wear loose clothing to promote air circulation and avoid sweating, which could exacerbate pain and itching. Distract the child with activities to keep his or her mind off of the discomfort.

Provide Education

Education about integumentary disorders should center on prevention and home care. Bacterial and viral skin infections are spread from person to person either via contact or droplets. Discuss with parents ways to prevent the spread of these types of infections. Tell parents of a child with an infection to inform the child's close contacts that they have been exposed to the viral or bacterial infection. Teach parents how to take care of both bacterial and viral rashes at home. Further prevention education emphasizes avoidance of causative agents (Patient Teaching 29.1).

Preventing Integumentary Disorders

- Teach the child to recognize and avoid poison ivy and poison oak.
- Avoid exposing the child to any other triggers of atopic and contact dermatitis.
- If the child will be spending time outdoors, apply sunscreen to all exposed areas to prevent sunburn.
- Learn to identify infestations such as lice, scabies, and bedbugs.
- Teach the child to recognize and avoid insect nests.
- Have the child wear insect repellent when outdoors for extended periods of time.
- Teach the child not to approach animals quickly or pet them unless the child is told it is okay, so as to minimize the risk of bites.

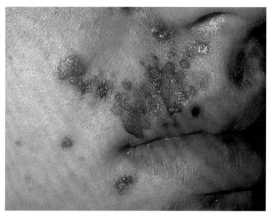

Figure 29.1. Impetigo. Impetigo most commonly occurs around the mouth and nose. Note the classic honey-colored crusted lesions. Reprinted with permission from Burkhart, C., Morrell, D., Goldsmith, L. A., Papier, A., Green, B., Dasher, D., & Gomathy, S. (Eds.). (2009). *VisualDx: Essential pediatric dermatology* (1st ed., Fig. 3.7). Philadelphia, PA: Lippincott Williams & Wilkins.

Bacterial Skin Infections

Bacterial skin infections are generally self-limiting and treated in the outpatient setting.

Impetigo

There are two types of impetigo: bullous and nonbullous. Bullous impetigo more commonly occurs in infants. Nonbullous impetigo accounts for over 70% of cases (Juern & Drolet, 2016a). Nonbullous impetigo is one of the most common skin infections among children 2 to 5 years old, although it can occur at any age (VanRavenstein, Durham, Williams, & Smith, 2017).

Etiology and Pathophysiology

Under normal circumstances, skin is colonized by bacteria. Overgrowth of bacteria can cause infection under certain conditions, such as moisture, breaks in skin integrity, poor hygiene, or age. *Staphylococcus aureus* is the most common cause of impetigo. The staphylococci bacteria spread from the nose to the skin, causing infection. The infection spreads easily from person to person through contact, especially with fingers, towels, and clothing. Complications are rare but include cellulitis and septicemia (VanRavenstein et al., 2017). Bullous impetigo is caused by strains of *S. aureus* that produce exfoliative toxins. The toxins cause blisters to form, which can rupture easily.

Clinical Presentation

Bullous impetigo is generally found on the trunk of infants. Other sites of infection include the face, buttocks, perineum, and extremities. Once the **bulla** (a large blister filled with clear fluid) ruptures, a shiny erythematous base appears and a thick, brown crust forms around the edges of the area.

Typical presentation of nonbullous impetigo begins as small vesicles, less than 2 cm in diameter (Fig. 29.1). The vesicles quickly develop into plaques with a characteristic honey-crusted appearance. Lesions are typically around the nose and mouth but can spread to other parts of the body. Nonbullous impetigo is not painful. Regional lymphadenopathy is present.

Assessment and Diagnosis

Ask the parents when the lesions appeared. Determine whether the child has been around others who are infected. Enquire whether there are any other symptoms, besides the visible lesions. Diagnosis is based on the clinical presentation.

Therapeutic Interventions

Impetigo is self-limiting. However, use of the topical antibiotic ointment mupirocin for 10 to 14 days is the treatment of choice (The Pharmacy 29.1). Oral antibiotics, such as cephalosporins, may be used in bullous impetigo and more severe cases of nonbullous impetigo. Nursing interventions include preventing secondary infection and providing education about the spread of impetigo. Teach parents to clean the lesions with soap and warm water and apply antibiotic ointment as directed.

Evaluation

Expected outcomes for a child with impetigo include the following:

- The presence of lesions decreases over 10 to 14 days.
- No secondary infections of primary lesions occur.
- Infection does not occur in the child's family members.

The Pharmacy 29.1   Mupirocin and Cephalexin

Medication	Classification	Route	Action	Nursing Considerations
Mupirocin	Antibiotic	Top.	• Bacteriostatic • Binds to bacteria to inhibit protein synthesis	• Apply a small amount to the affected area three to five times daily for 5–14 d. • Monitor for localized burning or stinging. • Monitor for anaphylaxis. • Avoid contact with eyes.
Cephalexin	Antibiotic	PO	• Bacteriostatic • Inhibits bacterial cell wall synthesis	• Administer 25–50 mg/kg/d divided every 6–8 h. • Check the child's allergies before administration. • Educate parents that the child should take all medication.

PO, by mouth; Top., topical.
Adapted from Taketomo, C. K., Hodding, J. H., & Kraus, D. M. (2018). *Pediatric & neonatal dosage handbook* (25th ed.). Hudson, OH: Lexicomp.

Discharge Planning and Teaching

Nurses play an important role in teaching parents how to prevent the spread of impetigo. If the child is in day care, notify the day care provider. The child should have a dedicated towel and washcloth until the infection clears. Teach proper hand washing techniques to the family. Inform the parents to call the healthcare provider if the lesions become red and warm to the touch or if the child develops a fever.

Folliculitis

Folliculitis is an infection of the hair follicle and can occur anywhere on the body, with the main sites being the scalp, extremities, and buttocks.

Etiology and Pathophysiology

Folliculitis is caused by infection with *S. aureus*, a common bacterium found on the skin, because of poor hygiene, drainage from wounds, exposure to contaminated water, and shaving.

Clinical Presentation

Folliculitis presents as small pustules with an erythematous base located at the base of the hair follicles (Fig. 29.2). The lesions generally do not cause pain or pruritus.

Assessment and Diagnosis

Enquire about when the lesions appeared. Ask whether the child has been swimming in a lake or hot tub. Inspect the child for cleanliness. Determine whether there are other symptoms. Diagnosis is made on the basis of clinical presentation.

Therapeutic Interventions

Folliculitis is self-limiting but is often treated with topical antibiotics. Preventing secondary infection is the primary goal of

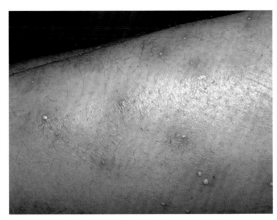

Figure 29.2. Folliculitis. Small, erythematous papules associated with folliculitis. Reprinted with permission from Burkhart, C., Morrell, D., Goldsmith, L. A., Papier, A., Green, B., Dasher, D., & Gomathy, S. (Eds.). (2009). *VisualDx: Essential pediatric dermatology* (1st ed., Fig. 3.11). Philadelphia, PA: Lippincott Williams & Wilkins.

nursing interventions. Wash the affected areas with soap and water and apply warm compresses several times daily.

Evaluation

Expected outcomes for a child with folliculitis include the following:

• The presence of lesions decrease over 10 to 14 days.
• No secondary infections of primary lesions occur.
• No new lesions appear.

Discharge Planning and Teaching

Teach parents the causes of folliculitis and how to avoid it, such as by avoiding extended exposure to dirty water, such as that found in hot tubs, and practicing daily hygiene. Tell the parents to call the healthcare provider if the lesions become bigger rather than smaller, feel warm to the touch, or have drainage.

Cellulitis

Cellulitis is localized inflammation and infection of the subcutaneous tissue.

Etiology and Pathophysiology

Cellulitis is a secondary infection preceded by some sort of trauma to the skin, such as an injury, insect bite, or some other primary skin lesion. The most common etiology is *Streptococcus pyogenes* or *S. aureus*.

Cellulitis can also be caused by community-acquired methicillin-resistant *S. aureus* (CA-MRSA). Lesions resulting from this type of cellulitis present similarly to those of other types of cellulitis but often are filled with purulent fluid.

Clinical Presentation

Children with cellulitis often have fever, chills, and lymphadenopathy. Infected areas are erythematous and warm to the touch and may be edematous and painful (Fig. 29.3).

Assessment and Diagnosis

During the health history, enquire about previous injuries or lesions at the site of infection. Ask when the signs and symptoms of infection began. Assess the child's vital signs to determine whether the child has a fever. Inspect the affected area. Palpate for warmth and tenderness.

Diagnosis is made on the basis of clinical presentation. An aspirate at the site of inflammation can identify the causative organism (Juern & Drolet, 2016a). As ordered, draw blood for culture for hospitalized or immunocompromised children.

Therapeutic Interventions

Children with mild cellulitis are treated on an outpatient basis with oral antibiotics, with cephalexin often being the drug of choice. Cephalexin is effective for treating most causative organisms of cellulitis, including CA-MRSA. Children with more extensive cellulitis or periorbital or orbital cellulitis are hospitalized. Obtain wound and blood cultures as ordered. Mark the edges of the affected area to monitor healing progress or spread of infection. Administer intravenous cephalosporin as ordered. Assess the affected area to determine the effectiveness of treatment.

Evaluation

Expected outcomes for a child with cellulitis include the following:

- Erythema and inflammation decrease at the site.
- The child is free of fever.
- The child is free of systemic signs and symptoms of infection.

Discharge Planning and Teaching

Educate parents to complete the full course of oral antibiotics as prescribed. Inform parents to call the healthcare provider if redness extends beyond the marked edges or if the child appears ill.

Viral Exanthems

Many viral infections cause a rash in addition to symptoms such as fever, rhinorrhea, and malaise. Most viral rashes are common in childhood and have no long-term effects. These include roseola, which is discussed in Chapter 15; erythema infectiosum, commonly known as fifth disease, which is discussed in Chapter 17; and Coxsackie virus, commonly known as hand-foot-and-mouth disease, which is also discussed in Chapter 17. (Similarly, note that fungal infections are covered elsewhere in the book; candidal diaper rash is discussed in Chapter 15 and tinea infections in Chapter 18.) However, some viruses, such as measles, mumps, rubella, and varicella, can have negative sequelae, and children should be vaccinated against them.

Rubeola (Measles)

Measles is highly contagious. However, owing to widespread vaccination, measles is no longer endemic in the United States. The current rate in the United States is less than one per one million (Mason, 2016). However, there are outbreaks in unvaccinated populations as of June 6, 2019 there were 1,022 cases

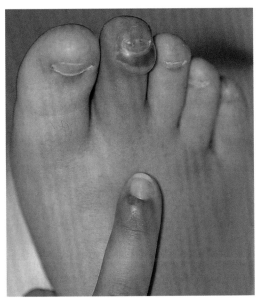

Figure 29.3. Cellulitis. Cellulitis of the toe with edema and erythema. Reprinted with permission from Fleisher, G. R., Ludwig, S., & Baskin, M. N. (Eds.). (2004). *Atlas of pediatric emergency medicine* (1st ed., Fig. 11.37). Philadelphia, PA: Lippincott Williams & Wilkins.

reported, up from a total of 372 cases in all of 2018 (CDC, 2019). There are occasional outbreaks in unvaccinated populations. In many other areas of the world, however, measles is still endemic and a threat to population health.

Etiology and Pathophysiology

The measles virus is a single-stranded RNA virus. The virus spreads easily through respiratory secretions and can survive on inanimate surfaces for up to an hour. The incubation period is 7 to 21 days, with an average time of 14 days. A child is contagious 4 days before and 4 days after the appearance of the rash (Alter, Bennett, Koranyi, Kreppel, & Simon, 2015).

Clinical Presentation

Children initially present in the **prodromal**, or early symptom, phase. During this phase, children experience mild fever, conjunctivitis, coryza, and cough. Conjunctival drainage is nonpurulent. **Koplik spots** (Fig. 29.4), which are clustered white lesions, may or may not be apparent on the oral mucosa at the time of presentation. However, Koplik spots appear within 4 days of the rash onset. Fever is highest 1 to 2 days before the appearance of the rash. The rash is maculopapular, beginning at the head and progressing down the trunk and upper extremities (Fig. 29.5). After 5 days, the rash begins to fade, leading to desquamation. Complications of measles commonly affect the respiratory system.

Assessment and Diagnosis

Obtain a thorough history of the current illness and immunization status. Ask whether the child has been exposed to anyone with measles. Determine the onset of symptoms and day of fever. Assess the child's vital signs. Inspect the child's mouth for Koplik spots. Inspect and palpate the skin. Document the distribution of the rash. Palpate for lymphadenopathy, noting

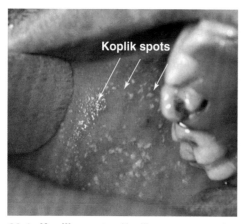

Figure 29.4. Koplik spots. Koplik spots associated with measles appear as clustered white lesions with an erythematous base on the buccal mucosa. Reprinted with permission from Harvey, R. A., & Cornelissen, C. N. (2012). *Lippincott illustrated reviews: Microbiology* (3rd ed., Fig. 34.10). Philadelphia, PA: Lippincott Williams & Wilkins.

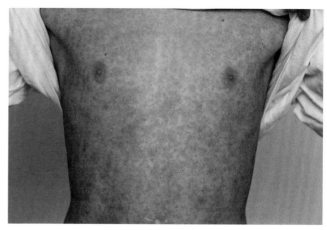

Figure 29.5. Measles. Maculopapular rash on the trunk of a child with measles.

the presence and location of swollen lymph nodes. Assess for adventitious lung sounds to determine whether any respiratory complications are present.

Diagnosis is confirmed with immunoglobulin (Ig) M titers. Titers become positive 2 to 4 days after the rash appears. Serology may not be needed in the case of a known measles outbreak (Mason, 2016).

Therapeutic Interventions

Management is supportive. Maintain fluid status, monitor oxygenation, and promote comfort. Monitor the child's status carefully to prevent secondary infections. Give acetaminophen and ibuprofen as ordered. Monitor respiratory status, and provide supplemental oxygen if needed. Promote oral hydration. Monitor hydration status and administer intravenous fluids as necessary. Place the hospitalized child on droplet precautions. Give antibiotics for secondary infections as needed.

In the immunocompromised patient, measles can be life-threatening. Ribavirin has been shown to have benefits against the measles virus. Ribavirin is often administered with intravenous gamma globulin (Mason, 2016).

Evaluation

Expected outcomes for a child with measles include the following:

- The child's O$_2$ saturation level remains at 95% or above.
- The child's fever decreases by day 6.
- The child's comfort is maintained.
- The child's hydration status is maintained.

For children who develop a secondary respiratory infection, monitor respiratory status and maintain oxygenation.

Discharge Planning and Teaching

Educate parents that the child is contagious up to 4 days after the rash appears. Have parents inform their child's contacts of exposure to the virus. Unimmunized people exposed to measles should receive the measles, mumps, and rubella (MMR) vaccine within 72 hours of exposure or Ig within 6 days of exposure (Alter et al., 2015). Explain to parents that the best treatment for measles is prevention of the disease with the MMR vaccine.

Mumps

Mumps is a self-limiting virus that has declined in prevalence in the United States because of widespread vaccination. However, large outbreaks have occurred in the United States in the past 10 years, mostly in unvaccinated 18- to 24-year-olds attending college (Alter et al., 2015).

Etiology and Pathophysiology

The mumps virus is spread by respiratory secretions. The virus settles in the respiratory tract, invades the epithelium, and spreads via the lymphatic system (Mason, 2016). Close contact is required for the virus to spread. The incubation period is 16 to 18 days. Children are infectious 7 days before parotid swelling and up to 8 days after the onset of parotid swelling (Alter et al., 2015). The virus targets the salivary glands, central nervous system (CNS), and the testes. The most common complications are meningitis and orchitis.

Clinical Presentation

Parotid gland swelling is the hallmark presentation of mumps (Fig. 29.6). A prodromal period of 1 to 2 days consists of fever, aches, and rhinitis. Once parotitis begins, the area is tender, often with ipsilateral ear pain. Fever and systemic symptoms last up to 5 days. Parotid swelling subsides within 7 days.

Assessment and Diagnosis

Obtain a thorough history of the illness and immunization status. Enquire about exposure and close contacts. Ask about pain. Assess vital signs. Inspect the jaw for parotid swelling. Palpate the parotid gland for tenderness. Assess for signs and symptoms of increased intracranial pressure to determine CNS involvement. Inspect the testes for swelling, indicating orchitis.

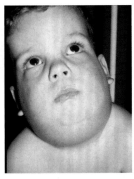

Figure 29.6. Mumps. Parotid swelling associated with mumps. Reprinted with permission from Kyle, T., & Carman, S. (2016). *Essentials of pediatric nursing* (3rd ed., Fig. 15.4). Philadelphia, PA: Wolters Kluwer.

Diagnosis is confirmed through increased mumps IgM antibodies. In the presence of a known outbreak, serology may not be needed.

Therapeutic Interventions

Management is supportive. Monitor for meningitis and orchitis. Promote comfort by administering pain medication as ordered. Administer acetaminophen or ibuprofen for fever. Monitor hydration status and encourage fluids.

Evaluation

Expected outcomes for a child with mumps include the following:

- The child is free of fever.
- Parotid swelling decreases.
- Pain is at an acceptable level for the child.
- No signs and symptoms of meningitis are present.
- Testicular swelling decreases.

Discharge Planning and Teaching

There are typically no long-term complications in children with mumps. Males with orchitis do not generally suffer sterility. Educate the family to inform close contacts. Teach the family about the prevention of mumps through the MMR vaccine.

Rubella

Rubella is often referred to as German measles or 3-day measles. The infection is mild in children. Endemic cases have been eliminated in the United States, but cases are brought into the country through travel. The major complication of rubella is congenital rubella syndrome (CRS), which occurs when a pregnant mother contracts the disease and passes it to the fetus. This discussion focuses on postnatal rubella.

Etiology and Pathophysiology

Rubella is transmitted via aerosolized particles. The virus is a single-stranded RNA virus that replicates in the respiratory epithelium. Spread is through the lymph system.

Clinical Presentation

The first presenting symptom in a child with rubella is the rash. A prodromal period consists of fever, malaise, headache, sore throat, and red eyes. The rash begins on the face and neck as irregular macules (Fig. 29.7). The rash on the face disappears as it spreads to the trunk and lasts no longer than 3 days. Anterior cervical, posterior cervical, and occipital lymphadenopathy is generally present.

Assessment and Diagnosis

Obtain a thorough history of the illness and immunization status. Determine when the child may have been exposed to the virus. Enquire about generalized symptoms such as malaise, fever,

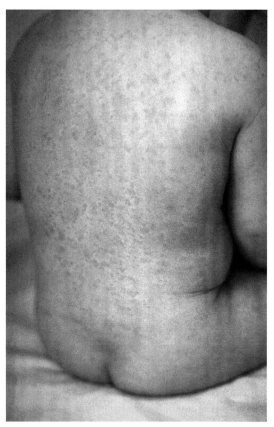

Figure 29.7. **Rubella.** Rash associated with rubella. From the Centers for Disease Control and Prevention Public Health Image Library.

and aches. Ask when the rash first appeared. Assess vital signs. Inspect the skin for a rash, noting the type and distribution. Palpate for lymphadenopathy.

The rash of rubella is nonspecific, and a diagnosis cannot be made on clinical presentation alone. Diagnosis is confirmed by elevated levels of rubella-specific serum IgM. Leukopenia and mild thrombocytopenia may be present (Mason, 2016).

Therapeutic Interventions

Management of postnatal rubella is supportive. Antipyretics may be given for fever. CRS requires a multidisciplinary pediatric healthcare team.

Evaluation

Expected outcomes for a child with postnatal rubella include the following:

- The child is free of fever.
- The child's symptoms are well managed.

Discharge Planning and Teaching

Educate parents on prevention of rubella through immunization with the MMR vaccine. Inform close contacts of exposure. Pregnant women exposed to rubella should have titers drawn to determine immune status.

Varicella

Varicella virus is a member of the herpes viruses. Primary infection is more commonly known as chickenpox. The virus can remain latent and become reactivated later in life as shingles. Varicella is most commonly a mild illness of childhood. Complications are more common in infants, adolescents, and immunocompromised children (LaRussa & Marin, 2016). The incidence of varicella has declined since the introduction of the two-step varicella vaccine. Immunized children may still contract a modified, milder form of the disease.

Etiology and Pathophysiology

Varicella virus is transmitted by contact with weeping lesions or nasopharyngeal secretions of an infected person. The incubation period is 10 to 21 days, during which the virus replicates in the lymph system. Children are contagious 1 to 2 days before the rash appears and continue to be contagious until there are no more new lesions and all lesions are crusted over. The virus is extremely contagious. The infection rate of household members of infected children is 90% (Alter et al., 2015). Complications include secondary infection of lesions with *S. aureus* and group A beta-hemolytic *Streptococcus*, as well as varicella pneumonia. More rare complications are meningitis, arthritis, hepatitis, and cerebellar ataxia.

Clinical Presentation

Prodromal symptoms include fever, malaise, and headache for 24 to 48 hours before the eruption of lesions. Skin lesions appear in various stages. New lesions appear as old ones scab over. The lesion begins as an erythematous macule and progresses to a pustule and finally a clear fluid-filled vesicle (Fig. 29.8). Lesions appear over a period of 6 days. Children with chickenpox typically experience severe pruritus. The average number of lesions is 300, but there may be more, especially in immunocompromised children. Immunized children may have a smaller number of lesions with infection.

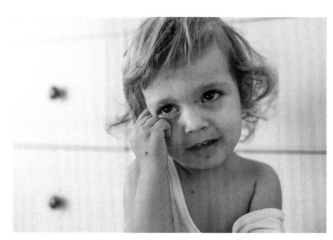

Figure 29.8. **Varicella.** Lesions of varicella on a young girl.

Assessment and Diagnosis

Obtain a thorough history of the illness and immunization status. Determine when exposure occurred. Ask when the prodromal symptoms began and when the lesions appeared. Enquire about close contacts and their immunizations status. Assess vital signs. Inspect the skin for lesions. Document the amount, distribution, and appearance of the lesions. Assess for signs and symptoms of secondary infection of the lesions. Auscultate for adventitious or decreased lung sounds, which indicate respiratory system involvement.

Diagnosis is made depending on clinical presentation. Hospitalized or immunocompromised patients may have the diagnosis confirmed via rapid varicella-zoster virus polymerase chain reaction.

Therapeutic Interventions

Most children with chickenpox require only supportive therapy. Antiviral therapy is not indicated for the typical child with chickenpox. However, treatment with acyclovir is indicated depending on the status of the child (The Pharmacy 29.2). If warranted, initiation of oral acyclovir within 72 hours of the start of symptoms may lessen the illness in healthy children. Children with severe disease or immunocompromised children should be started on intravenous acyclovir.

Symptomatic treatment involves promoting comfort and decreasing the itching associated with the lesions. Nursing management focuses on preventing secondary infection, promoting comfort, and maintaining skin integrity. Administer antipyretics for fever.

Evaluation

Expected outcomes for a child with a primary varicella-zoster infection include the following:

- No skin breakdown is present around primary lesions.
- No secondary infection occurs.
- The child's pain level is acceptable.
- Symptoms of infection decrease over time.
- Infection does not occur in others.

Discharge Planning and Teaching

Educate parents on how to identify signs and symptoms of secondary infection of the varicella lesions. Explain signs and symptoms of complications and when to contact the healthcare provider. Have parents inform close contacts. Discuss prevention of varicella through immunization.

Hypersensitivity Reactions

Hypersensitivity reactions include skin reactions such as atopic dermatitis (see Chapter 16), contact dermatitis, erythema multiforme, and urticaria.

Contact Dermatitis

Contact dermatitis can be divided into irritant contact dermatitis, allergic contact dermatitis, nickel dermatitis, and diaper dermatitis (see Chapter 15).

Etiology and Pathophysiology

Irritant dermatitis is caused by repetitive contact with an irritant. The irritant may be physical, mechanical, or chemical. Examples include household cleaners, detergents, soaps, saliva, sweat, rough fabric, or ill-fitting shoes.

Allergic dermatitis is a T cell–mediated reaction to an antigen that requires sensitization for a reaction to occur. The antigen enters through the skin, binds with a complement protein, and is distributed through sensitized T cells. First exposure to the allergen results in sensitization, and subsequent exposures result in dermatitis within a few hours. Each subsequent exposure may result in a more severe reaction. Distribution of the rash depends on the allergen. Airborne allergens cause a rash on the exposed areas, such as the face and arms, whereas other allergens elicit a rash at the point of contact (Dickey & Chiu, 2016a). Common causes of allergic dermatitis include jewelry, detergents, topical creams and lotions, and fabric dyes. An additional cause of allergic contact dermatitis is exposure to plants such as poison ivy, poison oak, and poison sumac. Oils in these plants elicit the allergic reaction, which only appears at the point of contact.

The Pharmacy 29.2 Acyclovir

Classification	Route	Action	Nursing Consideration

Antiviral	• PO
	• IV
		Inhibits DNA synthesis and viral replication	• IV administration:
			  ○ Give 10–15 mg/kg every 8 h for 5–10 d.
			  ○ Infuse each dose over 1 h.
			  ○ Continue for 48 h after the last new lesions appear.
			• PO administration:
			  ○ Give 20 mg/kg four times daily for 5–7 d.
			  ○ Give with or without food.

IV, intravenous; PO, by mouth.
Adapted from Taketomo, C. K., Hodding, J. H., & Kraus, D. M. (2018). *Pediatric & neonatal dosage handbook* (25th ed.). Hudson, OH: Lexicomp.

Nickel dermatitis is a T cell–mediated reaction specific to the nickel found in jewelry, buttons on pants, belt buckles, and other materials that contain nickel. More recently, cell phone cases, tablets, and laptops have become a source of nickel dermatitis (Tuchman, Silverberg, Jacob, & Silverberg, 2015).

Secondary infection from scratching, lichenification of the skin, and changes in pigmentation are all complications of any type of contact dermatitis.

Clinical Presentation

Children with contact dermatitis present with a rash at the point of contact. The rash is erythematous and causes intense pruritus. Lesions may be erythematous and vesicular in appearance (Figs. 29.9 and 29.10).

Assessment and Diagnosis

Differentiating between irritant, allergic, and nickel contact dermatitis is difficult based solely on clinical presentation. Obtain a thorough history of the reaction. Enquire about exposure to irritants, plants, and other possible sources of the dermatitis within the past 24 to 48 hours. Inspect the skin for lesions, noting the distribution. Eruptions at the navel, belt line, or earlobes suggest nickel contact dermatitis. Linear lesions on the hands, forearms, or legs suggest exposure to poison ivy or other plants. Diffuse lesions may indicate a reaction to soaps, detergents, or lotions.

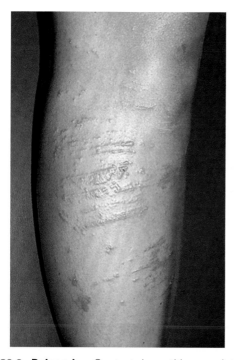

Figure 29.9. Poison ivy. Contact dermatitis associated with poison ivy. Note the pustules and erythema in a linear pattern. Reprinted with permission from Werner, R. (2012). *Massage therapist's guide to pathology* (5th ed., Fig. 2.31). Philadelphia, PA: Wolters Kluwer.

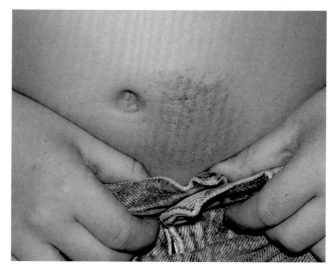

Figure 29.10. Nickel dermatitis. Contact dermatitis associated with a nickel button on jeans. Reprinted with permission from Werner, R. (2012). *Massage therapist's guide to pathology* (5th ed., Fig. 2.30). Philadelphia, PA: Wolters Kluwer.

Therapeutic Interventions

Management of contact dermatitis begins with elimination of exposure to the irritant or allergen. For exposure to one of the poisonous plants, wash the area vigorously with warm water and soap for at least 10 minutes. Topical corticosteroids are commonly used to treat contact dermatitis. If contact dermatitis is apparent on greater than 10% of the body or on the face, oral corticosteroids are prescribed. Antihistamines can be given to relieve the associated pruritus. Nursing management focuses on prevention of secondary bacterial infections of the lesions, maintenance of skin integrity, and promotion of comfort.

Evaluation

Expected outcomes for a child with contact dermatitis include the following:

- The child has no secondary bacterial infections.
- Pruritus associated with contact dermatitis decreases.
- The child remains free of further episodes of contact dermatitis.
- The parents and child verbalize understanding of triggers for contact dermatitis.

Discharge Planning and Teaching

Determine whether the parents and the child understand the mechanism for contact dermatitis. Explain that contact dermatitis is not infectious and cannot be spread to others. In addition, contact dermatitis cannot be spread from one part of the body to another by scratching. New lesions may appear days after the initial rash but are still from the primary contact. Help parents identify poison ivy, poison oak, and poison sumac so that they can eliminate them from the yard. Discuss with parents other ways to prevent contact dermatitis (Patient Teaching 29.2).

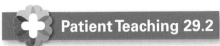

Patient Teaching 29.2

Preventing Contact Dermatitis

- Have the child wear long sleeves and pants when playing in areas known to have poison ivy, poison oak, or poison sumac.
- Wash clothes after plant exposure to get rid of the plant oils.
- Apply a commercially available precontact solution to exposed areas to minimize the risk of contact dermatitis.
- Identify the causative agent and have the child avoid it as much as possible.
- Read product labels to ensure that products contain no offending ingredients.
- Use fragrant- and dye-free products.

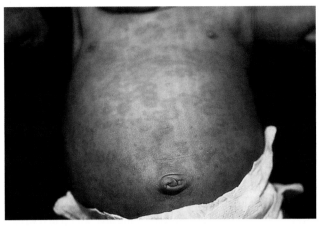

Figure 29.11. Erythema multiforme. Papules with an erythematous border and central clearing associated with erythema multiforme. Reprinted with permission from Kyle, T., & Carman, S. (2016). *Essentials of pediatric nursing* (3rd ed., Fig. 23.13). Philadelphia, PA: Wolters Kluwer.

Erythema Multiforme

Erythema multiforme is an acute hypersensitivity reaction that is more common in children older than age 10 years. Signs and symptoms of erythema multiforme often overlap or mimic signs and symptoms of Stevens-Johnson syndrome (SJS) and toxic epidermal necrolysis (TEN). It is important to distinguish between the different disorders. Erythema multiforme is self-limiting, whereas SJS and TEN require isolation and hospitalization (Sousa-Pinto, Araújo, Freitas, Correia, & Delgado, 2018).

Etiology and Pathophysiology

Although erythema multiforme was once thought to be a milder form of SJS, which is often related to sulfa drugs, continued research has shown that this is not the case. The most common cause of erythema multiforme is infection with the herpes simplex virus (HSV), with fewer than 10% of the cases being drug induced (Sousa-Pinto et al., 2018). The pathophysiology of erythema multiforme is not well known. It is thought that the rash of erythema multiforme is a cell-mediated immune response to HSV, resulting in the release of inflammatory cytokines.

Clinical Presentation

There are no prodromal symptoms associated with erythema multiforme. Erythema multiforme appears as an abrupt onset of lesions symmetrically distributed across the upper extremities, trunk, and, possibly, the oral mucosa. The lesions are characteristically doughnut shaped. Papules have an erythematous border with a central clearing, giving the appearance of a target or a bull's-eye (Fig. 29.11). On initial appearance, the lesions may resemble urticaria. However, the lesions of erythema multiforme do not disappear within 24 hours, as do those of urticaria. Lesions associated with erythema multiforme begin as macules and progress to the characteristic target lesions, which last for approximately 2 weeks.

Assessment and Diagnosis

Obtain a thorough history of the rash onset. Determine whether the child is on any medications that could possibly cause erythema multiforme. Enquire whether the child is experiencing pruritus. Assess vital signs. Inspect the skin, noting the stage and distribution of the lesions. Diagnosis is based on history and clinical presentation.

Therapeutic Interventions

Therapeutic management is supportive. Nursing interventions focus on preventing secondary infection of the lesions and maintaining skin integrity.

Evaluation

Expected outcomes for a child with erythema multiforme include the following:

- The child is free of secondary bacterial infection of the lesions.
- The child's comfort level is tolerable.

Discharge Planning and Teaching

Educate parents that some children have recurrent erythema multiforme. The lesions should resolve within 2 weeks. Tell parents that if the lesion recurs, they should notify the healthcare provider. There are no long-term sequelae associated with erythema multiforme, with the exception of hypopigmentation in individuals with darker skin.

Urticaria

Acute urticaria, more commonly known as hives, is a self-limiting reaction to an allergen.

Etiology and Pathophysiology

Urticaria is caused by an allergic trigger. The allergen stimulates an IgE reaction, activating the mast cells in the skin. The most common causes of urticaria include foods, medications, viral infections, and insect stings.

Clinical Presentation

Hives present acutely as erythematous wheals that blanch with pressure (Fig. 29.12). The lesions are transient and cause extreme pruritus. The distribution ranges from minimal to widespread. **Angioedema**, or swelling of the dermis and subcutaneous tissues, may be present. Each lesion only lasts a few hours. Most cases of hives resolve in a few days; however, some may last up to 6 weeks.

Assessment and Diagnosis

Obtain a thorough history of the onset of urticaria. Determine the causative agent depending on the history of exposure. Enquire whether the child is having any difficulty breathing, which would suggest a more systemic reaction. Assess vital signs. Inspect the skin for distribution of lesions. Palpate the lesions to determine blanching with pressure. Palpate the skin for increased warmth, particularly if angioedema is present. Observe the child's respiratory effort. Auscultate the lungs to determine respiratory involvement.

Diagnosis is based on history and clinical presentation. Children presenting with hives may be referred for allergy testing to determine triggers and prevent potential anaphylactic reactions.

Therapeutic Interventions

Acute urticaria is self-limiting. Therapeutic management focuses on identifying triggers and decreasing exposure to them. If medications are the cause, discontinue the medications immediately. Oral antihistamines are given to promote comfort. Instruct the parent and child to avoid scratching to prevent secondary infections.

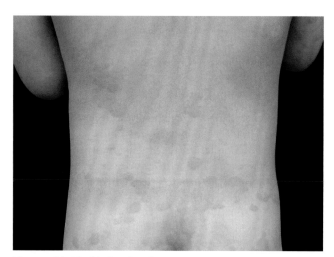

Figure 29.12. Urticaria. Erythematous wheals associated with urticaria on the lower back and buttocks of a child.

Evaluation

Expected outcomes for a child with urticaria include the following:

- Pruritus associated with urticaria is decreased.
- The child maintains normal respiratory rate and effort.
- The child has no signs or symptoms of secondary infection.
- The allergen that triggered the urticaria is identified.
- The child remains free of future episodes of urticaria.

Discharge Planning and Teaching

Educate parents and children on how to avoid triggers that elicit urticaria. If the child experiences a recurrence of urticaria, inform the family of signs and symptoms of anaphylaxis and when to call 911. For severe allergies, advise parents to have the child wear a medical alert bracelet.

Infestations

Lice, scabies, and bedbug bites are common reasons for parents to take children to see a healthcare provider. Although all of these infestations are treatable, they carry with them a stigma that may cause psychological stress for both the child and the parents.

Lice

Lice can be one of two types: head lice or body lice. Body lice are associated more with the homeless population and developing countries. This discussion focuses on head lice, which is more common in the pediatric population.

Etiology and Pathophysiology

Pediculus capitis is a head louse that commonly lays its eggs, also known as nits, at the base of human hair, close to the scalp. The common sites to lay eggs are the temple, occipital area, and postauricular area of the head (Alter et al., 2018). Lice lay approximately 7 to 10 eggs per day. Once the eggs hatch, the louse injects saliva into the scalp of the host. The saliva is the cause of the intense pruritus and excoriation associated with a head lice infestation. Lice live for 3 to 4 weeks and cannot survive off of a human head for more than 2 days (Alter et al., 2018).

The peak incidence of head lice infestation is from 3 to 12 years old. The infestation is spread through head-to-head contact, mainly through play. Sharing hair brushes, combs, hats, and towels contributes to the spread of lice, particularly in the summer months (Juern & Drolet, 2016b).

Clinical Presentation

Infestation with head lice results in a hypersensitivity reaction to the louse saliva. Head lice may be present for 2 to 6 weeks before symptoms occur (Alter et al., 2018). Most children present with intense pruritus of the scalp once the nits hatch and adult lice are present.

Assessment and Diagnosis

Obtain a health history to determine when the symptoms started. Enquire whether the child has been in contact with any children with known lice infestations. Inspect the scalp and hair shafts for nits and live head lice (Fig. 29.13). Diagnosis is made on the basis of visual identification of nits and live head lice.

Therapeutic Interventions

Treatment of head lice begins with pediculicidal agents. Permethrin is the treatment of choice and is an over-the-counter drug (The Pharmacy 29.3). One treatment is often not sufficient, and the treatment should be repeated in 7 days. Permethrin kills the live adult head lice but is not ovicidal, meaning that it does not

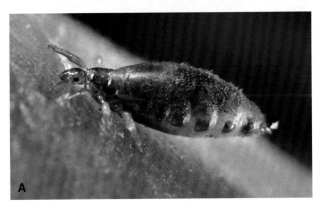

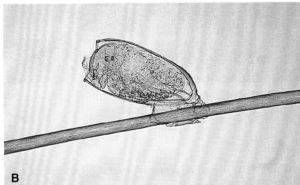

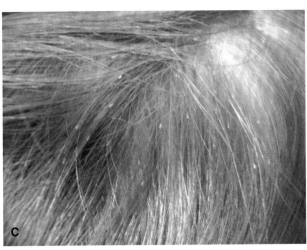

Figure 29.13. Head lice. (A) Adult louse. **(B)** Nit attached to a human hair. **(C)** Head lice infestation. Reprinted with permission from Nath, J. (2018). *Programmed learning approach to medical terminology* (3rd ed., Fig. 2.15). Philadelphia, PA: Wolters Kluwer.

The Pharmacy 29.3 Permethrin and Malathion

Medication	Classification	Route	Action	Nursing Considerations
Permethrin 1%	• Antiparasitic • Pediculicide	Top.	Inhibits sodium influx through the nerve cell membrane, resulting in paralysis and the death of the parasite	• Wash hair before application. • Apply to wet hair. • Apply enough cream to saturate the hair and scalp. • Apply behind the ears. • Leave on hair 10 min before rinsing. • Explain that itching may increase temporarily.
Malathion	• Antiparasitic • Pediculicide	Top.	Inhibits cholinesterase in head lice (used with head lice that are resistant to permethrin)	• Apply to dry hair and scalp. • Apply enough cream to saturate the hair and scalp. • Leave on overnight.

Top., topical.
Adapted from Taketomo, C. K., Hodding, J. H., & Kraus, D. M. (2018). *Pediatric & neonatal dosage handbook* (25th ed.). Hudson, OH: Lexicomp.

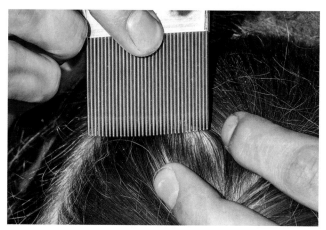

Figure 29.14. Nit comb for head lice. A parent using a nit comb to remove nits from a child's hair.

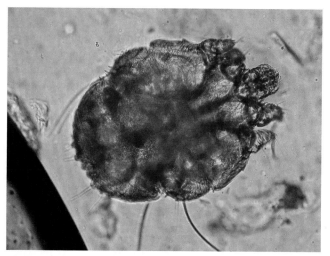

Figure 29.15. Scabies. Scabies mite. Reprinted with permission from Goroll, A. H., & Mulley, A. G. (2014). *Primary care medicine* (7th ed., Fig. 178.3). Philadelphia, PA: Wolters Kluwer.

kill the nits. Nits should be removed from wet hair with a specialized nit comb. It is important that parents section off areas of hair and remove the nits section by section.

For head lice infestations not responsive to permethrin, malathion is the drug of choice. This is a cream that is left on the scalp overnight. Malathion is ovicidal, but nit removal with a nit comb is still necessary.

In addition to applying the medicine as directed, parents must go through the child's hair nightly with a nit comb to remove the nits (Fig. 29.14). It is easier to see and remove the nits if the child's hair is wet. A lice infestation is not considered successfully treated until no more nits are seen.

Evaluation

Expected outcomes for a child with head lice include the following:

- The child is free of live head lice.
- The child is fee of nits.
- The child is free of scalp pruritus.

Discharge Planning and Teaching

When a child is diagnosed with lice, the child's parents should inform the parents of the child's closest friends, as well as the school. Children with lice often feel stigmatized because people may associate lice with uncleanliness. Educate parents and children that anyone can get lice and that there is nothing wrong with them. In addition to medication and nit removal, parents should wash the child's sheets and pillows in hot water. They should also place stuffed animals in garbage bags and seal them tightly for at least 72 hours to kill any live bugs. Remind children not to share combs or hats.

Scabies

Scabies is caused by the female mite *Sarcoptes scabiei* var. *hominis* (Alter et al., 2018; Fig. 29.15).

Etiology and Pathophysiology

The female mite burrows under the skin to lay her eggs and lays up to 25 eggs daily (Juern & Drolet, 2016b). Eggs hatch within 3 to 5 days, and the nymphs move to the surface of the skin to become mature adults and begin the cycle again. Spread of scabies is determined by the duration of physical contact. Scabies can live off of a human host for up to 3 days.

Scabies is common among those in crowded living conditions or those with poor sanitation (Alter et al., 2018). The infestation may be transmitted through contact with an infested individual's clothing or sheets, but this is a less common mode of transmission.

Clinical Presentation

Small pinpoint papules can be seen where the female mite begins her burrow. Leading away from the papule is a threadlike track that is the classic lesion of scabies (Fig. 29.16; Juern & Drolet, 2016b). Children with scabies experience intense pruritus. The most common sites include the spaces between the fingers and toes, the axillae, the buttocks, and the groin area. Secondary skin infections such as impetigo, folliculitis, or cellulitis may be present.

Scabies presents differently in infants, with papules and pustules being common. The track associated with the burrowing mite is generally not visible in infants. Common sites of scabies infestations of infants include the palms of the hands, the soles of the feet, and the scalp.

Assessment and Diagnosis

Obtain a thorough history of symptoms. Enquire about the family's living conditions. Ask about the child's participation in sports in which there is skin-to-skin contact, such as wrestling. Assess the areas of involvement. Inspect for the papules and

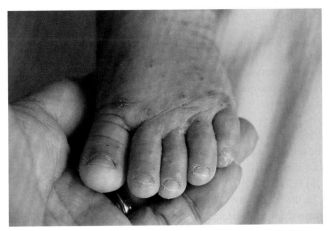

Figure 29.16. Scabies rash. Scabies rash on a child's foot.

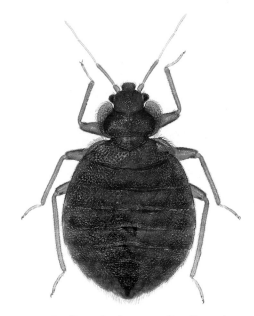

Figure 29.17. Bedbug. Bedbugs are 3 to 6 mm long.

tracks associated with scabies. Inspect for signs and symptoms of secondary infection such as erythema, edema, or drainage. Diagnosis is typically made on the basis of clinical presentation. Scrapings of skin can be examined under a microscope for a definitive diagnosis.

Therapeutic Interventions

Permethrin 5% is the treatment of choice for scabies and can be used in children 2 months and older. Teach parents to apply the cream to affected areas and rinse off 8 to 12 hours later. The treatment should be repeated in 1 to 2 weeks. Household contacts should be treated as well.

Promote comfort with oral antihistamines and topical corticosteroids. Teach parents and children the importance of avoiding scratching to prevent secondary infection of the scabies lesions.

Evaluation

Expected outcomes for a child with scabies include the following:

- The child is free of signs of scabies.
- The child is free of secondary infections.
- The child reports that pruritus is relieved.
- The child does not experience reinfestation.

Discharge Planning and Teaching

Teach parents to wash clothes and sheets in hot water. Any item that cannot be washed should be kept in a closed garbage bag for at least 72 hours.

Bedbugs

Bedbug infestations have increased in the United States over the past several years. This increase is attributed to growing worldwide travel and the bedbug's resistance to common pesticides (Alter et al., 2018).

Etiology and Pathophysiology

The common bedbug is 3 to 6 mm long, is reddish-brown, and has three legs on each side (Fig. 29.17). The lifespan of a bedbug is 6 to 12 months. Bedbugs are nocturnal insects that are difficult to detect because they live in inconspicuous places such as under mattresses, in crevices, or in furniture fabric. Bedbugs feed on mammalian blood but can live for several months without feeding (Alter et al., 2018).

Reaction to a bedbug bite is a result of the formation of antibodies to the insect's saliva. The initial bite may have no reaction. Once the antibodies are formed, however, reactions occur to subsequent bites.

Clinical Presentation

Bedbug bites cause erythematous papules on exposed areas such as the arms, neck, and trunk. The papules appear in either clusters or a linear fashion. When in a linear arrangement, the papules typically number three, giving rise to the phrase, "breakfast, lunch, and dinner" (Fig. 29.18). Bedbug saliva causes intense pruritus.

Assessment and Diagnosis

Obtain a history of present symptoms. Ask about the initial appearance of the bites. Enquire about recent travel and hotel stays. Ask whether the family has seen any bedbugs. Determine whether anyone else in the family has similar bites. Inspect the skin for lesions, noting the size, number, and location. Diagnosis is made on the basis of clinical presentation.

Therapeutic Interventions

Management focuses on promoting comfort, preventing secondary infection, and exterminating the bedbugs. Topical

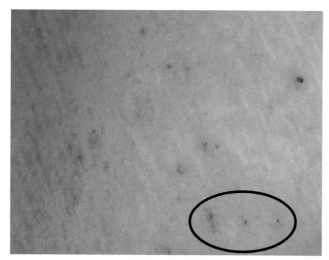

Figure 29.18. Bedbug bites. Note the linear bedbug bites in the typical "breakfast, lunch, and dinner" pattern, as indicated in the lower right corner of the photo. Modified with permission from Hall, J. C., & Hall, B. J. (2017). *Sauer's manual of skin diseases* (11th ed., Fig. 20.4). Philadelphia, PA: Wolters Kluwer.

corticosteroids and oral antihistamines are used to alleviate the pruritus associated with bedbug bites. Secondary infections from scratching are treated with topical antibiotic ointment.

Educate families to look for bedbugs at night with a flashlight under mattresses and box springs, around headboards, and in crevices in the child's bedroom. A professional exterminator is required to rid a house of bedbugs.

Evaluation

Expected outcomes for a child with bedbug bites include the following:

- The child's home has no signs of bedbugs.
- The child is free of secondary infections.
- The child reports that pruritus is relieved.

Discharge Planning and Teaching

Teach parents and children to inspect suitcases and other bags after travel. If there is any concern of bedbug exposure, wash all sheets and clothes in hot water or place items in the dryer on high heat for at least 30 minutes to kill any live bugs. Items that cannot be washed or dried in high heat should be placed in a closed garbage bag for at least 72 hours. Complete extermination is necessary to prevent reinfestation.

Injuries

Integumentary injuries are common in children and adolescents because of the nature of a child's skin and developmental stage. The most common injuries during childhood include burns, sunburn, frostbite, insect stings, spider bites, and human and animal bites.

Burns

Burns are common causes of unintentional injury in children and adolescents. According to the Centers for Disease Control and Prevention (CDC, 2016), about 300 children are treated daily in emergency rooms for unintentional burns. Of the children seen with burn injuries, about 15,000 are hospitalized per year, and approximately 1,000 of the hospitalized children and adolescents die from their injuries (Burn Foundation, 2018). Burns are the fifth leading cause of death in children 1 to 4 years old and the third leading cause of death in children 5 to 9 years old (CDC, 2018).

Although most burns sustained by children and adolescents do not result in death, even minor burns can cause significant pain. The more serious the burn is, the more significant the long-term sequelae are. If the burn extends beyond the superficial layers of the skin, there is potential for scarring. Disfigurement occurs if the deep layers of the integument are involved and skin grafts are required for healing.

Etiology and Pathophysiology

Thermal and chemical burns are among the most common types of burns in children and adolescents (Yin, 2017). Thermal burns occur after a child comes into contact with a hot surface, hot liquid, or fire. The most common type of thermal burns during the toddler years is scalding burns, which typically result from a child pulling a hot pan off of a stove or being immersed in bathwater that is too hot. Hot objects that cause thermal burn in children include irons, flat irons, curling irons, stoves, and ovens. During the school-age years, thermal burns are often caused by playing with matches, fireworks, or gasoline (Burn Foundation, 2018).

Chemical burns occur when chemicals come into contact with the skin, causing direct injury to the cells. Common causes of chemical burns are household cleaning agents such as drain cleaners, oven cleaners, toilet bowl cleaners, and detergents (Yin, 2017). Chemical burns to the airway occur when the child swallows a caustic substance and may cause significant esophageal swelling.

Burn injury causes coagulation to the exposed skin and underlying tissues. Areas of tissue adjacent to the burn area may also be affected by coagulation, vascular leakage, and inflammatory mediators, resulting in decreased tissue perfusion (Kaddoura, Abu-Sittah, Ibrahim, Karamanoukian, & Papazian, 2017). The extent of the damage depends on the type of injury, the temperature to which the skin is exposed, and the amount of time the skin is exposed. The longer the exposure or the higher the temperature, the deeper into the tissues the injury occurs. Even superficial burns cause some damage to the underlying tissue.

When burns exceed 30% of the total BSA, the child is at risk for hypovolemia and shock. There is decreased plasma volume, decreased cardiac output, and decreased urine output. Conversely, there is increased systemic vascular resistance (SVR) and decreased perfusion to the extremities (Kaddoura et al., 2017).

The inflammatory response creates increased capillary permeability. The increased permeability allows for fluid, electrolytes, and large molecules, such as protein, to leave the capillaries and enter the interstitial space, or **third space**, resulting in edema. The loss of capillary contents results in intravascular dehydration. Fluid loss occurs as a result of damaged skin. Partial-thickness and deeper burns cause the skin to lose protection against fluid loss until the skin is healed.

Severe burns increase the body's metabolic rate and glucose metabolism through the release of inflammatory mediators. The resting basal metabolic rate in a burn patient with burns covering 40% of total BSA is two times that of normal (Kaddoura et al., 2017). In addition, muscle is degraded at a higher rate because of the same inflammatory mediators, resulting in protein loss and a decrease in lean muscle mass.

Severe burns also significantly affect the cardiac and renal systems. Decreased cardiac output and increased SVR require increased workload of the heart. In addition, the decreased blood flow to the kidneys results in oliguria or anuria, putting the child at risk for renal failure.

Severe burns result in immunosuppression. Not only does damage to the skin decrease the body's mechanical barrier to infectious agents but overall impairment of the body's immune function also results in postburn bacterial and fungal infections (Kaddoura et al., 2017).

Clinical Presentation

Clinical presentation depends on the type and severity of the burn. Children with a superficial burn present with a painful, red area at the site of the burn. Blistering and edema are not present. Children with more severe burns may present with blistering, loss of skin, edema, and symptoms of burn shock (Fig. 29.19). If the child ingested a caustic agent, drooling and respiratory distress are present because of damage to the mucosal layer of the esophagus. When smoke inhalation is present, respiratory distress is caused as a result of esophageal edema.

In Chapter 11, Chase McGovern presented with burns over a third of his body. What were his presenting symptoms? What were the priority nursing interventions for Chase? What were the potential life-threatening consequences of his burns?

Assessment and Diagnosis

The first priority is to determine whether the child's condition is emergent through a primary survey. If the child's condition is emergent, obtain a quick health history if possible while providing emergency care. A primary survey of the child includes an assessment of airway, breathing, and circulation. Determine the child's respiratory status. If facial burns or smoke on the face is present, assume esophageal involvement and prepare for intubation. Determine perfusion status by assessing the color of the skin and strength of peripheral pulses. Assess the child's heart rate. Assess for edema, noting the location and amount.

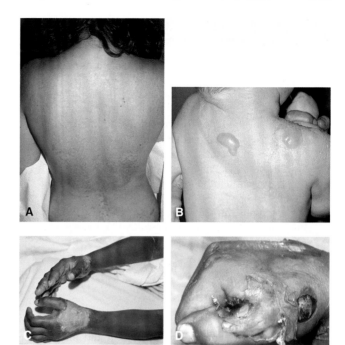

Figure 29.19. Types of burns. (A) Superficial burn. **(B)** Superficial partial-thickness burn with large blisters. **(C)** Deep partial-thickness burn. **(D)** Full-thickness burn with eschar. Part A reprinted with permission from Goodheart, H. P. (2003). *Goodheart's photoguide of common skin disorders* (2nd ed.). Philadelphia, PA: Lippincott Williams & Wilkins. Parts B and C reprinted with permission from Fleisher, G. R., Ludwig, S., & Baskin, M. N. (Eds.). (2004). *Atlas of pediatric emergency medicine* (1st ed.). Philadelphia, PA: Lippincott Williams & Wilkins. Part D reprinted with permission from Rubin, E., & Farber, J. L. (1999). *Pathology* (3rd ed.). Philadelphia, PA: Lippincott Williams & Wilkins.

If the child is not emergent, obtain a history of the injury from the parents. Determine whether the injury matches the mechanism of injury identified by the parents. If not, suspect child abuse. For example, a typical scald burn on a toddler has a splash pattern from hot liquid splashing on the skin. A well-demarcated burn on the hand that looks like a glove might indicate that the child's hand was held in scalding water, perhaps as a punishment. Furthermore, small, round burns may indicate cigarette burns inflicted by a parent or caregiver.

Once the child is stable, perform a secondary survey. The secondary survey includes assessment of the burn depth (see Table 11.1 and Fig. 11.1). Determine whether the wounded area is blistered or weeping and whether **eschar**, or dead skin tissue being sloughed off, is present. Determine whether there are any other injuries besides burns. Finally, estimate the total BSA covered in burns. The volume of fluid needed for fluid resuscitation is calculated on the basis of the depth of the burns and the total BSA involved. It is important to use age-appropriate tools to estimate the percentage of the body that is burned (see Box 11.1).

Diagnostic testing is used to determine systemic effects of the burns (Box 29.1).

Box 29.1 Diagnostic Testing for Burns

- Complete blood count with differential: to determine immune status
- Electrolyte panel: to monitor electrolyte disturbances and kidney function
- Albumin level: to monitor protein and nutritional status
- Arterial blood gases: to determine the presence of an acid/base imbalance
- Carboxyhemoglobin level: to detect carbon monoxide poisoning (used if the child was confined in a closed space)
- Electrocardiogram: to detect arrhythmia or damage to the heart due to electrical shock (used if the child has an electrical burn)

Therapeutic Interventions

Treatment of burns in children and adolescents is focused on proper wound care. Prevention of infection and maintaining fluid balance are priority interventions. The treatment regimen depends on the severity of the burns and whether the child is admitted to the hospital. The American Burn Association has established criteria for when children should be admitted to a burn center (Box 29.2).

Superficial burns and superficial partial-thickness burns that cover less than 10% of the total BSA can be treated on an outpatient basis. Only outstanding circumstances, such as suspected child abuse or the inability of the parents to adequately care for the child, would warrant hospitalization in children with these types of burns. If blisters are present, they should be left intact. Wash the area with lukewarm water. Dress the wound

Box 29.2 Criteria for the Admission of a Child to a Burn Center

- Partial-thickness burns affecting over 10% of the BSA
- Burns that involve the face, hands, feet, joints, or genitalia
- Full-thickness burns in a child of any age
- Inhalation injury, regardless of the type of burn
- Preexisting medical conditions that could complicate recovery, regardless of the type of burn
- Chemical burns
- Electrical burns
- Suspected child abuse
- Poor social situation
- Concomitant injuries
- Burns that will require extensive rehabilitation and emotional support

Adapted from Yin, S. (2017). Chemical and common burns in children. *Clinical Pediatrics, 55*(5S), 8S–12S and Antoon, A. Y., & Donovan, M. K. (2016a). Burn injuries. In R. M. Kliegman, B. F. Stanton, J. W. St. Geme III, N. F. Schor, & R. E. Behrman (Eds.), *Nelson's textbook of pediatrics* (20th ed.). Philadelphia, PA: Elsevier, Saunders.

with either bacitracin or sulfadiazine cream (see Chapter 11) and change the dressing once daily. If the blisters rupture, wash the area with warm water and continue daily dressing changes until healed (Antoon & Donovan, 2016a). Superficial partial-thickness burns are treated with a wound membrane saturated with silver iron, which promotes healing and pain control. This dressing is applied to the wound and covered with a dry, sterile dressing. The dressing is left on for a week at a time but checked twice a week (Antoon & Donovan, 2016a).

Children with full-thickness burns or burns over 10% of the BSA are admitted to a pediatric burn treatment center for care. Care for these children centers on airway management, fluid resuscitation, thermoregulation, pain control, monitoring of nutritional status, promotion of healing, prevention of infection, psychosocial support, and education (discussed in detail later). Children with deep partial- and full-thickness burns require skin grafts to promote healing (Box 29.3). Monitor for complications of skin grafts such as infection, rejection, and contractures. These children need physical therapy and occupational therapy to promote both gross and fine motor skill rehabilitation.

Maintain a Patent Airway and Adequate Oxygenation

During the primary survey, determine whether the airway is compromised or whether the child has a potential inhalation injury. Assist with intubation as needed. Monitor the child's O_2 saturation level and administer oxygen as ordered via a nonrebreather mask. Continue to monitor that child's airway closely as pulmonary edema can develop as late as 48 hours after the injury (Antoon & Donovan, 2016a).

Box 29.3 Types of Grafts

Allograft

- Is a graft of cadaver skin
- Is the graft of choice
- Stimulates epithelial growth
- Cannot be used with extensive burn injuries
- Requires immunosuppressive therapy
- Is short term
- May be rejected in the first 1–2 weeks (Dixit et al., 2017)

Xenograft

- Is a graft from a different species, often porcine
- Stimulates epithelial growth
- Is short term
- Requires frequent replacement

Bioengineered Skin

- Is grown using synthetic materials and living cells, the latter of which may be autologous or allogenic (Dixit et al., 2017)
- Allows for regeneration of the dermal layer
- May be short term or permanent
- Results in a decreased antigenic response, leading to a decreased risk of rejection (Dixit et al., 2017)

Assess the child's lung sounds frequently. Wheezes are common after an inhalation injury. Monitor for decreased breath sounds or crackles, which indicate a complication such as pneumonia.

Maintain Adequate Fluid Volume

Begin fluid resuscitation immediately with lactated Ringer solution. Determine the amount of fluid needed in the first 24 hours by using the Parkland formula (see Box 11.2). After 24 hours, add 5% glucose to the solution to prevent hypoglycemia. Weight initially increases because of increased interstitial fluid. Fluid begins to reabsorb after the first 24 hours, and the child has increased urinary output because of diuresis (Romanowski & Palmieri, 2017).

Monitor urine output via a Foley catheter, and notify the healthcare provider if output is less than 2 mg/kg/h. Assess daily weights to determine fluid status. Assess capillary refill and peripheral pulses to determine adequate circulation. Monitor sodium and potassium levels to detect hyponatremia and hypokalemia. Monitor blood urea nitrogen and creatinine levels to determine kidney function. Monitor arterial blood gas levels for acid-base imbalances.

Maintain Normal Body Temperature

Children have a larger BSA-to-volume ratio and thinner skin than adults, which puts them at increased risk for altered thermoregulation (Gill & Falder, 2017). Monitor the child's body temperature. Keep the room warm and the child covered to prevent heat loss.

Promote Pain Relief

Pain control is important to treat the pain associated with the burns as well as the pain caused by dressing changes. Children with superficial burns can typically manage pain with an oral analgesic such as acetaminophen or ibuprofen. Children hospitalized with more severe burns need extensive pain management. The injury itself is painful, unless the nerves are damaged, as occurs in a full-thickness burn. Adequately assess pain and administer intravenous pain medication as ordered. Once the child is stabilized, continue to assess pain at regular intervals using a developmentally appropriate pain tool.

Wound cleansing and dressing changes are painful procedures (How Much Does It Hurt? 29.1). Often, children require additional analgesics, or possibly sedatives, before these procedures. Assess the child's pain level before, during, and after dressing changes. Alert the healthcare provider if pain control is inadequate.

Maintain Adequate Nutrition

Burns can cause increased protein catabolism, leading to decreased lean muscle mass (Kaddoura et al., 2017). In addition, children with burns covering 30% or more of their BSA experience increased energy expenditure and increased metabolism (Antoon & Donovan, 2016a).

Interventions focus on meeting the energy needs of the child to promote adequate nutrition and healing. Ensure that the child is receiving calories equal to one-and-a-half times the

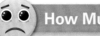
How Much Does it Hurt? 29.1

Burn Wound Dressing Changes

Burn wound dressing changes are extremely painful. Administering analgesics before the start of the procedure is imperative. Some dressing changes are so extensive that the child may require mild sedation to tolerate the procedure. Determine with the child, if appropriate, and the parents a tolerable pain level. Use an age-appropriate pain scale to assess the child's pain level both before and after the dressing change. If the agreed-upon tolerable pain level cannot be achieved with the ordered medications, notify the healthcare provider.

basal metabolic rate, along with 3 to 4 g/kg of protein per day. Nasogastric feedings may be necessary to ensure that the child is receiving adequate calories to promote healing.

Promote Wound Healing

Dressing changes with appropriate supplies are crucial to promote healing of burns. The type of dressing used depends on the type and location of the burn, the frequency of dressing changes, and the desired amount of continuous moisture. The dressing should prevent contamination of the wound, decrease physical damage to skin during dressing changes, and allow for adequate air flow and moisture retention. Many of commercial dressings are impregnated with silver, which helps prevent infection (Rowan et al., 2015; Analyze the Evidence 29.1). Synthetic

Analyze the Evidence 29.1

Dressings

Many commercial dressings are on the market to promote healing in children with burns. Most of the dressings are impregnated with silver, which helps prevent infection. However, many of these dressings adhere to the wound, causing damage to healing skin when removed for dressing changes.

Kee et al. (2015) conducted a randomized control trial of three different burn dressings for partial-thickness burns. The dressings tested were Acticoat; Acticoat with Mepitel; or Mepilex Ag. The researchers found that the dressing that was impregnated with silver and had a silicone interface, Mepilex Ag, promoted faster reepithelialization. The silicone interface allowed the dressing to adhere to the skin around the wound but not to the wound itself, thereby decreasing the amount of damage and pain during dressing changes.

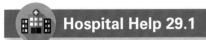

Hospital Help 29.1

Dressing Changes

Eliciting the child's cooperation during dressing changes and other interventions, as in the following ways, helps decrease pain and discomfort:

- Encourage children to be involved in their care at an age-appropriate level.
- Explain the dressing change procedure in age-appropriate terms.
- Allow the child to choose a means of distraction, such as television or music.
- Allow the child to determine on which area of the body to start the dressing change.
- Encourage the child to participate in the dressing change, if able.
- Provide positive feedback throughout the procedure.

skin coverings may be used with extensive wounds to minimize fluid loss, maintain temperature, and minimize pain (Antoon & Donovan, 2016a). No matter the type of dressing, involving the child in care of the dressing can improve outcomes (Hospital Help 29.1).

Prevent Infection

Preventing infection promotes healing and prevents further complications in the child with burns (Priority Care Concepts 29.1). If the child's immunization status is unknown or if it has been 5 years or more since the child's last tetanus shot, administer the tetanus vaccine or the tetanus Ig as ordered (Antoon & Donovan, 2016a).

Priority Care Concepts 29.1

Preventing Sepsis

Infection of burn wounds can quickly lead to sepsis. Nurses need to monitor the child's status closely and be alert for even minor changes in status. The following signs and symptoms indicate possible sepsis and should be reported to the healthcare provider immediately:

- Fever
- Decreased level of consciousness
- Lethargy
- Decreased capillary refill
- Diminished pulses
- Decreased bowel sounds
- Impaired wound healing
- Decreased white blood cell count

Perform dressing changes as ordered. Wear a gown, gloves, and a mask during dressing changes. When the dressings are off, assess the wounds for healing. Note any signs and symptoms of infection, such as drainage, foul odor, erythema, or edema. Note the color of the skin around the wounds. Notify the healthcare provider if the skin appears dark in color. Administer topical antibiotic ointments and parenteral antibiotics as ordered. Monitor for fever. Teach parents how to do proper dressing changes at home.

Promote Skin Integrity

Children with partial- and full-thickness burns experience a significant amount of scarring (Fig. 29.20). Scarring may interfere with range of motion; therefore, the child must participate in physical and occupational therapy. Physical and occupational therapy begin in the hospital and continue after discharge to

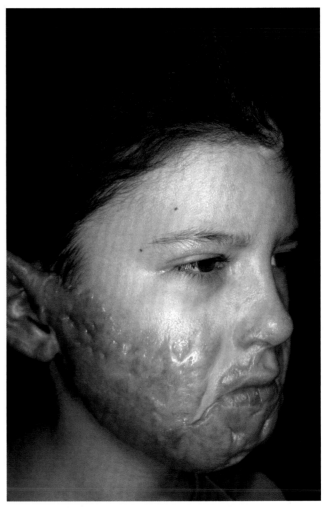

Figure 29.20. Scarring. Severe scarring from full-thickness burns on the face of a school-age child. Reprinted with permission from Thorne, C. H., Gurtner, G. C., Chung, K., Gosain, A., Mehrara, B., Rubin, P., & Spear, S. L. (2013). *Grabb and Smith's plastic surgery* (7th ed., Fig. 16.3A). Philadelphia, PA: Lippincott Williams & Wilkins.

prevent contractures and promote range of motion. Compression helps prevent excessive scarring by decreasing the blood flow to the forming scar tissue.

Healing burns often cause intense pruritus. Pruritus is treated with an oral antihistamine. In addition, application of moisturizers helps relieve any pruritus associated with wound healing. Massaging the scar tissue while applying moisturizer stretches the scar tissue and may help promote range of motion.

Provide Psychosocial Support

Families with children who have been burned need psychosocial support not only during hospitalization but also with long-term recovery. Parents' biggest stressors during the child's hospitalization include pain control, lengthy dressing changes, disfigurement, and uncertain outcomes for the child (Rimmer et al., 2015). Include parents in care decisions as part of their child's healthcare team throughout the child's hospital stay. Keep the family informed of the child's progress and what to expect with the next steps of care. The long hospital stays and multiple treatments can be a financial burden for families. Provide families with information on resources such as social workers and support groups to help navigate these stressors. Ensure there is an assessment of the home environment to determine what is needed for the family to care for the child at home. Develop a plan of care with the family and establish realistic expectations of recovery.

In addition to providing psychosocial support to the family, ensure that the child receives individual support. Involve the child in his or her care, if age appropriate (Growth and Development Check 29.1). Encourage children through positive reinforcement. Hypopigmentation of the burn site can last up to

6 months, and erythema of graft sites may last up to 12 months (Kee, Kimble, Cuttle, Khan, & Stockton, 2015). Multiple cosmetic surgeries are often necessary to maximize function and enhance the appearance of the grafts. Children, especially late school-age children and adolescents, need support to deal with the changes in body image.

Evaluation

Although care differs depending on the location and thickness of the burns, evaluation focuses on healing. Expected outcomes for a child with a burn injury include the following:

- O_2 saturation levels remain at or above 95%.
- The child maintains a patent airway.
- Pain is at a level designated as tolerable by the child.
- The child's urine output is adequate.
- The child demonstrates increased caloric and protein intake.
- Wound healing is in process.
- The child has no signs or symptoms of infection.
- No contractures are present.
- The parents demonstrate dressing changes.
- The parents and child voice concerns over the healing process and change in body image.

Discharge Planning and Teaching

When the child is in the hospital, educate the parents on how to change dressings and recognize signs and symptoms of infection. Before discharge, have parents demonstrate proper dressing change technique. Discuss signs and symptoms of infection and when to call the healthcare provider. Teach parents measures to prevent burn injuries (Patient Teaching 29.3). These measures include monitoring the temperature of the child's bathwater,

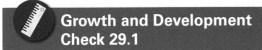

Growth and Development Check 29.1

Regression

Serious injuries, such as partial-thickness burns, interfere with growth and development at any age. Therefore, explain to parents that regression of development is also normal at any age. Toddlers, who are in the stage of autonomy versus shame and doubt, are no longer able to perform many tasks independently. School-age children, who are mastering tasks and becoming independent from parents, find themselves now relying on caregivers for activities of daily living. Scarring and loss of independence interferes with the adolescent's identity development.

Encourage age-appropriate involvement in care to help children and adolescents achieve developmental milestones. Ensure that children are given tasks they can master. Allow older children and adolescents to voice their frustration and anger. Provide information on support groups for adolescents with extensive burns.

Patient Teaching 29.3

Preventing Burns

- Keep the temperature of the hot water heater at 120°F (48.9°C) or lower (Fig. 29.21).
- Monitor the temperature of the child's bathwater.
- Keep the child away from hot liquids.
- Avoid drinking hot beverages while holding the child.
- Place all pots and pans on the back burner of the stove with the handles pointing toward the back.
- Never leave the child alone in the kitchen with the stove or oven on.
- Lock up matches or any other type of lighters.
- Lock up any cleaning fluids or other caustic agents.
- Ensure there are no frayed electrical wires in the home.
- Cover electrical outlets with safety covers, and teach the child not to touch the outlets.
- Have a fire escape plan.
- Teach the child, when old enough, to stop, drop, and roll.

Hot Water Burn & Scalding Graph

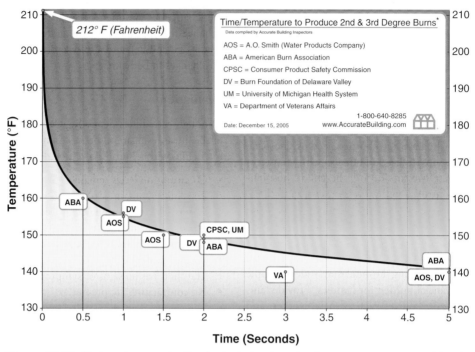

Figure 29.21. Hot water graph. Graph depicting length of water exposure resulting in burns based on water temperature. Used with permission of Accurate Building Inspectors. (2011). *Water temperature thermometry.* Retrieved June 5, 2011, from http://www.accuratebuilding.com/services/legal/charts/hot_water_burn_scalding_graph.html.

turning the pan handles toward the back of the stove, and locking up matches. Discuss with parents the temperature of the hot water heater and the potential for scald injuries in young children (Fig. 29.21). Also teach them how to care for minor burns at home (Patient Teaching 29.4).

Provide education on the therapies needed after discharge, as well as the potential healing time. Ensure that physical and occupational therapy appointments, as well as any other follow-up appointments, are scheduled.

Explain to parents that the child should return to school as quickly as possible after discharge, even if for only half the day.

Patient Teaching 29.4

Care of Minor Burns at Home

- Run cold water over the affected area.
- Do not apply ice to the affected area.
- If blisters form, leave them intact.
- Administer acetaminophen or ibuprofen for pain and discomfort.
- Pat the skin after bathing, do not rub it.
- Avoid having tight clothing over the affected area.

After discharge, work with parents to answer questions and ease the anxiety of teachers, school staff, and children. Explain to teachers that children may have decreased gross and fine motor skills, depending on the location of the injury (Pan et al., 2018).

Sunburn

Sunburn is similar to a thermal burn and can occur at any age, causing damage to the epidermis. This damage increases the risk of malignant melanoma in adulthood. Children and adolescents from 6 months to 18 years of age, especially those with fair skin, should minimize exposure to ultraviolet B (UVB) radiation to reduce their risk of skin cancer (Robinson & Jablonski, 2018).

Etiology and Pathophysiology

Sunburn is caused by exposure to UVB radiation. Effects from exposure to UVB radiation appear within 6 to 12 hours and peak at 24 hours (Dickey & Chiu, 2016b). Keratinocyte membrane damage occurs as a result of oxidative damage from UVB radiation exposure. The erythema associated with sunburn is mediated by prostaglandins and inflammatory cytokines. Sunburn is self-limiting. Desquamation occurs about 1 week after exposure. Scarring does not occur.

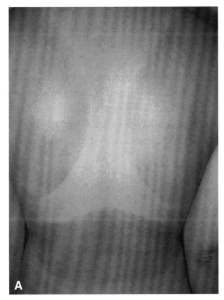
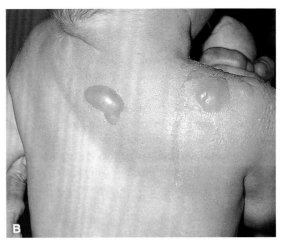

Figure 29.22. Sunburn. (A) First-degree sunburn on a child's back. **(B)** Second-degree sunburn with substantial blisters on a young child's back. Part A provided by Stedman's. Part B reprinted with permission from Fleisher, G. R., Ludwig, S., & Baskin, M. N. (Eds.). (2004). *Atlas of pediatric emergency medicine* (1st ed.). Philadelphia, PA: Lippincott Williams & Wilkins.

Clinical Presentation

Sunburn occurs on areas of the skin not covered with clothing or protected by sunscreen (Fig. 29.22). The areas are erythematous and tender and may blister depending on the extent of sun exposure. Fever, chills, nausea, and headache may occur with severe sunburn.

Assessment and Diagnosis

Obtain a history that includes the amount of time the child spent in the sun, the time of day of sun exposure, and whether sunscreen was used. Ask about pain level, presence of fever, chills, nausea, or headache. Inspect the skin for all areas of sun exposure. Note any blistering and document the location and size of the blisters. Diagnosis is made on the basis of clinical presentation.

Therapeutic Interventions

Promoting comfort and educating parents about prevention of future sunburns are the focus of treatment for the child with sunburn. Cool compresses to the affected areas and cool baths can help with the burning. Acetaminophen or ibuprofen helps relieve the pain associated with sunburn. Have the child wear loose clothing to promote comfort.

Severe sunburns, such as those over a large portion of the body or with significant blistering, are treated like a thermal burn. Children with severe sunburns may need fluid resuscitation and hospitalization.

Evaluation

The main expected outcome for a child with sunburn is comfort. Evaluate the child's pain level to determine whether it is at an acceptable level for the parent and child.

Discharge Planning and Teaching

Educate parents and children that the skin may itch as the sunburn begins to heal. Instruct the child not to pick at the skin once the burned areas begin to peel. Teach parents and children the best ways to prevent sunburn in the future (Patient Teaching 29.5).

Frostbite

Exposure to cold without proper attire or for extended periods of time places children and adolescents at risk of frostbite.

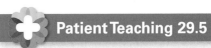
Patient Teaching 29.5

Preventing Sunburn

- Keep a child who is under 6 months old out of the sun.
- Keep a child who is 6 months or older out of the sun from 10:00 a.m. to 4:00 p.m.
- Have the child wear sun protective clothing such as a swim shirt with sun protective factor (SPF) in the material.
- Apply sunscreen of at least 15 SPF to all exposed areas.
- Only apply sunscreen to infants younger than 6 months old sparingly; keeping them out of the sun is best.
- Reapply sunscreen every 2 hours or after swimming or sweating.
- Have the child wear a wide-brimmed hat.
- Use umbrellas and tents for shade.

Those involved in winter sports, such as skiing and snowboarding, are at increased risk of cold injury. Children in homeless families are also at increased risk of cold injury during winter months in certain parts of the country.

Etiology and Pathophysiology

Frostbite occurs with exposure to extreme cold, less than 5°F (−15°C), for any duration or to temperatures below 32°F (0°C) for an extended period of time. Body heat is lost through wet clothing, through contact with cold metals, or when there is a strong wind chill. Dehydration, hunger, exhaustion, and anemia can exacerbate cold injury (Antoon & Donovan, 2016b). Any body part can be affected, but body parts that are exposed or covered with restrictive clothing are the most common areas of injury. The areas of the body most commonly affected are the hands, feet, ears, and nose.

When the skin is exposed to below-freezing temperatures, ice crystals begin to form in the extracellular and intracellular spaces (Laskowski-Jones & Jones, 2018). These ice crystals interfere with intracellular electrolytes. Blood is shunted to the core of the body to protect the major organs. The electrolyte disturbances and vasoconstriction cause tissue and nerve damage in the exposed areas. Damage can range from mild to severe.

Clinical Presentation

Clinical presentation depends on the degree of frostbite. First-degree frostbite symptoms include a stinging sensation in the skin, numbness, and edema. Frostbite that extends deeper into the tissues, or second-degree frostbite, results in skin that appears waxy, has a blue or white tint, and is hard to the touch. Either clear or hemorrhagic vesicles may appear over the affected areas with third-degree frostbite. Fourth-degree frostbite involves sloughing of the skin and gangrene (Laskowski-Jones & Jones, 2018).

Assessment and Diagnosis

Obtain a thorough history of the injury. Determine what the child was doing in the cold, the length of time of exposure, and the amount of clothing the child was wearing. Inspect the affected area for redness, edema, waxy and pale appearance, vesicles, or sloughing of the skin. Palpate the skin to assess temperature and texture. Conduct a pain assessment. Determine whether numbness is present. The diagnosis of frostbite is made on the basis of history and clinical presentation. Tissue damage is determined with diagnostic imaging.

Therapeutic Interventions

Initial treatment involves rewarming the affected areas. Rewarming is accomplished by placing the affected areas in warm water at a temperature of 37°C (98.6°F) to 39°C (102.2°F) for at least 30 minutes (Laskowski-Jones & Jones, 2018). Wound care specialists and plastic surgeons are involved in the care of children with more severe frostbite. Fourth-degree frostbite may require amputation.

Promoting comfort, promoting skin integrity, preventing secondary infection, and providing education are important nursing interventions for the child with frostbite. Do not massage the area because it may cause tissue damage. Rewarming is painful. Administer analgesics as ordered. Once the area is rewarmed, assess sensation and movement. Assess the color of the skin, which should be red to purple after rewarming. Continue to monitor the child's pain level and treat as ordered. Broken vesicles may need to be debrided to prevent secondary infection.

Evaluation

Expected outcomes for a child with frostbite include the following:

- The affected area remains warm.
- Sensation and movement are intact.
- The affected area functions optimally.
- The parents demonstrate an understanding of frostbite prevention.

Discharge Planning and Teaching

Children with third- and fourth-degree frostbite need follow-up with either the wound care specialist or the plastic surgeon. Ensure that follow-up appointments are scheduled as ordered. Educate parents on the causes of frostbite and how to prevent it (Patient Teaching 29.6).

Insect Stings and Spider Bites

Insect stings and spider bites produce mostly local reactions. Systemic reactions occur in only 0.4% to 0.8% of children in the United States (Wang & Sicherer, 2016). Systemic reactions include edema and airway compromise, leading to emergent situations. This discussion focuses on local reactions. Refer to the discussion on anaphylaxis in Chapter 34 for systemic reactions to insect stings.

Etiology and Pathophysiology

The order Hymenoptera includes the stinging insects, such as yellow jackets, hornets, wasps, honey bees, and bumblebees. Of

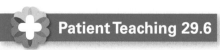

Patient Teaching 29.6

Preventing Frostbite

- Heed winter weather and wind chill advisories.
- When temperatures are below freezing, cover exposed skin on the hands, head, and ears.
- Wear layers that are waterproof and windproof.
- Do not wear multiple layers of socks and gloves, which may decrease circulation to the extremities.
- Exhaustion, dehydration, and poor nutrition increase the risk for frostbite.

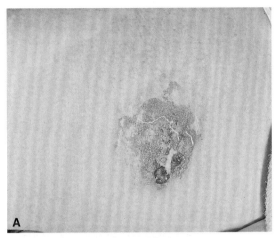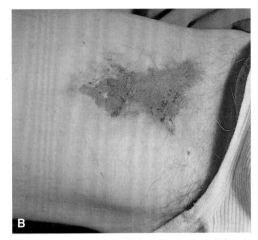

Figure 29.23. Spider bite. (A) Spider bite, with erythema, central necrosis, and blister formation. **(B)** Spider bite, with vertical extension of necrosis due to gravity. Reprinted with permission from Hall, J. C., & Hall, B. J. (2017). *Sauer's manual of skin diseases* (11th ed., Fig. 20.4). Philadelphia, PA: Wolters Kluwer.

these, yellow jackets are the most aggressive and most likely to sting. Honey bees are less aggressive but are the most likely to leave a barbed stinger in the skin. Localized responses are caused by vasoactive and irritant substances in the venom or other fluids of Hymenoptera (Wang & Sicherer, 2016).

Spiders inject venom into the skin with each bite. Most spider bites have a local reaction. The venom attacks the cell membrane and causes local tissue damage. The most serious reactions occur with brown recluse and black widow spiders. Black widow spider bites are neurotoxic, whereas brown recluse spiders cause a necrotizing reaction. The remainder of this discussion focuses only on local reactions to spider bites.

Clinical Presentation

Local reactions to insect stings and spider bites include pruritus, erythema, edema, and possibly pain (Figs. 29.23 and 29.24). Symptoms generally last for less than 24 hours. Large local reactions occur occasionally. These reactions may not appear for a day or two after the sting or bite, are larger than 10 cm, and can last for several days.

Assessment and Diagnosis

Obtain a history of the bite or sting. Enquire about when and where the bite or sting occurred. Ask the parent and child whether they saw the insect or spider, especially if a black widow or brown recluse spider bite is suspected. Assess pain level and pruritus. Inspect the affected area for erythema and edema. Note the size of the papule and whether the stinger is still present. Assess for systemic reaction. Auscultate the lungs bilaterally for wheezing to determine respiratory involvement. Diagnosis is made on the basis of history and clinical presentation.

Therapeutic Interventions

Management focuses on promoting comfort, preventing secondary infection, and providing prevention education. If the

stinger is still present, remove by scraping the skin. Do not pinch the skin because it may release more venom from the stinger. Use cold compresses for pain relief. Meat tenderizer or a baking soda paste may also be applied to promote comfort (American Academy of Pediatrics, 2018). Antihistamines and topical corticosteroids may be used if pain and itching are not relieved by other methods.

Teach children not to scratch the bite. Scratching may lead to secondary infection of the area.

Evaluation

Expected outcomes for a child with an insect sting or spider bite include the following:

- The child is free of signs and symptoms of a systemic reaction to the insect sting or spider bite.
- The child's pain is at a level acceptable to the parent and child.

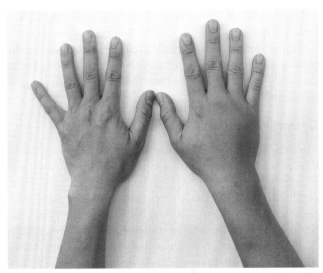

Figure 29.24. Insect sting. Erythema associated with an insect sting. Note the difference between the hands.

- The child is free of signs and symptoms of a secondary infection.
- The parents and child verbalize understanding of how to prevent insect stings and spider bites.

Discharge Planning and Teaching

The best way to manage insect stings and spider bites is to prevent them. Educate parents and older children to wear insect repellent when outside during the summer, especially in wooded areas. Teach children how to identify wasp nests, hornet nests, and bee hives and emphasize not to disturb them. Parents and children should inspect the inside of shoes that have been in storage or in the garage for spiders before putting them on.

Human and Animal Bites

Animal bites represent 1% of emergency room visits, or 4.7 million visits, per year in the United States (Hurt & Maday, 2018). Most animal bites occur to children 6 to 11 years old, and 75% are inflicted by animals the child knows. Fifty percent of animal bites are said to be unprovoked (American Academy of Pediatrics, 2015; Ginsburg & Hunstead, 2016).

Etiology and Pathophysiology

The most common animal bites are from dogs and cats, followed by rodents. Dog bites account for 80% to 90% of all animal bites in the United States, followed by cat bites at 5% to 15% and rodent bites at 2% to 5%. About 2% of dog bites require hospitalization, whereas 6% of cat bites require hospitalization (Ginsburg & Hunstead, 2016; Hurt & Maday, 2018). Dog bites cause approximately 10 to 20 deaths per year in children. The breeds most responsible for deadly bites are pit bulls and Rottweilers (Hurt & Maday, 2018).

Wounds from dog bites are contaminated with organisms such as *Streptococcus* and *Staphylococcus*. However, the risk of infection depends on the depth of the bite. Superficial bite wounds are less likely to become infected. Cat bite wounds are more likely to become infected because of the nature of the puncture wound. Infection from a cat bite is caused by *Pasteurella multocida*.

Human bites most commonly occur to children during the toddler and preschool years. Bites are most likely to occur in day care facilities and preschools. These bites do not typically inflict serious injury.

Clinical Presentation

Most dog bites occur on the face and hands. Dog bites can be divided into three categories: abrasions, puncture wounds, and lacerations with or without tissue avulsion (Ginsburg & Hunstead, 2016). Children may also sustain crushing injuries with more serious dog bites. Cat bites are almost always puncture wounds and typically occur on the hands and arms (Fig. 29.25).

Human bites result in an occlusion injury, which occurs from the upper and lower teeth coming into contact with skin. There may or may not be lacerations associated with human bites. Ecchymosis is generally present in the area of the bite.

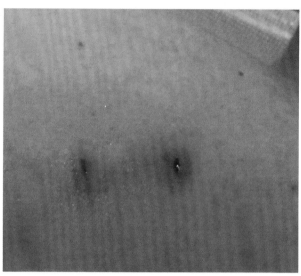

Figure 29.25. Cat bite. Puncture wounds associated with a cat bite. Reprinted with permission from Sherman, S. C., Ross, C., Nordquist, E., Wang, E., & Cico, S. (2015). *Atlas of clinical emergency medicine* (1st ed., Fig. 11.1). Philadelphia, PA: Wolters Kluwer.

Assessment and Diagnosis

Obtain a thorough history of the incident. If an animal bite, ask what type of animal, wild or domestic, and breed was involved, if known. Determine when the bite occurred, how the bite occurred, and whether the animal was provoked. Ask about the location of the attack and whether the animal has bitten before. Obtain the animal's vaccination history, if possible. Ask about the child's immunization status to determine whether he or she is up to date on the tetanus vaccine.

Inspect the bite wound, noting the size, type, and depth of injury. Inspect for any debris in the wound. Assess sensation and movement in the involved area. For more severe wounds, X-rays are needed to determine the extent of injury.

Therapeutic Interventions

Treatment begins with wound debridement and irrigation. Irrigate the wound with a povidone-iodine or 0.9% normal saline solution (Hurt & Maday, 2018). Dog bite wounds can be closed with sutures to promote cosmetic healing. Antibiotics are prescribed to prevent infection. Cat bite wounds are left open to heal by secondary intention because of the high rate of infections associated with these types of bites. More serious dog bites may require consultation with a surgeon, plastic surgeon, orthopedic surgeon, or other specialist.

Nursing management focuses on promoting comfort, promoting skin integrity, and preventing infection of the wounds. Assess the child's pain level and administer analgesics as ordered. Assess for signs and symptoms of wound infection (Fig. 29.26). Administer prophylactic antibiotics as ordered. Administer the tetanus vaccine if needed.

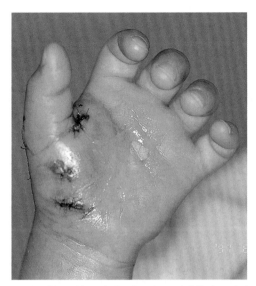

Figure 29.26. Dog bite. Infection in a child's hand that was sutured after a dog bite. Reprinted with permission from Fleisher, G. R., Ludwig, S., & Baskin, M. N. (Eds.). (2004). *Atlas of pediatric emergency medicine* (1st ed.). Philadelphia, PA: Lippincott Williams & Wilkins.

Evaluation

Expected outcomes for a child with a bite include the following:
- The child's pain is at a level acceptable to the child and parent.
- If sutured, the sutures remain intact with the skin edges approximated.

- The wound remains free of signs and symptoms of infection.
- Healing occurs with the least amount of scarring possible.

Discharge Planning and Teaching

Teach the parents and child how to care for the wound at home. If the wound is not sutured, explain to the family that it is to prevent infection of the wound. Explain how to either manage an open wound or to care for sutures. Antibiotics should be administered for the full length of time prescribed. Discuss with parents the best ways to prevent animal bites (Patient Teaching 29.7).

 Patient Teaching 29.7

Preventing Animal Bites

- Never leave a young child alone with animals.
- Teach the child not to play roughly with cats.
- Learn to identify dog breeds that are known for aggressive behavior.
- Teach the child to do the following when around dogs:
  - Never approach a strange dog abruptly.
  - Always ask before petting someone else's dog.
  - Initially approach a dog with a closed fist to smell.
  - Do not play aggressively with dogs.
  - Do not bother a dog that is sleeping or eating.
  - Do not scream around or run from dogs.

Think Critically

1. What special considerations should nurses take into account when educating parents about applying topical medications to infants?
2. Explain how poison ivy is and is not spread.
3. Explain the potential psychological effects of having lice, scabies, or bedbug bites and how nurses can mitigate these effects.
4. What are the most common types of burns in children?

5. What are priority nursing interventions for a child with a deep partial-thickness burn?
6. Discuss the potential long-term effects associated with burns.
7. Develop a teaching plan for sunburn prevention and treatment.
8. Why are young children most at risk for animal bites?

References

Alter, S. J., Bennett, J. S., Koranyi, K., Kreppel, A., & Simon, R. (2015). Common childhood viral infections. *Current Problems in Pediatric and Adolescent Health Care, 45,* 21–53.

Alter, S. J., Bennett, J. S., Koranyi, K., Kreppel, A., Simon, R., & Trevino, J. (2018). Common childhood and adolescent cutaneous infestations and fungal infections. *Current Problems in Pediatric and Adolescent Health Care, 48,* 3–25.

American Academy of Pediatrics. (2015). *Treatment for animal bites.* Retrieved from https://www.healthychildren.org/English/health-issues/conditions/from-insects-animals/Pages/Treatment-for-Animal-Bites.aspx.

American Academy of Pediatrics. (2018). *Insect sting allergies.* Retrieved from https://www.healthychildren.org/English/health-issues/conditions/from-insects-animals/Pages/Insect-Sting-Allergies.aspx.

Antoon, A. Y., & Donovan, M. K. (2016a). Burn injuries. In R. M. Kliegman, B. F. Stanton, J. W. St. Geme III, N. F. Schor, & R. E. Behrman (Eds.), *Nelson's textbook of pediatrics* (20th ed.). Philadelphia, PA: Elsevier, Saunders.

Antoon, A. Y., & Donovan, M. K. (2016b). Cold injuries. In R. M. Kliegman, B. F. Stanton, J. W. St. Geme III, N. F. Schor, & R. E. Behrman (Eds.), *Nelson's textbook of pediatrics* (20th ed.). Philadelphia, PA: Elsevier, Saunders.

Burn Foundation. (2018). *Pediatric burn fact sheet.* Retrieved from http://www.burnfoundation.org/programs/resource.cfm?c=1&a=12.

Centers for Disease Control and Prevention. (2016). *Protect the ones you love: Child injuries are preventable.* Retrieved from https://www.cdc.gov/safechild/burns/index.html.

Centers for Disease Control and Prevention. (2018). *10 Leading causes of injury deaths by age group highlighting unintentional injury deaths, United States - 2016.* Retrieved from https://www.cdc.gov/injury/wisqars/leadingcauses.html.

Centers for Disease Control and Prevention. (2019). *Measles Cases and Outbreaks.* Retrieved from https://www.cdc.gov/measles/cases-outbreaks.html

Dickey, B. Z., & Chiu, Y. E. (2016a). Contact dermatitis. In R. M. Kliegman, B. F. Stanton, J. W. St. Geme III, N. F. Schor, & R. E. Behrman (Eds.), *Nelson's textbook of pediatrics* (20th ed.). Philadelphia, PA: Elsevier, Saunders.

Dickey, B. Z., & Chiu, Y. E. (2016b). Photosensitivity. In R. M. Kliegman, B. F. Stanton, J. W. St. Geme III, N. F. Schor, & R. E. Behrman (Eds.), *Nelson's textbook of pediatrics* (20th ed.). Philadelphia, PA: Elsevier, Saunders.

Dixit, S., Baganizi, D. R., Sahur, R., Dosunmu, E., Chaudhari, A., Vig, K., . . . Dennis, V. A. (2017). Immunological challenges associated with artificial skin grafts: Available solutions and stem cells in future design of synthetic skin. *Journal of Biologic Engineering, 49*(11), 1–23. doi:10.1186/s13036-017-0089-9

Gill, P., & Falder, S. (2017). Early management of paediatric burn injuries. *Paediatrics and Child Health, 27*(9), 406–414.

Ginsburg, C. M., & Hunstead, D. A. (2016). Animal and human bites. In R. M. Kliegman, B. F. Stanton, J. W. St. Geme III, N. F. Schor, & R. E. Behrman (Eds.), *Nelson's textbook of pediatrics* (20th ed.). Philadelphia, PA: Elsevier, Saunders.

Hurt, J. B., & Maday, K. R. (2018). Management and treatment of animal bites. *Journal of the Academy of Physicians Assistants, 31*(4), 27–31.

Juern, A. M., & Drolet, B. A. (2016a). Cutaneous bacterial infections. In R. M. Kliegman, B. F. Stanton, J. W. St. Geme III, N. F. Schor, & R. E. Behrman (Eds.), *Nelson's textbook of pediatrics* (20th ed.). Philadelphia, PA: Elsevier, Saunders.

Juern, A. M., & Drolet, B. A. (2016b). Arthropod bites and infestations. In R. M. Kliegman, B. F. Stanton, J. W. St. Geme III, N. F. Schor, & R. E. Behrman (Eds.), *Nelson's textbook of pediatrics* (20th ed.). Philadelphia, PA: Elsevier, Saunders.

Kaddoura, I., Abu-Sittah, G., Ibrahim, A., Karamanoukian, R., & Papazian, N. (2017). Burn injury: A review of pathophysiology and therapeutic modalities in major burns. *Annals of Burns and Fire Disasters, 30*(2), 95–102.

Kee, E. L., Kimble, R. M., Cuttle, L., Khan, A., & Stockton, K. A. (2015). Randomized controlled trial of three burns dressings for partial thickness burns in children. *Burns, 41*, 946–955.

LaRussa, P. S., & Marin, M. (2016). Varicella-zoster virus. In R. M. Kliegman, B. F. Stanton, J. W. St. Geme III, N. F. Schor, & R. E. Behrman (Eds.), *Nelson's textbook of pediatrics* (20th ed.). Philadelphia, PA: Elsevier, Saunders.

Laskowski-Jones, L., & Jones, L. J. (2018). Frostbite: Don't be left out in the cold. *Nursing, 48*(2), 26–33.

Mason, W. H. (2016). Measles. In R. M. Kliegman, B. F. Stanton, J. W. St. Geme III, N. F. Schor, & R. E. Behrman (Eds.), *Nelson's textbook of pediatrics* (20th ed.). Philadelphia, PA: Elsevier, Saunders.

Pan, R., Domingos dos Santos, B., Nascimento, L. C., Rossi, L. A., Greenen, R., & Van Loey, N. E. (2018). School reintegration of pediatric burn survivors: An integrative literature review. *Burns, 44*, 494–511.

Rimmer, R. B., Bay, R. C., Alam, N. B., Sadler, I. J., Richey, K. J., Foster, K. N., . . . Rosenberg, D. (2015). Measuring the burden of pediatric burn injury for parents and caregivers: Informed burn center staff can help to lighten the load. *Journal of Burn Care & Research, 36*(3), 421–427.

Robinson, J. K., & Jablonski, N. G. (2018). Sun protection and skin self-examination and the US Preventive Services Task Force Recommendation on behavioral counseling for skin cancer prevention. *Journal of the American Medical Association, 319*(11), 1101–1102.

Romanowski, K. S., & Palmieri, T. L. (2017). Pediatric burn resuscitation: Past, present, and future. *Burns and Trauma, 5*(26), 1–9.

Rowan, M. P., Cancio, L. C., Elster, E. A., Burmeister, D. M., Rose, L. F., Natesan, S., . . . Chung, K. K. (2015). Burn wound healing and treatment: Review and advancements. *Critical Care*, 1–12. doi:10.1186/s13054-015-0961-2

Sousa-Pinto, B., Araújo, L., Freitas, A., Correia, O., & Delgado, L. (2018). Stevens–Johnson syndrome/toxic epidermal necrolysis and erythema multiforme drug-related hospitalisations in a national administrative database. *Clinical and Translational Allergy, 8*(2), 1–10.

Tuchman, M., Silverberg, J. I., Jacob, S. E., & Silverberg, N. (2015). Nickel contact dermatitis in children. *Clinics in Dermatology, 33*, 320–326.

VanRavenstein, K., Durham, C. O., Williams, T. H., & Smith, W. (2017). Diagnosis and management of impetigo. *The Nurse Practitioner, 42*(3), 41–44.

Wang, J., & Sicherer, S. H. (2016). Insect allergy. In R. M. Kliegman, B. F. Stanton, J. W. St. Geme III, N. F. Schor, & R. E. Behrman (Eds.), *Nelson's textbook of pediatrics* (20th ed.). Philadelphia, PA: Elsevier, Saunders.

Yin, S. (2017). Chemical and common burns in children. *Clinical Pediatrics, 55*(5S), 8S–12S.

Suggested Readings

American Academy of Pediatrics. (2015). *Treatment for animal bites.* Retrieved from https://www.healthychildren.org/English/health-issues/conditions/from-insects-animals/Pages/Treatment-for-Animal-Bites.aspx.

American Burn Association. (2018). *Prevention resources.* Retrieved from http://ameriburn.org/prevention/prevention-resources/#1493037731270-54b96b15-d6f6

Robinson, J. K., & Jablonski, N. G. (2018). Sun protection and skin self-examination and the US Preventive Services Task Force Recommendation on behavioral counseling for skin cancer prevention. *Journal of the American Medical Association, 319*(11), 1101–1102.

30 Alterations in Immune Function

Variations in Anatomy and Physiology

The immune system is made up of a variety of different cell types and proteins. These components act together to defend against infection and maintain a sense of equilibrium in the body through specific and nonspecific immune functions. An interruption in this balance can result in an immune system that either overfunctions or underfunctions. An **immunodeficiency** occurs when the immune system underfunctions, thus increasing the susceptibility of the body to infections. **Autoimmune disorders** occur when the immune system overfunctions, causing the body to produce antibodies against its own cells. The overfunctioning immune system can also result in a production of antibodies against external sensitizing agents, creating a basis for allergies and **hypersensitivity** reactions.

Nonspecific immune functions involve inflammation and phagocytosis, whereas specific immune functions involve humoral and cell-mediated immunity. Humoral immunity is an immune response involving B cells. The B cells recognize specific **antigens**, or foreign materials that provoke an immune response, and transform, secreting antibodies. These antibodies mark the antigens for destruction. Cellular immunity, also known as T-cell-mediated immunity, cannot identify antigens on its own but recognizes those marked for destruction and attacks them.

The organs of the immune system are immature at birth. The primary lymphoid organs are the thymus and bone marrow. The spleen, lymph nodes, and tonsils make up the secondary lymphoid organs (Fig. 30.1). The infant's thymus, spleen, and tonsils are large in proportion to the rest of the body. An infant's thymus reaches adult size at about 6 weeks of age and continues to grow in size until just before puberty, at which time cell-mediated immunity attains full function. After a child reaches puberty, the thymus begins to shrink in size as the tissue is replaced by adipose. The thymus shrinks because the majority of its role in producing T cells is completed during childhood; it produces very few new T cells after puberty. Peyer's patches increase in number until they peak between the ages of 15 and 25 years (Jung, Hugot, & Barreau, 2010). After peaking, they decline in number throughout the child's life. The spleen continues its growth throughout childhood and reaches full size when the child is an adult. Lymph node tissue in an infant is substantial and continues to grow until after puberty. Excessive swelling and enlargement of the lymphoid tissue tend to occur in response to an infection and may continue after the primary infection is gone (Patient Safety 30.1).

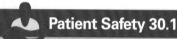

Patient Safety 30.1

Protecting Immune System Organs From Injury

A child's abdomen has less fat with which to protect the internal organs than an adult's. This decreased protection combined with an enlarged spleen puts the child at a higher risk for a traumatic injury, potentially resulting in splenic rupture.

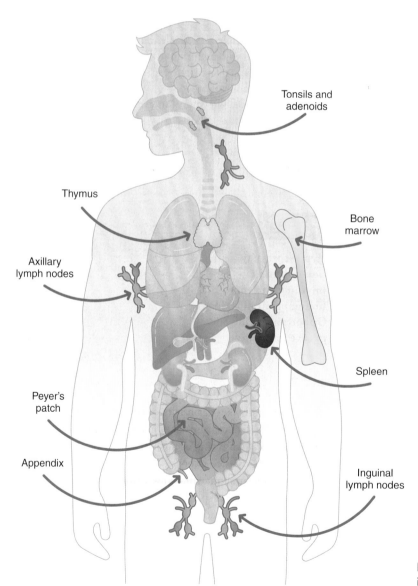

Figure 30.1. Major organs and tissues of the immune system.

Immune System Responses

The immune system functions the same in children as in adults but develops to maturity at varying stages of infancy and childhood, making it less effective than an adult system. Immune system disorders present differently in children than in adults. Primary immunodeficiency disorders (PIDs) tend to present within the first 6 months of life. Tests used for diagnosis are sometimes different for children, and the latency period for immunodeficiency infections is often shorter than is seen in adults.

The combination of an immature immune system and decreased amounts of **immunoglobulins (Igs)** available for immune responses places the child at a higher risk of developing more frequent infections throughout infancy and childhood. The younger the child or infant, the more susceptible he or she is to infections and harm. Diagnosis of infections is made more difficult because common signs and symptoms are not as prominent in children. The lack of an adequate immune response and the increased difficulty in recognizing the symptoms make it easier for infections to spread quickly and greatly increase the potential for sepsis.

Environments where children are in close contact with one another, such as in a day care or school, make it easier for infectious agents to spread. The most common routes for transmission are fecal–oral and respiratory. Infants and children have a tendency to place their hands in their mouths and on their faces, especially to rub their noses and eyes. Children, especially young children, do not always practice good hygiene behaviors that prevent transmission of communicable diseases. Poor practices include improper or unsupervised hand washing after toileting. Caretakers can also spread germs easily by not following good hygiene practices. Diapers can be a source of transmission, from leaking stool to improper handling and disposal. Many communicable diseases are contagious before symptoms occur, and other children and caretakers have usually already been exposed to the infectious agent by the time the contagious child becomes ill.

Immunoglobulins and Other Cells of Immunity

The body's ability to respond to infections develops over time as immunity is acquired. Immunity is acquired actively and passively. **Active immunity** is also called active acquired adaptive immunity. Active immunity is humoral (**antibody**-mediated) and cell-mediated immunity. An antigen-specific humoral function is stimulated to produce antibodies after exposure to an infectious disease in its natural state, or through **immunization**. This form of immunity typically lasts for many years, or a lifetime. The infant gradually develops acquired immunity over the first 6 years of life (Patient Teaching 30.1).

Passive immunity is also called passive acquired adaptive immunity. In passive immunity, an individual receives premade, fully formed antibodies against an antigen, either

Patient Teaching 30.1

Immunizations

- Although immunizations contain viruses in a weakened state, they still may cause infection.
- If your child has an immune disorder, he or she should not receive live virus vaccines.
- No live virus vaccines should be given to household members who reside with immunocompromised children.
- Discuss the risks and benefits of immunization with your healthcare provider.

Adapted from Centers for Disease Control and Prevention. (2018d). *Vaccines and preventable diseases. Who should NOT get vaccinated with these vaccines?* Retrieved from https://www.cdc.gov/vaccines/vpd/should-not-vacc.html; Immune Deficiency Foundation. (2015). *Diagnostic and clinical care guidelines for primary immunodeficiency diseases* (3rd ed.). Retrieved from https://primaryimmune.org/publication/healthcare-professionals/idf-diagnostic-clinical-care-guidelines-primary; Kroger, A. T., Duchin, J., & Vazquez, M. (2018). *General best practice guidelines for immunization. Best practices guidance of the advisory committee on immunization practices (ACIP).* Retrieved from https://www.cdc.gov/vaccines/hcp/acip-recs/general-recs/index.html. See the current recommendations for immunizations from the Centers for Disease Control and Prevention at https://www.cdc.gov/vaccines/vpd/should-not-vacc.html.

naturally, as in the transfer at birth of antibody (IgG) across the placenta from mother to infant, or artificially, as from antibody therapy. The individual is a passive recipient of the antibodies, and his or her body does not have to perform the actions needed to develop immunity. Passive immunity is immediate but short-term, usually diminishing within a few weeks or months.

At birth, natural immunity is passed from mother to infant via the transfer of IgG across the placenta (transplacental transfer) as well as through breast milk. A term infant receives an adult level of IgG, whereas a premature infant receives a lower level of IgG. The immunity from the IgG transfer provides protection for about 6 to 9 months, at which time the amount of IgG received from the mother drops significantly, rendering the infant more vulnerable to antigens and infections. However, the infant's own production of IgG increases during this time, and the infant reaches an adult level at 7 to 8 years of age.

Other Igs and cells important for immune responses reach adult levels at different ages (Table 30.1). Natural killer (NK) cells increase during gestation and are at about half the adult level at birth. During the first 2 to 3 days after birth, the level drops; then it increases until it reaches adult levels at around 5 years of age (Guilmot, Hermann, Braud, Carlier, & Truyens, 2011). Complement protein compounds are at low levels at birth, but some of the serum factors reach adult levels in 1 month (Simon, Hollander, & McMichael, 2015).

Table 30.1 Immunoglobulin Locations, Actions, and Significance Throughout Childhood

Ig	Location	Action/Significance
IgA	• Mucosal secretions (tears, saliva, sweat, colostrum) • Genitourinary, gastrointestinal, and respiratory tract secretions	• Defends against antigen invasion into mucosal barrier • Not present at birth; body begins to produce around 2 wk of age; reaches adult levels by age 6–7 y • Passed to newborns through breast milk
IgD	• Surfaces of mature B cells (with IgM) • Serum (less common)	• Function is still a mystery in immunology. • Not transferred across the placenta • Thought to signal B cells to be activated
IgE	• Plasma cells in mucous membranes and tonsils (site of production) • Surface membranes of basophils and mast cells (primarily in extravascular spaces)	• Not present at birth; body begins to produce around 2 wk of age; levels peak at 10–15 y of age • Important part of the first line of defense against pathogens entering epithelial barriers; protects against parasitic infections • Releases chemical mediators responsible for producing allergic responses
IgG	All body fluids	• Represents largest percentage of Igs produced • The only Ig to cross the placenta; also transferred through breast milk • Provides protection against bacteria, viruses, and fungi • Activates complement • Responsible for Rh reactions
IgM	• Spleen (major site of production) • Blood and lymph fluid	• Normally low levels at birth; increases until age 1 y • First Ig to appear in response to initial exposure to an antigen • Mediates cytotoxic response and activates complement

Ig, immunoglobulin.
Adapted from Rich, R. R., Fleisher, T. A., Shearer, W. T., Schroeder, H., Frew, A. J., & Weyand, C. M. (Eds.). (2018). *Clinical immunology. Principles and practice* (5th ed.). Beijing, China: Elsevier, Saunders; Sherwood, L. (2016). *Human physiology. From cells to systems* (9th ed., pp. 404–444). Boston, MA: Cengage.

Assessment of the Pediatric Immune System

Use the assessment guide in Table 30.2 and the questions in Growth and Development Check 30.1 to perform an in-depth nursing assessment of the pediatric patient with an altered immune system. Table 30.3 reviews abnormal assessment findings.

Common Laboratory and Diagnostic Tests of Immune Function

The common laboratory (lab) and diagnostic tests used for disorders of the immune system include bone marrow aspiration, white blood cell differentials, and allergy testing. Additional labs and diagnostics may be used for determining immune function.

Table 30.2 Assessment Guide: Pediatric Patient With an Altered Immune System

Component or System	Assessment
Health history	• Family history: allergies, HIV or other immune system disorder, maternal HIV • Child's history: relapsing or uncommon infections; response to treatments for infections; immunization status; other health disorders; delayed healing of lesions or wounds; additional infections associated with lesions; chronic cough; recurrent low-grade fever; recurrent deep skin or organ abscesses; persistent thrush in the mouth; allergies

Table 30.2   Assessment Guide: Pediatric Patient With an Altered Immune System (*continued*)

Component or System	Assessment
Skin and mucous membranes	• Skin integrity • Hives • Rash • Lesions (mucous membranes, skin) • Eczema (atopic dermatitis)
Eyes	• Pruritus • Drainage • Edema • Funduscopic exam (yearly) • Visual fields testing (yearly)
Nose, mouth, and throat	• Congestion or swelling • Rhinorrhea • Sneezing • Size of tonsils • Thrush • Pruritus
Lungs	• Adventitious sounds • Wheezing • Cough • Shortness of breath
Heart and blood vessels	• Blood pressure • Perfusion (color, pulses, edema, skin temperature, capillary refill)
Abdomen	Palpation • Enlarged liver • Enlarged spleen
Lymph nodes	Palpation • Palpable • Firm • Tender • Enlarged • Warm
Neurological function	• Gait • Unexplained ataxia • Level of consciousness

HIV, human immunodeficiency virus.

 Growth and Development Check 30.1

The Child With an Immune Disorder

Plot the child's weight, length, and height on growth charts and answer the following questions:

• Has the child met developmental milestones?
• Is the child's growth meeting expected standards?
• How is the child's appetite?
• What is the child's food intake?

Total Igs tend to be elevated in the early months and then decrease over the first year of life (Patient Safety 30.2). The names of the lymphocyte surface antigens are based on the "clusters of differentiation" (CDs). CD antigens on a leukocyte facilitate its identification. The two most commonly used surface antigens and their cell types are the CD4 helper T cells and the CD8 suppressor T cells. To determine the number of a particular type of cell, a complete blood count (CBC) must also be done at the same time (Fischbach & Fischbach, 2017). See Table 30.4 for additional information regarding labs and diagnostics used to test immune function.

Table 30.3 Abnormal Assessment Findings Related to Altered Immune Function

Finding(s)	Possible Reason
Growth failure (failure to thrive)	Immunodeficiency disorder
Ataxia	Neurological alterations (such as in HIV)
Adventitious lung sounds	Recurrent respiratory infections, pneumonia
Wheezing or whistling, cough, or shortness of breath	Inflammation/allergic reaction
Eczema, hives, rash, or other skin lesions	Allergic disorders, Wiskott–Aldrich syndrome
Thrush	Immunodeficiency
Enlarged, tender, firm, warm lymph nodes	Local or widespread inflammation
Fever	Infection or inflammation
Diminished LOC	Encephalopathy (HIV)
Hepatosplenomegaly	Immune disorder
Sneezing, congestion, swelling, rhinorrhea, and drainage in the nose and throat	Allergies
Hypotension	Allergies, other abnormalities affecting the cardiovascular system
Pruritus in the eyes, nose, and palate	Allergies
Abnormal results on the funduscopic exam or visual fields test	Ocular damage due to long-term use of antimalarial drugs or corticosteroids

HIV, human immunodeficiency virus; LOC, level of consciousness.

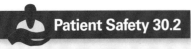

Patient Safety 30.2

Factors Affecting the Accuracy of Immune Tests

Serum immunoglobulin diagnostic test results can be affected by blood transfusions, tetanus antitoxin, immunizations, and toxoids received in the past 6 mo, and gamma globulin received in the past 6 wk. These should be noted on the lab requisition.

General Nursing Interventions for Immune Disorders

Priority nursing interventions for children with immune disorders include preventing infection, preventing and managing allergic reactions, and promoting pain relief, comfort, and rest. These and other general nursing interventions for immune disorders are discussed here.

Prevent Infection

Children with immunodeficiency disorders are particularly susceptible to infections. Routine hand washing and following basic infection control practices are the best ways to prevent the spread of organisms. Infection control is based on three principles: (1) prevent contact with infectious organisms, (2) create barriers if contact is necessary or unavoidable, and (3) kill organisms if there is contact. These principles can be carried out by interventions such as limiting exposure to individuals with infections and appropriately disposing of needles and contaminated materials or equipment. Another example of an intervention for basic infection control is to use sterile (aseptic) techniques when caring for all sites of invasive equipment or procedures, such as needles, catheters, central lines, endotracheal tubes, pressure-monitoring lines, or peripheral intravenous (IV) lines. Following current recommendations for immunizing the immunocompromised child is also an important part of infection prevention.

Table 30.4 Common Laboratory and Diagnostic Tests of Immune Function

Test	What Is Measured	Conditions Tested for	Nursing Considerations
Allergy skin prick test	Presence of activated T cells in response to certain substances	• Allergic reactions (immediate and delayed) • Immune disorders	• Common initial diagnostic tool • Yields result quickly. • Allergen is applied and skin is pricked or scratched. • Wheal indicates an allergy (but is not diagnostic alone). • Does not predict severity of an allergic reaction • Anaphylactic reaction is a risk; must have emergency equipment and medications on hand. • Reaction may occur immediately or after several minutes or hours.
ANA (FANA) test	Presence of autoantibodies that react against cellular nuclear material	Autoimmune disorders (SLE, JIA)	• Some medications and infections can result in a false positive. • Not used to monitor progression of SLE
Anergy skin test	Cell-mediated immune response to specific antigens	Immune function	• Antigens include mumps, tetanus, *Candida*. • Used to validate TB skin test results by ruling out false-negative findings
Bone marrow aspiration	• Quantity of cellular elements in the blood • Function of hematopoiesis	• Anemia • Blood disorders • Leukemia • Lymphoma • Multiple myeloma	• Not the same as bone marrow biopsy • Fluid-containing bone marrow cells aspirated from the iliac crest • Usually performed under local anesthesia • Does not represent all cells • Potential complications include bleeding and infection.
CBC with diff	• RBC count • Hemoglobin level • Hematocrit • RBC indices • WBC count • Platelet count • Percentage of each type of WBC to total	• Infection • Inflammatory process • Immune suppression	• Helpful in evaluating source of infection, especially the WBC count • WBC differential measures whether immune cells can ingest and destroy foreign substances. • May be affected by myelosuppressive drugs
CD4 count	Number of CD4 T lymphocytes in the blood	• HIV (viral load) • Response to HIV antiretroviral therapy (CD4 count is inversely related to virus count)	• Most valuable indicator of immune status of HIV-positive individuals • Low in HIV-positive children • See the latest National Institutes of Health (2018) guidelines for antiretroviral therapy in children at https://aidsinfo.nih.gov/guidelines/html/2/pediatric-arv/0.
Chest X-ray	Size of the thymus	Immune deficiency disorders	• Used with other tests (SCID)

(continued)

Table 30.4 Common Laboratory and Diagnostic Tests of Immune Function (*continued*)

Test	What Is Measured	Conditions Tested for	Nursing Considerations
Complement assay (C3, C4)	• Level of total complement in the blood • C3 and C4 levels in the blood	• SLE • Complement deficiency	• Decreased in SLE • Unstable at room temperature; send to lab immediately
ELISA	Presence of antibody or antigen	• HIV • Allergies	• Also known as EIA • Used for children at high risk for a strong reaction or anaphylaxis or with unstable health (cardiac condition or asthma) • Potential false positives in detecting HIV in infants and toddlers (antibodies from HIV-positive mothers may remain detectable up to 24 mo of age)
ESR	Presence of infection or inflammation	• Immune disorder (initial workup) • Autoimmune disease (ongoing monitoring)	• Send to lab immediately; if allowed to stand >3 h, falsely low result can occur.
HIV antibodies	Presence of antibodies to HIV	HIV (confirm infection)	• Not appropriate for high-risk infants <18–24 mo old because of circulating maternal antibodies • Autoimmune disease may cause false-positive results. • Requires serial testing
IgG subclasses	Blood levels of the four subclasses of IgG	Immune deficiency	• Normal levels vary with age. • Levels altered by IVIG and steroids • Conduct other tests first.
Intradermal skin test	Presence of activated T cells in response to certain substances	Drug or venom allergies	• Used if skin prick test is negative
Lymphocyte surface antigen	Percentage and numbers of lymphocyte types and subtypes in the blood (CD4, CD8, B cells, NK cells)	HIV (ongoing monitoring of CD cells)	• Do not refrigerate specimen. • Levels may be elevated by steroids and lowered by immunosuppressive drugs. • Most common use: to identify surface antigens and cell types for CD4 (helper T cells) and CD8 (suppressor T cells)
Patch test	Presence of activated T cells in response to certain substances	Contact dermatitis	• Allergen is placed on skin and covered with a bandage. • Patch is left in place for 48–96 h and then checked by physician. • Local rash develops if allergic to substance.
Physician-supervised challenge test	Presence of activated T cells in response to certain substances	Medication or food allergies	• Allergen inhaled or taken by mouth • Should be supervised by a physician, preferably an allergist, because of the risk of anaphylaxis

Table 30.4 Common Laboratory and Diagnostic Tests of Immune Function (*continued*)

Test	What Is Measured	Conditions Tested for	Nursing Considerations
RT-PCR	Presence of HIV RNA in the blood	HIV (confirm or rule out infection in infants as early as possible)	• Positive in infected infants older than 1 mo
RF	Level of RF in the blood	• JIA • SLE	• Only about 5% of children with JIA have a +RF. • +RF is also sometimes seen in chronic infectious disorders.
Serum antibody titer	Antibody level in the blood	Immune function (humoral)	• Tests antibody level to specific antigens
Serum Ig electrophoresis	Levels of individual Igs (IgA, IgD, IgE, IgG, IgM) in the blood	• Immune deficiency (humoral) • Autoimmune disorders	• Normal levels vary with age. • IVIG administration and steroids alter levels. • Total Igs high in early months, and then decline during the first year of life • May be unusually high in HIV early in the disease process, and then decline
Specific IgE blood tests (RAST, ImmunoCAP)	Allergen-specific IgE level in a blood sample	Allergies (in those with a history of a strong reaction, a higher risk for anaphylaxis, unstable heart disease, or asthma)	• More expensive than skin tests • Longer wait time for results, usually a few days • Carries no risk of anaphylaxis, but it is not as sensitive as skin testing • Often needs to be sent out to a reference laboratory • Used to aid diagnosis in conjunction with other clinical findings • The higher the level, the more likely the person has an allergy to the food or substance. • Associated with many false positives
Virological assay	Presence and levels of HIV RNA and DNA in the blood	HIV (diagnosis in children older than 2 wk and ongoing monitoring of viral load)	• HIV-1 RNA is the primary indicator for assessing antiretroviral treatment effectiveness. • Sensitive and specific for presence of HIV in blood • Sequential testing needed to determine perinatal transmission

ANA, antinuclear antibody; CBC, complete blood count; CD, cluster of differentiation; diff, differential; EIA, enzyme immunoassay; ELISA, enzyme-linked immunosorbent assay; ESR, erythrocyte sedimentation rate; FANA, fluorescent antinuclear antibody; HIV, human immunodeficiency virus; Ig, immunoglobulin; IVIG, intravenous immunoglobulin; JIA, juvenile idiopathic arthritis; NK, natural killer; RAST, radioallergosorbent test; RBC, red blood cell; RF, rheumatoid factor; RT-PCR, reverse transcriptase polymerase chain reaction; SCID, severe combined immune deficiency; SLE, systemic lupus erythematosus; TB, tuberculosis; WBC, white blood cell.
Adapted from Asthma and Allergy Foundation of America. (2015c). *Allergy Diagnosis.* Retrieved from http://www.aafa.org/page/allergy-diagnosis.aspx; Corbett, J. A., & Banks, A. D. (2013). *Laboratory tests and diagnostic procedures with nursing diagnoses* (8th ed.). Upper Saddle River, NJ: Pearson Education Inc.; Fischbach, F., & Fischbach, M. (2017). *Fischbach's. A manual of laboratory and diagnostic tests* (10th ed.). Philadelphia, PA: Lippincott Williams & Wilkins; Mayo Clinic. (2018). *Test ID: IGGS. IgG subclasses, serum.* Retrieved from https://www.mayomedicallaboratories.com/test-catalog/Clinical+and+Interpretive/9259; Quest Diagnostics. (2018). *ImmunoCap specific IgE blood test.* Retrieved from http://www.questdiagnostics.com/home/physicians/testing-services/by-test-name/immunocap.html?utm_medium=print&utm_campaign=allergy&utm_source=aafp

Teach families to reduce the risk of infection by doing the following:

- Practice safe food preparation, such as using different surfaces for meats and cleaning well after their preparation to avoid contamination of other foods or items.
- Do not share eating utensils, especially those used by the child.
- Use hot water and soap for washing eating utensils, including bottles, nipples, and pacifiers; a dishwasher can also be used for cleaning the items.
- Practice good hand hygiene, especially before handling or feeding the child and after changing diapers.
- Practice diligent skin care to avoid breakdown, change diapers frequently, and keep the diaper area clean and dry.
- If pets are part of the household, keep them and their items clean.
- Avoid people with known infections, including family members.
- As children become adolescents, discuss with them the infection risks associated with body piercing and tattooing.

Prevent and Manage Allergic Response

For children with allergies, reduce their risk of having an allergic response by teaching them and their families about triggers and how to avoid them. They need to have a plan in place for recognizing and managing reactions, including appropriate medications and actions to take for an emergency. The child should wear a medical alert bracelet and carry an epinephrine auto-injector (EpiPen) at all times. If a child is allergic to insect stings and will be in a high-risk area, teach the child and family guidelines on how to prevent stings, such the following:

- Wear only light-colored, fitted clothes, preferably long-sleeved and nondecorative.
- Only use unscented hygiene products.
- Apply insect repellant.
- Avoid areas of high insect activity, such as flowers and shrubs.

Provide instructions on how to allergy-proof the home. Help parents learn how to distinguish allergies from a cold.

Promote Skin Integrity

For many immunodeficient children, the skin may be their only intact defense. Provide frequent and thorough skin care, paying special attention to the perineal area. Oral mucous membranes break down with blisters, cracking, and discharge from recurrent *Candida* infections. Provide oral care with normal saline or another non–alcohol-based solution. A prescription mouthwash may be ordered. Monitor pressure areas closely for signs of breakdown or infection. The child should be repositioned frequently and encouraged to do range-of-motion exercises.

For children with autoimmune disorders, complications, such as mouth ulcers, can cause weakening of the tissues, leading to skin breakdown, which in turn increases a child's risk for

infection. Provide oral care instructions to prevent or minimize the skin breakdown. Mild soap is recommended for hand hygiene, and the use of cosmetics should be kept to a minimum. Teach adolescents the appropriate type of cosmetics and skin care items to avoid, such as oil-based ones. Encourage protection from the sun to prevent rashes from photosensitivity, such as by limiting time spent in the sun, wearing sunscreen that is sun protection factor 30 or higher, and wearing protective clothing.

Promote Pain Relief, Comfort, and Rest

Complications associated with immunological disorders and their treatments can be painful and uncomfortable and can disturb rest and sleep patterns. Pain can come from many sources, such as infections, adverse effects of medications, and medical procedures. Aggressive pain management using both pharmacological and nonpharmacological interventions may be required for an increased quality of life. Adequate pain assessment becomes challenging with younger and less verbal children. Be alert to nonverbal signs of pain, such as the child not wanting to participate in interactive play or displaying inconsolable irritability. Identification of the type of pain (e.g., musculoskeletal vs. nerve pain) is crucial to appropriate pain management, as each type requires the use of different medications for treatment. Teach parents, caretakers, and the child ways to identify signs of pain and promote pain relief, comfort, and rest.

Multiple factors can influence the pain and discomfort that children with autoimmune disorders experience: severity of the disorder, functional level, the child's tolerance of pain, family dynamics, and coping skills. Even aggressive pain management using both pharmacological and nonpharmacological interventions may not provide complete pain relief. The goal is to minimize the pain to a tolerable level so the child can participate in activities of daily living and obtain adequate rest. Anti-inflammatory medications are a large part of the management regimen, along with other therapies such as relaxation. The use of opioids is not a routine therapy for the chronic pain associated with autoimmune disorders. The child may need referrals to someone specializing in pain management as well as to counseling.

Children with allergies and their families may experience increased anxiety because of the seriousness of the allergic response and the unknown potential of experiencing future reactions. Allergy testing and shots may cause stress and pain for the child. Use age-appropriate techniques for explaining procedures and reducing pain and stress. Normal family processes are interrupted when dealing with the disorder. Provide referrals as needed for support, counseling, or other services.

Maintain Adequate Hydration and Nutrition

Failure to thrive and nutritional deficiencies may occur as a result of the progression of an immunological disorder or as a result of treatments. Children may experience recurrent illnesses, diarrhea, and other physical problems, making it difficult to manage their nutrition. Monitor growth and weight, and implement aggressive measures if signs of slow growth or weight loss are noted. Encourage the child to consume adequate fluids and nutrition. Consider the child's food preferences, and provide foods with a high nutritional value. Offer small, frequent meals of high-calorie, protein-rich foods. The family and child may need a referral to a dietician for guidance in planning a diet and meals. Vitamin C and other antioxidants have been shown to enhance general immune system function (Carr & Maggini, 2017). The dietician can guide the parents on how to ensure that children are receiving adequate amounts of antioxidants in their diet. Parents can also make the environment conducive to healthy eating during meals by eliminating unpleasant stimuli and odors.

Although autoimmune disorders themselves typically do not require dietary restrictions, children with autoimmune disorders may have other conditions requiring a special diet, such as renal involvement, weight gain, or weight loss. Inactivity during painful exacerbations and treatments involving the use of steroids place the child at a higher risk for weight gain. Include calcium and vitamin D supplements in the child's diet, as they support bone density. Encourage adequate hydration.

Maintain Effective Gas Exchange and Airway Clearance

Frequent secondary, opportunistic, and respiratory infections, especially pneumonia, are common occurrences for the child with an immunodeficiency disorder. Encourage both physical activity to promote lung aeration and periods of rest to prevent fatigue, conserve energy, and decrease the body's demand for oxygen. While the child is in the hospital or during illnesses, encourage the child to cough and perform deep breathing exercises every 2 to 4 hours and to frequently change position.

Manage Medication Therapy

Medications used long-term to treat immunodeficiency disorders often have many side effects; therefore, closely monitor children who are taking them. Evaluate drug toxicity and treatment response with periodic blood work. Instruct parents on the type and frequency of specialized examinations needed to monitor for problems, such as ophthalmic evaluations for macular inflammatory problems. Conduct age-appropriate teaching and counseling about the medications. Parents and children need to understand the potential interactions of medications with other medications, supplements, and, at times, food products. Sexually active adolescents need counseling about the effects of medications on birth control and pregnancy and may need referrals to specialists.

Provide Emotional and Psychosocial Support and Referrals

Immunodeficiency disorders can be anxiety-provoking, life-threatening, and overwhelming for a child and loved ones. Encourage and support the family and child as they experience anticipatory grieving and discuss their concerns and fears. Make referrals to support groups, a counselor, and any other appropriate services as needed. Evaluate the family's coping skills and ability to care for the child at home. Assess the need for education about the disorder, prevention of complications, and treatment measures. Promote normal family processes and activities, and include siblings and other significant friends and family members in the support process. As the disorder progresses, provide the family with information regarding palliative and end-of-life care as appropriate.

Children with autoimmune disorders may experience chronic pain and decreased mobility that impact their psychological and emotional status significantly, during both childhood and adulthood. Clinical manifestations of the autoimmune disorder, such as rash, alopecia, and arthritic changes in the joints, along with the side effects experienced from medications, can alter the child's perception of his or her body image. Assist children in setting and achieving goals to increase their sense of hopefulness. Encourage children and families to become involved with local support groups so that they can see that they are not alone. Referrals to counseling or social services may also be needed.

Promote Growth and Development

Growth and development can be altered by the effects of an immune disorder, its chronicity, treatment regimens, and frequent hospitalizations. Children need support because they experience body image changes due to treatments, such as weight gain caused by corticosteroid therapy. Encourage and provide support for safe social interactions with peers and family by discussing the stigma of diagnosis, the potential for infection, and how to manage bleeding. Provide referrals as needed for support groups and counseling.

To prevent social isolation in children with autoimmune disorders, encourage them to attend school and ensure that teachers, the school nurse, and classmates are educated about the child's disease and any limitations on activity. Modifications, such as allowing the child to leave the classroom early to get to the next class on time, may seem small but can have a significant impact on the child's life. Encourage adequate sleep, because sleep disturbance contributes to daytime sleepiness and fatigue, which interfere with the child's ability to cope with symptoms and to function at school.

For children with allergies, educate their school personnel about how to recognize and manage an allergic reaction. The teachers and school nurse can monitor the child for behavior changes or drowsiness while on medications, such as antihistamines. Encourage the parents and the child to have teachers provide homework if the child is unable to attend school. Also encourage the child to participate in social activities with peers.

Promote Compliance With Treatment

Treatment regimens for children with immune disorders may be complex, time consuming, costly, and an overwhelming challenge for the child and family to maintain compliance with. The statistical rates for nonadherence are alarming for some diagnoses. An estimated 40% of pediatric patients experience treatment failure within the first 2 years of a prescribed medication regimen, with noncompliance being reported as the primary reason (Agwu et al., 2017). In some cases, such as with a retroviral regimen, not adhering to the prescribed regimen could result in worsening of the disease.

Frequency of dosing, interruptions in daily routines, taste and side effects of medications, and dietary restrictions are some of the more common reasons families give for noncompliance. For children with autoimmune disorders, providing adequate pain relief and promoting compliance with the disease-modifying medication regimen may allow children to have a more normal life in the present as well as in the future. Parents, caretakers, and the child need education regarding the purpose and benefits of treatment regimens, as well as the consequences of not adhering to them. Collaborate with the family and adapt treatment regimens to the family's routine as much as possible. Positive reinforcement techniques can help modify behaviors of the child, as well as support the family in their compliance. Explore reasons for noncompliance, such as cultural beliefs, and discuss alternative options and solutions. Provide referrals as needed for support, counseling, financial, or other services.

Primary and Secondary Immunodeficiency Disorders

Immunodeficiency disorders are classified as either primary or secondary. The primary disorders consist of over 300 chronic disorders, which are further classified according to defects: B-cell deficiencies (antibody), T-cell deficiencies (cellular), phagocytic disorders, complement defects, and cytokine defects (Grubbs, 2015; Sharma, Jindal, Rawat, & Singh, 2017). Primary immunodeficiencies are also known as congenital or hereditary disorders and have a genetic cause. The inherited defects affect the immune system's ability to make antibodies to defend against infections. Children with a PID remain susceptible to infections throughout their life, experience recurring health problems, and often develop a serious, incapacitating illness (Immune Deficiency Foundation [IDF], 2018a).

Etiology and Pathophysiology

PIDs occur as the result of defects in the development of the immune system components, resulting in an ineffective or nonfunctioning system. Humoral immune deficiencies are caused by defects in B cells, resulting in impaired antibody production. Cellular, or cell-mediated, immune deficiencies are caused by defects in T cells. Depending on the type and severity of the defect, patients can present at any age; however, the most common age is infancy and early childhood.

Clinical Presentation

Children with PIDs have an increased susceptibility to infections in infancy and early childhood. Highly indicative signs of PIDs are repeated or persistent respiratory tract infections, otitis and sinusitis, severe bacterial infections, **opportunistic infections,** and a poor response to appropriate therapies. Other signs include frequent skin lesions, failure to thrive, chronic diarrhea, thrush, anemia, thrombocytopenia, neutropenia, and small or absent lymph nodes, tonsils, and adenoids. PIDs often present first with skin manifestations, such as eczematous dermatitis and warts. In addition to the increased susceptibility to infectious agents, children with PIDs are also vulnerable to several noninfectious complications, such as autoimmune diseases and malignancies (IDF, 2018a; Sharma et al., 2017).

Assessment and Diagnosis

Conduct a comprehensive family history. Significant diagnostic clues to a possible PID can be discovered from a comprehensive family history, as well as from a health history on the child. There are warning signs that indicate a child may have a PID. One of the first physical signs involves the skin, such as a rash, recurrent skin infections, or nonhealing ulcers (Sharma et al., 2017). Additional signs include recurrent pneumonia; ear, sinus, fungal, or deep-seated infections; limited response to antibiotics; failure to gain weight or grow normally; required IV antibiotics to clear infections; and a family history of a PID (Jeffrey Modell Foundation, 2016). For a more detailed description of the warning signs, see the educational materials provided by the Jeffrey Modell Foundation at http://www.info4pi.org/library/educational-materials/10-warning-signs. These educational materials can be shared with families and healthcare providers. Diagnostic labs include a CBC and serum Ig level.

Therapeutic Interventions

Advancements in treatment have made it possible to do more than just manage the infection. Hematopoietic stem cell transplantation (HSCT; also called bone marrow or stem cell transplantation) offers a possible cure for many PIDs, in which stem cells from a donor are transplanted into the recipient (Morgan, Gray, Lomova, & Kohn, 2017; Negrin, Chao, & Rosmarin, 2017). Once a patient receives healthy bone marrow from a donor, the transplanted cells can then develop into functional B and T cells. Gene therapy and thymus transplantation are examples of other new therapies being developed (American Academy of Allergy Asthma & Immunology [AAAAI], 2018). If appropriate for the diagnosis, encourage genetic counseling if the parents plan to have more children.

Intravenous immune globulin (IVIG) therapy is given prophylactically to decrease infections, especially while waiting to undergo a transplantation (Bonilla et al., 2015). Follow safe protocols for administration of the IVIG and do not mix with other medications for infusion. IVIG is prepared from human plasma and contains globulin, primarily IgG; therefore, monitor the child for signs of adverse reactions, side effects, and anaphylaxis. Signs to watch for include a local inflammatory reaction, fever, chills, flushing, nausea, vomiting, joint pain, headache, difficulty breathing, and pain in the back or abdomen. Be prepared for an emergency by having medications and equipment readily available. An antipyretic and antihistamine may be administered prophylactically before the infusion (Perez et al., 2016).

Additional support is required for the family of a child undergoing a stem cell transplantation (see Chapter 26). If the family's home is far from the medical facility where the transplantation will take place, they may require support to be able to visit the child during the hospitalization while maintaining a job or caring for other members of the family. Assess the family's situation and make appropriate referrals to social services and support groups. The Immune Deficiency Foundation (2018b) offers many free educational materials, including a guide on stem cell transplantation, which can be accessed at https://primaryimmune.org/resource-center?f[]=type:publication#search.

Evaluation

Expected outcomes for a child with a PID include the following:

- The child is free of signs of infection.
- The child's skin remains free of preventable breakdown.
- The child has adequate nutritional intake, as determined by growth patterns and weight being within normal limits.
- The family adapts to and copes with the demands of a chronic illness and does not demonstrate knowledge deficits related to the care of their child.
- The child performs tasks that are developmentally appropriate for the child's age.

Discharge Planning and Teaching

Prevention of infection, as well as the importance of compliance with the prescribed therapy regimen, has been identified as major educational needs for the child and family. Assess the family's knowledge regarding the disorder, care of the child, expected growth and development, and prescribed treatment regimens (Growth and Development Check 30.2). Identify knowledge deficits and provide the needed education. Encourage families to follow the recommendations of the Centers for Disease Control and Prevention (CDC) regarding immunizations. If applicable, inform the family to notify any healthcare providers administering immunizations to the child that the child is receiving IVIG therapy, because it alters the recommendations for immunizations (IDF, 2015).

 Growth and Development Check 30.2

Developmental Delay

Children with chronic illnesses are at risk for developmental delay. Make sure to include teaching about normal growth and development during discharge planning and teaching. Refer as necessary children exhibiting signs of developmental delay.

Wiskott–Aldrich Syndrome

Wiskott–Aldrich syndrome (WAS) is a congenital X-linked recessive disorder and a form of congenital thrombocytopenia. The syndrome affects only males and is associated with a triad of characteristic abnormalities: (1) thrombocytopenia with small platelets, (2) eczema, and (3) immunodeficiency involving selective functions of B and T lymphocytes (Ochs, 2017).

Etiology and Pathophysiology

In WAS, phagocytes (macrophages) are unable to process foreign antigens, particularly polysaccharides. This results in immunologically competent cells failing because they are unable to produce normal Ig patterns. Although the exact defect for this disorder is unknown, the abnormal gene responsible for the disorder is named the Wiskott–Aldrich syndrome protein (Ochs, 2017). Patients diagnosed with WAS develop complications such as autoimmunity, chronic arthritis, inflammatory bowel disease, renal disease, and an increased risk of malignancy. The most common malignancy in patients with WAS is non–Hodgkin lymphoma (Mortaz et al., 2016).

Clinical Presentation

The three basic clinical features of WAS are as follows:

1. An increased tendency to bleed
2. Recurrent bacterial, viral, and fungal infections
3. Eczema of the skin

An infant may present with bleeding manifestations, such as petechiae, purpura, hematuria, bloody diarrhea, and hematemesis, along with a history of recurrent infections. The bleeding manifestations are associated with thrombocytopenia and small platelets and are life-threatening in about 30% of patients (Sharma et al., 2017). Eczema is a common skin manifestation and usually appears early in life (Fig. 30.2). Other features associated with WAS include lymphoma, autoimmune disease, and IgA nephropathy.

Assessment and Diagnosis

Note a history of petechiae, bloody diarrhea, or bleeding within the first 6 months of life (Patient Teaching 30.2). Also note any history of hematemesis, intracranial hemorrhage, or conjunctival hemorrhage. A history of eczema, which worsens over time and leads to secondary infections, is significant, especially in a male infant or child. Investigate the family history for incidence of X-linked inheritance.

The most important initial lab assessment is platelet size; patients with WAS have microthrombocytopenia (small platelets). A metabolic defect in platelet synthesis could be the reason the platelets are unusually small and have a reduced lifespan. Other lab findings include low platelet volume, nonfunctional B cells, low IgM, elevated IgA and IgE, and normal IgG levels (AAAAI, 2018; Buckley, 2016; Sharma et al., 2017).

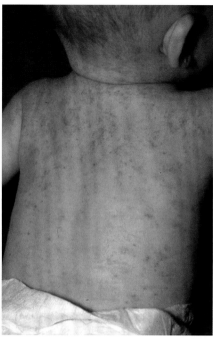

Figure 30.2. Wiskott–Aldrich syndrome. Eczema associated with Wiskott–Aldrich syndrome. Reprinted with permission from Kyle, T., & Carman, S. (2016). *Essentials of pediatric nursing* (3rd ed., Fig. 25.2). Philadelphia, PA: Wolters Kluwer.

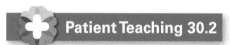

Patient Teaching 30.2

Signs of Wiskott–Aldrich Syndrome

Prolonged bleeding after a circumcision or at the umbilical stump may be the first sign of Wiskott–Aldrich syndrome in a newborn infant (Ochs, 2017).

Therapeutic Interventions

Advances in treatments have improved the prognosis for children with WAS; however, HSCT remains the only cure (IDF, 2013). Other therapies are currently under investigation (The Pharmacy 30.1). Children with WAS differ from other children with PIDs because not only are they at increased risk for infections but they are also at risk for bleeding because of the thrombocytopenia associated with this disorder. Management is supportive and involves treating the developing complications. If a child with WAS develops an autoimmune disorder, the treatment regimen changes to include high-dose steroids, immunosuppressive agents, or chemotherapy.

Measures need to be taken to prevent and control bleeding episodes. To correct thrombocytopenia, a splenectomy may be performed. Perform good skin care and frequent assessments of eczematous areas to detect signs of secondary infections. Because there is a genetic component of the disorder, parents need support to deal with feelings of guilt they may be experiencing, especially when dealing with the difficulties of treatment.

Evaluation

Expected outcomes for a child with WAS include the following:

* Risk of injury to the child is decreased by preventing and controlling bleeding episodes.
* Pain is managed to promote comfort and rest.
* Normal growth and development is promoted.
* The child and family have adequate knowledge about disease management and how to recognize signs of bleeding or infections.

Discharge Planning and Teaching

Parents need to be educated on prevention and management of bleeding. In the case of a child who undergoes a splenectomy, take care to prevent infection due to the increased risk of infection. Provide patients and families with information on appropriate referral services, such as that on the website of the Wiskott–Aldrich Foundation, available at http://www.wiskott.org/. This website provides information about the syndrome, the latest research, and an overview of financial resources (IDF, 2018a).

Severe Combined Immune Deficiency

PIDs exhibit a wide range of T- and B-cell abnormalities. The most severe form of immunodeficiency is severe combined

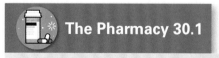

The Pharmacy 30.1	Intravenous Immune Globulin to Treat Wiskott-Aldrich Syndrome		
Classification	**Route**	**Action**	**Nursing Considerations**
Immune globulin	IV	Provides exogenous IgG antibodies Used to treat patients with PIDs or HIV	• Do not mix with other IV medications or fluids • Only administer via the IV route • Frequently monitor for adverse reactions during infusion • Have epinephrine available • Antipyretics and antihistamines may be administered

HIV, human immunodeficiency virus; IgG, immunoglobulin G; IV, intravenous; PID, primary immunodeficiency disorder.
Adapted from Taketomo, C. K., Hodding, J. H., & Kraus, D. M. (2018). *Pediatric & neonatal dosage handbook* (25th ed.). Hudson, OH: Lexicomp.

immune deficiency (SCID). SCID cases are characterized by absent T-cell and B-cell function and typically present within the first 6 months of life. SCID is life-threatening and requires careful medical and nursing management.

Etiology and Pathophysiology

SCID is a rare X-linked or autosomal recessive disorder and can occur in girls or boys. There are at least five different types, which are classified according to the exact genetic defect, and they involve deficiencies of both humoral and cell-mediated immune responses. SCID is a potentially fatal disorder, and emergency treatment with HSCT is needed at the time of diagnosis (Bonilla et al., 2015).

Clinical Presentation

Infants with SCID usually present within the first 6 months of life with serious bacterial, viral, and fungal infections. The other common presenting clinical manifestations are chronic infections, pneumonia, otitis media, persistent diarrhea, sepsis, oral thrush (candidiasis), meningitis, severe diaper rash, and failure to thrive (Capriotta & Frizzell, 2016).

Assessment and Diagnosis

Note a history of persistent candidiasis (oral thrush), chronic infections that began early in infancy, chronic diarrhea, failure to thrive, and severe diaper rash. Inspect the mouth for thrush. Auscultate the lungs, noting any adventitious sounds (Hogan, Wagner, White, & Johnson, 2013; Capriotti & Frizzell, 2016). Lab tests show signs of a complete absence of T-cell, B-cell, and NK immunity. Leukocyte counts are usually reduced; levels of circulating T cells are significantly decreased; levels of circulating B cells are normal or increased; levels of NK cells are decreased; and serum levels of the Igs are very low.

Therapeutic Interventions

Management is very similar to that for WAS. The current treatment for SCID is to manage the infection and replace abnormal components through HSCT (Priority Care Concepts 30.1; Abbas, Lichtman, & Pillai, 2014). Additional treatments may be needed, such as long-term antibiotic therapy. In the hospital setting, the child should be placed in a positive-pressure isolation room to reduce exposure to infectious individuals. The prognosis for these children is poor if they do not receive an HSCT, even with other aggressive therapies.

Evaluation

Expected outcomes for a child with SCID include the following:

- The child remains free of infection.
- The family demonstrates appropriate coping methods related to the diagnosis and prognosis.
- Interruptions in growth and development are decreased.
- The child maintains balanced nutrition and hydration.

Priority Care Concepts 30.1
Blood Transfusions

Blood or platelets to be used for transfusion should be irradiated and negative for cytomegalovirus (CMV). CMV-positive blood could cause an infection, and T lymphocytes in blood products can lead to fatal graft-versus-host disease (Bonilla et al., 2015).

Discharge Planning and Teaching

Protecting the child from infection is of primary importance. Teach the family about good hand washing as well as how to prevent exposure to infected people. Teach about prophylactic antibiotics, if prescribed, as well as appropriate immunization guidelines. The current recommendation is that a child with SCID should not receive live vaccines; encourage the family to discuss immunization administration with the child's primary care provider. Some children may have a poor appetite and require supplemental enteral feedings. Teach the family about the feedings and how to maintain adequate nutrition. Administer IVIG therapy as prescribed. Provide posttransplantation care and teaching if the child receives a bone marrow transplant (see Chapter 26). The therapies required for SCID are lifelong, and families need ongoing support. Refer the family for genetic counseling.

Hypogammaglobulinemia

Hypogammaglobulinemia refers to a group of B-cell disorders in which Igs are either present in inadequate numbers or absent. Hypogammaglobulinemia is the most common PID, accounting for about 50% of cases (Chin, 2014). Selective IgA deficiency, X-linked agammaglobulinemia, X-linked hyper-IgM syndrome, and IgG subclass deficiency are all different types of hypogammaglobulinemia. Transient hypogammaglobulinemia of infancy is a temporary decrease in the serum levels of Igs and is not considered a PID. The condition is fairly common, usually asymptomatic, and resolves itself (Fernandez, 2016; Chin, Windle, Jyonouchi, & Georgitis, 2014).

Etiology and Pathophysiology

During the first few months of life, newborns are protected from infection by maternal antibodies. Around 3 months of age, maternal antibodies begin to decline in the infant and, if hypogammaglobulinemia is present, symptoms of this condition start to appear. Infants with this disorder experience frequent bacterial infections and failure to thrive, but with treatment most children survive into adulthood. The prognosis depends on the degree of antibody deficiency.

Clinical Presentation

See Table 30.5 for the associated features of the clinical presentation for the different types of hypogammaglobulinemia.

Assessment and Diagnosis

Note a history of recurrent infections, especially respiratory, gastrointestinal (GI), or genitourinary. Palpate for enlarged lymph nodes and spleen. In children presenting for routine administration of IVIG, determine whether any infections have occurred since the previous infusion. Lab findings for the different types of hypogammaglobulinemia are listed in Table 30.6.

Therapeutic Interventions

The current treatment for hypogammaglobulinemia is to manage the infection and replace abnormal elements. Replacement therapy of most types involves periodic administration of IVIG (Table 30.7). Before IVIG infusion, obtain baseline measures of serum blood urea nitrogen (BUN) and creatinine. A potential adverse reaction to IVIG is acute renal insufficiency. Assess for risk factors for thromboembolism, although it is a less common complication of IVIG infusion in children than in adults (Taketokmo, Hodding, & Kraus, 2017).

Evaluation

Expected outcomes for a child with hypogammaglobulinemia include the following:

- The child has not suffered from an overwhelming infection.
- The child is demonstrating appropriate growth and progress toward developmental milestones.
- The child and family are exhibiting healthy coping skills and effectively managing the disorder.

Table 30.5   Clinical Presentation of Select Types of Hypogammaglobulinemia

Type	Clinical Features
Selective IgA deficiency	- The child may be asymptomatic. - IgA offers mucosal protection, and, therefore, a deficiency makes the child more inclined to develop allergies and experience recurrent respiratory, GI, and GU infections. - The child is also more susceptible to developing an autoimmune disorder.
X-linked agammaglobulinemia	- Only males are affected. - The child typically has a history of recurrent respiratory and GI infections.
X-linked hyper-IgM syndrome	- Only males are affected. - The child typically has a history of recurrent respiratory infections, diarrhea, and malabsorption. - The child also develops neutropenia and autoimmune disorders.
IgG subclass deficiency	- The child has a history of recurrent respiratory infections. - Some children outgrow this condition.

GI, gastrointestinal; GU, genitourinary; Ig, immunoglobulin.

Table 30.6   Laboratory Findings of Select Types of Hypogammaglobulinemia

Type	Clinical Features
Selective IgA deficiency	- Serum IgA level is decreased. - IgG and IgM levels are normal.
X-linked agammaglobulinemia	- IgG, IgM, and IgA levels are markedly reduced or absent. - B cells are absent.
X-linked hyper-IgM syndrome	A defect occurs in the protein found on the T-cell surface, resulting in decreased IgG and IgA levels and significantly increased IgM levels.
IgG subclass deficiency	Levels of one or more of the subclasses of IgG are low.

Ig, immunoglobulin.

Table 30.7 Therapeutic Interventions for Select Types of Hypogammaglobulinemia

Type	Clinical Features
Selective IgA deficiency	• No specific gammaglobulin treatment is available; manage infections or autoimmune disorders. • A severe anaphylactic reaction can occur if the child receives a blood transfusion containing IgA and IgA antibodies.
X-linked agammaglobulinemia	• Administer routine IVIG infusions; manage infections.
X-linked hyper-IgM syndrome	• Administer routine IVIG and subcutaneous G-CSF when the child is neutropenic; assist with bone marrow transplantation; treat autoimmune disorders.
IgG subclass deficiency	• Treat respiratory infections; administration of IVIG has been found to be beneficial in some children.

G-CSF, granulocyte colony-stimulating factor; Ig, immunoglobulin; IVIG, intravenous immune globulin.

Discharge Planning and Teaching

Provide education and support to the child and family. Include in the teaching the need for periodic screenings to evaluate for lymphomas due to long-term Ig therapy. An excellent book for children with an immune deficiency is *Our Immune System* (1993) by Sara LeBien, which is provided free of charge from the Immune Deficiency Foundation at https://primaryimmune.org/publication/patients-and-families/our-immune-system.

Human Immunodeficiency Virus

Secondary immunodeficiency disorders, also known as acquired immunodeficiencies, are acquired by infection, malignancy, or therapy and are more common than are the primary disorders. They are classified by cause. Human immunodeficiency virus (HIV) is a disorder caused by an infectious agent and is the most well-known acquired immunodeficiency disease. HIV has been identified as the main secondary immunodeficiency disorder seen in children (Abbas et al., 2014, 2018; Grubbs, 2015). There are two types of HIV: HIV-1 and HIV-2. HIV-2 is primarily confined to West Africa. HIV-1 is the type most prevalent worldwide, most referred to in the literature, and discussed here.

Etiology and Pathophysiology

Children acquire HIV either vertically or horizontally. The mode of infection for an infant is usually via vertical transmission from the mother. The virus can be transferred in utero, during birth, or via breast milk. Horizontal transmission occurs from using nonsterile needles (as in IV drug use or tattooing) or from sexual contact. Acquiring HIV from transfused blood products has become very rare. Infants primarily acquire the virus through their mothers, whereas adolescents primarily acquire it through sexual activity or IV drug use. According to the latest CDC (2018b) statistics, 22% of all newly diagnosed HIV cases in the United States during the year 2015 were young

people aged 13 to 24 years. Globally, the rate of new HIV cases among children declined by 47% from 2010 to 2016 (Joint United Nations Programme on HIV/AIDS, 2017).

HIV causes a wide range of illnesses in children. Symptoms can range from none to mild, moderate, or severe. Acquired immune deficiency syndrome (AIDS), also known as acquired immunodeficiency syndrome, represents the most severe form of the illness. After a person contracts the virus, the blood does not exhibit any HIV antibody for 2 weeks to 6 months. During this time, the virus is replicating itself by infecting the CD4 (T helper) cells, causing them to become dysfunctional. The T helper cells demonstrate a decline in function even in asymptomatic infants and children who have not experienced large decreases in their CD4 cell count. Gradually, the number of CD4 cells declines, which weakens both humoral and cell-mediated immunity. When the number of CD4 cells is low, immune deficiency occurs and the patient becomes susceptible to opportunistic infections. Once a patient's CD4 cell count drops to less than 200 cells/μL and the patient has developed an opportunistic infection, he or she is diagnosed with AIDS (Capriotti & Frizzell, 2016).

HIV also causes B-cell defects, leading to high rates of serious bacterial infections. These defects impair the B cells' response to antigens, resulting in defective antibody production. NK cells play a critical role in protecting the newborn infant while the body is developing its own T-cell defense system. The NKs depend on the CD4 cells to secrete cytokines, which is important for their development of functionality. Thus, the functionality of the NKs can also be affected by HIV because the CD4 cells become dysfunctional. The monocytes and macrophage functions are also affected, thus contributing further to the state of immunodeficiency. Children with HIV become infected with normal organisms more frequently than do children not infected with HIV, and the infections are more severe. As in adults with HIV, the children are vulnerable to opportunistic infections (Siberry, Abzug, & Nachman, 2013). HIV can progress rapidly and invade the central nervous system, progressing to HIV encephalopathy. The encephalopathy causes children to regress and lose previously achieved developmental milestones. Other neurological and motor deficits may occur. In children with encephalopathy, the neurological symptoms may develop faster than do the immunosuppressive symptoms.

Clinical Presentation

Children with HIV may be asymptomatic. Presenting symptoms include chronic diarrhea, failure to thrive, and delayed development. Later symptoms may include frequent infections, including symptoms of opportunistic infections. Infants with HIV develop illnesses and symptoms of AIDS disease within a shorter time frame than is seen in adults (i.e., the latency period is shorter).

Assessment and Diagnosis

During the health history, make note of any reports of the more common signs and symptoms: failure to thrive, recurrent bacterial infections, opportunistic infections, chronic or recurrent diarrhea (from GI infections and lactose intolerance), recurrent or persistent fever, developmental delay, and prolonged candidiasis. Look for risk factors in the medical history such as maternal HIV infection or AIDS, receipt of blood transfusions, sexual abuse, substance use or abuse, or participation in sexual behaviors without the use of a condom. Determine level of consciousness. Upon physical exam, note any presence of fever, plot growth on the standard growth chart, and assess for any growth or developmental delays. Inspect the oral cavity for candidiasis (thrush). Assess respirations and observe for work of breathing; auscultate for adventitious sounds. Palpate for enlarged lymph nodes or swollen parotid glands. Palpate the abdomen, making note of an enlarged spleen or liver.

The incidence of HIV-2 in the United States is so low that the CDC does not recommend routine testing for HIV-2. Testing for HIV-2 in children is considered only if the mother had risk factors for HIV-2 or a known HIV-2 infection or if the child is exhibiting signs of HIV but the results of diagnostic tests for HIV-1 have been negative (Nyamweya et al., 2013). Therefore, the tests discussed here are for HIV-1.

The tests used to diagnose HIV in children are different from those used in adults. In adults antibodies are measured, whereas in infants an aspect of the virus, not antibodies, is measured. Serum Ig levels may be unusually high early in HIV infection and then decrease. A child is diagnosed with AIDS when the child has developed an opportunistic infection, the serum shows signs of HIV antibody, and the CD4 count is 200 or less. The reverse transcriptase polymerase chain reaction, enzyme-linked immunosorbent assay, and CD4 counts are the common lab and diagnostic studies ordered to assess for HIV infection in infants and children.

Refer to Table 30.4 for additional information about these tests.

Therapeutic Interventions

Nursing care of an infant or a child diagnosed with HIV can be very challenging. The primary focus of care is on taking measures to recognize early signs of infection to avoid the

development of HIV encephalopathy and AIDS. The number of children being diagnosed with HIV encephalopathy drastically declined after highly active antiretroviral drug therapy (HAART) was initiated. Care includes promoting normal growth and development; preventing infections; promoting compliance with the medication regimen; promoting nutrition; providing pain management and comfort measures; promoting respiratory and other organ function; educating the child, family, and caregivers; and providing ongoing psychosocial support. Instruct women with HIV who are pregnant on measures they can take to prevent transmitting the virus to the infant. Offer all pregnant women the opportunity to be tested and to receive any needed counseling services. If a pregnant woman is HIV positive, treatment depends on the stage of pregnancy. Once infants are born, they should receive treatment per the current guidelines. Breastfeeding is discouraged in mothers with HIV, so educate the mother on safe alternatives to breastfeeding (Avert, 2018). During delivery, protect the infant from the infected maternal secretions. After delivery, bathe the newborn as soon as possible and wash the eyes and face before administering prophylactic eye medication. Invasive procedures should be avoided if possible in the newborn.

In 2017, the Department of Health and Human Services (DHHS) Panel on Antiretroviral Therapy (ART) and Medical Management of Children Living with HIV published updated guidelines for treatment (a link to the website and the document is located in the reference list at the end of the chapter). The treatment regimen prescribed should be based on consideration of patient characteristics (such as age and severity of illness), results of viral resistance testing, and characteristics of the proposed medications (DHHS, 2017 a-e; Van Dyke et al., 2016). The recommendations include the use of a combination of antiretroviral drugs. Often, this type of therapy is referred to as HAART and is described as an anti-HIV cocktail (Thompson & Shalit, 2014).

Although there is no cure for HIV infection, treatment with HAART has improved survival rates, growth, neurodevelopment, and immune function (The Pharmacy 30.2). Before HAART became a treatment option, neurocognitive complications, such as progressive HIV encephalopathy, were devastating. A diagnosis meant a terminal prognosis, usually within 2 years (Lazarus, Rutstein, & Lowenthal, 2015). Aggressive prophylactic antibiotic therapy in combination with ART or HAART has been successful in preventing opportunistic infections (Capriotti & Frizzell, 2016). Currently there is no evidence to indicate that starting treatment earlier than 14 days of life improves outcomes, but it remains an option (DHHS, 2017d). The therapy is adjusted as needed.

Many children with HIV experience failure to thrive, frequent diarrhea, and lactose intolerance, making it a challenge to maintain adequate nutrition and hydration. Treatments could include total parenteral nutrition, a special diet or formula, tube feedings, and vitamin supplements. Be aware of and avoid potential interactions between supplements and the child's prescribed antiretroviral medications. Antidiarrheal medications are not recommended for infants, but they may be prescribed

The Pharmacy 30.2 — Medications Used to Treat Human Immunodeficiency Virus

Medications	Classification	Route	Action	Nursing Considerations
Abacavir, lamivudine, zidovudine	NRTIs	• PO • IV	• Inhibit reverse transcription of viral DNA chain • Used in a three-drug regimen to treat HIV-1 • Zidovudine: also used to prevent perinatal HIV transmission	• Notify physician of muscle weakness, shortness of breath, headache, insomnia, rash, or unusual bleeding. • Zidovudine: administer IV over 1 h • Abacavir: risk of fatal hypersensitivity reaction
Amprenavir, atazanavir, indinavir, lopinavir, nelfinavir, ritonavir, saquinavir	Protease inhibitors	PO	• Used in a three-drug regimen to treat HIV-1 • Inhibit protease activity in the HIV-1 cell, giving rise to immature, noninfectious viral particles	• Risk of multiple drug interactions • Before administration, review adverse effects and administration implications for each drug.
Efavirenz, nevirapine	NNRTIs	• PO • IV	• Disrupt the virus life cycle by binding to HIV-1 reverse transcriptase, blocking DNA polymerase activity • Used in a three-drug regimen to treat HIV-1	Efavirenz: • May cause drowsiness Nevirapine: • Avoid St. John's wort. • Gently shake suspension before administration. • Monitor for symptoms of Stevens–Johnson syndrome.

HIV, human immunodeficiency virus; IV, intravenous; NNRTIs, nonnucleoside analog reverse transcriptase inhibitors; NRTIs, nucleoside analog reverse transcriptase inhibitors; PO, oral.
Adapted from Taketomo, C. K., Hodding, J. H., & Kraus, D. M. (2018). *Pediatric & neonatal dosage handbook* (25th ed.). Hudson, OH: Lexicomp.

for older children. Carefully monitor hydration status, skin turgor, and urine output.

Evaluation

Expected outcomes for a child with HIV include the following:

- The child has adequate respiratory function and remains well oxygenated and perfused.
- The child has sufficient nutritional intake and hydration to maintain normal growth patterns and weight.
- The child's skin remains free of preventable breakdown.
- The child and family demonstrate appropriate coping methods related to the diagnosis and prognosis.
- The child and family are able to adhere to the prescribed treatment regimens.

Discharge Planning and Teaching

Teach parents and caretakers how to watch for signs of infection and when to call the healthcare provider. Counsel adolescents about the methods and risk of transmission and how to decrease their risk if they are sexually active or involved in risky behaviors, such as drinking alcohol or using IV drugs. Preventative measures and early treatment of infection are vital and include practicing good hand washing and hand hygiene, avoiding contact with

individuals who are known to be infected, practicing good skin care, promoting a sanitary environment, receiving immunizations as scheduled, and following prescribed drug regimens. Regarding immunizations, it is important to keep on schedule. The administration of live virus vaccines depends on the CD4 count and level of immunosuppression. Children with HIV may receive the measles and varicella vaccines if they have mild-to-moderate immunosuppression (Kroger, Dutchin, & Vazquez, 2018).

Families of children infected with HIV face many stressors. These include coping with the diagnosis of an incurable disease, costly treatments and healthcare bills, possibly more than one family member being infected (mother and child), public stigma associated with HIV, confidentiality issues, and the amount of time needed to devote to multiple medical appointments and hospitalizations. Parents and family members may experience anticipatory grieving, guilt, anger, or denial. The nurse can help support the family's coping by encouraging participation in support groups and allowing them to express their feelings using therapeutic communication.

Educate the family regarding the importance of compliance with the HAART medication regimen. Work with the caregivers to develop a medication administration schedule that fits the family's routine. Educate personnel at the child's day care center or school regarding the disease, how it is transmitted, and how to handle having the child in the school setting. Eventually, as children with HIV get older, they will have to learn about their illness and how to care for themselves. Demonstrate acceptance of the child and model the behavior to others.

Adolescents with HIV must deal with not only the growth and developmental tasks of adolescence but also the challenges of HIV stigma, compliance with the ART or HAART regimen, concerns about sharing HIV status with others, limited social support, worries about HIV transmission, transitioning from pediatric to adult health care, and living with a chronic illness (Evangeli, 2018). Provide children, adolescents, and their families with appropriate referrals and information regarding available resources, such as the Elizabeth Glaser Pediatric AIDS Foundation at www.pedaids.org.

Autoimmune Disorders

When the immune system breaks down and does not function appropriately, the result can be an autoimmune disorder. When this happens, the body produces T cells and antibodies against its own cells and organs, known as autoantibodies. Although the exact cause of autoimmune disorders is unknown, potential factors include the following: changes in the immune system triggered by microorganisms or drugs; hormones; hereditary elements; exposure to environmental chemicals and solvents; dietary influences; and a lack of exposure to germs as a result of vaccines and antiseptics (Watson, 2017).

Systemic Lupus Erythematosus

Systemic lupus erythematosus (SLE), frequently referred to as lupus, is a chronic autoimmune disease. The highest incidence of SLE occurs among women of childbearing age, but children younger than 16 years can also develop SLE. The pediatric version of SLE is sometimes referred to as childhood-onset lupus or juvenile-type SLE (Tarr et al., 2015). SLE can affect any organ system and usually affects multiple organ systems. Diagnosis usually occurs after the age of 5 years, with the peak incidence of diagnosis occurring during the preadolescent years. The highest incidence occurs in non-Caucasian females, with African American and Hispanic females experiencing the most severe effects. Those living with SLE experience remissions and exacerbations (flares) throughout their life. Exacerbations can involve fever, skin rash, joint inflammation, and damage to the kidney and serosal membranes.

Etiology and Pathophysiology

The etiology is unknown, but identified risk factors include genetic predisposition and exposure to environmental, hormonal, and immunological triggers. Chromosomal regions linked to SLE have been identified, with chromosomes 1 and 6 being the most commonly documented (Capriotti & Frizzell, 2016). The inflammatory response in the tissues and organs is a result of the accumulation of immune complexes, which are formed when autoantibodies react with the body's self-antigens. The inflammation causes pain and injury to the tissues and microvasculature within the affected organ. Drug reactions, infections, and too much exposure to the sun are examples of factors that can trigger the inflammatory response.

Clinical Presentation

Initially, in children, the most common symptoms seen are in the hematological, cutaneous, and musculoskeletal systems. The skin appears to be one of the organs most affected by SLE. Changes in vision, neurological problems (such as cerebrovascular accidents, seizures, and transverse myelitis), kidney disease, cardiac problems, and mental psychosis are common complications. Symptoms vary depending on the organ system affected. The most common symptoms are listed in Box 30.1 and are shown in Figure 30.3.

Box 30.1 Common Symptoms of Systemic Lupus Erythematosus

- Classic butterfly rash across the bridge of the nose and the cheeks (can be used to make diagnosis; Fig. 30.3)
- Fever
- Joint inflammation and swelling and musculoskeletal symptoms (occur in 90% of patients)
- Fatigue
- Weight loss
- Splenic enlargement
- Pleural effusion
- Vasculitis
- Pericarditis
- Leukopenia
- Anemia
- Thrombocytopenia
- Nephrotic syndrome (effects on the kidney tend to be the most damaging)
- Raynaud phenomenon

Adapted from Capriotti, T., & Frizzell, J. P. (Eds.). (2016). *Pathophysiology. Introductory concepts and clinical perspectives.* Philadelphia, PA: F. A. Davis.

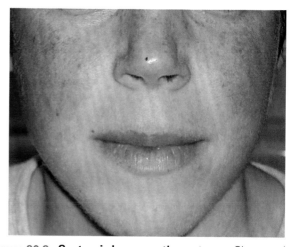

Figure 30.3. Systemic lupus erythematosus. Characteristic butterfly rash associated with systemic lupus erythematosus. Reprinted with permission from Kyle, T., & Carman, S. (2016). *Essentials of pediatric nursing* (3rd ed., Fig. 25.2). Philadelphia, PA: Wolters Kluwer.

Assessment and Diagnosis

Obtain a description of the current illness and chief complaint. During the health history, make note of any reports of the more common signs and symptoms: history of fatigue, fever, weight changes, pain or swelling in the joints, numbness, tingling or coolness of extremities, or prolonged bleeding. Look for risk factors in the medical history, such as the following: female sex; family history; African, Native American, or Asian descent; recent infection; drug reaction; or excessive sun exposure.

On physical exam, note any presence of fever. Measure the blood pressure, because hypertension can indicate renal involvement. Inspect the skin for the presence of a rash or lesions, specifically looking for the characteristic butterfly-shaped rash over the cheeks and for lesions on the face, scalp, or neck. Also make note of any changes in skin pigmentation, scarring, and areas of alopecia. Inspect the mouth for oral ulcerations (these tend to be painless). Assess the joints for pain and swelling. Auscultate the lungs, noting the presence of any adventitious sounds, which may indicate pulmonary system involvement and potential pleural effusion. Palpate the abdomen for areas of tenderness and splenic enlargement (abdominal involvement is more common in children than in adults).

SLE is diagnosed on the basis of a combination of clinical findings and lab evidence. The American College of Rheumatology (2017a) has identified criteria for diagnosing SLE. At least four physical symptoms and/or blood test abnormalities must be present to make the diagnosis (Box 30.2).

Box 30.2 Criteria for Diagnosis of Systemic Lupus Erythematosus

- Rash
  - Malar (butterfly-shaped and over the cheeks)
  - Discoid (red, with raised round or oval patches)
  - From sun exposure
- Sores in the mouth or nose (lasting from a few days to more than a month)
- Arthritis: two or more joints affected with tenderness and swelling lasting for a few weeks
- Pulmonary or cardiac inflammation (deep breathing causes chest pain due to the swelling of tissue lining the lungs and heart)
- Renal problems: blood or protein in the urine, or other tests indicating poor kidney function.
- Neurological problems: seizures, strokes, or psychosis (mental health issue)
- Abnormal blood tests
  - Low blood cell counts (hemoglobin, hematocrit, white blood cell, and platelet)
  - Positive antinuclear antibody (not specific to systemic lupus erythematosus but is usually present in children with the disorder)
  - The presence of autoantibodies
  - Decreased complement levels (C3 and C4)

Therapeutic Interventions

Children with SLE experience episodes of fatigue, especially during a flare-up. As a result, they do not get adequate rest or exercise. Additional rest is needed for healing during an exacerbation. Encourage daily activity and exercise to minimize the effects of complications from the disorder and side effects from corticosteroid therapy. Weight management, cardiovascular health, and prevention of osteoporosis are also benefits of daily activity and exercise. Teach the child and family how to balance exercise with comfort and rest.

Help the child and family recognize signs of impending flare-ups and identify what triggers them. Potential triggers include sunlight, stress, illness, and medications. Teach the child and family to protect against cold weather by dressing appropriately and how to inspect the toes and fingers for discoloration. Instruct them to avoid exposing the child to tanning beds, because they produce ultraviolet light, which can cause or worsen skin lesions, and unprotected fluorescent lighting, which has been reported to trigger exacerbations. Instruct patients who experience alopecia as a clinical manifestation on how to care for the head. Teach stress-reducing behaviors, which may benefit the child and lessen exacerbations. Smoking and use of alcohol or drugs, as well as use of birth control pills containing estrogen, increase the risk of a flare-up. Inform the adolescent of these risk factors and discuss options regarding birth control if they are sexually active.

A therapeutic management approach is used to treat the inflammatory response and prevent damage to the tissue and organ system. The dosing of drugs and types of treatments used depend on the severity of the disorder, which may be classified as mild-to-moderate, severe, or end-stage renal failure. Monitor for signs of nephritis, evaluating blood pressure, urine output, urine composition (i.e., assessing for hematuria and proteinuria), and serum BUN and creatinine levels. Children with mild-to-moderate SLE are treated with nonsteroidal anti-inflammatory drugs (NSAIDS), corticosteroids, and antimalarial agents (The Pharmacy 30.3). Children with severe SLE or those who experience frequent flare-ups are treated with high-dose (pulse) corticosteroid therapy or immunosuppressive drugs. Children with end-stage renal failure are placed on dialysis.

Evaluation

Expected outcomes for a child with SLE include the following:

- The child shares feelings about appearance.
- The child participates in activities.
- The child experiences minimal pain and discomfort.
- The child and family comply with prescribed treatment regimens.

Discharge Planning and Teaching

Care of the child with SLE is primarily supportive and requires long-term planning. The focus is on the prevention of complications. Infections are a leading cause of death for children with SLE. Teach parents the importance of informing other healthcare providers of the disorder so that they can take the necessary

The Pharmacy 30.3 Medications Used to Treat Systemic Lupus Erythematosus

Medication	Classification	Route	Action	Nursing Considerations
Hydroxychloroquine sulfate	Antimalarial	PO	• Impairs complement-dependent antigen-antibody reactions • Prevents skin problems and flare-ups in SLE and swelling and pain in JIA	Requires funduscopic eye exam and visual field testing every year
Cyclophosphamide	Cytotoxic	IV	• Interferes with normal DNA function by alkylation • Used to treat severe SLE	• Causes bone marrow suppression • Monitor for signs of infection. • Administer in the morning. • Provide adequate hydration. • Have child void frequently during and after infusion (risk of hemorrhagic cystitis).

IV, intravenous; JIA, juvenile idiopathic arthritis; PO, oral; SLE, systemic lupus erythematosus.
Adapted from Taketomo, C. K., Hodding, J. H., & Kraus, D. M. (2018). *Pediatric & neonatal dosage handbook* (25th ed.). Hudson, OH: Lexicomp.

precautions and prescribe prophylactic antibiotics, such as for dental work or surgical procedures. Educate the child and family regarding the importance of maintaining a healthy lifestyle, involving proper diet, exercise, sleep, and rest. Encourage yearly vision exams to monitor for any visual degeneration or ocular changes. Teach the child and parents to administer medications as ordered and to report any signs of possible complications related to treatment (Patient Safety 30.3). Recommend to adolescents with SLE genetic counseling about the risks of autoantibody transmission to the fetus during pregnancy. Refer the family to support services such as the Lupus Alliance of America and the Lupus Foundation of America for help in dealing with a chronic illness, which can be very challenging.

Juvenile Idiopathic Arthritis

Juvenile idiopathic arthritis (JIA) is an autoimmune disorder characterized by inflammation primarily affecting the joints. The disorder was formerly termed juvenile rheumatoid arthritis, but only a few types of juvenile arthritis produce a positive rheumatoid factor. A child with JIA may experience periods of

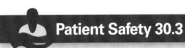

Patient Safety 30.3

Complications of Corticosteroid Therapy

Long-term or high-dose use of corticosteroids places patients with systemic lupus erythematosus at risk for developing avascular necrosis (osteonecrosis). Educate the child and family about the signs and what to report to their primary care practitioner, such as a new onset of pain or limited range of motion in the joints, especially with weight bearing (Mont et al., 2015).

being healthy that alternate with periods of joint inflammation flare-ups. Milder cases of the disorder have been reported to resolve as children reached adulthood. Other children may experience a more severe form of the disorder, causing them to deal with joint inflammation throughout their adulthood.

Etiology and Pathophysiology

As the term idiopathic in its name indicates, the cause of this condition is unknown. Factors such as infection, trauma, and stress have been discussed as possible triggers, but it has proved difficult to scientifically demonstrate a causal relationship. Scientists have also suggested that there is a genetic component making the child more susceptible, and research continues to look for a possible connection with human leukocyte antigens. Twice as many females as males are diagnosed with JIA (U.S. Department of Health & Human Services, 2018a).

Autoantibodies primarily target the synovial joints, resulting in decreased mobility, swelling, and pain. Normal synovial fluid acts as a cushion and helps lubricate cartilage, allowing for smooth joint movement. Once the synovium is inflamed, excessive thin, watery fluid is produced, diminishing the lubricating and cushion effects. Structures outside the joints may also become involved in the process, leading to further damage and deterioration. Potential complications include tendinitis, adhesions between joint surfaces, ankylosis of the joints, and soft-tissue contractures.

Clinical Presentation

The typical symptoms seen in JIA involve manifestations of joint inflammation, such as pain, redness, warmth, stiffness, and swelling (Fig. 30.4). Inactivity increases the stiffness and pain, and thus people with JIA tend to be very stiff in the morning after a night of sleep and decreased activity. Other forms of the disorder can involve the eyes and other organs. JIA is classified according to the number of joints involved and the presence of systemic manifestations, as shown in Table 30.8.

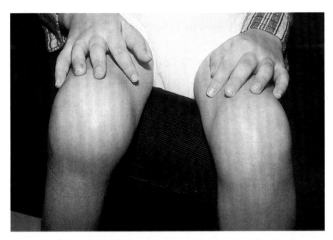

Figure 30.4. Juvenile idiopathic arthritis. Swollen knees associated with juvenile idiopathic arthritis. Reprinted with permission from Kyle, T., & Carman, S. (2016). *Essentials of pediatric nursing* (3rd ed., Fig. 25.2). Philadelphia, PA: Wolters Kluwer.

Assessment and Diagnosis

Note any history of irritability as an infant or a young child, because this may be the first sign of inflammation. Note any history of the child complaining of pain or not wanting to play or get out of bed in the morning. Ask whether the child has a history of fever. Assess for delayed growth and development and signs of current systemic disease, such as fever, rash, limping, or guarding of a joint or extremity. Inspect and palpate joints for edema, redness, warmth, tenderness and preferred position of comfort.

Common lab results consistent with a diagnosis with JIA include mild-to-moderate anemia and elevated erythrocyte sedimentation rate. Other lab results are associated with the different types, such as a positive antinuclear antibody with the pauciarticular form and a positive rheumatoid factor with the polyarticular form.

Therapeutic Interventions

The focus of nursing care is on promotion of a normal lifestyle by managing the inflammation, pain, and mobility issues (resulting from pain and swelling in the joints) of the disorder. The medication regimen includes NSAIDS, corticosteroids, and antirheumatic medications (The Pharmacy 30.4). Encourage parents to promote the child's sleep by providing a warm bath at bedtime, warm compresses to affected joints, or massage. Refer the child to a specialist in pediatric rheumatology. Refer the family to appropriate websites and groups, such as the Childhood Arthritis and Rheumatology Research Alliance, where they can obtain up-to-date information regarding clinical research and available treatments.

Evaluation

Expected outcomes for a child with JIA include the following:

- The child is able to move joints and complete activities of daily living with minimal pain and discomfort.
- The child is able to demonstrate appropriate growth and development.
- The child and family know how to recognize and manage the signs and symptoms of complications, such as avascular necrosis.

Discharge Planning and Teaching

A primary goal for these children and families is to learn how to effectively manage pain and maintain mobility. Evaluate their knowledge about the disorder and the treatment regimen.

Table 30.8 Types of Juvenile Idiopathic Arthritis

Type	Common Features
Pauciarticular (oligoarticular)	• Most common type • Involves up to four joints • Knee is often involved. • *Nonjoint manifestations:* eye inflammation, malaise, poor appetite, and poor weight gain • *Complications:* iritis, uveitis, and asymmetrical leg bone growth
Polyarticular	• Involves five or more joints • Frequently involves small joints • Usually affects the body symmetrically • *Nonjoint manifestations:* malaise, lymphadenopathy, organomegaly, and poor growth • *Complications:* rapidly progressing, severe form of arthritis; results in joint damage and rheumatoid nodules
Systemic	• May have fever and rash in addition to the joint involvement • *Nonjoint manifestations:* spleen, liver, and lymph node enlargement; myalgia; and severe anemia • *Complications:* pericarditis, pericardial effusion, pleuritis, and pulmonary fibrosis

Adapted from Hersh, A., & Prahalad, S. (2015). Immunogenetics of juvenile idiopathic arthritis: A comprehensive review. *Journal of Autoimmunity, 64*, 113–124. doi:10.1016/j.jaut.2015.08.002

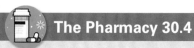

The Pharmacy 30.4   Medications Used to Treat Juvenile Idiopathic Arthritis

Medication	Classification	Route	Action	Nursing Considerations
Corticosteroids	Corticosteroids	• IV • PO	• Anti-inflammatory • Immunosuppressive	• Administer with food to decrease GI upset. • May mask signs of infection • Monitor blood pressure, urine (for glucose). • Monitor for Cushing syndrome, hypertension (during IV pulse infusion). • Do not stop treatment abruptly (risk of acute adrenal insufficiency). • May taper doses over time
Methotrexate, etanercept	DMARDS	• IV • PO	Methotrexate (antimetabolite): • Depletes DNA precursors • Inhibits DNA and urine synthesis Etanercept: • Binds to TNF, rendering it ineffective • Used for severe polyarticular juvenile arthritis	Methotrexate: • Do not give PO with dairy products. • Effects take 3–6 wk. • Salicylates may delay clearance. • Protect IV drug from light. • Labs to monitor: CBC, renal and liver function • Monitor for infection. Etanercept: • Monitor for infection. • Do not administer live vaccines. • Effects take 1 wk to 3 mo.

CBC, complete blood count; DMARDS, disease-modifying antirheumatic drugs; GI, gastrointestinal; IV, intravenous; PO, oral; TNF, tumor necrosis factor.
Adapted from Taketomo, C. K., Hodding, J. H., & Kraus, D. M. (2018). *Pediatric & neonatal dosage handbook* (25th ed.). Hudson, OH: Lexicomp.

Administer medications as prescribed to control inflammation and prevent disease progression. Refer to The Pharmacy 30.4 for information related to corticosteroids and disease-modifying antirheumatic drugs. Encourage the child to maintain joint range of motion and muscle strength via exercise (physical or occupational therapy). Swimming is a particularly useful exercise to maintain joint mobility without placing pressure on the joints. Teach families appropriate use of splints prescribed to prevent joint contractures. Monitor for pressure areas or skin breakdown with splint or orthotic use. Having two sets of books (one at school and one at home) allows the child to do homework without having to carry heavy books home. Health promotion includes educating the family about regular vision screening for the child to identify potential visual changes early and prevent further damage. Special summer camps for children with juvenile arthritis allow the child to socialize and belong to a group and have been shown to promote self-esteem in the child with chronic illness. Encourage appropriate family functioning and refer the family to support groups such as those sponsored by the American Juvenile Arthritis Organization.

Allergic Disorders

An allergy, also known as an allergic or hypersensitivity reaction, is an immune-mediated response that results in an adverse physiological reaction. Environmental and host factors, the duration and rate of exposure to the **allergen** (a foreign substance that triggers an allergic reaction), and the amount of the allergen all influence the allergic response type and severity. According to the CDC (2017), the number of cases of allergies being diagnosed in children has risen. Box 30.3 denotes common allergens in children. Careful assessments and teaching help to identify those at risk, as well as promote successful management of reactions (Capriotti & Frizzell, 2016).

Environmental Allergies

Environmental allergies result from exposure to allergens such as dust, mold, pollen, and pet dander.

Etiology and Pathophysiology

When a person is first exposed to an antigen, the body produces antibodies (usually IgE). Later exposures to the same antigen

Box 30.3   Common Allergens in Children

- Food allergens: cow's milk, eggs, wheat, chocolate, citrus fruits
- Inhalant allergens: mold, pollen, house dust, pet dander
- Drug allergens: oral and injectable
- Contact allergens: plants, dyes, chemicals
- Other: animal serum/venom, insect stings

Adapted from AAFAb, 2015.

cause an antigen–antibody reaction, which results in cell damage, release of histamine into the bloodstream, and allergic symptoms.

Clinical Presentation

The severity of symptoms during an allergic reaction can vary widely. Box 30.4 lists common symptoms of an allergic reaction.

Assessment and Diagnosis

There are three steps used to diagnose allergies: personal and medical history, physical exam, and diagnostic tests. Obtain a health history, noting any reports of signs of allergies or adverse reactions or any past testing and results. Assess the child's ears, nose, throat, eyes, skin, chest, and lungs for signs of inflammation or allergic reaction, such as nasal swelling and drainage, atopic dermatitis, or adventitious sounds and wheezing on auscultation of lungs. An X-ray of the lungs and sinuses may be obtained to look for signs of inflammation (Asthma and Allergy Foundation of America [AAFA b,c], 2015).

Additional tests may be conducted to rule out other disorders, such as lung function tests for asthma. Allergy tests help identify the specific antigens causing reactions (Priority Care Concepts 30.2). Allergy testing involves a variety of labs, including IgE skin prick tests, intradermal injections of allergens, blood tests, CBC differential, total eosinophil count, nasal smear, serum IgE level, and antigen-specific IgE radioallergosorbent test (RAST; AAAAI, 2018). The appearance of urticarial wheals on the skin half an hour after administration of selected potential allergens is considered a positive allergy result from skin testing. The reaction can be immediate or delayed.

Box 30.4 Common Symptoms of an Allergic Reaction

- Itchy, watery eyes
- Itchy, runny nose and sneezing
- Rashes, hives
- Stomach cramps, bloating, vomiting, diarrhea
- Swelling, redness, pain
- Tongue swelling, throat closing
- Cough, wheezing, chest tightness, shortness of breath
- Feeling faint, light-headed, or "blacking out"
- A sense of "impending doom"

Adapted from AAFA b, 2015.

Priority Care Concepts 30.2

Allergy Testing

In skin testing, an anaphylactic reaction is rare but can still occur, even if the exposure to the allergen is minimal. Keep emergency equipment and medications immediately available.

Therapeutic Interventions

Medication therapy for environmental allergies includes antihistamines, bronchodilators, corticosteroids, preventative inhaled medications, such as cromolyn sodium for asthma, and epinephrine. See The Pharmacy 30.5 for additional drug information.

Evaluation

Expected outcomes for a child with an allergy disorder include the following:

- The child has adequate nutritional intake, as determined by growth patterns and weight being within normal limits.
- The child and family have adequate knowledge about recognizing and managing episodes of hypersensitivity.
- The child and family demonstrate appropriate coping methods related to the diagnosis.

Discharge Planning and Teaching

The goals of treatment interventions and therapy are to decrease the exposure to allergens, increase a child's tolerance to allergens, and prevent or treat symptoms of reactions to exposure. Immunotherapy, also called hyposensitization or allergy shots, is used to increase the child's tolerance to allergens.

Food Allergies

A food allergy, or food hypersensitivity, is an IgE-mediated immunological reaction to ingestion of a food or food additive. About 4% to 6% of children in the United States are affected by food allergies (CDC, 2018a). The most common food allergies acquired during childhood are allergies to milk, eggs, peanuts, tree nuts, fish, shellfish, wheat, and soy. Peanut, tree nut, fish, and shellfish allergies tend to be the only ones that continue into adulthood.

Etiology and Pathophysiology

There are two categories of food allergies: IgE-mediated and non–IgE-mediated. In IgE-mediated allergies, the IgE antibodies react to certain foods. In non–IgE-mediated allergies, other parts of the immune system react to the food. This reaction still causes symptoms but does not involve IgE. A person can have both types of allergies (Kids with Food Allergies, 2014).

Clinical Presentation

Allergic reactions can involve the skin, mouth, eyes, lungs, heart, gut, and brain. Signs and symptoms include hives, flushing, facial swelling, mouth and throat itching, runny nose, and GI reactions, such as vomiting, abdominal pain, and diarrhea. In severe reactions, the tongue, uvula, pharynx, or upper airway may swell. Wheezing indicates that edema is occurring in the airway and is considered a serious sign of respiratory complications. Although it is rare, collapse of the cardiovascular system can occur.

The Pharmacy 30.5 Medications Used to Treat Allergies

Medication	Classification	Route	Action	Nursing Considerations
Various	Antihistamine	• PO • IV • PR	Competes with histamine on receptor sites during a hyper-sensitivity reaction	• Give before or early in a hy-persensitivity reaction • Ineffective if given late in a reaction
Various	Bronchodilator	INH	Given for lower respiratory symptoms and to decrease inflammation	• Short-acting: used to imme-diately open airway passages (rescue inhaler) • Long-acting: used with in-haled steroid to manage the disorder
Cromolyn sodium	Mast cell stabilizer	INH	Anti-inflammatory; used to prevent bronchospasms and bronchial asthma attacks	• Not approved for use in chil-dren <2 y of age • Not a rescue inhaler; will not help the patient during an asthma attack
Epinephrine (EpiPen)	Bronchodilator	• IM • SQ	Used for severe asthma and allergy attacks, including anaphylaxis	• EpiPen Jr: up to 65 lb • EpiPen Adult: over 65 lb

IM, intramuscular; INH, inhalational; IV, intravenous; PO, oral; PR, rectal; SQ, subcutaneous.
Adapted from Taketomo, C. K., Hodding, J. H., & Kraus, D. M. (2018). *Pediatric & neonatal dosage handbook* (25th ed.). Hudson, OH: Lexicomp.

Assessment and Diagnosis

Immediately assess airway, breathing, and circulation to identify potential serious reactions. Once a child is determined to be sta-ble, complete the rest of the assessment. Obtain a detailed food history and details about reactions, including the suspected food, quantity consumed, length of time between ingestion and symptoms, description of the symptoms, treatments received, and response to treatments. The detailed food history can help determine whether the reactions are a result of a food intoler-ance or a true food allergy. Make note of any reported GI symp-toms, such as burning in the mouth or throat, bloating, nausea, and diarrhea. Identify potential risk factors such as a previous exposure to the suspected food, a history of asthma that has not been appropriately managed and controlled, or a report of eczema flare-ups related to food. Inspect the skin, observing for color and signs of a rash, hives, or edema. Auscultate the heart and lungs, making note of the heart and respiratory rates and any wheezing.

Diagnostic testing involves allergy skin prick tests, RASTs, blood tests, IgE tests, and challenge tests. Challenge tests are done for suspected food and medication allergies. During a challenge test, a very small amount of an allergen is inhaled or taken by mouth. A physician, preferably an allergist, should be supervising the tests (AAAAI, 2018).

Therapeutic Interventions

Therapeutic and nursing management should be focused on avoiding and alleviating the child's immunological response to food allergens. Medications used include histamine blockers and epinephrine. An important first step is to determine the difference between a food intolerance and a true food allergy.

Food intolerance can occur when certain foods or additives cause an abnormal physiological, but not immunological, re-sponse. An example is milk allergy, which is often misperceived as lactose intolerance. Determining the difference helps ensure that the child receives appropriate treatment (Analyze the Evi-dence 30.1).

Evaluation

Expected outcomes for a child with a food allergy include the following:

• The child has not experienced harm from a hypersensitivity reaction due to the ability to successfully prevent or manage a reaction.
• The child is maintaining adequate nutrition and hydration, as evidenced by achieving growth and development patterns appropriate for age.

Discharge Planning and Teaching

Parents need much teaching and support, because having a child with a food allergy can cause anxiety and fear. Educate the parents, child, day care personnel, school teachers, friends, and others involved in the child's daily activities on the signs of an allergic reaction. Children with allergies are at risk for anaphy-laxis, so teach parents and caregivers to be alert to the signs of an anaphylactic reaction. Refer families to the Food Allergy and Anaphylaxis Network for additional information and support. Teaching should include how and when to use the medications, especially during an allergic reaction (Patient Teaching 30.3; Fig. 30.5). The family should have a written emergency plan in case of severe reactions.

Analyze the Evidence 30.1 Peanut Oral Immunotherapy

Current treatment for peanut allergy includes peanut desensitization through peanut oral immunotherapy. Much like desensitization to animal dander through allergy shots, peanut oral immunotherapy desensitizes allergic children through exposure to peanuts in scheduled doses. In a study conducted by Nachshon, Goldberg, Katz, Levy, and Elizer (2018), the researchers found that oral immunotherapy was effective even in children with prior anaphylactic reactions or associated asthma as long as the guidelines for maintenance therapy were followed. Children beginning oral immunotherapy should be monitored in a clinic or hospital setting during the buildup phase because of the risk of an allergic reaction.

Patient Teaching 30.3

Using an Epinephrine Auto-injector

Children who have been identified as being at risk for severe reactions are prescribed an epinephrine auto-injector (EpiPen), which they should carry on their person at all times. To use an epinephrine auto-injector, the child should do the following:

1. Hold the leg steady.
2. Place the orange tip of the auto-injector in the middle of the thigh (Fig. 30.5).
3. Hold the auto-injector at a right angle to the thigh.
4. Push the auto-injector firmly until a "click" is heard.

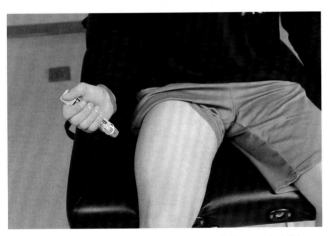

Figure 30.5. Using an epinephrine auto-injector. A child getting ready to use an epinephrine auto-injector. The orange tip is placed in the middle of the thigh at a 90° angle. Reprinted with permission from Miller, M., & Berry, D. (2015). *Emergency response management for athletic trainers* (2nd ed., Fig. 20.2). Philadelphia, PA: Wolters Kluwer.

Dietary teaching should include how to read food labels, information about hidden allergens in food, and what foods are safe substitutes. A list of hidden food allergens can be accessed from the Kids with Food Allergies (2015) website at http://www.kidswithfoodallergies.org/page/top-food-allergens.aspx. A referral to a dietician may be helpful for the family to learn additional ways of avoiding the food allergens and how to manage the child's nutrition.

Latex Allergy

Latex refers to the protein in the sap of the Brazilian rubber tree (*Hevea brasiliensis*) and to the natural rubber products made from the sap. Latex can be found in many everyday household products, such as balloons, rubber bands, rubber balls, and bandages (AAFA, 2015).

The development of an allergy to latex products has become a common occurrence among children, healthcare workers, and the general population worldwide (Wu, McIntosh, & Liu, 2016). Millions of consumer and commercial products containing latex are produced and are not required to include on the label whether the product contains latex. This lack of identification of latex content makes it difficult to completely prevent contact with the allergen. Gloves are an example of a very common item used in health care that contains latex and exposes patients and healthcare workers alike to this potential allergen. Many health institutions have now eliminated the use of latex gloves, but the gloves are still being sold in stores and used in other industries, so the risk of exposure remains high for those with an allergy. Children at the highest risk for latex allergy are those with spina bifida and those who undergo frequent medical procedures and surgeries in which they are exposed to products containing latex.

Etiology and Pathophysiology

Latex allergy and food allergy have a similar pathophysiology. A person can have a reaction from breathing in latex fibers in the air or from skin contact with a latex product. Not all reactions are a true allergy. There are three types of reactions to natural rubber latex:

- *IgE-mediated latex allergy*: This type involves the immune system, is considered a true allergic reaction, and can be life-threatening. This type of reaction occurs when IgE antibodies react with latex proteins.
- *Cell-mediated contact dermatitis*: This type causes skin inflammation but is not life-threatening. This type of reaction is more of a sensitivity to the chemicals used in the making of the product rather than to the rubber protein. The dermatitis can spread but usually resolves on its own. Four out of five people who develop an IgE-mediated allergy are reported to have had contact dermatitis first; thus, such a diagnosis should be taken as a warning sign and the child should be monitored closely for development of a true allergy.

- *Irritant dermatitis*: This type is a common reaction but not an allergy. A red, itchy rash develops where the skin comes into contact with a natural rubber product. Healthcare workers who wear powdered gloves often develop this condition. Again, any contact dermatitis should be taken seriously and the person monitored for the development of a true allergy (AAFA, 2015).

Clinical Presentation

A child who has come into contact with latex can present with any of the symptoms of an allergic reaction: hives, wheezing, cough, shortness of breath, nasal congestion, rhinorrhea, sneezing, pruritus in the nose, palate or eyes, and hypotension.

Assessment and Diagnosis

All children who go to healthcare facilities need to be screened for latex allergy. Obtain the child's health history, making note of reported allergy to rubber items, such as gloves, or any symptoms of a reaction after exposure, such as hives, rash, coughing, wheezing, or shortness of breath. Additional questions and signs to look for in the health history include the following:

- Swelling or itching of the mouth after a dental examination
- Allergic symptoms after eating foods known to have cross-reactivity to latex (e.g., pears, peaches, passion fruit, plums, pineapple, kiwi, figs, grapes, cherries, melons, nectarines, papaya, apples, apricots, bananas, chestnuts, carrots, celery, avocados, tomatoes, or potatoes)

On physical exam, assess the child for signs and symptoms of a reaction and implement appropriate interventions.

Therapeutic Interventions

The focus of nursing management is to prevent exposure to latex products. Once exposed, remove the allergen and cleanse the area with soap and water. Assess the child for reaction signs, and prepare to intervene as needed, such as by resuscitation, if the reaction is severe. Latex allergy should be documented as an alert on the child's chart, identification band, medication administration record, and physician's order sheet.

Evaluation

Expected outcomes for a child with a latex allergy include the following:

- The child and family have taken measures to reduce the child's exposure potential triggers of allergic reaction.
- The child, family, and school personnel understand the signs and symptoms of a reaction and have created an emergency plan.

Discharge Planning and Teaching

Teach the child and family about foods with a known cross-reactivity to latex. Parents should receive information about signs and symptoms of latex hypersensitivity and create an emergency treatment plan. Provide resource information, such as websites and the names of organizations for people with latex allergy.

Anaphylaxis

Anaphylaxis is an acute, immediate, and severe IgE-mediated response to an allergen. Any allergen, whether it is from food, latex, an insect sting, or drugs, has the potential to trigger a severe reaction that results in anaphylaxis. The most common triggers for anaphylaxis are listed in Box 30.5.

Etiology and Pathophysiology

An anaphylactic response is an exaggerated allergic reaction in which the entire body is affected by an excessive release of chemical mediators. The response can be triggered by an allergen that has induced a response in the past or by one that has never evoked a response in the child before. Because anaphylaxis involves many organ systems and may be life-threatening, it is considered a medical emergency. Once contact is made with an allergen, a severe reaction usually starts within 5 to 10 minutes. B cells are triggered to produce plasma cells. The plasma cells secrete Igs. The IgE, mast cells, and eosinophils release a large amount of histamines and other inflammatory mediators, leading to tissue edema. Cutaneous, cardiopulmonary, GI, and neurological symptoms occur as a result. Plasma volume rapidly decreases from vasodilation, placing the body at risk for circulatory collapse. The child may need prolonged resuscitation, and there is a risk of death.

Clinical Presentation

Clinical manifestations include pruritic urticaria (itchy hives), coughing, stridor, asthma attack, extreme anxiety, and loss of consciousness. Additional manifestations include lip, tongue, or palate pruritus and swelling; nasal pruritus; congestion; sneezing; stridor; tachycardia; and chest pain.

Assessment and Diagnosis

Note the child's level of consciousness. In the health history, obtain information about prior exposure to the allergen, including any medications the child received and the response to treatment. Symptoms seen on examination include the following: urticaria; edema of tongue; bronchospasm; laryngeal edema; facial edema (angioedema); hypotension; tingling of the palms of the hands, soles of the feet, or lips; light-headedness; and tightness of the chest (CDC, 2017). If prompt treatment is not received, these symptoms can progress to seizures, cardiac arrhythmia, shock, respiratory distress, and, ultimately, death (Priority Care Concepts 30.3).

Diagnostic testing involves obtaining lab tests to check for elevated IgE and eosinophils levels in nasal and bronchial secretions. Check vital signs to assess for severe hypotension.

Box 30.5   Common Triggers for Anaphylaxis

- Food, such as nuts, shellfish, and eggs
- Insect stings, such as by a bee or wasp
- Drugs, such as penicillin and nonsteroidal anti-inflammatory drugs
- Radiopaque dyes
- Latex

Therapeutic Interventions

The focus of nursing management for children with anaphylaxis is on supporting the airway, breathing, and circulation. Determine whether the airway is patent and breathing and circulation are sufficient. This is a medical emergency, and therefore the child should be treated with IV antihistamine, IV epinephrine, and IV corticosteroids (Capriotti & Frizzell, 2016). The focus of therapeutic management is to assess and provide ongoing support of the airway, breathing, and circulation. The initial goal is to maintain a patent airway. Sometimes endotracheal intubation is needed to meet this goal. After establishing a patent airway, administer epinephrine as ordered. Administer supplemental oxygen as needed. If bronchospasms occur, administer a bronchodilator inhalation treatment. Administer IV fluids to provide volume expansion and corticosteroids to prevent late-onset reactions. Monitor the child for at least 2 hours after an anaphylactic reaction.

Priority Care Concepts 30.3

Anaphylaxis

- Observe children with allergic urticaria carefully for signs of anaphylaxis.
- Anaphylaxis is a medical emergency and requires immediate injection of epinephrine.
- Children experiencing an anaphylactic reaction can quickly progress to shock.
- Monitor the child's airway, breathing, and circulation.
- Assess for hypotension.
- Assess for cardiac arrhythmia.
- Have emergency equipment ready in case of cardiac arrest.
- Administer emergency medications as ordered.

Evaluation

Expected outcomes for a child with anaphylaxis include the following:

- The child is able to maintain a patent airway and adequate oxygenation and perfusion.
- The child has not experienced harm from a severe hypersensitivity reaction.
- The child and family demonstrate appropriate coping skills.
- The child is able to meet growth and developmental milestones appropriate for age.

Discharge Planning and Teaching

Priority education for the family is how to prevent and manage future episodes of an anaphylactic reaction. An emergency plan should be in place at home and at the child's school or day care center with up-to-date contact information. Teach the family, caretakers, and child, if age-appropriate, how to use injectable epinephrine, usually in the form of an EpiPen, in the case of allergen exposure. The child should carry the epinephrine at all times and wear a medical alert identification bracelet or necklace. Instruct the child and family to call emergency personnel (911) as soon as possible after the EpiPen has been administered. To help prevent future episodes, teach the child and family how to avoid known allergens. Immunotherapy (allergy shots) or desensitization treatments may be indicated for certain types of allergies, such as a hypersensitivity to stinging insects or a severe penicillin allergy. Families need to understand the treatments and what is involved; for example, desensitization typically requires the child to spend a few days in the intensive care unit while the treatment is being administered. Make referrals as needed to support groups, counseling, and other services.

Think Critically

1. The nurse is providing discharge teaching to the parents of an infant newly diagnosed with an immunodeficiency disorder. What kinds of lifestyle changes should the nurse encourage the family to make?
2. A mother who is positive for HIV wants to breastfeed her infant. What does the evidence-based research indicate regarding the practice of allowing HIV-positive mothers to breastfeed their infants?
3. A family needs assistance developing a safe nutrition plan for their child, who has just been diagnosed with food allergies. What is important to include in the dietary teaching concerning how to shop for and identify safe food choices?
4. The goal of pain management for a child with an autoimmune disorder is to minimize the pain to a tolerable level. How does living with a child with chronic pain affect the quality of life of the family?
5. An 18-year-old female with a chronic immunological disorder has graduated from high school and is preparing to move away from home and enter college. The healthcare team is working with her on a transition preparation plan. What is important to include in the plan as she transitions to adult life and the adult healthcare system?
6. A child diagnosed with HIV needs to see a dentist, but the mother is concerned about sharing the child's diagnosis with the dentist's staff. What are the risks associated with disclosure vs. nondisclosure of the child's diagnosis?

References

Abbas, A. K., Lichtman, A. H., & Pillai, S. (2014). *Basic immunology. Functions and disorders of the immune system* (4th ed.). Philadelphia, PA: Elsevier.

Abbas, A. K., Lichtman, A. H., & Pillai, S. (2018). *Cellular and molecular immunology* (9th ed.). Philadelphia, PA: Elsevier.

Agwu, A. L., Warshaw, M. G., McFarland, E. J., Siberry, G. K., Melvin, A. J., Wiznia, A. A., . . . & Carey, V. J. (2017). Decline in CD4 T lymphocytes with monotherapy bridging strategy for non-adherent adolescents living with HIV infection: Results of the IMPAACT P1094 randomized trial. *PLoS One, 12*(6), e0178075. doi:10.1371/journal.pone.0178075

American Academy of Allergy Asthma & Immunology (AAAAI). (2018). *Primary immunodeficiency disease.* Retrieved from http://www.aaaai.org/conditions-and-treatments/primary-immunodeficiency-disease

American College of Rheumatology. (2017a). *Patient fact sheet. Systemic lupus erythematosus (juvenile).* Retrieved from https://www.rheumatology.org/Portals/0/Files/Systemic-Lupus-Erythematosus-Juvenile-Fact-Sheet.pdf

Asthma and Allergy Foundation of America. (2015a). *Allergies. Latex allergy.* Retrieved from http://www.aafa.org/page/latex-allergy.aspx

Asthma and Allergy Foundation of America. (2015b). *Allergies. What are the symptoms of an allergy?* Retrieved from http://www.aafa.org/page/allergy-symptoms.aspx

Asthma and Allergy Foundation of America. (2015c). *Allergy diagnosis.* Retrieved from http://www.aafa.org/page/allergy-diagnosis.aspx

Avert. (2018). *Pregnancy, childbirth & breastfeeding and HIV.* Retrieved from https://www.avert.org/hiv-transmission-prevention/pregnancy-childbirth-breastfeeding?gclid=Cj0KCQjwvqbaBRCOARIsAD9s1XAvKJHUNiDtAeXxU3u0RZoZDCUyg4GF8Uw0tU3JB1AtDQUiRb87DzUaAmi9EALw_wcB

Bonilla, F. A., Khan, D. A., Ballas, Z. K., Chinen, J., Frank, M. M., Hsu, J. T., . . . & Wallace, D. (2015). Practice parameter for the diagnosis and management of primary immunodeficiency. *The Journal of Allergy and Clinical Immunology, 136*(5), 1186–1205.e78. doi:10.1016/j.jaci.2015.04.049

Buckley, R. H. (2016). T lymphocytes, B lymphocytes, and natural killer cells. In R. M. Kliegman, B. F. Stanton, J. W. St. Geme, & N. F. Schor (Eds.), *Nelson textbook of pediatrics* (20th ed., pp. 1006–1012). Philadelphia, PA: Elsevier.

Capriotti, T., & Frizzell, J. P. (Eds.). (2016). *Pathophysiology. Introductory concepts and clinical perspectives.* Philadelphia, PA: F. A. Davis.

Carr, A., & Maggini, S. (2017). Vitamin C and immune function. *Nutrients, 9*(11), 1211. doi:10.3390/nu9111211

Centers for Disease Control and Prevention. (2017). *Allergies.* Retrieved from https://www.cdc.gov/healthcommunication/toolstemplates/entertainmented/tips/Allergies.html

Centers for Disease Control and Prevention. (2018a). *Food allergies in schools.* Retrieved from https://www.cdc.gov/healthyschools/foodallergies/index.htm

Centers for Disease Control and Prevention. (2018b). *HIV among youth.* Retrieved from https://www.cdc.gov/hiv/group/age/youth/index.html

Chin, T. (2014). *Agammaglobulinemia.* Retrieved from https://emedicine.medscape.com/article/884942-overview?pa=Yms3TCMXY7j3ZX-G9URlVsQIpDi1Gs0g3q0827Od%2FiasHLXhVFL26iTxUpOTGjiIo-90HykujeBj583Ixuq11RHKbXa1aj0VoWN5%2BW19QIDeU%3D#a5

Chin, T., Windle, M., Jyonouchi, H., & Georgitis, J. (2014). IgA and IgG subclass deficiencies. Retrieved from https://emedicine.medscape.com/article/885348-overview#showall

Department of Health and Human Services (DHHS) Panel on Antiretroviral Therapy and Medical Management of Children Living with HIV. (2017a). *Guidelines for the use of antiretroviral agents in pediatric HIV infection. Diagnosis of HIV infection in infants and children.* Retrieved from https://aidsinfo.nih.gov/guidelines/html/2/pediatric-arv/59/clinical-and-laboratory-monitoring-of-pediatric-hiv-infection

Department of Health and Human Services (DHHS) Panel on Antiretroviral Therapy and Medical Management of Children Living with HIV. (2017b). *Guidelines for the use of antiretroviral agents in pediatric HIV infection. Clinical and laboratory monitoring.* Retrieved from https://aidsinfo.nih.gov/guidelines/html/2/pediatric-arv/55/diagnosis-of-hiv-infection-in-infants-and-children

Department of Health and Human Services (DHHS) Panel on Antiretroviral Therapy and Medical Management of Children Living with HIV. (2017c). *Guidelines for the use of antiretroviral agents in pediatric HIV infection. Management of children receiving antiretroviral therapy.* Retrieved from https://aidsinfo.nih.gov/guidelines/html/2/pediatric-arv/438/recognizing-and-managing-antiretroviral-treatment-failure

Department of Health and Human Services (DHHS) Panel on Antiretroviral Therapy and Medical Management of Children Living with HIV. (2017d). *Guidelines for the use of antiretroviral agents in pediatric HIV infection. Treatment recommendations.* Retrieved from https://aidsinfo.nih.gov/guidelines/html/2/pediatric-arv/62/treatment-recommendations

Department of Health and Human Services (DHHS) Panel on Antiretroviral Therapy and Medical Management of Children Living with HIV. (2017e). *Guidelines for the use of antiretroviral agents in pediatric HIV infection. When to initiate therapy in antiretroviral-naive children.* Retrieved from https://aidsinfo.nih.gov/guidelines/html/2/pediatric-arv/70/when-to-initiate-therapy-in-antiretroviral-naive-children

Evangeli, M. (2018). Mental health and substance use in HIV-infected adolescents. *Current Opinion in HIV & AIDS, 13*(3), 204–211. doi:10.1097/COH.0000000000000451

Fernandez, J. (2016). *Transient hypogammaglobulinemia of infancy.* Retrieved from https://www.merckmanuals.com/professional/immunology-allergic-disorders/immunodeficiency-disorders/transient-hypogammaglobulinemia-of-infancy

Fischbach, F., & Fischbach, M. (2017). *Fischbach's. A manual of laboratory and diagnostic tests* (10th ed.). Philadelphia, PA: Lippincott Williams & Wilkins.

Grubbs, L. (2015). Nonspecific complaints. Immunodeficiency disorders. In M. J. Goolsby, & L. Grubbs (Eds.), *Advanced Assessment. Interpreting findings and formulating differential diagnoses* (3rd ed., pp. 487). Philadelphia, PA: F. A. Davis Company.

Guilmot, A., Hermann, E., Braud, V., Carlier, Y., & Truyens, C. (2011). Natural killer cell responses to infections in early life. *Journal of Innate Immunity, 3*(3), 280–288. doi:10.1159/000323934

Hogan, M. A., Wagner, N. H., White, J. E., & Johnson, T. (Eds.). (2013). *Child health nursing. Reviews & rationales* (3rd ed.). Upper Saddle River, NJ: Pearson Prentice Hall.

Immune Deficiency Foundation. (2013). *Patient and family handbook for primary immunodeficiency diseases* (5th ed.). Towson, MD: Immune Deficiency Foundation. Retrieved from https://primaryimmune.org/wp-content/uploads/2016/03/IDF-Patient-Family-Handbook-5th-Edition-2015-Reprint-Web.pdf

Immune Deficiency Foundation. (2015). *Diagnostic and clinical care guidelines for primary immunodeficiency diseases* (3rd ed.). Retrieved from https://primaryimmune.org/publication/healthcare-professionals/idf-diagnostic-clinical-care-guidelines-primary

Immune Deficiency Foundation. (2018a). *About primary immunodeficiencies.* Retrieved from https://primaryimmune.org/about-primary-immunodeficiencies

Immune Deficiency Foundation. (2018b). *Guide to hematopoietic stem cell transplantation.* Retrieved from https://primaryimmune.org/resourcecenter?f%5B%5D=type%3Apublication#search

Jeffrey Modell Foundation. (2016). *10 warning signs of primary immunodeficiency.* Retrieved from http://www.info4pi.org/library/educational-materials/10-warning-signs

Joint United Nations Programme on HIV/AIDS. (2017). *Fact sheet-World AIDS day 2017.* Retrieved from http://www.unaids.org/sites/default/files/media_asset/UNAIDS_FactSheet_en.pdf

Jung, C., Hugot, J. P., & Barreau, F. (2010). Peyer's patches: The immune sensors of the intestine. *International Journal of Inflammation, 2010*, 823710. doi:10.4061/2010/823710

Kids with Food Allergies. (2014). *Living with food allergies. What is a food allergy? There are different types of allergic reactions to foods.* Retrieved from http://www.kidswithfoodallergies.org/page/what-is-a-food-allergy.aspx

Kids with Food Allergies. (2015). *Living with food allergies. Allergen avoidance lists.* Retrieved from http://www.kidswithfoodallergies.org/page/top-food-allergens.aspx

Kroger, A. T., Duchin, J., & Vazquez, M. (2018). *General best practice guidelines for immunization. Best practices guidance of the advisory committee on immunization practices (ACIP).* Retrieved from https://www.cdc.gov/vaccines/hcp/acip-recs/general-recs/index.html

Lazarus, J. R., Rutstein, R. M., & Lowenthal, E. D. (2015). Treatment initiation factors and cognitive outcome in youth with perinatally acquired HIV infection. *HIV Medicine, 16*(6), 355–361. doi:10.1111/hiv.12220

Mont, M., Pivec, R., Banerjee, R., Issa, K., Elmallah, R. K., & Jones, L. C. (2015). High-dose corticosteroid use and risk of hip osteonecrosis: Meta-analysis and systematic literature review. *The Journal of Arthroplasty, 30*(9), 1506–1512. doi:10.1016/j.arth.2015.03.036

Morgan, R., Gray, D., Lomova, A., & Kohn, D. (2017). Hematopoietic stem cell gene therapy: Progress and lessons learned. *Cell Stem Cell, 21*(5), 574–590. doi:10.1016/j.stem.2017.10.010

Mortaz, E., Tabarsi, P., Mansouri, D., Khosravi, A., Garssen, J., Velayati, A., & Adcock, I. M. (2016). Cancers related to immunodeficiencies: Update and perspectives. *Frontiers in Immunology, 7*, 365. doi:10.3389/fimmu.2016.00365

Nachshon, L., Goldberg, M. R., Katz, Y., Levy, M. B., & Elizer, A. (2018). Long-term outcome of peanut oral immunotherapy—Real-life experience. *Pediatric Allergy and Immunology, 29*, 519–526.

National Institutes of Health. (2018). *Guidelines for the use of antiretroviral agents in pediatric HIV infection.* Retrieved from https://aidsinfo.nih.gov/guidelines/html/2/pediatric-arv/0

Negrin, R., Chao, N., & Rosmarin, A. (2017*). Patient education: Hematopoietic cell transplantation (bone marrow transplantation). Beyond the basics.* Retrieved from https://www.uptodate.com/contents/hematopoietic-cell-transplantation-bone-marrow-transplantation-beyond-the-basics

Nyamweya, S., Hegedus, A., Jaye, A., Rowland-Jones, S., Flanagan, K., & McCallan, D. (2013). Comparing HIV-1 and HIV-2 infection: Lessons for viral immunopathogenesis. *Reviews in Medical Virology, 23*(4), 221–240. doi:10.1002/rmv.173

Ochs, H. D. (2017). *Wiskott-Aldrich syndrome.* Retrieved from https://www.uptodate.com/contents/wiskott-aldrich-syndrome

Perez, E., Orange, J., Bonilla, F., Chinen, J., Chinn, I., Dorsey, M., . . . & Ballow, M. (2016). Update on the use of immunoglobulin in human disease: A review of evidence. *The Journal of Allergy and Clinical Immunology, 139*(3), S1–S46. doi:10.1016/j.jaci.2016.09.023

Sharma, D., Jindal, A., Rawat, A., & Singh, S. (2017). Approach to a child with primary immunodeficiency made simple. *Indian Dermatology Online Journal, 8*(6), 391–405. doi:10.4103/idoj.IDOJ_189_17

Siberry, G., Abzug, M., & Nachman, S. (2013). Executive summary: 2013 update of the guidelines for the prevention and treatment of opportunistic infections in HIV-exposed and HIV-infected children. *Pediatric Infectious Disease Journal, 32*(12), 1303–1307. doi:10.1097/INF.0000000000000080

Simon, A., Hollander, G., & McMichael, A. (2015). Evolution of the immune system in humans from infancy to old age. *Proceedings of the Royal Society Biological Sciences, 282*(1821), 20143085. doi:10.1098/rspb.2014.3085

Taketokmo, C., Hodding, J., & Kraus, D. (2017). *Lexi-comp's pediatric & neonatal dosage handbook* (24th ed.). Hudson, OH: Lexi-comp.

Tarr, T., Dérfalvi, B., Győri, N., Szántó, A., Siminszky, Z., & Malik, A. (2015). Similarities and differences between pediatric and adult patients with systemic lupus erythematosus. *Lupus, 24*(8), 796–803. doi:10.1177/0961203314563817

Thompson, G., & Shalit, P. (2014). *HIV: Antiretroviral therapy (ART)-Topic overview.* Retrieved from https://www.webmd.com/hiv-aids/tc/hiv-highly-active-antiretroviral-therapy-haart-topic-overview

U.S. Department of Health & Human Services. (2018a). *Human leukocyte antigens.* Retrieved from https://ghr.nlm.nih.gov/primer/genefamily/hla

Van Dyke, R. B., Patel, K., Kagan, R. M., Karalius, B., Traite, S., Meyer, W., III, . . . & Willen, E. (2016). Antiretroviral drug resistance among children and youth in the United States with perinatal HIV. *Clinical Infectious Diseases, 63*(1), 133–137. doi:10.1093/cid/ciw213

Watson, S. (2017). Autoimmune diseases: Types, symptoms, causes and more. *Healthline Newsletter.* Retrieved from https://www.healthline.com/health/autoimmune-disorders

Wu, M., McIntosh, J., & Liu, J. (2016). Current prevalence rate of latex allergy: Why it remains a problem. *Journal of Occupational Health, 58*, 138–144.

Suggested Readings

Fisher, C., Fried, A., Ibrahim Puri, L., Macapagal, K., & Mustanski, B. (2018). "Free Testing and PrEP without Outing Myself to Parents:" Motivation to participate in oral and injectable PrEP clinical trials among adolescent men who have sex with men. *PLoS One, 13*(7), e0200560. doi:10.1371/journal.pone.0200560

Nickels, A., Myers, G., Johnson, L., Joshi, A., Sharp, R., & Lantos, J. (2016). Can parents refuse a potentially lifesaving transplant for severe combined immunodeficiency? *Pediatrics, 138*(1). doi:0.1542/peds.2016-0892

Rachid, R., & Keet, C. (2018). Current status and unanswered questions for food allergy treatments. *Journal of Allergy and Clinical Immunology. In Practice, 6*(2), 377–382. doi:10.1016/j.jaip.2017.10.023

31

Alterations in Endocrine Function

After completing this chapter, you will be able to:

1. Compare and contrast anatomical and physiological characteristics of the endocrine systems of children and adults.
2. Relate pediatric assessment findings to the child's endocrine status.
3. Discuss the pathophysiology of common pediatric endocrine disorders.
4. Differentiate between signs and symptoms of common pediatric endocrine disorders.
5. Outline the therapeutic regimen for each of the pediatric endocrine disorders.
6. Describe the pharmacological management of common pediatric endocrine disorders.
7. Apply the principles of growth and development to the care of a child with an endocrine disorder.
8. Create a nursing plan of care for each of the common pediatric endocrine disorders.

Key Terms

Bone age
Diabetic ketoacidosis (DKA)
Enuresis
Exophthalmos
Glycosuria
Goiter
Hemoglobin A1C (HbA1C)

Hyperglycemia
Nocturia
Polydipsia
Polyphagia
Polyuria
Thyrotoxicosis
Water intoxication

Variations in Anatomy and Physiology

Similar to that of an adult, a child's endocrine system consists of the hypothalamus, thyroid gland, pituitary gland, adrenal glands, thymus, pancreas, and gonads (Fig. 31.1). Unlike the adult endocrine system, which has its reproductive organs in place, the pediatric endocrine system must allow for the gonads to develop over time. The gonads differentiate into testes or ovaries early in pregnancy, by the 10th week of gestation. At that time, the male embryo begins to secrete testosterone, whereas the female begins to secrete estrogen, causing the gonads to develop into the testes and ovaries, respectively. These hormones also allow the ducts to develop into the vas deferens in males and to the uterus and fallopian tubes in females (Snyder, 2016).

The endocrine system plays an integral role in growth and development from conception to adulthood. In early childhood, sex hormone levels are very low. These levels increase as the gonads begin to secrete estrogen and androgen during puberty for girls and boys, respectively (see Chapter 19 for a discussion of the physical changes that occur in males and females during puberty). Although the age of puberty varies from person to person, this time of sexual maturation occurs concurrently with skeletal growth.

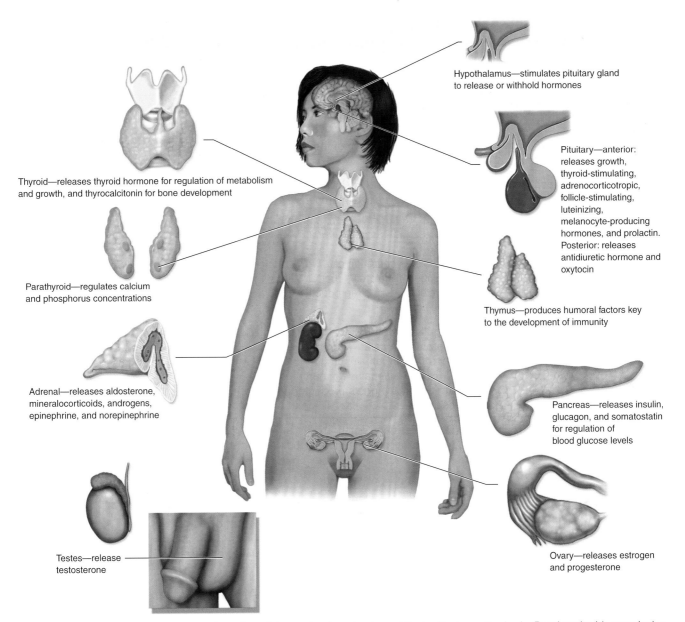

Hypothalamus—stimulates pituitary gland to release or withhold hormones

Pituitary—anterior: releases growth, thyroid-stimulating, adrenocorticotropic, follicle-stimulating, luteinizing, melanocyte-producing hormones, and prolactin. Posterior: releases antidiuretic hormone and oxytocin

Thyroid—releases thyroid hormone for regulation of metabolism and growth, and thyrocalcitonin for bone development

Parathyroid—regulates calcium and phosphorus concentrations

Thymus—produces humoral factors key to the development of immunity

Adrenal—releases aldosterone, mineralocorticoids, androgens, epinephrine, and norepinephrine

Pancreas—releases insulin, glucagon, and somatostatin for regulation of blood glucose levels

Testes—release testosterone

Ovary—releases estrogen and progesterone

Figure 31.1. The endocrine system. Location of the endocrine glands and their effects on the body. Reprinted with permission from Kyle, T., & Carman, S. (2013). *Essentials of pediatric nursing* (2nd ed., Fig. 27.1). Philadelphia, PA: Lippincott Williams & Wilkins.

The various glands of the endocrine system excrete **hormones**, or chemical messengers, throughout the body to assist in controlling cells in the body (Table 31.1). Endocrine disorders occur when there is too much (hyperfunction) or too little (hypofunction) of a hormone being produced. These abnormalities may result in delays in growth and development, intellectual disabilities, and even death. Treatment with hormone supplementation and inhibiting substances, as needed, can help children with endocrine disorders lead full and healthy lives.

Assessment of the Pediatric Endocrine System

Much like other pediatric assessments, your assessment of the pediatric endocrine system must change because the signs and

symptoms of endocrine disorders vary from age to age. For instance, congenital hypothyroidism may manifest as a protuberant tongue and a dull appearance in a newborn but as hypotonia, umbilical hernia, and constipation in an older infant. In an older child, this condition may manifest as continued constipation, along with dry skin, thin hair, brittle nails, or cold intolerance. Assess for growth issues (too fast or too slow), which are common complaints of patients with an endocrine disorder. Pair subjective complaints with objective findings to help identify endocrine disorders.

In addition to the physical findings associated with an abnormal endocrine system, assess for alterations in social, emotional, and cognitive development, which also may be present with an endocrine disorder. Having the patient or the parent describe a 24-hour recall of diet, elimination, and daily activities may assist in distinguishing an endocrine issue. For example, excessive

Table 31.1 Endocrine Hormones and Their Actions

Gland	Hormone	Actions	Hypofunction Conditions	Hyperfunction Conditions
Anterior pituitary	Growth hormone	Regulates metabolic actions related to growth	Growth hormone deficiency	Hyperpituitarism
	Thyroid-stimulating hormone	Stimulates secretion of the thyroid hormones	Hypothyroidism	Hyperthyroidism
	Adrenocorticotropic hormone	Stimulates secretion of glucocorticoids and androgens	Adrenal insufficiency	Cushing syndrome
	Prolactin	Stimulates breast development and triggers lactation	No concern	Hyperprolactinemia
	Follicle-stimulating hormone	Stimulates secretion of estrogen; regulates pubertal development and reproductive processes	Fertility issues	Fertility issues
	Luteinizing hormone	Regulates reproductive systems: in males, androgen secretion; in females, triggers ovulation, maintains the corpus luteum, and triggers progesterone secretion	Secondary hypogonadism	Women: primary ovarian failure, polycystic ovarian syndrome; men: testicular failure
Posterior pituitary	Antidiuretic hormone	Decreases urine output by reabsorbing water into the blood	Diabetes insipidus	Syndrome of inappropriate antidiuretic hormone secretion
	Oxytocin	Stimulates breast milk ejection reflex and uterine contractions	Decreased milk production	No concern
Thyroid	Thyroxine and triiodothyronine	Regulate the metabolic and heart rate, digestive and muscle functions, and body temperature	Hypothyroidism	Hyperthyroidism
	Calcitonin	Regulates calcium and phosphate in the blood; works with parathyroid hormone	No concern	No concern
Parathyroids	Parathyroid hormone	Regulates calcium and phosphate in the blood; works with calcitonin	Hypoparathyroidism	Hyperparathyroidism
Adrenal medulla	Epinephrine	Stimulates systemic vasoconstriction (increase in blood pressure) and relaxation of the gastrointestinal system	No concern	Hypertension
	Norepinephrine	Stimulates increased heart rate and blood flow to muscles and releases glucose into the blood; is released under stressful circumstances	No concern	Hypertension

(continued)

Table 31.1 Endocrine Hormones and Their Actions (*continued*)

Gland	Hormone	Actions	Hypofunction Conditions	Hyperfunction Conditions
Adrenal cortex	Cortisol	Regulates the use of energy (carbohydrates, fats, and protein), blood pressure, and sleep cycles; assists in handling stressful situations	Adrenal insufficiency (Addison disease)	Cushing syndrome; congenital adrenal hyperplasia
	Aldosterone	Regulates blood pressure by controlling the sodium-potassium pump in the kidneys; water follows increase in sodium retention, thereby increasing blood pressure	Primary adrenal insufficiency	Congenital adrenal hyperplasia
Pancreas	Insulin	Regulates use of glucose; stimulated by high glucose levels	Diabetes mellitus type I	Hypoglycemia
	Glucagon	Increases concentration of glucose; stimulated by low glucose levels	Hypoglycemia	Hyperglycemia
Testes	Testosterone	Stimulates sperm production and development of secondary sex characteristics: i.e., muscle mass and hair growth	In men: bone density issues	In women: polycystic ovarian syndrome
Ovaries	Estrogens	Stimulate the development of female secondary sexual characteristics: i.e., breast development; cause changes in the endometrium during the menstrual cycle	Delayed puberty	In males: gynecomastia
	Progesterone	Stimulates breast development; produced by the placenta to help maintain pregnancy	Irregular menses	Congenital adrenal hyperplasia
Thymus	Thymosin	Stimulates the creation of T cells	Decreased immune function	Immune system dysfunction
Pineal	Melatonin	Regulates sleep-wake cycles	No concern	Insomnia and depression

fatigue may indicate an underactive thyroid, whereas unprecedented weight loss may suggest diabetes. For this reason, your assessment of the endocrine system must go beyond examining growth charts and physical findings.

General Nursing Interventions for Endocrine Disorders

A child with an endocrine disorder requires a team of healthcare providers. Many of these are lifelong conditions, requiring both nurse-led teaching for the outpatient and pristine nursing care for the inpatient child.

Promote Self-management in Patients With Chronic Conditions

Owing to the chronic nature of many endocrine conditions, the parents of young children with these conditions must manage their medications, medical appointments, and blood draws for many years. As the children get older, it is important that they learn to manage their own illness. Doing so creates positive self-esteem and empowerment.

Some illnesses, such as diabetes mellitus, require constant monitoring and an understanding of how medications and foods affect the child and the condition (e.g., the effect of insulin and carbohydrates consumed on blood glucose level). For these patients, who will not have a parent with them at all times, it is important to teach them about the illness and how to manage it as early as possible.

Administer and Manage Medications

Patients with endocrine disorders require specific management of their medications. Depending on the illness, these medications can be given by mouth or as injection. As the children get older, they should be given opportunities to participate in their own care. In some cases, this may be as simple as letting them choose which drink to have with the medication. In other cases, patients may choose their injection sites. As patients mature, they should be given the responsibility to give their own medications and, eventually, manage their own care.

Provide Emotional and Psychosocial Support to the Child and Family

Many of these lifelong illnesses affect the day-to-day lives of the patient and the patient's family. For this reason, it is important to address all of their concerns. A chronic illness, such as diabetes, may be isolating to a young child or an adolescent. Offer these patients support groups consisting of patients of similar age.

Depending on the illness, parents may feel at fault or have guilt about a patient's condition. These parents may request access to their own support group or individual therapy.

Siblings of the patient should also not be ignored. While the patient and parents are focused on the patient's illness, the sibling may feel ignored. When possible, include siblings in day-to-day activities related to the patient's care. If the siblings are mature enough, give them an age-appropriate explanation of what the patient is being treated for.

Promote Growth and Development and a Healthy Body Image

Endocrine conditions are caused by a variety of hormone imbalances. Many of these conditions, such as hyper- and hypothyroidism, result in weight gain or loss. Other endocrine conditions, such as type 2 diabetes mellitus, are believed to occur partially due to obesity. Therefore, it is important to help children with endocrine disorders manage their length or height, weight, and body mass index (BMI) while promoting a positive body image.

Pediatric nurses must document patients' growth on standardized growth charts, and therefore be familiar with how to plot and interpret these numbers. These values may be some of the earliest indicators of a growth issue. When you note concerning data regarding a child's growth and development, share your concerns with healthcare providers and parents, because doing so may prevent an illness from progressing.

Pituitary Gland Disorders

Alterations in pituitary gland function include deficiency, excess, early-onset release, and late-onset release of the various hormones secreted by this gland, including growth hormone ([GH]; GH deficiency, gigantism, and acromegaly), gonadotropins (precocious puberty and delayed puberty), and antidiuretic hormone ([ADH]; diabetes insipidus [DI] and syndrome of inappropriate antidiuretic hormone [SIADH]).

Growth Hormone Deficiency

Growing to one's full potential depends on the appropriate production of human GH. A deficiency of this hormone,

sometimes called hypopituitarism, results in children being smaller than other children of the same gender and age. Treated early, children can fall within normal parameters of the growth curve. Without treatment, children remain proportional in size but are unlikely to meet their full growth potential.

Etiology and Pathophysiology

Causes of hypopituitarism include genetic defects, brain trauma, and cystic tumors that compress the pituitary gland.

Clinical Presentation

At birth, children with GH deficiency tend to be of normal length and weight. As their growth is assessed in the early years, however, it begins to fall below the third percentile for gender and age. The child's mandible and nose are small for the child's age, and the teeth may not fit appropriately into the mouth. The development of puberty features, such as pubic, facial, and genital hair, as well as genital growth, is delayed.

Assessment and Diagnosis

Monitor children's growth at each primary care visit. If a child starts falling more than 2 standard deviations below the mean or below the fifth percentile on the growth curve, anticipate laboratory testing of the child's hormone levels. A low GH level indicates GH deficiency. Assessing family growth patterns may also help to determine nonpituitary-related causes of growth delays.

In addition to genetic factors, consider chronic illnesses as a cause for slowed growth. Assess for conditions affecting the pituitary gland, such as a pituitary tumor or recent head trauma causing increased intracranial pressure. As ordered, obtain blood for laboratory tests to assess for hypothyroidism, hypoadrenalism, and hypoaldosteronism. Analysis of growth factor–binding proteins, as well as imaging, such as computerized tomography, magnetic resonance imaging, X-ray skull series, or ultrasound, can help detect lesions and tumors. During physical assessment, assess for any signs of child abuse or neglect, such as abnormal or excessive bruising, which may also cause slowed growth.

Therapeutic Interventions

Recombinant human growth hormone (rhGH) can be given to treat GH deficiency (The Pharmacy 31.1). rhGH is given intramuscularly at bedtime to simulate the normal peaks of GH (Graber & Rapaport, 2012). To assist with continued bone growth and prevent premature epiphyseal closure, some children require suppression of luteinizing hormone (LH)-releasing hormone.

Evaluation

Expected outcomes for a child with GH deficiency include the following:

- The child achieves and maintains normal growth according to standardized growth charts.
- The child demonstrates appropriate skeletal growth.
- The child expresses feelings of self-worth and self-esteem.

The Pharmacy 31.1 Somatropin

Classification	Route	Action	Nursing Considerations
Recombinant human growth hormone	• IM • SQ	Assists in the growth of linear bone, skeletal muscle, and organs	• Monitor urine for glucose. • Monitor the child's growth on the growth curve. • Monitor for thyroid dysfunction. • Monitor for progression of scoliosis, if present

IM, intramuscular; SQ, subcutaneous.
Adapted from Taketomo, C. K., Hodding, J. H., & Kraus, D. M. (2018). *Pediatric & neonatal dosage handbook* (25th ed.). Hudson, OH: Lexicomp.

Discharge Planning and Teaching

The introduction of injectable medication is likely to be life altering not only for the child but also for the entire family. For this reason, include the family in the discussion of the importance of this medication. As early as possible, teach the patient how to draw up and self-administer this medication, which helps the patient establish a feeling of control over the disorder. Work with families to establish a schedule for administering medications that will not interfere with the child's life. Schedule medication administration around meals, school, activities, and sleep so that it is less disruptive. For children prescribed injectable medications, teach as many of their family members as possible how to inject the medication in case they must perform this action.

GH Excess

Too little GH may result in diminished growth, whereas an excess of this hormone, or hyperpituitarism, can cause inappropriately increased growth in children. Depending on the onset time of oversecretion of GH, a child with unfused growth plates can grow to 7 to 8 ft in height, whereas those with fused growth plates can experience acromegaly, or enlargement of one's bones.

Etiology and Pathophysiology

The most common cause of hyperpituitarism is pituitary adenoma. When evaluating excessive linear growth in children, consider a family history of tall stature as a factor but also assess for other causes, as needed.

Clinical Presentation

Although rare in children, excess GH secretion can occur at any point in childhood. Measure the child's height (or length, for those children < 2 years old) at each physical exam and at episodic visits as needed. If growth accelerates excessively in a school-aged or teenaged child and the child begins to increase more than 2 standard deviations on the growth chart, consider excess GH. As the child matures and epiphyseal fusion begins to occur, linear growth may not be as prevalent, but widening or coarseness of facial features, as well as excessive foot and/or finger growth may be noted.

Assessment and Diagnosis

A thorough family history and review of the child's growth charts are integral to determining the cause of abnormal increased growth. Further evaluation includes assessing levels of insulin-like growth factor 1 (IGF-1), which are increased in hyperpituitarism. X-rays may be used to determine the state of growth plate closure to anticipate whether the child will continue to grow taller or exhibit signs of acromegaly.

Therapeutic Interventions

The most common management for GH excess is removal of the pituitary adenoma. The removal is often curative; however, postsurgical complications include transient DI and recurrent pituitary adenoma. DI would have to be managed appropriately, whereas the recurrent pituitary adenoma may have to be surgically excised in the future.

Evaluation

Expected outcomes for a child with GH excess include the following:

- The child's acceleration of growth slows.
- The child demonstrates normal growth according to standardized growth charts.
- The child demonstrates appropriate skeletal growth.
- The child achieves normal levels of IGF-1.

Discharge Planning and Teaching

Much like delayed growth, excessive early growth can be stressful for the child and the family. Adolescents may need support with self-image, particularly if they feel they are being treated as if they were older than their chronological age. Remind families to interact with their children depending on the developmental age as opposed to the age that may be associated with their height. Teach patients and families about the surgical process of the removal of the pituitary adenoma, including preoperative and postoperative care.

Precocious Puberty

When the usual secondary sex characteristics occur earlier than expected, the patient is diagnosed with precocious puberty. Puberty includes the onset of sexual characteristics that occur when the gonads produce sex hormones.

Etiology and Pathophysiology

Girls tend to reach puberty about 1 to 2 years before boys, from about 10 to 12 years of age, compared with 11 to 14 years of age in boys. When any sex characteristic develops in girls before 8 years of age or boys before 9 years of age, it is classified as precocious puberty (Harrington & Palmert, 2018). Precocious puberty is more common in females than in males and is more likely to be idiopathic (of unknown cause) in females than in males (Bulcao Macedo, Nahime Brito, & Latronico, 2014). In males, it often occurs as a result of a central nervous system (CNS) abnormality (Garibaldi & Chemaitilly, 2017).

On the basis of its etiology, precocious puberty may be classified as either central or peripheral. Central precocious puberty occurs when the hypothalamic–pituitary–gonadal axis is activated prematurely, resulting in early production of gonadotropin-releasing hormone (GnRH), which stimulates the pituitary to produce the gonadotropins LH and follicle-stimulating hormone (FSH). In turn, LH and FSH stimulate the gonads to produce estrogen or testosterone at an earlier age than expected. This causes pubertal changes such as secondary sex characteristics, bone closure, and the ability to reproduce in children earlier than in their peers. In most cases, the underlying cause of the premature production and release of GnRH is not known. In other cases, CNS abnormalities, genetic defects, or brain tumors may be implicated.

Peripheral precocious puberty occurs when a cause other than premature activation of the hypothalamic–pituitary–gonadal axis leads to the early development of secondary sex characteristics. These causes include genetic syndromes and tumors within endocrine glands outside of the brain.

Clinical Presentation

Children with precocious puberty present with early onset of secondary sex characteristics specific to their gender, such as thelarche (onset of breast development), menarche (onset of vaginal bleeding), testicular growth, and/or adrenarche (onset of development of pubic and axillary hair). Adrenarche is considered premature when it occurs before the age of 8 years in girls or 9 years in boys. They may also present with acne or adult-like body odor.

Assessment and Diagnosis

Assessment of height may demonstrate that these children are growing taller faster than expected. However, owing to circulating hormones, growth plates fuse prematurely, resulting in shorter stature. Much like older adolescents going through these changes, these children may experience emotional lability and mood swings.

Laboratory studies associated with this condition include blood levels of LH, FSH, testosterone, and estradiol. The GnRH stimulation test is used to confirm the diagnosis of precocious puberty. This test assesses the response of the pituitary gland to an injection of GnRH. X-rays are used to assess for advanced **bone age**, a hallmark of precocious puberty. Evaluations using magnetic resonance imaging, computerized axial tomography, and ultrasound are done to assess for tumors or cysts of the CNS, abdomen, pelvis, or testes.

Therapeutic Interventions

For precocious puberty caused by a CNS tumor, excision, radiation, and/or chemotherapy is required. With central precocious puberty, the most common type, GnRH agonist administration is required. Initial administration of this agonist causes gonadotropin release. With continuous use, however, it suppresses gonadotropin release, causing the child's growth rate to slow and halting the progression of secondary sex characteristics. When it is deemed appropriate for the child to be progressing through puberty, the medication is stopped, and the body resumes its development. Forms of GnRH agonist include daily subcutaneous injections, intranasal spray (two or three times per day), a monthly depot injection, a quarterly depot injection, or a subcutaneous implant, which is changed yearly (Carel & Leger, 2008).

Evaluation

Expected outcomes for a child with precocious puberty include the following:

- The child's acceleration of growth slows.
- Levels of LH, FSH, and estrogen or testosterone normalize.
- The child achieves appropriate physical development.
- The child achieves appropriate progression of pubertal development for age.

Discharge Planning and Teaching

Nursing care should focus on teaching the patient and family about the diagnosis and the physical changes that they should expect. On the basis of the child's age, explain that these changes are normal but are occurring prematurely and that the child's friends will also go through these changes in due time. Remind parents that although their child has physical attributes that make the child appear older, all other aspects of development, including social and emotional, are age appropriate and that the parents should treat the child accordingly.

It is important to provide support for a child's mental health with the diagnosis of precocious puberty. At times, these children may feel ostracized by their classmates. Provide them with a safe space to discuss changes that are occurring in their body. Owing to their advanced physical characteristics, these children may need to have counseling about issues of sexuality earlier than normal.

Delayed Puberty

When the usual secondary sex characteristics occur significantly later than expected, the patient is diagnosed with delayed puberty. In contrast to delayed puberty, stalled puberty refers to patients who start having symptoms of sexual maturation but do not complete all pubertal development within 4 years.

Etiology and Pathophysiology

As mentioned earlier, girls tend to reach puberty at about 10 to 12 years of age and boys around 11 to 14 years. If the first expected sex characteristics do not develop in girls (breast development) by 12 years old or boys (increase in testicular size) by 14 years old, it is classified as delayed puberty, or hypogonadism (Argente, 1999).

Delayed puberty occurs because of a variety of causes. Primary hypogonadism can be caused by gonadal diseases, including Turner and Klinefelter syndromes. Other causes of primary hypogonadism include gonadal injuries resulting from chemotherapy, radiotherapy, autoimmune disease, or infection. Secondary hypogonadism results from decreased secretion of FSH and LH from the anterior pituitary gland secondary to deficient GnRH. The most common cause of these hormonal changes is constitutional delay of growth and puberty, which causes a decrease in GnRH secretion from the hypothalamus.

Clinical Presentation

Children with delayed puberty present with late onset of secondary sex characteristics specific to their gender, such as thelarche (onset of breast development), menarche (onset of vaginal bleeding), testicular growth, and/or adrenarche (onset of development of pubic and axillary hair; Growth and Development Check 31.1). Thelarche is considered delayed when it occurs after the age of 12 years. Failure to menstruate by 15 years old is another sign of delayed puberty in females. In boys, delayed puberty is diagnosed if pubic hair does not develop by age 15 or testicles do not enlarge by age 14.

Assessment and Diagnosis

Physical assessment is an important component to any pediatric exam. Assessment of height and arm span may demonstrate that these children are growing more slowly than expected. If arm span exceeds height by greater than 5 cm, there is concern of delayed growth plate closure due to hypogonadism, or delayed puberty.

Children with delayed growth should be evaluated for a potential of thyroid abnormalities or nutritional issues, including anorexia nervosa, bulimia nervosa, and chronic inflammatory bowel disease, as well as celiac disease. This evaluation includes laboratory studies associated with these conditions, such as the following: a complete blood count, erythrocyte sedimentation rate, liver function tests, thyroid function tests, and blood levels of urea nitrogen, creatinine, LH, FSH, testosterone, estradiol, prolactin, and IGF-1. In cases of primary hypogonadism, LH and FSH levels are elevated. These elevated levels may also be indicative of Turner syndrome, so female patients with elevation of LH and FSH should be evaluated further. Low levels of testosterone or estradiol paired with low or normal levels of LH and FSH are associated with constitutional delayed growth and puberty. X-rays are used to assess for delayed bone age.

Therapeutic Interventions

For constitutional delayed growth and puberty, the most common cause of hypogonadism, the initial management includes watchful waiting. These patients require more frequent well-child visits and plotting on the standardized growth chart.

Short-term hormonal therapy may also be necessary in patients with constitutional delayed growth and puberty and no signs of pubertal development in girls by age 12 or boys by age 14. The goal of the short-term therapy is to initiate linear growth and the development of secondary sex characteristics.

Evaluation

Expected outcomes for a child with delayed puberty include the following:

- Linear growth increases without premature closure of the growth plates.
- Levels of LH, FSH, and estrogen or testosterone normalize.
- The child achieves appropriate physical development.
- The child achieves appropriate progression of secondary sex characteristics.

Discharge Planning and Teaching

Nursing care should focus on educating the patient and family about the diagnosis, treatment of this condition and the physical changes that they should expect with delayed puberty and its treatment. Explain to the patient that treatment will promote secondary sex characteristic development. The patient should understand what changes to expect (breast or testicular development, pubic hair, etc.) and verbalize understanding and any concerns.

It is important to provide support for an adolescent's mental health with the diagnosis of delayed puberty. These patients may feel as though their friends' physical maturity is distancing them. Discuss their concerns and provide them with an expected timeline for their secondary sex characteristic development.

Growth and Development Check 31.1

Delayed Puberty in Competitive Athletes

Delayed puberty may be concerning to many teenagers, whereas to others it can be a sign that they are more passionate about their sport. Commonly, female gymnasts and dancers are perceived to have a competitive edge if they remain smaller. In some female teen athletes, intense diet control (some with anorexia nervosa or bulimia nervosa) can prevent menstruation. Keep these concerns in mind when assessing teenagers' weights, BMIs, and secondary sex characteristics.

Diabetes Insipidus

DI is a disorder in which the kidneys cannot concentrate urine because of decreased sensitivity to or a lack of the hormone vasopressin, also known as antidiuretic hormone (ADH; Gonzalez et al., 2018).

Etiology and Pathophysiology

Two types of DI exist: nephrogenic and central (neurogenic). Nephrogenic DI, which is extremely rare, is caused by a decreased responsiveness of the kidneys to ADH, whereas central DI is caused by a lack of production of vasopressin. In both conditions, fluid is not reabsorbed into the circulation from the distal convoluted tubules of the kidneys, which causes an increased volume of urine (**polyuria**). Because the body is releasing water rather than retaining what it needs, dehydration occurs (Bockenhauer & Bichet, 2015).

Nephrogenic DI is most often an acquired illness and is unrelated to the pituitary gland. Its frequent causes include damage to the kidneys from drug toxicity or an adverse drug reaction, although it can also be passed on genetically. Whatever the underlying cause, this condition results in decreased renal sensitivity to vasopressin (Bichet, 2019).

Central DI is the most common form of DI. It may be caused by a lesion, tumor, or an injury to the posterior pituitary gland and, in some cases, is idiopathic. Because central DI is the most common form of DI in children, it is the focus of this section.

Clinical Presentation

Classically, DI presents with polyuria and **polydipsia** (excessive thirst). Because the body does not understand that there is a vasopressin deficiency, it prompts the person to consume more liquid by increasing thirst to compensate for the fluid loss. Owing to the increase in volume of urine produced, **nocturia** (nighttime waking to urinate) and **enuresis** (involuntary urination) are common. The increased urination and lack of fluid absorption will result in dehydration and irritability if that patient is not given fluids when requested.

Assessment and Diagnosis

Patients with DI may present with signs and symptoms of dehydration, and their serum sodium levels and serum osmolality are typically increased (145 mEq/L and >300 mOsm/kg, respectively). Other laboratory findings consistent with DI include a low specific gravity of urine (<1.005) and decreased urine osmolality (<300 mOsm/kg). To confirm diagnosis of DI, a fluid deprivation test must be performed, in which the ability of the patient to concentrate urine while fasting from fluids is assessed.

Therapeutic Interventions

The goals of treatment for a child with central DI are to control dehydration and decrease urinary symptoms. In doing so, constant thirst and nocturia decrease, as well. Treatment includes a low-sodium, low-protein diet paired with administration of intranasal or oral desmopressin acetate, a long-acting vasopressin analog (Bichet, 2019).

Evaluation

Expected outcomes for a child with DI include the following:
- The child achieves appropriate intake and output of fluid.
- Laboratory values normalize, including serum osmolality, serum sodium, and urine specific gravity.
- The child achieves normal blood pressure for age, size, and gender.
- The child and parents demonstrate an understanding of the signs and symptoms of **water intoxication**.

Discharge Planning and Teaching

Ensure that families of children with DI are well versed in the signs and symptoms of dehydration. Provide the family with teaching on medication administration and monitoring of urine intake and output, which should help them manage the child's DI appropriately. Teach parents to make fluids readily available to the child at all times and to encourage the child to drink. If the child requires nasogastric or gastrostomy feedings, provide teaching to the family on this, as well.

Inform the child and the parents that the child must wear a medical alert bracelet at all times because of the risk of DI complications arising very quickly. The information provided on the bracelet, including the diagnosis of DI, can save a lot of time in an emergency, allowing treatment to be started immediately.

Syndrome of Inappropriate Antidiuretic Hormone

SIADH is a condition involving excessive secretion of ADH.

Etiology and Pathophysiology

SIADH can be the result of CNS changes caused by head trauma, brain tumors, or CNS infections such as meningitis. In addition, SIADH can occur secondary to pulmonary illnesses such as cystic fibrosis and asthma, specifically in cases requiring positive-pressure ventilation.

Whatever the underlying etiology, SIADH occurs when the feedback mechanism that regulates ADH does not function properly, resulting in increased secretion of ADH from the posterior pituitary gland. This causes ADH to be continuously secreted and water to be reabsorbed, causing decreased urine output. This fluid retention results in decreased serum sodium levels due to hemodilution.

Clinical Presentation

Water intoxication, or extreme water intake, and hyponatremia are acute signs of SIADH. This water intoxication causes increased blood pressure, jugular vein distension, fluid in the lungs, sudden weight gain, fluid and electrolyte imbalance, and decreased urine output with concentrated urine. As SIADH progresses because of decreasing serum sodium levels, headaches, confusion, change in mental status, coma, and death may occur.

Assessment and Diagnosis

Testing is done in patients who present with signs of water intoxication and includes serum sodium levels, urine osmolality, and serum osmolality. Findings consistent with SIADH include decreased serum sodium levels, high urine osmolality, and low serum osmolality.

Therapeutic Interventions

Nursing responsibility includes monitoring for worsening symptoms of SIADH. Fluid monitoring and restriction is necessary to prevent further dilution of the blood, resulting in decreased serum sodium levels. In addition, demeclocycline is given to reduce reabsorption of water from the renal tubules by blocking the action of ADH.

Monitor intake and output strictly in these patients. Continuously assess laboratory test results to monitor the child's serum sodium levels and urine osmolarity and specific gravity.

Evaluation

Expected outcomes for a child with SIADH are similar to those for a child with DI. Refer to the section Evaluation under Diabetes Insipidus, earlier. Additional expected outcomes include the following:
- The child achieves normal urea, creatinine, uric acid, and albumin levels.
- The child achieves and maintains a normal weight without signs or symptoms of edema.

Discharge Planning and Teaching

Provide parent and patient teaching on water restriction and which foods contribute significantly to water intake. In addition, encourage families to monitor these patients at home for sudden increases in weight.

Although some cases of SIADH resolve, others require lifelong management. Encourage these patients to wear a medical alert bracelet. Those on demeclocycline must have follow-up care because of potential renal side effects.

Thyroid Gland Disorders

Thyroid gland disorders can be either congenital or acquired. These disorders cause the thyroid to produce either too little or too much thyroid hormone.

Table 31.2 indicates the differences in the clinical presentation of hyperthyroidism and hypothyroidism.

Congenital Hypothyroidism

Congenital hypothyroidism is a condition of deficient production of thyroid hormones that exists from birth. It is a common

Table 31.2	**Hypothyroidism Versus Hyperthyroidism: Clinical Presentation**
Hypothyroidism	**Hyperthyroidism**
• Fatigue	• Anxiousness
• Constipation	• Diarrhea
• Weight gain	• Weight loss
• Dry skin	• Velvety skin
• Cold intolerance	• Feelings of overheating

illness, occurring in approximately 1 in 3,000 live births. It is more common in Hispanic and Native American populations than in Black populations (Rastogi & LaFranchi, 2010).

Etiology and Pathophysiology

Congenital hypothyroidism occurs when an autosomal recessive trait causes one of the following to occur: failure of the thyroid gland to develop properly during fetal development, failure of the CNS-thyroid feedback mechanism to develop, or pituitary dysfunction. Any of these defects can cause the thyroid to decrease production of the thyroid hormones, which are needed to help promote the body's physical and intellectual growth. This slowed production leads to low circulating levels of the thyroid hormones triiodothyronine (T_3) and thyroxine (T_4). Without treatment, this condition can result in intellectual disability, short stature, and growth failure that are irreversible (Rastogi & LaFranchi, 2010).

Clinical Presentation

Often, children with congenital hypothyroidism present with few to no clinical signs in the first weeks of life. In time, however, these children develop clinical signs such as persistent open posterior fontanelle, thickened protuberant tongue, dull expression, hypotonia, hypoactivity, and poor sucking response. Skin may appear cool and dry. The baby's heart rate may be lower than expected and abdominal palpation may reveal a mass consistent with an umbilical hernia or stool (due to constipation; Fig. 31.2). In addition, children with congenital hypothyroidism may not follow the same percentile on their growth charts as they did when they were born.

Assessment and Diagnosis

Patients presenting with a combination of signs and symptoms as listed earlier should have their circulating levels of thyroid hormones assessed. Neonatal screening for congenital hypothyroidism is required in all 50 states before discharge from the hospital, which allows detection of this disease before symptom development in nearly all cases (Shapira et al., 2015). If the results of neonatal screening are positive, the infant undergoes blood tests that assess the circulating levels of the thyroid hormones T_3, T_4, and thyroid-stimulating hormone (TSH) as an outpatient. In hypothyroidism, the T_4 level is decreased, with a normal T_3 level

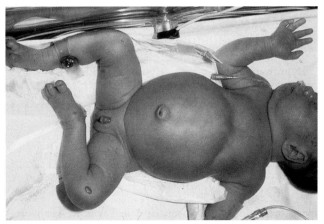

Figure 31.2. Congenital hypothyroidism. A newborn exhibiting a protruding abdomen as a result of constipation due to congenital hypothyroidism. Reprinted with permission from Kyle, T., & Carman, S. (2017). *Essentials of pediatric nursing* (3rd ed., Fig. 26.3). Philadelphia, PA: Wolters Kluwer.

and an elevated TSH level. This elevated TSH level is significant because it indicates that the lack of T_4 hormone is a thyroid issue as opposed to a pituitary issue.

Therapeutic Interventions

Synthetic thyroid hormone (sodium levothyroxine; The Pharmacy 31.2) is started for newborns with low T_4 and elevated TSH levels at a dosage of 8 to 12 µg/kg/d (Signh, 2017). Thyroid hormone levels are measured frequently, with the standard routine calling for monitoring every 1 to 2 weeks until the dose is stabilized, then every 1 to 3 months until the child is 1 year old, then every 2 to 3 months until the child is 3 years old, and then less frequently as the child ages (Adis Medical Writers, 2018). Monitoring of this frequency is necessary because of the rapid growth of the child and, therefore, the likelihood of the dose being insignificant quickly.

Evaluation

Expected outcomes for a child with congenital hypothyroidism include the following:
- The child achieves and maintains appropriate growth.
- TSH and T_4 blood levels normalize.
- Symptoms of temperature instability are relieved.
- Bowel movements normalize.

Discharge Planning and Teaching

As the child's growth slows, less frequent monitoring is necessary. However, T_4 and TSH levels will have to be measured throughout life to assess for excess or low levels of thyroid hormones. Teach the family the importance of daily medication adherence to encourage normal growth and development.

Monitor growth charts closely to ensure that the child is meeting growth goals throughout the lifespan. Teach families the signs and symptoms of excessive thyroid hormone, such as sweating, increased heart rate, and weight loss or plateauing, as well as of deficient thyroid hormone, such as chills, constipation, and fatigue. Encourage parents to communicate any concerns they have regarding their child's condition or treatment to the pediatric endocrinologist (Whose Job Is It, Anyway? 31.1).

Acquired Hypothyroidism

Hypothyroidism can also occur later in life because of an autoimmune disorder (Hashimoto thyroiditis); late-onset thyroid dysfunction; isolated TSH deficiency due to pituitary or hypothalamic dysfunction; drugs; or idiopathic causes.

Etiology and Pathophysiology

Acquired hypothyroidism can occur because of an autoimmune disorder (Hashimoto thyroiditis), late-onset thyroid dysfunction,

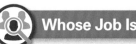

Whose Job Is It, Anyway? 31.1
Endocrinologist and Nurse Specialists

Children with congenital hypothyroidism require the care and vigilant assessment of several healthcare team members. An endocrinologist is needed to determine correct doses of synthetic thyroid hormone (sodium levothyroxine) depending on the patient's levels of TSH and thyroxine. Neonatal nurses must conduct newborn screening of the child in the hospital or birth center. Pediatric endocrinology and primary care nurses should recognize signs and symptoms of hypothyroidism in both hypothyroid children as well as in previously healthy children who may verbalize complaints or exhibit physical abnormalities during a well-child exam or sick visit.

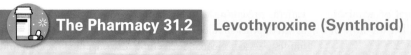

The Pharmacy 31.2 Levothyroxine (Synthroid)

Classification	Route	Action	Nursing Considerations
Thyroid product	• PO • IV	As a synthetic form of thyroxine, counteracts the deficit caused by the lack of endogenous hormone secreted by the thyroid gland	• Monitor TSH, T_4, and blood pressure levels. • Monitor for clinical signs of hyper- or hypothyroidism.

IV, intravenous; PO, oral; T_4, thyroxine; TSH, thyroid-stimulating hormone.
Adapted from Taketomo, C. K., Hodding, J. H., & Kraus, D. M. (2018). *Pediatric & neonatal dosage handbook* (25th ed.). Hudson, OH: Lexicomp.

isolated TSH deficiency due to pituitary or hypothalamic dysfunction, drug toxicity, or an unknown cause. Hashimoto thyroiditis is one of the most common forms of acquired hypothyroidism and is believed to be caused by an autosomal dominant gene that leads to the development of thyroid antibodies (LaFranchi, 2011). These antibodies cause the thyroid to be overrun by lymphocytes, resulting in an autoimmune reaction characterized by an enlarged thyroid, low levels of T_4, and increased levels of TSH.

Clinical Presentation

Symptom presentation greatly depends on how long the child has had this condition. Patients may present with increased fatigue and/or weight gain, which may have been ignored because of other factors, such as school, activities, and puberty. The child and the parents may report vague symptoms of weakness, cold intolerance, and skin and hair changes. Slowed height acquisition may also be noted if the hormone imbalance has been long-standing. Young women may present with changes in their menstrual cycle, whereas any patient may have a **goiter**, or enlargement of the thyroid gland, on physical exam.

Assessment and Diagnosis

Much like that of congenital hypothyroidism, diagnosis of acquired hypothyroidism is based on the levels of thyroid hormones and TSH.

Therapeutic Interventions

As with congenital hypothyroidism, treatment of acquired hypothyroidism includes administration of the supplemental thyroid hormone sodium levothyroxine, except at a lower starting dosage of 2 to 6 µg/kg/d depending on the patient's age. Instruct families to avoid administering this medication near a time of food consumption to aid in the uptake of the supplemental hormone. The child should take levothyroxine at least 60 minutes before or after food intake and at a different time of day than when vitamins are taken.

Evaluation

Expected outcomes for a child with acquired hyperthyroidism are similar to those for a child with congenital hypothyroidism. Refer to the section Evaluation under Congenital Hypothyroidism, earlier.

Discharge Planning and Teaching

Because acquired hypothyroidism is diagnosed later in life than is congenital hypothyroidism, it is unlikely that a child with this condition would be growing as rapidly. For this reason, thyroid hormone levels only need to be monitored every 3 to 6 months until stabilized and then every 6 months thereafter.

Monitor the child's height and weight to assure that they are following the same growth chart percentiles. Also monitor the child's developmental milestones to assure that the child is reaching age-appropriate milestones.

Hyperthyroidism

Hyperthyroidism, or **thyrotoxicosis**, occurs when too much thyroid hormone is secreted.

Etiology and Pathophysiology

Although uncommon in childhood, its peak incidence is due to Graves disease during the adolescent period. With Graves disease, the thyroid hormone T_4 is produced in excess because of immunoglobulins produced by the B lymphocytes (Lafranchi, 2011). Family inheritance is believed to be a factor in this autoimmune illness.

Clinical Presentation

Early in the illness, hyperthyroid symptoms can present as similar to behavioral problems such as decreased performance in school, hyperactivity, and becoming easily distracted. As with hypothyroidism, when the thyroid gland enlarges, a goiter is present. As the disease progresses and an excessive amount of T_4 is circulating in the body, other symptoms occur, including the following: weight loss despite a history of appropriate eating, hot flashes, tachycardia, fine tremors, and ocular changes such as **exophthalmos** (bulging of the eye out of the orbit anteriorly), proptosis, lid lag, staring expression, periorbital edema, and diplopia (Fig. 31.3).

An abrupt release of thyroid hormones, or thyroid storm, is a life-threatening emergency. These high levels of thyroid hormone are manifested by sudden onset of irritability, fever, tremors, anxiety, diaphoresis, and tachycardia. This condition can quickly progress to heart failure and shock.

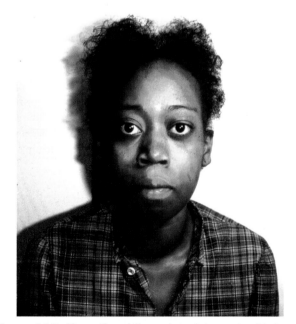

Figure 31.3. Hyperthyroidism. An adolescent with hyperthyroidism exhibiting exophthalmos. Reprinted with permission from Kyle, T., & Carman, S. (2017). *Essentials of pediatric nursing* (3rd ed., Fig. 26.4). Philadelphia, PA: Wolters Kluwer.

Assessment and Diagnosis

In addition to observing for the signs and symptoms described earlier, assessment of hyperthyroidism includes laboratory testing of thyroid hormone levels. Findings consistent with hyperthyroidism include increased serum levels of T_4 and T_3 and a decreased serum level of TSH. The presence of thyroid autoantibodies, such as antithyroglobulin (anti-TG) and antithyroid peroxidase (anti-TPO), is also monitored for, because they are usually seen in Graves disease and Hashimoto thyroiditis. A thyroid scan is performed to assess the thyroid and its size. When Graves disease is suspected, the thyroid scan will also be used to study the uptake of radioactive iodine.

Therapeutic Interventions

The goal of hyperthyroidism treatment is to achieve a **euthyroid** state, meaning a state of normal serum thyroid hormone levels in the body. Treatment is multifaceted and can include a thyroidectomy (surgical removal of the thyroid gland), radioactive iodine therapy, and antithyroid medication. Methimazole is the drug of choice for children with hyperthyroidism (The Pharmacy 31.3). It lowers thyroid hormone levels while posing less of a risk of causing liver disease than its competitor, propylthiouracil (Rivkees, Stephenson, & Dinauer, 2010).

If necessary, beta-adrenergic blocking agents (i.e., propranolol, atenolol, or metoprolol) are used to assist with extreme hyperthyroidism symptom management (Bahn et al., 2011; LaFranchi, 2011). For children older than 10 years, radioactive therapy is becoming increasingly common for the treatment of hyperthyroidism (LaFranchi, 2011).

A thyroidectomy provides an immediate cure to hyperthyroidism while avoiding the side effects associated with hyperthyroid medication and radioactive iodine therapy. However, without a thyroid, the patient becomes hypothyroid, which, in turn, requires lifelong treatment with hormone replacement therapy (sodium levothyroxine). In addition, surgical excision of the thyroid may result in the release of parathyroid hormone, which can cause hypercalcemia. For this reason, in addition to frequent thyroid hormone monitoring, a child who has undergone a thyroidectomy must also have his or her calcium levels monitored.

Evaluation

Expected outcomes for a child with hyperthyroidism are similar to those for a child with hypothyroidism. Refer to the section Evaluation under Congenital Hypothyroidism, earlier. Additional expected outcomes include the following:
- Tachycardia resolves.
- Adverse drug effects do not occur or are addressed appropriately.

Discharge Planning and Teaching

Nursing care for a child with hyperthyroidism depends on the treatment choice for the patient. Educate families and patients on the use and side effects of any medications prescribed. For medications requiring multiple doses per day, encourage the family to use a reminder system such as a pill dispenser or an alarm feature on their phone. Teach families that children taking thyroid medications need to be monitored closely by blood draws to assess whether the medication is bringing the thyroid levels into the normal range. For children requiring a thyroidectomy, provide thorough and age-appropriate preoperative and postoperative teaching and care. Immediately after surgery, elevate the head of the child's bed to promote a patent airway and make sure emergency medical supplies are available in the event of respiratory compromise.

As thyroid hormone levels become more stable and as the child ages, less frequent blood monitoring is necessary. Once stabilized, and in the absence of abnormal thyroid symptoms, thyroid hormone levels need only be assessed via blood testing one or two times per year. Remind families that this monitoring is lifelong and that medication titration may be needed at any time. All patients and families require extensive teaching on the signs and symptoms of abnormal thyroid hormone levels, because they may indicate the need for an unscheduled thyroid hormone level assessment.

Adrenal Gland Disorders

Adrenal gland disorders can be acute or chronic and caused by too much or too little production of adrenal hormones. Note that adrenal gland disorders that have a clinical presentation in children that is similar to that in adults, such as pheochromocytoma, are not covered here; rather, those that have a clinical

---

The Pharmacy 31.3 Methimazole

Classification	Route	Action	Nursing Considerations
Antithyroid agent	PO	Inhibits the synthesis of thyroid hormones	• Monitor for signs of hyper- or hypothyroidism. • Monitor thyroxine level. • Monitor liver function. • Monitor complete blood count.

PO, oral.
Adapted from Taketomo, C. K., Hodding, J. H., & Kraus, D. M. (2018). *Pediatric & neonatal dosage handbook* (25th ed.). Hudson, OH: Lexicomp.

presentation that differs significantly from that in adults are covered.

Adrenal Insufficiency (Addison Disease)

Adrenal insufficiency is defined as a deficiency of glucocorticoids (cortisone) and, in some cases, mineralocorticoids (aldosterone). Also known as Addison disease, this glucocorticoid deficiency causes the body to have difficulty managing stress, including that resulting from infection or surgery.

Etiology and Pathophysiology

There are believed to be numerous causes for Addison disease, the most common of which is an autoimmune disorder. Tuberculosis, fungal infections, and human immunodeficiency virus are believed to be other triggers of adrenal insufficiency in children.

Clinical Presentation

Over time, adrenal insufficiency presents with vague symptoms, including fatigue, skin changes, and abdominal symptoms, such as nausea, vomiting, and diarrhea. Stressors such as dehydration, illness, and trauma can cause adrenal crisis. During an adrenal crisis, children are at risk for lethargy, weight changes, and, most significantly, hypoglycemia.

Assessment and Diagnosis

The symptoms of adrenal insufficiency are suggestive of the illness, and laboratory tests are confirmatory. In children with adrenal insufficiency, initial test results show evidence of inappropriately low cortisol secretion in the morning. To determine whether the adrenal insufficiency is caused by primary or central causes, adrenocorticotropic hormone (ACTH) level is assessed. In those patients with primary adrenal insufficiency, the ACTH level is elevated. These patients are also at risk for other abnormalities, including mineralocorticoid deficiency, which is evidenced by decreased aldosterone and sodium levels as well as elevated plasma renin activity and potassium level. A patient diagnosed with primary adrenal insufficiency should receive further testing to find the cause, including assessments of antiadrenal antibody levels and for tuberculosis and adrenoleukodystrophy.

In contrast, central adrenal insufficiency is marked by low levels of ACTH. These patients do not have electrolyte abnormalities, because their ACTH secretion is impaired and their mineralocorticoid levels are normal. Instead, they often have abnormalities in other pituitary hormones (GH, TSH, LH, and/or FSH). Early monitoring of these levels could prevent additional complications with growth and the thyroid.

Therapeutic Interventions

Close monitoring for the signs and symptoms as listed is an important component of the management of adrenal insufficiency. All deficient hormones must be replaced. These patients receive oral hydrocortisone titrated depending on the patient's response. Those with primary adrenal insufficiency also receive

Priority Care Concepts 31.1

Taking Your Medication

Vomiting in children with adrenal insufficiency is not an excuse to skip a dose of medication. Injectable hydrocortisone should be available for these patients during illness. It is important that the patient continues to take the prescribed doses of medications at the specified times because the drugs mimic a healthy body's secretion of steroids.

fludrocortisone acetate to replace mineralocorticoids, which, in turn, help regulate the electrolytes.

In cases in which an adrenal crisis is triggered, additional interventions are needed. Because these patients are susceptible to hypoglycemia, they are treated with intravenous (IV) fluid administration, glucose, and hydrocortisone. When stressful events are anticipated (e.g., surgery), steroid doses are increased for days leading up to the event as well as for the stressful time after the event (Priority Care Concepts 31.1).

Evaluation

Expected outcomes for a child with adrenal insufficiency include the following:

- The child reaches appropriate pubertal development.
- The child and parents demonstrate an understanding of the use of stress dosing in times of illness.
- The child does not experience side effects resulting from overdosed steroids, such as inappropriate weight gain or a puffy face.

Discharge Planning and Teaching

Nursing care for a child with adrenal insufficiency includes extensive teaching about medication administration. Educate families and patients on the use and side effects of any medications prescribed. In an effort to mimic the body's natural secretion of steroids, oral hydrocortisone is commonly dosed three times a day, with doses in the morning being higher than those in the afternoon and evening. Encourage the family to use a reminder system for taking medication, such as the alarm feature on a smartphone, where they can also include a note about what dose is required at that time. Owing to the importance of not missing doses, remind patients and families to always have backup doses of medication (not expired) with them at work, school, and while on vacation.

Medication compliance, particularly during times of stress and illness, is critical to the treatment of these patients. As children mature, teach them, along with their parents, how to increase dosing during times of stress and when it is time to go to the emergency department (Patient Safety 31.1). In times of vomiting or gastrointestinal upset, IV fluids, glucose, and steroids are often necessary. Encourage families to have a healthcare provider evaluate such symptoms, should they occur. Remind

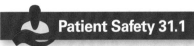

Patient Safety 31.1

Medical Alert Bracelet

Many endocrine disorders, including diabetes mellitus, DI, and adrenal insufficiency, are life-threatening illnesses. To ensure that children with these conditions receive the immediate medical attention they need, encourage them to wear a medical alert bracelet at all times.

families that this treatment is lifelong and that medications will need to be modified as the child grows. A close relationship with a pediatric endocrinologist is ideal so that treatment and monitoring can be evaluated over time.

Congenital Adrenal Hyperplasia

Congenital adrenal hyperplasia (CAH) is an autosomal recessive disorder resulting in insufficient enzymes for the synthesis of cortisol and aldosterone. Although not common, it is the most frequently occurring type of adrenocortical insufficiency, with an incidence rate of 1 in 16,000 live births (Yang & White, 2017). Because the vast majority of CAH cases are related to 21-hydroxylase (21-OH) enzyme deficiency, which causes inadequate production of aldosterone and cortisol, this section focuses on this specific type of CAH (White & Bachega, 2012).

Etiology and Pathophysiology

21-OH is an autosomal recessive disease that blocks production of adrenal mineralocorticoids and glucocorticoids and thus cortisol, causing the pituitary to continue secretion of ACTH. Although the adrenal glands become hyperplastic because of the increased production of ACTH, they still lack the ability to produce cortisol because of the defective gene. The elevated ACTH level instead triggers the body to overproduce androgen.

Clinical Presentation

Overproduction of androgen in utero can affect the external genitalia of both male and female fetuses. The male fetus with CAH tends to have an enlarged penis with appropriately sized testicles, whereas the female fetus with CAH may have ambiguous genitalia, including an enlarged clitoris, which may be mistaken for a penis, and fused labia, which may be mistaken for undescended testes (Fig. 31.4). Because CAH is the most common cause of ambiguous genitalia, any abnormal appearance of the genitalia should prompt the healthcare provider to look further into the cause.

As the male child with CAH ages, his penis may grow to be disproportionately large for his age while his testes remain appropriately sized. In both genders with 21-OH, the increase in androgen production may cause precocious puberty, as evidenced by increased height velocity early in life and the early onset of pubic hair, acne, and closure of the epiphyseal plates.

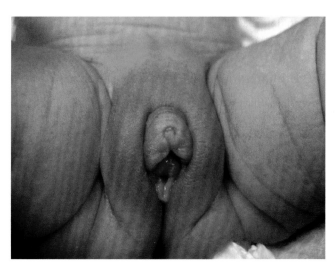

Figure 31.4. Congenital adrenal hyperplasia. An infant with congenital adrenal hyperplasia. Note the difficulty in determining whether the child has a clitoris or a penis. Reprinted with permission from Kyle, T., & Carman, S. (2017). *Essentials of pediatric nursing* (3rd ed., Fig. 26.6). Philadelphia, PA: Wolters Kluwer.

Long-term disturbances of 21-OH include short adult stature and a high likelihood of infertility. Aldosterone insufficiency can lead to hyponatremia, hyperkalemia, and hypotension due to extracellular fluid depletion. Cortisol insufficiency can lead to hypoglycemia. Therefore, it is important to diagnose and treat CAH immediately after birth.

Assessment and Diagnosis

In utero detection of CAH is possible at 6 to 8 weeks of gestation using maternal serum analysis. Follow-up testing can be done using amniocentesis at 15 weeks of gestation. If prenatal testing is not done, the newborn physical assessment may provide the first indication that the patient has CAH.

The presence of 21-OH is detected on the newborn metabolic screening, which is performed within 48 to 72 hours of birth. Alternatively, the ACTH stimulation test may be performed to assess how the adrenal glands respond to ACTH. In older children, X-rays may be performed to assess for advanced bone age by assessing for premature closure of epiphyseal plates.

Therapeutic Interventions

Much like that for other endocrine disorders, the treatment goal for CAH is to normalize the level of the hormone in question. In the case of CAH, cortisol must be replaced to decrease ACTH production, which, in turn, will normalize adrenal size and androgen production. This will prevent the advancement of sexual maturation and bone growth. Because cortisol, which is not produced in CAH, is necessary for life, children with CAH must be given a synthetic form of this hormone for life.

Providing a corticosteroid agent, such as hydrocortisone or fludrocortisone, regulates stimulation by ACTH and restores the production of androgen to normal levels. This corticosteroid therapy, too, is lifelong, and the child's serum cortisol levels must be closely monitored. Teach the child and the parents the importance of this lifelong therapy to manage symptoms.

Evaluation

Expected outcomes for a child with CAH include the following:
- Androgen and serum cortisol levels normalize.
- The child and the parents demonstrate an understanding of the use of stress dosing in times of illness.
- The child achieves and maintains appropriate growth for age.

Discharge Planning and Teaching

Periods of increased stress, such as times of illness or surgery, may require an increased dose (stress dosing) of the baseline corticosteroid therapy for CAH. Teach families that the under-dosing or overdosing of corticosteroids may have adverse effects on the patient's growth. Low levels of cortisol can result in adrenal crisis, which can be life-threatening. Signs and symptoms include persistent vomiting, dehydration, hyponatremia, hyperkalemia, hypotension, tachycardia, and shock. Adrenal crisis requires immediate IV steroids to prevent irreversible damage.

Cushing Syndrome

Cushing syndrome results from overproduction of the hormone cortisol by the adrenal cortex and is associated with a set of distinctive physical traits.

Etiology and Pathophysiology

Cushing syndrome is most commonly caused by increased levels of glucocorticoids, specifically cortisol, which results from a small ACTH-producing pituitary adenoma (Broersen, Jha, Biermasz, Pereira, & Dekkers, 2018). In addition, Cushing syndrome can occur from prolonged exposure to corticosteroid therapy, most commonly for CAH, chronic respiratory illness, cancer therapy, or severe eczema (involving a high-potency steroid cream).

Clinical Presentation

The overproduction of cortisol encourages glucose production, which, in turn, produces some cardinal clinical features of Cushing syndrome. This glucose production causes fat to accumulate in specific areas of the body while avoiding other areas. For this reason, obesity, a rounded (moon) face, prominent cheeks, a pendulous abdomen, and abdominal striae are common. As compared with the trunk, the child's extremities appear thin because of protein wasting caused by cortisol (Fig. 31.5; Van Haalen et al., 2018). Cortisol may also suppress the immune system and cause vasoconstriction, which may progress to hypertension. Increased cortisol levels may also put patients at risk for depression and/or anxiety (Santos, Resmini, Pascual, Crespo, & Webb, 2017).

Assessment and Diagnosis

Children who present with the physical characteristics described should undergo further assessment, including laboratory testing of 24-hour urinary level of free cortisol and nighttime salivary

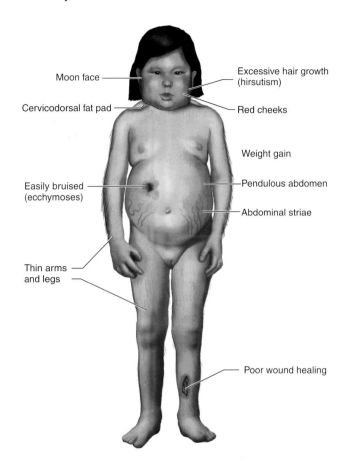

Figure 31.5. Cushing syndrome. Different effects of Cushing syndrome on the child. Reprinted with permission from Kyle, T., & Carman, S. (2017). *Essentials of pediatric nursing* (3rd ed., Fig. 26.5). Philadelphia, PA: Wolters Kluwer.

cortisol levels, as well as a glucose tolerance test (GTT). Findings of increased levels of cortisol and blood glucose on these tests indicate Cushing syndrome. Further testing might include assessment of the adrenal cortisol level by providing an additional dose of dexamethasone before bedtime to assess for dexamethasone suppression (Nieman, 2018).

Magnetic resonance imaging, computed tomography scan, or ultrasound is used to assess for adrenal and/or pituitary tumors.

Depression screening should also be performed, because depression and other psychiatric disorders have been associated with Cushing syndrome and its treatment (Santos et al., 2017).

Therapeutic Interventions

In some patients, medication alone can normalize cortisol levels, whereas others require surgical removal of the pituitary adenoma. Combination therapy with medication and irradiation of the pituitary is often successful, as well (Broersen et al., 2018). Removal of the adrenal glands is necessary if cortisol continues to be excreted at high levels. In this case, cortisol supplementation must be provided indefinitely. When Cushing syndrome is caused by long-term steroid therapy, the dosage of this therapy must be decreased to the lowest possible while still treating the illness.

Management of associated psychiatric conditions may include therapy for body image disturbance and medications for depression and anxiety (Santos et al., 2017).

Evaluation

Expected outcomes for a child with Cushing syndrome include the following:

- Hormone balance normalizes.
- Symptoms of Cushing syndrome resolve.
- Any tumor present is removed.
- If due to long-term steroid therapy, steroids are titrated while still effectively treating the original condition that required steroid therapy.

Discharge Planning and Teaching

Teach families of children with Cushing syndrome about this condition and its management. Provide both preoperative and postoperative teaching for patients undergoing surgery. Address any concerns that the child or parents have about the child's cushingoid appearance, and explain that these physical attributes are reversible with proper treatment. Address nutritional concerns by referring the family to a nutritionist, who can encourage healthy ways to maintain an appropriate weight.

Cortisol replacement therapy is necessary for all patients with bilateral adrenal gland removal. As ordered, instruct patients and families to administer cortisol early in the morning or every other day to reduce side effects and mimic the normal daily cycle of cortisol secretion, and emphasize to them the importance of consistent administration. Hydrocortisone is available in many forms, including liquid, tablet, and injectable. The liquid form is bitter and can cause stomach irritation. Explain that providing food or antacids with the medication may reduce these irritations. Most importantly, impress upon families the importance of cortisol administration in times of illness; skipping doses because a child is sick can result in severe illness and cardiovascular compromise.

Pancreas Disorders

The pancreas works to titrate insulin for the body depending on glucose intake. When insulin is not produced because of beta-cell destruction or insulin is unable to be used, glucose builds up in the body, causing diabetes.

Diabetes mellitus is a chronic disease that can develop at any point in the lifespan. It involves impaired insulin secretion or action or a combination of the two, resulting in **hyperglycemia** in the body. The major types of diabetes are type 1 and type 2. Because the clinical presentations and progressions of these two types can be similar, determining which type a child has can be difficult. Because type 1 is the more common pediatric illness, it is the focus of this chapter.

Type 1 Diabetes Mellitus

Type 1 diabetes mellitus is a disorder of the pancreas that develops during childhood and requires lifelong monitoring and treatment. For additional information regarding type 1 diabetes mellitus, refer to Chapter 10.

Etiology and Pathophysiology

Type 1 diabetes is caused by an autoimmune condition that causes pancreatic beta-cell damage, impairing the secretion of insulin. Although there is a genetic predisposition for this condition, its incidence is equal in the sexes, and it affects about 0.2% of the childhood population (Sherr & Weinzimer, 2012).

It is believed that those who are genetically susceptible to type 1 diabetes have a high frequency of human leukocyte antigens. When such individuals are exposed to certain environmental or acquired factors, the immune system's T lymphocytes are activated and mistakenly identify the beta cells of the pancreas as antigens, or foreign invaders, and attack and destroy them. The beta cells normally produce the hormone insulin, which is required to transport glucose from the blood into the cells of the body. Without the beta cells, insulin is no longer secreted, which, in turn, leads to excess circulating glucose in the blood (hyperglycemia). With more circulating glucose outside the cells and less glucose in the cells, the kidneys start excreting the glucose into the urine (**glycosuria**), which leads to an excessive amount of fluid entering the urine, a process known as osmotic diuresis (Alemzadeh & Ali, 2011). This diuresis causes large amounts of fluid to be excreted in the urine, a condition known as polyuria. With the excess urine production comes increased thirst, also known polydipsia, a cardinal sign of diabetes.

Because insulin is not available to transport glucose into cells, the cells must turn to new sources of energy, including protein and fat. In an effort to obtain energy, muscle breaks down protein into amino acids. These amino acids are converted to glucose, causing more circulating glucose. This glucose pulls water out of the cells, resulting in dehydration and increased urination.

Fat is broken down into fatty acids, which results in highly acidic ketone bodies being formed, a condition known as **diabetic ketoacidosis (DKA)**. Ketone bodies accumulate in the blood, significantly decreasing the pH level, and may spill into the urine. Potassium and phosphate attempt to neutralize the blood, moving from cells into the bloodstream. Ultimately, this chain of physiological events, if not corrected, can lead to coma or even death.

Clinical Presentation

The excessive use of fat and protein for energy causes the child to lose significant weight. In addition, diabetes often causes a combination of polydipsia, **polyphagia** (increased hunger), polyuria, fatigue, blurred vision, and mood changes. The chief complaints of polydipsia and polyuria are often paired with an ill appearance. If DKA is present, the patient may also present with vomiting, tachycardia, Kussmaul respirations, acetone breath, confusion, and, potentially, coma.

Remember Sophia Carter from Chapter 10? Sophia was a 7-year-old girl who was diagnosed with type 1 diabetes mellitus. What symptoms of diabetes did Sophia initially develop that caused her mother to take her to see her pediatrician, Dr. Hall? What assessment findings concerned Dr. Hall after he had examined Sophia? What was Sophia's blood glucose level at diagnosis? What blood glucose level indicates diabetes?

Assessment and Diagnosis

In addition to observing for the signs and symptoms described, assessment of a child with suspected type 1 diabetes includes bloods tests, such as a random plasma glucose level. Diagnosis of diabetes is confirmed in a patient with symptoms and a random plasma glucose level of greater than 200 mg/dL, a fasting blood glucose level of greater than 126 mg/dL, a 2-hour plasma glucose level greater than 200 mg/dL during a 75-g oral GTT or a **hemoglobin A1C (HbA1C)** level of greater than or equal to 6.5%.

Conducting the GTT proves to be difficult in this population because of the steps necessary, including ingesting a large quantity of glucose in a limited amount of time, undergoing multiple venous punctures (fasting, 1-hour, and 2-hour), and staying relatively still for 2 hours. Findings from urinalysis consistent with type 1 diabetes include a low specific gravity and glycosuria. The presence of islet cell autoantibodies is suggestive of type 1 diabetes, but they are not present in approximately 15% of cases of type 1 diabetic (T1DB) children.

During acute illness, including DKA, many other blood tests must be performed, including assessments of pH level, partial pressure of carbon dioxide, sodium and potassium levels, and white blood cell count.

In Chapter 10, Sophia Carter's nurse, Annie, determined that Sophia was in DKA. What laboratory test results led Annie to this conclusion? How severe was Sophia's ketoacidosis?

Therapeutic Interventions

Management of diabetes is multifaceted and includes insulin therapy, maintaining proper nutrition, and patient and family education on all aspects of this disease.

Insulin Therapy

Upon initial diagnosis of diabetes and as ordered, acutely manage hyperglycemia by administering short-acting IV insulin at a dose of 0.1 to 0.2 units per kilogram of body weight per hour. Closely monitor the patient's blood glucose level, and, as the level falls, very cautiously titrate down the dosage of insulin accordingly, per orders. As insulin is administered, the

body quickly becomes ready to utilize glucose. Without readily available glucose, the body continues to break down fat and protein, causing worsening acidosis. For this reason, glucose is often given concurrently with the insulin.

As glucose levels normalize in the body, IV glucose is replaced with carefully monitored food intake. Subcutaneous injections of rapid-acting insulin are continued for a few days (How Much Does It Hurt? 31.1). In the days following initial presentation, intermediate-acting insulin is added to help with the long-term management of diabetes.

Where on her body did Sophia Carter (in Chapter 10) receive her first insulin injection, given by her nurse, Annie? When did Sophia first self-administer an injection of insulin? If Sophia had been younger, how could she have helped be in control of her insulin injections? What changes in diet did the dietitian, Brett, recommend to Sophia and her parents to help manage her diabetes?

Glucose Monitoring

A patient's blood glucose level must be monitored for both the short and long terms. Blood glucose monitoring allows the patient, family, and medical team to assess the efficacy of short-term management of glucose and to titrate insulin up or down as needed to correct or prevent hyperglycemia or hypoglycemia, respectively. The frequency of monitoring depends on the patient, situation, and goals of therapy. Initial management during a time of diabetic crisis requires hourly monitoring.

Patients using subcutaneous insulin require their blood glucose level to be checked before meals and at bedtime, plus more frequently if symptoms of hypoglycemia or hyperglycemia appear. Teach the patient and family how to properly perform a finger-stick glucose test, and involve the child in his or her own care as early as possible (Fig. 31.6), preferably from the time of diagnosis. By school age, children should be able to learn how to perform a finger puncture on themselves and read the results of the blood glucose monitor. Although many home blood glucose monitors can save the dates, times, and blood glucose levels

How Much Does It Hurt? 31.1

Subcutaneous Injections

Understanding that subcutaneous injections are painful is important when teaching children with diabetes and their parents. Teach them that using distraction methods, such as having the child sing, watch a show, or play on a smart phone, may help alleviate some of the pain and anxiety associated with daily injections.

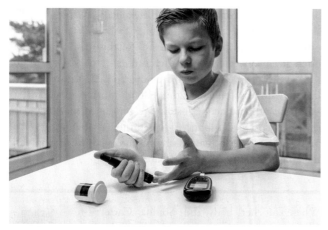

Figure 31.6. Blood glucose monitoring. A child is using a glucometer to check his blood glucose level.

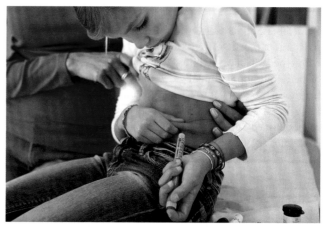

Figure 31.7. Subcutaneous insulin injection. It is important to have the child pinch the adipose tissue when giving an insulin injection.

of readings, it is valuable to write down this information, as well as the child's activity level and diet for the day. These data help establish how a patient is reacting to therapy (American Diabetes Association, 2018).

In some cases, finger-stick glucose monitoring is being replaced by a continuous glucose monitoring system, in which a sensor is placed subcutaneously in the child and readings are sent directly to the patient and/or family's smartphone. This is one of the simplest ways to monitor blood glucose level and assess for extreme highs and lows. However, before insulin administration, it is still recommended to test the blood glucose level using a traditional blood glucose monitor.

Although frequent monitoring with a blood glucose meter is the best way to assess the short-term need for insulin, the HbA1C test is used to assess long-term management of glucose. The HbA1C test monitors the amount of glucose that binds to hemoglobin molecules in the blood, which directly correlates with the amount of glucose circulating in the blood. Although prevention of hyperglycemia is the goal of therapy, it is critical to avoid hypoglycemia in the patient, as well. For this reason, the standard upper limit value for normal HbA1C level in children with diabetes tends to be higher than that for adults with diabetes (Table 31.3).

The American Diabetes Association (2018) recommends that all pediatric patients have an HbA1C of less than 7.5%.

Insulin Education

Different types of insulin are used in conjunction with one another to control blood glucose levels depending on the onset, peak action, and function of action of the insulin (see The Pharmacy 10.1). Dosing is specific to the child's needs, and insulin is administered subcutaneously into adipose tissue over large muscle masses using an insulin syringe or an insulin pen in divided doses (Fig. 31.7).

In Chapter 10, how did Sophia learn to give herself a shot? How did that method help decrease Sophia's anxiety? Would the teaching method have been different if Sophia had been 14 years old?

Rapid-acting insulin can be administered using an insulin pump. The pump includes a reservoir of rapid-acting insulin, thin tubing to deliver the insulin, and a small needle to insert into the subcutaneous tissue. These pumps work like the pancreas do by releasing small amounts of insulin continuously. Then, depending on the results of blood glucose testing, a bolus of rapid-onset insulin can be given at mealtimes or if glucose levels are found to be elevated. Providing insulin in this manner decreases the number of injections needed. In addition, the medication is titrated depending on the individual needs of the day, related to the child's food intake and activity level.

Oftentimes, patients require a combination of different types of insulin, including rapid-acting, short-acting, intermediate-acting, and long-acting types. No single combination is used for every patient. Instead, the patient and family work closely with the healthcare team to establish which insulins best manage the patient's blood glucose level (Analyze the Evidence 31.1).

Table 31.3   Recommended Blood Glucose and Hemoglobin A1C Levels

	Children Without Diabetes	Children/ Adolescents With Diabetes
Blood glucose level		
Before meals (mg/dL)	<100	90–130
At bedtime (mg/dL)	<100	90–150
HbA1C level (%)	<5.7	<7.5

HbA1C, hemoglobin A1C.

Analyze the Evidence 31.1 Parenting Styles and Glucose Control

Hannonen, Aunola, Eklund, and Ahonen (2019) conducted a study to analyze how maternal parenting styles affect diabetic glycemic control in their school-aged children. The study compared 63 T1DB children and their mothers with 83 children without diabetes and their mothers. The three parenting styles that were compared included parental warmth (warmth, acceptance, and involvement between child and parent), behavioral control (limit setting), and psychological control (guilt induction, manipulation, and love withdrawal).

Parenting styles were compared to determine whether parents of T1DB children used different parenting styles than those with healthy children, and also to determine whether a particular parenting style resulted in better diabetic control with the child. It is notable that because of the risk of severe illness, mothers of children with diabetes may be more fearful than are their counterparts about their children's health. The study concluded that children with T1DB were more likely than were their healthy peers to be managed by their mothers using psychological control. In those boys with T1DB, it was found that maternal use of psychological control was associated with poorer concurrent glycemic control. In girls with T1DB, poor glycemic control early in the disease resulted in the maternal use of psychological control. Although it is unlikely that one parenting method is best for all families, it is important to consider the best way to address important healthcare concerns at home with both the parent and the child.

Nutritional Education

Nutritional management by a patient with diabetes requires more than following a list of "good" and "bad" foods. Instead, the medical team must work closely with a nutritionist and the family to address cultural, socioeconomic, and lifestyle needs. It is important to consider the necessary caloric intake of a growing child while still working to maintain normal glucose levels.

Carbohydrate counting is a mainstay of diabetes management in children. A carbohydrate-to-insulin ratio is established per patient to help manage insulin administration. Commonly, 10 g of carbohydrates is covered by 1 unit of insulin. For example, an injection of 5 units of insulin is administered for 50 g of carbohydrates. In addition to carbohydrate counting, timing of meals and snacks should be consistent to help maintain glucose levels. Three large, high-fiber meals should be spaced out by smaller snacks.

Psychosocial Education

Type 1 diabetes is a lifelong illness that will likely have difficult times to manage. Stressful situations may cause changes in glucose levels and thus require a titration of insulin. Hospital admission is necessary at the time of diagnosis so that intensive teaching can be performed for both the patient and the family (Patient Teaching 31.1). Parents may have feelings of guilt after ignoring symptoms of diabetes such as polyphagia, polyuria, and polydipsia for days or weeks before presentation to the hospital. Enquire about the family's support system to assess their ability to care for this new, chronic illness.

Ask children in private how they are dealing with managing diabetes at school. At times, patients may feel embarrassed to have to perform finger-stick glucose monitoring or insulin injections, unlike their classmates who do not have diabetes. Children may begin to act out or have difficulty in classes as they adjust to the management of diabetes. Families should work with teachers, school nurses, and school administrators to find ways for patients to manage stress.

Patient Teaching 31.1

Education for Families Caring for Children With Diabetes

- Provide written information regarding the child's diagnosis.
- Ensure that the family has a written treatment plan that discusses medications, monitoring, and other necessary information.
- Discuss how to monitor blood glucose level.
  - Perform blood glucose checks before each meal and at bedtime.
  - Complete additional monitoring at times of stress: illness, prolonged exercise, eating more or less than usual, or feeling symptomatic.
  - Perform calibrations on the glucometer as noted by the manufacturer.
  - Monitor for consistencies at particular times of day. If levels are constantly low, the child may need an increase in food intake or a decrease in insulin administration.
  - Base insulin dosing on individual responses.
- Discuss how to identify signs and symptoms of hypoglycemia or hyperglycemia (Table 31.4).
- Instruct parents to go to the emergency room in the following situations:
  - Ketones are found in the urine.
  - Their child seems confused.
  - Vomiting occurs.

Evaluation

Expected outcomes for a child with type 1 diabetes mellitus include the following:

- The HbA1C level is reduced to less than 7.5%.
- Blood glucose levels are less than 130 mg/dL before meals and less than 150 mg/dL at bedtime most of the time.

Table 31.4 Comparison of Hypoglycemia and Hyperglycemia: Clinical Presentation

Hypoglycemia	Hyperglycemia
• Confusion	• Abdominal cramping
• Slurred speech	• Vomiting
• Tremors	• Fruity breath
• Palpitations	• Blurred vision
• Diaphoresis	• Flushed skin
• Seizures	• High serum glucose level
• Low serum glucose level	• Glucose in urine

- There is no need for emergency room visits.
- The child achieves and maintains appropriate weight gain for age.

Discharge Planning and Teaching

Managing diabetes is a lifelong endeavor that requires thorough teaching for both the patient and the family. The patient will require regular follow-up visits with an endocrinologist in addition to any acute visits to the emergency department. A child's blood glucose monitoring, medication administration, dietary intake, and exercise must be accounted for at school just as they are in the home setting. The school nurse should be an active member of the medical team for the child.

Family teaching is the cornerstone of diabetes management. Teaching should be tailored to the needs and education level of the family and patient. This often requires different teaching sessions: sessions for patients for 10 to 20 minutes at a time, and sessions for the parents for 45 to 60 minutes at a time. Families must learn how to perform blood glucose monitoring, carbohydrate counting, and subcutaneous insulin injection and/or insulin pump use, as well as to recognize the signs and symptoms of hypoglycemia and hyperglycemia (Table 31.4).

The family must understand the proper treatments for both high and low blood glucose levels as well as how to monitor for complications of abnormal blood glucose levels. Extremely low blood glucose levels may need to be treated with glucagon via the subcutaneous or intramuscular route. With mild hypoglycemia, it is recommended that that the patient be given glucose paste or tablets. If these are unavailable, foods containing simple sugars, such as orange juice, can be given followed by a complex carbohydrate, such as crackers. The occurrence of high blood glucose levels may require administration of additional insulin, above the basal rate. In severe hyperglycemia, the patient may progress into DKA. DKA is a common complication from diabetes and often is the result of incorrect insulin administration or dosing, illness, trauma, or surgery. It commonly appears with the initial presentation of diabetes.

It is important for patients to understand these symptoms so that they can be better prepared to prevent a potentially fatal progression from occurring.

Ensure that children and their families feel supported throughout the care. Refer them to online and in-person support groups for both the patients and their families. Refer children to play groups of other children with diabetes to help make their diabetic management more normalized. At times, families may need individual or family counseling to manage this new stressor. Do not assume that families are managing the diagnosis well. Rather, engage families by asking questions and reviewing the teaching.

Type 2 Diabetes Mellitus

Type 2 diabetes was previously thought of as "adult-onset diabetes." However, owing to the increase in childhood obesity, type 2 diabetes now often occurs in school-aged and teenaged children.

Etiology and Pathophysiology

Unlike in type 1 diabetes, the pancreas of a person with type 2 diabetes produces insulin, but the insulin produced is unable to be utilized by the body (**insulin resistance**). As a result, the pancreas works harder to produce more unusable insulin (**hyperinsulinemia**). In time, the pancreas can no longer produce insulin, and the result is a body with no insulin, similar to that of a person with type 1 diabetes. The onset of puberty is believed to contribute to type 2 diabetes because of the change in sex hormones and thus the need for more insulin production.

Clinical Presentation

The progression of illness is slower in type 2 diabetes than it is in type 1. During a routine or sick visit, the provider may notice **acanthosis nigricans**, or shiny, velvet-like patches most often seen on the back of the neck, inner thighs, or axillae, that occurs because of insulin resistance (Fig. 31.8). Families might mistake this darkening of the skin for dirt and believe that the child is simply not practicing proper hygiene. Use this as a time to teach the family and perform further assessment for type 2 diabetes.

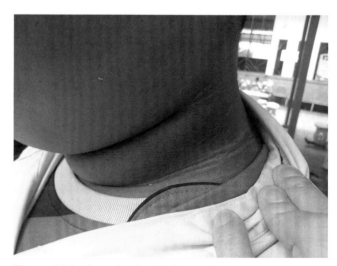

Figure 31.8. Acanthosis nigricans. Note the darkening of the skin on the back of the neck.

The patient is also likely to have a weight for age in the obese category, a high BMI, and a large waist circumference.

Assessment and Diagnosis

Diagnosis of type 2 diabetes is similar to that of type 1. When diabetes is recognized, it is important to determine whether the cause is lack of insulin (type 1) or insulin resistance (type 2) by assessing islet cell autoantibodies. Abnormal blood glucose test results, as described (Type 1 Diabetes: Assessment and Diagnosis), and normal levels of islet cell autoantibodies is suggestive of type 2 diabetes. Nonetheless, initial classification of diabetes is difficult, and confounding factors, such as clinical appearance, lipid levels (dyslipidemia is common), and blood pressure (hypertension is common), must be assessed as well to help diagnose type 2 diabetes.

Therapeutic Interventions

The initial presentation of symptoms determines whether the child needs to be hospitalized. Depending on the level of hyperglycemia, the child may need to be admitted to the hospital to manage the blood glucose level and potential ketoacidosis. During an outpatient visit or before discharge from the hospital, review information on the child's growth and development, diet, exercise, and understanding of diabetes. Diet and exercise are recommended (as described later) for the initial treatment of type 2 diabetes. If diet and exercise alone do not control blood glucose levels, treatment of type 2 diabetes progresses to include use of metformin (The Pharmacy 31.4). Metformin improves sensitivity to target cells to insulin in the liver and muscle cells. Metformin also slows the production of glucose by the liver.

Evaluation

Expected outcomes for a child with type 2 diabetes mellitus are similar to those for a child with type 1 diabetes mellitus. Refer to the section Evaluation under Type 1 Diabetes Mellitus, earlier. Additional expected outcomes include the following:

- Acanthosis nigricans resolves.
- BMI normalizes.

Discharge Planning and Teaching

Teaching is the most important portion of managing this lifelong illness. Increasing exercise and creating habits for a more

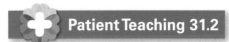

Patient Teaching 31.2
Let's Get Physical

- Encourage the child to engage in 60 minutes of physical activity per day.
- Divide the physical activity into 10- to 15-minute increments, to make it more manageable.
- Adopt a positive attitude about the child's progress toward exercise goals.
- Make activity time fun for the child.
- Limit the child's screen time to < 2 hours per day.
- Suggestions for activities include the following:
  o Having a fit kit available, including such items as a jump rope, hand weights, and resistance bands.
  o Taking walks together.
  o Planning outings together, such as biking and hiking.
  o Encouraging children to join teams, such as for sports or dance.
  o Finding ways to incorporate moving into daily activities, such as raking leaves, gardening, or playing in the snow.
  o Turning household activities into fun: seeing how quickly the child can make the bed or having races to move things from upstairs to downstairs.

active lifestyle are important components of managing type 2 diabetes (Patient Teaching 31.2).

Consider ethical concerns and a family's socioeconomic status when discussing changes to the patient's and family's diet. Making food changes as a family makes it more likely that the child will stick with the changes. Suggestions might include replacing sports drinks and juices with water and cooking at home rather than eating fast food (Patient Teaching 31.3).

Monitoring height, weight, and BMI at each visit helps assess how the patient is managing the aforementioned lifestyle changes. When the patient is still growing, it is recommended to describe weight management as "growing" into the child's healthy weight. By doing this, positive body image can be maintained, and the focus is shifted from weight loss to growing into the child's desired size.

The Pharmacy 31.4 — Metformin

Classification	Route	Action	Nursing Considerations
Antidiabetic agent	PO	Decreases glucose production in the liver, which decreases intestinal absorption of glucose; increases uptake and use of glucose	• Administer with meals. • Monitor blood glucose levels. • Monitor HbA1C level.

HbA1C, hemoglobin A1C; PO, oral.
Adapted from Taketomo, C. K., Hodding, J. H., & Kraus, D. M. (2018). *Pediatric & neonatal dosage handbook* (25th ed.). Hudson, OH: Lexicomp.

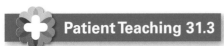

Patient Teaching 31.3

Eating "Right" Makes the Wallet Tight

When teaching families about appropriate dietary changes to help improve glycemic control in their newly diagnosed children, it is important to recognize the potential financial strain on families. Nuts and berries are often pricier than chips and cookies. Try to think of affordable alternatives or resources to share with families of children with diabetes.

Home glucose monitoring is standard practice for children with type 2 diabetes. By monitoring blood glucose levels, families can assess the effects of lifestyle changes they are making. At primary care and endocrine healthcare provider visits, HbA1C tests are performed to measure the efficacy of blood glucose control over the preceding 2 to 3 months.

When metformin is prescribed, review and enforce the same diet and exercise suggestions. Annual assessment of lipid levels, blood pressure, liver function, and renal function, as well as eye examinations, should be performed to assess for complications and progression of type 2 diabetes. As with type 1 diabetes, poor management of type 2 diabetes puts the child at risk for long-term vascular complications.

Parathyroid Gland Disorders

Parathyroid hormone is secreted by the parathyroid gland. This hormone helps regulate calcium and phosphate in the body. Cases of too much or too little of this hormone are rare in pediatric patients.

Hypoparathyroidism

Hypoparathyroidism is a condition of deficient secretion of the parathyroid hormone from the four small parathyroid glands, which are located on the back of the thymus gland in the neck. This hormone helps regulate the level of calcium in the blood to ensure sufficient levels to maintain bones and perform other vital functions in the body.

Etiology and Pathophysiology

Hypoparathyroidism, a rare illness, is most commonly caused by the accidental removal of the parathyroid gland during a thyroidectomy or other surgeries of the neck. Other causes include congenital disorders (such as DiGeorge syndrome), diseases that affect the parathyroid glands (such as autoimmune illnesses), and/or medications (such as asparagine and cytosine). In some cases, the cause of this disease is not known. Whatever the cause, this condition results in hypocalcemia and hyperphosphatemia.

Clinical Presentation

In infancy, hypoparathyroidism presents with symptoms of hypocalcemia including hyperirritability, poor eating, and seizures.

Assessment and Diagnosis

A classic assessment for hyperirritability of the face, which occurs in hypocalcemia, is the **Chvostek sign**, which may be elicited by tapping on the facial nerve (cranial nerve VII) just anterior to the earlobe and below the zygomatic arch (Fig. 31.9). A positive response is indicated by a spasm of the facial muscles surrounding the eye, nose, and mouth.

Blood tests are performed to confirm the diagnosis of hypoparathyroidism and include assessments of serum calcium, parathyroid hormone, and phosphorus levels. Positive findings include low calcium and parathyroid hormone levels and elevated phosphorus levels.

Therapeutic Interventions

Children experiencing severe symptoms of hypoparathyroidism—particularly hypocalcemia—may require hospitalization. Inpatient management of hypocalcemia may be very aggressive. IV calcium gluconate is often necessary for initial management, followed by intramuscular or oral calcium (The Pharmacy 31.5).

The Pharmacy 31.5   Calcium Gluconate

Classification	Route	Action	Nursing Considerations
Calcium supplement	• PO • IV	Controls nerve and muscle reactions through the regulation of action potentials	• Monitor for signs of hyper- and hypocalcemia. • PO: administer with plenty of fluids. • IV: monitor for extravasation and tissue necrosis. • Monitor calcium levels. • Monitor electrocardiogram.

IV, intravenous; PO, oral.
Adapted from Taketomo, C. K., Hodding, J. H., & Kraus, D. M. (2018). *Pediatric & neonatal dosage handbook* (25th ed.). Hudson, OH: Lexicomp.

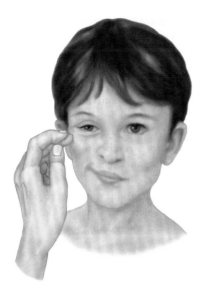

Figure 31.9. Chvostek sign. Tapping on the facial nerve results in spasms of the muscles around the mouth, nose, and eyes. Reprinted with permission from Hinkle, J. L., & Cheever, K. H. (2017). *Brunner & Suddarth's textbook of medical-surgical nursing* (14th ed., Fig. 13-7A). Philadelphia, PA: Lippincott Williams & Wilkins. Adapted from Bullock, B. A., & Henze, R. J. (2000). *Focus on pathophysiology* (p. 173). Philadelphia, PA: Lippincott Williams & Wilkins.

Nursing care includes monitoring and managing calcium levels closely to avoid a cardiac arrhythmia. Maintain seizure precautions and keep the patient on a cardiorespiratory monitor. Keep an airway tray at the bedside in case it is needed to stabilize the airway. Establish and maintain an IV line to administer calcium supplementation. Closely monitor the IV site for any signs of infiltration, because infiltrated calcium can cause tissue extravasation and sloughing.

Children with less severe symptoms may only require outpatient care. In such cases, oral calcitriol and calcium are prescribed and foods high in phosphorus are limited. Serum blood levels of calcium and phosphorus are monitored periodically. The duration of treatment depends on the patient's response to therapy; in some cases, it may need to be lifelong.

Evaluation

Expected outcomes for a child with hypoparathyroidism include the following:
- The child achieves and maintains normal calcium levels.
- The child achieves and maintains normal cardiac rhythms.
- The child and the parents demonstrate appropriate administration of calcium and vitamin D before discharge.
- The child exhibits no signs of weakness, headache, vomiting, or diarrhea.

Discharge Planning and Teaching

Teach the family and the patient the importance of daily adherence to calcium and vitamin D administration. Explain that the increased vitamin D intake aids in the absorption of the

abnormally high level of calcium. Without sufficient amounts of vitamin D, the calcium will not be properly absorbed.

Hyperparathyroidism

Hyperparathyroidism is a condition of excess secretion of the parathyroid hormone.

Etiology and Pathophysiology

Hyperparathyroidism is rare in childhood and most commonly caused by a parathyroid adenoma or chronic renal failure. In the case of renal failure, the kidneys stop converting vitamin D to its active form. Because vitamin D is necessary for absorbing calcium from the food we eat into the bloodstream, a decrease in usable vitamin D results in a decrease in absorption of calcium into the bloodstream, and therefore a decrease in the blood level of calcium. This low level of calcium in the blood stimulates the parathyroid glands to continuously secrete parathyroid hormone in an attempt to increase the serum calcium level to normal.

Clinical Presentation

Hyperparathyroidism can cause hypercalcemia and hypophosphatemia. Symptoms include bone pain and fractures and kidney stones.

Assessment and Diagnosis

Blood tests are performed to confirm the diagnosis of hyperparathyroidism and include assessments of serum calcium, parathyroid hormone, and phosphorus levels. Positive findings include elevated calcium and parathyroid hormone levels and decreased phosphorus levels.

Therapeutic Interventions

When hyperparathyroidism is the result of a tumor, surgical excision of the affected parathyroid gland is performed. In addition, the other parathyroid gland on the same side must be biopsied.

In kidney failure, the goal of treatment of hyperparathyroidism is to maintain normal calcium levels using vitamin D supplementation and phosphorus binders.

Evaluation

Expected outcomes for a child with hyperparathyroidism include the following:
- The child's intake of dietary calcium is restricted.
- If renal rickets develops, the child begins using long-term braces and undergoes physical therapy.
- The child increases fluid intake to assist in the reduction of renal calculi formation.

Discharge Planning and Teaching

Provide preoperative and postoperative teaching for patients who require surgical removal of the parathyroid. After the surgery, review with the patient and family the guidelines regarding calcium supplementation and the monitoring of serum calcium and phosphorus levels.

Think Critically

1. A previously healthy adolescent female is complaining of cold intolerance, weight gain, and brittle nails. What abnormal laboratory values would you expect to see? How might they be corrected?

2. DI causes decreased urine specific gravity as noted on a urinalysis and an increased serum osmolality. What subjective complaints might this patient have?

3. When treating a patient for hypothyroidism, what signs and symptoms may be a signal that the patient is taking too much thyroid hormone supplement?

4. Monitoring growth is an essential part of the nurse's job. What findings would alert you to potential problems when plotting length or height, weight, head circumference, and/or BMI? What follow-up questions would you ask the patient related to the abnormal findings?

5. Many endocrine disorders require injections of medications. What administration techniques would you use when caring for a toddler versus a school-aged versus an adolescent patient?

6. Psychosocial considerations must be included when caring for a patient with a chronic illness. What nursing diagnoses should be included when caring for a patient with a lifelong illness?

References

Adis Medical Writers (2018). Diagnose and treat paediatric hypothyroidism promptly to achieve optimal growth and developmental outcomes. *Drugs & Therapy Perspectives, 34*, 116–120.

Alemzadeh, R., & Ali, O. (2011). Diabetes mellitus. In R. M. Kliegman, B. F. Stanton, J. W. St. Geme III, N. F. Schor, & R. E. Behrman (Eds.), *Nelson's textbook of pediatrics* (19th ed., pp. 1968–1997). Philadelphia, PA: Elsevier Saunders.

American Diabetes Association. (2018). Standards of medical care in diabetes-2018. *Diabetics Care, 41*(Suppl. 1), S1–S156. Retrieved from https://diabetesed.net/wp-content/uploads/2017/12/2018-ADA-Standards-of-Care.pdf

Argente, J. (1999). Diagnosis of late puberty. *Hormone Research, 51*(Suppl 3), 95.

Bahn, R. S., Burch, H. B., Cooper, D. S., Garber, J. R., Greenlee, M. C., Klein, I., Laurberg, P., McDougall, I.R., Montori, V.M. & Rivkees, S. A. (2011). Hyperthyroidism and other causes of thyrotoxicosis: management guidelines of the American Thyroid Association and American Association of Clinical Endocrinologists. *Thyroid, 21*(6), 593–646.

Bichet, D. G. (2019). *Treatment of central diabetes insipidus.* Retrieved (June 10, 2019) from https://www.uptodate.com/contents/treatment-of-central-diabetes-insipidus?search=diabetes%20insipidus&source=search_result&selectedTitle=2-150&usage_type=default&display_rank=2#H144709921.

Bockenhauer, D., & Bichet, D. G. (2015). Pathophysiology, diagnosis and management of nephrogenic diabetes insipidus. *Nature Reviews Nephrology, 11*(10), 576.

Broersen, L. H., Jha, M., Biermasz, N. R., Pereira, A. M., & Dekkers, O. M. (2018). Effectiveness of medical treatment for Cushing's syndrome: A systematic review and meta-analysis. *Pituitary, 21*, 1–11.

Bulcao Macedo, D., Nahime Brito, V., & Latronico, A. C. (2014). New causes of central precocious puberty: The role of genetic factors. *Neuroendocrinology, 100*(1), 1–8. doi:10.1159/000366282.

Carel, J. C., & Leger, J. (2008). Clinical practice. Precocious puberty. *New England Journal of Medicine, 358*(22), 2366–2377.

Garibaldi, L., & Chemaitilly, W. (2017). Disorders of pubertal development. In R. Kliegman, B. Stanton, J. St. Geme, & N. Schor (Eds.), *Nelson's textbook of pediatrics* (20th ed., Chapter 562, pp. 2565–2662). Philadelphia, PA: Elsevier Saunders.

Gonzalez, C. L., Mesa, E. M., Huerta, Y. Z., Marquez, M. P. O., Arranz, M. T. H., & Abizanda, E. P. (2018, May). Diabetes insipidus as first clinical manifestation of pineal tumor. In *20th European Congress of Endocrinology* (Vol. 56). Barcelona, Spain: BioScientifica.

Graber, E., & Rapaport, R. (2012). Growth and growth disorders in children and adolescents. *Pediatric Annals, 41*(4), e65–e72.

Hannonen, R., Aunola, K., Eklund, K., & Ahonen, T. (2019). Maternal parenting styles and glycemic control in children with type 1 diabetes. *International Journal of Environmental Research and Public Health, 16*(2), 214.

Harrington, J., & Palmert, M. R. (2018). *Definition, etiology, and evaluation of precocious puberty.* Retrieved from https://www.uptodate.com/contents/definition-etiology-and-evaluation-of-precocious-puberty?search=Definition,%20etiology,%20and%20evaluation%20of%20precocious%20puberty&source=search_result&selectedTitle=1-134&usage_type=default&display_rank=1

Nieman, L. K. (2018). Diagnosis of Cushing's syndrome in the modern era. *Endocrinology and Metabolism Clinics of North America, 47*(2), 259–273.

Rastogi, M. V., & LaFranchi, S. H. (2010). Congenital hypothyroidism. *Orphanet Journal of Rare Diseases, 5*, 17.

Rivkees, S. A., Stephenson, K., & Dinauer, C. (2010). Adverse events associated with methimazole therapy of graves' disease in children. *International Journal of Pediatric Endocrinology, 2010*(1), 176970.

Santos, A., Resmini, E., Pascual, J. C., Crespo, I., & Webb, S. M. (2017). Psychiatric symptoms in patients with Cushing's syndrome: Prevalence, diagnosis and management. *Drugs, 77*(8), 829–842.

Shapira, S. K., Hinton, C. F., Held, P. K., Jones, E., Harry Hannon, W., & Ojodu, J. (2015). Single newborn screen or routine second screening for primary congenital hypothyroidism. *Molecular Genetics & Metabolism, 116*(3), 125–132.

Sherr, J., & Weinzimer, S. (2012). Diabetes types 1 and 2 in the pediatric population. *Pediatric Annals, 41*(2), 1–7.

Singh, R. (2017). Determinants of levothyroxine dose required to achieve euthyroidism in pediatric population-a hospital-based prospective follow-up study. *European Journal of Pediatrics, 176*(8), 1027–1033.

Snyder, C. K. (2016). Puberty: An overview for pediatric nurses. *Journal of Pediatric Nursing: Nursing Care of Children and Families, 31*(6), 757–759.

Van Haalen, F. M., van Dijk, E. H., Dekkers, O. M., Bizino, M. B., Dijkman, G., Biermasz, N. R., . . . Pereira, A. M. (2018). Cushing's syndrome and hypothalamic–pituitary–adrenal axis hyperactivity in chronic central serous chorioretinopathy. *Frontiers in Endocrinology, 9*, 39.

White, P. C., & Bachega, T. A. S. S. (2012). Congenital Adrenal Hyperplasia Due to 21 Hydroxylase Deficiency: From Birth to Adulthood. *Seminars in Reproductive Medicine, 30*(5), 400–409.

Yang, M., & White, P. C. (2017). Risk factors for hospitalization of children with congenital adrenal hyperplasia. *Clinical Endocrinology, 86*(5), 669–673.

Suggested Readings

Chiang, J. L., Maahs, D. M., Garvey, K. C., Hood, K. K., Laffel, L. M., Weinzimer, S. A., . . . Schatz, D. (2018). Type 1 diabetes in children and adolescents: A position statement by the American Diabetes Association. *Diabetes Care, 41*(9), 2026–2044.

Di Dalmazi, G., & Reincke, M. (2018). Adrenal surgery for Cushing syndrome: An update. *Endocrinology and Metabolism Clinics of North America, 47*(2), 385–394.

Jones, N. H. Y., & Rose, S. R. (2018). Congenital hypothyroidism. In *Pediatric endocrinology* (pp. 371–383). Cham, Switzerland: Springer.

32 Genetic Disorders

After completing this chapter, you will be able to:
1. Identify and distinguish among specific genetic disorders affecting children.
2. Discuss the pathophysiology of specific genetic disorders affecting children.
3. Identify common diagnostic procedures associated with diagnosis of specific genetic disorders affecting children.
4. Describe the role and responsibility of the nurse caring for a child diagnosed with a genetic disorder.
5. Apply principles of growth and development to the care of a child with a genetic disorder.
6. Create a nursing plan of care for each pediatric genetic disorder.

Key Terms

Fragile X syndrome
Genetic counseling
Genetic testing
Inborn errors of metabolism
Newborn screening

Phenylketonuria (PKU)
Trisomy 13
Trisomy 18
Trisomy 21
Turner syndrome

Overview of Genetic Disorders in Children

A genetic disorder is a disease caused by an abnormality in an individual's genetic material. Genetic disorders can be categorized into monogenic (Mendelian), multifactorial, nontraditional inheritance, or chromosomal disorders. Monogenic disorders occur when a single gene is defective. Monogenic disorders may be autosomal dominant, autosomal recessive, X-linked dominant, or X-linked recessive. Multifactorial inheritance disorders are thought to be caused by multiple gene and environmental factors. Many common congenital malformations such as cleft lip, cleft palate, clubfoot, and cardiac defects are attributed to multifactorial inheritance.

Nontraditional inheritance disorders do not follow the typical patterns of dominant, recessive, X-linked, or multifactorial disorders. One type, mitochondrial disorders, is usually passed from the mother to the offspring because mitochondrial genes are inherited almost exclusively from the mother. With nontraditional inheritance disorders, abnormalities are often seen in one or more organs, such as the brain, skeletal muscle, or eyes. These disorders have a variable age of onset, from infancy to adulthood, and can have extreme variability in symptoms even within a family. Examples of these disorders include carnitine deficiency, Kearns–Sayre syndrome (a multisystem disorder), and leukodystrophy (a neurological disorder).

Chromosomal abnormalities do not follow a straightforward pattern of inheritance. Most chromosomal abnormalities occur due to an error in the sperm or egg, often during the process of cell division, leaving the sperm or egg with too few or too many chromosomes. Abnormalities can occur in the number or structure of autosomal chromosomes or in sex chromosomes.

Examples of abnormalities in the chromosome number include trisomy 21 (Down syndrome), trisomy 18 (Edwards syndrome), and trisomy 13 (Patau syndrome). In trisomies, there are three copies of a chromosome instead of the usual two. Chromosome structure abnormalities occur when a portion of one or more chromosomes breaks and, during repair, the chromosomes are rejoined incorrectly, leading to too much or too little genetic material. Parts of chromosomes can be missing (deletions) or have extra segments or components (duplications). Clinical findings vary depending on the amount of chromosome material involved. Sex chromosome abnormalities occur when there is a missing or extra sex chromosome. Abnormalities in sexual development, fertility, and growth and deficits in behavior and learning are common. These disorders include Turner syndrome and Klinefelter syndrome.

Children with genetic disorders often have complex medical needs, and care often involves the assessment and treatment of multiple organ systems. Genetic disorders do not have specific treatments or cures; treatment focuses on symptomatic care, supportive care, and prevention of complications related to the disorder. A wide variety of treatments and interventions, along with a multidisciplinary approach, are necessary in the treatment of genetic disorders.

General Nursing Interventions for Genetic Disorders

Provide Emotional and Psychosocial Support to the Child and Parents

Families caring for a child with a genetic disorder often have interrupted family processes because of the child's frequent illnesses and hospitalizations, increased care needs at home, abnormal growth and development patterns, and concerns about survival. Assist the family in recognizing and maintaining a functional support system and developing adequate coping mechanisms while caring for their child. Encourage families to verbalize concerns about their child's diagnosis, illness, and prognosis. Identify areas where further education may be needed, and assist families in gaining the knowledge and skills to adequately care for their child. Explain all therapies, procedures, and plans of care to the parents. Accurate and thorough explanations decrease anxiety and help families cope more effectively. Encourage parents to actively participate in care and decision making for their child. Teach parents to be advocates for their child. Provide information about support groups and resources for children and families with genetic disorders. Knowledge and use of available resources help parents develop a wide array of support in dealing with the challenges that may occur when caring for a child with a genetic disorder.

Promote Growth and Development

Children with genetic disorders are often at risk for delayed growth and development related to cognitive deficits, physical disabilities, and activity restrictions secondary to their genetic disorder. Nurses play an important role in helping children achieve their highest potential for growth and development and in teaching parents ways to help their child achieve milestones within age parameters and limits of disease. Screening for developmental capabilities to determine a child's current level of functioning is important. Regular monitoring of height and weight is essential to identify growth patterns and deviations from growth trends. Encourage parents to participate in early intervention programs available for their child. Early intervention refers to a variety of programs and resources that are available to infants and young children with developmental delays and cognitive impairments. Early intervention services may include physical therapy, occupational therapy, speech therapy, and special education.

Offer children age-appropriate toys and activities to encourage development. Help parents and families understand that their child's developmental progress may be slower than normal because of immobility and extremity deficits or cognitive delays. Teach parents to maximize potential for growth and development by providing a stimulating environment when possible. Encourage parents to praise their child for accomplishments and emphasize the child's abilities to improve the child's feelings of confidence, competence, and self-esteem.

Prevent and Manage Complications

Children with genetic disorders often have an increased risk of health complications such as cardiac, gastrointestinal, respiratory, immune, or musculoskeletal problems. For example, congenital heart disease occurs more frequently in children with Down syndrome, and children with Turner syndrome are more prone to kidney and thyroid complications, as well as skeletal disorders. Children with genetic disorders need the usual immunizations, well-child care, and regular screenings recommended by the American Academy of Pediatrics. Encourage parents to keep well-child visits and stay up to date on immunizations as recommended by their provider. Hearing and vision problems are common in many genetic disorders; therefore, regular evaluation of vision and hearing is essential. For children with immune dysfunction related to a genetic disorder, preventing infection is a priority in their care. Teach parents proper hand washing and ways to reduce the risk of or prevent infection in their susceptible child. Children with musculoskeletal complications may require physical therapy and orthotics or braces. Encourage parents to seek regular follow-up for mobility devices, particularly as the child grows and outgrows devices. Encourage families to seek regular dental care for children and to support proper oral hygiene.

Promote Nutrition

Children with genetic disorders may have trouble swallowing, sucking, or feeding because of lack of muscle tone or lack of coordination of reflexes needed to suck and swallow. Some children with genetic disorders have an abnormally developed oral cavity, which can lead to feeding difficulties. Children with Down syndrome, for example, tend to have small mouths and a flat, smooth, large tongue, in addition to lack of muscle tone. These characteristics lead to difficulty sucking, swallowing, and feeding. Adaptive devices, such as special nipples and eating utensils, are often used. Special positioning, such as supporting the head, chin, and throat when feeding, is often necessary. Some children with genetic disorders may need a gastrostomy tube or jejunostomy tube to be safely fed and achieve an adequate caloric intake.

A special diet may be necessary for some genetic disorders; for example, a child with Down syndrome is more likely to have celiac disease or other gastrointestinal disorders. In such cases, special formulas or diets are necessary. Teach parents which types of foods should be avoided and which foods are tolerated for these children. Children with **inborn errors of metabolism**, such as phenylketonuria (PKU), require a special diet. Parents need teaching geared toward the specific genetic disorder and the dietary restrictions and requirements associated with the disorder.

Genetic Disorders

Fragile X Syndrome

Fragile X syndrome is an inherited, genetic condition and is the most common cause of intellectual disability (Centers for Disease Control and Prevention [CDC], 2017b; National Institutes of Health [NIH], 2018b). Fragile X syndrome occurs in approximately 1 in 4,000 boys and 1 in 6,000 to 8,000 girls, with boys experiencing more severe symptoms due to having only one X chromosome (CDC, 2017b).

Etiology and Pathophysiology

Fragile X syndrome follows an X-linked dominant inheritance pattern (Fig. 32.1). Although it is X-linked, fragile X syndrome has some unique features of inheritance. For instance, unaffected males who carry the gene in premutation form may not have any symptoms themselves (National Fragile X Foundation, 2018). A protein called FMRP is responsible for regulating the production of other proteins and plays a role in developing synapses. A gene called *FMR1* provides instructions for making this protein, and mutations in this gene are the cause of fragile X syndrome (NIH, 2018b). In individuals with a full mutation, the *FMR1* gene "shuts down" (National Fragile X Foundation, 2018).

Clinical Presentation

Clinical presentation is usually subtle during childhood, with minor dysmorphic features and developmental delay. In adolescence, boys may present with features such as a large head, long face, and prominent ears, chin, and forehead, as well as flexible joints, flat feet, and enlarged testicles (CDC, 2017b). Children may present with a range of cognitive deficits, such as trouble with learning, solving problems, and speaking, as well as behavioral problems, such as biting, hand flapping, short attention span, and trouble making eye contact (Fig. 32.2; CDC, 2017b).

Assessment and Diagnosis

Many times, the first signs include problems with sensation and people touching them, being anxious around crowds and in new situations, and behavior problems (CDC, 2017b). A delay in meeting developmental milestones may be the first assessment finding. Diagnosis is confirmed with **genetic testing.**

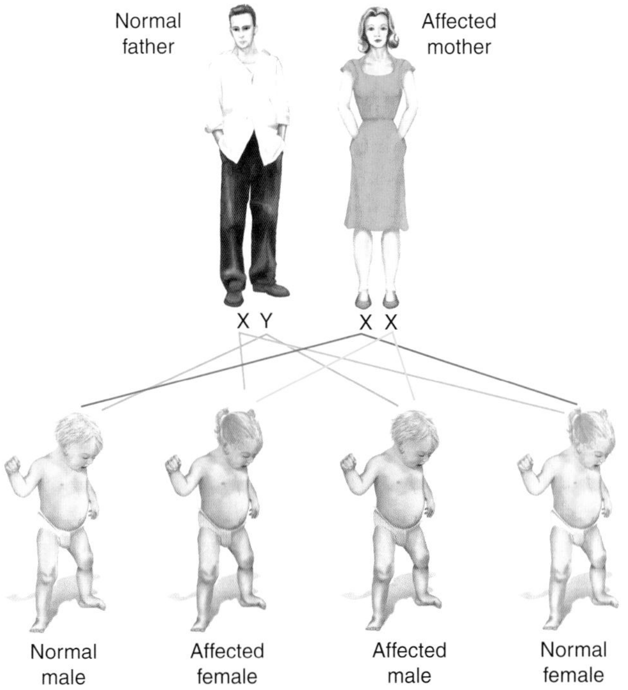

Figure 32.1. X-linked dominant inheritance pattern. Reprinted with permission from Kyle, T., & Carman, S. (2016). *Essentials of pediatric nursing* (3rd ed., Fig. 27.4). Philadelphia, PA: Wolters Kluwer.

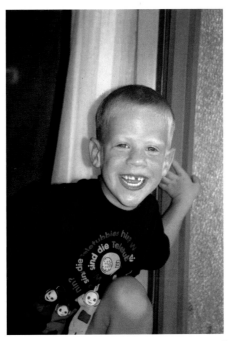

Figure 32.2. A child with fragile X syndrome. Reprinted with permission from Schaaf, C. P., Zschocke, J., & Potocki, L. (2011). *Human genetics* (1st ed., Fig. 31.7A). Philadelphia, PA: Wolters Kluwer.

Therapeutic Interventions

Nursing management should focus on developmental therapies such as those for children with intellectual disabilities.

Evaluation

Although there is no cure for fragile X syndrome, the prognosis is good, with a normal life span expected. Expected outcomes for a child with fragile X syndrome include the following:

- The child remains free from injury to self.
- The child receives referrals for appropriate developmental therapies.
- Caregivers receive education and support for managing the condition.

Discharge Planning and Teaching

The National Fragile X Foundation (https://fragilex.org/# 1476180604782-5feb1bfb-8dc5) can provide families with education about the diagnosis as well as support through advocacy and community resources.

During the child's initial presentation, assessment, and diagnosis, parents may require much reassurance and support. If the child is hospitalized, explain to the parents the hospital environment, equipment, and monitors. The child may not be able to communicate pain or needs without difficulty. Provide developmentally appropriate means of communication for the child and support for the parents.

Phenylketonuria

Phenylketonuria (PKU) is a rare, inherited, metabolic disorder. It is an inborn error of metabolism and is detected during the first few days of life by **newborn screening** (NIH, n.d.a). Approximately 10,000 to 15,000 babies are born with PKU yearly. This disorder affects males and females equally and occurs in all ethnic groups, although it is more common in individuals who are Native American or Northern European (March of Dimes, 2013).

Etiology and Pathophysiology

PKU follows an autosomal recessive inheritance pattern (Fig. 32.3).

PKU results from a deficiency of a liver enzyme, leading to the inability of the body to process the essential amino acid phenylalanine (NIH, n.d.a). Elevated levels of phenylalanine in the bloodstream can result in irreversible brain damage unless PKU is detected and treated.

Clinical Presentation

Usually there are no symptoms at birth, but if PKU is undetected and untreated, infants can soon begin to show signs. Initial signs and symptoms may include irritability, vomiting of protein feedings, musty body smell, increased reflex action, and seizures (March of Dimes, 2013). If left untreated or with dietary

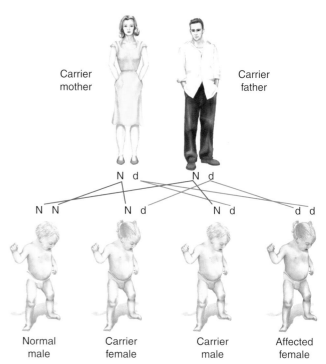

Figure 32.3. Autosomal recessive inheritance pattern. Reprinted with permission from Kyle, T., & Carman, S. (2016). *Essentials of pediatric nursing* (3rd ed., Fig. 27.2). Philadelphia, PA: Wolters Kluwer.

noncompliance, symptoms may include skin rashes, microcephaly, developmental delays, intellectual disabilities, and behavior problems such as hyperactivity (March of Dimes, 2013).

Assessment and Diagnosis

Newborn screening for PKU is required for all infants in the United States, and testing is completed 24 to 48 hours after protein feeding. The infant needs to ingest enough formula or breast milk to raise the phenylalanine levels for the screening test to identify PKU accurately. This is completed with a heel stick in the hospital (March of Dimes, 2013). If the screening results aren't normal, a diagnostic test is required to determine whether the infant has PKU.

Therapeutic Interventions

Nursing management should focus on meal plans low in phenylalanine (low protein). Formulas that are low in phenylalanine are available, and infants can have some breast milk (mothers must work closely with the provider; March of Dimes, 2013). Individuals with PKU can eat vegetables, fruits, some grains, and other foods that are low in phenylalanine. Foods to avoid include dairy products, eggs, meat and poultry, fish, nuts, beans, and foods that contain aspartame.

Testing for phenylamine levels is part of the lifetime treatment of an individual with PKU. As an infant, testing may need to be done once a week or more often. Through childhood, testing may be done once or twice a month (March of Dimes, 2013).

Evaluation

Although there is no cure for PKU, the prognosis is good as long as the child complies with a diet low in phenylalanine and maintains blood levels of phenylalanine in the therapeutic range. Expected outcomes for a child with PKU include the following:

- The child complies with a diet low in phenylalanine.
- The child complies with phenylalanine level testing.
- Phenylamine levels remain in the therapeutic range.
- The child receives referrals for appropriate developmental therapies as needed.
- Caregivers receive education and support for managing the condition.

Discharge Planning and Teaching

Several organizations provide families with education about PKU and support through advocacy and community resources; their websites are as follows:

- https://www.marchofdimes.org/complications/phenylketonuria-in-your-baby.aspx
- https://pkunews.org
- http://pkunetwork.org

After the child's diagnosis, parents may require much reassurance and support. If the child is hospitalized, explain the hospital environment, equipment, and monitors to the parents and the child. Dietary compliance is essential to prevent complications, and if the child hospitalized, this diet must be maintained in the hospital, as well. Provide developmentally appropriate means of communication and pain assessment for the child and support for the parents.

Trisomy 13

Trisomy 13, also called Patau syndrome, is a noninherited chromosomal condition. Trisomy 13 occurs in about 1 in 16,000 newborns, with the prevalence increasing with maternal age (NIH, 2018c).

Etiology and Pathophysiology

Trisomy 13 results from random events that occur during the formation of eggs and sperm causing an error in cell division, leading to an abnormal number of chromosomes—in this case, three copies of the chromosome 13 in each cell (NIH, 2018c; Fig. 32.4). Trisomy 13 can also occur with two normal copies of chromosome 13 and one extra copy of chromosome 13 attached to another chromosome in the cells.

Clinical Presentation

Characteristic anomalies associated with trisomy 13 include cleft lip and palate and extra digits (Fig. 32.5), as well as clenched hands (with outer fingers on top of inner fingers), close-set eyes, hernias, low-set ears, scalp defects (such as missing skin), a single palmar crease, limb abnormalities, microcephaly, micrognathia (small lower jaw), and undescended testicles (NIH, n.d.b).

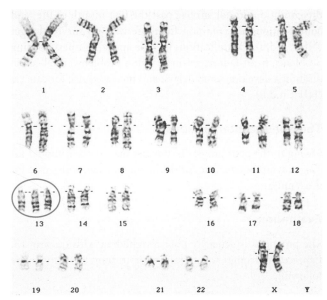

Figure 32.4. Patau syndrome karyotype. Note the third chromosome located at chromosome 13. Reprinted with permission from Stephenson, S. R., & Dmitrieva, J. (2017). *Obstetrics and gynecology* (4th ed., Fig. 31.25B). Philadelphia, PA: Wolters Kluwer.

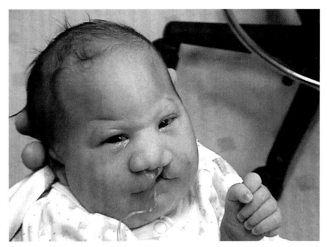

Figure 32.5. Clinical characteristics of trisomy 13. A cleft lip and malformed digits are common clinical characteristics in trisomy 13. Reprinted with permission from Baum, V. C., & O'Flaherty, J. E. (2015). *Anesthesia for genetic, metabolic, and dysmorphic syndromes of childhood* (3rd ed., unnumbered figure in Chapter 19). Philadelphia, PA: Wolters Kluwer.

Assessment and Diagnosis

Nursing assessment for trisomy 13 includes observation for the characteristic anomalies. Prenatal testing or screening for the condition is available, and thus it can be diagnosed prenatally. If not diagnosed prenatally, it is usually diagnosed in the first few days of life depending on the physical anomalies. Trisomy 13 involves multiple abnormalities, many of which are life-threatening (NIH, n.d.b). Most infants with the condition do not survive past the first month of life, and complications are common for those who do survive longer (NIH, n.d.b). Complications include apnea, deafness, feeding problems, heart failure, seizures, vision problems, intellectual disability, developmental delays, and increased risk for cancers (NIH, n.d.b).

Therapeutic Interventions

Owing to the poor prognosis, nursing management should focus on symptomatic care for the infant and supportive care for the family.

Evaluation

The prognosis is generally poor for children with trisomy 13. Expected outcomes for a child with trisomy 13 include the following:

- The child receives comfort care.
- The child receives symptomatic care as needed.
- Caregivers receive supportive care.
- Caregivers receive **genetic counseling**.

Discharge Planning and Teaching

SOFT is a support organization for families who have a child with a chromosome abnormality. The website is https://trisomy.org/.

Trisomy 18

Trisomy 18, also called Edwards syndrome, is a chromosomal condition that, in most cases, is not inherited. Trisomy 18 occurs in about 1 in 5,000 live-born infants, with the prevalence increasing with maternal age (NIH, 2018d).

Etiology and Pathophysiology

Trisomy 18 results from random events that occur during the formation of eggs and sperm causing an error in cell division, leading to an abnormal number of chromosomes—in this case, three copies of the chromosome 18 in each cell (NIH, 2018d). Trisomy 18 can also occur with two normal copies of chromosome 18 and one extra copy of chromosome 18 attached to another chromosome in the cells. Partial trisomy 18 can be inherited and involves an unaffected person carrying a rearrangement of genetic material between chromosome 18 and another chromosome. Such a person does not have signs of trisomy 18 but is at an increased risk of having children with the syndrome (NIH, 2018d).

Clinical Presentation

Individuals with trisomy 18 may have intrauterine growth retardation and a low birth weight (NIH, 2018d). Characteristic anomalies for trisomy 18 include a small, abnormally shaped head; a small jaw and mouth; low-set ears; short eyelid fissures; and clenched, overlapping digits (Fig. 32.6); as well as a prominent occiput, severe hypotonia, hypoplasia of the fingernails, narrow hips with limited abduction, and a short sternum (NIH, 2018d).

Assessment and Diagnosis

Nursing assessment for trisomy 18 includes observation for the characteristic anomalies. Prenatal testing or screening is available for the condition, and thus it can be diagnosed prenatally. If not diagnosed prenatally, it is usually diagnosed in the first few days of life based on the physical anomalies. Trisomy 18 involves multiple abnormalities, many that are life-threatening. Most infants with the condition do not survive past the first month of life, and complications are common for those who do survive longer (NIH, 2018d). Five to ten percent live past the

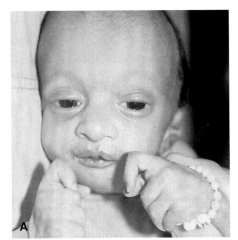
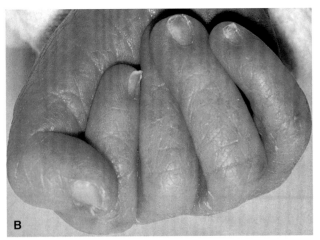

Figure 32.6. Clinical characteristics of trisomy 18. Note the abnormally shaped head and low-set ears **(A)** and clenched, overlapping digits **(B)**. Reprinted with permission from Kyle, T., & Carman, S. (2016). *Essentials of pediatric nursing* (3rd ed., Fig. 27.9). Philadelphia, PA: Wolters Kluwer.

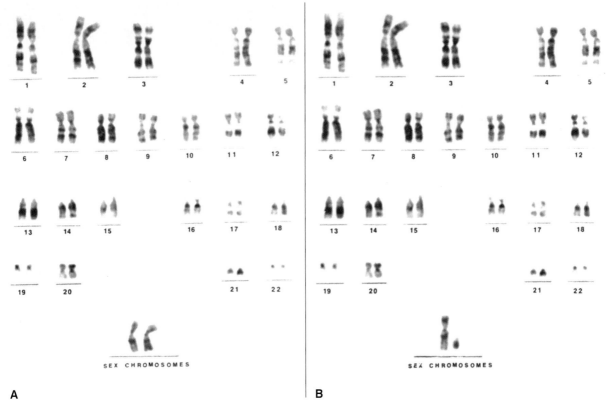

Figure 32.7. Normal chromosomes in a karyotype. Photomicrographs of human chromosome karyotypes. **A.** A normal female karyotype. **B.** A normal male karyotype. Reprinted with permission from Silbert-Flagg, J., & Pillitteri, A. (2018). *Maternal and child health nursing: Care of the childbearing and childrearing family* (8th ed., Fig. 8.1). Philadelphia, PA: Lippincott Williams & Wilkins.

first year but often have severe intellectual disability. Complications include heart defects and abnormalities of other organs (NIH, 2018d).

Therapeutic Interventions

Owing to the poor prognosis, nursing management should focus on symptomatic care for the infant and supportive care for the family.

Evaluation

Expected outcomes for a child with trisomy 18 include the following:

- The child receives comfort care.
- The child receives symptomatic care as needed.
- Caregivers receive supportive care.
- Caregivers receive genetic counseling.

Discharge Planning and Teaching

SOFT is a support organization for families who have a child with a chromosome abnormality; the website is https://trisomy.org/.

Trisomy 21

Trisomy 21, also called Down syndrome, is a chromosomal condition that, in most cases, is not inherited. Trisomy 21 occurs in about 1 in 700 newborns (~6,000 babies are born with the condition in the United States each year), with the prevalence increasing with maternal age (CDC, 2018b).

Etiology and Pathophysiology

Trisomy 21 results from random events that occur during the formation of reproductive cells (usually the egg cells) causing an error in cell division, leading to an abnormal number of chromosomes—in this case, three copies of the chromosome 21 in each cell (NIH, 2018a; Figs. 32.7 and 32.8). Mosaic Down syndrome, a variant of this condition, is also not inherited and occurs because of a random event during cell division, resulting in some of the body's cells having two copies of chromosome 21 and others having three copies of chromosome 21 (NIH, 2018a). Trisomy 21 is the most common genetic chromosomal disorder and cause of intellectual disabilities in children (Mayo Clinic, 2018a). The degree of intellectual disability and the degree of developmental delays vary in severity depending on the person.

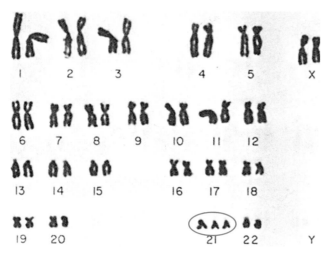

Figure 32.8. Down syndrome karyotype. Note the third chromosome located at chromosome 21. Reprinted with permission from Kyle, T., & Carman, S. (2016). *Essentials of pediatric nursing* (3rd ed., Fig. 27.7). Philadelphia, PA: Wolters Kluwer.

Clinical Presentation

Most individuals with trisomy 21 have mild-to-moderate cognitive impairment with developmental delays and short- and long-term memory effects (Mayo Clinic, 2018a). Not all individuals with trisomy 21 have the same features. Some common characteristics include facial features, such as a flattened bridge of the nose and almond-shaped eyes that slant up, and other complications, such as cardiac defects, hearing and vision impairment, and increased mobility of the cervical spine (Fig. 32.9; CDC, 2018b). See Box 32.1 for other common clinical manifestations.

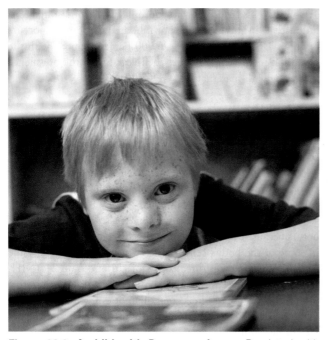

Figure 32.9. A child with Down syndrome. Reprinted with permission from Kyle, T., & Carman, S. (2016). *Essentials of pediatric nursing* (3rd ed., Fig. 27.8). Philadelphia, PA: Wolters Kluwer.

Box 32.1 Clinical Manifestations of Down Syndrome

- Short stature
- Small head
- Flat occiput
- Flat face, including a flat nasal bridge and a small nose
- Almond-shaped eyes, with an upward slant and epicanthal folds (small skin folds in the inner corners of the eyes)
- Tiny white spots on the iris of the eye
- Small, abnormally shaped, and low-set ears
- A small mouth with an arched palate and a large, protruding tongue
- A short neck, with abundant skin at the nape
- Small hands with broad, short fingers; pinky fingers tend to curve toward the thumb
- A single deep crease on the palm of each hand (palmar crease)
- Congenital heart defect
- Small feet, with excessive space between the large toe and the second toe
- Lack of muscle tone
- Excessively flexible and loose joints

Assessment and Diagnosis

Prenatal screening tests can indicate the chances of a baby having trisomy 21. They often include a blood test and an ultrasound, conducted to assess for fluid behind the baby's neck (CDC, 2018b). Diagnostic tests, including chorionic villus sampling, amniocentesis, and percutaneous umbilical blood sampling, are used after a screening test to confirm a diagnosis of trisomy 21. If not diagnosed prenatally, trisomy 21 is usually diagnosed within the first few days of life depending on the physical characteristics associated with the syndrome. Upon assessment, the infant may have poor muscle tone and loose joints, with a floppy appearance.

Developmental screening is also important for the child with trisomy 21. Table 32.1 lists developmental milestones and the average age of acquisition of each milestone for children with trisomy 21 and for typical children. For children with trisomy 21, it may be more important to focus on the order of developmental milestones instead of the age at which each is acquired, because these children progress through the same developmental stages as typical children, just at their own pace.

Therapeutic Interventions

The prognosis for children with trisomy 21 has been improving in recent decades, and nursing management should focus on supportive care and preventing complications.

Many services are available to help accelerate development and/or prevent developmental delays in children with trisomy 21. Refer children to these services, which include speech, occupational, and physical therapy, early on (CDC, 2018b).

Table 32.1 Average Age of Skill Acquisition in Children With Down Syndrome

Developmental Milestone	Average Age of Acquisition, Children With Down Syndrome (mo)	Average Age of Acquisition, Typical Children (mo)
Smile	2	1
Roll over	6	4
Sit alone	9	7
Crawl	11	9
Feed self with fingers	12	8
Speak words	14	10
Use a spoon	20	13
Walk	21	13
Speak in sentences	24	21
Undress	40	32
Bowel training	42	29
Bladder training	48	32
Put on clothes	58	47

Adapted from Pueschel, S. M. (2011). *A parent's guide to Down syndrome: Toward a brighter future* (rev. ed.). Baltimore, MD: Paul H. Brookes Publishing Company, Inc.

Individuals with Down syndrome can have a variety of complications, some of which worsen or become more prominent as they age. Potential problems include heart defects, gastrointestinal anomalies, immune disorders, obesity, dental issues, and hearing and vision problems. Table 32.2 lists potential problems, complications from these problems, and diagnostic tests to determine whether these problems are present. See Patient Teaching 32.1 for guidelines for educating parents and caregivers on how to prevent complications.

Table 32.2 Potential Complications in Individuals With Down Syndrome

Problem	Complications	Diagnostics
Heart defects	Congenital heart defects (atrioventricular canal defect is common in trisomy 21)	Echocardiogram
GI defects	• GI abnormalities of the intestines, esophagus, trachea, anus • Can cause GI blockage, gastroesophageal reflux, celiac disease	Ultrasound to assess for GI malformations
Immune disorders	Autoimmune disorders, some forms of cancer (leukemia), infectious diseases (pneumonia), recurrent or chronic respiratory infections, otitis media	Laboratory values
Sleep apnea	Soft-tissue and skeletal changes, leading to obstruction of the airway	Sleep apnea test, polysomnogram
Spinal problems	• Atlantoaxial instability of the first and second cervical vertebrae • Risk of serious injury to the spinal cord from overextension of the neck	Cervical X-rays
Endocrine problems	Hypothyroidism	Thyroid hormone level

GI, gastrointestinal.
Adapted from Centers for Disease Control and Prevention, Division of Birth Defects and Developmental Disabilities. (2018b). *Facts about Down syndrome.* Retrieved from https://www.cdc.gov/ncbddd/birthdefects/DownSyndrome.html; Global Down Syndrome Foundation. (2017). *Facts and FAQ about Down syndrome.* Retrieved from https://www.globaldownsyndrome.org/about-down-syndrome/facts-about-down-syndrome/?gclid=Cj0KCQjw45_bBRD_ARIsAJ6wUXQQVotwABOh1Yie3_H-gF59qhNXkz6kC2LzdoINPBusqGMmxP1PsuUaAg1pE ALw_wcB; National Institutes of Health, U.S. National Library of Medicine, Genetics Home Reference. (2018a). *Down syndrome.* Retrieved from https://ghr.nlm.nih.gov/condition/down-syndrome

Patient Teaching 32.1

Health Guidelines for Children With Down Syndrome

- General
    - Begin early interventions, therapy, and education as soon as possible.
    - Have your child follow a regular diet and exercise routine.
    - Make sure your child brushes his or her teeth daily and visits the dentist every 6 mo.
    - Make sure your child gets regular medical care, including recommended immunizations and a thyroid test at 6 and 12 mo and then yearly.
- Heart
    - Have your child evaluated by a pediatric cardiologist.
    - Have your child undergo an echocardiogram.
- Eyes and Ears
    - Take your child for routine vision and hearing tests.
    - By 6 mo, have your child visit a pediatric ophthalmologist.
- Immune System
    - Make sure all family members perform proper hand hygiene to prevent infection.
    - Monitor for signs and symptoms of respiratory infections, such as pneumonia and otitis media.
    - Discuss with your physician the use of pneumococcal, respiratory syncytial virus, and influenza vaccines.
- Bones and Joints
    - Make sure the child gets a cervical X-ray between 3 and 5 y of age to screen for atlantoaxial instability.
    - Report any changes in gait or use of arms and hands, weakness, changes in bowel or bladder function, complaints of neck pain or stiffness, head tilt, torticollis, or generalized changes in function.
    - Ensure that cervical spine positioning precautions (to avoid overextending or overflexing of the neck) are used during procedures, such as those involving anesthesia, surgery, or X-rays.

Adapted from Bull, M. J., & Committee on Genetics. (2011). From the American Academy of Pediatrics: Clinical report: Health supervision for children with Down syndrome. *Pediatrics, 128*(2), 393–406. Retrieved from http://pediatrics.aappublications.org/content/128/2/393.full

Evaluation

The average lifespan of an individual with trisomy 21 is approximately 60 years, and the prognosis has dramatically improved over the past few decades (Global Down Syndrome Foundation, 2017). Expected outcomes for a child with trisomy 21 include the following:

- The child receives routine vision and hearing tests.
- The child receives regular medical care.

- The child receives referrals for appropriate developmental therapies.
- Caregivers receive education and support for managing the condition.
- The child and caregivers receive supportive measures.
- The child's growth and development are promoted.
- The child is free of complications.
- The child receives sufficient nutrition.

Discharge Planning and Teaching

Provide families with resources that offer education about trisomy 21 as well as support through advocacy and community resources. Websites for some key Down syndrome support organizations include the following:

- https://www.globaldownsyndrome.org
- https://www.nads.org/
- https://www.ndss.org/

During the child's initial presentation, assessment, and diagnosis, parents may require much reassurance and support. Provide developmentally appropriate means of communication for the child and support for the parents.

Turner Syndrome

Turner syndrome, which affects only females, is a chromosomal condition caused by the complete or partial absence of the second sex chromosome in some or all of the cells of the body (Fig. 32.10; Turner Syndrome Society of the United States, 2018). It occurs in approximately one out of every 2,000

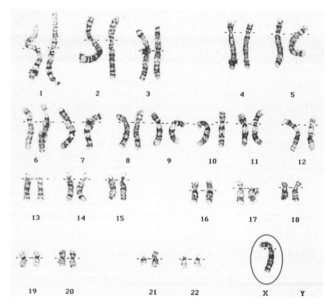

Figure 32.10. Turner syndrome karyotype. Note the loss of the second sex chromosome. Reprinted with permission from Stephenson, S. R., & Dmitrieva, J. (2017). *Obstetrics and gynecology* (4th ed., Fig. 31.18B). Philadelphia, PA: Wolters Kluwer.

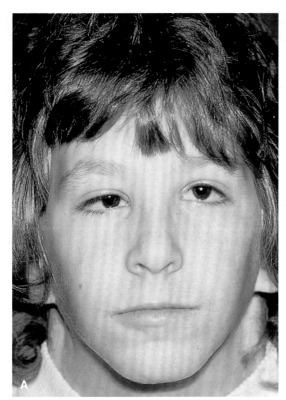 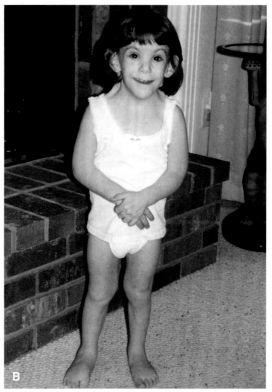

Figure 32.11. Children with Turner syndrome. A. Webbed neck. **B.** Webbed neck, short stature, edema of the hands and feet. Reprinted with permission from Kyle, T., & Carman, S. (2016). *Essentials of pediatric nursing* (3rd ed., Fig. 27.11). Philadelphia, PA: Wolters Kluwer.

to 4,000 female live births (Turner Syndrome Society of the United States, 2018), although it is much more common in pregnancies that do not survive to term (NIH, 2018e).

Etiology and Pathophysiology

Individuals with Turner syndrome have either monosomy X, with only one copy of the X chromosome, or X chromosome mosaicism, with chromosomal change in only some of their cells (NIH, 2018e). Most cases are not inherited.

Clinical Presentation

Signs and symptoms vary among girls and women with Turner syndrome (Fig. 32.11). Signs may first appear before birth, at birth, during infancy, or later in childhood, the teens, or in adulthood. See Table 32.3 for clinical manifestations at various time periods (Mayo Clinic, 2018b).

Assessment and Diagnosis

Turner syndrome may be suspected prenatally if fetal edema on the back of the neck, heart abnormalities, or abnormal kidneys are seen on ultrasound (Mayo Clinic, 2018b). If not suspected prenatally, the first indication is usually short stature and/or slow growth during infancy or childhood (Turner Syndrome Society of the United States, 2018). Diagnosis is confirmed using genetic testing.

Therapeutic Interventions

Nursing management should focus on health issues that arise because of the condition. Medical concerns can include chronic middle ear infections, hearing loss, autoimmune disorders, and heart, liver, and kidney abnormalities. Individuals with Turner syndrome may also experience difficulty with nonverbal communication skills, spatial relationships, and executive functions (Turner Syndrome Society of the United States, 2018).

The primary treatments required for almost all girls and women with Turner syndrome include growth hormone and estrogen therapy (Mayo Clinic, 2018b).

Evaluation

Although there is no cure for Turner syndrome, the prognosis is good, and care focuses on managing the health issues that may occur with the syndrome. Expected outcomes for a child with Turner syndrome include the following:

- The child is monitored closely for growth and development.
- The child receives referrals for appropriate developmental therapies.
- The child sees specialists as needed for health concerns that arise due to the syndrome.
- Caregivers receive education and support for managing the condition.

Table 32.3 Clinical Manifestations of Turner Syndrome

Time Period	Clinical Manifestations
Before birth	• Large fluid collection on the back of the neck or other abnormal fluid collections (edema) • Heart abnormalities • Abnormal kidneys
At birth or during infancy	• Wide or weblike neck (Fig. 32.11) • Low-set ears • Broad chest with widely spaced nipples • High, narrow roof of the mouth (palate) • Arms that turn outward at the elbows • Fingernails and toenails that are narrow and turned upward • Swelling of the hands and feet, especially at birth • Slightly smaller than average height at birth • Slowed growth • Cardiac defects • Low hairline at the back of the head • Receding or small lower jaw • Short fingers and toes
Childhood, teens, and adulthood	• Slowed growth • No growth spurts at expected times in childhood • Adult height significantly less than might be expected for a female member of the family • Failure to begin sexual changes expected during puberty • Sexual development that "stalls" during teenage years • Early end to menstrual cycles not due to pregnancy • For most women with Turner syndrome, inability to conceive a child without fertility treatment

Discharge Planning and Teaching

The Turner Syndrome Society of the United States can provide families with education about the diagnosis as well as support through advocacy and community resources. The website is https://www.turnersyndrome.org/about-turnersyndrome.

During the child's initial presentation, assessment, and diagnosis, parents may require much reassurance and support. Counsel the parents about possible learning disabilities and infertility in the child. Provide resources for the parents and child related to peer groups and social networks.

Think Critically

1. What assessment findings would the nurse most expect to find in a male child who has been diagnosed with fragile X syndrome?
2. Newborn screening for PKU is required for all infants in the United States within 24 to 48 hours of a protein feeding. What is the significance of this time frame and dietary requirement?
3. A diet low in phenylalanine is vital to children with PKU. Which foods must be avoided to prevent developmental delays, intellectual disabilities, and behavior problems?
4. What are some characteristic anomalies associated with trisomy 13?
5. An infant is suspected to have either trisomy 13 or trisomy 18 due to the many complications experienced after birth. What should the focus of nursing management be for this infant and family?
6. The nurse is caring for a 3-year-old with trisomy 21 and is reviewing health promotion information with the parents. What are some health guidelines to include for a child of this age?
7. The nurse is caring for a child with trisomy 21 who has feeding difficulties due to the small mouth and large tongue with lack of muscle tone. What are some adaptive devices and positioning techniques the parents may need?
8. The nurse is creating a plan of care for the parents of a 3-year-old with Turner syndrome. What medical concerns should the parents be aware of?

References

Centers for Disease Control and Prevention, Division of Birth Defects and Developmental Disabilities. (2018b). *Facts about Down syndrome*. Retrieved from https://www.cdc.gov/ncbddd/birthdefects/DownSyndrome.html

Centers for Disease Control and Prevention, National Center on Birth Defects and Developmental Disabilities, Division of Human Development and Disability. (2017b). *Facts about Fragile X syndrome*. Retrieved from https://www.cdc.gov/ncbddd/actearly/pdf/parents_pdfs/fragile_x.pdf

Global Down Syndrome Foundation. (2017). *Facts and FAQ about Down syndrome*. Retrieved from https://www.globaldownsyndrome.org/about-down-syndrome/facts-about-down-syndrome/?gclid=Cj0KCQjw45_bBRD_ARIsAJ6wUXQQVotwABOh1Yie3_H-gF59qhNXkz6kC2Lzdo-INPBusqGMmxP1PsuUaAg1pEALw_wcB

March of Dimes. (2013). *PKU (Phenylketonuria) in your baby*. Retrieved from https://www.marchofdimes.org/complications/phenylketonuria-in-your-baby.aspx

Mayo Clinic. (2018a). *Down syndrome*. Retrieved from https://www.mayoclinic.org/diseases-conditions/down-syndrome/symptoms-causes/syc-20355977

Mayo Clinic. (2018b). *Turner syndrome*. Retrieved from https://www.mayoclinic.org/diseases-conditions/turner-syndrome/symptoms-causes/syc-20360782

National Fragile X Foundation. (2018). *Fragile X prevalence*. Retrieved from https://fragilex.org/learn/prevalencegenetics-and-inheritance/

National Institutes of Health, U.S. Department of Health and Human Services, Eunice Kennedy Shriver National Institute of Child Health and Human Development. (n.d.a). *Introduction to the NIH consensus development conference on Phenylketonuria (PKU): Screening & management*. Retrieved from https://www1.nichd.nih.gov/publications/pubs/pku/Pages/sub2.aspx

National Institutes of Health, U.S. Department of Health and Human Services, National Center for Advancing Translational Sciences, Genetic and Rare Diseases Information Center. (n.d.b). *Trisomy 13*. Retrieved from https://rarediseases.info.nih.gov/diseases/7341/trisomy-13

National Institutes of Health, U.S. National Library of Medicine, Genetics Home Reference. (2018a). *Down syndrome*. Retrieved from https://ghr.nlm.nih.gov/condition/down-syndrome

National Institutes of Health, U.S. National Library of Medicine, Genetics Home Reference. (2018b). *Fragile X syndrome*. Retrieved from https://ghr.nlm.nih.gov/condition/fragile-x-syndrome

National Institutes of Health, U.S. National Library of Medicine, Genetics Home Reference. (2018c). *Trisomy 13*. Retrieved from https://ghr.nlm.nih.gov/condition/trisomy-13

National Institutes of Health, U.S. National Library of Medicine, Genetics Home Reference. (2018d). *Trisomy 18*. Retrieved from https://ghr.nlm.nih.gov/condition/trisomy-18

National Institutes of Health, U.S. National Library of Medicine, Genetics Home Reference. (2018e). *Turner syndrome*. Retrieved from https://ghr.nlm.nih.gov/condition/turner-syndrome

Turner Syndrome Society of the United States. (2018). *About Turner syndrome*. Retrieved from https://www.turnersyndrome.org/about-turnersyndrome

Suggested Readings

American Academy of Pediatrics. Management guidelines for patients with genetic and genetic-related conditions. Retrieved from https://www.aap.org/en-us/advocacy-and-policy/aap-health-initiatives/genetics-in-primary-care/Genetics-in-Your-Practice/Pages/Patient-Management-Guidelines.aspx

Centers for Disease Control and Prevention. *National Center on Birth Defects and Developmental Disabilities*. Retrieved from https://www.cdc.gov/ncbddd/sitemap.html

Global Down Syndrome Foundation. Retrieved from https://www.globaldown-syndrome.org

March of Dimes. *Birth defects and other health conditions*. Retrieved from https://www.marchofdimes.org/complications/birth-defects-and-health-conditions.aspx

Support Organization for Trisomy 18, 13, and Related Disorders. Retrieved from https://www.trisomy.org

The National Fragile X Foundation. Retrieved from https://fragilex.org/#1476180604782-5feb1bfb-8dc5

33 Alterations in Cognition and Mental Health

Variations in Anatomy and Physiology

The World Health Organization (WHO) defines **mental health** as the "state of well-being in which every individual realizes his or her own potential, can cope with the normal stresses of life, can work productively and fruitfully, and is able to make a contribution to her or his community" (WHO, 2014). For children, mental health involves an overall sense of well-being and the attainment of appropriate social relationships. **Cognition** is the process of thought and knowing that is acquired through experiences and maturation (Chaney, 2013). Although the definitions are consistent among age groups, children differ from adults in the scope, presentation, and progression of mental and cognitive disorders.

Both pediatric mental health issues and cognitive disorders often result from a combination of genetics, physiological changes, and environmental exposures. Chromosomal alterations and genetic syndromes play a role in cognitive disorders such as intellectual disability. Anatomical changes to the fetal brain, either as a part of a larger genetic syndrome or as a result of teratogenic damage during embryonic development, can yield cognitive and behavioral deficits in the child. In addition, larger socioeconomic constructs, such as access to good nutrition and safe housing, as well as interpersonal relationships that foster nurturing and progression through normal growth and development, can impact the development of both mental illness and cognitive disability (World Health Organization and Calouste Gulbenkian Foundation, 2014).

Assessment of Pediatric Cognition and Mental Health

Careful attention to both subjective and objective data at each well-child visit is essential in the identification of cognitive and behavioral abnormalities (Tables 33.1 and 33.2). Early identification, referral, and intervention are key to the success of future treatment and optimization of cognitive and behavioral development.

Table 33.1	Subjective Data to Assess for in Relation to Pediatric Cognition and Mental Health
Area of History	**Assessment Items**
Birth	• Problems during the prenatal period • Gestational age at delivery • Delivery complications and APGAR scores • Newborn hospital course
Past medical	• Neurological disorders • Mental health disorders • Cognitive disorders • Genetic disorders • Central nervous system infections • Traumatic brain injuries • Medications • Past hospitalizations • Past surgeries
Family	• Mental health disorders • Cognitive disorders • Alcohol or substance abuse • Neurological disorders • Genetic disorders
Social	• Type and age of dwellings • Neighborhood • Inhabitants of the home • Exposure to chemicals, toxins, and second-hand smoke • Grade level • Life events: trauma, change in family structure, death, major illness, divorce
Behavioral	• School performance • Extracurricular activities • Sleep habits • Dietary patterns • Sibling interaction • Friendships • Risk-taking behaviors

APGAR, Appearance, Pulse, Grimace, Activity, and Respiration.

Table 33.2	Objective Data to Assess for in Relation to Pediatric Cognition and Mental Health
Assessment	**Assessment Items**
Developmental screening	Screening and monitoring using validated tools to assess multiple domains of development, including language, motor, and sensory function Examples: • Ages and Stages Questionnaire (Squires & Bricker, 2009) • Child Development Inventory (Ireton, 1992)
Physical examination	• General appearance (including dress) • Affect, mood, eye contact • Facial symmetry • Ear alignment • Cranial nerves • Deep tendon reflexes • Gait and muscle strength • Hearing • Vision • Caregiver/child interaction
Diagnostic tests[a]	• Complete blood count • Thyroid-stimulating hormone • Urine drug analysis • Magnetic resonance imaging • Electroencephalogram

[a]Not all tests are indicated for every child.

The *Diagnostic and Statistical Manual of Mental Disorders (DSM-5)* lists the diagnostic criteria for a multitude of mental health conditions and cognitive disorders for both adults and children (American Psychiatric Association [APA], 2013). This clinical resource book is of paramount importance in the correct diagnosis of mental and cognitive issues.

General Nursing Interventions for Cognitive and Mental Health Disorders

Providing supportive care, such as play therapy and art therapy, and maintaining a safe care environment are key nursing interventions for children with cognitive and mental health disorders.

Provide Supportive Care

Pediatric cognitive and mental health disorders are usually treated by psychiatric or mental health specialists and/or developmental pediatricians. Nurses support and educate the child

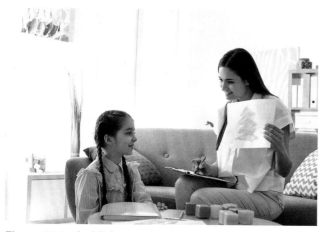

Figure 33.1. A child engaging in play therapy.

and family and link them to available community resources. Nurses may also assist in the delivery of certain forms of therapy under the guidance of mental health specialists. Although there are numerous forms of therapy appropriate for the treatment of childhood cognitive and mental health disorders, some of the more common types include play therapy and art therapy.

Play therapy should not be confused with the use of therapeutic play, which is a technique employed by child life specialists for hospitalized children. Play therapy is a form of psychotherapy that is conducted by specialized mental health providers. During play therapy, children are encouraged to express their feelings and emotions through a variety of traditional play (Fig. 33.1). A wide variety of problems can be addressed through play, including anxiety, physical or sexual abuse, conduct disorder, and grief. This form of therapy is most appropriate for children from 3 to 12 years of age (Association for Play Therapy, 2018).

Art therapy is another specialized form of psychotherapy and incorporates creativity in the understanding of childhood emotions and healing. In addition to its use in the diagnosis and treatment of mental health disorders, this form of therapy is used as a treatment modality for those with cognitive deficits including sensorimotor issues. Art therapy can be used in children and adolescents of all ages (American Art Therapy Association, 2017).

Maintain a Safe Environment

Safety of the child is one of the most crucial nursing responsibilities for children with mental or cognitive health issues. In the initial stages, this responsibility includes ensuring the safety of the child from self-harm. A careful environmental assessment of the inpatient hospital setting may yield multiple threats to child safety. As such, any objects that could be used to inflict harm should be removed from the room. Do not leave extra supplies such as tourniquets, needles, and tubing in the room. Children with cognitive deficits may have difficulty acclimating to a new environment and become disoriented, thereby increasing their risk for falls. Institute standard safety measures such as keeping the hospital bed in the lowest position with the wheels locked. Ensuring adequate lighting and placing the child in a room close to the nursing station can also decrease the chance of injury.

Adult supervision should be provided at all times, which may include parent, guardian, or dedicated medical staff observation.

Although self-harm prevention is an important factor in the outpatient nursing management of children with cognitive and mental health disorders, the safety of the home environment is of paramount importance. The nurse has a legal responsibility to report suspected or confirmed child abuse to child protective services.

Developmental and Behavioral Disorders

Developmental and behavioral disorders common among children include learning disabilities, autism spectrum disorders (ASDs), attention-deficit/hyperactivity disorder (ADHD), and anxiety disorders.

Learning Disabilities

Learning disabilities are a varied group of disorders that involve difficulties in receiving and processing information and generating appropriate responses. These disorders usually manifest in difficulties with reading, listening, writing, spelling, and performing mathematical calculations (Handler & Fierson, 2011). Approximately 7% to 8% of children 3 to 17 years of age in the United States are affected by a learning disability. Learning disabilities are more common in boys, non-Hispanic blacks, and children living in families below the federal poverty level (Boyle et al., 2011).

Etiology and Pathophysiology

The most common learning disability is dyslexia, which accounts for 80% of all learning disabilities. Dyslexia is primarily a disorder of receptive language, in which the child has difficulty using letters to decode written language. As a result, dyslexia is often referred to as a "reading disorder." There appears to be an environmental and genetic relationship in the development of dyslexia. Almost 40% of family members of an affected person also have dyslexia. Furthermore, twin studies indicate that only about 50% of the difficulties experienced by children with dyslexia have a genetic factor. The environment appears to play a more significant role among children with lower intelligence quotient scores (Handler & Fierson, 2011).

Clinical Presentation

The clinical presentation of learning disorders varies depending on the area of learning affected. In addition, signs and symptoms may not be apparent until a child enters the formal school setting.

For dyslexia, common symptoms include the slower acquisition of language skills and difficulty in recognizing letters and numbers. These children may also exhibit a lower-than-expected reading level and problems with reading comprehension. This disorder may also manifest as difficulty in spelling and writing. Consequently, these children often avoid activities that include reading and writing (Fig. 33.2).

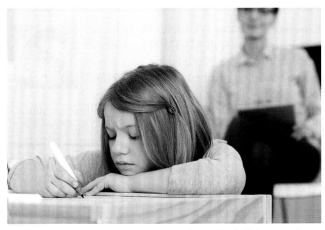

Figure 33.2. Children with learning disabilities such as dyslexia may avoid reading vs. writing or be uninterested in these activities.

Assessment and Diagnosis

The nurse plays an important role in the both the screening for and treatment of learning disabilities. In particular, assess the child at each visit for the presence of appropriate developmental milestones and collect information about educational progress. Conduct a standardized developmental evaluation with a validated screening tool at 9, 18, and 24 to 30 months of age (Engorn & Flerlage, 2015). Also conduct hearing and vision screening tests to evaluate for possible sensory impairments. Formal diagnostic testing for specific learning disabilities is conducted by a developmental pediatrician, a clinical psychologist, or other mental health specialists.

Therapeutic Interventions

If assessment reveals deficiencies, assist the family in locating appropriate testing and treatment facilities. In addition, assist the family in working with the school to develop an **individualized education plan (IEP)** that will foster appropriate growth and development of the child (Handler & Fierson, 2011).

Evaluation

Expected outcomes for a child with a learning disability include the following:
- An IEP is developed and implemented for the child.
- The child maintains a healthy self-image and self-esteem.
- The child and family are satisfied with the learning environment, and the child acquires age-appropriate knowledge and skills.

Autism Spectrum Disorder

Autism spectrum disorder (ASD), as newly termed in the *DSM-5*, is a continuum of neurobiological symptoms that result in difficulty with communication, behavior, and social interaction. ASD encompasses what were four separate autism-related disorders in the *DSM-IV*: autistic disorder, Asperger disorder,

childhood disintegrative disorder, and pervasive developmental disorder not otherwise specified. The presentation of ASD is varied and exists along a spectrum of manifestations (Johnson & Myers, 2007). ASD is also a relatively common diagnosis, with approximately 1 in 59 children affected, with the majority being boys. According to the American Academy of Pediatrics (AAP, 2018), the incidence of ASD is 5 times greater in males than females.

Etiology and Pathophysiology

The exact etiology of ASD is unclear at this time. However, there is clear evidence to suggest a genetic basis for the disorder. In families with an older sibling with ASD, the recurrence risk for future children is from 2% to 8%. Research is ongoing to pinpoint the genes responsible for the development of ASD. In addition to a genetic basis, environmental factors may be responsible for some of the variability of disease manifestations. Despite robust public campaigns touting a causal link between the measles, mumps, and rubella vaccine, as well as other thimerosal-containing vaccines, and the development of ASD, there is no evidence to support this claim. On the basis of the pathological evaluation of the brain tissue of people with ASD, the early period of brain development (20–24 days post-conception) is indicated in the development of autism (Johnson & Myers, 2007).

Clinical Presentation

The clinical presentation of ASD involves deficits in communication, behavior, and social interaction that are usually present by the age of 3 years. Repetitive movements and obsessive behaviors are also characteristic of ASD. This feature is known as **stereotypy** and may include hand flapping, head banging, and self-biting. Children with ASD also have difficulty with sensory integration and may have problems tolerating loud noises, bright environments, and touching or hugging. These children may also avoid eye contact and avoid social interaction. Communication difficulties are also a hallmark of this disorder. Children with ASD often have difficulty mastering spoken language and may exhibit some characteristic speech-related symptoms, such as **echolalia**. Most communication deficits are clinically apparent by 18 months of age (Johnson & Myers, 2007).

Assessment and Diagnosis

As with other cognitive and mental health disorders, pay special attention to the achievement of appropriate developmental milestones by children with ASD at every office visit. In addition, given the heritability of ASD, conduct a thorough family history to determine the presence of additional siblings or other family members with ASD. As previously described, the Ages and Stages Questionnaire is an excellent tool for evaluating normal growth and development achievement. In addition to this routine screening, every child should receive specific ASD screening at the 18- to 24-month wellness visit with the Modified Checklist for Autism in Toddlers tool. Hearing evaluation, as well as advanced diagnostic imaging such as magnetic resonance imaging and computed tomography (CT) scan, may be conducted to rule out other causes of the child's symptoms. Final diagnosis is based on the criteria delineated in the *DSM-5* (APA, 2013); these are available at the following website of the Centers for Disease Control and Prevention (CDC): https://www.cdc.gov/ncbddd/autism/hcp-dsm.html.

Therapeutic Interventions

The cornerstone of effective treatment for ASD is the early iden-tification of children affected with the disorder and referral to an **early intervention program**. Assist the child and family in planning educational activities that will limit overstimulation of the senses, collaborating with school personnel, as needed, to align the child's needs for maximal learning and limited distress. Consultation with a speech therapist can also help the child improve communication skills. A multidisciplinary team with behavioral health specialists and a developmental pediatrician should be utilized whenever possible.

Evaluation

Expected outcomes for a child with ASD include the following:
- The child is able to manage his or her behavior safely and effectively.
- The child is able to communicate effectively.
- The child is able to progress steadily in development.

Attention Deficit Hyperactivity Disorder

As previously discussed in Chapter 13, ADHD is a neurobe-havioral disorder characterized by inattentiveness with or with-out hyperactivity and impulsivity. ADHD affects about 11% of school children and is much more common in boys than in girls (Soreff, 2018).

Etiology and Pathophysiology

Although the exact cause of ADHD is not understood at this point, the neurotransmitters dopamine and norepineph-rine have been implicated. There also appears to be a slower progression of brain maturation in individuals with ADHD (Soreff, 2018).

In addition, there is an increased incidence of ADHD in families, often with multiple members of a family (parents and siblings) being affected. There has been no single gene linked to ADHD. Environmental exposure to lead as well as prenatal exposure to alcohol and cigarette smoke may contribute to the development of ADHD. Furthermore, there is evidence sup-porting the association of significant traumatic brain injury with the subsequent development of ADHD (AAP, 2017).

Clinical Presentation

Children with ADHD usually present with symptoms of short-ened attention span, impulsivity, and/or difficulties with move-ment. Girls with ADHD tend to exhibit much less impulsivity than boys.

Remember Jack Wray in Chapter 13? Jack was an 8-year-old boy with ADHD. What behav-iors did Jack initially exhibit that caused his parents to suspect that he might have ADHD? What process did Jack go through to receive his diagnosis of ADHD? What problems did Jack encounter in school as a result of his ADHD?

Assessment and Diagnosis

The initial evaluation of a child with suspected ADHD should include laboratory assessment of blood counts and serum lead levels to rule out an organic cause of the symptoms. In addition, hearing and vision assessments are fundamental to ensure that inattentiveness is not caused by an inability to receive accurate sensory inputs. In most cases, radiographic imaging is not indi-cated. Formal evaluation and psychological testing is conducted by a developmental pediatrician and/or child psychologist. In-formation should be sought from not only the child and family but also the child's school teachers to obtain the most com-prehensive assessment. The full *DSM-5* (APA, 2013) diagnos-tic criteria are available at the following website of the CDC: https://www.cdc.gov/ncbddd/adhd/diagnosis.html.

Therapeutic Interventions

Clinical therapy for ADHD often centers on parental educa-tion about the condition, development of IEPs with the school system, and the use of pharmacotherapy for the child. The most widely used type of medications are stimulants, such as methylphenidate (Ritalin), dextroamphetamine (Adderall), or dexmethylphenidate (Focalin). Refer to The Pharmacy 13.1 for medication specifics. These medications are considered con-trolled substances and, as such, have more stringent prescribing restrictions than most medications. They also have potential side effect profiles that include appetite suppression, weight loss, tachycardia, and elevated blood pressure (Soreff, 2018). Perform accurate height, weight, pulse, and blood pressure measurements at each visit of a child with ADHD.

If you'll recall, Jack Wray in Chapter 13 ex-perienced a side effect related to his ADHD medication that concerned his mom. Which medication was he taking? What was the side effect? What measures did his pediatrician, Dr. Mario, recommend to further evaluate the side effect?

Some medications also require the measurement of serum liver function tests before initiation and periodically through-out treatment (Soreff, 2018). These medications have the po-tential for diversion and abuse among individuals who do not have a clinical indication for them.

Evaluation

Expected outcomes for a child with ADHD include the following:
- The child achieves his or her full academic potential.
- The child's self-esteem is maximized.
- The child and parents demonstrate an accurate understanding of the safe and effective use of stimulant medications.

Anxiety Disorders

Anxiety is a normal part of life across all age groups. Anxiety is necessary for human survival in times of challenge and in learning how to anticipate dangerous situations (fight-or-flight response). However, when worry, fear, and anxiety extend past normal adaptive coping mechanisms and cause stress significant enough to impact daily life, a pathological anxiety disorder is present. Anxiety disorders affect up to 10% of children and are thereby classified as the most common psychiatric illness of childhood (Bagnell, 2011).

Etiology and Pathophysiology

As with the majority of childhood mental health issues, a combination of genetic predisposition and environmental triggers is implicated in the development and manifestation of anxiety disorders. Most childhood anxiety develops during the school-age years, and females are twice as likely to develop anxiety symptoms as are males. In addition, the presence of anxiety disorders in adults has been linked to the development of these disorders in adolescence (Bagnell, 2011). This underscores the need for early identification and management of symptoms to maximize psychosocial development and mitigate the progression of the disorder.

The activation of the normal stress response (fight or flight) in traditionally nonstressful situations or the overexpression of the stress response and inability to appropriately regulate it during times of challenge produces the characteristic physical symptoms of anxiety and the associated behavioral manifestations. The physical symptoms may include abdominal pain, nausea, headaches, palpitations, dizziness, and dyspnea. The desire to avoid these manifestations often leads to behavioral changes in the child, such as aggression, defiance, and avoidance of certain situations. In fact, anxiety may not be the chief complaint associated with parents seeking medical advice. Assistance is often sought for the management of frequent somatic complaints and associated behavioral changes (Bagnell, 2011).

Anxiety disorders in childhood include generalized anxiety disorder, separation anxiety disorder (SAD), and panic disorder. SAD, which is one of the most common anxiety disorders present in childhood, is the primary focus of this section. It includes school phobia, also known as school avoidance or school refusal.

Separation anxiety is a normal occurrence from late infancy to the early preschool years. As a result, early cases of SAD and school phobia may be mistaken for normal growth and development. The peak age for symptom onset is 7 to 9 years, but this disorder can occur any time before the age of 18 years. SAD and school phobia are characterized by recurrent, persistent distress and worry related to separation from an attachment figure. Children may have a fear that a catastrophic event such as kidnapping or becoming lost may occur (Bagnell, 2011).

Clinical Presentation

Physical symptoms of SAD include headaches, abdominal pain, nausea, vomiting, palpitations, and dizziness. SAD onset may occur after an acute life stressor or an extended time away from school, such as summer vacation or a leave due to medical illness (Hanna, Fischer, & Fluent, 2006). These worries and fear then often manifest as a persistent pattern of school avoidance or extreme stress associated with the attendance of school (Fig. 33.3; Bagnell, 2011).

Assessment and Diagnosis

The nurse may find that the use of a standardized anxiety rating scale can help in the diagnosis of SAD in children. One such tool, the Screen for Child Anxiety Related Emotional Disorders (SCARED), includes both child self-report and parental report. This 41-item tool is free, quick to administer (10 minutes), and has a high degree of psychometric certainty. The SCARED tool is appropriate for use in children from 8 to 18 years of age (Birmaher et al., 1999).

Conduct a complete history and physical exam on children exhibiting characteristics of school refusal and separation anxiety. For best results, incorporate structured diagnostic interviewing, using a tool such as the Diagnostic Interview Schedule for Children or the Anxiety Disorders Interview Schedule for Children and Parents (Hanna et al., 2006).

Therapeutic Interventions

The treatment of choice for children with SAD and school refusal is exposure-based **cognitive behavioral therapy**. Children are also taught to recognize the physiological sensations associated with fear and anxiety and how to cope and modulate these sensations. Pharmacological therapy may be indicated.

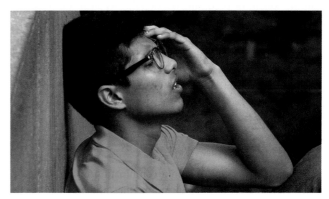

Figure 33.3. A teenager exhibiting signs of anxiety.

The Pharmacy 33.1 Fluoxetine

Classification	Route	Action	Nursing Considerations
Selective serotonin reuptake inhibitor	PO	Blocks the reuptake of serotonin in the central nervous system	Monitor for changes in behavior, worsening of anxiety, and development of suicidality

PO, oral.

Adapted from Engorn, B., & Flerlage, J. (2015). *The Harriet Lane handbook* (20th ed.). Philadelphia, PA: Elsevier Publishing.

Although the Food and Drug Administration has not approved the use of selective serotonin reuptake inhibitors (SSRIs) for the treatment of childhood anxiety disorders (The Pharmacy 33.1), extensive evidence supports their beneficial use in treatment of these disorders (Ipser, Stein, Hawkridge, & Hoppe, 2009). In rare cases, SSRIs have been shown to increase suicidal thoughts and behaviors in adolescents. In general, tricyclic antidepressants and benzodiazepines should be avoided in the treatment of SAD and school refusal (Hanna et al., 2006).

Evaluation

Expected outcomes for a child with separation anxiety or school phobia include the following:
- The child is able to identify coping strategies to handle feelings of stress and anxiety.
- The self-reported severity of anxiety is decreased.
- The somatic complaints associated with anxiety are reduced.
- The avoidance of social situations and school absenteeism are decreased.

Eating Disorders

This chapter focuses on two of the most prevalent eating disorders among children and adolescents: anorexia nervosa and bulimia nervosa.

Anorexia Nervosa

Anorexia nervosa is an eating disorder characterized by fear of gaining weight or becoming overweight. As such, this disorder usually manifests as an extremely low body weight. Although anorexia nervosa can occur in a wide range of ages (including adults), the typical age of onset is in late adolescence (18–19 years of age). Females are much more likely than are males to be affected by anorexia nervosa, and the lifetime prevalence of the disorder is 0.9% (National Association of Anorexia Nervosa and Associated Disorders, 2018).

Etiology and Pathophysiology

Anorexia nervosa results from a combination of physiological and psychological factors, including the influence of societal pressures and ideals. Data from studies involving twins suggest a strong genetic component to this disorder. Risk factors for the development of anorexia nervosa include the following:
- Female gender
- Low self-esteem
- Family history of anorexia nervosa or other eating disorders
- Perfectionist personality
- Adolescence

Clinical Presentation

Individuals with anorexia nervosa may begin at a normal weight and attempt to lose weight to obtain an unrealistic body image due to ever-increasing societal pressures. Or, they may begin as overweight or obese, lose weight through dieting and exercise, and then, in response to the praise they receive for their success, become preoccupied with continued weight loss. People with anorexia nervosa also have a higher risk of other comorbid mental health issues, such as mood disorders and anxiety. One-third to one-half of people with an eating disorder also have a disorder affecting mood, such as major depressive disorder. In addition, up to 50% also have an anxiety disorder (National Association of Anorexia Nervosa and Associated Disorders, 2018). The emotional distress related to weight and food leads to behavior change, which in turn can manifest in multiple physical signs and symptoms. Therefore, the clinical presentation can encompass many facets of health (Table 33.3; Fig. 33.4).

Assessment and Diagnosis

Careful attention to the presence of the abovementioned emotional, behavioral, and physical manifestations is crucially important. This involves the accurate measurement of height, weight, and vital signs. Individuals suspected of having anorexia nervosa undergo laboratory evaluation to assess for signs of poor nutrition and fluid and electrolyte abnormalities. They may also undergo body composition assessment using skin-fold measurement, waist-to-hip ratio, or bioelectrical impedance. The *DSM-5* (APA, 2013) provides clear criteria for the diagnosis of anorexia nervosa; these are available at the following website of the National Eating Disorders Association: https://www.nationaleatingdisorders.org/learn/by-eating-disorder/anorexia.

Therapeutic Interventions

Although nutritional support is paramount to the treatment of anorexia nervosa, the underlying psychological issues must be

Table 33.3	Clinical Manifestations of Anorexia Nervosa
Type	**Manifestations**
Emotional	• Anxiety • Depression • Poor self-esteem • Disturbed body image • Obsessive thoughts • Suicidal thoughts
Behavioral	• Preoccupation with weight (Fig. 33.4) • Preoccupation with food and the associated caloric content • Crying • Avoidance of social situations • Compulsive exercising
Physical	• Low body mass index • Loss of subcutaneous fat • Low body fat percentage • Amenorrhea • Dehydration • Electrolyte imbalances • Poor bone density • Lanugo • Cold intolerance • Hypotension • Bradycardia

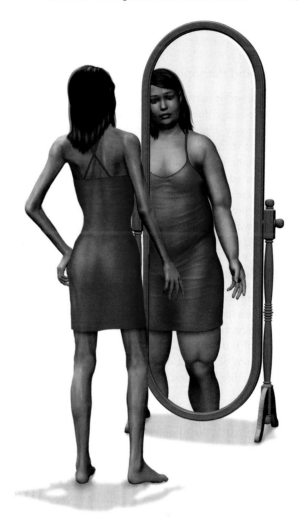

Figure 33.4. Children and teens with anorexia have an intense and irrational fear of being overweight. Reprinted with permission from Werner, R. (2015). *Massage therapist's guide to pathology* (6th ed., Fig. 4.15). Philadelphia, PA: Wolters Kluwer.

addressed, as well. Clinical therapy may be conducted in the outpatient or inpatient setting depending on the degree of severity of the disorder. The choice of treatment setting can depend on the degree of weight loss and the presence and type of complications, including, but not limited to, fluid and electrolyte imbalances and cardiovascular involvement (Harvard Health Publishing, 2009a).

A multidisciplinary team composed of pediatricians, behavioral health specialists, and registered dietitian nutritionists is more likely to achieve the desired treatment outcomes than is a lone practitioner. The importance of involving the family in the counseling and support of the adolescent with anorexia nervosa cannot be overemphasized.

Proper nutrition is fundamental to successfully addressing the underlying emotional issues and thought process of the child with anorexia nervosa. Therefore, initial stages of treatment focus on the optimization of nutrition and the correction of the weight deficit. In the inpatient setting, a gradual weight gain of 2 to 3 lb/wk is appropriate. Depending on the degree of severity, this caloric support may include nasogastric feedings. In the outpatient setting, a goal of 0.5 to 1 lb/wk is appropriate (Harvard Health Publishing, 2009a).

Evaluation

Expected outcomes for an adolescent with anorexia nervosa include the following:

- The adolescent attains and maintains appropriate weight, fluid status, and electrolyte balance.
- The adolescent demonstrates an accurate understanding of the fundamentals of healthy nutrition.
- The adolescent achieves and maintains a healthy body image and self-esteem.

Bulimia Nervosa

Bulimia nervosa is an eating disorder characterized by periods of binge eating followed by periods of purging. Binge eating involves the consumption of large amounts of food in a short time frame and usually in secret. Purging is the compensatory mechanism used to relieve the uncomfortable physical sensation of overeating and the guilt and emotional distress caused by the binge habit, as well as to prevent weight gain. Purging may be accomplished in many ways, including self-induced vomiting, diuretics, or laxatives. As with anorexia nervosa, this disorder is more prevalent in female adolescents but may extend into young adulthood, as well (National Eating Disorders Association, 2018).

Etiology and Pathophysiology

Similar to anorexia nervosa, bulimia nervosa is usually the result of poor self-image due to societal pressures to look or behave in a certain way. Unlike in anorexia nervosa, in which family involvement tends to be overwhelming to the adolescent and may contribute to the disorder, bulimia nervosa is more likely to be associated with a family dynamic that is disorganized and distant. There is also a significant link between bulimia nervosa and depression. However, there is not enough evidence to determine which disorder precedes the other (National Eating Disorders Association, 2018).

Clinical Presentation

Unlike those with anorexia nervosa, individuals with bulimia nervosa often have a normal weight or are only slightly underweight, which can delay or prevent the timely diagnosis and treatment of this disorder. Emotional, behavioral, and physical manifestations of bulimia nervosa are delineated in Table 33.4 (National Eating Disorders Association, 2018).

Assessment and Diagnosis

The *DSM-5* (APA, 2013) provides clear criteria for the diagnosis of bulimia nervosa; these are available at the following website of the National Eating Disorders Association: https://www.nationaleatingdisorders.org/learn/by-eating-disorder/bulimia.

Table 33.4 Clinical Manifestations of Bulimia Nervosa

Type	Manifestations
Emotional and behavioral	• Distress or avoidance of eating in a social situation • Food rituals • Immediate trips to the restroom following a meal • Repeated fad dieting • Labile mood
Physical	• Low, normal, or above average weight • Gastrointestinal bloating and discomfort • Esophageal irritation or tearing • Poor dentition (including caries and erosion of tooth enamel) • Thinning hair • Dry skin and brittle nails • Hypokalemia • Anemia • Calluses on the backs of hands or fingers (from self-induced vomiting) • Bradycardia

Careful attention to fluid and electrolyte status is of extreme importance. In particular, monitor serum potassium levels. In addition, perform cardiovascular evaluation, including an electrocardiogram. Also evaluate individuals with bulimia nervosa for the presence of other mental illnesses, such as depression and suicidality.

Therapeutic Interventions

Clinical therapy focuses on the establishment of healthy dietary choices and patterns. As these are established, the individual will also develop a sense of control over food, which should help mediate the overwhelming feeling of lack of control that drives binge eating. Establishing a routine for meals and snacks also helps prevent anxiety related to food consumption. Food diaries or journals are helpful tools in establishing normal dietary patterns. Cognitive behavioral therapy, an extremely important treatment strategy for this disorder, involves reframing the way people with bulimia nervosa think and behave around food. In conjunction with cognitive behavioral therapy, the use of the SSRI fluoxetine (Prozac) has been shown to be beneficial. Fluoxetine dosage for eating disorders is considerably higher than that usually prescribed for the treatment of depression alone (Harvard Health Publishing, 2009b).

Evaluation

Expected outcomes for an adolescent with bulimia nervosa are very similar to those for an adolescent with anorexia nervosa. Refer to the section Evaluation under Anorexia Nervosa, earlier. An additional expected outcome is the following:

• Depressive or anxious thoughts and behaviors associated with food, weight, and body image resolve.

Abuse and Violence

The Federal Child Abuse Prevention and Treatment Act (Child Welfare Information Gateway, 2019) defines child abuse as: "Any recent act or failure to act on the part of a parent or caretaker which results in death, serious physical or emotional harm, sexual abuse or exploitation; or an act or failure to act which presents an imminent risk of serious harm." Child physical and sexual abuse exist within the larger context of child maltreatment, which may include emotional abuse, neglect (both medical and physical), and exposure to domestic violence.

Physical and Sexual Abuse

Physical abuse may manifest in many different ways, including the presence of fractures, bruises, burns, and inflicted traumatic brain injuries. Childhood sexual abuse can involve sexual acts such as orogenital contact, vaginal or anal penetration, fondling, genital exposure, prostitution, and pornography. Physical and sexual abuse can occur at any age, with the majority of cases occurring in infancy and early childhood (Flaherty & Stirling, 2010).

Analyze the Evidence 33.1

Infant Crying as a Trigger for Shaken Baby Syndrome

A study of 26 cases of shaken baby syndrome (SBS) requiring hospital management from 1997 to 2003 were examined to determine the relationship, if any, of the occurrence of SBS to the trigger of infant crying. Infant crying begins and increases in intensity along a relatively well-documented curve based on age. As the emergence of the normal crying curve began, there was a matching increase in the number of cases of SBS. Review of outpatient medical records indicated that 88.5% of parents of the child with SBS had contacted a healthcare professional about excessive infant crying or irritability before the abuse (Talvik, Alexander, & Talvik, 2008).

Table 33.5 Caregiver and Environmental Risk Factors for Child Abuse

Caregiver Factors	Environmental Factors
• Depression and/or other mental illness • Lack of knowledge about normal growth and development • Poor self-esteem • History of being a victim of abuse • Alcohol abuse • Substance abuse • Young parental age • Poor coping skills	• Low income • Unemployment • Domestic violence • Presence of a nonrelated male figure in the home • Low educational attainment • Lack of support system

Adapted from Flaherty, E. G., & Stirling, J., Jr. (2010). The pediatrician's role in child maltreatment prevention. *Pediatrics, 126,* 833–841.

Etiology and Pathophysiology

Crying is one of the most common triggers for physical child abuse (Analyze the Evidence 33.1). In addition, other normal developmental behaviors of infancy and childhood are associated with increased risk of abuse (Flaherty & Stirling, 2010). These include but are not limited to the following:
• Nighttime awakenings
• Picky eating
• Toilet training opposition
• Independence-seeking behaviors

In addition to the risk factors associated with the child, factors specific to the caregiver and the socioeconomic environment place the child at increased risk for physical abuse (Table 33.5).

Clinical Presentation

The clinical manifestations of pediatric physical and sexual abuse can be vague or explainable by normal childhood illness and injuries. Multiple fractures in various staging of healing coupled with a fracture type that does not match the stated mechanism of injury (e.g., a spiral fracture purported to have been caused by a simple fall) should prompt suspicion of abuse. Bruising is one of the most common manifestations of abuse (Fig. 33.5). However, bruises are also a normal result of unintentional injuries. Suspicious bruising is heralded by (Boos, Lindberg & Wiley, 2019) the following:

• Occurrence in a child younger than 6 months
• Occurrence of more than one or two bruises at a time in a young child
• Location on the trunk, head, or buttocks
• Presence of an object pattern (loops, belt, rope)

Pediatric sexual abuse is often manifested with genital complaints such as redness, pain, itching, vaginal discharge, or the presence of a sexually transmitted infection. The presence of blood in the underwear or diaper is also a warning sign. Children may also manifest vague somatic complaints such as abdominal pain or headaches. The development of enuresis in a previously toilet-trained child should prompt suspicion (Kellog, 2005).

Assessment and Diagnosis

The successful assessment and diagnosis of suspected abuse hinges on a detailed history and physical exam. Often, the general pediatric nurse is not the healthcare provider conducting

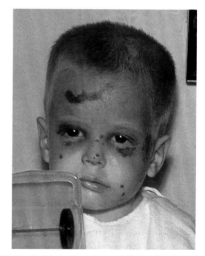

Figure 33.5. Facial injuries in a child who has been physically abused. Reprinted with permission from Bickley, L. S., & Szilagyi, P. (2003). *Bates' guide to physical examination and history taking* (8th ed.). Philadelphia, PA: Lippincott Williams & Wilkins.

this detailed data collection. To limit the amount of emotional trauma to a child and to comply with legal requirements regarding the collection and processing of samples, a forensic medical team often performs the history and physical. However, nurses in emergency departments, urgent care centers, or school-based settings may be the initial point of contact for children who have been abused. In such cases, the nurse should take special care in describing the history of how the injury occurred and the location and appearance of lesions and deformities. This information will be vital in determining whether the injury is attributable to an unintentional cause.

Advanced diagnostics may also be performed at the discretion of the medical team, including, but not limited to, radiographs (often referred to as a skeletal survey), CT scans, electroencephalograms, slit-lamp ophthalmological evaluations, and genital examinations. Whenever possible, genital examinations and specimen collection should be performed by a specially trained pediatric Sexual Assault Nurse Examiner.

Therapeutic Interventions

Cases of abuse that involve internal injuries or extensive external damage, such as lacerations or burns, often require hospitalization for proper treatment. Hospitalization may also be appropriate when the safety of the home environment is in question or when safe alternative placement cannot be achieved.

In the United States, the nurse is a mandatory reporter of suspected abuse and neglect. The importance of this role cannot be overemphasized. It is the nurse's professional duty to notify child protective services of any potential or confirmed cases of abuse and neglect.

The best treatment for pediatric abuse is the prevention of the abuse. Conduct a careful evaluation of the child, family, and environment at each office visit. In addition, providing targeted anticipatory guidance is paramount in equipping parents with the skills and strategies they need to cope with their role as caregiver.

Evaluation

Expected outcomes for a child who has experienced physical or sexual abuse include the following:
- The child's physical and emotional needs are met.
- The child is in a safe environment.
- The child achieves normal growth and developmental milestones.
- The child has no more experiences with abuse.

Munchausen Syndrome by Proxy

Munchausen syndrome by proxy (MBP), also known as factitious disorder imposed on another, is a form of medical child abuse. In the case of children, this imposer is often the mother but may be any parent or caregiver. MBP involves the misinterpretation or presentation of exaggerated or absent symptoms in a child to gain entry into the medical setting (Roesler & Jenny, 2018).

Etiology and Pathophysiology

MBP is fundamentally an underlying psychological disorder affecting the perpetrator. A clear cause for this is not readily apparent, but potential contributing factors include a past history of abuse (the perpetrator was victim) as well as other comorbid psychiatric conditions, such as personality disorders, somatic symptom disorder, or pathological lying (Brannon, 2015).

Clinical Presentation

The presentation of MBP is varied and can include frequent medical visits for fictitious symptoms, purposeful inducement of physical symptoms (medication-induced vomiting, intentional bruising, etc.), or manipulation of laboratory tests to produce clinical signs of disease (adding blood to a urine sample). In extreme forms of the disorder, serious harm or death may result from suffocation or poisoning (Stirling, 2007).

Assessment and Diagnosis

The diagnosis of MBP can be extremely difficult to determine, because organic causes of signs and symptoms must be excluded. The nurse plays an integral role in the diagnosis of this disorder through careful observation and documentation. In particular, when a parent or caregiver reports the presence of a symptom, such as vomiting, the nurse should take care to report whether the nurse witnessed the complaint or it was merely reported by the caregiver. In cases that are difficult to determine, video surveillance has proved to be an important tool in promoting child safety (Stirling, 2007).

Therapeutic Interventions

The hallmark of MBP treatment involves ensuring the child's current and future safety and facilitating the appropriate level of management for the child and the caregiver (Stirling, 2007). This strategy involves multiple members of the healthcare team, including the following:

- Pediatricians
- Forensic medicine specialists
- Mental health specialists
- Child protective services agency personnel
- Social workers
- Nurses

Treatment may include in-home treatment, inpatient admission, foster home placement, individual and family counseling, or caregiver incarceration depending on the degree of severity. Regardless of treatment modality, the nurse's role is in maximizing child safety and promoting normal growth and development.

Evaluation

Expected outcomes for a child who has experienced abuse in the form of MBP include the following:
- Further harm to the child is prevented.
- The family unit is preserved, when feasible.

Think Critically

1. When evaluating a child for potential learning disorders, what sensory evaluations should the nurse conduct?
2. How should the nurse respond to a parent's concerns about the association of vaccinations and autism?
3. When counseling the child and parent about ADHD medications, which side effects should the nurse instruct them to report to the healthcare provider?

4. On the basis of the evidence provided in Analyze the Evidence 33.1, what role could the pediatric nurse play in the prevention of physical child abuse?
5. During an exam, the nurse discovers several burns in multiple stages of healing along both arms of a preschool child. The parent states that the child bumped into the iron this morning. After assuring the safety of the child, what is the best action of the nurse?

References

American Academy of Pediatrics. (2018). *Autism spectrum disorder*. Retrieved from https://www.healthychildren.org/English/health-issues/conditions/Autism/Pages/Autism-Spectrum-Disorder.aspx

American Academy of Pediatrics. (2017). *Causes of ADHD: What we know today*. Retrieved from https://www.healthychildren.org/english/health-issues/conditions/adhd/pages/causes-of-adhd.aspx

American Art Therapy Association. (2017). *About art therapy*. Retrieved from https://arttherapy.org/about-art-therapy

American Psychiatric Association. (2013). *Diagnostic and statistical manual of mental disorders* (5th ed.). Arlington, VA: American Psychiatric Association.

Association for Play Therapy. (2018). *Why play therapy?* Retrieved from https://www.a4pt.org/page/WhyPlayTherapy

Bagnell, A. L. (2011). Anxiety and separation disorders. *Pediatrics in Review, 32*(10), 440–446.

Birmaher, B., Brent, D. A., Chiappetta, L., Bridge, J., Monga, S., & Baugher, M. (1999). Psychometric properties of the Screen for Child Anxiety Related Emotional Disorders (SCARED): A replication study. *Journal of the American Academy of Child and Adolescent Psychiatry, 38*(10), 1230–1236.

Boos, S.C., Lindberg, D.M., & Wiley, J.F. (2019). *Physical child abuse: Recognition*. Retrieved from: https://www.uptodate.com/contents/physical-child-abuse-recognition

Boyle, C. A., Boulet, S., Schieve, L. A., Cohen, R. A., Blumberg, S. J., Yeargin-Allsopp, M., . . . & Kogan, M. D. (2011). Trends in the prevalence of developmental disabilities in US children, 1997–2008. *Pediatrics, 127*(6), 1034–1042.

Brannon, G. E. (2015). *Factitious disorder imposed on another (Munchausen by proxy)*. Retrieved from https://emedicine.medscape.com/article/295258-overview

Chaney, D. W. (2013). An overview of the first use of the terms cognition and behavior. *Behavioral Sciences, 3*, 143–153.

Engorn, B., & Flerlage, J. (2015). *The Harriet Lane handbook* (20th ed.). Philadelphia, PA: Elsevier Publishing.

Flaherty, E. G., & Stirling, J., Jr. (2010). The pediatrician's role in child maltreatment prevention. *Pediatrics, 126*, 833–841.

Handler, S. M., & Fierson, W. M. (2011). Learning disabilities, dyslexia, and vision. *Pediatrics, 127*(3), e818–e856.

Hanna, G. L., Fischer, D. J., & Fluent, T. E. (2006). Separation anxiety disorder and school refusal in children and adolescents. *Pediatrics in Review, 27*(2), 56–63.

Harvard Health Publishing. (2009a). *Treating anorexia nervosa*. Retrieved from https://www.health.harvard.edu/newsletter_article/Treating-anorexia-nervosa

Harvard Health Publishing. (2009b). *Treating bulimia nervosa*. Retrieved from https://www.health.harvard.edu/newsletter_article/Treating-bulimia-nervosa

Ireton, H. (1992). *Child development inventory manual*. Minneapolis, MN: Behavior Science Systems.

Ipser, J. C., Stein, D. J., Hawkridge, S., & Hoppe, L. (2009). Pharmacotherapy for anxiety disorders in children and adolescents. *Cochrane Database of Systematic Reviews*, (3), CD005170. doi:10.1002/14651858.CD005170.pub2

Johnson, C. P., & Myers, S. M. (2007). Identification and evaluation of children with autism spectrum disorders. *Pediatrics, 120*, 1183–1215.

Kellog, N. (2005). The evaluation of sexual abuse in children. *Pediatrics, 116*(2), 506–512.

National Association of Anorexia Nervosa and Associated Disorders. (2018). *Eating disorder statistics*. Retrieved from: http://www.anad.org/education-and-awareness/about-eating-disorders/eating-disorders-statistics/

National Eating Disorders Association. (2018). *Bulimia nervosa*. Retrieved from https://www.nationaleatingdisorders.org/learn/by-eating-disorder/bulimia

Roesler, T. A., & Jenny, D. (2018). Medical child abuse: Munchausen syndrome by proxy. *UpToDate*. Retrieved from https://www.uptodate.com/contents/medical-child-abuse-munchausen-syndrome-by-proxy

Soreff, S. (2018). *Attention deficit hyperactivity disorder (ADHD)*. Retrieved from https://emedicine.medscape.com/article/289350-overview

Squires, J., & Bricker, D. (2009). *Ages and stages questionnaires* (3rd ed.). Baltimore, MD: Brooks Publishing Company.

Sterling, J.S. (2007). Beyond Munchausen Syndrome by Proxy: Identification and treatment of child abuse in a medical setting. *Pediatrics, 119*: 1026-1030.

Talvik, I., Alexander, R. C., & Talvik, T. (2008). Shaken baby syndrome and a baby's cry. *Acta Paediatrica, 97*(6), 782–785.

Child Welfare Information Gateway. (2019). *About CAPTA: A legislative history*. Washington, DC: U.S. Department of Health and Human Services, Children's Bureau. Retrieved from: https://www.childwelfare.gov/pubpdfs/about.pdf

World Health Organization. (2014). *Mental health: A state of well-being*. Retrieved from http://www.who.int/features/factfiles/mental_health/en/

World Health Organization and Calouste Gulbenkian Foundation. (2014). *Social determinants of mental health*. Geneva: World Health Organization.

Suggested Readings

Child Welfare Information Gateway. (2019). *About CAPTA: A legislative history*. Washington, DC: U.S. Department of Health and Human Services, Children's Bureau. Retrieved from: https://www.childwelfare.gov/pubpdfs/about.pdf

Healthychildren.org. *Vaccine safety: Examine the evidence*. Retrieved from https://www.healthychildren.org/English/safety-prevention/immunizations/Pages/Vaccine-Studies-Examine-the-Evidence.aspx

34 Pediatric Emergencies

Emergencies in the pediatric population can occur in any setting and include respiratory arrest, submersion injury, shock, and poisoning. Nurses must be able to identify subtle changes and warning signs of a child in an impending emergency so they can quickly and effectively intervene to prevent deterioration and cardiopulmonary arrest. Early intervention, particularly in cases of impending shock, sepsis, and respiratory failure can save lives and result in favorable outcomes (de Caen et al., 2015). Assessment and management of the most common types of pediatric emergencies are discussed in this chapter.

Pediatric Assessment in an Emergency

Care of the child during an emergency includes a rapid cardiopulmonary assessment. Initially, assessment and resuscitation should address life-threatening injuries that affect ventilation, oxygenation, and perfusion (Priority Care Concepts 34.1). Essential measures to perform in a pediatric emergency include assessment for a patent airway and adequate breathing; if needed, prompt establishment of an airway to achieve effective oxygenation and ventilation, ensuring adequate breaths per minute to support ventilation; and establishing adequate perfusion to ensure circulation.

A rapid cardiopulmonary assessment is used to evaluate the status of a child in an emergency. The 2015 Pediatric Advanced Life Support guidelines recommend an order of interventions based on the acronym CAB-D when assessing a patient who is found unresponsive or in a life-threatening emergency (de Caen et al., 2015). CAB-D stands for cardiovascular, airway, breathing, and disability. However, the initial rapid assessment proceeds in the order of safety, airway, breathing, circulation, and disability. On finding a pediatric patient in distress

Priority Care Concepts 34.1

Protect the Cervical Spine

If a cervical spine injury is a possibility, avoid using the head-tilt chin-lift maneuver, as shown in part A below. Instead, use the jaw-thrust technique for opening the airway, as shown in part B below.

A. Head-tilt chin-lift maneuver

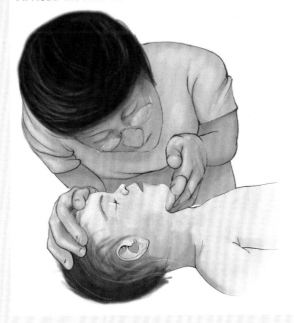

B. Jaw-thrust maneuver

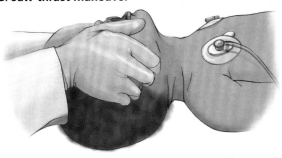

Part A reprinted with permission from Kyle, T., & Carman, S. (2016). *Pediatric nursing clinical guide* (2nd ed., Fig. 1.13). Philadelphia, PA: Wolters Kluwer; part B reprinted with permission from Kyle, T., & Carman, S. (2016). *Essentials of pediatric nursing* (3rd ed., Fig. 29.4). Philadelphia, PA: Wolters Kluwer.

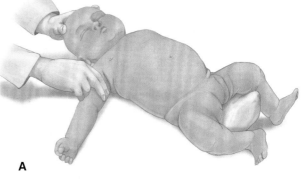

A

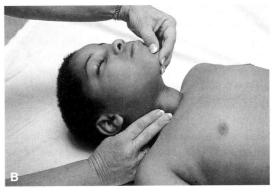

B

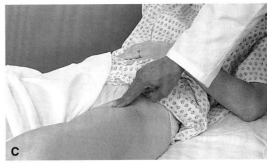

C

Figure 34.1. Location of pediatric pulses. A. Brachial pulse. **B.** Carotid pulse. **C.** Femoral pulse. Part A modified with permission from Ateah, C. A., Scott, S. D., & Kyle, T. (2012). *Canadian essentials of pediatric nursing* (1st ed., Fig. 10.26). Philadelphia, PA: Lippincott Williams & Wilkins. Part B reprinted with permission from Bowden, V. R., & Greenberg, C. S. (2011). *Pediatric nursing procedures* (3rd ed., Fig. 21.2). Philadelphia, PA: Wolters Kluwer. Part C: Photo by B. Proud. Reprinted with permission from Taylor, C., Lillis, C., & Lynn, P. (2014). *Fundamentals of nursing* (8th ed., unnumbered figure in Chapter 25). Philadelphia, PA: Lippincott Williams & Wilkins.

cardiopulmonary resuscitation (CPR) by first checking for responsiveness. If the victim is unresponsive and not breathing or is only gasping for breath, take no more than 10 seconds to assess for a pulse (Fig. 34.1).

A systematic approach is used when assessing a child in an emergency or a life-threatening situation. Assessment of the airway is done by performing a head-tilt, chin-lift maneuver, except in infants and small children and in children with suspected spinal cord

or who has suffered a traumatic injury, first assess the scene for safety before approaching the victim and providing care. Once a safe environment is established, assesses the need for

injury or an unwitnessed injury. In these children, tilting the head back too far can actually occlude the airway. In these scenarios, a jaw-thrust maneuver is best used to open the airway. Positioning the child's airway in a neutral position is essential in opening the small passages of the upper airway and glottic region. Assessment of breathing includes monitoring for adequate chest rise, adequate number of respirations per minute for the child's age, and adequate effort to ensure enough minute ventilation. Minute ventilation is the number of breaths per minute times the volume per breath. A rapid cardiovascular assessment includes locating a central pulse (brachial or femoral in infants and toddlers) and assessing the adequacy of pulses along with number of beats per minute.

Once airway, breathing, and circulation are established, a more in-depth assessment of the cardiovascular system includes assessing capillary refill, determining bleeding and blood loss, assessment of peripheral pulses and skin color, and assessment of blood pressure. Placing the child on a cardiopulmonary monitor is helpful for continuous monitoring of heart rate, respiratory rate, and noninvasive blood pressure monitoring.

Children in life-threatening emergencies often have an altered mental status. In some emergencies, a child may need to be intubated to protect the airway if the child is neurologically compromised. A neurological assessment includes assessing level of consciousness; presence of irritability or lethargy; pupils for equal size, roundness, and reactivity to light and accommodation; and, in older children, orientation to person, place, and time. The Glasgow Coma Scale is often used in the emergency department or trauma center to determine the patient's neurological status. A Glasgow Coma Score of less than 8 is an indication to intubate a child in an emergency situation.

General Nursing Interventions for Pediatric Emergencies

Emotional Impact

In the event of a life-threatening event such as a respiratory arrest, near drowning, or poisoning, perform a rapid assessment of the airway, breathing effort, circulation status, and neurological state, as described earlier, and immediately provide any intervention needed. Assisting with or providing resuscitative measures to a pediatric patient can be emotionally overwhelming. Be aware of your own feelings regarding critically ill and dying children and prepare yourself to be "present" with the family and child during such a crisis. The death of a child is, in general, traumatic not only for parents and families but also for healthcare providers and clinicians. No matter how many times a nurse intervenes in, assists with, or is involved in the care of a child with a life-threatening event, the emotional impact still exists.

Administer Medications and Intravenous Fluids

The nurse is responsible for administering life-saving medications and intravenous (IV) fluids in the event of a pediatric emergency (The Pharmacy 34.1). Medications are weight based. IV fluid boluses, either 0.9% normal saline or lactated Ringer's solution, are given in 10- to 20-mL/kg increments and over a short period of time, such as 20 minutes or even less, using a push–pull technique to administer the fluids as quickly as possible. In some cases, the IV fluids are warmed or cooled, depending on the events leading up to the emergency.

Medications to speed up the heart rate or increase blood pressure are often administered in an emergency. Give meticulous attention to dosing in an emergency, because medications are weight based and too much of a medication can have detrimental effects. Be aware of the side effects of medications, such as dilation of the pupils after administration of atropine. Emergency doses of epinephrine can quickly increase the heart rate and blood pressure, but if the underlying cause is not treated, **bradycardia** (a slow heart rate) and hypotension may resume. Once the patient is stabilized, infusions of inotropes such as dopamine, dobutamine, and epinephrine may be administered to maintain an adequate blood pressure and perfusion.

Be aware of two additional medications often used in pediatric emergencies: dextrose and naloxone. Dextrose 25% is administered for hypoglycemia. Naloxone is administered for opioid overdose. Alarmingly, the annual rate of hospitalizations for opioid poisoning almost doubled from 1997 to 2012, with the highest increase in children aged 1 to 4 years and 12 to 17 years (Gaither, Leventhal, Ryan, & Camenga, 2016). Naloxone may need to be administered multiple times in a short period, because the antidote has a very short half-life compared with many opioids.

Provide Emotional and Psychological Support to the Child and Family

Nurses who work with parents and families of a child who is critically ill play an important role in helping them adapt to the situation and promote coping and family functioning. Parents of an acutely ill or injured child may feel sadness, fear, guilt, or anger and may be concerned that their child might die. In an emergency or a critical situation, parents need up-to-date information, open and honest communication, and ongoing emotional support throughout the event. Provide information in simple terms, and explain interventions as they are being performed.

Offer empathy and support to the family. Avoid providing false reassurance, because the outcome is never certain. Provide information in an honest manner while respecting each family's diversity and cultural needs. Even when the emergency may be a result of abuse or neglect, remain nonjudgmental in all interactions with the child and family. During an emergency, parental control is often taken away and parents feel helpless and no longer the expert in their child's care. Allow parents to hold the child's hand and be present for procedures (according to the hospital guidelines), and encourage them to

The Pharmacy 34.1 Medications Used in Pediatric Emergencies

Medication	Classification	Route	Action	Nursing Considerations
Atropine	Anticholinergic	• IV • IO • ET	• Increases heart rate • Increases cardiac output • Dries secretions	• Do not mix with sodium bicarbonate (incompatible). • Monitor heart rhythm following administration. • Causes pupil dilation
Dextrose	Hypoglycemic	• IV • IO	Increases blood glucose levels	• Monitor blood glucose levels closely. • When administering peripherally, dilute with 1:1 sterile water to make D25%.
Dobutamine	Beta-adrenergic agonist (primarily affects beta-1 receptors)	• IV • IO	• Increases myocardial contractility • Increases heart rate	• Titrate infusion depending on BP and cardiac output. • Monitor for ventricular arrhythmias. • Administer via central line, preferably.
Dopamine	Beta-adrenergic agonist	• IV • IO	• Increases cardiac output and BP • Increases renal perfusion	• Monitor for ventricular arrhythmias. • Administer via central line, preferably.
Epinephrine	Alpha- and beta-adrenergic agonist	• IV • IO • ET	• Increases heart rate • Increases systemic vascular resistance	• Repeat every 3 min during CPR. • Monitor for ventricular arrhythmias. • High risk for extravasation and tissue necrosis; administer via central line, preferably.
Naloxone	Narcotic antagonist	• IV • IO • SC • IN • ET	Reverses respiratory depression and hypotension related to narcotic effects	• Narcotic effects outlast therapeutic effects. • May repeat dose as necessary for opiate-induced apnea, bradypnea

BP, blood pressure; CPR, cardiopulmonary resuscitation; ET, endotracheal; IN, intranasal; IO, intraosseous; IV, intravenous; SC, subcutaneous.
Adapted from Taketomo, C. K., Hodding, J. H., & Kraus, D. M. (2018). *Pediatric & neonatal dosage handbook* (25th ed.). Hudson, OH: Lexicomp.

provide information about their child that may help the team provide care.

A social worker or chaplain is often present when a child is receiving life-saving interventions. These interdisciplinary staff are often skilled in communicating with families who are scared, overwhelmed with the situation, or fearing the child's death. If possible, use these team members during life-saving interventions when the family is present so that you can focus on providing skilled nursing care.

Respiratory Arrest

Respiratory arrest is a state of cessation of breathing (apnea) or respiratory dysfunction so severe that adequate ventilation and oxygenation cannot be maintained. It occurs as a result of inadequate ventilation, inadequate oxygenation, or a combination of the two. A respiratory arrest is generally preceded by respiratory distress or impending respiratory failure. Respiratory arrest eventually leads to cardiopulmonary arrest if left untreated.

Etiology and Pathophysiology

The causes of respiratory arrest in children are numerous. Determining the cause is important to not only treat the cause but also provide appropriate interventions for establishing an airway and maintaining adequate respiratory support. Table 34.1 reviews potential causes of respiratory arrest in children.

Clinical Presentation

Signs and symptoms of respiratory arrest occur because the oxygen deficit is beyond spontaneous recovery. Cerebral oxygenation is dramatically affected, and changes in the central nervous system are ominous. Infants and children in respiratory arrest may appear tachypneic (but have very shallow chest rise), bradypneic (low respiratory rate), or apneic. The child is often lethargic or unresponsive to stimuli. Cyanosis may be present.

Table 34.1   Causes of Respiratory Arrest in Children

Condition Category	Cause
Upper airway disorder	• Croup • Epiglottitis • Foreign body aspiration • Strangulation • Tracheal stenosis • Tracheomalacia
Lower airway disorder	• Asthma • Bronchitis • Pertussis • Pneumonia • Pneumothorax
Upper and lower airway disorder	• Burns • Foreign body aspiration • Reflux
Neurological disorder	• Central nervous system infection • Guillain–Barré syndrome • Seizures • Sleep apnea • Spinal cord trauma • Sudden infant death syndrome
Shock	All types
Chronic illness	Cystic fibrosis
Metabolic or endocrine disorder	• Diabetic ketoacidosis • Mitochondrial disorders
Cardiac disorder	• Acquired heart problems (i.e., Kawasaki, heart failure) • Arrhythmias • Congenital heart defects
Traumatic injury	• Asphyxia • Child abuse (nonaccidental trauma) • Drowning • Electrocution • Gunshot wound • Motor vehicle–related trauma • Poisoning via ingestion

Adapted from Sarnaik, A., Clark, J., & Sarnaik, A. (2016). Respiratory distress and failure. In R. Kliegman, B. Stanton, J. St. Geme, N. Schor, & R. Behrman (Eds.), *Nelson textbook of pediatrics* (20th ed., pp. 528–536). Philadelphia, PA: Elsevier.

Assessment and Diagnosis

Signs of impending respiratory arrest in children include gasping, agonal breathing, cyanosis, paradoxical breathing, use of accessory muscles, and a slowed respiratory rate.

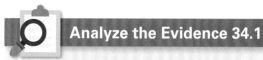

Analyze the Evidence 34.1

Parent Presence During Resuscitation

Parent presence is an important concept of family-centered care, a key theme in pediatric care that ensures holistic care of the child and family. Several questions often arise from healthcare clinicians during the discussion of family presence during life-saving measures and invasive procedures.

1. How do parents feel about being present during the resuscitation or while life-saving measures are being performed on their child?
2. How do parents who are present during the resuscitation cope compared with parents who are not present during resuscitation or life-saving measures?

In a systematic review (McAlvin & Carew-Lyons, 2014), findings indicate that parents do wish to be present during invasive procedures and would choose to be present again if in a similar situation. Parents would also recommend being present to others who may encounter their child receiving life-saving measures.

Parents and family members experience a great deal of distress and often have difficulty coping when their child is hospitalized with life-threatening conditions or critical illnesses. McAlvin and Carew-Lyons (2014) also found that parents who were present during life-saving measures and invasive procedures had better coping and adjustment in the case of the child dying vs. parents who were not present. Parents who were not present reported more distress.

Children may also appear confused or excessively sleepy if carbon dioxide levels are high or oxygen levels are low. A rapid cardiopulmonary assessment is necessary. Once an open airway is established and oxygen is being delivered, a determination of the cause of respiratory arrest should be quickly established to optimize treatment and prevent further respiratory arrest.

Therapeutic Interventions

Immediate interventions for a child in respiratory arrest include opening the airway and assisting with breathing to ensure that adequate oxygen can be delivered (Analyze the Evidence 34.1). The use of a bag and mask may be necessary to deliver oxygen and assist the child in breathing. Use of an appropriately sized mask is essential for ensuring a proper fit around the mouth and nose. Initial interventions should be aimed at ensuring adequate oxygenation, because hypoxemia is life-threatening compared with hypercapnia (Sarnaik, Clark, & Sarnaik, 2016).

If the child does not resume adequate respiratory effort and number of breaths per minute for age and condition, intubation and mechanical ventilation may be necessary. Endotracheal **intubation** is a medical procedure in which a breathing tube is placed via the mouth or nose into the trachea. Intubation allows the child to be mechanically ventilated. Mechanical ventilation is used to assist or replace spontaneous breathing via a machine that allows for oxygen and carbon dioxide to move in and out of the lungs. In this case, the child will need intensive care monitoring.

Evaluation

Expected outcomes for a child experiencing respiratory arrest include the following:

- The child's airway and breathing are adequately supported.
- Carbon dioxide and oxygen levels are within normal limits or return to baseline.
- Emotional support is provided to parents and family.

Discharge Planning and Teaching

When a child who has experienced a respiratory arrest is ready for discharge, teaching and discharge planning are based on the cause of the respiratory arrest. Review with parents what to do in the event of a future respiratory arrest or if their child has difficulty breathing. Review the signs and symptoms of respiratory distress and when to contact the child's provider versus when to call 911. Parents are often worried that a similar situation will occur again. Allow parents to talk through these feelings. Encourage parents to take a CPR class. Community CPR classes are often held at local firehouses or community centers. Provide resources for locating community CPR classes, such as the number to the American Red Cross.

Trauma

Injuries are the most common cause of death in all children older than 1 year (Daley, Raju, & Lee, 2015). Unintentional injuries account for approximately 30% of deaths in children and young adults aged 1 to 24 years (Rivara & Grossman, 2016). There are numerous mechanisms of injury or trauma in the pediatric patient, including motor vehicle accidents; head trauma (Chapter 22); multiple organ trauma; severe lacerations, burns, and other integumentary injuries (Chapter 29); musculoskeletal injuries (Chapter 27); spinal cord injury (Chapter 28); and gunshot wounds. This chapter covers submersion injury (near drowning), shock, and poisoning.

Submersion Injury

A **submersion injury** is trauma caused by near drowning, or survival after suffocation and respiratory impairment by submersion in a liquid medium (Martinez & Hooper, 2014).

Etiology and Pathophysiology

Drowning is the leading cause of unintentional injury deaths in children aged 1 to 4 years and the second leading cause of death in children aged 1 to 16 years (Rivara & Grossman, 2016). For each fatal drowning victim, five patients receive emergency care for near-drowning events (Centers for Disease Control and Prevention [CDC], 2016).

Risk factors for drowning include lack of swimming ability, lack of barriers, lack of close supervision, and location (Fig. 34.2). At highest risk are males, children aged 1 to 4 years, and minorities (CDC, 2016). In the United States, children of racial and ethnic minorities have more than 4 times the rate of near-fatal drownings as do Caucasian children (Felton, Myers, Liu, & Davis, 2015). In 2016, drowning was responsible for more deaths among children aged 1 to 4 years than any other diagnosis except congenital anomalies (CDC, 2018). For children of all ages, near drowning most commonly occurs in swimming pools, followed by natural waterways such as ponds (Felton et al., 2015).

Drowning begins when the airway is submerged in water. Breath holding, panic, swallowing of water, aspiration, and laryngospasm occur following submersion. Unconsciousness ensues from hypoxia and hypercapnia. As the child becomes unconscious, the larynx relaxes and fluid is aspirated into the lungs. Hypoxia worsens and metabolic and respiratory acidosis begins. Aspirated fluid may be contaminated with debris, sand, mud, or vomit (Martinez & Hooper, 2014).

Submersion injuries often have long-term consequences as a result of prolonged hypoxia and brain damage. Hypoxic brain injury, which begins within 5 minutes of inadequate cerebral oxygenation, is the leading cause of morbidity and mortality in drowning (Martinez & Hooper, 2014). Other complications include acute respiratory distress syndrome (ARDS) and lung infection. ARDS occurs in up to 70% of symptomatic survivors of drowning (Martinez & Hooper, 2014). Lung infection occurs in up to 50% of drownings as a result of aspiration of contaminated fluid (Martinez & Hooper, 2014).

Clinical Presentation

Children who have experienced a near-drowning event are at risk for respiratory compromise up to 8 hours after the event,

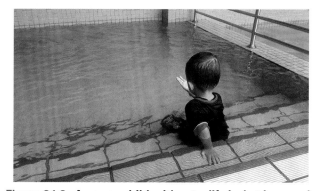

Figure 34.2. A young child without a life jacket in a pool.

even if they arrive at the emergency department asymptomatic or minimally symptomatic (Caglar & Quan, 2016). Following return of spontaneous breathing or resuscitation, tachypnea, labored breathing, shortness of breath, wheezing, and hypoxemia are often present as a result of aspirating water. Children who had a prolonged time without oxygen and required CPR may be hemodynamically unstable and have decreased capillary refill, decreased peripheral pulses, and hypotension or arrhythmias.

Assessment and Diagnosis

On arrival at the emergency department, a systematic physical assessment should focus on the respiratory, cardiovascular, and neurological systems. Dyspnea, wheezing, and crackles are indicative of aspiration. A chest X-ray may be obtained to assess for atelectasis, pneumonia, or lung insult. Cardiovascular status, including heart rate, blood pressure, capillary refill, and peripheral pulses are examined. A thorough neurological exam is completed, particularly in children who are unresponsive or received CPR for an extended period of time. Core temperature should be obtained. Near-drowning victims may be hypothermic. Temperature is closely monitored.

Therapeutic Interventions

Initially, rapid rescue from the water and the provision of basic life support are essential. Because hypoxia is the underlying cause of cardiac arrest and neurological compromise, resuscitation should focus on restoring oxygenation, ventilation, and perfusion. When administering CPR, clear the airway of foreign material such as vomit before providing rescue breaths. If the child is pulseless, start CPR and include rescue breaths. Observe spinal precautions in children with suspected spinal cord injury from a diving accident or fall. However, spinal cord injury is rare in this population; only about 0.5% of drowning victims have cervical spine injuries (Caglar & Quan, 2016).

Management of the child who survives a submersion injury includes close monitoring of the child's respiratory, cardiovascular, and neurological status. Treatment is focused on optimizing oxygenation and cardiac output and controlling temperature (Martinez & Hooper, 2014). The awake, neurologically appropriate child with mild respiratory distress should be placed on oxygen and continuously monitored for 6 to 8 hours after a submersion injury. Serial monitoring of O_2 level, electrocardiogram (ECG), heart rate, respiratory rate, blood pressure, and neurological status are indicated. Most children who are alert and present with mild respiratory symptoms respond to oxygen therapy within 4 to 6 hours, and their respiratory rate and O_2 level return to normal, despite an initial abnormal chest X-ray (Caglar & Quan, 2016).

For children who have been resuscitated, the level of respiratory support required may vary. Perform frequent respiratory assessments, and pay attention to the child's oxygenation and ventilation. Children may need noninvasive ventilatory support (if conscious) or intubation and mechanical ventilation (if unconscious). Hypercarbia should be avoided in children with

neurological compromise, because increased carbon dioxide levels can accelerate brain injury (Caglar & Quan, 2016). Up to 70% of symptomatic drowning survivors develop pulmonary edema and ARDS resulting from aspirated fluid, increased capillary permeability, negative pressure, and neurogenic pulmonary edema (Martinez & Hooper, 2014).

Fluid resuscitation and inotropic support are often necessary. Significant hypovolemia may be present from capillary leak and the onset of the systemic inflammatory response syndrome (Martinez & Hooper, 2014). As ordered, administer crystalloids in 20-mL/kg increments to restore intravascular volume and inotropes, such as epinephrine, to maintain a blood pressure within normal limits for the child's age.

Temperature control is often necessary when caring for the near-drowning child. Uncontrolled hypothermia initially causes hyperventilation, tachycardia, and shivering, which collectively increase oxygen consumption (Martinez & Hooper, 2014). Hyperthermia can also occur and should be controlled with antipyretics and cooling mechanisms such as a cooling blanket. Almost half of all drowning victims have a fever within the first 48 hours of the submersion incident (Caglar & Quan, 2016). Increased temperature is not usually caused by infection, so prophylactic antibiotics are not generally recommended. However, hyperthermia can increase the risk of mortality and ischemic brain injury, so establishing normothermia or slight hypothermia is paramount to reducing further brain injury after a near drowning (Caglar & Quan, 2016).

Evaluation

Expected outcomes for a child who has experienced near drowning include the following:

- The child regains consciousness following CPR measures.
- Signs of respiratory distress or mental status change are quickly detected and managed.
- Oxygenation and ventilation are restored and optimized.
- Hemodynamic stability is achieved.
- Parents and family members learn drowning-prevention strategies.

Discharge Planning and Teaching

Parents can reduce the risk of drowning or near drowning. Teach parents to clear the pool area or swimming area of all toys, floats, and balls when not in use so that children are not tempted to play with them and enter the pool unsupervised. Swimming pools should be surrounded by fences on all sides, with the fence being at least 4 ft high (Fig. 34.3). Encourage parents to install self-closing or self-latching locks on gates and fences to the pool that open outward and are out of the reach of children.

Encourage parents to teach children to swim. Formal swimming lessons, although not a substitute for close supervision, can protect young children from drowning. An adult or a responsible older child or adolescent should be designated to closely watch any child who is in the bathtub or around water.

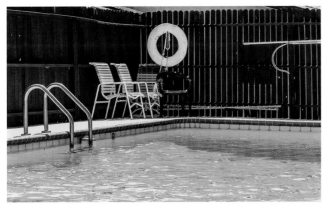

Figure 34.3. A fenced swimming pool with safety equipment available.

Shock

Shock is defined as a reduction in tissue perfusion resulting in decreased oxygen delivery to the tissues and decreased removal of harmful by-products of metabolism such as lactate (Waltzman, 2015). The effects of decreased tissue perfusion are initially reversible. However, prolonged oxygen deprivation leads to cellular hypoxia and ultimately to cell death.

Etiology and Pathophysiology

Shock can be categorized in various ways. For the following discussion, four categories of shock are described: hypovolemic, distributive, obstructive, and cardiogenic. Distributive shock includes neurogenic shock, septic shock, and anaphylactic shock.

Hypovolemic shock, the most common category of shock in children, results from loss of plasma or blood in the intravascular space. In children, etiologies of hypovolemic shock include acute diarrhea, severe vomiting, dehydration, and hemorrhage associated with significant injury or surgery. Hypovolemic shock can also occur in diabetic ketoacidosis as a result of associated fluid and electrolyte loss. Burns, nephrotic syndrome, and sepsis can lead to a large volume of plasma loss and, in turn, to hypovolemic shock.

Distributive shock occurs when there is an abnormal distribution of blood volume or maldistribution of blood flow, often resulting from decreased systemic vascular resistance, vasodilation, or capillary permeability (Fig. 34.4). Preload drops as a result of less blood returning to the heart, and cardiac output diminishes. Decreased cardiac output results in insufficient blood flow to tissue beds. Causes of distributive shock include neurogenic shock, sepsis, and anaphylactic shock. Neurogenic shock, or injury to the spinal cord with associated autonomic dysregulation, results in massive vasodilation, with loss of vasomotor tone. Autonomic dysregulation is due to the loss of sympathetic tone with unopposed parasympathetic response. Spinal cord injury, particularly cervical and high-thoracic injury, is the most common cause of neurogenic shock (Dave & Choo, 2018). Other causes of neurogenic shock include

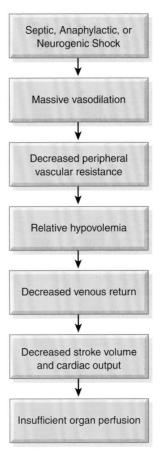

Figure 34.4. Pathophysiological progression of distributive shock. Distributive shock states (anaphylactic, septic, or neurogenic shock) are caused by decreased venous return as a result of displacement of blood volume away from the heart due to enlargement of the vascular compartment and loss of blood vessel tone. Reprinted with permission from Morton, P. G., & Fontaine, D. K. (2017). *Critical care nursing: A holistic approach* (11th ed., Fig. 54.6). Philadelphia, PA: Lippincott Williams & Wilkins.

Guillain–Barré syndrome, transverse myelitis, and other neuropathies (Dave & Choo, 2018).

Sepsis, a life-threatening inflammatory reaction to the invasion of bacteria and their toxins into the blood and tissues, can lead to septic shock. Organisms commonly involved in sepsis include *Neisseria meningitidis, Streptococcus pneumoniae, Staphylococcus aureus, Pseudomonas, Haemophilus influenzae* type b, and *Candida*. During sepsis, endotoxins are released and overwhelming inflammatory processes occur. Macrophages produce and release cytokines, resulting in massive vasodilation, with increased capillary permeability and fluid leak. Capillaries are damaged by the presence of multiplying neutrophils, ending in further capillary leak and fluid shifts. If left untreated or treatment is not begun soon enough, multisystem organ failure can result from tissue hypoxia and ischemia and disseminated intravascular coagulation (Fig. 34.5).

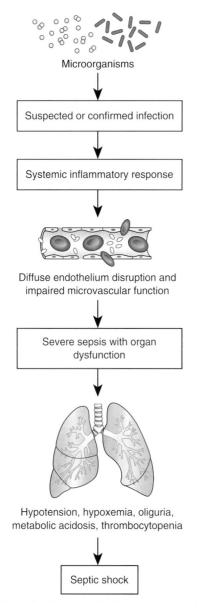

Figure 34.5. **Pathophysiological progression leading to septic shock.** Reprinted with permission from Porth, C. M. (2014). *Essentials of pathophysiology: Concepts of altered health states* (4th ed., Fig. 20.10). Philadelphia, PA: Lippincott Williams & Wilkins.

Anaphylactic shock occurs when mediators from tissue mast cells in an immediate hypersensitivity reaction cause vasodilation from loss of vasomotor tone and capillary leak. Systemic response to anaphylaxis includes vasodilation, increased capillary permeability, bronchoconstriction, increased mucus production, and increased inflammatory mediators released to the site of antigen interaction. Without treatment, circulatory collapse occurs.

Obstructive shock occurs when there is reduced or blocked blood flow from the heart to the great vessels. Pulmonary embolism, tension pneumothorax, pleural effusions, pericardial tamponade, and congenital heart defects can cause obstructive shock in children.

Cardiogenic shock occurs when the heart is unable to adequately pump blood to the rest of the body. The heart cannot maintain adequate cardiac output; therefore, tissue perfusion is decreased. In cardiogenic shock, there is an impairment of the right or left ventricle's pumping ability. In children, cardiogenic shock can result from obstructive congenital heart disease such as hypoplastic left heart, cardiomyopathy, myocarditis, endocarditis, and severe Kawasaki disease (Brissaud et al., 2016). Table 34.2 reviews the categories of shock and associated etiologies.

In Chapter 5, Maalik Abdella developed gastroenteritis after being infected with norovirus. As a result, he had many episodes of vomiting and diarrhea. Which type of shock was Maalik at risk for developing? What complication of gastroenteritis did Maalik develop that put him at risk for this type of shock? What interventions did his nurses implement to prevent him from going into shock?

Shock may be further classified as compensated, decompensated, or irreversible (refractory; Table 34.3). Compensated shock occurs during the early stages, when the body is able to compensate for inadequate oxygen delivery to the cells. The body compensates by using the adrenergic and renal mechanisms. In the initial stages of shock, catecholamine and cortisol levels increase significantly, resulting in an increased heart rate, blood pressure, and myocardial contractility. When kidney perfusion is reduced, the renin-angiotensin-aldosterone system is set into motion, resulting in sodium and intravascular fluid retention. Antidiuretic hormone is released by the hypothalamus, resulting in water retention and increased vascular volume. The respiratory centers are activated, and the respiratory rate increases to improve oxygenation and blow off carbon dioxide in an attempt to improve blood pH. The liver releases glucagon into the bloodstream to increase blood glucose levels for energy and to support vital functions. Peripheral vasoconstriction occurs to maintain systemic vascular resistance. In addition, hydrostatic pressure falls, allowing fluid into the intravascular space to increase intravascular blood volume. Figure 34.6 depicts the compensatory mechanisms.

Clinical Presentation

The clinical presentation of a child in shock varies depending on the type of shock and whether the child is in compensated or decompensated shock. Early signs of shock include unexplained tachycardia and tachypnea. The child may appear mildly ill in the early stages of shock and very toxic in the later stages of shock. The child may present with fever, malaise, or a recent history of illness. Progressing shock and late signs of shock include altered mental status, extreme tachycardia or bradycardia, hypotension, and a significantly delayed capillary refill.

Table 34.2   Categories of Shock and Associated Etiologies

Category	General Cause	Specific Etiologies
Hypovolemic	• Loss of blood or plasma in the intravascular space • A "volume" problem	• Diarrhea • Dehydration • Severe vomiting • Hemorrhage from injury or surgery (i.e., splenic laceration, liver laceration, ruptured vessels) • Burns (excessive plasma loss) • Sepsis • Diabetic ketoacidosis
Distributive	• Abnormal distribution of blood volume secondary to vasodilation and/or capillary permeability; less blood is returned to the heart • A "vessel" problem	• Anaphylaxis • Sepsis • Spinal cord injury
Obstructive	• A mechanical blockage of blood into the heart and major vessels • A "blockage" problem	• Pericardial tamponade • Tension pneumothorax • Pulmonary embolism • Pleural effusion • Congenital heart disease with outflow obstruction • Compression of the vena cava
Cardiogenic	• Impaired myocardial function; the heart is not able to maintain cardiac output and tissue perfusion • A "pump" problem	• Cardiomyopathy • Myocarditis • Severe obstructive congenital heart disease • Severe electrolyte or acid–base imbalance

Table 34.3   Stages of Shock and Associated Clinical Manifestations

Stage	Description	Clinical Manifestations
Compensated	Homeostatic mechanisms compensate for decreased perfusion, helping to maintain blood pressure in a normal range.	• Tachycardia • Tachypnea • Warm or cool skin
Decompensated	Compensatory mechanisms fail to meet metabolic demands; once hypotension develops, rapid deterioration and cardiovascular collapse ensue if left untreated.	• Early: Cool skin, decreased peripheral pulses, decreased urine output • Extremely elevated heart rate • Hypotension begins • Altered neurological status (evidence of poor perfusion to the brain)
Irreversible (refractory)	The shock process is irreversible despite resuscitative efforts; death is imminent.	• Bradycardia • Hypotension (very low blood pressure), often unresponsive to inotropic agents • Evidence of end-organ damage

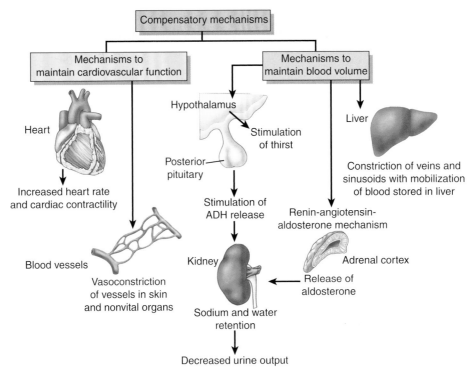

Figure 34.6. Compensatory mechanisms in shock. Adapted with permission from Norris, T. L., & Lalchandani, R. (2018). *Porth's pathophysiology* (10th ed., 27.37). Philadelphia, PA: Wolters Kluwer.

Assessment and Diagnosis

Initial assessment of the child in shock, regardless of the cause or classification, includes an assessment of airway, breathing, and circulation to recognize a life-threatening situation and intervene immediately. Obtain a history while interventions are provided to stabilize the child (Box 34.1). Obtain vital signs initially and monitor them frequently throughout the stabilization of the child.

Laboratory values for the child in shock vary, depending on the cause of shock. Common laboratory tests used in the evaluation of children in shock include blood glucose, complete blood count, blood cultures, C-reactive protein, procalcitonin, lactate, urinalysis, and urine culture. Lumbar puncture may be performed to evaluate the cerebral spinal fluid for culture, white blood cell count, red blood cell count, protein level, and glucose level to assess for meningitis.

Diagnosis of shock is based on the presenting symptoms, initial assessment, and recent health concerns of the child. It is imperative that an early diagnosis is determined to accurately treat the specific type of shock. For example, a child with hypovolemic shock resulting from severe vomiting and diarrhea needs fluid resuscitation, whereas a child with anaphylactic shock may also need fluid resuscitation but needs intramuscular epinephrine, diphenhydramine, and hydrocortisone too.

Therapeutic Interventions

Early, goal-directed therapy in which an aggressive systematic approach to resuscitation targets improvements in perfusion and vital organ function is strongly recommended when treating a child with shock, particularly septic shock (Rhodes et al., 2017).

Interventions are determined by the degree of illness and response to initial treatment within the first hour of care (Rhodes et al., 2017). Physiological parameters that should be targeted during the treatment of shock include heart rate, central and peripheral

---

Box 34.1 Pertinent Health History Questions for the Child in Shock

1. Has the child been vomiting or had diarrhea? If so, for how long?
2. Has the child had decreased oral intake? If so, for how long?
3. Has the child had blood loss? If so, from where and what is the mechanism?
4. When did the child last urinate? For children in diapers, how many wet diapers has the child had in the past 24 h?
5. Has the child had a fever or rash?
6. Has the child had a headache?
7. Has the child been exposed to anyone with a fever, rash, or headache?
8. Does the child have a congenital heart defect or heart problems?
9. Does the child have severe allergies or a history of anaphylaxis?
10. Has the child possibly ingested any medications or substances?

pulses, perfusion (capillary refill time), blood pressure, mental status, and urine output (Turner & Cheifetz, 2016).

Administering IV fluids to restore circulating volume is considered the priority treatment in pediatric shock (Waltzman, 2015). Establish IV access as soon as possible. Multiple IV lines may be necessary. Administer isotonic crystalloids, such as normal saline or lactated Ringer's solution, in increments of 20 mL/kg over 5 minutes if the child is hypotensive (Waltzman, 2015). For children in compensated shock, administer fluid boluses over 5 to 20 minutes if cardiogenic shock is not a factor. In cases of cardiogenic shock or diabetic ketoacidosis, be cautious with fluid administration, because the condition may worsen with increased fluid volume. Following the initial fluid bolus, reassess heart rate, blood pressure, central and peripheral pulses, perfusion, mental status, and urine output. Additional fluid boluses may be given, up to a total of 60 to 80 mL/kg (Turner & Cheifetz, 2016). Goals of fluid therapy include a heart rate normal for age, blood pressure within age parameters, urine output of 1 mL/kg/h, capillary refill time of less than 2 seconds, and a baseline mental status (Turner & Cheifetz, 2016). Before administration of each bolus, assess the child for signs of fluid overload, such as crackles, hepatomegaly, gallops, or decreased oxygenation (Waltzman, 2015).

For children who have not responded to fluid resuscitation, inotropic support may be necessary. Epinephrine and norepinephrine (common inotropes used in treatment of shock) are titrated as ordered to maintain a blood pressure within normal limits for the child's age.

Anaphylactic shock is treated with fluid resuscitation and inotropic support (when necessary). In addition to fluid administration, intramuscular epinephrine, diphenhydramine, and hydrocortisone are also administered.

For children in septic shock, IV antibiotic therapy should begin within the first hour of diagnosis. Early administration of antibiotic therapy is associated with decreased mortality (Turner & Cheifetz, 2016). Antibiotic agents are chosen on the basis of predisposing factors and clinical presentation.

Cardiogenic shock is treated with smaller fluid boluses, 5 to 10 mL/kg, to maintain preload and replace any fluid losses. Use caution when administering additional fluid. Children in cardiogenic shock are often treated with epinephrine or dopamine to improve cardiac output (Turner & Cheifetz, 2016). Vasodilators such as milrinone may also be used to decrease systemic vascular resistance, which is often elevated in cardiogenic shock.

In cases of obstructive shock, the underlying cause must be quickly determined and treated. Fluid boluses may temporarily maintain cardiac output and the child may briefly appear to be improving, but the underlying cause must be addressed (Turner & Cheifetz, 2016). For a tension pneumothorax, a chest tube is placed. In cases of a pericardial effusion, a pericardial drain is placed. Pulmonary emboli may require a thrombectomy or thrombolysis.

For all categories of shock, additional treatment and interventions include monitoring and replacing electrolytes such as calcium, potassium, and sodium. Administration of blood products when bleeding is causing hypovolemic shock may lead to decreased calcium levels and increased potassium levels. Administration of too much fluid may alter sodium and chloride levels. Lactate levels are also trended as an indicator of adequate resuscitation. Lactate levels rise when anaerobic metabolism occurs, such as in cases of inadequate perfusion, leading to hypoxemia and ischemia. Lactate levels fall when tissues are perfused and receiving oxygen.

Evaluation

Expected outcomes for a child with shock include the following:

- Progression to uncompensated shock is prevented by early recognition and intervention.
- The child's vital signs, including heart rate, blood pressure, and respiratory rate are maintained at age-appropriate values.
- The child is free of tissue injury and organ damage as a result of shock.
- Parents understand and cope with the stress of their child having shock.

Discharge Planning and Teaching

Teaching regarding shock varies depending on the type of shock the child was diagnosed with. For children diagnosed with hypovolemic shock, particularly related to vomiting, diarrhea, or dehydration, teach parents how to avoid or lessen the risk of recurrence. Parents should understand the appropriate amount of fluid intake and number of wet diapers per day for an infant or toddler. Teach parents the early signs and symptoms of dehydration, such as increased thirst, sleepiness, decreased wet diapers or voids, irritability, and sunken fontanels (in infants). Teach parents methods of rehydrating a child who is vomiting or has severe diarrhea. Instruct parents to offer several teaspoons or up to two tablespoons of liquid at a time rather than an entire bottle to children 1 year and older and to not offer water to children younger than age 1 year. For breastfed babies, mothers should allow the baby to breastfeed for shorter periods of time, such as 5 to 10 minutes every 2 hours, until the child has not vomited for 8 hours (Ben-Joseph, 2015). Teach parents to offer small amounts of fluid spaced out over 15 to 20 minutes and to offer electrolyte replacement drinks (e.g., Pedialyte), gelatin, broth, or sips of water for children 1 year or older.

Teach parents of a child who has experienced septic shock ways to reduce the risk of infection in and around the home, school, and play areas. Teach parents and children (when appropriate) proper hand washing techniques and the importance of hand washing. Teach parents the early signs of sepsis. Provide education about fever and the importance of seeking treatment early, particularly for neonates and infants younger than 3 months of age. Teach parents to contact the provider when fever is accompanied by lethargy or extreme sleepiness or if the child is difficult to arouse. Signs and symptoms of sepsis can be vague and vary from child to child. Encourage parents to contact their healthcare provider if they believe their child is not acting right or if they have a suspicion something is not right with their child.

Poisoning

Poisoning is the number-one cause of injury deaths in the United States (Kostic, 2016). Over 90% of poisonings occur in private residences and involve a single substance (Kostic, 2016). In 2012, carbon monoxide, acetaminophen, and salicylates were the leading causes of death by poisonings in children younger than age 6 years (Kostic, 2016).

Etiology and Pathophysiology

The consequences of ingesting a toxic or poisonous substance are determined by several factors, including the child's weight and age, the type and toxicity of the substance ingested, the adult response time in finding the child, and the treatment provided (Schwebel et al., 2017). The most common substances that lead to poisoning in children when ingested (Table 34.4) are cosmetics and personal care products, analgesics such as acetaminophen, household cleaning products, pesticides, cardiovascular medications, art/craft supplies, and alcohols (Glenn, 2015; Gummin et al., 2017).

Clinical Presentation

The clinical presentation of a child who has ingested a toxic substance varies depending on the substance ingested. Often, there is a delay from the time of ingestion to the onset of symptoms. Many ingestions are not witnessed, and parents may be unaware, until symptoms begin, that the child has ingested a poison or toxin.

Assessment and Diagnosis

Assessment of the child with suspected poisoning initially includes a rapid cardiopulmonary assessment to ensure that an adequate airway, breathing, and pulse are present. A neurological exam to assess alertness is necessary because many poisons alter the central nervous system and can cause confusion, lethargy, and even coma.

Determining what substance and how much was ingested is critical in prioritizing care for a child who has ingested a toxic substance. Also, understanding the half-life (when medications have been ingested) is important for knowing when peak symptoms may occur. Many medications are extended-release ones, so symptoms may not be evident immediately.

Table 34.4 Commonly Ingested Toxic Agents

Type	Source	Clinical and Laboratory Manifestations	Priorities of Care
Acetaminophen	Over-the-counter products, including: • Pain relievers • Cold medicines	• Nausea • Vomiting • Anorexia • Sweating • Pallor • Right upper quadrant pain • Increased bilirubin • Increased liver enzymes	• Administer antidote N-acetylcysteine. • Administer activated charcoal. • Monitor liver function tests.
Opioids	• Fentanyl • Morphine • Methadone • Heroin	• Slowed respiratory rate, apnea • Altered mental status • Bradycardia • Hypotension	• Administer naloxone as ordered. • Repeated doses of naloxone may be necessary.
Salicylates	Over-the-counter products containing aspirin, including medications for: • Migraines • Colds • Premenstrual syndrome	• Nausea • Vomiting • Tachypnea • Increased salicylate level	• Administer activated charcoal. • Replace electrolytes. • Administer sodium bicarbonate IV (to alkalinize urine). • Monitor for bleeding.
Cardiac medications	• Beta blockers • Calcium channel blockers • Digoxin	• Bradycardia • Hypotension • Arrhythmias, heart block • Dizziness • Altered mental status, seizures • Nausea, vomiting	• Monitor EKG for arrhythmias • Frequent monitoring and evaluation of blood pressure, heart rate, pulse quality and perfusion • Monitor potassium (digoxin toxicity) • Monitor glucose (beta blocker and calcium channel blocker) • Administer calcium salts for calcium channel blocker toxicity • Administer antidotes as ordered: • Betablockers: glucagon • Calcium channel blockers: insulin • Digoxin: Digifab or Digibind

Table 34.4 Commonly Ingested Toxic Agents (*continued*)

Type	Source	Clinical and Laboratory Manifestations	Priorities of Care
Antidepressants	Prescription medications: • Tricyclics • SSRIs	• Tricyclics: delirium, dry mucous membranes, tachycardia, hyperthermia, urinary retention, lethargy, coma, seizures, tachycardia, arrhythmias • SSRIs: lethargy, tachycardia, prolonged QT, serotonin syndrome	• Monitor for lethargy, altered mental status, ability to maintain airway and adequate respiratory rate • Continuous EKG monitoring • Tricyclics: Administer sodium bicarbonate as ordered • SSRIs: monitor for serotonin syndrome; administer benzodiazipenes as ordered
Hypoglycemic agents	• Sulfonylurea • Meglitinides	• Hypoglycemia • Dizziness, tremors, irritability • Lethargy, difficult to arouse • Pale, clammy skin, sweating • Tachycardia	• Administer glucagon and dextrose-containing fluids as ordered. • Monitor blood sugar frequently; effects of toxin may be long-lasting.
Corrosives	• Batteries (particularly button batteries found in toys, watches) • Drain cleaners • Toilet bowl cleaners	• Respiratory distress, stridor • Redness, irritation around/in mouth • Drooling • Abdominal pain, vomiting • Pain in mouth, throat • Difficulty swallowing	• Do not induce vomiting, which can cause further damage. • Give milk or water to dilute corrosive. • X-ray or imaging to visualize battery.
Hydrocarbons	• Gasoline • Lighter fluid • Paint thinners • Kerosene • Furniture polish	• Difficulty breathing • Tachypnea, retractions, cyanosis • Coughing • Altered mental status • Fever, leukocytosis • Nausea, vomiting	• Do not induce vomiting. • Support patient with oxygen, mechanical ventilation.

IV, intravenous; SSRIs, selective serotonin reuptake inhibitors.
Adapted from Kostic, M. (2016). Poisonings. In R. Kliegman, B. Stanton, J. St. Geme, N. Schor, & R. Behrman (Eds.), *Nelson textbook of pediatrics* (20th ed., pp. 447–467). Philadelphia, PA: Elsevier.

Therapeutic Interventions

Initial therapeutic interventions include assessment of airway, breathing, circulation, and neurological function. Substances such as corrosives can quickly cause respiratory compromise due to oropharyngeal and tracheal erosion and swelling. Ingestion of cardiac medications can cause life-threatening arrhythmias, circulatory compromise, or bradycardia. Ingestion of opioids can cause extreme neurological compromise and lead to respiratory arrest. Following stabilization of the child's airway, breathing, and circulation, interventions are based on the substance ingested and the possible complications of that substance.

Providers contact poison control centers to understand what alterations an ingested medication or poison may cause. Poison control centers are staffed by providers who are toxicology specialists and can provide expert poison and treatment advise. There are 55 poison control centers in the United States, all of which are staffed 24 hours a day, 365 days a year.

Children may need to be monitored in the hospital setting either in the acute care setting or in the intensive care unit.

Continuous ECG monitoring, frequent blood pressure monitoring, and frequent neurological assessment are often necessary when an ingestion has occurred. When respiratory distress is present (in the case of corrosives, hydrocarbons, and substances causing severe lethargy or altered mental status leading to respiratory failure), the child may need to be intubated and mechanically ventilated to establish a patent airway or ensure adequate oxygen delivery and ventilation.

Evaluation

Expected outcomes for a child with poisoning include the following:

• The child maintains a patent airway, effective ventilation, and effective gas exchange.
• The child's heart rate and blood pressure remain stable.
• The child's neurological status remains appropriate for age.
• Parents demonstrate effective measures to prevent future episodes of accidental ingestions.

Patient Safety 34.1

Strategies to Prevent Accidental Poisonings

In the Home

- Practice safe storage: Store medications, chemicals, oils, detergents, cleaning supplies, alcohol, and personal care products up, away, and out of the sight of children. Consider locking medications in cabinets with child-resistant locks.
- Practice safe food handling: To avoid food poisoning, cook meats to proper temperatures, clean surfaces and utensils used in preparing raw meat with hot, soapy water, and avoid cross-contamination.
- Install carbon monoxide detectors. Carbon monoxide is a colorless, odorless gas that can lead to death with even a short period of exposure without adequate ventilation.
- Read all labels of hazardous or toxic chemicals and follow directions for use, storage, and disposal.
- Keep substances in their original containers for easy identification and product information should an accidental poisoning occur.
- Teach preadolescents and teens about over-the-counter medication safety: ensure the correct dosage and use, follow the instructions on the label, and ask an adult before taking.

- Dispose of medications that are expired or no longer needed in the proper way. Many communities have drug take-back days to assist with proper disposal. Ask your local pharmacist for proper ways to dispose of medications.

Outdoors

- Reduce the risk of snake bites by wearing protective clothing.
- Use a stick while walking in tall grass to scare snakes away.
- Do not handle or pick up a snake.
- If bitten, do not apply a tourniquet or attempt to suck the venom out of the wound. Call your local poison control center immediately for assistance and seek immediate medical attention.
- Be aware of other poisonous creatures native to your area, such as jellyfish in coastal areas and poisonous spiders in the southwest United States.

Adapted from American Association of Poison Control Centers. *Prevention and education.* Retrieved from https://www.aapcc.org/Prevention

Discharge Planning and Teaching

Education regarding prevention of poisoning begins at well-child visits as part of anticipatory guidance teaching. For parents of a child who has experienced a poisoning, education regarding child proofing the home and ways to reduce poison exposure is necessary before discharge. Patient Safety 34.1 reviews strategies to prevent accidental poisoning.

Think Critically

1. Upon entering the hospital room of a 3-month-old infant who was admitted for bronchiolitis, you find that the infant is breathing at a rate of 3 to 5 breaths/min and has dusky lips. There is no one else in the room. What are your priorities of care for this infant?
2. You are preparing discharge instructions for the parents of a 2-year-old who has recovered from a near-drowning episode in the family pool. What teaching points regarding drowning prevention for a 2-year-old should you include in the discharge instructions?
3. A 3-year-old girl is admitted for osteomyelitis of her left knee and to rule out sepsis. She has been on antibiotics for 24 hours. Her mother calls you in the room because she feels her child is getting sicker. You assess the child for signs of sepsis. What is included in your assessment?

4. A 12-year-old has been brought to the emergency room following an automobile accident. His heart rate is 156 beats/min, his blood pressure is 75/48 mm Hg, and his respiratory rate is 36 breaths/min. He is actively bleeding from a large wound in his left leg. What type of shock is this child at risk for? What are three priority interventions for this child?
5. An 18-month-old has been admitted for acetaminophen poisoning. The grandmother states that she accidently left the bottle of acetaminophen on the living room end table and only left the room for a minute. When she returned, the toddler was putting pills into his mouth. The parents, clearly distraught, begin asking you what will happen to their child. What organ systems are affected by an acetaminophen overdose? Explain to the parents, in simple terms, what you will be assessing for while the child is hospitalized.

References

Ben-Joseph, E. P. (2015). Vomiting. *KidsHealth from Nemours.* Retrieved from https://kidshealth.org/en/parents/vomit.html

Brissaud, O., Botte, A., Cambonie, G., Dauger, S., de Saint Blanquat, L., Durand, P., . . . & Mauriat, P. (2016). Experts' recommendations for the management of cardiogenic shock in children. *Annals of Intensive Care, 6*(1), 14.

Caglar, D., & Quan, L. (2016). Drowning and submersion injury. In R. Kliegman, B. Stanton, J. St. Geme, N. Schor, & R. Behrman (Eds.), *Nelson textbook of pediatrics* (20th ed., pp. 561–568). Philadelphia, PA: Elsevier.

Centers for Disease Control and Prevention (CDC). (2016). *Unintentional drowning: Get the facts.* Retrieved July 28, 2018 from https://www.cdc.gov/homeandrecreationalsafety/water-safety/waterinjuries-factsheet.html

Centers for Disease Control and Prevention, National Center for Injury Prevention and Control. (2018). *Web-based Injury Statistics Query and Reporting System (WISQARS).* Retrieved August 3, 2018 from http://www.cdc.gov/injury/wisqars

Daley, B., Raju, R., & Lee, S. (2015). *Considerations in pediatric trauma.* Retrieved August 1, 2018 from https://emedicine.medscape.com/article/435031

Dave, S., & Cho, J. (2018). *Shock, neurogenic.* StatPearls [Internet]. Treasure Island, FL: StatPearls Publishing.

de Caen, A., Berg, M., Chameides, L., Gooden, C., Hickey, R., Scott, H., . . . & Schexnayder, S. (2015). Part 12: Pediatric advanced life support: 2015 American Heart Association guidelines update for cardiopulmonary resuscitation and emergency cardiovascular care. *Circulation, 132*(18 suppl 2), S526–S542.

Felton, H., Myers, J., Liu, G., & Davis, D. (2015). Unintentional, non-fatal drowning of children: US trends and racial/ethnic disparities. *BMJ Open, 5*(12), e008444.

Gaither, J., Leventhal, J., Ryan, S., & Camenga, D. (2016). National trends in hospitalizations for opioid poisonings among children and adolescents, 1997 to 2012. *JAMA Pediatrics, 170*(12), 1195–1201.

Glenn, L. (2015). Pick your poison: What's new in poison control for the preschooler. *Journal of Pediatric Nursing, 30,* 395–401.

Gummin, D., Mowry, J., Spyker, D., Brooks, D., Fraser, M., & Banner, W. (2017). 2016 Annual Report of the American Association of Poison Control Centers' National Poison Data System (NPDS): 34th Annual Report. *Clinical Toxicology, 55*(10), 1072–1254.

Kostic, M. (2016). Poisonings. In R. Kliegman, B. Stanton, J. St. Geme, N. Schor, & R. Behrman (Eds.), *Nelson textbook of pediatrics* (20th ed., pp. 447–467). Philadelphia, PA: Elsevier.

Martinez, F., & Hooper, A. (2014). Drowning and immersion injury. *Anaesthesia & Intensive Care Medicine, 15*(9), 420–423.

McAlvin, S., & Carew-Lyons, A. (2014). Family presence during resuscitation and invasive procedures in pediatric critical care: a systematic review. *American Journal of Critical Care, 23*(6), 477–485.

Rhodes, A., Evans, L., Alhazzani, W., Levy, M., Antonelli, M., Ferrer, R., . . . & Rochwerg, B. (2017). Surviving sepsis campaign: International guidelines for management of sepsis and septic shock: 2016. *Intensive Care Medicine, 43*(3), 304–377.

Rivara, F., & Grossman, D. (2016). Injury control. In R. Kliegman, B. Stanton, J. St. Geme, N. Schor, & R. Behrman (Eds.), *Nelson textbook of pediatrics* (20th ed., pp. 40–47). Philadelphia, PA: Elsevier.

Sarnaik, A., Clark, J., & Sarnaik, A. (2016). Respiratory distress and failure. In R. Kliegman, B. Stanton, J. St. Geme, N. Schor, & R. Behrman (Eds.), *Nelson textbook of pediatrics* (20th ed., pp. 528–536). Philadelphia, PA: Elsevier.

Schwebel, D., Evans, W., Hoeffler, S., Marlenga, B., Nguyen, S., Jovanov, E., . . . & Sheares, B. (2017). Unintentional child poisoning risk: A review of causal factors and prevention studies. *Children's Healthcare, 46*(2), 109–130.

Turner, D., & Cheifetz, I. (2016). Shock. In R. Kliegman, B. Stanton, J. St. Geme, N. Schor, & R. Behrman (Eds.), *Nelson textbook of pediatrics* (20th ed., pp. 516–528). Philadelphia, PA: Elsevier.

Waltzman, M. L. (2015). Pediatric shock. *Journal of Emergency Nursing, 41*(2), 113–118.

Suggested Readings

Friedman, M. L., & Bone, M. F. (2014). Management of pediatric septic shock in the emergency department. *Clinical Pediatric Emergency Medicine, 15*(2), 131–139.

Lowe, D. A., Vasquez, R., & Maniaci, V. (2015). Foreign body aspiration in children. *Clinical Pediatric Emergency Medicine, 16*(3), 140–148.

Glossary

A

Abduction: The movement of a body part away from the body's midline

Absence: A type of mild seizure in which the person stares blankly for less than 30 seconds

Absolute neutrophil count (ANC): A measure of the number of neutrophils in the blood, which indicates the ability of the body to fight infection

Acrocyanosis: A condition in which the hands or feet of an infant appear bluish as a result of immature circulation

Active immunity: A type of immunity in which the body develops antibodies to a specific antigen after exposure to it via natural disease or immunization; also called active acquired adaptive immunity

Acute chest syndrome (ACS): A life-threatening pulmonary complication of sickle cell disease triggered by an occlusion in the pulmonary blood vessels, leading to symptoms of chest pain, fever, and difficulty breathing and typically manifesting as a new infiltrate on a chest X-ray

Acute splenic sequestration: An acute complication of sickle cell disease in which sickled cells pool in the spleen, causing enlargement of the spleen, a decrease in hemoglobin level, and a significant trapping of circulatory blood volume, leading to shock

Afterload: The resistance against which the ventricle must pump to eject blood

Airway resistance: The opposition to airflow in the airways during inspiration and expiration; the amount of force required to move air in and out of the lungs

Allergen: Any foreign antigen or agent capable of stimulating an antibody-mediated hypersensitivity reaction (allergic reaction)

Alopecia: Hair loss

Alveoli: Small sacs at the end of each bronchiole that assist with the exchange of oxygen and carbon dioxide between the bloodstream in the capillaries and the air in the lungs

Anaphylaxis: A severe and potentially life-threatening hypersensitivity reaction

Anasarca: Generalized or massive edema

Anencephaly: A neural tube defect resulting in the absence of major portions of the brain, scalp, and skull

Angioedema: Swelling that affects the deeper layers of the skin, including the dermis and subcutaneous tissues

Animism: The attributing of lifelike qualities to inanimate objects

Aniridia: The absence of an iris

Anterior fontanelle: The opening between the frontal and parietal bones of the skull, just above the forehead, which normally closes between 12 and 18 months of age; often called the "soft spot"

Antibody: A protein produced by the immune system capable of binding to specific antigens (infectious agents) for destruction and elimination from the body; also known as immunoglobulin

Anticipatory guidance: Education provided to parents and caregivers about what to expect with regard to their child's growth, development, and needs in the coming months

Antigen: A substance that the body recognizes as foreign and triggers a response from the immune system

Antipyretic: A medication that reduces fever

Anuria: Failure of the kidneys to produce urine

Apocrine gland: A type of sweat gland that secretes an odor and is located in the armpits, groin, and around the nipples

Apoptosis: Normal cell death, which occurs as a result of biochemical mechanisms

Ascites: Accumulation of fluid in the peritoneal cavity, often caused by cirrhosis

Atelectasis: A condition in which a lung or a lobe of the lung collapses because of deflation of the alveoli, leading to difficulty breathing and manifesting as diminished lung volume on a chest X-ray

Atonic: A type of seizure characterized by a loss of muscle tone

Atresia: Absence or closure of a normal body orifice

Attention-deficit/hyperactivity disorder (ADHD): A chronic neurobehavioral disorder marked by a persistent pattern of inattention and/or hyperactivity and impulsivity that interferes with functioning and development

Aura: A perceptual disturbance that occurs just before a seizure, such as an unpleasant smell, change in light perception, or confusing thoughts

Autoimmune disorder: A condition in which the immune system no longer differentiates between self and nonself and produces antibodies against the cells of the body (autoantibodies); characterized by tissue injury from the attack on self

Azotemia: Accumulation of nitrogenous wastes in the blood

B

Balanitis: Inflammation or infection of the glans penis

Basal insulin: A type of insulin used to continually meet the body's insulin need between boluses

Body image: Perception of one's own body with regard to looks and sexual appeal

Body mass index (BMI): A method of assessing body composition and associated health that involves dividing one's mass in kilograms by the square of one's height in meters; for children and teens, age- and gender specific

Bolus insulin: A type of fast-acting insulin used to cover carbohydrate consumption or for blood glucose correction

Bone age: The degree of maturity of a child's bones

Bradycardia: A heart rate less than normal for age and condition; in general, a heart rate less than 90 beats/min (bpm) for infants and toddlers and less than 60 bpm for children and adolescents

Bronchioles: The smallest of the airways that branch off the mainstem bronchi, each of which ends in small sacs called alveoli

Buckle fracture: A type of fracture in which one side of the bone buckles or bends inward in response to excessive pressure being applied to it without disrupting the other side of the bone; common in children because of the soft, more flexible nature of a child's bones; also called a torus fracture

Bulla: A large blister filled with clear fluid

C

Cardiac output: The amount of blood flowing out of the left ventricle into the systemic circulation; determined by heart rate × stroke volume (amount of blood pumped with each beat)

Cardiomegaly: Abnormal enlargement of the heart

Cardiopulmonary resuscitation (CPR): A life-saving method for restoring normal heart function and breathing in an unresponsive person

Central venous catheter (CVC): A long, thin, flexible tube inserted through the chest into a large vein for the infusion of fluids, medications, and blood products

Cephalocaudal: A pattern of development in which the infant acquires skills beginning at the head and then moving downward to the legs

Chloroma: A solid collection of leukemic cells forming a tumor outside of the bone marrow; typically associated with acute myelogenous leukemia

Cholesterol: A waxy, fat-like substance produced by the body, found in certain foods, and required by the body for the production of hormones and vitamin D and for digestion of food

Chordee: Congenital defect in which the penis curves sharply upward or downward

Cisternogram: A medical imaging study that involves injecting a radionuclide into the spinal canal through a lumbar puncture to determine whether there is an abnormality or leakage of the cerebrospinal fluid

Clonic: A type of seizure characterized by the jerking of body parts

Cognition: The process of thought and knowing that is acquired through experiences and maturation

Cognitive behavioral therapy: A form of psychotherapy used to change thinking patterns and behaviors

Comedone: A small papule associated with acne; can be open or closed

Compartment syndrome: A condition in which pressure within a muscle compartment builds to such a degree that blood supply can become decreased or absent, depriving tissues and cells of oxygen and nourishment

Conjunctivitis: An inflammation of the conjunctiva, the transparent membrane that covers the eyeball and lines the inner eyelid; also known as "pink eye"

Conservation: The understanding that quantity stays the same even though appearance changes

Craniosynostosis: A condition of premature closure of one or more of the cranial sutures

Croup: Inflammation of the upper airway, most often caused by viruses

Cryptorchidism: Undescended testes

Cyclic vomiting: Repeated episodes of severe nausea and vomiting that often have no apparent cause

Cystitis: Inflammation or infection of the urethra or bladder

D

Dactylitis: A condition of severe inflammation of the fingers or toes

Deceleration: A sudden stopping of movement; a type of traumatic brain injury in which the brain continues in motion within the skull because of inertia after the skull has been forcibly stopped, leading to brain injury as it hits the skull

Deep partial-thickness burn: A burn that extends deep into the skin, is painful with deep pressure, almost always forms blisters, does not turn white with pressure, takes more than 21 days to heal, and develops scarring; also known as a third-degree burn

Deformational plagiocephaly (DP): Asymmetry and flattening of an infant's head on one side caused by external forces applying pressure to the skull

Development: A process in which a child attains various fine motor, gross motor, language, and cognitive skills

Developmental milestone: The attainment of a skill, such as sitting, walking, or talking, by an expected age that indicates positive growth and development of the child

Developmental reflexes: Primitive reflexes that are present at birth but normally disappear within the first few months of life as the nervous system matures

Diabetes type 1: An autoimmune condition in which the beta cells of the pancreas are destroyed, leading to decreased production of insulin

Diabetic ketoacidosis (DKA): A condition that occurs when the body does not produce enough insulin, resulting in the use of fat for energy, which causes high levels of blood acids called ketones

Diaphysis: The shaft of a long bone

Diurnal enuresis: Enuresis occurring during the day

Ductus arteriosus: The fetal vascular connection between the pulmonary artery and the proximal descending aorta

Dysmenorrhea: A condition of painful uterine cramps that occurs before the onset of menses

Dysphagia: Difficulty swallowing

Dysphonia: Difficulty speaking; in the pediatric respiratory patient, often due to swelling or obstruction

Dysplasia: Abnormal development or growth

Dyspneic: Having difficult or labored breathing

E

Early intervention program: A special program designed to help children achieve developmental milestones

Eccrine gland: A type of sweat gland that releases water to the skin surface and is important in the body's temperature control

Echolalia: A meaningless repetition of words, often occurring in early speech development; also known as parroting

Effusion: An accumulation of fluid within the body

Egocentrism: A focus on self and inability to understand another's perspective

Emesis: The act of vomiting

Encephalitis: Inflammation of the brain, typically caused by a viral infection and resulting in cerebral edema

Encephalocele: A neural tube defect in which the skull fails to properly fuse during the third or fourth week of gestation, resulting in a protrusion of the brain and cranial membranes anywhere along the midline of the skull, from the nose to the back of the neck

Encopresis: Fecal incontinence

Enuresis: Spontaneous, involuntary voiding of urine at an age in which bladder control is expected

Epilepsy: A condition in which a person has two or more seizures without a proximal cause (unprovoked) more than 24 hours apart

Epiphysis: The end of a long bone, which sits on top of the physis (growth plate) and is separated from it by cartilage

Epispadias: A congenital anomaly in males in which the urethral meatus is located on the dorsal surface of the penile shaft

Erythropoiesis: The production of red blood cells by the bone marrow

Eschar: Dead tissue that sloughs off from the surface of the skin

Exophthalmos: A condition of the eyes bulging out of the orbit anteriorly, commonly indicative of Graves disease, a type of hyperthyroidism

Expressive language: Verbal and nonverbal communication skills related to conveying meaning to others

F

Fine motor: The development of small muscle coordination, such as in the hands and fingers

Focal seizure: A seizure in which the abnormal electrical activity originates in only one hemisphere of the brain

Food jag: A phenomenon in which a child only eats one type of food meal after meal

Foramen ovale: An opening in the fetal heart between the right and left atria

Fragile X syndrome: An inherited, genetic condition that is caused by a mutation in the X chromosome and that is the most common known cause of intellectual disability

Full-thickness burn: A burn that extends through all layers of the skin, usually does not hurt, has a waxy white to leathery gray or black color, is dry, does not blanch when touched, and cannot heal without surgical treatment; also known as a fourth-degree burn

G

Galactagogue: A herb or drug that increases milk supply in breast-feeding mothers

Gallop: A third heart sound (S_3), which produces a rhythm similar to that of a galloping horse

Gastroschisis: A congenital malformation in which an infant's intestines extend outside the abdomen through a hole in the abdominal wall

Gender dysphoria: The feeling that one's gender identity as either male or female does not match with the biological sex

Gender identity: One's personal experience of gender, which may or may not match one's biological sex

Generalized seizure: A seizure in which the abnormal electrical activity originates in both hemispheres of the brain

Genetic counseling: Counseling provided to women who would like to conceive and their partners regarding genetic disorders, associated risk factors, and genetic testing

Genetic testing: A series of tests conducted during pregnancy that assess for genetic changes, or mutations, in the fetus indicative of a genetic disorder

Genu: Referring to the knee

Glomerulonephritis: Inflammation of the glomeruli of the kidney

Glucometer: A machine used to measure blood glucose levels

Glycated hemoglobin A1c (HgbA1c): A hemoglobin level that indicates average blood glucose concentration over a 3-month period

Glycosuria: A condition in which glucose is excreted in the urine

Goiter: An enlargement of the thyroid gland

Gross motor: The development of large muscle coordination, such as in the arms, trunk, and legs, to accomplish full-body motion, as in walking, running, and skipping

Growth: An increase in physical size

Grunting: Making a deep, short sound during exhalation, particularly as a compensatory response to respiratory distress to prevent end-expiratory alveolar collapse by helping to keep the alveoli open at the end of expiration

H

Heart failure: A condition that occurs when the heart does not pump enough blood to the rest of the body to meet the body's demand

Hematopoiesis: The production of blood components by the bone marrow

Hemochromatosis: An iron overload resulting from an inherited condition that causes tissue and organ damage because of excessive iron storage

Hemoglobin A1C (HbA1C): A laboratory test that measures the amount of glucose that binds to hemoglobin molecules in the blood as an indicator of the amount of glucose circulating in the blood; used to diagnose types 1 and 2 diabetes mellitus and to assess long-term management of blood glucose level in these diseases

Hemosiderin: An iron-containing pigment that is released during the breakdown of hemoglobin

Hemosiderosis: An iron overload disorder resulting from excessive hemosiderin buildup in the organs and tissues without producing damage to the organs or localized iron absorption

Hemostasis: Stoppage of bleeding

Hepatosplenomegaly: Enlargement of the liver and spleen

High-density lipoprotein (HDL): A complex containing lipids and protein that carries cholesterol to the liver so that it may be excreted in bile; often known as "good cholesterol" because of its protein-to-lipid ratio

Hijab: A head covering worn by women of the Islamic faith in the presence of men other than their immediate family

Hydrocephalus: A condition involving the excessive accumulation of cerebrospinal fluid in the ventricles of the brain

Hydronephrosis: Dilation of the renal calyces and pelvis with urine as a result of an obstruction of outflow of urine from the kidney

Hyperbilirubinemia: Elevated levels of bilirubin in the blood

Hypercapnia: A condition of excessive carbon dioxide in the blood stream, usually caused by hypoventilation; defined as carbon dioxide greater than 45 mm Hg on an arterial blood gas test

Hyperglycemia: A condition of excessive circulating glucose in the blood

Hypersensitivity: An extreme response of the immune system to an antigen leading to inflammation and tissue injury; responsible for extreme allergic reactions

Hypertension: Persistent high arterial blood pressure

Hypertonia: Increased muscular tone, often to the point of spasticity and/or rigidity

Hypoplastic: Small, underdeveloped, and often dysfunctional

Hypospadias: A congenital anomaly in which the urethral meatus is located anywhere along the course of the anterior urethra on the ventral surface

Hypotonia: Decreased muscular tone, often to the point of flaccidity and weakness, making movement difficult

Hypoxia: A condition of inadequate oxygen to the tissues

I

Idiopathic: Occurring without a known cause

Immunization: A medication containing an infectious organism in a weakened, nondisease-producing form that is administered to stimulate the immune system for future protection against exposure to a virulent form of the organism; also known as a vaccine

Immunodeficiency: A state of weakened or absent immune system function leading to ineffective responses to antigens and increased susceptibility to infections

Immunoglobulins (Igs): Proteins produced by the immune system capable of binding to specific antigens (infectious agents) for destruction and elimination from the body; classified as IgM, IgG, IgA, IgD, and IgE; also known as antibodies

Impulsivity: A tendency to act without thinking of the consequences of the action

Inborn errors of metabolism: Mutations (or alterations) in the genes that direct our cells on how to make the enzymes and cofactors necessary for metabolism

Incarceration: A hernia that cannot be reduced, resulting in compromised blood flow to entrapped tissues

Individualized education plan (IEP): A written educational plan adapted to a child's individual needs

Inotropic: Altering the force or strength of a muscle contraction, whether weakening (negative inotropes) or strengthening (positive inotropes)

Insulin pump: A subcutaneous pump that is programmed to deliver a continuous basal insulin dose; can be programmed to give bolus doses of insulin, as well

Intercostal retractions: The inward movement of soft tissue in the intercostal space during inspiration, which can be an indication of moderate respiratory distress

Intrathecal: Referring to a route of drug administration involving injection of a medication directly into the spinal column

Intubation: The insertion of a tube into the trachea to secure a patent airway

Intuitive thinking: A substage of Piaget's preoperational stage in which preschoolers learn about their world by asking questions

Intussusception: An abdominal emergency in which a segment of the intestine slides into an adjacent segment, much like a telescope

Irreversibility: The belief that processes cannot be reversed

Ischemia: The absence of oxygen in the tissues, which can lead to necrosis or cellular death

Isotonic fluid: A fluid that expands volume in the blood vessels without altering the electrolyte balance in the body

J

Jargon: Speech that is difficult to understand

K

Kerion: A severe inflammatory response that may occur with tinea capitis that results in a boggy, granulomatous mass on the scalp

Ketoacidosis: A condition that occurs when the body does not produce enough insulin, resulting in the use of fat for energy, which causes high levels of blood acids called ketones

Ketones: Weak acids that are the by-products of the breakdown of fat and, in diabetes, indicate a lack of insulin when present

Koplik spots: Clustered white lesions on the buccal mucosa associated with the onset of measles

L

Laryngospasm: A brief spasm of the vocal cords, which makes air entry into the trachea difficult

Lethargic: A state in which a child has extreme lack of energy and is sluggish

Leukocoria: A white reflection from the retina; also known as "cat's eye" reflex

Ligament: A type of fibrous tissue that connects bone to bone

Low-density lipoprotein (LDL): A complex containing mostly lipids and few proteinaceous elements; often known as "bad cholesterol"

Lymphadenopathy: Swelling of one or more lymph nodes

Lymphoblast: An immature lymphocyte, typically found in the bone marrow, that is not able to fight infection and is found circulating in large numbers in the peripheral blood in children with leukemia

M

Magical thinking: A preschooler's belief that he or she can make things happen as a result of his or her thoughts

Meconium: The first stool of a newborn, which consists of materials ingested in utero

Medicine man: A spiritual leader and traditional healer for the American Indian community

Menarche: The onset of menstruation

Meningitis: Inflammation of the meninges (the protective membranes covering the brain and spinal cord), typically caused by a bacterial (septic) or viral (aseptic) infection

Mental health: A state of well-being that includes the ability to realize one's potential, cope with stress effectively, work productively, and contribute to one's community

Metaphysis: The narrow portion of the bone, which contains the growth plate

Microcephaly: A congenital defect resulting from abnormal brain development in which the infant's head is smaller than normal

Muscular atrophy: The wasting of muscle from lack of use, which can be caused by nerve, muscle, or cellular damage

Myoclonic: A type of seizure characterized by muscular jerking

N

Nasal flaring: A widening of the nostrils, which in infants often represents a physiologic attempt to increase the diameter of the air passages to allow more air into the body and to decrease airway resistance, possibly in response to respiratory distress

Navajo Nation: An area of the United States occupied by the Navajo tribe, encompassing portions of Utah, Arizona, and New Mexico

Neoplasm: An abnormal growth of cells that can occur anywhere in the body

Nephrotic syndrome: An alteration in kidney function secondary to increased glomerular basement membrane permeability to plasma protein

Neural tube defect (NTD): A defect of the spine, spinal cord, or brain that develops in the first month of pregnancy

Neurogenic bladder: Impairment of bladder voiding function due to an interrupted nerve supply that leads to incomplete bladder emptying

Newborn screening: Routine screening performed on every infant born in the United States shortly after birth using heel-stick blood spots to detect a variety of congenital conditions

Nocturia: Nighttime waking to urinate

Nocturnal enuresis: Enuresis occurring during the night

Nonorganic failure to thrive: A pediatric condition in which a child has a weight less than the third percentile or unexplained weight loss due to a lack of sufficient caloric intake; also known as weight faltering

O

Obesity: A condition of excessive body fat, indicated by having a body mass index at or above the 95th percentile

Oliguria: Less than normal amounts of urine; in children, less than 0.5 to 1 mL/kg/h

Omphalocele: A congenital malformation in which the intestines, liver, and other abdominal organs are outside the abdominal wall in a sac

Oncogenesis: The process by which normal cells mutate into cancer cells

Opportunistic infection: A type of infection caused by normally nonpathogenic, low-virulence organisms in people with weakened immune systems

Organic failure to thrive: A pediatric condition in which a child has a weight less than the third percentile or unexplained weight loss due to an underlying medical cause

Osteoblasts: Cells that are responsible for making bone and that work with osteoclasts, which break down bone, to heal and keep bones strong

Otoacoustic emissions: Sound generated from the inner ear

O_2 saturation: A measure of the amount of oxygen being carried by hemoglobin in the blood

P

Palsy: A weakness that impairs the ability to move muscles properly

Pancytopenia: A condition of simultaneous anemia, leukopenia, and thrombocytopenia; all blood cellular components are low or absent

Parallel play: A type of play typically occurring in the toddler years in which children play alongside of each other but not with each other

Paraphimosis: A condition in which the foreskin cannot be returned to its normal position over the glans, causing constriction of the penis, swelling of the glans, and obstruction of penile blood flow

Paroxysmal: A sudden recurrence or intensification of symptoms

Passive immunity: Immediate, short-term immunity provided by the transfer of fully formed antibodies either from a person with active immunity or via administration of immunoglobulin therapy; also called passive acquired adaptive immunity

Periorbital cellulitis: An infection of the eyelid and soft tissues surrounding the eye, characterized by acute edema of the tissues

Periosteum: A type of connective tissue that covers bone

Petechiae: A condition of pinpoint red spots on the skin that indicate bleeding under the skin

Phenylketonuria (PKU): An inherited condition in which the body cannot break down an amino acid called phenylalanine

Phimosis: A condition in which the foreskin over the glans penis cannot be retracted

Photophobia: Hypersensitivity to light

Physiological anorexia: A stage in which toddlers have a decrease in caloric need and therefore have a decrease in appetite

Physis: The region in the bone between the epiphysis and diaphysis where growth occurs; the growth plate

Pneumothorax: Air in the pleural space as a result of tears in the trachea, bronchial tree, chest wall, or esophagus; also known as air-leak syndrome

Poikilothermia: Inability to regulate body temperature; loss of normal thermoregulation

Polycythemia: A greater-than-normal number of red blood cells in the circulation due to increased production by the bone marrow to increase the amount of hemoglobin available in response to chronic hypoxemia

Polydipsia: Increased thirst as a result of disease

Polyphagia: Excessive hunger

Polyuria: Producing large volumes of dilute urine

Posterior fontanelle: The small, triangular opening that is between the two parietal bones and the occipital bone on the back of the infant's head, which normally closes between 2 and 3 months of age

Postictal: The phase of a seizure that occurs after the active phase of a seizure, lasting minutes to hours, during which the person may have an altered level of consciousness

Posturing: An abnormal body posture resulting from brain injury

Precocious puberty: A condition in which signs of puberty begin before the appropriate age

Preload: The volume of blood in the ventricle at the end of diastole

Preoperational thought: The ability to use words and pictures to convey thoughts

Primitive reflexes: Reflexes that are present at birth but normally disappear within the first few months of life as the nervous system matures; also known as developmental reflexes

Prodromal: Relating to vague, mild initial symptoms that precede the manifestation of distinctive symptoms associated with an illness

Projectile vomiting: Forceful vomiting in which the contents are propelled over a distance, often several feet; a hallmark symptom of pyloric stenosis

Proto-oncogene: A gene that causes a normal cell to mutate into a cancer cell and that can regulate either cell division or cell death

Proximodistal: A pattern of development in which the infant acquires skills beginning proximally in the trunk (gross motor function of the limbs), and then moving distally to the extremities (fine motor function)

Puberty: The process of physiological changes through which a child's body develops into that of an adult

Pulmonary vascular resistance: The resistance encountered when blood flows from the right ventricle into the pulmonary bed; the vascular resistance of the pulmonary bed

Pyelonephritis: Inflammation of the kidney tissues, renal calyces, and renal pelvis, commonly caused by a bacterial infection

Pyeloplasty: A procedure involving removal of an obstructed segment of the ureter and reimplantation in the renal pelvis

R

Receptive language: The ability to understand words

Regression: A loss of acquired developmental skills due to stress, change in routine, or major illness

Respiratory arrest: A state of cessation of breathing (apnea) or respiratory dysfunction so severe that ventilation and oxygenation cannot be maintained

Reversibility: The understanding that objects or numbers can change and then return to their original state

S

Sepsis: A life-threatening inflammatory reaction to the invasion of bacteria and their toxins into the blood and tissues

Shock: A state of inadequate tissue perfusion, resulting in decreased oxygen delivery to and waste removal from the tissues; caused by low blood volume (hypovolemic), abnormal distribution of blood volume or maldistribution of blood flow (distributive), reduced or blocked blood flow from the heart to the great vessels (obstructive), or impaired pumping by the heart (cardiogenic)

Shunt: A diversion of blood from one blood vessel to another through an abnormal anatomical or surgically created opening

Solitary play: A type of play in which the infant is unaware of what others are doing

Spina bifida: A neural tube defect in which the spine and membranes around the spinal cord do not close completely, resulting in minor or major neurological and physical problems

Status epilepticus: A medical emergency involving a seizure that lasts longer than 5 minutes or a series of seizures occurring within a 5-minute period

Steatorrhea: A condition in which the stool contains excessive amounts of fat, possibly making it bulky and foul smelling

Steeple sign: A condition of narrowing of the subglottic area (on a neck X-ray), which indicates swelling and in which the trachea appears to be in the shape of a church steeple on the X-ray

Stenosis: Abnormal narrowing of a blood vessel

Stereotypy: Repetitive movement

Stomatitis: Inflammation in the mouth characterized by small, painful ulcers

Strabismus: Misalignment of the eyes

Stridor: A condition of audible harsh, high-pitched, musical sound on inspiration produced by turbulent airflow through a partially obstructed upper airway

Stroke volume: The amount of blood ejected with each contraction of the heart

Submersion injury: Trauma resulting from a near drowning, in which water is aspirated into the lungs or laryngospasm occurs, leading to respiratory distress, failure, or arrest

Substance use disorder (SUD): Recurrent use of alcohol or illicit drugs that consistently interferes with one's daily life; classified as mild, moderate, or severe

Superficial burn: A burn that involves only the top layer of skin; does not form blisters; is painful, dry, and red; and turns white when pressed; also known as a first-degree burn

Superficial partial-thickness burn: A burn that involves the top two layers of skin, is painful with air movement or temperature changes, reddens the skin, forms blisters, and turns white when pressed; also known as a second-degree burn

Syncope: A loss of consciousness related to transient cerebral hypoxia; also known as fainting

Systemic vascular resistance: The resistance blood encounters in the vessels as it travels throughout the body

T

Tachypnea: Increased respiratory rate; a respiratory rate above age-specific normal values

Tanner stages: A scale of physical development for children and adolescents

Telegraphic speech: Speech that includes only words vital to being understood

Temporal thermometer: A device that measures a person's core body temperature by capturing and quantifying the heat emitted from the superficial temporal artery when the device is swiped over the side of the head

Tendon: A type of fibrous tissue that connects muscle to bone

Teratogen: An agent or factor—such as a medication, chemical, or maternal infection—that can cause malformation in the developing embryo or fetus

Terminal hair: Mature hair in humans, typically thick, coarse, and pigmented

Thelarche: The onset of female breast development

Third space: The nonfunctional interstitial (between cells) space in the body, as opposed to the functional intracellular (within a cell) and intravascular (within a blood vessel) spaces, in which excess fluid can accumulate, resulting in edema

Thyrotoxicosis: A condition of excessive secretion of thyroid hormones; also known as hyperthyroidism

Tonic: A type of seizure characterized by the stiffening of body parts

Tonic-clonic seizure: A type of seizure in which the body stiffens (tonic) and there is loss of consciousness, followed by rhythmic jerking (clonic); also known as a convulsion

Transductive reasoning: The belief that two unrelated events are related

Triglycerides: A type of fat that is formed by glycerol esterified at each of its three hydroxyl groups by a fatty acid

Tripod position: A position in which the person is sitting upright and leaning forward with hands on knees; a sign of respiratory distress in children

Trisomy 13: A genetic disorder that results from a mutation in the 13th chromosome and that is associated with severe intellectual disability and physical abnormalities in many parts of the body; also known as Patau syndrome

Trisomy 18: A genetic disorder that results from a mutation in the 18th chromosome and that is associated with abnormalities in many parts of the body

Trisomy 21: A genetic disorder that results from a mutation in the 21st chromosome in which a person has an extra chromosome and that results in intellectual disability, distinctive facial features, and health complications; also known as Down syndrome

Tumor suppressor gene: A gene that helps prevent cells from mutating; abnormal function of this gene can result in tumor growth

Turner syndrome: A genetic disorder that results from a mutation in the X sex chromosome and that affects development in females

U

Uremia: Excessive amounts of nitrogenous wastes in the blood, which leads to fluid, electrolyte, and hormone imbalances and metabolic abnormalities

V

Valgus: An abnormal position in which the distal portion of a bone is bent laterally, away from the body's midline

Vaping: The use of an electronic cigarette, which simulates the feeling of smoking

Varus: An abnormal position in which the distal portion of a bone is bent medially, toward the body's midline

Vasoocclusive crisis: A complication of sickle cell disease in which blood vessels become obstructed by sickled cells, leading to ischemic injury to organs and pain

Vellus hair: Fine, nonpigmented hair that covers most of the human body

Ventilation: The movement of air into and out of the lungs; breathing

Ventricular septal defect (VSD): A hole or defect in the septum (wall) that divides the left and right ventricles and results in a communication between the left and right sides of the heart

Ventricular septum: The wall that separates the right and left ventricles, the upper portion of which is thinner and more membranous and the lower portion of which is composed of muscle

Vesicoureteral reflux: A condition in which urine flows backward from the bladder into the kidneys

Voiding cystourethrogram: A test to examine the function of the bladder and urethra while a patient voids, using fluoroscopy and a contrasting agent to visualize the lower urinary tract

Volvulus: A twisting of the intestine around itself and the mesentery that supports it, creating an obstruction

W

Water intoxication: A condition of severe electrolyte disturbance caused by excessive water intake

Weight faltering: A pediatric condition in which a child has insufficient weight gain or unexplained weight loss; also known as nonorganic failure to thrive

Wheezing: A high-pitched whistling sound heard in the lungs that occurs as a result of obstructed or narrowed airways

Index

Note: Page numbers followed by *f* and *t* indicate figures and tables respectively.